ADVANCED MEDICAL NUTRITION THERAPY

Kelly Kane, MS, RD, LDN, CNSC
Director of Nutrition and Business Operations
Tufts Medical Center
Assistant Professor
Friedman School of Nutrition Science and Policy
Tufts University
Boston, Massachusetts

Kathy Prelack, PhD, RD, LDN
Director of Clinical Nutrition
Shriners Hospitals for Children
Assistant Professor
School of Nursing and Health Sciences
Simmons College
Boston, Massachusetts

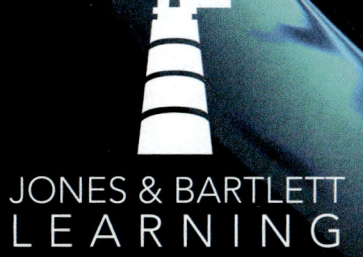

JONES & BARTLETT
LEARNING

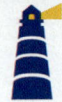

World Headquarters
Jones & Bartlett Learning
5 Wall Street
Burlington, MA 01803
978-443-5000
info@jblearning.com
www.jblearning.com

Jones & Bartlett Learning books and products are available through most bookstores and online booksellers. To contact Jones & Bartlett Learning directly, call 800-832-0034, fax 978-443-8000, or visit our website, www.jblearning.com.

Substantial discounts on bulk quantities of Jones & Bartlett Learning publications are available to corporations, professional associations, and other qualified organizations. For details and specific discount information, contact the special sales department at Jones & Bartlett Learning via the above contact information or send an email to specialsales@jblearning.com.

Copyright © 2019 by Jones & Bartlett Learning, LLC, an Ascend Learning Company

All rights reserved. No part of the material protected by this copyright may be reproduced or utilized in any form, electronic or mechanical, including photocopying, recording, or by any information storage and retrieval system, without written permission from the copyright owner.

The content, statements, views, and opinions herein are the sole expression of the respective authors and not that of Jones & Bartlett Learning, LLC. Reference herein to any specific commercial product, process, or service by trade name, trademark, manufacturer, or otherwise does not constitute or imply its endorsement or recommendation by Jones & Bartlett Learning, LLC and such reference shall not be used for advertising or product endorsement purposes. All trademarks displayed are the trademarks of the parties noted herein. *Advanced Medical Nutrition Therapy* is an independent publication and has not been authorized, sponsored, or otherwise approved by the owners of the trademarks or service marks referenced in this product.

There may be images in this book that feature models; these models do not necessarily endorse, represent, or participate in the activities represented in the images. Any screenshots in this product are for educational and instructive purposes only. Any individuals and scenarios featured in the case studies throughout this product may be real or fictitious, but are used for instructional purposes only.

The authors, editor, and publisher have made every effort to provide accurate information. However, they are not responsible for errors, omissions, or for any outcomes related to the use of the contents of this book and take no responsibility for the use of the products and procedures described. Treatments and side effects described in this book may not be applicable to all people; likewise, some people may require a dose or experience a side effect that is not described herein. Drugs and medical devices are discussed that may have limited availability controlled by the Food and Drug Administration (FDA) for use only in a research study or clinical trial. Research, clinical practice, and government regulations often change the accepted standard in this field. When consideration is being given to use of any drug in the clinical setting, the health care provider or reader is responsible for determining FDA status of the drug, reading the package insert, and reviewing prescribing information for the most up-to-date recommendations on dose, precautions, and contraindications, and determining the appropriate usage for the product. This is especially important in the case of drugs that are new or seldom used.

02584-2

Production Credits

VP, Product Management: David D. Cella
Director of Product Management: Cathy L. Esperti
Product Manager: Sean Fabery
Associate Production Editor: Alex Schab
Director of Marketing: Andrea DeFronzo
Production Services Manager: Colleen Lamy
VP, Manufacturing and Inventory Control: Therese Connell
Composition: SourceHOV LLC
Cover Design: Michael O'Donnell

Text Design: Michael O'Donnell
Director of Rights & Media: Joanna Gallant
Rights & Media Specialist: Merideth Tumasz
Media Development Editor: Shannon Sheehan
Cover Image (Title Page, Part Opener, Chapter Opener):
    © Mina De La O/Getty Images
Printing and Binding: LSC Communications
Cover Printing: LSC Communications

Library of Congress Cataloging-in-Publication Data

Names: Kane, Kelly, 1969- author, editor. | Prelack, Kathy, author, editor.
Title: Advanced medical nutrition therapy / Kelly Kane and Kathy Prelack.
Description: Burlington, Massachusetts : Jones & Bartlett Learning,
    [2019] | Includes bibliographical references.
Identifiers: LCCN 2017058457 | ISBN 9781284042634
Subjects: | MESH: Nutrition Therapy
Classification: LCC RM216 | NLM WB 400 | DDC 615.8/54–dc23
LC record available at https://lccn.loc.gov/2017058457

6048

Printed in the United States of America
22 21 20 19 18   10 9 8 7 6 5 4 3 2 1

Dedication

To Dana, Patrick, and Jake for their unending patience and support, and to the staff and students of the Frances Stern Nutrition Center for their insight and encouragement.
—Kelly

To my students who inspire me to work hard every day; to my colleagues and mentors who bring me perspective and keep me humble; and to my family who gives me strength, love, and purpose.
—Kathy

Contents

Foreword   xiii
Preface   xiv
Features of This Text   xvi
Acknowledgments   xix
About the Authors   xx
Contributors   xxi
Reviewers   xxiii

Section 1   Fundamentals in Practice

1   Nutrition Assessment **3**
  Overview of the Nutrition Care Process **4**
    The Purpose of Nutrition Assessment   5
  Nutrition Screening **7**
    The Role of Nutrition Screening in NCPM   7
    Screening in Acute Care   7
    Nutrition Screening Tools   8
    Final Comparison of Screening
      Tools for Acute Care   12
  Nutrition Assessment **14**
    Anthropometric Measurements   14
    Biochemical Data, Medical Tests, and Procedures   27
    Client History   27
    Nutrition-Focused Physical Findings   28
    Food/Nutrition-Related History   36
    Energy Balance   39
  Chapter Summary **39**
  Key Terms **39**
  References **40**

2   Biochemical Assessment **45**
  Introduction **46**
  Specimen Types **46**
  Assay Types **48**
  Routine Medical Laboratory Tests **48**
    Fluid and Electrolytes   48
    Acid–Base Physiology   64
    Endocrine Function: Glucose and
      Glycosylated Hemoglobin   69
    Protein Assessment   70
    Enzymes   75
    Lipid Profile   77
    Hematology   78
    Interpretation of Anemia   83
  Chapter Summary **89**
  Key Terms **89**
  References **89**

3   Enteral Nutrition **91**
  Introduction **92**
  The Evolution of Enteral Nutrition **92**
  **Determining the Route of
    Enteral Nutrition** **92**
    Short-term Placement   94
    Long-term Placement   95
  Types of Enteral Tubes **96**
  Gastric Versus Small-Bowel Feeding **96**
    Gastric Feeding   96
    Small-bowel Feeding   97
  Formula Delivery Methods **97**
    Continuous   98
    Intermittent   98
    Bolus Feedings   98
  Enteral Formula Compositions **99**
    Carbohydrates   100
    Fats   101
    Protein   102
    Vitamins and Minerals   102
    Fiber   102
    Pre- and Probiotics   102
  Disease-Specific Formulas **103**
    Renal Dysfunction   103
    Pulmonary Dysfunction   104
    Liver Dysfunction   104
    Diabetes   104
    Trauma/Wound Healing   104
  Developing an EN Feeding Plan **104**
  Complication Monitoring **104**
    Aspiration   104
    Nausea/Vomiting   106
    Abdominal Distention   106
    Gastroparesis (Delayed Gastric Emptying)   106
    Constipation   107
    Diarrhea   107
  Early Enteral Nutrition **107**
  Immunonutrition **108**
    Gastrointestinal Tract as an Immune Organ   108
    The Gut and Systemic Inflammatory
      Response System   109
    Conditionally Essential Amino Acids   109
  Chapter Summary **112**
  Key Terms **112**
  References **112**

4   Parenteral Nutrition Therapy **115**
  Introduction **116**
  Brief History of Parenteral Nutrition **116**
  Parenteral Nutrition Administration **116**
    Venous Access   116
    Central Parenteral Nutrition   118
    Peripheral Parenteral Nutrition   120

Indications and Contraindications   120

Parenteral Nutrition Formulation........................ 122
Carbohydrate   123
Amino Acids   123
Lipids   125
Electrolytes   126
Multivitamins   126
Trace Elements   126
Other Additives   129

Initiation and Progression of Parenteral Nutrition.............. 130
Safety Check of Macronutrient Infusion Rates   134
Electrolyte Requirements   134
Vitamin and Trace Element Requirements   134
Progression of PN   135
Transitional Feeding   135

Parenteral Nutrition Monitoring..................... 135
Anthropometrics   136
Vital Signs   136
Biochemistry   136
Nutrition-Focused Physical Exam   137

Central Venous Access Complications and Their Management............. 137
Mechanical Complications   137

Metabolic Complications............... 140
Hyper- and Hypoglycemia   140
Electrolyte Abnormalities   140
Hyper- and Hypovolemia   140
Overfeeding   140
Essential Fatty Acid Deficiency   140
Hepatobiliary Complications   141

Home Parenteral Nutrition............ 142
Indications and Access   142
Prognosis of HPN   142

Chapter Summary.................. 143
Key Terms....................... 143
References...................... 143

5 Energy Expenditure and Body Composition in Metabolic Stress...................... 147

Introduction...................... 148

Characteristics of the Inflammatory Response......................... 148

Ebb and Flow Phases................ 148

Alterations in Metabolism Associated with the Inflammatory Response....... 150
Energy Cost Associated with Altered Metabolism   150
Hormonal and Metabolic Response to Stress Versus Starvation   150
Glucose Metabolism and Stress Hyperglycemia   151
Protein Catabolic State   152
Fat Metabolism and Lipolysis   153

Determination of Energy Expenditure During Normal and Stressed Conditions........................ 154
Total Energy Expenditure and Its Components   154

Estimating Total Energy Expenditure..... 155
Factorial Approach to Determining Energy Requirements Under Normal Conditions   155
Factorial Approach in Determining TEE in Hospitalized, Metabolically Stressed Patients   156

Measuring Energy Expenditure—Direct and Indirect Calorimetry............ 157
Use of Indirect Calorimetry to Prevent Over- and Underfeeding   162
Interpretation of Respiratory Quotient   162

Determination of Body Composition and Its Components During Metabolic Stress................... 163
Traditional Assessment of Nutritional Status   163
Models of Body Composition   164
Anthropometry   164
Two Compartment Model   164
Methods Relying on Measures of Total Body Water   165
The Effect of Catabolic Disease on Body Composition   165

Multi-Compartmental Models........... 166
Combined Isotope Dilution Studies   166
Dual Energy X-ray Absorptiometry   166
Imaging Techniques   167

Metabolic Support Aimed at Preserving Body Cell Mass.......... 167

Chapter Summary.................. 168
Key Terms....................... 169
References...................... 169

Section 2   Nutrition in Disease States

6 Nutrition in Critical Illness: A Burn Injury Model.......................... 175

Introduction...................... 176

Pathophysiology of the Catabolic Response Following Acute Burn Injury........................ 176

Medical Treatment/Clinical Course....... 180

Medical Treatment/Clinical Course Specific to Burn Patients........ 180
Oxandrolone   182
Propranolol   183

Nutritional Management............. 183
Assessment   183
Treatment   190

Chapter Summary.................. 192
Key Terms....................... 192
References...................... 192

vi Contents

7 Nutrition in Wound Healing 195

Introduction 196

Pathophysiology of Wounds and Wound Healing 196
Inflammation   196
Proliferation   198
Remodeling   198

Chronic Wounds 198
Pathophysiology of the Chronic Wound   199
Chronic Venous Ulcers   199
Diabetic Ulcers   199
Pressure Ulcers   200
Alterations in Physiological State and Metabolism During Wound Healing   201

Medical Treatment of Wounds 203

Medical Nutrition Therapy for Wound Healing 204
Screening   204
Assessment   204
Nutritional Requirements   204
Diet and Nutrition Intervention   212
Monitoring   214

Chapter Summary 214
Key Terms 214
References 214

8 Nutritional Management of Obesity 217

Introduction 218

Prevalence 218

Classification of Obesity: Is Obesity a Disease? 220

Causes and Contributions to the Obesity Epidemic 221
Genetic Factors   221
Environmental Factors   221
Social Factors   221
Biological Factors   222
Developmental Factors   223
Hormonal Factors   223
Orexigenic Hormones   224
Anorexigenic Hormones   225

Alterations in Body Composition in Obesity 225

Nutrition Assessment in Obesity 226
Anthropometric Assessment   226
Body Mass Index (BMI)   227
Waist Circumference   227
Waist-to-Hip Ratio   227
Weight History   227

Biochemical Assessment 227

Clinical Assessment 227
Medical and Psychosocial History   227
Nutrition-Focused Physical Exam   227

Dietary Assessment 227
Dietary History   227
Nutrition Patterns   227

Other Considerations 227
Physical Activity   227
Sleep Patterns   228
Readiness/Motivation   228
Support System   228
Cultural and Socioeconomic Factors   228
Other   228
Assessment of Energy Requirement   228

Pathophysiology Associated with Obesity 229
Weight-Related Comorbidities   229
Cardiovascular System   229
Metabolic/Endocrine System   230
Gastrointestinal System   231
Immune System   232
Musculoskeletal System   232
Respiratory System   232

Obesity Management 233
Comprehensive Lifestyle Intervention   233
Dietary   233
Behavior   234
Physical Activity   235
Pharmacotherapy   235
Bariatric Surgery   236
Comorbidity Outcomes   239

Micronutrient Concerns 241

Emerging Treatment Options 241

Chapter Summary 247
Key Terms 247
References 247

9 Nutritional Management of Diabetes Mellitus 251

Introduction: Incidence and Scope 252

Pathophysiology of Diabetes 252
Type 1 Diabetes   252
Type 2 Diabetes   254
Gestational Diabetes   257

Screening, Risk Factors, and Diagnosis of Diabetes 258
Diabetes Screening and Risk Factors   258
Diagnostic Criteria and Staging   258

Nutritional Requirements in Diabetes 259
Carbohydrate   259
Fiber   261
Sucrose and Other Nutritive Sweeteners   262
Protein   262
Fat   262
Nonnutritive Sweeteners   263
Alcohol   263
Micronutrients   263
Herbal and Dietary Supplements   264
Cinnamon   265

Medical Nutrition Therapy for Diabetes 266
Nutrition Assessment   266
Nutrition Intervention   267
Advanced Carbohydrate Counting or Matching Insulin to Carbohydrate Method   268

Exercise 270
Type 1 Diabetes   270
Type 2 Diabetes   271
Carbohydrate Adjustment   271

Glycemic Targets and Self-Monitoring of Blood Glucose. 272

Acute and Chronic Complications of Diabetes 273
Acute Complications   273
Chronic Complications   275

Medical Treatment of Diabetes 280
Insulin   280

Surgical Treatment Options 285
Metabolic Surgery   285

Hospitalization and Illness for Patients with Diabetes.............. 285
Noncritical Patients with Diabetes Admitted to the Hospital   286
Management of Patients with Diabetes Requiring Nutrition Support   286

Chapter Summary................... 287
Key Terms 287
References 287

10 Nutrition in Cardiovascular Disease... 293

Introduction 294

Cardiac Physiology in Health and Disease 294

CVD Clinical Course................. 298
Dyslipidemia   299

Nutritional Management in CVD 300
Nutrition Assessment in CVD   300
Medications in CVD   301
Energy Needs in CVD   302
Nutrition Intervention in CVD   302
Replacement of Saturated/Trans Fats with Other Fats or Carbohydrates   303
Omega-3 Fatty Acids   303
Fiber   304
Nuts   304
Plant Stanols and Sterols   304
Added Sugar   305
Physical Activity   305
Antioxidant Supplements   305
Alcohol   305
Smoking Cessation   305
Nutrition Monitoring/Evaluation in CVD   305

Hypertension Clinical Course 305

Nutritional Management in Hypertension 306
Nutrition Assessment in Hypertension   306
Medications in Hypertension   307
Energy Needs in Hypertension   307
Nutrition Intervention in Hypertension   307
DASH Diet and Sodium Reduction   307
Potassium Supplementation   309
Alcohol Intake   309
Physical Activity   310

Smoking Cessation   310
Nutrition Monitoring/Evaluation in Hypertension   310

Obesity and CVD Clinical Course 310
CVD Outcomes   311
Advanced Coronary Artery Disease Diagnosis and Surgical Treatment   311

Heart Failure Clinical Course 312

Nutritional Management in Heart Failure 316

Nutrition Assessment in Heart Failure................... 316
Medications in Heart Failure   316
Assessing for Obesity   317
Assessing for Cardiac Cachexia   317
Nutrition Intervention in Heart Failure   319
Sodium and Fluid Restrictions   319
Heart-healthy Eating   320
Blood Glucose Management   320
Dietary Supplements   320
Nutrition Intervention in the Case of Cardiac Cachexia   322
Nutrition Monitoring/Evaluation in Heart Failure   322

Nutrition Support in CVD 322

Chapter Summary................... 325
Key Terms 325
References 325

11 Nutrition in Oral Health 329

Introduction 330
Background...................... 330

Nutrition and Oral Health Interrelationships.................. 330

Nutrition and Development of the Oral Cavity 330
Effect of Oral Health on Diet and Nutrition   331
Effect of Systemic Nutrition Deficiency or Excess on the Oral Cavity   332

Effects of Diet and Dietary Habits on Common Oral Diseases 333
Dental Caries   333
Periodontal Disease   341
Edentulism and Dentures   343
Oral Infections   344

Oral Health During the Life Cycle 345
Pregnancy   345
Infancy and Early Childhood   345
Adolescence   347
Adulthood   348
Geriatrics   349

Chapter Summary................... 350
Key Terms 350
References 350

12 Nutritional Management of Gastrointestinal Maldigestion..... 353

Introduction 354

Functional Anatomy of the Digestive
  System 354
Overview of Digestion and Absorption 356
  Pathophysiological Distinction:
    Maldigestion versus Malabsorption 356
Key Mechanisms of Digestion 356
Medical Nutrition Therapy
  for Disorders of Digestion. 357
  Gastric Surgery 357
  Pancreatitis 360
  Gastroesophageal Reflux Disease 368
Chapter Summary. 371
Key Terms 371
References 371

13 Nutrition Management of Gastrointestinal Malabsorption . . . 373

Introduction 374
Key Mechanisms of Absorption 374
  Absorption Sites 374
Medical Nutrition Therapy
  for Disorders of Absorption 375
  Celiac Disease (CD) 375
  Irritable Bowel Syndrome (IBS) 378
  Non-Celiac Gluten Sensitivity 382
  Inflammatory Bowel Disease (IBD) 383
  Leaky Gut 393
  Helicobacter pylori 395
  Small Intestinal Bacterial Overgrowth (SIBO) 396
  Bowel Surgery and Short Bowel Syndrome
    (SBS) 400
Chapter Summary. 408
Key Terms 409
References 409

14 Nutrition in Kidney Disease 413

Introduction 414
Renal Physiology in Health and Disease . . . 414
Functions of the Kidney 417
Diseases of the Kidney. 418
  Acute Kidney Injury 420
  Chronic Kidney Disease 422
  End-Stage Renal Disease 431
  Renal Replacement Therapy 431
  Kinetic Modeling 433
Monitoring Nutritional Adequacy
  During Dialysis. 436
Nutrition Support in Kidney Disease. 437
  Indications for Nutrition Support 437
Nephrotic Syndrome 438
  Medical Nutrition Therapy for
    Nephrotic Syndrome 439
Chapter Summary. 439
Key Terms 439
References 440

15 Nutrition in Liver Disease 443

Introduction to the Liver 444
  Liver Structure and Functions 444
  Overview and Pathophysiology
    of Liver Disease 445
  Malnutrition in Liver Disease 449
Acute Liver Disease. 451
  Acute Viral Hepatitis 451
  Acute Drug-Induced Hepatitis 451
  Acute Liver Failure 452
  Nutrition Management 453
Chronic Liver Disease. 453
  Alcoholic Liver Disease 453
  Nonalcoholic Fatty Liver Disease 455
  Inherited Diseases 456
Alterations in Metabolism 457
  Carbohydrate Metabolism 457
  Protein Metabolism 457
  Fat Metabolism 459
Nutrition Assessment 459
  Body Composition 459
  Functional Capacity 460
Nutrition Therapy for Cirrhosis 461
  Energy Requirements 461
  Protein Requirements 461
  Vitamin D 461
  Zinc 462
  Oral Nutrition 463
  Enteral Nutrition 463
  Parenteral Nutrition 464
Summary 465
Key Terms 466
References 466

16 Nutrition in Pulmonary Disease 471

Introduction 472
Pulmonary Physiology in Health
  and Disease 472
  Asthma 472
  Chronic Obstructive Pulmonary Disease 472
  Body Composition 475
  Nutrition Intervention 476
Acute Respiratory Distress Syndrome. 477
Nutrition Support
  and Pulmonary Disease 478
Immunonutrition 479
Micronutrients 480
  Antioxidants 480
  Vitamins and Minerals 481
Quality of Life and Psychosocial Support. . . 481
Chapter Summary. 481
Key Terms 481
References 482

17 Nutrition in Cystic Fibrosis. 487

Introduction 488

Diagnosis 488
Clinical Manifestations of CF 488
CF and the Lungs 488
Relationship between Lung Function
   and Nutritional Status 491
Nutrition Assessment 492
   Energy and Protein Needs   493
   Anthropometrics   494
   Biochemical Assessment   494
   Diet Assessment   494
Pancreatic Insufficiency 494
Nutrition Management in Patients
   with Cystic Fibrosis 497
   Macronutrients   497
   Infants   497
   Micronutrients   498
   Sodium Chloride   498
   Nutrition Support   498
Nutrition-related Complications of
   Cystic Fibrosis 499
   Gastrointestinal Complications   499
   CF-related Diabetes   499
   CF-related Bone Disease   500
Summary 500
Key Terms 500
References 500

18 Nutrition in Solid Organ Transplantation 503

Introduction 504
Background 504
Indications and Contraindications
   for Transplantation 506
   Kidney Transplant Indications   506
   Pancreas Transplant Indications   506
   Liver Transplant Indications   506
   Heart Transplant Indications   506
   Lung Transplant Indications   506
   Small-bowel Transplant Indications   506
   Contraindications to Transplantation   506
Medical Treatment 508
   Organ Donation and Matching   508
   Complicating Factors   508
Nutritional Management 509
   Pretransplant Phase   509
   Acute Posttransplant Phase   511
   Dietary Therapy   515
   Chronic Posttransplant Phase   516
Chapter Summary 518
Key Terms 518
References 518

19 Nutrition in Oncology and Hematopoietic Stem Cell Transplant ... 521

Background/Etiology 522
Epidemiology 524

Cancer Staging 524
Medical Treatment of Cancer 524
   Radiation Therapy   525
   Chemotherapy   526
   Surgery   527
   Biotherapy   527
   Hormone Therapy   527
Nutrition Screening and Assessment
   in Cancer Patients 527
   Nutrition Screening   527
   Nutrition Assessment   528
   Estimating Nutrition Needs in Cancer Patients   529
Cancer Cachexia and Metabolic Changes
   Associated with Cancer 529
   Cancer Cachexia   529
   Approaches to Management in Cancer Cachexia   530
Overview of Nutritional Support in
   the Cancer Patient 531
Nutritional Management of Specific
   Solid Tumors 532
   Head and Neck Cancers   532
   Esophageal Cancer   533
   Gastric Cancer   533
   Intestinal Cancers   534
   Pancreatic Cancer   534
   Lung Cancer   535
Nutritional Management of Hematological
   Cancers Undergoing Hematopoietic
   Stem Cell Transplant 535
   Estimating Energy Needs   536
   Nutritional Support During Acute Phase
      of HSCT   537
   Graft Versus Host Disease   537
   Glutamine and Nutrition Support   539
   Low-Microbial Diets   539
Nutrition Support in the Advanced
   Cancer Patient 540
Complementary and Alternative
   Medicine, Integrative Medicine,
   and the Cancer Patient 540
Chapter Summary 540
Key Terms 541
References 541

20 Nutrition in HIV/AIDS 545

Introduction 546
HIV Infection 546
Epidemiology 547
Medical Management 548
   Antiretroviral Treatment   548
Food Insecurity 548
   Primary Care   549
Pathophysiology and Alterations
   in Physical State 550
   Energy and Protein Metabolism   550
   Lipid Metabolism   551
   Bone Loss   552

Contents

Gastrointestinal Function, Inflammation, and Micronutrient Deficiencies 552
Breastfeeding 552
Nutritional Management 552
Medical History and Antiretroviral Treatment Adherence 553
Nutritional Assessment 553
Nutritional Management of HIV Wasting 558
Nutritional Management of Unintentional Weight Loss 558
Nutritional Management of Lipodystrophy 559
Nutritional Management of Bone Loss 559
Micronutrient Supplementation 559

Chapter Summary 560
Key Terms 560
References 560

Section 3 Nutrition in the Lifecycle

21 Nutrition in Pregnancy and Lactation ... 565

Introduction: Nutrition in Pregnancy 567
Maternal Health and Birth Outcome 567
Physiological Alterations Throughout Pregnancy 568

Nutrition Therapy Throughout Pregnancy 571
Nutrition Assessment During Pregnancy 571
Preconception/Prenatal Care 572
Gestational Weight Gain 575
Macronutrient Requirements 575
Physical Activity Recommendations 581
Dietary Restrictions During Pregnancy 581
Food Cravings and Aversions 582
Gastroenterologic Symptoms During Pregnancy 582
Nutrition Therapy in Unique Pregnancies 582

Nutritional Management of Preexisting Diseases in Pregnancy 584
Eating Disorders During Pregnancy 584
Diabetes (Nongestational) 584
HIV Infection 585
Pregnancy-Induced Diseases 586

Nutrition Support in Pregnancy 591
Enteral Nutrition 592
Parenteral Nutrition 592

Summary: Nutrition in Pregnancy 593
Introduction: Nutrition in Lactation 594
Physiology of Lactation 594
Human Milk Composition 596
Nutritional Composition of Breast Milk 596
Practice of Lactation 598
Breastfeeding Initiation and Techniques 599
Special Cases and Contraindications 603

The Lactating Mother: Nutritional Considerations 604
Nutrition Assessment of a Lactating Mother 604
Nutritional Requirements for Lactation 605

The Registered Dietitian's Role in Breastfeeding Promotion 606
Promoting Breastfeeding as an RD 606
Current Trends and Breastfeeding Assistance Programs 606

Summary: Nutrition in Lactation 606
Key Terms 607
References 607

22 Nutrition in Neonatology 613

Introduction 614
Background 614
Goals of Growth and Nutrition for Premature Infants 616
Metabolism and Body Composition in Prematurity 616
Energy Requirements 616
Protein Requirements 617
Carbohydrate Requirements 618
Fat Requirements 619
Fluid Requirements 619
Electrolyte Requirements 621

Methods of Feeding 624
Parenteral Nutrition (PN) 624
Vascular Access 625
Energy Requirements 625
Enteral Nutrition 628

Feeding Selection 630
Breast Milk, Breastfeeding, and Donor Milk 630
Preterm and Transitional Formulas 632
Preparing for Discharge 632

Chapter Summary 633
Key Terms 633
References 633

23 Nutrition in Pediatrics 637

Introduction 638
Growth and Development 638
Physical Growth and Its Characteristics 638
Body Composition During Growth 639

Nutrition Screening and Assessment 641
Anthropometric Measures 641
Evaluating Growth Using Standardized Growth Charts 643
Diet Interview and History 652
Nutrition-focused Physical Exam 654
Biochemical Data 655
Medical and Social History 656

Assessing Patterns of Growth and Etiology 657
Interpreting Changes in Weight-for-Age 657

Normal Pediatric Nutrition 660
Nutrient Requirements 660
Introduction of Food and Developmental Cues 666

Pediatric Malnutrition 669
Failure to Thrive 669

Calculating Energy Needs
for Catch-Up Growth 670
Nutrition Support During Times
of Illness or Chronic Disease 671
Enteral Nutrition   671
Parenteral Nutrition   675
Immunonutrition in Nutrition
Support of Children 678
Glutamine   679
Arginine   679
Omega-3 Fatty Acids   679
Chapter Summary 679
Key Terms 679
References 680

24 Nutritional Management of Childhood Obesity 683

Introduction 684
Prevalence 684
Defining Childhood Obesity 684
Childhood Obesity and Medical
Comorbidities 687
Left Ventricular Hypertrophy,
Hypertension, and Epicardial Fat   687
Metabolic Syndrome   688
Insulin Resistance and Type 2 Diabetes   689
Asthma   690
Sleep Apnea   691
Other Comorbidities: Orthopedic, Dental,
and Nonalcoholic Fatty Liver 691
Psychological Effects
of Childhood Obesity 691
Depression and Obesity Stigma   692
Peer Relationships   693
Family Relationships   693
Cognitive Impairment   693
Health-Related Quality of Life   693
Factors Associated
with Childhood Obesity 693
Low Socioeconomic Status   693
Family Patterns   694
Genetic Factors   694
Assessment, Management,
and Intervention 695
Nutrition Assessment of Childhood
Obesity   695
Primary and Secondary Prevention:
Approaches to Weight Loss   695
Behavioral Intervention   698
Dietary Intervention   699
Physical Activity   699
Intervention Approaches 699
Group Based   699
Motivational Interviewing   699
Positive Reinforcement   700
Stimulus Control   701
Goal Setting   701
Surgical Intervention 702

Indications for Surgical Intervention   702
Weight Loss Procedures   702
Nutritional Considerations   703
Postoperative Care   705
Chapter Summary 705
Key Terms 705
References 705

25 Nutrition in Eating Disorders 707

Introduction 708
Background and Etiology 708
Anorexia Nervosa   708
Bulimia Nervosa   710
Binge Eating Disorder   710
Other Specified Feeding or Eating Disorder   711
Unspecified Feeding or Eating Disorder   711
Avoidant Restrictive Food Intake Disorder
and Orthorexia   711
Prognosis 711
Anorexia Nervosa   711
Bulimia Nervosa   713
Binge Eating Disorder   714
Psychological Treatment 715
Pharmacotherapy 716
Nutrition Assessment 716
Anthropometric Assessment   716
Dietary Assessment   716
Biochemical Assessment   718
Medical Nutrition Therapy 719
Goals and Guidelines 719
Anorexia Nervosa   719
Bulimia Nervosa   722
Binge Eating Disorder   722
Counseling 723
Nutrition Education   724
Patient Monitoring and
Evaluation 724
Chapter Summary 725
Key Terms 725
References 725

26 Nutrition in Developmental Disabilities 727

Introduction 728
Prader Willi 729
Anthropometrics   730
Biochemical and Clinical   731
Assessment of Energy Needs   734
Long-term Monitoring and Evaluation   735
Spina Bifida 735
Anthropometrics   736
Biochemical and Clinical   737
Assessment of Energy Needs   738
Feeding Difficulties   739
Weight Challenges   739
Long-term Monitoring and Evaluation   739

Cerebral Palsy **740**
Anthropometrics   740
Biochemical and Clinical   741
Assessment of Energy Needs   742
Feeding Difficulties   742
Weight Challenges   743
Long-term Monitoring and Evaluation   744

Down Syndrome. **744**
Anthropometrics   746
Biochemical and Clinical   746
Assessment of Needs   747
Long-term Monitoring/Evaluation   747

Autism Spectrum Disorders **747**
Anthropometrics   749
Biochemical and Clinical   749
Feeding Difficulties   749
Assessment of Needs   750
Long-term Monitoring and Evaluation   750

Chapter Summary. **750**

Key Terms **750**

References **750**

27 Nutrition in Geriatrics 753

Introduction **754**

Background and Etiology. **754**

**Changes in Body Composition
    in the Geriatric Population** **756**
Sarcopenia   757
Frailty   758

Pressure Injury   759
Sarcopenic Obesity   759

Malnutrition Risk in Geriatrics **760**

Physiologic Factors **760**
Overall Health Status   762
Psychological/Neurocognitive Status   762
Functional Status   763
Dysphagia   763
Social Factors   765

**Nutrition Screening and Assessment
    in Geriatrics** **765**

Nutrient Needs. **766**
Energy Requirements   768
Protein Requirement   769
Recommendations for Fiber Intake   769
Fluid Requirements   770

**Physiologic Alterations Effecting
    Micronutrient Metabolism** **770**
Vitamin B_{12} 771
Vitamin D   771
Calcium   773

Nutrition Management **773**
Nutrition Support   774

Chapter Summary. **775**

Key Terms **776**

References **776**

Glossary   781
Index   793

Foreword

It is a pleasure to introduce *Advanced Medical Nutrition Therapy* by Kelly Kane, MS, RD and Kathy Prelack, PhD, RD to readers. I can testify that they are both master clinicians who bring readers the wisdom they have accumulated after several decades of clinical experience in academic medical centers in Boston, Massachusetts. I am also well-acquainted with their ability to teach at both the graduate and undergraduate levels.

The setting in which the authors practice is unique; Boston has long been known for the excellence of its education in the health sciences, and the text draws heavily on the resources of colleagues in the city. Among their many affiliations, both of the authors are faculty members of the Friedman School of Nutrition Science and Policy at Tufts University and the Department of Nutrition at Simmons College, which sponsors a didactic program in dietetics and combined dietetic internship/Master's degree programs. Their clinical associations include Shriners Hospitals for Children, a pediatric burn and surgical specialty hospital; Massachusetts General Hospital; and the Frances Stern Nutrition Center at Tufts Medical Center, the oldest ambulatory nutrition service in the United States. The authors have used their access to excellent resources in the nutritional aspects of clinical medicine at both theoretical and practical levels to produce a text that is unique in that it reflects both the science and the art of the nutritional care of patients and members of the larger community.

Their text uses a practice-oriented, case-based approach that draws heavily on problem-based learning to engage the reader. The chapters include *Clinical Controversies* and *Clinical Roundtable* features on difficult topics. At the end of each chapter, the reader will have mastered both the theoretical basis and the core clinical skills needed to deliver medical nutrition therapy and treat the patient.

The first section of the text provides a review of core concepts of clinical nutrition that are relevant to nutrition screening, assessment, and nutrition support. This is followed by a number of chapters that focus on various organ systems as well as infectious disease and the complications that are involved in critical illness. Chapters on various points during the lifecycle are also included.

The great strength of the text is that it is written by clinicians for clinicians. While it does not stint to provide the pathophysiology of the diseases and illnesses discussed, it spends most of its time in helping the reader develop and apply practical clinical nutrition expertise.

The chapter on nutrition in oncology and transplantation offers a good example of the strengths of the approach the authors have taken. The chapter begins with a brief review of why the topic is important and clearly states learning objectives. Next, core concepts and some background on the epidemiology and causation of common cancers are presented, along with methods for cancer staging and typical medical treatments of cancer. This is followed by an extensive section on clinical nutrition that includes screening and assessment of the cancer patient and nutritional support of different forms of cancers, including solid tumors, hematological cancers, and advanced cancers, as well as cancer cachexia. Complementary and alternative medicine is discussed in an evidence-based context. The chapter is interlarded with practical points and clinical case studies, heavily referenced with up-to-date citations, and concludes with a brief summary.

Instructors will welcome the Instructor's Manual, a Test Bank with examination questions, and slides in PowerPoint format that may ease their teaching burdens.

I am acquainted with most of the authors of this text, and I can assure readers that they will find that this distillation of their wisdom is a welcome guide to mastering medical nutrition therapy.

Johanna Dwyer, DSc, RD

Professor of Medicine and Community Health
Tufts University School of Medicine
Gerald J. and Dorothy R. Friedman School of Nutrition
Science and Policy at Tufts University

Senior Scientist
Jean Mayer USDA Human Nutrition Research Center
on Aging
Boston, Massachusetts

Preface

Advanced Medical Nutrition Therapy is designed as the primary text for an upper-level undergraduate or graduate-level Medical Nutrition Therapy or Clinical Nutrition course for nutrition majors. The text is designed to be a current, evidence-based, and practical nutrition resource for nutrition students, dietetic interns, nutrition professionals, and nonnutrition clinicians. Other trainees, such as medical students or students enrolled in graduate programs in biomedical science, may also have an interest in such a text. This text will present information that meets the needs of those at the graduate nutrition level, as well as those who have advanced academic backgrounds, but limited clinical experience, or clinicians of other disciplines (nurses, physicians, physician assistants, etc.).

Conceptual Approach

Advanced Medical Nutrition Therapy utilizes a practice-oriented, case-based approach that incorporates problem-based learning and engages the reader in various clinically based scenarios that guide the narrative text. This approach is designed to encourage the reader to digest the didactic scientific information while applying it to a patient-based clinical situation. The cases in the text provide the framework around which the didactic information is presented. By understanding the importance of the subject matter through application, the reader will look beyond the rote memorization approach that can be typical of science courses and integrate the science with the clinical scenario to gain a more complete understanding.

The text is practice-oriented with a strong clinical focus highlighting the treatment of the medical condition while incorporating the latest guidelines and research, with an emphasis on current topics. Commonly used formulas and equations are included to emphasize clinical application.

Organization

The first section of the text introduces the core concepts of nutrition, highlighting nutrition and biochemical assessment, nutrition support, and energy expenditure. These chapters provide the framework of the text. The next section provides an overview of various disease states, including critical illness, wound healing, obesity, diabetes mellitus, cardiovascular disease, oral health, gastrointestinal conditions, kidney disease, liver disease, pulmonary disease, cystic fibrosis, solid organ transplantation, oncology/bone marrow transplantation, and HIV/AIDS. The last section provides an overview of nutrition in the lifecycle, outlining content on pregnancy, lactation, neonatology, pediatrics, pediatric obesity, eating disorders, developmental disabilities, and geriatrics, thus providing a comprehensive overview of medical nutrition therapy.

Features

Each chapter is designed to provide the reader the comprehension and skills to render effective nutrition care plans based on the fundamentals of diet and disease and existing research evidence. Each chapter introduces *Core Concepts*, which are important principles or themes that will be identified and highlighted to encourage functional learning. *Learning Objectives* are included at the beginning of each chapter to better assess student learning. A *Case Study* or clinical scenario introduces each topic and stimulates critical thinking by developing questions that are subsequently expanded upon in the text. Reliance on evidence-based practice via a *Clinical Controversy* is fostered through the introduction of research concepts in journal review. Discussion of clinical scenarios that do not have one clear, correct answer is covered in the *Clinical Roundtable*. *Practice Points* of useful clinical information are presented throughout each chapter to identify how it works "in the real world." *Key Terms* also help to familiarize the reader with new concepts in an organized fashion.

Benefits

The text is designed for students and practitioners who are fairly new to the clinical environment, as well as those who are new to addressing nutrition in the clinical environment and who have more recently studied and learned the basics of metabolism (anatomy; physiology; and carbohydrate, protein, and fat metabolism, for example). It incorporates a clinical case presentation, with discussion throughout each chapter calling upon details of the case in order to reinforce the didactic science information, thus challenging the student to think outside of the classroom. This approach will allow the student to apply this information and reinforce learning.

The text more broadly covers nutrition in the lifecycle by integrating aspects of both adult and pediatric nutrition. This strong pediatric focus is reflected in chapters on general pediatrics, neonatology, pediatric obesity, developmental disabilities, and eating disorders. Presentation of both states allows for a more complete reference, and it provides an opportunity to better discuss the similarities and difference in various adult and pediatric states. The text also incorporates more specialized chapters on topics such as oral health, and it also features chapters on maldigestion and malabsorption, historically covered through content related to "upper gastrointestinal" and "lower gastrointestinal" disorders.

The text offers the versatility for use as both a classroom text as well as a clinical practice resource to integrate lectures with application and journal review. The text ties the clinical information directly with instruction in one text. Reliance on evidence-based practice is fostered through introduction of research concepts and exercises in journal review.

Supplement Package

Instructors using *Advanced Medical Nutrition Therapy* will have access to a full suite of supplemental resources, including the following:
- Test Bank, providing examination questions for each chapter as well as Midterm and Final Exam
- Slides in PowerPoint format, including bulleted notes that can be easily customized
- Instructor's Manual, containing an array of useful instructor tools
- Image Bank, collecting photographs and illustrations that appear in the text

Kelly Kane
Kathy Prelack

Features of This Text

Advanced Medical Nutrition Therapy incorporates a number of engaging pedagogical features in order to emphasize how the content can be applied in practice.

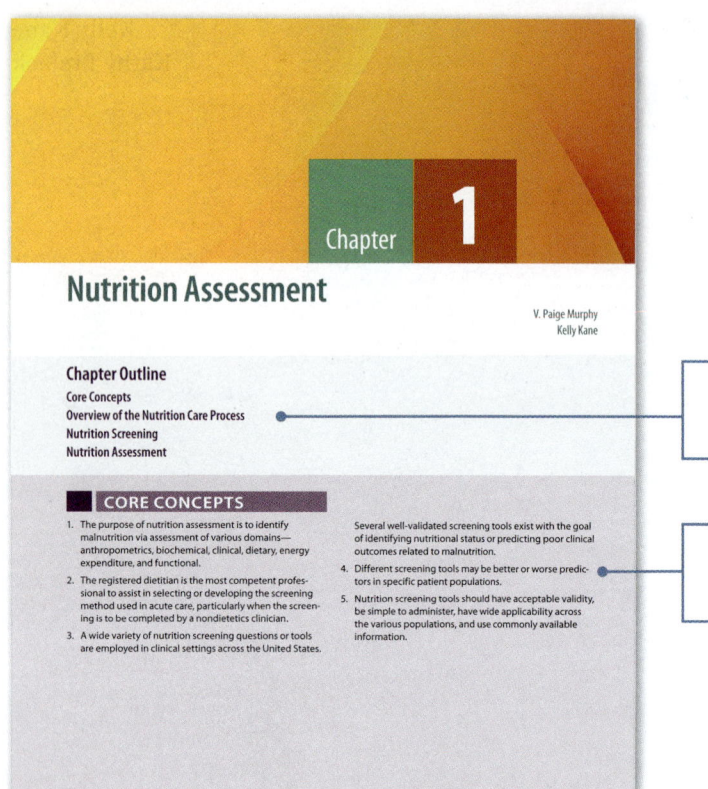

Each chapter opens with a **Chapter Outline** previewing the topics to be covered.

Core Concepts establish important principles that will be explored in the chapter; they later reappear within the chapter text once the relevant content has been broached.

Learning Objectives establish what the reader can expect to learn from the chapter.

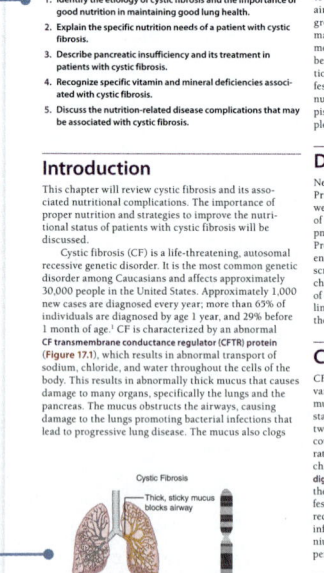

A comprehensive and instructional **art package** includes color photographs and illustrations throughout this text to add a visual dimension to the content being presented.

Features of This Text   xvii

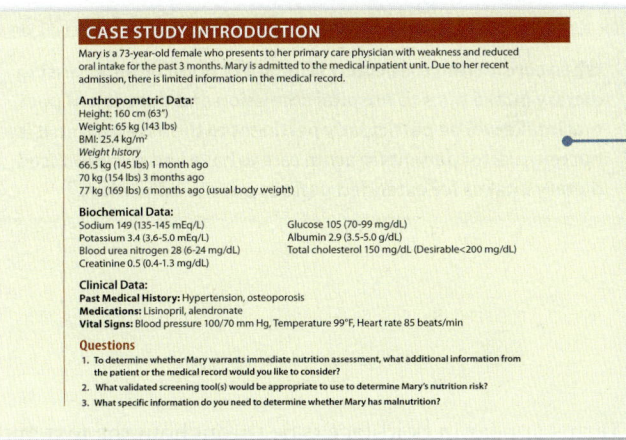

Each chapter begins with a **Case Study**, illustrating how topics discussed in the text might appear in practice. These case studies are revisited throughout the chapter, building in concert with the foundational material. Questions are incorporated to encourage active engagement with the scenarios.

Clinical Controversy boxes emphasize engagement with evidence-based content by highlighting areas where there may be disagreements in the literature.

⚠ **Clinical Controversy**

Is BMI a reliable indicator of cardiometabolic risk across various racial and ethnic groups?

Obesity as measured by BMI is associated with increased cardiometabolic risk, such as increased risk of cardiovascular disease and type 2 diabetes mellitus. BMI is an imperfect tool; it is limited in its ability to differentiate body composition or body fat distribution. The applicability of BMI as a disease risk indicator across different racial and ethnic groups has been more closely examined. In a study of a cardiometabolic risk phenotype described as "metabolic abnormality but normal weight" (MAN), Gujral et al. conducted a cross-sectional analysis of two community-based normal-weight cohorts to evaluate the prevalence of MAN in five racial/ethnic groups. BMI classification cut-offs can be noted in Table 1.7. BMI for South Asian and Chinese American participants was classified according to WHO Asian cut-off points: normal weight BMI 18.5 to 22.9 kg/m^2; overweight BMI 23.0 to 24.7 kg/m^2; obese BMI ≥27.5 kg/m^2. The authors found that Indians and other South Asians had more than double the prevalence of MAN, followed by Hispanics, Chinese Americans, and African Americans, who had greater prevalence of MAN compared to whites. It was estimated that the BMI values at which the expected equivalent numbers of metabolic abnormalities would equal those among whites at an overweight BMI of 25 kg/m^2, after adjusting for age, sex, and race-BMI interactions, were as follows:

1. >22.9 kg/m^2 for African Americans
2. 21.5 kg/m^2 for Hispanics
3. 20.9 kg/m^2 for Chinese Americans
4. 19.6 kg/m^2 for South Asians

These findings suggest that standard BMI categories may not be a useful screen for cardiometabolic risk in the non-white population.

Questions

1. How might BMI confound cardiometabolic screening in racial/ethnic minority groups?
2. What metabolic differences could be hypothesized to account for some of these risk variations?
3. How might these findings influence a clinician's ability to utilize BMI classification of overweight and obesity to identify cardiometabolic risk in a racially and ethnically diverse population?

References

1. Gujral UP, Vittinghoff E, Mongraw-Chafflin M, et al. Cardiometabolic abnormalities among normal-weight persons from five racial/ethnic groups in the United States: a cross-sectional analysis of two cohort studies. *Ann Intern Med*. 2017;166:628–636.
2. WHO Expert Consultation. Appropriate body-mass index for Asian populations and its implications for policy and intervention strategies. *Lancet*. 2004;363:157–163.

🩺 **Clinical Roundtable**

Topic: Nutrition Assessment in the Intensive Care Unit (ICU)[13,68,127,154-158]

Background: Patients treated in the intensive care units are some of the highest acuity patients in the hospital. Many of the typical assessment criteria (weight status, dietary intake, biochemical markers, etc.) are difficult to reliably obtain or are confounded by factors like metabolic stress. Anthropometric measurements, which are fundamental to any nutrition assessment, may not be easily acquired from the intubated and sedated critically ill patient who may be both unable to be moved for measurement and unable to provide self-reported data. Other factors related to clinical status, like fluid shifts or edema, will further confound this assessment.

To help clinicians better assess those who are critically ill, Heyland et al.[155] developed and validated a novel risk assessment tool based directly on the ICU patient population. This tool, the NUTrition Risk in the Critically ill (NUTRIC score), is based on variables that are easy to obtain in the critical care setting. Patients receive a score of 1 to 10 based on an algorithm that considers six variables: age; Acute Physiology and Chronic Health Evaluation scores (APACHE II); Sequential Organ Failure Assessment scores (SOFA); number of comorbidities; days from hospital to ICU admission; and serum interleukin-6 (IL-6). The following table outlines the NUTRIC score variables as they apply to the final evaluation:

Variable	Range	Points
Age (years)	<50	0
	50-74	1
	≥75	2
APACHE II	<15	0
	15-19	1
	20-28	2
	≥28	3
SOFA	<6	0
	6-9	1
	≥10	2

(continues)

Variable	Range	Points
Number of Comorbidities	0-1	0
	≥2	1
Days from Hospital to ICU Admission	<1	0
	≥1	1
IL-6	0-399	0
	≥400	1

Modified from Heyland DK, Dhaliwal R, Jiang X, Day AG. Identifying critically ill patients who benefit the most from nutrition therapy: the development and initial validation of a novel risk assessment tool. *Crit Care*. 2011;15(6):R268.

To be most clinically applicable, the NUTRIC score provides interpretation guidelines based on whether or not the IL-6 marker is available (the other markers are routinely obtainable from the medical record of an ICU patient):

If IL-6 is available:
- High score (6-10 points): associated with worse clinical outcomes (i.e., mortality); these patients are most likely to benefit from aggressive medical nutrition therapy
- Low score (0-5 points): low malnutrition risk

If IL-6 is *not* available:
- High score (5-9 points): associated with worse clinical outcomes (i.e., mortality); these patients are most likely to benefit from aggressive medical nutrition therapy
- Low score (0-4 points): low malnutrition risk

In general, the higher the sum of the scores from each component, the greater the likelihood of nutritional risk and anticipated benefit of nutrition intervention.

Roundtable Discussion

1. Given the difficulties with nutritional assessment in the critical care setting, how might the NUTRIC score be a valuable tool for clinicians in this setting?
2. Due to its validation, should the NUTRIC score supersede standard nutrition assessment in this setting? Why or why not?
3. What are the advantages and disadvantages of using a nutrition assessment tool, such as the NUTRIC score, in the critical care setting?

Clinical Roundtable boxes highlight clinical scenarios that invite a multitude of possible approaches.

Brief **Practice Points** provide additional details relevant to clinical dietetics practice.

> **PRACTICE POINT**
>
> When considering the acutely ill inpatient population, assessing dietary intake prior to hospital admission and duration of poor oral intake will be particularly pertinent to the assessment. It is not unusual for patients in acute care to have had compromised dietary intakes for extended periods prior to admission.[13]

Key Terms

nutrition care process and model (NCPM), nutrition care process terminology (NCPT), malnutrition, nutrition screening, nutritional risk screening (NRS-2002), malnutrition universal screening tool (MUST), short nutritional assessment questionnaire (SNAQ), malnutrition screening tool (MST), anthropometry, height, stadiometer, self-reported height (SRH), knee-height, total arm span (TAS), half arm span (HAS), actual body weight, usual body weight (UBW), percent usual body weight (%UBW), percent weight change (%weight change), ideal body weight (IBW), percent ideal body weight (%IBW), adjusted body weight, dry weight, body mass index (BMI), skinfold anthropometry, triceps skinfold (TSF), mid-upper arm circumference (MUAC), mid-arm muscle circumference

Key Terms appear in bold-face type throughout the text and are collected at the end of each chapter.

Acknowledgments

We sincerely thank the contributors of this text who have devoted their time, energy, and passion to share their expertise. We could not have done this without you!

In addition, we would like to thank the following people:

- Lisa Brown, PhD, RD, LDN, Associate Professor of Nutrition at Simmons College, for reviewing the chapters on Nutrition in Pregnancy and Lactation and Nutrition in Geriatrics
- Haewook Han, PhD, RD, CSR, Renal Nutrition Specialist at Atrius Health/Harvard Vanguard and Tufts Medical Center, for reviewing the chapter on Nutrition in Kidney Disease
- Grace Phelan, MS, RD, LDN, CNSC, Nutrition Support Coordinator at Tufts Medical Center, for reviewing the chapters on Nutrition in Kidney Disease and Parenteral Nutrition Therapy
- Yvette Penner, RD, CNSC, Neonatal Dietitian at the Floating Hospital for Children at Tufts Medical Center, for reviewing the chapter on Nutrition in Neonatology
- Rachel Wilkinson, MS, RD, LDN, Practice Manager and Dietitian at the Boston Food Allergy Center, for contributions to the chapters on Nutrition in Diabetes Mellitus and Nutritional Management of Developmental Disabilities
- Lauren Fialkoff, MS, RD, Clinical Bariatric Dietitian at Tufts Medical Center, for reviewing and contributing to the chapter on Nutrition in Oral Health

About the Authors

Kelly Kane, MS, RD, LDN, CNSC, is the Director of Nutrition and Business Operations and Dietetic Internship Director at Tufts Medical Center and Assistant Professor in the Gerald J. and Dorothy R. Friedman School of Nutrition Science and Policy at Tufts University. She has been a Registered Dietitian for more than 20 years, over which time she has worked in the clinical setting providing medical nutrition therapy for acutely ill adults and children as well as educating patients on ways to improve their health with nutrition. She has taught nutrition to health professionals including dietetic interns, physician assistants, and medical students for over 10 years. She also works as a nutrition consultant with various business and physician groups. She is a Certified Nutrition Support Clinician, member of the Academy of Nutrition and Dietetics, and member of the American Society of Parenteral and Enteral Nutrition.

Kathy Prelack, PhD, RD, LDN, is an Assistant Professor at Simmons College and Adjunct Associate Professor at Tufts University with a primary academic focus on clinical nutrition, medical nutrition therapy, and interprofessional learning. She has taught advanced medical nutrition at Tufts University for over 10 years. Her research interests include energy expenditure and protein metabolism using isotope methodology, and methods of body composition analysis in a clinical setting. Kathy is a Registered Dietitian and is currently the Director of Clinical Nutrition at Shriners Hospitals for Children, a pediatric burn hospital. She has worked in the field of pediatric burn injury for over 20 years. She also serves as the Chair of the Research Council at the hospital. She enjoys mentoring young investigators interested in clinical research. Kathy is a member of the Academy of Nutrition and Dietetics, the American Society of Parenteral and Enteral Nutrition, and the American Burn Association.

Contributors

Deena Altschwager, MS, RD, LDN
Clinical Dietitian
Boston Children's Hospital
Boston, Massachusetts
Chapter 19: Nutrition in Oncology and Hematopoietic Stem Cell Transplant

Katelyn Castro, MS, RD
Nutrition Fellow
Boston Children's Hospital
Boston, Massachusetts
Chapter 2: Biochemical Assessment

Jennifer Cho, MS, RD
Clinical Dietitian
University Hospital
Newark, New Jersey
Chapter 27: Nutrition in Geriatrics

Maggie Dylewski, PhD, RD, LD
Clinical Assistant Professor
Department of Agriculture, Nutrition, and Food Systems
Durham, New Hampshire
Chapter 6: Nutrition in Critical Illness: A Burn Injury Model

Natalie Faella, MS, RD
Registered Dietitian
Metrowest Nutrition
Waltham, Massachusetts
Chapter 25: Nutrition in Eating Disorders

Katie Fort, MS Candidate
Tufts Medical Center
Boston, Massachusetts
Chapter 4: Parenteral Nutrition Therapy

Sonja Goedkoop, MSPH, RD
Manager of Nutrition and Wellness
Zesty, Inc.
San Francisco, California
Chapter 8: Nutritional Management of Obesity

Adi Goldberg, MS Candidate
Simmons College
Boston, Massachusetts
Chapter 24: Nutritional Management of Pediatric Obesity

Angela Goscilo, MS, RDN, CDN
Registered Dietitian
Nutrition Energy
New York City, New York
Chapter 23: Nutrition in Pediatrics

Laura Grande, MS, RD, CSP, LDN
Clinical Dietitian
Children's Hospital of Philadelphia
Philadelphia, Pennsylvania
Chapter 16: Nutrition in Pulmonary Disease

Jennifer Hall, MS, RD
Clinical Dietitian
Shriners Hospital for Children
Boston, Massachusetts
Chapter 19: Nutrition in Oncology and Hematopoietic Stem Cell Transplant
Chapter 26: Nutrition in Developmental Disabilities

Haley Hooks, MS, RD
Clinical Dietitian
Cook Children's Health Care System
Fort Worth, Texas
Chapter 11: Nutrition in Oral Health

Andrea Hurwitz, MS Candidate
Simmons College
Boston, Massachusetts
Chapter 27: Nutrition in Geriatrics

Grace Ling, MS
Tufts Medical Center
Boston, Massachusetts
Chapter 4: Parenteral Nutrition Therapy

Alexis Madej, MS, RD
Registered Dietitian
Show Low, Arizona
Chapter 10: Nutrition in Cardiovascular Disease

Isadora Nogueira, MS, RD, CDN
Clinical Dietitian
SUNY Downstate Medical Center
Brooklyn, New York
Chapter 8: Nutritional Management of Obesity

Nusheen Orandi, BS
Dietetic Intern
UCSF Medical Center
San Francisco, California
Chapter 3: Enteral Nutrition

V. Paige Murphy MS, RD
Pediatric Clinical Dietitian
Johns Hopkins Hospital
Baltimore, Maryland
Chapter 1: Nutrition Assessment
Chapter 12: Disorders of Digestion
Chapter 13: Disorders of Absorption

Carole Palmer, MEd, EdD, RD
Professor
School of Dental Medicine
Tufts University
Professor and Head of the Master's Component of the Frances Stern Combined Dietetic Internship Master's Program
Friedman School of Nutrition Science and Policy
Tufts University
Tufts Medical Center Hospital
Boston, Massachusetts
Chapter 11: Nutrition in Oral Health

Lauren Parsly, RD
Transplant Dietitian
Tufts Medical Center
Boston, Massachusetts
Chapter 18: Nutrition in Solid Organ Transplantation

Antoinette Pert, MS, RD, CSP, LDN
Neonatal Dietitian and Dietetic Internship Coordinator
Children's Hospital of Philadelphia
Philadelphia, Pennsylvania
Chapter 22: Nutrition in Neonatology

Grace Phelan, MS, RD, LDN, CNSC
Nutrition Support Coordinator
Tufts Medical Center
Boston, Massachusetts
Chapter 16: Nutrition in Pulmonary Disease

June N. Pierre-Louis, PhD, MPH, CDN
Nutrition Consultant
Former Health Program Administrator
NYSDOH AIDS Institute
New York City, New York
Chapter 20: Nutrition in HIV and AIDS

Poonhar Poon, MS, RD
Dietitian
DCI Dialysis Clinic, Inc.
Boston, Massachusetts
Chapter 14: Nutrition in Kidney Disease

Jillian Reece, RD, LDN, CSOWM
Clinical Bariatric Dietitian
Tufts Medical Center
Boston, Massachusetts
Chapter 8: Nutritional Management of Obesity

Alicia Romano, MS, RD
Ambulatory Nutrition Support Dietitian
Tufts Medical Center
Boston, Massachusetts
Chapter 19: Nutrition in Oncology

Nora Saul, MS, RD
Registered Dietitian
Diabetes Nutrition Consultant
Boston, Massachusetts
Chapter 9: Nutritional Management of Diabetes Mellitus

Jenna Stefin, MS, RD
Clinical Dietitian
Northwest Community Hospital
Chicago, Illinois
Chapter 18: Nutrition in Solid Organ Transplantation

Sarah Trautman, MS, RD, LDN
Clinical Dietitian
Tufts Medical Center
Boston, Massachusetts
Chapter 21: Nutrition in Pregnancy and Lactation

Emily Trussler, MS Candidate
Simmons College
Boston, Massachusetts
Chapter 21: Nutrition in Pregnancy and Lactation

Molly Uebele, MS, RD
Registered Dietitian
Arlington, Virginia
Chapter 15: Nutrition in Liver Disease

Rachel Wilkinson, MS, RD, LDN
Dietitian
Boston Food Allergy Center
Boston, Massachusetts
Chapter 12: Disorders of Digestion
Chapter 13: Disorders of Absorption

Kathryn Wilson, MS Candidate
Tufts Medical Center
Boston, Massachusetts
Chapter 14: Nutrition in Kidney Disease

Caitlin Wong, MS, RD
Nutrition Education Specialist
Henry M. Jackson Foundation
Bethesda, Maryland
Chapter 7: Nutrition in Wound Healing

Reviewers

Joseph C. Bonilla, PhD, RD
Associate Professor
Department of Nutrition
University of the Incarnate Word
San Antonio, Texas

Detri M. Brech, PhD, RD, LD, CDE
Professor
Department of Dietetics
Ouachita Baptist University
Arkadelphia, Arkansas

Matthew Durant, PhD, PDt, MEd, CDE, FDC
Associate Professor
School of Nutrition and Dietetics
Acadia University
Wolfville, Nova Scotia, Canada

Ann Gaba, EdD, RD, CDN, CDE
Assistant Professor
CUNY Graduate School of Public Health and Health Policy
Hunter College
New York, New York

Andrea M. Hutchins, PhD, RD
Associate Professor
Department of Health Sciences
University of Colorado, Colorado Springs
Colorado Springs, Colorado

Kristine Jordan, PhD, MPH, RD
Associate Professor
Department of Nutrition and Integrative Physiology
University of Utah
Salt Lake City, Utah

Patricia Z. Marincic, PhD, RDN, LDN, CLE
Associate Professor
Department of Nutrition, Dietetics, and Hospitality Management
Auburn University
Auburn, Alabama

Catherine Morley, PhD, PDt, FDC
Assistant Professor
School of Nutrition and Dietetics
Acadia University
Wolfville, Nova Scotia, Canada

Lisa M. Morse, MS, RDN, CNSC
Clinical Assistant Professor
School of Nutrition and Health Promotion
Arizona State University
Gilbert, Arizona

Shaekira L. Niehuser, MS, RD, CNSC
Clinical Assistant Professor
Department of Nutrition and Exercise Physiology
Washington State University
Spokane, Washington

Kevin Pietro, MS, RD, LD
Clinical Assistant Professor
Department of Agriculture, Nutrition, and Food Systems
University of New Hampshire
Durham, New Hampshire

SeAnne Safaii-Waite, PhD, RDN
Associate Professor
Margaret Ritchie School of Family and Consumer Sciences
University of Idaho
Boise, Idaho

Vicki S. Schwartz, DCN, RD, LDN, CNSC
Assistant Clinical Professor
College of Nursing and Health Professions
Drexel University
Philadelphia, Pennsylvania

Bettina Taylor, PhD, RD
Assistant Professor
Department of Agriculture and Natural Resources
Delaware State University
Dover, Delaware

Peggy Turner, MS, RD/LD, FAND
Associate Professor
College of Allied Health
University of Oklahoma Health Sciences Center
Oklahoma City, Oklahoma

Mary Width, MS, RD
Director and Senior Lecturer
Coordinated Program in Dietetics
Wayne State University
Detroit, Michigan

Stanley R. Wilfong, MS, RD, LD, FAND
Lecturer
Department of Family and Consumer Sciences
Baylor University
Waco, Texas

Linda Yarrow, PhD, RDN/LDN, CDE
Assistant Professor
Department of Food, Nutrition, Dietetics, and Health
Kansas State University
Manhattan, Kansas

Section 1

Fundamentals in Practice

Chapter 1   Nutrition Assessment
Chapter 2   Biochemical Assessment
Chapter 3   Enteral Nutrition
Chapter 4   Parenteral Nutrition Therapy
Chapter 5   Energy Expenditure and Body Composition in Metabolic Stress

Chapter 1

Nutrition Assessment

V. Paige Murphy
Kelly Kane

Chapter Outline

Core Concepts
Overview of the Nutrition Care Process
Nutrition Screening
Nutrition Assessment

CORE CONCEPTS

1. The purpose of nutrition assessment is to identify malnutrition via assessment of various domains—anthropometrics, biochemical, clinical, dietary, energy expenditure, and functional.

2. The registered dietitian is the most competent professional to assist in selecting or developing the screening method used in acute care, particularly when the screening is to be completed by a nondietetics clinician.

3. A wide variety of nutrition screening questions or tools are employed in clinical settings across the United States. Several well-validated screening tools exist with the goal of identifying nutritional status or predicting poor clinical outcomes related to malnutrition.

4. Different screening tools may be better or worse predictors in specific patient populations.

5. Nutrition screening tools should have acceptable validity, be simple to administer, have wide applicability across the various populations, and use commonly available information.

SECTION 1 FUNDAMENTALS IN PRACTICE

Learning Objectives

1. Describe the purpose of nutrition assessment as part of the Nutrition Care Process and Model.
2. Define and differentiate between nutrition screening and nutrition assessment.
3. Identify the screening tools applicable to clinical practice.
4. Explain the components of anthropometric assessment and their purposes, and recognize which have greater relevance to clinical practice and which should be used with caution.
5. Describe appropriate components of a clinical assessment and why that information may be pertinent to the overall nutrition assessment.
6. State the benefits and limitations of dietary assessment and the dietary recall methods.
7. Identify the purpose and relevant components of a functional assessment of muscle strength.

Nutritional status affects virtually every individual's response to illness.[1] Those in a malnourished state benefit most if malnutrition is quickly identified. The importance of thorough and appropriate nutrition assessment is critical in both the prevention and treatment of illness. The process of assessment will provide the foundation from which any necessary nutrition-related intervention is built. The purpose of this chapter is to identify the specific components of recognizing and evaluating at-risk adult patients as the integral backbone of dietetics practice.

Overview of the Nutrition Care Process

In order to facilitate the provision of the highest quality of care, the Academy of Nutrition and Dietetics (AND; formerly known as the American Dietetic Association, or

CASE STUDY INTRODUCTION

Mary is a 73-year-old female who presents to her primary care physician with weakness and reduced oral intake for the past 3 months. Mary is admitted to the medical inpatient unit. Due to her recent admission, there is limited information in the medical record.

Anthropometric Data:
Height: 160 cm (63")
Weight: 65 kg (143 lbs)
BMI: 25.4 kg/m²
Weight history
66.5 kg (145 lbs) 1 month ago
70 kg (154 lbs) 3 months ago
77 kg (169 lbs) 6 months ago (usual body weight)

Biochemical Data:
Sodium 149 (135-145 mEq/L)
Potassium 3.4 (3.6-5.0 mEq/L)
Blood urea nitrogen 28 (6-24 mg/dL)
Creatinine 0.5 (0.4-1.3 mg/dL)

Glucose 105 (70-99 mg/dL)
Albumin 2.9 (3.5-5.0 g/dL)
Total cholesterol 150 mg/dL (Desirable<200 mg/dL)

Clinical Data:
Past Medical History: Hypertension, osteoporosis
Medications: Lisinopril, alendronate
Vital Signs: Blood pressure 100/70 mm Hg, Temperature 99°F, Heart rate 85 beats/min

Questions
1. To determine whether Mary warrants immediate nutrition assessment, what additional information from the patient or the medical record would you like to consider?
2. What validated screening tool(s) would be appropriate to use to determine Mary's nutrition risk?
3. What specific information do you need to determine whether Mary has malnutrition?

ADA) adopted the **Nutrition Care Process and Model (NCPM)** as a systematic framework to recognize, diagnose, and intervene upon nutrition-related problems for which a nutrition intervention is the primary treatment. The NCPM (**Figure 1.1**) was designed to provide a methodical structure for critically assessing patients across the wide spectrum of health and disease. The process consists of four steps to be completed in sequence—assessment, diagnosis, intervention, and monitoring and evaluation—each of which is linked to corresponding standardized terminology, called the **Nutrition Care Process Terminology (NCPT)**, for consistent documentation. In all cases, assessment is preceded by screening, a separate but supportive task that triggers the entry of a patient into the NCPM.[2-6]

Nutrition assessment serves as the essential first step that provides a comprehensive evaluation of an individual's nutrition-related history. It is a systematic approach to collecting, recording, and interpreting all relevant data for the purpose of accurately diagnosing a nutrition-related problem. As part of the NCPM, nutrition assessment is organized into five domains: anthropometric measurements; biochemical data, medical tests, and procedures; client history; nutrition-focused physical exam; and food/nutrition-related history. This information may be obtained from a number of sources, including, but not limited to, the patient, family members, caregivers, medical care team, or medical record, depending upon the specific situation. The process of assessment is not stagnant; instead, it should be viewed as an ongoing and continual analysis of an individual's nutritional status.[2,4,6]

The Purpose of Nutrition Assessment

The purpose of nutrition assessment is straightforward: to identify the presence of any nutrition-related problems, particularly malnutrition. However, over the past several decades, the topic of assessment has been surrounded by ongoing discussion, research, reworking, and redefining. Although researchers, clinicians, and public policy makers have invested significant energy into a unified approach for the identification and evaluation of malnutrition, no universally accepted approach has been determined. This may be attributed to the wide variation in existing definitions of the malnourished state.[8-10]

Defining Malnutrition

A clear definition of the components of clinical malnutrition is imperative to the assessment process. It would be difficult to identify the malnourished state without a

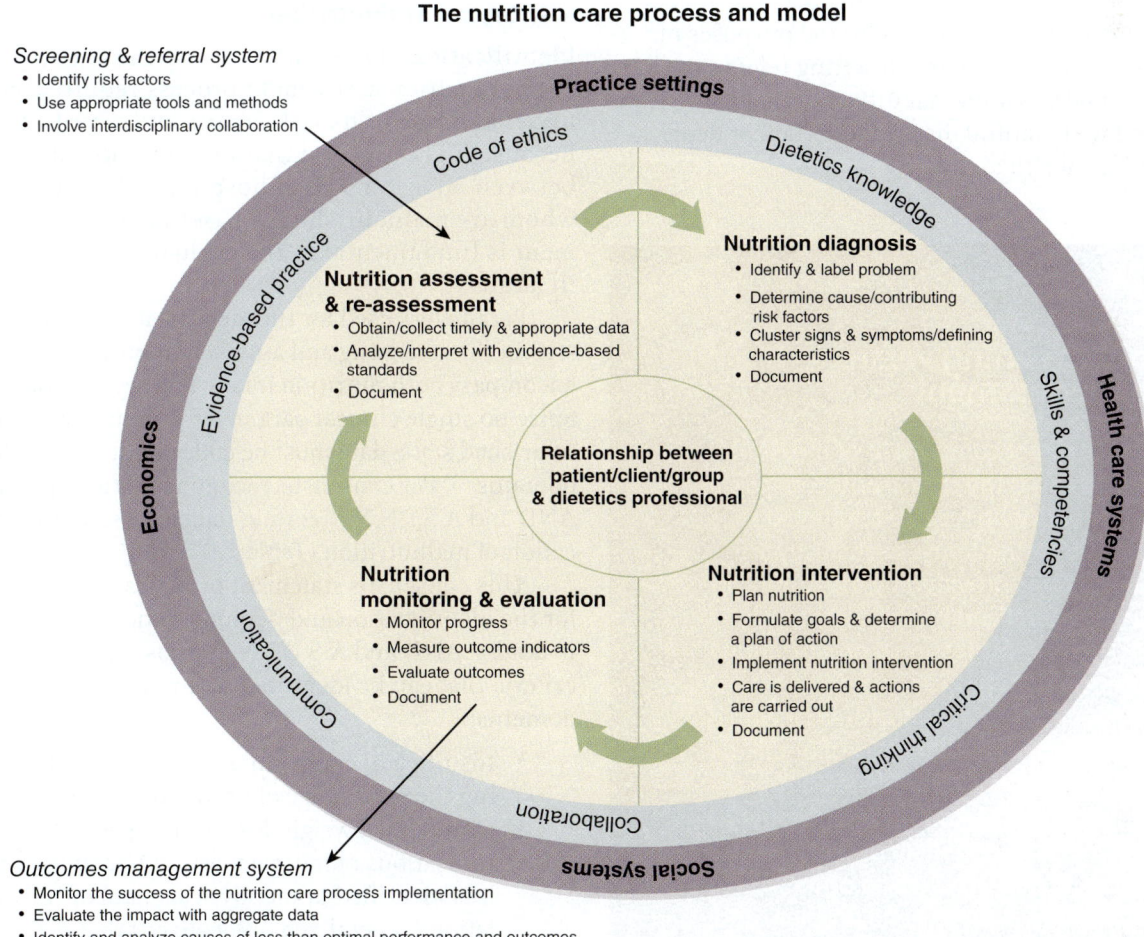

FIGURE 1.1 The Nutrition Care Process and Model
Reproduced from Hammond MI, Myers EF, Trostler N. Nutrition care process and model: An academic and practice odyssey. *J Acad Nutr Diet*. 2014;114(12):1879–1894.

known set of risk factors and/or manifestations for which to probe. One may assume that defining such a common and well-researched phenomenon would be relatively simple. Unfortunately, the nutrition community lacks a universal agreement; every organization, every publication, and every practitioner claims its own (slightly different) definition of the state.[11-13]

The relationship between malnutrition and nutrition assessment is critical. Any elements that influence the development of malnutrition and the manifestations that result should both comprise the steps of assessment and provide reliable identifiers for nutrition screening. Solidifying a transparent definition of the malnourished state is vital to understanding what and why specific signs and symptoms are assessed.

Consider the general concept of nutritional adequacy—the state of equilibrium in which an individual's dietary intake matches his or her requirements. In theory, malnutrition will occur when intake falls below (or exceeds) what is required. In practice, this process is significantly more complex. It is marked by a resulting succession of metabolic abnormalities, physiologic changes, reduced organ and tissue function, and loss of critical body mass. For these reasons, malnutrition can be identified as any alteration in physiology, composition, or function attributable to a diet or to a disease that affects nutritional outcomes. Malnutrition for the purposes of nutrition assessment in the clinical setting refers to a disease-related malnutrition that differs dramatically from that associated with natural disaster, conflict, or deprivation in the public health arena.[8,9,11,14]

Current research indicates that varying degrees of acute or chronic inflammation as part of the disease state are key factors in the pathogenesis of malnutrition. In clinical practice, malnutrition should be considered within one of three subcategories as defined by a joint International Guidelines Committee of A.S.P.E.N. and the European Society for Clinical Nutrition and Metabolism (ESPEN):

1. Chronic starvation without inflammation (e.g., anorexia nervosa)
2. Chronic disease–associated malnutrition, when inflammation is chronic and of mild-to-moderate degree (e.g., organ failure, pancreatic cancer)
3. Acute disease- or injury-associated malnutrition, when inflammation is acute and of severe degree (e.g., sepsis, burns, trauma, or closed head injury)[11-13,15,16]

With these considerations in mind, one definition serves as a solid framework for the purposes of identifying and assessing clinical malnutrition: "**Malnutrition** is a subacute or chronic state of nutrition, in which a combination of varying degrees of overnutrition or undernutrition and inflammatory activity has led to a change in body composition and diminished function."[17]

Identifying Malnutrition

Identification of malnutrition and the entire purpose of the nutrition assessment process require a general understanding of its risk factors and manifestations.[16,18] Because it is estimated that malnutrition affects between 30% and 55% of hospitalized patients, many of whom are malnourished at baseline, nutrition assessment is fundamental to the evaluation of the acutely ill adult.[5,19-21]

Parameters used for the identification of malnutrition within the screening and assessment processes should encompass both nutrition intake and severity of disease. Since no single clinical parameter is indicative of the malnourished state, data must be collected from a variety of domains.[7,16] Per consensus recommendations published by AND and A.S.P.E.N.,[10] certain data are useful in the identification of malnutrition (**Table 1.1**).

This consensus statement provides further guidance for the identification and documentation of malnutrition in adults. AND and A.S.P.E.N. propose specific diagnostic criteria that can be identified within the aforementioned domains:

- Insufficient energy intake, established by determining the percentage of needs consumed
- Unintended weight loss over a specific period of time
- Indications of muscle mass and/or subcutaneous fat loss identified upon physical exam or fluid accumulation (generalized or localized) that may mask any recent weight loss
- Diminished functional status as measured by handgrip strength

---

Box 1.1

Nutrition Screening versus Nutrition Assessment

Although not a direct component of the NCPM, nutrition screening is the critical antecedent step to identify patients who require additional assessment. This distinction is best illustrated using the definitions provided by the American Society for Parenteral and Enteral Nutrition (A.S.P.E.N.). This interprofessional organization defines nutrition screening as "a process to identify an individual who is malnourished or who is at risk for malnutrition to determine if detailed nutrition assessment is indicated." In contrast, the longer, more detailed nutrition assessment process evaluates the patient in detail to identify a nutrition-related problem. In other words, screening determines the *risk* of a problem and assessment determines the *presence* of a problem.[5,7]

TABLE 1.1 DATA USEFUL IN THE IDENTIFICATION OF MALNUTRITION

Domain	Specific Data
Anthropometric	Standard measures of height, weight, and body composition, with particular focus on unintended weight loss
Biochemical	Biochemical assessment involves use of laboratory tests of patients' blood, urine, feces, and tissue samples to help determine nutritional status and organ function
Clinical	Nutrition-focused past medical history and clinical diagnosis, as well as a nutrition-focused physical exam that may reveal the presence of several diagnostic characteristics of malnutrition
Dietary	Information regarding food and nutrient intake will indicate the presence of any inadequacies or imbalances
Energy	Estimation of energy requirements and comparison to current intake; determining ability to meet needs, particularly when increased by disease state
Functional	Declines in function measured via muscle strength and/or physical performance

A positive finding of any two characteristics indicates malnutrition. Purposeful examination for these features should be present in every nutrition assessment.[10,12]

Consequences of Malnutrition

The importance of an appropriate assessment for the identification of malnutrition can be attributed to prevention of its far-reaching and damaging clinical impacts. It has long been understood that patients with poor nutritional status have inferior outcomes compared to their well-nourished counterparts. In the acute care setting, malnutrition is a major contributor to increased morbidity and mortality, increased lengths of stay and rates of readmission, decreased function and quality of life, and higher healthcare costs. The presence of malnutrition alters the function and recovery of virtually every organ system, which can manifest as the development of pressure injuries, increased rates of infection, impaired wound healing, surgical complications, and increased ventilatory requirements, among others. Assessment of nutritional status in critically ill patients should evaluate for the presence of malnutrition in its many domains to prevent clinical deterioration.[5,9,10,18,22-25]

> **CORE CONCEPT 1**
>
> The purpose of nutrition assessment is to identify malnutrition via assessment of various domains—anthropometrics, biochemical, clinical, dietary, energy expenditure, and functional.

Nutrition Screening

The Role of Nutrition Screening in NCPM

Prior to the introduction of the NCPM, nutrition screening was recommended by AND as an integral component of care.[26] The process to identify those individuals at nutritional risk who would benefit from further assessment and intervention has evolved into a critical antecedent step of the NCPM. AND currently defines **nutrition screening** as "the process of identifying patients, clients, or groups who may have a nutrition diagnosis and benefit from nutrition assessment intervention by a registered dietitian (RD)."[5] The initial screen may not always be completed by a dietetics practitioner and is not actually considered to be part of the NCPM.[4,12]

AND supports nutrition screening as the preliminary step that triggers entrance into the NCPM. Given the impracticality of conducting a full assessment of all patients, practitioners rely upon an appropriate screen to identify individuals who are either already malnourished or at risk of becoming malnourished. The goal in this case is not necessarily to *diagnose* malnutrition, but instead to identify the known characteristics associated with the malnourished state or other nutritional issues that would warrant a more thorough evaluation and potential intervention.[5,12,27]

Screening in Acute Care

The Joint Commission (JC) is the independent entity responsible for the accreditation and certification of healthcare organizations in the United States. In 1995, the JC mandated that the nutrition screen be performed when warranted by the patient's needs and conditions based upon organizational criteria. When applicable to a patient's condition, the screen must be completed within 24 hours of an inpatient admission.[7,28] The JC does not require that a specific tool or criteria be used; the guidelines instead specify that each organization must have "defined criteria that identify when nutritional plans are developed."[28] In other words, there are no clear standards that dictate the screening tool itself, only that each organization screens within the designated time frame. As such, the methods used between sites vary considerably.[5,28,29]

The vast majority of acute care centers have incorporated screening into the admission process in order to help prioritize hospital resources, although the screening methods used to meet JC's mandate will vary from center to center. Several common denominators prevail among the multitude of tools utilized: validity and reliability, ease of use and convenience, speed (typically requiring less than 5 minutes), avoidance of complicated calculations or laboratory data, minimal expense, and noninvasiveness. In order to meet each of these characteristics, initial screening in most hospitals is based, at least in part, on height and weight collected upon admission.[5,12,26,28,30]

Any screening tool a hospital employs will be unable to account for the extreme variability seen in patients within an acute care setting. Other aspects of the disease state must be considered, in addition to nutritional measurements, to determine if and when intervention is warranted or is likely to be beneficial. Screening is not meant to replace the training and clinical judgment of the RD, but instead to assist in initiating the NCPM.[7,20]

Selecting a Screening Method

A number of existing screening tools are available for use as is or with slight modification in the clinical setting. These tools, which will be described in detail in the following sections, serve as exceptional resources for implementing a new, or revamping an existing, screening method. When selecting the tool or criteria to be used in acute care, there are two important considerations:

1. The screening of patients in the clinical setting differs greatly from that of the community setting. The primary purpose in this context is to identify those patients who will require further assessment of need for nutrition support. Given that many of the developed tools were intended for use in the community setting, it is important to ensure that the tool selected has been validated within the specific inpatient population in which it will be used.[5]
2. Given the complexity of the malnourished state, there is no single parameter that is both sensitive and specific for malnutrition. Screening patients in acute care must be ongoing and should consider the routes for development of malnutrition (deficient intake, excessive losses, increased metabolic demand, etc.) in order to identify those who increase in risk over time.[5,19,30]

Overall, the screening tool selected should identify all individuals at risk. In order to ensure this validity, a screening tool will have a high sensitivity (meaning that patients identified as at risk of malnutrition are actually generally malnourished) *and* a high specificity (patients not identified as at risk are, in fact, not malnourished). Furthermore, a screening tool should be reliable in that it consistently reproduces the same or similar results. The use of an inappropriate tool—or one that has not been validated or has been validated in a different population than the one for which it is currently being used—will negatively influence patient care and risk misdiagnosis of malnutrition.[5,30]

> **CORE CONCEPT 2**
>
> The registered dietitian is the most competent professional to assist in selecting or developing the screening method used in acute care, particularly when the screening is to be completed by a nondietetics clinician.[12]

Nutrition Screening Tools

Nutrition screening allows all patients at risk to receive the appropriate individualized nutrition care they require. The consensus of literature and clinical practice demonstrates that when appropriate screening leads to appropriate intervention, outcomes are dramatically improved including reduced readmissions, shorter lengths of hospital stays, and lower mortality rates.[12] Given this insight, a number of screening tools have been developed and validated for use in the acute care setting. Most validated tools will address four basic areas of nutrition risk: recent weight loss, recent dietary intake, current body mass index (BMI), and current disease state. Depending on the tool, various other measurements of nutritional status may be included to further assist in the prediction of malnutrition risk.[20,31,32]

Although some screening tools have been endorsed by international nutrition societies, there is no universal or empirical agreement on a single best tool. The four most well-known and widely used examples include Nutritional Risk Screening (NRS-2002), Malnutrition Universal Screening Tool (MUST), Short Nutritional Assessment Questionnaire (SNAQ), and Malnutrition Screening Tool (MST). Please note that while some of these tools were developed by professional groups outside of the United States, they are used widely across clinical practice.[20,28]

Nutritional Risk Screening (NRS-2002)

When the **Nutritional Risk Screening (NRS-2002)** tool was developed by a working group of ESPEN, the goal was to establish a screening system based on the nutrition criteria or characteristics used in the current clinical trials. The developers relied on the assumption that nutritional status and indication for nutrition support (based on undernutrition and/or increased nutritional requirements) relate directly to severity of disease. The tool measures disease impact in addition to the markers of current or potential malnutrition. It has been validated to identify not only patients who are malnourished at the time of screening, but also those at risk for malnutrition secondary to the disease state or associated treatment, thus emphasizing the need for preventing further deterioration of nutritional status as the clinical course progresses.[21,30-32]

The purpose of the NRS-2002 system is to detect either existing or anticipated malnutrition in the hospital setting. The initial screening tool consists of four simple, but strategic, questions (**Figure 1.2**) that consider weight loss, BMI, and dietary intake history in the setting of illness. If there is a positive response to any of the questions in the initial screen, a second, more detailed screen is conducted. This final screen calculates two scores: one for current nutritional status and another for severity of disease as a reflection of the increase in metabolic demand it may cause. These scores are then combined and adjusted for age (with age older than 70 years as a risk factor) to result in a final evaluation of nutrition risk. Ultimately, this score is linked to an example intervention, although the content of the nutrition care plan is determined by the clinician.[9,12,18,20,28,30]

Nutritional Risk Screening (NRS 2002)

Table 1	Initial screening		
		Yes	No
1	Is BMI <20.5?		
2	Has the patient lost weight within the last 3 months?		
3	Has the patient had a reduced dietary intake in the last week?		
4	Is the patient severely ill ? (e.g. in intensive therapy)		
Yes: If the answer is 'Yes' to any question, the screening in Table 2 is performed. **No**: If the answer is 'No' to all questions, the patient is re-screened at weekly intervals. If the patient e.g. is scheduled for a major operation, a preventive nutritional care plan is considered to avoid the associated risk status.			

Table 2	Final screening			
	Impaired nutritional status		**Severity of disease ($\approx$ increase in requirements)**	
Absent **Score 0**	Normal nutritional status	Absent **Score 0**	Normal nutritional requirements	
Mild **Score 1**	Wt loss >5% in 3 mths or Food intake below 50–75% of normal requirement in preceding week	Mild **Score 1**	Hip fracture* Chronic patients, in particular with acute complications: cirrhosis*, COPD*. *Chronic hemodialysis, diabetes, oncology*	
Moderate **Score 2**	Wt loss >5% in 2 mths or BMI 18.5 – 20.5 + impaired general condition or Food intake 25–60% of normal requirement in preceding week	Moderate **Score 2**	Major abdominal surgery* Stroke* *Severe pneumonia, hematologic malignancy*	
Severe **Score 3**	Wt loss >5% in 1 mth (>15% in 3 mths) or BMI <18.5 + impaired general condition or Food intake 0-25% of normal requirement in preceding week in preceding week.	Severe **Score 3**	Head injury* Bone marrow transplantation* *Intensive care patients (APACHE>10).*	
Score:	+	Score:	=Total score	
Age	if ≥70 years: add 1 to total score above	=age-adjusted total score		
Score ≥3: the patient is nutritionally at-risk and a nutritional care plan is initiated **Score <3**: weekly rescreening of the patient. If the patient e.g. is scheduled for a major operation, a preventive nutritional care plan is considered to avoid the associated risk status.				

NRS-2002 is based on an interpre-tation of available randomized clinical trials. *indicates that a trial directly supports the categorization of patients with that diagnosis. Diagnoses shown in *italics* are based on the prototypes given below.
Nutritional risk is defined by the present **nutritional status** and risk of impairment of present status, due to **increased requirements** caused by stress metabolism of the clinical condition.

A nutritional care plan is indicated in all patients who are

(1) severely undernourished (score = 3), or (2) severely ill (score = 3), or (3) moderately undernourished + mildly ill (score 2 + 1), or (4) mildly undernourished + moderately ill (score 1 + 2).
Prototypes for severity of disease
Score = 1: a patient with chronic disease, admitted to hospital due to complications. The patient is weak but out of bed regularly. Protein requirement is increased, but can be covered by oral diet or supplements in most cases.
Score = 2: a patient confined to bed due to illness, e.g. following major abdominal surgery. Protein requirement is substantially increased, but can be covered, although artificial feeding is required in many cases.
Score = 3: a patient in intensive care with assisted ventilation etc. Protein requirement is increased and cannot be covered even by artificial feeding. Protein breakdown and nitrogen loss can be significantly attenuated.

FIGURE 1.2 The Nutritional Risk Screening (NRS-2002) System
Reproduced from: Kondrup J, Allison SP, Elia M, Vellas B, Plauth M. ESPEN guidelines for nutrition screening 2002. *Clin Nutr*. 2003;22(4):415-421.

The current ESPEN Screening Guidelines recommend the sole use of the NRS-2002 in the hospital setting.[20] This system yields unsurpassed predictive validity when compared to other screening tools in the adult population. A number of studies have validated the NRS-2002 across a range of hospitalized patients—from surgical to cardiovascular to gastrointestinal—with strong inter-rater reliability (i.e., can be used by various professionals with similar results). This system can be applied in the acute care setting without concern for impracticality or inaccuracy.[9,20,30,32-37]

Malnutrition Universal Screening Tool (MUST)

In an effort to identify both undernutrition and overnutrition in adults of different ages and diagnoses, the Malnutrition Advisory Group, a standing committee of the British Association for Parenteral and Enteral Nutrition (BAPEN), convened to develop the **Malnutrition Universal Screening Tool (MUST)**. Similar to the NRS-2002, the MUST tool considers current weight status as BMI, unintentional changes in weight, and the presence of an acute disease that influences, or is likely to influence, dietary intake. Each of these three components can individually influence clinical outcome, serving as a powerful predictor of nutrition risk when combined. To assess these variables, the MUST framework utilizes a simple five-step process to arrive at an overall score for risk of malnutrition—either low, medium, or high risk (**Figure 1.3**). The tool then refers clinicians to management, which can be modified according to the specific healthcare setting and patient population.[12,24,27,28,30,31,38]

MUST has been deemed valid and reliable across a wide spectrum of adult patients, even among those requiring special interpretation for fluid disturbances, amputations, or inability to be measured for height and weight. In these situations, the MUST framework supplies instructions for alternative measurements that ensure reliability nearly identical to that of the original tool. Although originally developed

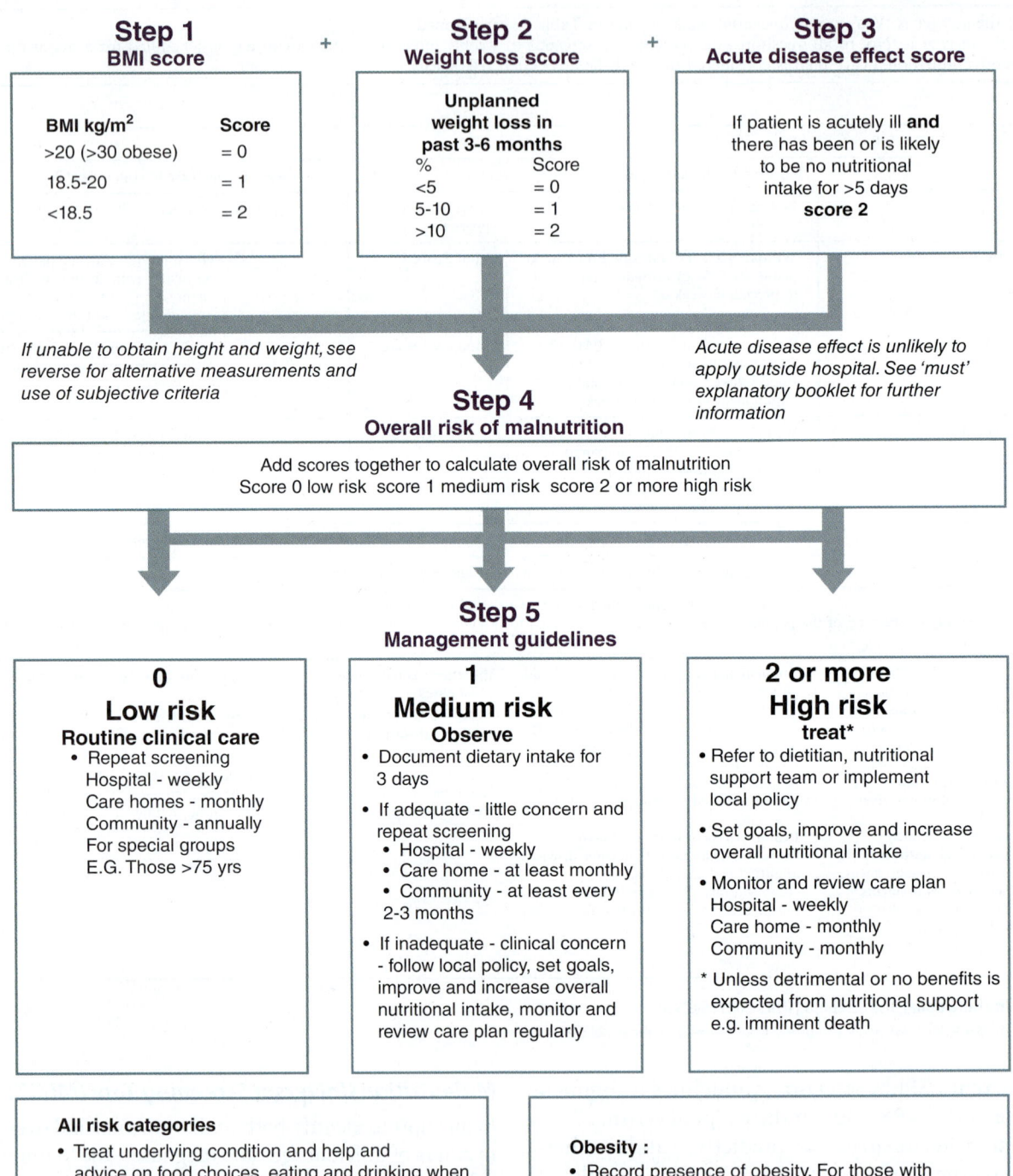

FIGURE 1.3 The Malnutrition Universal Screening Tool (MUST) with inclusion of Alternative Measurements Guidelines

Reproduced from Professor Marinos Elia. The 'MUST' report. Nutritional screening of adults: a multidisciplinary responsibility. Development and use of the malnutrition universal screening tool (MUST) for adults. *BAPEN*; 2003. ISBN 1-899467-70-X.

Alternative measurements: instructions and tables

If height cannot be obtained, use length of forearm (ulna) to calculate height using tables below.
(see the 'MUST' explanatory booklet for details of other alternative measurements (knee height and demispan) that can also be used to estimate height).

Estimating height from ulna length

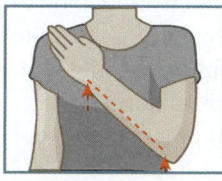

Measure between the point of the elbow (olecranon process) and the midpoint of the prominent bone of the wrist (styloid process) (left side if possible).

Height (m)														
men (< 65 years)	1.94	1.93	1.91	1.89	1.87	1.85	1.84	1.82	1.80	1.78	1.76	1.75	1.73	1.71
men (≥ 65 years)	1.87	1.86	1.84	1.82	1.81	1.79	1.78	1.76	1.75	1.73	1.71	1.70	1.68	1.67
Ulna length (cm)	32.0	31.5	31.0	30.5	30.0	29.5	29.0	28.5	28.0	27.5	27.0	26.5	26.0	25.5
women (< 65 years)	1.84	1.83	1.81	1.80	1.79	1.77	1.76	1.75	1.73	1.72	1.70	1.69	1.68	1.66
women (≥ 65 years)	1.84	1.83	1.81	1.79	1.78	1.76	1.75	1.73	1.71	1.70	1.68	1.66	1.65	1.63
men (< 65 years)	1.69	1.67	1.66	1.64	1.62	1.60	1.58	1.57	1.55	1.53	1.51	1.49	1.48	1.46
men (≥ 65 years)	1.65	1.63	1.62	1.60	1.59	1.57	1.56	1.54	1.52	1.51	1.49	1.48	1.46	1.45
Ulna length (cm)	25.0	24.5	24.0	23.5	23.0	22.5	22.0	21.5	21.0	20.5	20.0	19.5	19.0	18.5
women (< 65 years)	1.65	1.63	1.62	1.61	1.59	1.58	1.56	1.55	1.54	1.54	1.51	1.50	1.48	1.47
women (≥ 65 years)	1.61	1.60	1.58	1.56	1.55	1.53	1.52	1.50	1.48	1.47	1.45	1.44	1.42	1.40

Estimating BMI category from mid upper arm circumference (MUAC)

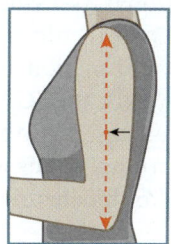

The subject's left arm should be bent at the elbow at a 90 degree angle, with the upper arm held parallel to the side of the body. Measure the distance between the bony protrusion on the shoulder (acromion) and the point of the elbow (olecranon process). Mark the mid-point.

Ask the subject to let arm hang loose and measure around the upper arm at the mid-point, making sure that the tape measure is snug but not tight.

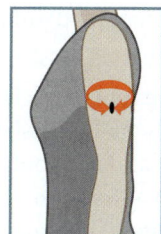

If MUAC is < 23.5 cm, BMI is likely to be < 20 kg/m^2
If MUAC is > 32.0 cm, BMI is likely to be > 30 kg/m^2

The use of MUAC provides a general indication of BMI and is not designed to generate an actual score for use with 'MUST'. For further information on use of MUAC please refer to *The 'MUST' Explanatory Booklet*.

FIGURE 1.3 *(Continued)*

for use in the community setting and supported by ESPEN as the preferred screening tool in this context, MUST has been shown suitable for use across the continuum of health care. When extended to the acute setting, this framework demonstrates concurrent validity with other tools and strong predictive validity in terms of lengths of hospital stay, discharge destination, and mortality. MUST can be utilized by all members of the interdisciplinary team without concern for inter-rater variation. Overall, this tool is simple, evidence-based, valid, and reliable, with a practicability supported by literature and clinical practice.[12,20,30,38-43]

Short Nutritional Assessment Questionnaire (SNAQ)

The publication of the first ESPEN Screening Guidelines prompted international reevaluation of hospital-wide screening processes. Upon assessment of the tools available for use, many nations found that their current frameworks failed to meet the criteria recommended by the guidelines. In response, a committee of dietitians in the Netherlands developed the **Short Nutritional Assessment Questionnaire (SNAQ)**, a "quick and easy" screening tool intended for use during admission to an acute care facility. The development of

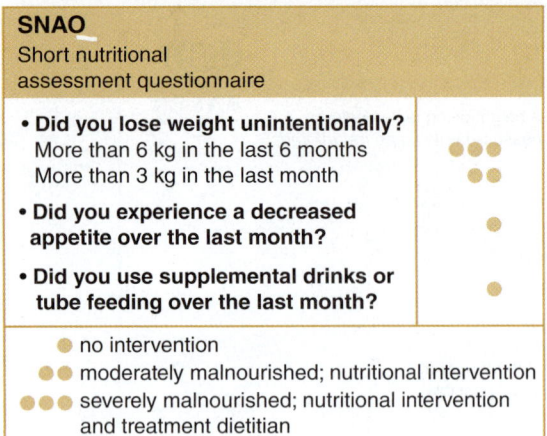

FIGURE 1.4 The Short Nutritional Assessment Questionnaire
Reproduced from Dutch Malnutrition Steering Group. SNAQ tools in english. Fight Malnutrition Web site. www.fightmalnutrition.eu. Updated 2017. Accessed February 10, 2017.

SNAQ was based on an evaluation of mixed hospitalized medical and surgical adult patients. Following a statistical analysis of 26 questions related to nutritional status and disease state, the 3 questions identified with the highest predictive validity were included in the tool (see **Figure 1.4** for the complete tool):[30,31]

1. Did you lose weight unintentionally? (scored according to the amount of weight loss)
2. Did you experience a decreased appetite over the last month?
3. Did you use supplemental drinks or tube feeding over the last month?

Based on response, the tool then classifies patients as well nourished, moderately malnourished, or severely malnourished. Using the validated tool, malnourished patients are recognized on admission and receive necessary intervention at an early stage. This early identification and intervention has been associated with reduced length of hospital stay. The SNAQ screening tool has been validated in both outpatient and inpatient populations, with a simplicity that allows easy inclusion into the admission process.[12,30,44-48]

Malnutrition Screening Tool (MST)

Similar in concept to the SNAQ, the **Malnutrition Screening Tool (MST)** is a three-question tool that was developed and validated for use based on general medical and surgical hospitalized patients. It was created based on the need for a framework that used routinely available data, was noninvasive and convenient for nondietetics staff, and could be employed across a heterogeneous adult population. In a process similar to that used for the development of SNAQ, 21 screening questions were selected based on the literature and clinical experience. Those with the highest sensitivity and specificity in predicting nutrition status were included in the final tool.[30]

Two questions—"Have you lost weight recently without trying?" and "Have you been eating poorly because of a decreased appetite?"—were deemed the best predictors of nutrition risk. In addition, a third question was incorporated to assess the degree of weight loss, if present. A score is allocated based on patient or caregiver response, which will categorize the patient as "not at risk" or "at risk" (**Figure 1.5**). The scoring system can then be used to prioritize patient care, with those receiving the highest scores requiring the earliest intervention.[28,49,50]

The MST is an attractive choice when selecting a screening tool due to its simplicity and ability to be completed without additional calculations. Despite its minimal nature, the MST is an acceptable screening tool secondary to its relative validity, inter-rater reliability, sensitivity, and specificity. In the literature and in practice, the tool is lauded as a strong predictor of nutritional status.[12,28,30,31,49,51,52]

> **CORE CONCEPT 3**
>
> A wide variety of nutrition screening questions or tools are employed in clinical settings across the United States. Several well-validated screening tools exist with the goal of identifying nutritional status or predicting poor clinical outcomes related to malnutrition.[28]

Assessment Tools Confused For Screening Tools

Two additional tools—the Subjective Global Assessment (SGA) and the Mini-Nutritional Assessment (MNA)—are often grouped with the list of screening tools previously discussed. These tools, however, function as a means of nutrition assessment. In other words, the SGA and MNA should most readily be used as to assess, not to screen, because they combine data on nutritional status with clinical observations, disease status, and/or biochemical values.[5,31]

Final Comparison of Screening Tools for Acute Care

As previously mentioned, there is no universal agreement on a "gold standard" in terms of nutrition screening tools. Comprehensive tools, like NRS-2002 and MUST, will require slightly more time and skill from the screening clinician because of the need for measurements, calculations, and evaluation of disease severity. In many studies, these tools (particularly the NRS-2002) outperform all others in the clinical population.[53,54] Conversely, the "quick and easy" tools, such as SNAQ and MUST, are often supported in the literature due to the adequate availability of screening components. The questions used in these tools are not only simple to complete, but have been shown to identify malnutrition risk with similar accuracy as the comprehensive tools without the need for additional calculations.[48,55] Yet another study found each of the four tools to be adequate for screening malnutrition at a nearly identical level. The bottom line is that each of the four screening tools may be employed based on individual hospital or clinical preferences (**Table 1.2**). Because each is well validated and considered reliable, the RD must be careful to recommend the most appropriate tool for the specific setting, patient population, and/or screening goals.[11,18,30,55]

Malnutrition screening tool (MST)

Step 1: screen with the MST

① Have you recently lost weight without trying?

No	0
Unsure	2

If yes, how much weight have you lost?

2-13 lb	1
14-23 lb	2
24-33 lb	3
34 lb or more	4
Unsure	2

Weight loss score: ☐

② Have you been eating poorly because of a decreased appetite?

No	0
Yes	1

Appetite score: ☐

Add weight loss and appetite scores

MST SCORE: ☐

Step 2: score to determine risk

MST = 0 OR 1
NOT AT RISK
Eating well with little or no weight loss

If length of stay exceeds 7 days, then rescreen, repeating weekly as needed.

MST = 2 OR MORE
AT RISK
Eating poorly and/or recent weight loss

Rapidly implement nutrition interventions. Perform nutrition consult within 24-72 hrs, depending on risk.

Step 3: intervene with nutritional support for your patients at risk of malnutrition.

Notes: _____

Abbott nutrition

FIGURE 1.5 The Malnutrition Screening Tool (MST)

Reproduced from: Ferguson M, Capra S, Bauer J, Banks M. Development of a valid and reliable malnutrition screening tool for adult acute hospital patients. *Nutrition*. 1999;15(6):458-464.

TABLE 1.2 COMPARISON OF MALNUTRITION RISK SCREENING TOOLS*

Screening Tool	NRS-2002	MUST	SNAQ©	MST
Complexity	Comprehensive	Comprehensive	Abbreviated	Abbreviated
Intent	Developed for use in acute care settings.	Developed for use in the community setting.	Developed for use during admission to acute care facility.	Developed based on general medical and surgical inpatients.
Brief Description	Two-part tool that relates nutritional status to existing disease state.	Five-step framework that scores nutritional status in the setting of acute illness.	Three question tool that assesses simple and common indicators of malnutrition.	Two question tool that requires no measurements or additional calculations.
Parameters	• Unintentional weight loss • BMI • History of dietary intake • Disease acuity • Age	• Unintentional weight loss • BMI • Presence of an acute illness that may affect dietary intake	• Unintentional weight loss • Decreases in appetite • Need for supplemental or enteral nutrition	• Unintentional weight loss • Decreases in appetite

Modified from Jensen GL, Compher C, Sullivan DH, Mullin GE. Recognizing malnutrition in adults: Definitions, characteristics, screening, assessment, and team approach. *JPEN J Parenter Enteral Nutr*. 2013;37(6):802-807.

> ### CASE STUDY REVISITED
>
> After completing a nutrition screen, Mary is identified as being at high nutrition risk. You initiate a nutrition assessment for Mary, who is now on bedrest. When you seek to confirm Mary's height, she states that she used to be 5'3" tall, but she is now shorter than that and is uncertain of her actual height.
>
> #### Questions
> 1. Given the discrepancy in Mary's reported height, how do you proceed with your anthropometric evaluation?
> 2. Calculate Mary's percent usual body weight and percent weight loss.
> 3. What are Mary's nutritional risk factors?
> 4. Based on the information you have gathered so far, how would you describe Mary's nutritional status?

> **CORE CONCEPT 4**
>
> Different screening tools may be better or worse predictors in specific patient populations.

> **CORE CONCEPT 5**
>
> Nutrition screening tools should have acceptable validity, be simple to administer, have wide applicability across the inpatient population, and use commonly available information.

Nutrition Assessment

Following the identification of nutrition risk via screening, a thorough assessment of a patient's nutrition status is the critical next step in identifying malnutrition. As there is neither a single parameter nor gold standard that can determine nutritional status or the degree of malnutrition in an individual, a comprehensive nutrition assessment includes a review of the nutrition "ABCDEFs"—anthropometrics, biochemical, clinical, dietary, energy, and functional assessment. The remainder of this chapter will discuss the components of nutrition assessment as they are subdivided by the NCPM terminology. AND defines nutritional assessment as the process "to obtain, verify, and interpret data needed to identify nutrition-related problems, their causes, and significance."[5] It establishes the foundation for all other steps of the NCPM by providing the information necessary for determining a nutrition diagnosis and its etiology. The true purpose of the nutrition assessment is to collect all relevant information to identify nutrition-related problems and their causes[5,8,12,16,56]

Anthropometric Measurements

One of the most obvious and indispensible components of nutrition assessment is the use of **anthropometry**, the assessment of measures and proportions of the human body.[57] Regardless of the setting, anthropometric assessment will involve obtaining and interpreting physical measurements as part of a comprehensive evaluation of nutritional status. These measures are essential to either determining the need for or monitoring the progress of an intervention. In this context, all anthropometric measures obtained should be compared to both of the following:

1. Population-specific standards that help reflect the current condition of the patient
2. The patient's previous measures to identify the loss or gain of body components

> **PRACTICE POINT**
>
> Trending anthropometric data points provide the most useful information. A patient whose measurements begin above or at the upper end of the normal range may still be considered "normal" by comparative standards despite significant individual change.

Height, weight, skinfold measures, and circumferences provide the most readily used data points, although there are a number of additional assessment methods available for use. It is up to the clinician to determine which measures are most appropriate to the individual circumstance.[13,14,58,59]

> **PRACTICE POINT**
>
> Anthropometric measurements are only one piece of the nutrition assessment puzzle. Although changes in these measures are reliable predictors of nutritional outcome,[22] they should always be considered in the context of the overall status of the patient.

Assessing Height

Measures of **height** (stature) are not particularly useful for assessing nutritional status without context. Body height remains an essential measure because it provides a necessary variable for calculating other useful parameters (including ideal body weight and BMI). Several important decisions, both nutrition related (i.e., the estimation of energy needs) and not nutrition related (i.e., medication dosing), depend on the collection of an accurate measure of height.[19,59-62]

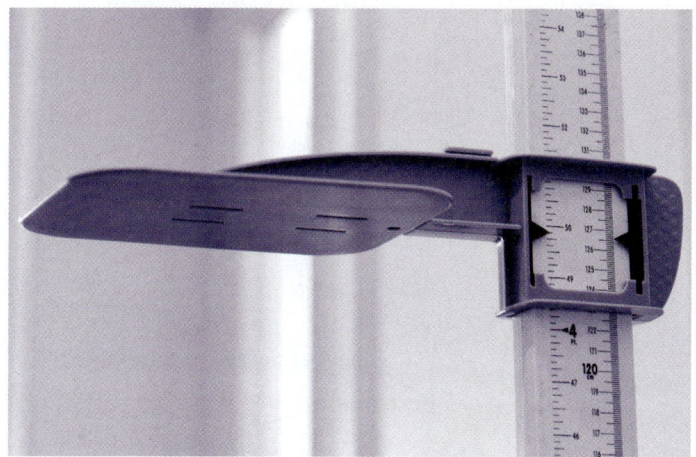

FIGURE 1.6 Stadiometer
© ChameleonsEye/Shuttertstock.

the supine position attached to several intravenous lines, for example, must instead rely upon an alternate technique.[13,59-62]

> **PRACTICE POINT**
>
> For those able, height is measured in the upright position. To be most accurate, the individual should stand with bare feet flat on the floor and heels together; arms should hang loosely to the side with legs and back straight. The head should be in the Frankfort plane (i.e., outer corners of the eyes and tops of the ears parallel to the floor); height is measured after a deep in-breath, ensuring that the head remains in the correct position. Three points of contact—heels, scapula, and buttocks—should be touching the wall.[13,59] (Figure 1.7)

Ideally, height is measured with the patient in the standing position using either a wall-mounted or freestanding calibrated **stadiometer**, a piece of equipment designed to measure height constructed of a ruler and sliding horizontal headpiece adjusted to rest on the top of the head (**Figure 1.6**). Upright measures are not always feasible in the critical care setting due to the limitations of bed confinement or difficulties in maintaining the erect position. Obtaining an accurate measurement of the hospitalized patient who remains in

Alternate Measures to Assess Height For all patients, an accurate measure of height must be obtained. Given the impracticability of the upright measure because of a number of conditions, such as immobility due to contractures, kyphosis, amputations, or quadriplegia, alternatives for estimating this value are often employed in the clinical setting. These surrogate measures use the length of other body segments in order to predict or estimate standing height.[60,61,63-65]

A large percentage of adult height records in the acute setting are based on verbal information provided by the patient instead of an actual measurement. Although this

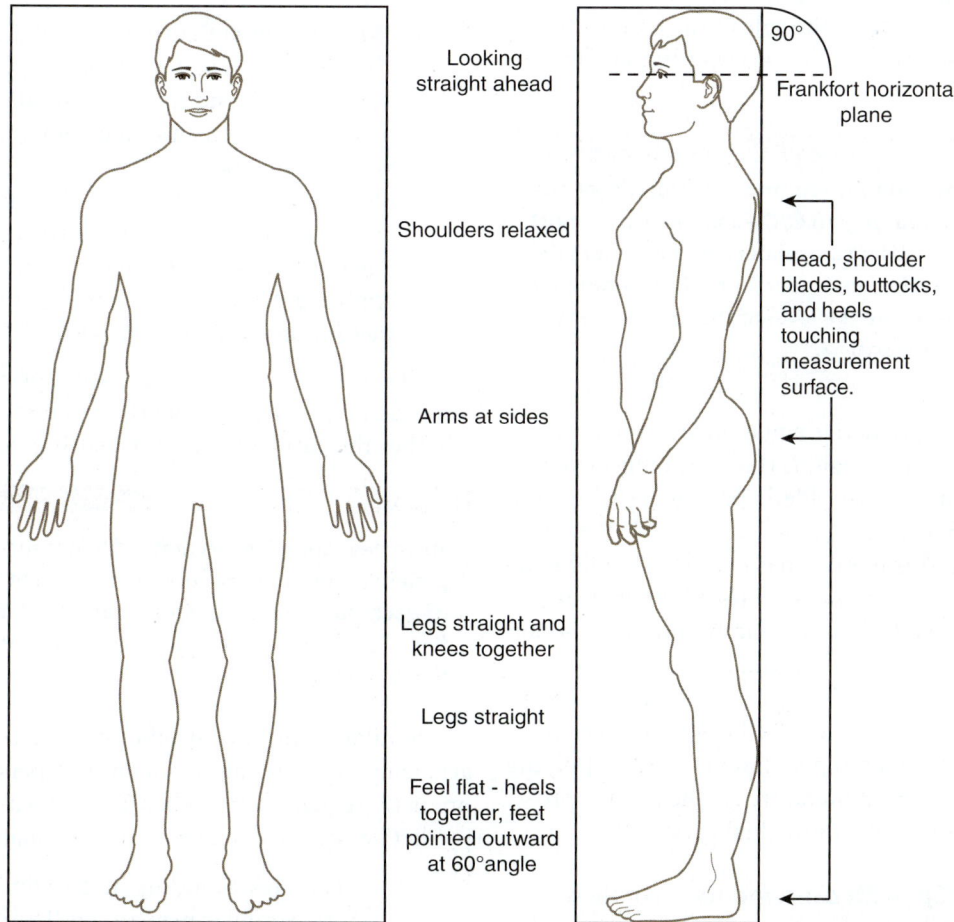

FIGURE 1.7 Upright Position for Accurate Measure of Adult Body Height
Reproduced from Center for Disease Control and Prevention (CDC). National health and nutrition examination survey (NHANES): Anthropometry procedures manual. 2007.

may appear to be an inaccurate substitute for assessing height, several studies have illustrated that the reliability of **self-reported height** (SRH) is comparable to, or often surpasses, other alternative measures. Given the ease and practicably of obtaining a SRH, it is much more likely to see this surrogate measure than any other in the clinical setting. Despite the significant room for error, clinicians can feel comfortable using SRH as long as it is taken with the caveat that most individuals tend to overestimate height.[59,60,66,67]

When neither standing height nor SRH is available (or in an effort to confirm an unlikely SRH), height can be estimated using one of the three most common surrogate measures—knee height, arm span, or arm length. These methods rely on the measurement of one or more long bones that do not lose length with aging in the same manner as the spine. Thereafter, a predictive equation specific to the body segment measured can be used to arrive at an estimate of stature. The available literature is in strong support of the use of any of these three measures; each has been shown to have a reproducible and reliable correlation to standing height.[64,68]

Knee-Height Measurement
Of the many available alternate measures of stature, measurement of **knee-height** using a caliper device is perhaps the most acceptable and widely used in the clinical setting.[13,61] Due to its high correlation with upright height, this technique is often selected to assess the critically ill patient given the ability to complete the measure while the patient is recumbent. The measurement itself is easily taken from the sole of the foot to the anterior surface of the thigh while the lower limb is flexed (**Figure 1.8**).[19,60]

> **PRACTICE POINT**
>
> Measurement of knee-height requires positioning of the patient's lower limb at a 90° angle (i.e., the ankle and thigh must be flexed to this degree). Using the caliper device, measure the distance from the sole of the foot (under the heel) to the anterior surface of the thigh—above the level of the condyles of the femur and proximal to the patella.[19,68]

The most accurate predictive equation for estimating standing height from knee-height is that originally developed for use in nonambulatory elderly patients by Chumlea et al., otherwise known as the Chumlea method.[69] Despite its original intention, this method has been cross-validated for use in acute care patients and for those of other ethnic and age groups (such as the Korean elderly and/or immobile patient populations).[61,62,68,70] The original predictive equations are outlined in **Table 1.3**. Since its development, variations of the Chumlea equation(s) have been published that allow for its use in a number of populations. Before applying this method, consult current literature for the most appropriate equation specific to the individual patient.[69,71]

Total and Half Arm Span Measurements
For those adults who cannot safely stand and are unable to position the lower limb in the angle necessary for measurement of knee-height, measurement of arm span can be used as a surrogate

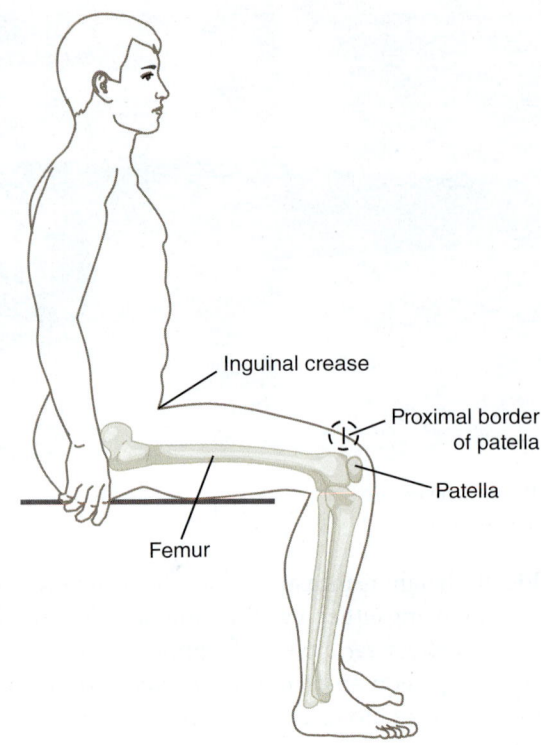

FIGURE 1.8 Positioning for the Measurement of Knee-Height

Reproduced from Center for Disease Control and Prevention (CDC). National health and nutrition examination survey (NHANES): Anthropometry procedures manual. 2007.

marker of standing height at maturity. Depending on the capacity of the patient, one of two measures can be taken:

1. With the patient's arm horizontal and in line with the shoulders, the length between the middle of the sternal notch and tip of the middle finger for each side is measured and then combined; this is called the **total arm span** (TAS).
2. With one of the patient's arms extended horizontally, measure the extension from the tip of the middle finger to the sternal notch, maintaining the superior limb at a 90° angle to the body; this is called the **half arm span** (HAS; or arm length).

These measures, which are appropriate for use in adolescents, adults, and the elderly, can be accurately obtained whether the patient is standing, sitting, or recumbent.[13,62,65]

> **PRACTICE POINT**
>
> To achieve the most accurate TAS measurement, both of the patient's arms must be spread in a straight line; the fingertips of each hand must be equidistant from and parallel to the floor. For measuring HAS, only one arm must remain extended horizontally in a 90° angle.[65]

Similar to the knee-height estimate, the accuracy of an arm length or span measurement is dependent on the use of a predictive equation.[65,66] When TAS is measured, the following predictive equation can be used to estimate standing height[62]:

Females: Standing height (cm) = [1.35 × total arm span (cm)] + 60.1*

Males: Standing height (cm) = [1.40 × total arm span (cm)] + 57.8*

TABLE 1.3 EQUATIONS FOR PREDICTING STATURE FROM KNEE-HEIGHT*

White Men	Predicted height (cm) = [knee height (cm) × 1.88] + 71.85
Black Men	Predicted height (cm) = [knee height (cm) × 1.79] + 73.42
White Women	Predicted height (cm) = [knee height (cm) × 1.87] − [0.06 × age (y)] + 70.25
Black Women	Predicted height (cm) = [knee height (cm) × 1.86] − [0.06 × age (y)] + 68.10

*For use in those aged 18 to 60 years
Data from Chumlea WC, Guo SS, Steinbaugh ML. Prediction of stature from knee height for black and white adults and children with application to mobility-impaired or handicapped persons. *J Am Diet Assoc.* 1994;94(12):1385-1388.

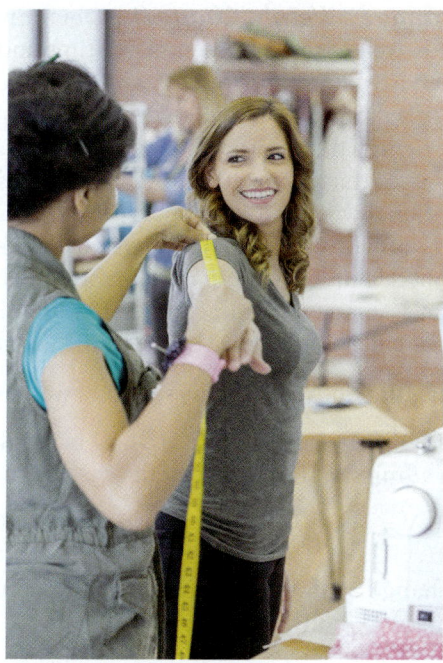

FIGURE 1.9 Measurement of Armspan
© Steve Debenport/E+/Getty Images.

HAS (arm length) is recommended by the World Health Organization (WHO) for estimating the height of non-ambulatory patients (**Figure 1.9**). The value obtained from this measure can either be multiplied by two to provide an estimate of TAS (and then plugged into the TAS predictive equation mentioned above) *or* can be used to estimate stature using the WHO equation[60]:

$$\text{WHO Equation: Standing height (cm)} = 0.43 + [0.73 \times (2 \times \text{HAS (cm)})]*$$

Overall, practicality is a critical factor in determining the alternate measure of standing height to be used: While some patients may have difficulty raising one or both arms, which would suggest knee-height as the most appropriate method, others may be unable to bend the lower limb in the necessary angle and would be better assessed using an arm

---

*Of note, both the TAS and HAS equations may overestimate height when used in the elderly population. This occurs because arm measurements tend to give an estimate of maximal height rather than current height, which may change as in the aging process progresses.[60,64]

measurement. Given that the literature does not support one surrogate measure over the other, clinicians are advised to consider all estimates of height and select the most appropriate for the individual circumstance.[59]

> **PRACTICE POINT**
>
> In all cases, when standing height cannot be obtained, the clinician must use the SRH, a surrogate measure, or both. Supine length measurement, which uses a flexible measuring tape to determine the length between the vertex of the head and the heel, has been proven inaccurate and unreliable (and as such should be used as a last resort).[61,62] Instead, utilize TAS, HAS, or knee-height, depending on the individual circumstance.

Assessing Weight

The assessment of **actual body weight (ABW)** or body cell mass measurement, which represents the unadjusted sum of all body compartments without distinction between fat and fat-free mass, is fundamental to determining nutritional status. From a nutritional standpoint, an individual weight value provides limited information. Ideally, the value will be contextualized using an additional parameter. This may include the identification of individual trends, as in percent changes from a usual body weight, or relation to appropriate standards, like ideal body weight. Given that ABW is representative of muscle, fat, and fluid combined, the true value of the measure is found in its comparison to other criteria in the setting of the whole medical picture. A number of conditions, such as those that induce fluid retention, will complicate the assessment of an ABW.[58,59] The various adjustments to or calculations that involve ABW measures will be discussed throughout this section.

Weight should be measured upon admission to any acute and chronic care facility and monitored throughout the length of stay. Serial measures are necessary for tracking trends in weight that may relate to nutritional and/or overall clinical status. The most accurate measure of current ABW is that obtained from actually weighing the patient (**Figure 1.10**) instead of relying upon self-reported values, which tend to be underestimated. For those in the inpatient setting, this often requires the use of bed scales for those unable to transfer to the standing scale.[10,13,16,67]

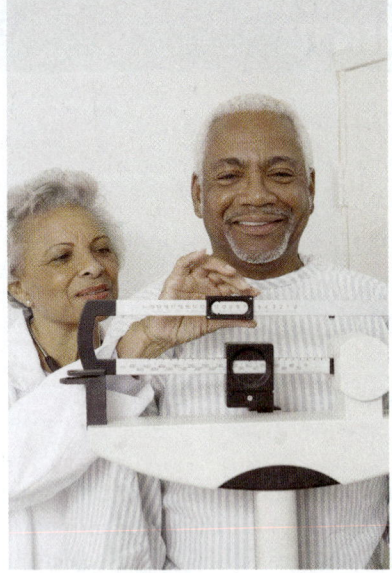

FIGURE 1.10 Measurement of Weight
© sirtravelalot/Shutterstock.

> **PRACTICE POINT**
>
> Height and weight should never be visually estimated; an inaccurate weight may compromise application of effective medical nutrition therapy when used to assess energy and protein needs. Instead, employment of one of the surrogate measures to provide the best approximation is recommended.

> **PRACTICE POINT**
>
> Patients who can stand should be weighed on a standing digital or balanced-mechanism scale without overgarments or shoes. To obtain an accurate ABW measure, the patient should first remove all outer garments and empty pockets of loose change and/or keys. The patient will then step onto the digital or balanced mechanism scale with feet together in the center and arms hanging loosely at each side.[16,59]

> **PRACTICE POINT**
>
> For hospitalized patients, an appropriately calibrated bed scale may be utilized instead of a standing scale. Standardized procedures (i.e., all of the bedding be removed except for the bottom sheet and one pillow, along with any catheter bags, etc.) are often difficult to maintain for patients in acute care.[16,59]

Usual Body Weight (UBW) In order to identify weight trends, it is necessary to have an understanding of a patient's normal weight range to compare to the current ABW. This value, which can be obtained during the patient interview or estimated using serial measures documented in the medical record, is referred to as **usual body weight (UBW)**. In most cases, the UBW value is a self-reported measure of what the individual has weighed for the majority of his or her adult life. This is a critical comparison used to determine whether any change in weight has occurred. The deviation is quantified as percent UBW and/or percent weight change.

> **PRACTICE POINT**
>
> The majority of patients can respond appropriately to the question, "What have you weighed for most of your adult life?" It may also be helpful to speak with family members or refer to documentation from primary care or past hospital admissions. If weight change is evident, always note the time frame in which the deviation from UBW occurred and if the change was intentional versus unintentional.

Percent Usual Body Weight (%UBW) and Percent Weight Change (%Weight Change) Obtaining repeated body weight measurements over time and/or comparing an ABW measure to UBW are recommended for the identification of weight changes. In the clinical setting, these comparisons are made with specific attention to any losses that occurred unintentionally. Although any unintentional weight loss is concerning, it must be quantified as either **percent usual body weight (%UBW)** or **percent weight change (%weight change)** in order to be used as a nutrition assessment parameter; %UBW and %weight change can be calculated using the following equations[10,16]:

$$\%UBW = (\text{actual body weight}/\text{usual body weight}) \times 100\%$$

For example, a male with a UBW of 91 kg is weighed as 85 kg upon admission to the hospital:

$$\%UBW = (85 \text{ kg}/91 \text{ kg}) \times 100\% = 93.4\% \text{ UBW}$$

$$\%\text{weight change} = (\text{amount of weight lost or gained}/\text{usual body weight}) \times 100\%$$

For this same patient, who has lost 6 kg:

$$\% \text{ weight change} = (6 \text{ kg}/91 \text{ kg}) \times 100\% = 6.6\% \text{ weight loss}$$

These values as measures of unintentional weight loss are the best-validated indicators for both the recognition of weight changes and malnutrition. Clinical significance of these values can be determined by the degree and duration of weight loss. The time frame in which the loss occurred is necessary for interpretation of the data. For example, a 5% unintentional weight loss over 1 year may not be considered significant, but a 5% weight loss over the course of 1 month certainly would be. One of the six key indicators of the AND/A.S.P.E.N. consensus statement for malnutrition identification is interpretation of %weight loss in the context of the patient's clinical status and a specified length of time (**Table 1.4**).[10,13,18]

Additional parameters exist for the interpretation of %UBW alone:

- 85% to 90% UBW: mild malnutrition
- 75% to 84% UBW: moderate malnutrition
- <74% UBW: severe malnutrition[72]

As with any nutrition-related parameter, the interpretation of weight loss must also be considered in the context

TABLE 1.4 INTERPRETATION OF %WEIGHT LOSS AS KEY INDICATOR OF MALNUTRITION

	Malnutrition in the Context of							
	Acute Illness or Injury				**Chronic Illness**			
	Nonsevere (Moderate) Malnutrition		Severe Malnutrition		Nonsevere (Moderate) Malnutrition		Severe Malnutrition	
	%	Time	%	Time	%	Time	%	Time
Interpretation of Weight Loss	1–2	1 week	>2	1 week	5	1 month	>5	1 month
	5	1 month	>5	1 month	7.5	3 months	>7.5	3 months
	7.5	3 months	>7.5	3 months	10	6 months	>10	6 months
	–		–		20	1 year	>20	1 year

Data from White JV, Guenter P, Jensen G, et al. Consensus state of the Academy of Nutrition and Dietetics/American Society of Parenteral and Enteral Nutrition: Characteristics recommended for the identification and documentation of adult malnutrition (undernutrition). *JPEN J Parenter Enteral Nutr.* 2012;36(3):275–283.

of the overall clinical picture. Weight changes often reflect more than just nutritional status. Loss may be an indication of the severity of underlying disease or inflammatory condition, while gains often represent a positive fluid status. This will be important beyond the assessment period when later determining the appropriate intervention.[16]

Ideal Body Weight (IBW) In the clinical setting and beyond, comparisons of weight-to-height measures are the most commonly used anthropometric parameters. **Ideal body weight (IBW)**, a metric that adjusts weight-for-height for comparison of weight status and/or weight-associated health risks, was originally defined according to the weights associated with lowest mortality for the respective heights. Ideal body weight was first based on historical data that compared the relative disease risk and life expectancy of individuals of different height-weight combinations. IBW has historically been the weight-for-height that correlated with the lowest mortality. Today, there are numerous formulas and published height-weight tables available for the determination of IBW. These algorithms are based on the notion that height defines weight as a linear function.[58,73,74]

Ideal body weight is determined using either a predictive equation (most often the Hamwi method) or via a height-weight table (as in the Metropolitan Life Ideal Weight Tables). There is controversy as to which provides the most appropriate or accurate calculation, although an equation is often selected for ease of use.[14,58]

Height-Weight Tables Although a number of height-weight tables exist for the estimation of IBW, the most recognized and widely used are the Metropolitan Life Ideal Weights Tables, which were initially developed by the Metropolitan Life Insurance Company in 1943 based on data obtained from policy holders between the ages of 25 and 59 years. The most recent update of the table, published in 1983, reports IBW as a range for respective height and frame size. The frame size must first be deemed small, medium, or large based on elbow breadth measurements taken from National Health and Nutrition Examination Survey (NHANES) data. Note that this method of assessment is largely outdated and is not routinely used in clinical practice.[58,73]

> **PRACTICE POINT**
>
> The use of height–weight tables (like those developed by Metropolitan Life Insurance Company) is not recommended due to their limited sample size, lack of applicability to a number of age and/or ethnic groups, and inconvenience. These data should not be considered representative of the entire population.[19]

Predictive Equations Given the impracticality of calculating IBW using height–weight tables, equations for predicting weight as a linear function of height have been developed (**Table 1.5**). The most frequently used is the Hamwi method; this equation is generally thought to be the "rule of thumb" in calculating IBW. The Hamwi method is often described as the most appropriate measure for use in the clinical setting.[19,58,75,76]

The Hamwi Method:

Females: IBW = 100 lbs for a height of 5 feet plus 5 lbs for each additional inch

Male: IBW = 106 lbs for a height of 5 feet plus 6 lbs for each additional inch

Adjust for large (+10%) and small (–10%) frames to derive the final IBW calculation

TABLE 1.5 SUMMATION OF IDEAL BODY WEIGHT EQUATIONS FOR MEN AND WOMEN[58,75]

Source	Equation
Broca (1871)	IBW (kg) = height (cm) − 100
Hamwi (1964)*	IBW (females) = 100 lbs + 5 lbs/inch over 5 feet IBW (males) = 106 lbs + 6 lbs/inch over 5 feet
Devine (1974)	IBW (females) = 45.5 kg + 2.3 kg/inch over 5 feet IBW (males) = 50 kg + 2.3 kg/inch over 5 feet
Robinson et al. (1983)	IBW (females) = 49 kg + 1.7 kg/inch over 5 feet IBW (males) = 52 kg + 1.9 kg/inch over 5 feet
Miller et al. (1983)†	IBW (females) = 53 kg + 1.33 kg/inch over 5 feet IBW (males) = 55.7 kg + 1.39 kg/inch over 5 feet
Hammond (2000)*	IBW (females) = 45 kg for 150 cm + 0.9 kg/cm IBW (males) = 48 kg for 150 cm + 1.1 kg/cm
Peterson et al. (2016)	IBW (kg) = 2.2 × BMI + 3.5 × BMI (Height (m) − 1.5 m)

*For Hamwi and Hammond methods, the calculated weight may be subtracted by 10% to account for a small frame or increased by 10% for a large frame.
†The Miller et al. formula is calculated for a medium frame.

Data from Shah B, Sucher K, Hollenbeck CB. Comparison of ideal body weight equations and published height-weight tables with body mass index tables for healthy adults in the United States. *Nutr Clin Pract*. 2006;21(3):312–319; Peterson CM, Thomas DM, Blackburn GL, Heymsfield SB. Universal equation for estimating ideal body weight and body weight at any BMI. *Am J Clin Nutr*. 2016;103(5):1197–1203.

TABLE 1.6 IDEAL BODY WEIGHT DETERMINED FROM BMI OF 22 KG/M²

Height	IBW
58 in/147 cm	105 lbs/47.7 kg
59 in/150 cm	109 lbs/49.5 kg
60 in/152 cm	112 lbs/50.9 kg
61 in/155 cm	116 lbs/52.7 kg
62 in/158 cm	120 lbs/54.5 kg
63 in/160 cm	124 lbs/56.4 kg
64 in/163 cm	128 lbs/58.2 kg
65 in/165 cm	132 lbs/60 kg
66 in/168 cm	136 lbs/61.8 kg
67 in/170 cm	140 lbs/63.6 kg
68 in/173 cm	144 lbs/65.5 kg
69 in/175 cm	149 lbs/67.7 kg
70 in/178 cm	153 lbs/69.5 kg
71 in/180 cm	157 lbs/71.4 kg
72 in/183 cm	162 lbs/73.6 kg
73 in/185 cm	166 lbs/75.5 kg
74 in/188 cm	171 lbs/77.7 kg
75 in/191 cm	176 lbs/80 kg
76 in/193 cm	180 lbs/81.8 kg

IBW = BMI 22 kg/m² × [height in m]²

Data from Shah B, Sucher K, Hollenbeck CB. Comparison of ideal body weight equations and published height-weight tables with body mass index tables for healthy adults in the united states. *Nutr Clin Pract*. 2006;21(3):312-319.

IBW can be determined using an equation based on the BMI that is associated with the lowest morbidity (22 kg/m², the middle value within the normal range). Current literature suggests that estimates made using BMI [i.e., 22 kg/m² × height in meters²] are comparable to what is determined from other predictive equations and is desirable in the clinical setting due to the simplicity of the calculation.[58] Refer to **Table 1.6** for a reference table generated using this calculation.

Applications of Ideal Body Weight

Similar to the use of %UBW as an indicator of weight status, **percent ideal body weight (%IBW)** can be used to compare current ABW to the IBW value specific to the patient's height.

%IBW = (actual body weight/ideal body weight) × 100%

For example, a male who measures as 183 cm (72 in) tall would have an IBW of 81 kg (178 lbs) based on the Hamwi method. If this patient actually weighs 97 kg (213 lbs), %IBW is calculated as:

%IBW = (97 kg/81 kg) × 100% = 120% IBW

Because IBW was standardized using healthy adult populations, %IBW should never be used as the sole basis for determination of nutritional status. Percent IBW is used much more infrequently in the clinical setting when compared to the use of %UBW. Instead, IBW can be useful when assessing the energy needs of an obese patient requiring nutrition support. It is important to recognize how the different anthropometric parameters can be applied within the nutrition care process.[74]

Adjusted Body Weight (Adjusted BW) In addition to assessment of body weight as a measure of nutritional status, weight is an important component in the determination of energy expenditure. A body weight at the extremes (i.e., obese) complicates this calculation by resulting in a possible underestimation or overestimation of needs. Although this practice is significantly less common now, utilizing **adjusted body weight** (adjusted BW) was a common method of preventing under- or overfeeding in the past. Adjusted BW can be calculated for those with an ABW greater than 115% of the calculated IBW.[77-79]

$$\text{Adjusted BW} = [(\text{actual body weight} - \text{ideal body weight}) \times 0.25] + \text{IBW}^{79}$$

For example, consider a 170 cm (67 in) female with an IBW of 61 kg (135 lbs; per Hamwi method) and an ABW of 95.5 kg (210 lbs):

$$\text{Adjusted BW} = [(95.5 \text{ kg} - 61 \text{ kg}) \times 0.25] + 61 \text{ kg} = 70 \text{ kg}$$

Use of adjusted BW was first recommended in order to account for the percentage of obese weight that is most metabolically active (i.e., lean mass) instead of feeding based on ABW. The underlying rationale is that subcutaneous fat is significantly less metabolically active than lean tissue and thus using ABW to calculate needs will result in overprediction. It is important to note that adjusted BW, although sometimes used in practice, is *not* an evidence-based assessment. Recent studies have illustrated that utilizing adjusted BW actually results in a vast underestimation of energy needs. A.S.P.E.N. and AND both urge against the use of adjusted BW despite its previous longstanding use in the clinical setting, recommending instead the use of ABW and IBW based on the severity of obesity.[78,80,81]

Body Weight Modifications for Special Circumstance As previously mentioned, body weight must always be considered in the setting of the overall clinical picture. There are two notable (and common) conditions that require special assessment of body weight measures: amputations and chronic fluid retention.

Adjusting Body Weight for Amputations For those with extremity amputation(s), special weight adjustments are necessary in order to account for the body compartment that has been lost. An adjusted BW is calculated based on an estimate of the proportion of total body weight that the lost body segment represents (**Figure 1.11**). Using this technique, known as the Osterkamp method, the proportion that represents the missing limb is added back to the individual's current ABW. This new adjusted BW can be used in other calculations or for comparison to population targets, such as body mass index (BMI).[19,82,83]

$$\text{Adjusted BW (Osterkamp)} = \text{actual body weight}/(100 - \%\text{amputation}) \times 100$$

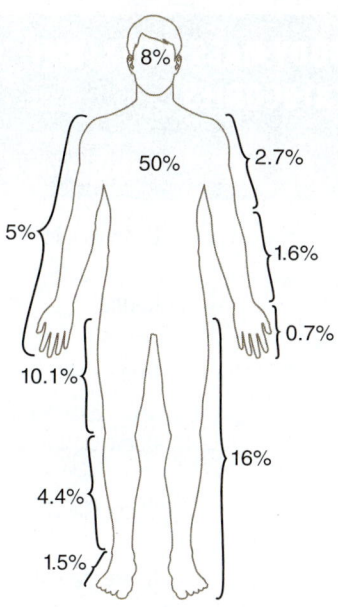

FIGURE 1.11 Body Segment Contribution (%) to Total Body Weight (Osterkamp Method)

Reproduced from Osterkamp LK. Perspective on assessment of human body proportions of relevance to amputees. *J Am Diet Assoc.* 1995;95(2):215-218.

For example, consider a male who weighs 91 kg (200 lbs) with a total leg amputation:

$$\text{Adjusted BW (Osterkamp)} = 91 \text{ kg}/(100 - 16) \times 100 = 108 \text{ kg}$$

The Osterkamp method, when completed correctly, will yield an adjusted BW that provides a better basis for most nutritional assessments when compared to the use of post-amputation ABW. Some measures (most notably the calculation of energy requirements) will be best completed using the new ABW and not the adjusted BW.[82,84]

Calculating Dry Weight for Chronic Fluid Overload For many hospitalized patients, including those with liver disease, renal failure, or malignancy, fluid overload precludes the use of ABW. Increases in weight will often reflect overhydration, edema, ascites, or dialysate in the abdomen, instead of providing an accurate picture of actual body compartments. An estimate of **dry weight** is used to represent an individual's ABW without the excess fluid. For those with chronic and fluctuating retention, dry weight may be estimated based on the UBW of the patient prior to onset of fluid retention *or* based on other clinical parameters, like the achievement of a normotensive blood pressure.[14,85]

Calculating Body Mass Index (BMI)

The Quetelet's Index, better known as **body mass index (BMI)**, is the most common anthropometric comparison of body weight to body height independent of frame size. Defined by the equation weight (kg)/(height [m])², BMI offers a simple measure of body composition that can be read (with caution) as an indirect measure of fat mass. The BMI classifications for interpretation of the adult patient population are outlined in **Table 1.7**, although all clinicians should be aware of the many caveats associated with this measure. Although sex, body type, and ethnicity influence

TABLE 1.7 BODY MASS INDEX (BMI) CATEGORIES

BMI (kg/m²)	Classification
<18.5	Underweight
18.5–24.9	Normal
25.0–29.9	Overweight
30.0–34.9	Obese Class I
35.0–39.9	Obese Class II
>40.0	Obese Class III

Data from National Heart, Lung, and Blood Institute. Classification of Overweight and Obesity by BMI, Waist Circumference, and Associated Disease Risks. https://www.nhlbi.nih.gov/health/educational/lose_wt/BMI/bmi_dis.htm.

BMI results, these factors are neither taken into account nor reflected in the measure. For example, BMI will often overestimate body fat for the muscular athlete and underestimate fat stores in the elderly. As with any method of nutrition assessment, interpretation of the measure should be made in the context of the individual situation.[16,18,19]

Despite the known limitations of BMI, it remains widely used due to both its efficiency and its relatively high correlation with estimates of body fatness.[59] Although malnutrition can occur in individuals of any BMI, measures at either extreme represent an increased likelihood of poor nutritional status and are associated with increased risk of mortality. This phenomenon is represented by a J-shaped relationship between mortality and BMI. Relative to normal weight, BMI values categorized as overweight or obese are associated with increased risk of cardiovascular disease and some cancers, while measures representing the underweight classification are associated with increased postsurgical complications, infection rates, and length of hospital stay.[10,59,86,87]

> **PRACTICE POINT**
>
> Interpretation of BMI should involve consideration of age, sex, body type, and common confounders of body weight in the clinical setting, such as edema or ascites.

> **PRACTICE POINT**
>
> Use caution when applying BMI to patients with amputations. Refer to the Osterkamp method (as previously mentioned) for a more appropriate weight assessment.

Body Composition Measures

Classic anthropometric measurements, such as height, weight, and BMI, are extremely useful in the clinical setting but are unable to accurately represent body composition. As understanding of body composition and its impact on health risk and clinical outcome increases, so does the importance of obtaining its accurate measure. Clinicians turn to skinfold anthropometry and circumference measures for the most feasible representation of an individual's fat and muscle stores.[13,16,59]

Skinfold Anthropometry Skinfold anthropometry, often referred to as skinfold thickness, involves the measure of one or more anatomical sites using a skinfold caliper device to estimate body fat stores. The measures of skinfold thickness are representative of subcutaneous fat stores in the triceps, biceps, subscapular, and suprailiac regions (**Figure 1.12**). This measure is the most widely used method of indirectly estimating body fat percentage and, when used in an additional calculation, can provide an approximation of muscle stores.[59,88]

> **PRACTICE POINT**
>
> A "skinfold" measure represents the subcutaneous fat layer. Clinicians should take caution to avoid including the underlying muscle in this measure. Anatomic sites often used in this context are the biceps, triceps, subscapular, and suprailiac regions.

The procedure itself requires noncomplex portable equipment and can be applied to most clinical and public health settings. A variety of calipers—ranging from precision-engineered to plastic and disposable—are available for use. Validity of skinfold thickness depends less on the caliper used and more on the measurement technique

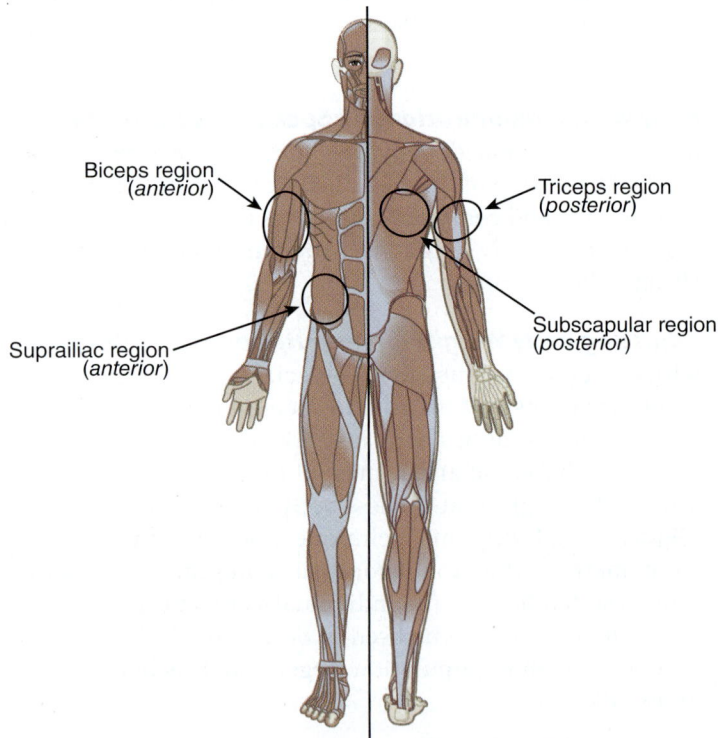

FIGURE 1.12 Common Body Sites for Skinfold Anthropometry

and repetition over time. As with any anthropometric measure, differences in equipment can account for differences in measures. When used for serial measurements of the same individual, the same caliper tool should be used for each measure to best represent any changes (or lack thereof) in body composition.[59,89]

> **PRACTICE POINT**
>
> Follow the procedures that accompany the skinfold caliper for the most accurate instructions on use. In general, at the given site, a lengthwise skinfold should be grasped and slightly lifted between the index and thumb of the hand (without including underlying muscle). The caliper is applied approximately 1 cm below the finger grasping the skinfold. All measurements should be repeated three times and averaged for the final value.

> **PRACTICE POINT**
>
> Accuracy of the skinfold measure decreases with increasing obesity. This technique is more useful in lean individuals (i.e., those with smaller fat stores) because skinfold caliper devices are unable to assess intra-abdominal adipose tissue.[59]

Triceps Skinfold For clinicians in the inpatient and outpatient settings, **triceps skinfold (TSF)** is the most common skinfold measure used for nutritional assessment. As with any other anatomic location mentioned above, TSF measures the amount of subcutaneous body fat, which represents ~50% of total body fat stores. TSF is the site found to be most reflective of actual body fatness when performed with strict adherence to measurement protocols by a trained professional. This site is not only the most convenient and accessible, but can be accurately measured in the supine position for patients unable to sit or stand (**Figure 1.13**).[19,59,89-91]

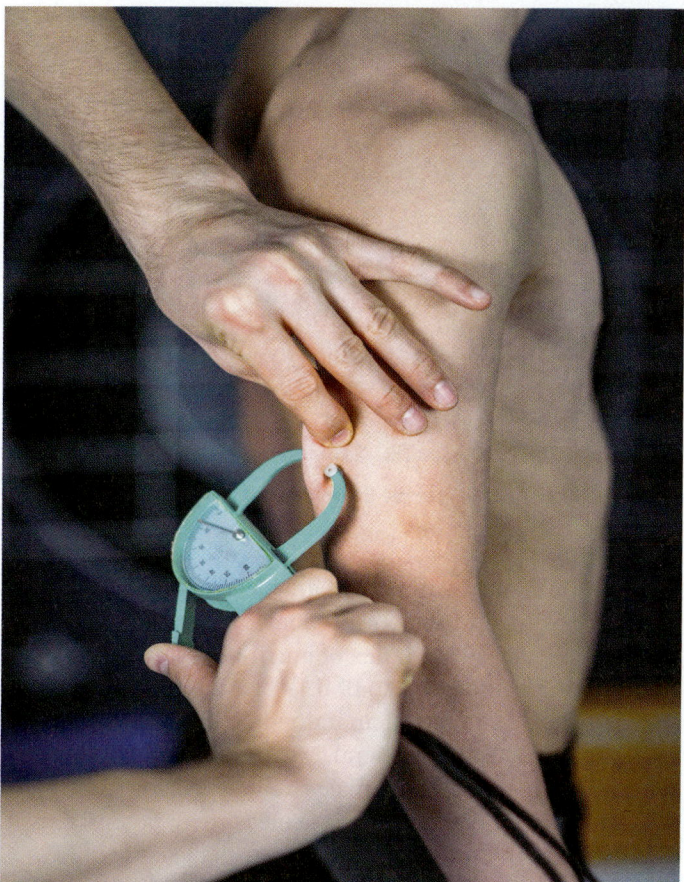

FIGURE 1.13 Measurement of Triceps Skinfold
© Microgen/Shutterstock.

> **PRACTICE POINT**
>
> Triceps skin fold measurements are taken using skinfold calipers on the nondominant arm of the individual, midway between the olecranon process and the acromion process (i.e., midway between the shoulder and the elbow). This measure may be difficult to implement in the critically ill if, for example, impeded by wound dressings or edema.[19,91]

TSF measurements are interpreted in one of two ways: the measure can be compared against population standards due to abundant reference table availability or (preferably) by using serial measurements to assess change in the individual. Serial measures allow for estimates in body fat store changes and are more useful for assessment purposes than population comparisons. Depletion of this compartment can reflect chronic inadequate intake or nutrient depletion, which would be a critical consideration in determining future interventions. As with any other measure of assessment, TSF will be impacted by fluid retention; if edema is present, TSF measures cannot be considered reliable.[59,89]

Circumference Measurements Depending on the anatomic location where the value is obtained, circumference measurements are used to measure skeletal muscle and/or fat mass. For example, mid-upper arm circumference can be used as an index of somatic protein stores (particularly when compared to other measures, like the TSF), whereas waist circumference provides a measure of central adiposity that is considered to be a significant marker of metabolic and cardiovascular risk.[89,92]

Mid-Upper Arm Circumference (MUAC) **Mid-upper arm circumference (MUAC)** is a measure of total arm circumference and provides a measure of both muscle and fat area (**Figure 1.14**). Measures of limb circumference, such as the MUAC, are used as indicators of nutrition status; in other words, MUAC is most often used to estimate malnutrition risk rather than as a marker of obesity. The measure is simple, noninvasive, and feasible (even in the acutely ill patient population) because it can be completed in the supine position (if necessary) using only a tape measure. MUAC becomes particularly useful when height and weight measurements are inappropriate or impossible to obtain on a consistent basis.[1,19,93-95]

> **PRACTICE POINT**
>
> To measure MUAC, a nonstretch tape measure is used at the midpoint between the acromion and olecranon processes.[96]

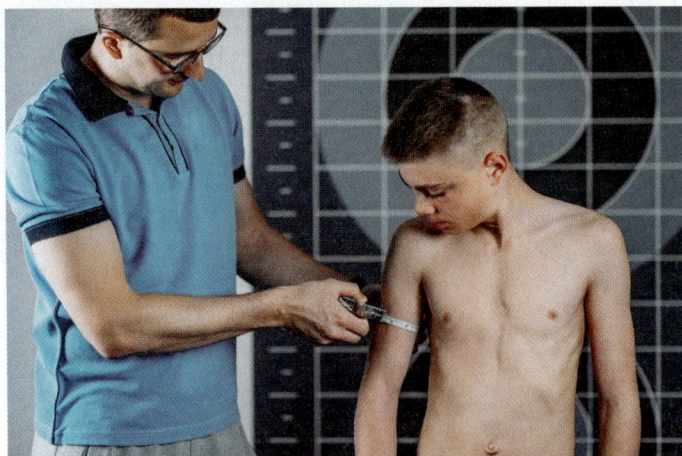

FIGURE 1.14 Measurement of Mid-Upper Arm Circumference
© Microgen/Shutterstock.

For the critically ill patient unable to assume the supine position for other anthropometric measures, MUAC provides an alternative index of nutritional status that is accurate and comparable to BMI.[89,96-98] MUAC can be used to calculate an estimate of an individual's BMI through a predictive equation; in general, MUAC measures of <25 cm for males and <24 cm for females will correlate with a BMI <20 kg/m², providing a substitute measure of potential adult undernutrition. Similarly, if a serial measure of MUAC changes by >10%, it can be assumed that the BMI has also changed by >10%. This solidifies the applicability of MUAC in identifying chronic energy deficiency and as a predictor of mortality in the acutely ill.[95,99,100]

Predicting BMI with MUAC:

$$\text{Males: BMI (kg/m}^2) = 1.01 \times \text{MUAC (cm)} - 4.7$$
$$\text{Females: BMI (kg/m}^2) = 1.10 \times \text{MUAC (cm)} - 6.7$$

MUAC can be used in combination with a TSF measure to calculate **mid-arm muscle circumference (MAMC)**, a surrogate measure of lean body mass. MAMC cannot be measured directly by anthropometry but is instead obtained from the predictive equation: MAMC (cm) = MUAC (cm) − [TSF (mm) × 0.3142]. The value obtained provides an indication of muscle mass. Note that the equation provided will include the bone as well as the muscle; this should be considered in your assessment. MAMC equations that do correct for bone are available, although these are not routinely used due to inherent issues with adjusting for bone size. Similar to other measures of body composition, interpretation of MAMC requires either comparison to reference standards specific to age, sex, and ethnicity or in the context of changes in serial measures. In general, lower MAMC values (MAMC <90% the reference value for the specific individual)[101] are associated with adverse outcomes including increased risk of mortality.[14,59,89]

Waist Circumference In contrast to limb circumference measures like the MUAC, **waist circumference** is utilized as an assessment of excess abdominal fat. This measure provides an indication of central adiposity, which can be interpreted in terms of obesity-related health risk, that is easily obtainable in the general population.[19,59,92] Waist circumference is more strongly associated with visceral adipose tissue and thus cardiometabolic risk than any other anthropometric measure.[102-105]

The literature describes several different anatomical sites for measuring waist circumference. Four measurement sites are common, including the WHO's recommendation for measuring the midpoint between the iliac crest and costal margin of the lowest rib (WC-mid) and the National Institutes of Health's (NIH) recommendation for measuring in the horizontal plane of the superior border of the iliac crest (WC-IC). Other cited locations include the level of the umbilicus and the minimal waist, regardless of where on the abdomen it occurs. Studies indicate that a waist circumference measured mid-abdominally (WC-mid) is the most accurate measure available for defining central obesity (**Figure 1.15**).[106] Because the various sites will yield drastic differences in interpretation of the measure, the clinician must be sure to document the location utilized in order to obtain accurate serial changes in the long term.[59,92,102,106,107]

> **PRACTICE POINT**
>
> Waist circumference is measured using nonstretch tape placed directly on the skin, midway between the iliac crest and costal margin of the lowest rib at end expiration.[19,59,92]

Abdominal obesity is associated with significantly greater health risks than fat deposited below the abdomen. For those with an android ("apple") body shape, a waist measurement >40 inches (102 cm) for males and >34 inches (88 cm) for females has been illustrated to be an independent risk factor for type 2 diabetes mellitus, hypertension, and cardiovascular disease—even for individuals who are of normal weight by BMI standards. This risk has not been demonstrated for those with a gynoid ("pear") shape, indicating fat deposits below the

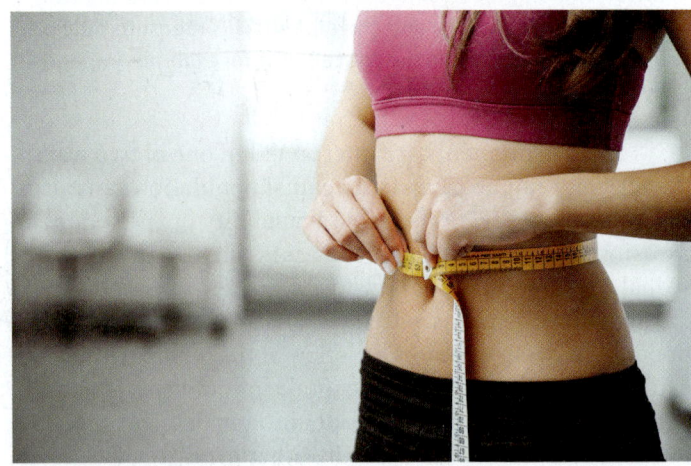

FIGURE 1.15 Measurement of Waist Circumference
© Stock-Asso/Shutterstock.

⚠ Clinical Controversy

Is BMI a reliable indicator of cardiometabolic risk across various racial and ethnic groups?

Obesity as measured by BMI is associated with increased cardiometabolic risk, such as increased risk of cardiovascular disease and type 2 diabetes mellitus. BMI is an imperfect tool; it is limited in its ability to differentiate body composition or body fat distribution. The applicability of BMI as a disease risk indicator across different racial and ethnic groups has been more closely examined. In a study of a cardiometabolic risk phenotype described as "metabolic abnormality but normal weight" (MAN), Gujral et al. conducted a cross-sectional analysis of two community-based normal-weight cohorts to evaluate the prevalence of MAN in five racial/ethnic groups. BMI classification cut-offs can be noted in Table 1.7. BMI for South Asian and Chinese American participants was classified according to WHO Asian cut-off points: normal weight BMI 18.5 to 22.9 kg/m^2; overweight BMI 23.0 to 24.7 kg/m^2; obese BMI ≥27.5 kg/m^2. The authors found that Indians and other South Asians had more than double the prevalence of MAN, followed by Hispanics, Chinese Americans, and African Americans, who had greater prevalence of MAN compared to whites. It was estimated that the BMI values at which the expected equivalent numbers of metabolic abnormalities would equal those among whites at an overweight BMI of 25 kg/m^2, after adjusting for age, sex, and race-BMI interactions, were as follows:

1. >22.9 kg/m^2 for African Americans
2. 21.5 kg/m^2 for Hispanics
3. 20.9 kg/m^2 for Chinese Americans
4. 19.6 kg/m^2 for South Asians

These findings suggest that standard BMI categories may not be a useful screen for cardiometabolic risk in the non-white population.

Questions

1. How might BMI confound cardiometabolic screening in racial/ethnic minority groups?
2. What metabolic differences could be hypothesized to account for some of these risk variations?
3. How might these findings influence a clinician's ability to utilize BMI classification of overweight and obesity to identify cardiometabolic risk in a racially and ethnically diverse population?

References

1. Gujral UP, Vittinghoff E, Mongraw-Chafflin M, et al. Cardiometabolic abnormalities among normal-weight persons from five racial/ethnic groups in the United States: a cross-sectional analysis of two cohort studies. *Ann Intern Med*. 2017;166:628–636.
2. WHO Expert Consultation. Appropriate body-mass index for Asian populations and its implications for policy and intervention strategies. *Lancet*. 2004;363:157–163.

---

waist (**Figure 1.16**).[19,59,108–111] The measurement of waist circumference has evolved into a key diagnostic criterion for metabolic syndrome; according to the U.S. National Cholesterol Education Program and the International Diabetes Federation, the aforementioned sex-specific thresholds (>102 cm for males and >88 cm for females) are practical indicators of elevated risk.[107,109]

Hip Circumference Similar to waist circumference, hip circumference will also provide an indication of adiposity, although its value in predicting disease risk and/or mortality is of significantly less importance. Although some studies do indicate a significant and inverse relationship between hip circumference and cardiometabolic disease risk, this protective effect is not present in all ethnicities. Instead of using a direct measure of hip circumference as a marker of nutritional status, this value is typically interpreted as part of a **waist–hip ratio (WHR)**. WHR, the waist circumference value divided by the hip circumference value, provides an additional measure of body fat distribution as an index of both subcutaneous and intra-abdominal adipose tissue. In general, a WHR value ≥0.90 in men and ≥0.85 in women is associated with increased risk of cardiometabolic complications, although ethnic-specific cutoffs do exist. While these cutoffs are not well researched, they may provide a general guideline for assessing different patient populations (examples of those acceptable for use are outlined in **Table 1.8**).[59,103,108,112,113]

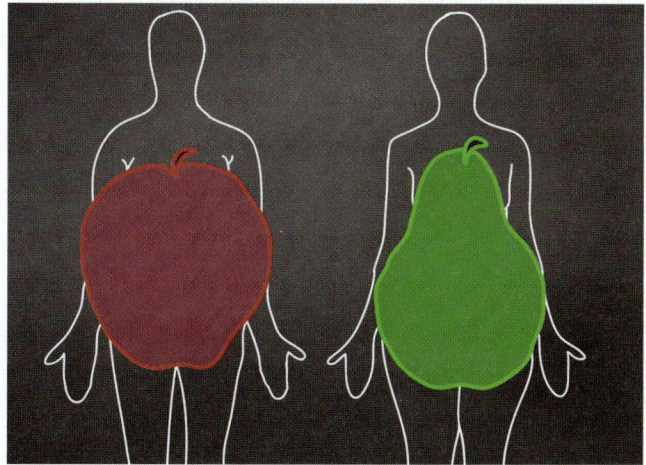

FIGURE 1.16 Android ("apple") versus Gynoid ("pear") Body Shapes
© ssimone / Shutterstock.

TABLE 1.8 SUGGESTED WAIST-TO-HIP RATIO ETHNIC CUTOFFS FOR CENTRAL OBESITY[113]

Ethnicity	Male	Female
Asian	≥0.90	≥0.80
African American	≥0.90	≥0.85
European	≥0.90	≥0.85
Hispanic	≥0.90	≥0.85
Middle Eastern	≥0.90	≥0.85

Data from Lear SA, James PT, Ko GT, Kumanyika S. Appropriateness of waist circumference and waist-to-hip ratio cutoffs for different ethnic groups. *Eur J Clin Nutr.* 2010;64:42-61

> **PRACTICE POINT**
>
> When measuring hip circumference, the measuring tape should be positioned at the widest part over the buttocks and below the iliac crest. The subject should be asked not to contract his or her gluteal muscles before the measurement is taken.[59,108]

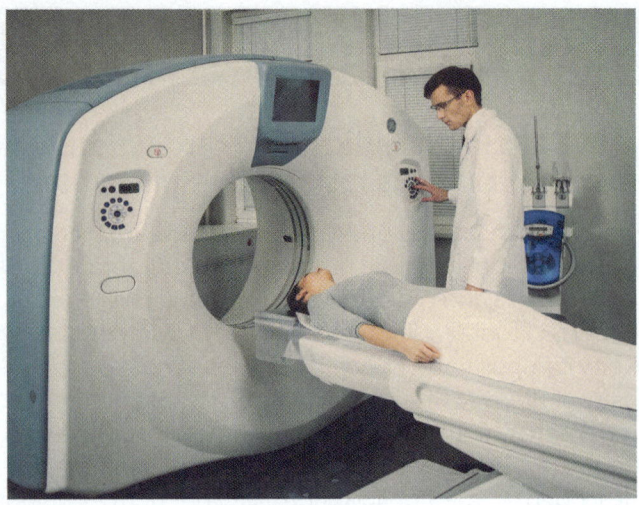

FIGURE 1.17 Computed Tomography Machine
© Nejron Photo/Shutterstock.

Imaging Technologies Imaging techniques represent the most precise and reliable assessments of muscle mass when determining body composition; however, these methods are rarely applicable in the clinical setting.[16] The most common methodologies—bioelectrical impedance analysis, dual-energy x-ray absorptiometry, computerized tomography, and magnetic resonance imaging—will be discussed briefly in this section.

Computed Tomography (CT) A **computed tomography (CT)** scan utilizes x-ray technology to provide quantitative data on muscle composition and distribution (**Figure 1.17**). CT scans are valuable due to the ability to measure fat and muscle content within a single abdominal cross-sectional slice; thereafter, the images obtained can be used to distinguish between fat mass, fat-free mass, and skeletal muscle, and even further between visceral and subcutaneous fat. The CT scan will provide an accurate quantification of whole body composition. Although this technique may be routinely used for diagnosis and evaluation of a number of medical conditions, its application for nutrition assessment in the clinical setting is limited. CT scans are *not* recommended for the sole purpose of determining body composition due to expense and radiation exposure.[114,115]

Magnetic Resonance Imaging (MRI) Body composition analysis can also be accomplished using **magnetic resonance imaging (MRI)**, utilizing what is referred to as a free-ionizing radiation technique. Following either a whole-body or regional scan, an MRI will illustrate adipose tissue and lean mass (including skeletal muscle) distribution. Although widely used in research, the utility of MRI for assessing body composition in the clinical setting is limited due to long scan duration and extreme expense.[115,116]

Bioelectrical Impedance Analysis (BIA) Of the available technologies, **bioelectrical impedance analysis (BIA)** is perhaps the most widely used for body composition estimation. By measuring the resistance of a high-frequency, low-amplitude electrical current passed through the body, BIA allows for the distinction between fat-free mass (through determination of total body water) and fat mass. The scientific basis for this two-compartment model is based on conductivity of an electrical current, which is greater in compartments rich in fluid and electrolytes such as the fat free mass. Conversely, bone and fat have poor conductivity and greater resistance to the electrical signal. Through conductivity and resistance, fat and fat-free mass can be differentiated. These values can be converted into body fat percentages using a variety of available regression equations. Within the realm of body composition analysis, this method can also be used to assess hydration status. BIA can only be applied to those without significant fluid or electrolyte abnormalities; in addition, a valid BIA equation appropriate to age, sex, and race must be available for the specific patient. When compared to other methods, BIA is attractive due to its relative simplicity, low cost, and portability (**Figure 1.18**). Previous research also suggests that changes in body composition as measured by BIA correlate directly with levels of energy and protein intake.[117] BIA cannot be recommended for use in the acutely ill patient population, for subjects at either BMI extreme, or for those with an abnormal hydration status (including renal disturbances).[14,18,117-123]

Dual Energy X-ray Absorptiometry (DXA) Developed originally for the measurement of bone density and bone mass, **dual energy x-ray absorptiometry (DXA)** has quickly

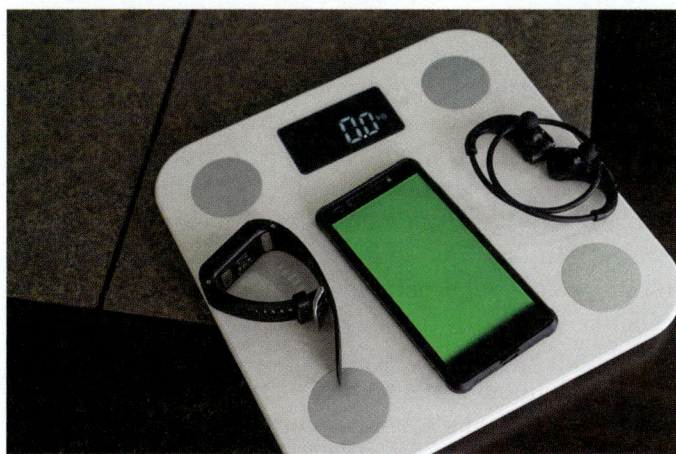

FIGURE 1.18 Bioelectrical Impedance Machine
© Syafiq Adnan/Shutterstock.

become a reference method for body composition assessment. Due to technological advancements, DXA can now be used to quantify soft-tissue composition, thus introducing the possibility for measuring total and regional body composition. In sum, the DXA scan divides the body into three compartments: bone, lean body mass, and fat mass. This method relies on the attenuation characteristics of tissues exposed to radiation at two peak energies, which are then converted into body assessment percentages using a number of available equations. Although DXA is not widely used in clinical practice for the assessment of body composition, DXA remains the method of choice for measuring bone mineral density, which, if available, may be an important consideration in a complete nutrition assessment.[14,18,114,115,121,123]

> **PRACTICE POINT**
>
> Although often cited in current literature and research papers, imaging techniques are generally not applicable to the clinical setting for nutrition assessment.

Biochemical Data, Medical Tests, and Procedures

A number of critical biochemical values are important to consider as part of a complete nutrition assessment. Note that a variety of other tests and procedures, including gastric emptying time and resting metabolic rate, may also fall into this category of assessment. Please refer to the chapter on biochemical assessment for information on biochemical assessment and its application to nutritional status.

Client History

A patient's nutritional status must be considered in the context of the overall clinical status. For that reason, a thorough nutrition assessment should always include an evaluation of client history, which includes personal as well as familial past medical history.

Nutrition-Focused Past Medical History

The relevance of the clinical picture to nutrition assessment cannot be overstated. Knowledge of an individual's medical and/or surgical history and current disease state(s) are particularly helpful in identifying a nutritional concern. Begin with an overview of the clinical diagnosis and its accompanying symptoms, particularly those that may affect intake. Note that any ongoing complaints or relevant past medical history (PMH) may represent a significant metabolic stressor or provide etiology behind poor appetite, decreased oral intake, or weight loss, all of which can indicate risk of malnutrition.[10,16,18] As a general guideline, a nutrition-focused PMH may include the following factors:

1. Demographic data: age, sex, occupation, family history, education level, any other personal history the clinician deems relevant
2. Chief complaint: a subjective statement of the problem, including onset and duration
3. History of present illness: note all nutritionally relevant data, including recent diet and/or weight changes, UBW, appetite changes, gastrointestinal symptoms (nausea, vomiting, diarrhea, and/or constipation), abdominal pain, etc.
4. PMH: surgical history, previous acute or chronic illnesses, allergies, eating disorders, disease or complication risk, psychosocial health, and/or cognitive disabilities
5. Medication history: evaluate for medications with strong nutrition interactions (such as drugs that may promote anorexia or interfere with the absorption, metabolism, or excretion of nutrients), including steroids, immunosuppressants, chemotherapy

CASE STUDY REVISITED

As you continue your interview, you learn that Mary is a retired school teacher who lives alone in her single-family home since her husband died 6 months ago.

Questions

1. How might Mary's social history impact her nutritional status?
2. What further information might you seek to obtain from Mary?

agents, antibiotics, diuretics, etc.; this section should also include any herbal or dietary supplement use
6. Family medical history: note the presence of any familial or genetic disorder that may impact nutritional status (cardiovascular disease, diabetes mellitus, cancer, etc.)
7. Social history: socioeconomic status, social and medical support, relevant cultural and religious beliefs, and/or living situation

In general, note any chronic disease state, episode of acute critical illness, and/or surgical procedure that may affect the nutritional status of the patient. Any number of conditions may increase the likelihood that the individual is malnourished. This may take the form of significantly increased metabolic demand, decreased appetite, comprised ability to ingest food by mouth (PO), and/or impaired nutrient absorption.[10,13,16,18,19]

> **PRACTICE POINT**
>
> A number of conditions, injuries, and/or complications cause significant metabolic demands.

Nutrition-Focused Physical Findings

Although often underused in clinical practice, a **nutrition-focused physical exam (NFPE)** is an instrumental and informative component of nutrition assessment. The NFPE is a system-based examination of each region of the body that aids in the evaluation of nutrition status by identifying markers of malnutrition and/or nutrient deficiencies. The goal is to identify whether the fat, muscle, fluid, and/or micronutrient status of a patient has diminished due to inflammation, chronic disease, and/or poor nutrient intake. Because physical signs tend to be nonspecific, any findings should be considered in the context of other clinical parameters (including biomarkers) and the patient interview. Although the NFPE is only one component of a comprehensive nutrition assessment, it can provide the necessary supportive data to identify and/or diagnose malnutrition.[56,124-127]

To assist the clinician in clinical practice, AND/A.S.P.E.N. have published a joint consensus statement with recommended characteristics for the identification and documentation of malnutrition. When diagnosing adult malnutrition, four out of the six necessary components include an evaluation of muscle and fat stores as part of the NFPE. In addition, the NFPE is included as part of the Standards of Practice for dietitians working in both adult and pediatric populations. If the NFPE is not performed, the nutrition assessment is incomplete.[126,127]

Techniques of the NFPE

The NFPE is performed following the review of the PMH and any pertinent laboratory data using four techniques: inspection, palpation, percussion, and auscultation. The bulk of the examination employs the technique of **inspection**, which involves the visual observation of color, shape, texture, and size. **Palpation** is used to evaluate and assess texture, size, temperature, tenderness, and mobility; here, the tips and pads of the fingers should be used to assess pulsations and areas of sensitivity, whereas the back of the hand is used to assess temperature. **Percussion** describes the tapping of fingers against body surfaces for sounds that reflect solids, fluids, or gas. This technique provides minimal nutrition information but is important for abdominal assessment and/or feeding tube placement for advanced practice dietetics. **Auscultation** involves the assessment of sounds that reflect

CASE STUDY REVISITED

As you continue your interview, you complete a nutrition-focused physical examination on Mary. Your findings are as follows:

Mary is alert but appears pale and tired. Her hair is thin, dry, and easily plucked. Her face is notable for dark circles under both eyes, narrow facial appearance, and temporal muscle depression. Her eyes appear normal. Mary's oral exam is notable for dry oral mucosa and angular stomatitis. She has good dentition with no missing teeth and normal tongue. She has evident clavicular muscle wasting. Her biceps reveal muscle wasting and triceps demonstrate subcutaneous fat loss with loose and slightly hanging arm skin. Rib fat loss is evident. Mary's skin is dry with poor skin turgor. No wounds are evident. Abdominal exam is unremarkable. No lower extremity or pedal edema is evident. Nails are thin with slow capillary refill. Interosseous muscle is mildly wasted.

Questions

1. How would you assess Mary's nutrition-focused physical exam findings?
2. Can you corroborate your findings with Mary's anthropometric data and diet history?
3. Based on the nutrition-focused physical exam findings, what specific nutrients are of concern for Mary?
4. Based on these findings, how would you describe Mary's nutritional status?

movement of fluid or air through organs and viscera using a stethoscope. Auscultation may provide useful information about the dietary status of the patient (for example, bowel sounds in the intestines as an indication of return of function following a postoperative ileus).[56,128]

> **PRACTICE POINT**
>
> The examination techniques most commonly used for identifying malnutrition as part of the NFPE include observation and palpation.[56]

Using these techniques, the physical examination should begin with observation (i.e., inspection) of the general appearance of the patient, including body type, mobility, skin color, and hair condition. Before initiating any hands-on assessment, the clinician should explain what the assessment will entail and request permission from the patient or healthcare proxy (if applicable) before proceeding. As previously mentioned, the clinician will look to identify any signs of poor nutritional status, including any physical manifestation of deficiency or malnutrition. Any notable observations are then compared to the nutrition-related concerns that were identified when reviewing the patient's PMH.[124,125]

> **PRACTICE POINT**
>
> In order to complete a thorough NFPE, it is recommended that the clinician follow a systematic approach. For example, the cephalocaudal order of examination is a guide to head-to-toe physical examination and includes these nutritionally relevant areas:
>
> - Head, eyes, ears, nose, throat (HEENT)
> - Neck
> - Upper extremities
> - Chest and back
> - Breast and axillae
> - Abdomen
> - Lower extremities
>
> *Note: Skin is checked throughout the assessment.*

Components of the NFPE

A system-based evaluation of body should include the following regions: general inspection, skin, hand and nails, head and hair, eyes and nose, oral cavity, neck and upper body, and musculoskeletal and lower extremities. Although the sections to follow will offer helpful hints on inspecting each region, refer to **Table 1.9** for general guidelines on the NFPE components and to **Table 1.10** for the specific deficiency that can be associated with physical findings.[128]

TABLE 1.9 COMPONENTS OF THE NUTRITION-FOCUSED PHYSICAL EXAM[56,128]

General Inspection	Observe overall appearance. Evaluate level of consciousness, demeanor, facial expression, body positioning, alterations in motor skills, body habitus, contractures, and/or amputations. Observe for wasting, cachexia, or obesity.
Skin	Observe for redness, pallor, cyanosis, jaundice or yellowing, bruising, and/or dark areas. Monitor for dry/moist skin, sweating, and temperature. Assess texture, thickness or hyperkeritosis, wounds or lesions, and turgor.
Hand and Nails	Inspect the hand and nails for color, texture, shape, and/or presence of lesions. Assess for transverse ridge, koilonychia. Observe and palpate the interosseous muscle for fullness and distribution.
Head and Hair	Inspect the scalp and hair for quantity, distribution, texture, and color. Evaluate for thinning, dryness, depigmentation, and corkscrew appearance. Assess temporalis muscle.
Eyes and Nose/Face	Interview to assess for changes in dryness of eyes or night vision. Observe the color of the sclera and conjunctiva. Evaluate corners of eyes for fissures or redness. Assess fullness and color around the orbital region.
Oral Cavity	Evaluate lips for pallor, dryness, or redness. Inspect corners of the mouth for dryness or redness. Observe tongue for inflammation and atrophic lingual papilla. Assess mucous membranes for moisture or dryness. Observe gums for swelling or bleeding. Evaluate teeth for caries, loose/missing teeth, discoloration, or eroded dentition.
Neck and Upper Body	Inspect the neck for distention or masses. Assess for muscle and subcutaneous fat loss in these regions: clavicles, shoulders, scapula, fat overlying the ribs, and triceps. Note sagging skin. Evaluate for edema.
Musculoskeletal and Lower Extremity	Observe overall muscle appearance. Note size and shape of quadriceps and calf muscles. Rate fluid accumulation around ankles. Assess for atrophy.

Data from Pogatshnik C, Hamilton C. Nutrition-focused physical examination: Skin, nails, hair, eyes, and oral cavity. *Support Line*. 2011;33(2):7-13; and Esper DH. Utilization of nutrition-focused physical assessment in identifying micronutrient deficiencies. *Nutr Clin Pract*. 2015;30(2):194-202.

TABLE 1.10 PHYSICAL ASSESSMENT NUTRIENT CHART

Region	Abnormal Findings	Possible Deficiency or *Excess (in italics)*
Skin	Pallor: paleness Cyanosis: bluish discoloration	Iron Folate or vitamin B$_{12}$ Biotin Copper
	Yellowing of skin	*Carotone or bilirubin (excess related)*
	Dermatitis Follicular hyperkeratosis: rough, cone-shaped, elevated papules around hair follicles	B-complex vitamins Vitamin A Vitamin C Zinc
	Poor wound healing	Vitamin A Vitamin C Zinc
	Xerosis: abnormal dryness	Vitamin A Essential fatty acid
	Perifolliculosis: pigmented plaques (thorax, abdomen, thighs, legs)	Vitamin C
	Pellagrous dermatitis: dermatitis with hyperpigmentation of areas exposed to sunlight	Niacin Tryptophan
	Flaky paint dermatitis: hyperpigmented patches, usually on backs of thighs/buttocks, that peel to reveal hypopigmented skin	Protein
	Edema (**Figure 1.19**) Poor turgor or tenting (**Figure 1.20**)	*Fluid (hydration) in excess* Fluid (hydration)
	Acanthosis nigricans: dark patches of skin	*Insulin excess due to insulin resistance*
Hand and Nails	Clubbing (**Figure 1.21**) Raised edges (spoon-shape) Koilonychia: thin, concave nails	Iron
	Excessive dryness Dark color of nails Curved nail ends	Vitamin B$_{12}$
	Lackluster or dull nails Pallor or white coloring Ridging, transverse on 2+ extremities	Protein
	Mottled, pale, poor blanching	Vitamin A Vitamin C
	Splinter hemorrhages on distal ends of nails	Vitamin C

(continues)

TABLE 1.10 PHYSICAL ASSESSMENT NUTRIENT CHART (continued)

Region	Abnormal Findings	Possible Deficiency or *Excess* (in italics)
Head and Hair	Dull, lackluster color or depigmentation	Protein Copper
	Easily plucked Thinness Sparseness Alopecia	Protein Biotin Copper Essential fatty acids
	Scaly and/or flaky scalp	Essential fatty acids
	Corkscrew, coiled hairs	Vitamin C Copper
Eyes and Nose/Face	Vision changes, particularly at night Excessive dryness Bitot spots: shiny gray spots on conjunctiva Keratomalacia: hazy, dry, softened cornea	Vitamin A
	Itching Burning Corneal inflammation	Riboflavin Niacin
	Pallor conjunctiva	Iron Folate Vitamin B_{12}
	Yellowish icterus (**Figure 1.22**)	*Bilirubin in excess*
	Diffuse pigmentation	Protein Energy
	Nasolabial seborrhea: scaling around nostrils	Riboflavin Niacin Vitamin B_6
	Temporal wasting (bilateral)	Protein Energy
Oral Cavity	Angular stomatitis (swollen corners of the mouth)	Riboflavin Niacin Vitamin B_6 Iron
	Glossitis (beefy red tongue, magenta color) (**Figure 1.24**) Atrophied papillae	Riboflavin Niacin Folate Vitamin B_{12} Iron (severe)

(continues)

TABLE 1.10 PHYSICAL ASSESSMENT NUTRIENT CHART (continued)

Region	Abnormal Findings	Possible Deficiency or *Excess* (in italics)
Oral Cavity	Pallor and generalized inflamed mucosa	Iron Vitamin B_{12} Folate B-complex
	Bleeding gums and poor dentition	Vitamin C
	Dysgeusia: distorted taste Hypogeusia: diminished taste	Zinc
	Cheilosis: dry, swollen, or ulcerated lips	Riboflavin Vitamin B_6 Niacin Iron (severe)
	Stomatitis: general inflammation of oral mucosa	B-complex Iron Vitamin C
	Edematous tongue	Niacin
	Atrophic filiform papillae: tongue is smooth or slick	Niacin Folate Riboflavin Iron Vitamin B_{12}
	Mottled teeth: whitish opaque-to-severe brown discoloration	*Fluoride excess*
	Caries: tooth decay	Fluoride Vitamin C
Neck and Upper Body	Enlarged thyroid	Iodine
	Enlarged parotid	Protein Bulimia
	Muscle and fat wasting with prominent bony chest region	Calorie and protein depletion
Musculoskeletal and Lower Extremity	Poor muscle control (ataxia) Numbness or tingling	Thiamin Vitamin B_{12} Copper
	Rickets, bowed legs	Vitamin D Calcium Phosphate
	Pitting edema	Protein Thiamin Vitamin C *Fluid excess*
	Swollen, painful joints	Vitamin C

Data from Pogatshnik C, Hamilton C. Nutrition-focused physical examination: Skin, nails, hair, eyes, and oral cavity. *Support Line*. 2011;33(2):7-13;

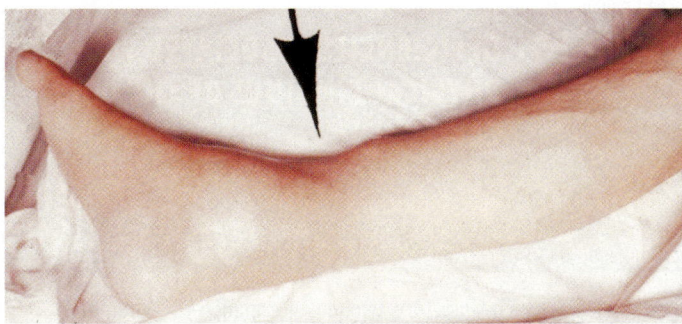

FIGURE 1.19 Lower Extremity Edema

Skin

Findings of the skin examination are considered to be accurate reflections of nutrient deficiencies because rapidly proliferating tissues, such as the skin, are thought to change simultaneously with developing nutritional abnormalities. Although a number of factors may affect the appearance of the skin, alterations in nutrition are often the culprit behind changes in fluid distribution (**Figure 1.19**), pigmentation, poor wound healing, development of dermatitis, and changes in turgor (**Figure 1.20**). These manifestations may be noted on the trunk or extremities, or on less obvious locations (as in the lips, mucous membranes, fingernails, and/or palms of hands and feet).[56,128]

> **PRACTICE POINT**
>
> When observing the skin, inspect the entire skin surface for changes in color, texture, temperature, moisture, lesions, mobility, and turgor.[128]

Hands and Nails A healthy nail plate should be firmly adhered to the nail bed, feel smooth to the touch, and appear uniformly thick and symmetric. The nail itself should be flat or slightly convex with translucent with a pink hue that is derived from the capillary system located underneath the nail plate. When palpating the nail by gently squeezing between the thumb and forefinger, the

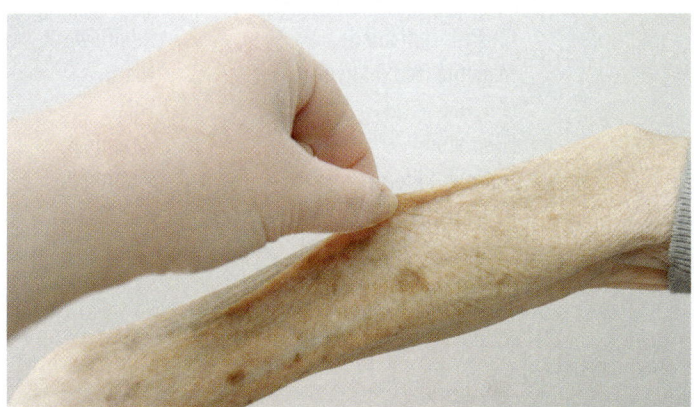

FIGURE 1.20 Poor Skin Turgor (Tenting)
©Libby Welch/Alamy Stock Photo.

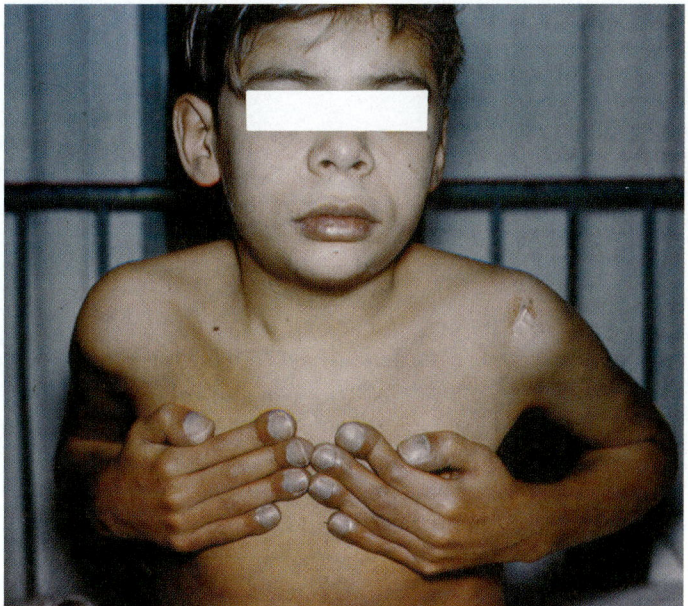

FIGURE 1.21 Child with Cyanosis and Clubbing of Fingernails

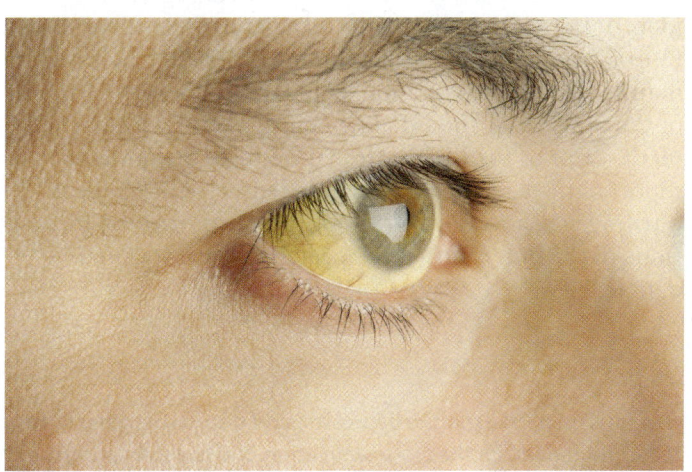

FIGURE 1.22 Scleral Icterus
© Oktay Ortakcioglu/Getty Images.

nail should blanch white and return to its pink color almost immediately (indicating normal capillary refill time indicating adequate hydration and blood flow to tissue). Any abnormalities in color or structure may represent nutritional deficiency and/or dehydration and should be considered in the context of the overall clinical picture.[56]

> **PRACTICE POINT**
>
> Inspect the nails for color, length, configuration, symmetry, and cleanliness; nail hygiene often reflects a patient's self-care and emotional order.[56]

Head and Hair Inspection and palpation of the head, scalp, and hair should be performed to assess for shape, quantity, distribution, and texture. Healthy scalp hair is shiny, smooth, resilient, and not easily plucked. Any abnormalities may indicate nutrient deficiency.[56]

> **PRACTICE POINT**
>
> Inspect the hair for color, pigmentation, distribution pattern, shine, texture, and quantity.[56]

Eyes and Nose/Face In general, the structure of the face should appear symmetric. Facial shape, particularly in regard to the temporal region, can also indicate deficiency in the form of protein-energy malnutrition. Be sure to note any temporal wasting upon inspection.[56]

The most common variations in eye health secondary to nutritional etiology include vitamin A deficiency, which manifests as night blindness or may be observed as Bitot spots in the eye conjunctiva (shiny gray spots). During the patient interview, note changes in night vision, dryness, and/or inability to produce tears.[56]

Oral Cavity The oral cavity is a critical region for identifying malnutrition. Due to the rapid turnover (3 to 5 days) of cells in the oral mucosa, deficiencies often manifest in the lips, tongue, gingiva, or mucosa. NFPE of the oral cavity should also include assessment of the teeth. Prior to the oral examination, note any patient report of taste changes, pain or bleeding gums, and/or burning sensations. Refer to **Table 1.11** for specific locations of the oral cavity to inspect and the associated deficiencies.[56,125]

> **PRACTICE POINT**
>
> A small penlight, tongue depressor, and disposable gloves are recommended for the oral examination. Start by examining the lips, then assess the inside of the mouth, including the tongue, gums, and teeth.[56,125]

Neck and Upper Body, Musculoskeletal and Lower Extremities The most important physical finding to identify on the trunk and extremities is that of muscle and/or fat wasting as an indicator of malnutrition. Incorporating the characteristics of malnutrition into the NFPE requires the evaluation of physical changes, including overt weight loss, shifts in body composition, loss of subcutaneous fat, and muscle wasting. Note that fluid retention in the form of edema or ascites may mask weight loss for many acutely ill patients. In addition, note that the AND/A.S.P.E.N. Consensus Statement on Identifying Adult Malnutrition[10] refers to several specific body areas that require assessment of fat, muscle, and/or fluid status. Per these guidelines, loss of subcutaneous fat is best identified in the orbital region, triceps, and/or overlying the ribs; muscle mass depletion manifests as wasting of the temples (temporalis muscle, clavicles

TABLE 1.11 DEFICIENCIES ASSOCIATED WITH PHYSICAL FINDINGS OF THE ORAL CAVITY[125]

Location	Signs/Symptoms	Possible Deficiency
Lips	Cheilosis (dry, swollen, ulcerated)	Vitamin B_6
	Angular cheilosis (fissures in the corners of the mouth)	Folate Riboflavin Niacin Vitamin B_{12} Iron
Mouth	Xerostomia (dry mouth)	Zinc
	Aphthous stomatitis (canker sores) (**Figure 1.23**)	Vitamin B_{12} Folate
	Candidiasis (thrush)	Vitamin C Iron
	Pale tissues	Iron
	Stomatopyrosis (painful, inflamed mouth)	Iron
	Dysesthesia (burning mouth syndrome)	Vitamin B_{12} Folate Magnesium
Teeth & Gums	Bleeding Gums	Vitamin C
	Tooth Loss	Vitamin C
	Dental Carries	Fluoride Vitamin C Vitamin B_{12}
Tongue	Glossitis (inflamed) Magenta (red colored) (**Figure 1.24**) Edematous Atrophic filiform Papillae (flattened protrusions on tongue, giving it a smooth, slick appearance)	Riboflavin Niacin Folate Vitamin B_6 Vitamin B_{12} Iron

Data from Radler DR, Lister T. Nutrient deficiencies associated with nutrition-focused physical findings of the oral cavity. *Nutr Clin Pract*. 2013;28(6):710-721.

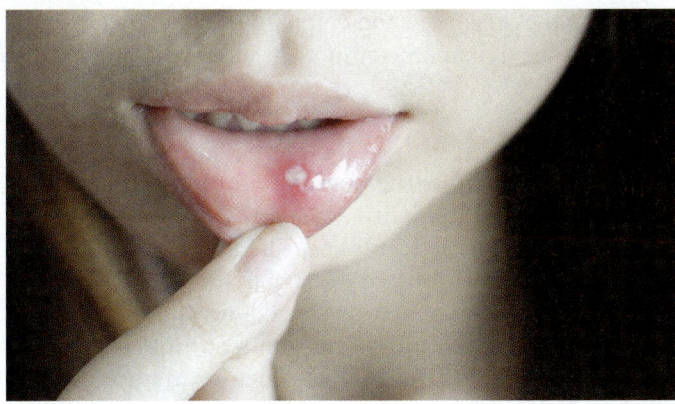

FIGURE 1.23 Aphthae on Lip
© C.PIPAT/Shutterstock.

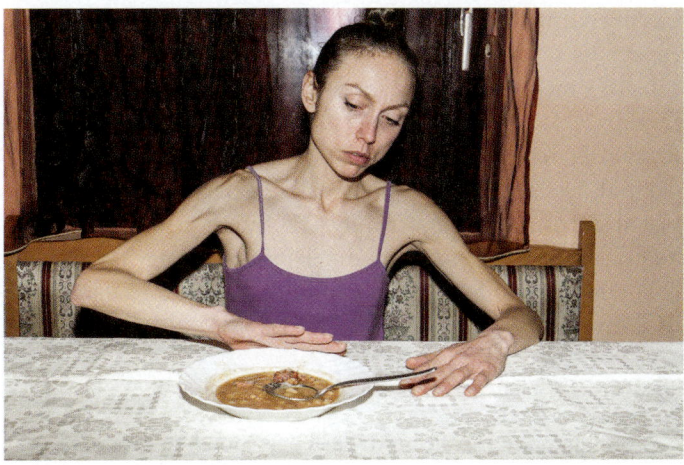

FIGURE 1.25 Clavicular Muscle Wasting
© Bony shoulders/Shutterstock.

(pectoralis and deltoids; **Figure 1.25**), shoulders (deltoids), interosseous muscles, scapula (latissimus dorsi, trapezious, deltoids), thigh (quadriceps), and calf (gastrocnemius); and generalized or localized fluid accumulation can be seen in the extremities, vulvar/scrotal region, or abdomen (as in ascites).[10,124]

Functional Assessment

Advanced malnutrition, often related to a decline in clinical status, is associated with loss of muscle mass and function that leads to measurable declines in strength and/or physical performance. The relationship is reciprocal: malnutrition can impair functioning and impaired functioning can lead to poor nutritional status through a number of avenues (e.g., inability to prepare meals, etc.). A functional assessment can be used to evaluate the degree of baseline impairment and should be repeated regularly thereafter for comparison of improvements with intervention or later declines in status. This assessment may include any abnormalities in body composition that interfere with normal function—including muscle strength and function. The functional assessment becomes particularly important when assessing the geriatric patient population. Both physical performance and the ability to perform **activities of daily living** (ADLs; routine activities that most individuals complete on a daily basis including eating, bathing, dressing, toileting, and walking) have important nutritional implications for older adults.[8,16,17,129]

Muscle Function and Strength: Handgrip Strength Declines in muscle strength will accompany loss of muscle mass—the body's largest protein reserve—that results from advanced malnutrition. The most practical measure for the clinical assessment of muscle strength is that of **handgrip strength** using a simple **handgrip dynamometer** (**Figure 1.26**). Other physical performance batteries include measures such as a timed gait, chair stands, and stair steps, although these measures are generally outside the dietetics scope of practice.[16,17,129,130]

Muscle function reacts quickly to nutritional deprivation; changes in muscle function may manifest prior to visual depletions. Because the function most easily measured is muscle force, handgrip strength, which is the simplest to measure and has been correlated with overall muscle strength,[131,132] can be used as a surrogate for voluntary muscle strength. A decline in handgrip strength

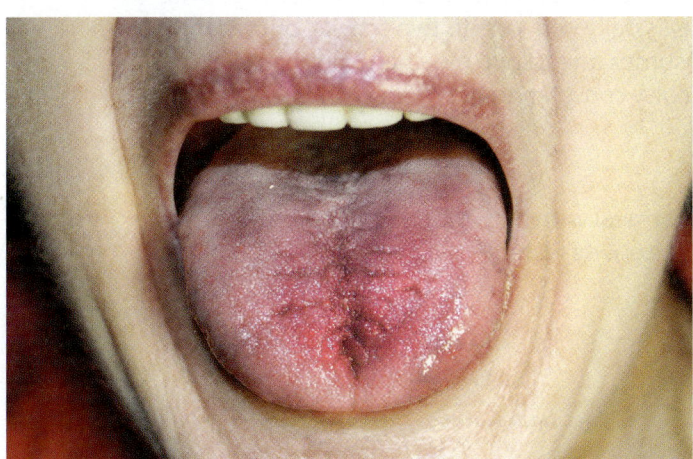

FIGURE 1.24 Inflamed, Magenta Tongue
© Timonina/Shutterstock.

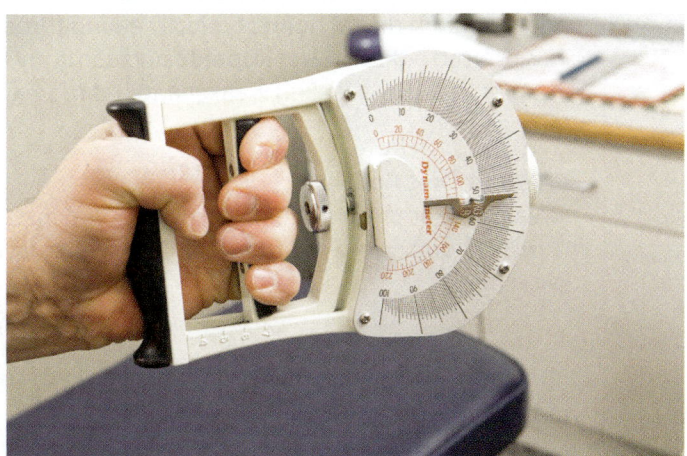

FIGURE 1.26 Handgrip Dynamometer
© BanksPhotos/Getty Images.

has been directly related to declines in nutrition status, especially in the elderly,[30,133] and can be relied upon as a sensitive measurement of short-term response to nutritional therapy.[134] It has also been deemed a relevant predictor of prognosis, hospital length of stay, and re-admission rates. In general, handgrip strength provides information on nutritional status, muscle mass, physical function, and overall health status. Moreover, handgrip dynamometry is rapid, cost-effective, and user-friendly with high test, re-test, and inter-rater reliability.[8,17,129-131,135-140]

> **PRACTICE POINT**
>
> Although handgrip strength has been shown to be a reliable marker of declining nutrition status, for some patients, declines in handgrip strength may be attributable to frailty with old age instead of overt malnutrition.

Procedure In regard to technique, there is some evidence that posture, choice between dominant/nondominant hand, and different dynamometer models produce varying results. These factors can be avoided by following standardized procedures. The patient should perform the test while sitting comfortably with shoulder adducted and forearm neutrally rotated, elbow flexed to 90°, and wrist in a neutral position. Ideally, the patient will be seated on a chair or at the side of the bed with feet on the floor. The grip on the dynamometer should be adjusted for hand size so that the dynamometer rests on the middle of four fingers. The grip should be held for about 3 to 5 seconds with the patient being instructed to perform a maximal isometric contraction and exhaling during grip exertion. The test should be repeated, alternating hands (for example, left hand then right hand then left hand, etc.) with about 15 seconds between each hand with a total of three tests per hand. An average value of the three tests should be recorded and compared to reference ranges specific to the dynamometer model that have been stratified by age and sex.[133,137,140,141]

Food/Nutrition-Related History

Dietary assessment is the portion of nutrition assessment that is used to identify inadequate, excessive, or imbalanced nutrient intakes. The most frequently used method for obtaining dietary history in both acute and outpatient care is the 24-hour dietary recall, although each of the most common techniques will be discussed later in this section. If dietary history cannot be obtained from direct patient interview, then medical records, family members, or caregivers can provide insight. It is not unusual for patients in the clinical setting to have compromised dietary intake for extended periods of time prior to assessment (particularly for those with acute medical events superimposed on chronic health conditions). The diet history can help to identify reasons behind changes in dietary intake, including disease-related symptoms.[13,16]

The diet history is also useful for providing average macronutrient and micronutrient intakes, as well as a depiction of general diet variety and eating patterns. When malnutrition is of concern, the current dietary recall should be compared to a normal dietary recall to provide the current percentage of normal intake. The dietary history will objectivize the contribution of poor dietary intake to the malnourished state.[8,16]

In general, a thorough food and nutrition history should address a number of areas.

Food Intake

Assess for diet composition, adequacy of food and nutrient intake, meal and snack patterns, as well as any allergies or intolerances, food preferences, environmental cues to

---

CASE STUDY REVISITED

As you continue to interview Mary, you ask about her dietary history. Mary states that she follows a low-sodium diet at home, typically eating three meals daily with one to two snacks, but recently has noticed a decrease in appetite and currently consumes one to two meals and no snacks. She reports that she is feeling weaker and has more difficulty completing her grocery shopping and meal preparation.

24-hour Diet Recall:
Breakfast 8 am: 8 oz coffee black with ½ cup instant oatmeal with 2 oz added skim milk
Lunch 12 pm: ½ low-salt tuna sandwich with mayonnaise, 6 oz water
No dinner

Questions

1. How is Mary's intake influencing her nutritional status?
2. What other assessments can be conducted to assess Mary's functional status?
3. Does Mary classify as malnourished?

eating, and current diets and/or food modifications; note that underreporting or overreporting are both common occurrences. Also note any influences on appetite, which should be assessed as within normal limits or for any relevant changes. Consider the current disease state or medication use as sources for symptoms that affect intake (e.g., taste changes, gastrointestinal symptoms, swallowing ability, requirements for assistance or feeding, etc.). This assessment should also address the use of dietary supplements.[16,18]

Nutrition Support

Assess whether a patient requires nutrition support in the form of oral nutrition supplements, tube feeding, or parenteral support. If so, note the home regimen. In the acute care setting, dietary assessment must continue when nutrition support is initiated in order to monitor adequacy of nutrient provision. If a patient is receiving nutrition support in addition to oral feeding, it is important to track the adequacy of oral feeds in order to adjust the nutrition support provided.[13,16]

Cultural Background

In all settings, assess and consider any cultural or religious influence on eating habits and perception of healthy weight status.

Nutrition and Health Awareness

Assess knowledge and beliefs about nutrition recommendations, including self-monitoring principles and past nutrition experience, particularly in the outpatient setting. Look to identify attitudes toward food or eating patterns.

Food Availability, Economics, Home Life

Food availability and economics will have a significant impact on dietary habits for many patients. Attempt to assess food planning, purchasing, and preparation abilities; limitations; nutrition program utilization; and/or food insecurity. Tailor counseling to income and availability, but always be sensitive to the individual situation.

Within this arena, consider the number of people in the household, the individual who does the shopping and/or cooking, food storage and cooking facilities, and type of housing—each of these factors will certainly impact dietary habits.

Physical Activity and Exercise

Physical activity and exercise habits should be assessed as part of the dietary history. Other pertinent information includes functional status, activity patterns, amount of sedentary time, sleep habits, and occupation. If applicable, also note any handicaps that would impact physical activity and decrease energy need.

Allergies, Intolerances, Food Avoidances

As part of the dietary history, note foods that are avoided and the reason for the avoidance (including allergies and intolerances), description of associated symptoms, length of time of avoidance, and foods used to replace the avoided item.

> **PRACTICE POINT**
>
> When considering the acutely ill inpatient population, assessing dietary intake prior to hospital admission and duration of poor oral intake will be particularly pertinent to the assessment. It is not unusual for patients in acute care to have had compromised dietary intakes for extended periods prior to admission.[13]

Dietary Recall Methods/Methods of Obtaining Intake Data

The accurate assessment of dietary intake is an integral component of nutrition assessment. Self-reporting of intake via 24-hour dietary recalls, food records diary, and/or food frequency questionnaires are the most common methods for assessment. Because diet is inherently complicated to measure, any self-reported data are prone to errors attributed to memory, estimation of portion size, underreporting or overreporting, and distortion to socially desirable responses. These methods may be limited for use in the acutely ill or elderly patients who may be unable to self-report dietary intake. An additional observational method, the calorie count, is useful in the clinical setting but is often cumbersome, reliant on an accurate record, and cannot be applied to the outpatient setting. Despite these difficulties, assessment of nutrient intake is crucial to identifying individuals at risk for malnutrition and to estimating the contribution on decreased oral intake to the malnourished state.[8,17,142-146]

24-Hour Dietary Recall The 24-hour dietary recall is a retrospective tool that requires the client to recite all food intake during the previous 24 hours. To improve patient recall, a multiple-pass method is often employed; this involves multiple passes through the day ([1] collecting a quick list of foods; [2] assessing time, meal, and place; [3] reviewing a foods forgotten list; [4] revising food details; [5] final review) to provide additional memory cues. This method was developed to minimize underreporting of data by providing respondents with numerous opportunities to recall dietary intake. Visual aids may be used to assist subjects in estimating more accurate portion sizes.[142,144,147-149]

The 24-hour dietary recall is practical, quick, inexpensive, is independent of literacy ability, and has a low respondent burden. With this type of recall, the patient or client is more likely to be honest about their dietary behavior. The known limitations include reliance on respondent memory, tendency to underestimate portion sizes, and high inter-rater variability. The 24-hour recall has several

Clinical Roundtable

Topic: Nutrition Assessment in the Intensive Care Unit (ICU)[13,68,127,154-158]

Background: Patients treated in the intensive care units are some of the highest acuity patients in the hospital. Many of the typical assessment criteria (weight status, dietary intake, biochemical markers, etc.) are difficult to reliably obtain or are confounded by factors like metabolic stress. Anthropometric measurements, which are fundamental to any nutrition assessment, may not be easily acquired from the intubated and sedated critically ill patient who may be both unable to be moved for measurement and unable to provide self-reported data. Other factors related to clinical status, like fluid shifts or edema, will further confound this assessment.

To help clinicians better assess those who are critically ill, Heyland et al.[155] developed and validated a novel risk assessment tool based directly on the ICU patient population. This tool, the NUTrition Risk in the Critically ill (NUTRIC score), is based on variables that are easy to obtain in the critical care setting. Patients receive a score of 1 to 10 based on an algorithm that considers six variables: age; Acute Physiology and Chronic Health Evaluation scores (APACHE II); Sequential Organ Failure Assessment scores (SOFA); number of comorbidities; days from hospital to ICU admission; and serum interleukin-6 (IL-6). The following table outlines the NUTRIC score variables as they apply to the final evaluation:

Variable	Range	Points
Age (years)	<50	0
	50-74	1
	≥75	2
APACHE II	<15	0
	15-19	1
	20-28	2
	≥28	3
SOFA	<6	0
	6-9	1
	≥10	2

(continues)

Variable	Range	Points
Number of Comorbidities	0-1	0
	≥2	1
Days from Hospital to ICU Admission	<1	0
	≥1	1
IL-6	0-399	0
	≥400	1

Modified from Heyland DK, Dhaliwal R, Jiang X, Day AG. Identifying critically ill patients who benefit the most from nutrition therapy: the development and initial validation of a novel risk assessment tool. *Crit Care*. 2011;15(6):R268.

To be most clinically applicable, the NUTRIC score provides interpretation guidelines based on whether or not the IL-6 marker is available (the other markers are routinely obtainable from the medical record of an ICU patient):

If IL-6 is available:

- High score (6-10 points): associated with worse clinical outcomes (i.e., mortality); these patients are most likely to benefit from aggressive medical nutrition therapy
- Low score (0-5 points): low malnutrition risk

If IL-6 is *not* available:

- High score (5-9 points): associated with worse clinical outcomes (i.e., mortality); these patients are most likely to benefit from aggressive medical nutrition therapy
- Low score (0-4 points): low malnutrition risk

In general, the higher the sum of the scores from each component, the greater the likelihood of nutritional risk and anticipated benefit of nutrition intervention.

Roundtable Discussion

1. Given the difficulties with nutritional assessment in the critical care setting, how might the NUTRIC score be a valuable tool for clinicians in this setting?
2. Due to its validation, should the NUTRIC score supersede standard nutrition assessment in this setting? Why or why not?
3. What are the advantages and disadvantages of using a nutrition assessment tool, such as the NUTRIC score, in the critical care setting?

limitations to its use in the inpatient clinical setting; be sure to clarify whether the recall depicts a typical day and, if not, determine what makes it atypical. As with any 24-hour recall, engage in a discussion on how that intake compares to usual intake. Bear in mind that this method of recall portrays a snapshot in time; it will be beneficial to combine the information obtained from the recall with information on typical intake to better understand eating habits and any changes in usual patterns. The reliability of dietary assessment increases when 24-hour dietary recalls are repeated on several occasions.[8,17,142,143,150]

Food Records Diary The food records diary is applicable only to the outpatient setting. As a prospective tool, this method requires the client to record food intake for a specific time period (usually several days to 1 week). The diary provides greater precision than the 24-hour dietary recall and is not reliant on client memory. It can be considered more reflective of an "actual intake" because it will typically encompass several days, including weekdays and weekend days. The most notable limitation is that participants tend to modify eating behavior based on what they feel is an "acceptable" dietary intake for the duration of the food record. This method has a much higher client burden when compared to the 24-hour dietary recall and is dependent on literacy and numeracy with knowledge of portion sizes.[143]

Food Frequency Questionnaire (FFQ) The food frequency questionnaire (FFQ) is utilized most often in the outpatient setting or for national survey data collection, although modified versions may be useful for assessing intake patterns of the hospitalized patient. The FFQ is a retrospective tool that requires the client to complete a survey about food intake over a specific period of time in an attempt to depict "usual" intake. This method has several benefits, including low client burden, ease of administration, low cost, ease of standardization, and ability to examine specific nutrients. The data provided are qualitative. The tool also requires that the client be literate and numerate, and is significantly memory-dependent. The tool may be cognitively difficult because it relies on a foods list and is not meal-based.[143,151,152]

Observation of Food Intake: "Calorie Counts" Observation of food intake in the form of "calorie counts" can only be employed in controlled settings (like an inpatient hospital unit). This method will not represent usual intake, but instead a picture of current intake that is often useful when diagnosing malnutrition or assessing need for nutrition support in the clinical setting. Observation methods have a low client burden (i.e., the client is generally unaware of the dietary assessment) and is not memory or literacy dependent. In addition to increasing staff burden, this tool is intrusive and may be difficult to implement and interpret. This tool should not serve as the first choice for dietary assessment method and should be saved for instances when other dietary recall methods are not feasible.[143,146]

Technological Advancements for Tracking Dietary Intake

Technological advancements have begun to change the way dietary assessment is implemented in the outpatient setting. Innovative dietary assessment technologies using smartphones and web-based platforms have grown in popularity and now tend to replace traditional pen-and-paper versions of dietary assessment. The application of technology in this setting has recently been shown to reduce issues associated with accuracy, client burden, and time of data collection. Being aware of the current technologies and their function may help facilitate better data collection when compared to the traditional methods.[144,145,148,153]

Energy Balance

Assessment of current dietary intake and the influencing factors should be made in the context of energy needs. These needs will vary greatly depending on disease state (among many other factors). Refer to Chapter 5, *Energy Expenditure and Body Composition in Metabolic Stress* for additional information.

Chapter Summary

Nutrition assessment is an integral part of patient care because it involves obtaining and interpreting information needed to identify and then treat nutrition-related issues, such as malnutrition. It is a multifactorial process that utilizes various data sources including anthropometric, biochemical, clinical, dietary, energy balance, and functional information in order to compare to specific criteria. Although there is a broad range of evaluation parameters, assessment of nutritional status requires interpretation of data compared to standards made within the context, interpreted, and adjusted for the individual clinical situation. Nutrition assessment is supported by, but does not include, nutrition screening, which seeks to identify individuals who would benefit most from a complete assessment.

Key Terms

nutrition care process and model (NCPM), nutrition care process terminology (NCPT), malnutrition, nutrition screening, nutritional risk screening (NRS-2002), malnutrition universal screening tool (MUST), short nutritional assessment questionnaire (SNAQ), malnutrition screening tool (MST), anthropometry, height, stadiometer, self-reported height (SRH), knee-height, total arm span (TAS), half arm span (HAS), actual body weight, usual body weight (UBW), percent usual body weight (%UBW), percent weight change (%weight change), ideal body weight (IBW), percent ideal body weight (%IBW), adjusted body weight, dry weight, body mass index (BMI), skinfold anthropometry, triceps skinfold (TSF), mid-upper arm circumference (MUAC), mid-arm muscle circumference

(MAMC), waist circumference, waist-hip ratio (WHR), computed tomography (CT), magnetic resonance imaging (MRI), bioelectrical impedance analysis (BIA), dual energy x-ray absorptiometry (DXA), nutrition-focused physical exam (NFPE), inspection, palpation, percussion, auscultation, activities of daily living handgrip strength, handgrip dynamometer, 24-hour dietary recall, food records diary, food frequency questionnaire

References

1. Ravasco P, Camilo ME, Gouveia-Oliveira A, Adam S, Brum G. A critical approach to nutritional assessment in critically ill patients. *Clin Nutr.* 2002;21(1):73-77.
2. Charney P, Peterson SJ. Practice papers of the Academy of Nutrition and Dietetics: critical thinking skills in nutrition assessment and diagnosis. *J Acad Nutr Diet.* 2013;115(11):1545-1558.
3. Hammond MI, Myers EF, Trostler N. Nutrition care process and model: an academic and practice odyssey. *J Acad Nutr Diet.* 2014;114(12):1879-1894.
4. Writing Group of the Nutrition Care Process/Standardized Language Committee. Nutrition care process and model part I: the 2008 update. *J Am Diet Assoc.* 2008;108(7):1113-1117.
5. Field LB, Hand RK. Differentiating malnutrition screening and assessment: a nutrition care process perspective. *J Acad Nutr Diet.* 2015;115(5):824-828.
6. Lacey K, Pritchett E. Nutrition care process and model: ADA adopts road map to quality care and outcomes management. *J Am Diet Assoc.* 2003;103(8):1061-1072.
7. Mueller C, Compher C, Ellen DM. American Society for Parenteral and Enteral Nutrition (A.S.P.E.N.) Board of Directors. A.S.P.E.N. clinical guidelines: nutrition screening, assessment, and intervention in adults. *JPEN J Parenter Enteral Nutr.* 2011;35(1):16-24.
8. Soeters PB, Reijven PLM, van Bokhorst-de van der Schueren MA, et al. A rational approach to nutrition assessment. *Clin Nutr.* 2008;27(5):706-716.
9. Lawson CM, Daley BJ, Sams VG, Martindale R, Kudsk KA, Miller KR. Factors that impact patient outcome: nutrition assessment. *JPEN J Parenter Enteral Nutr.* 2013;37(Suppl 1):30S-38S.
10. White JV, Guenter P, Jensen G, et al. Consensus state of the academy of nutrition and dietetics/american society for parenteral and enteral nutrition: characteristics recommended for the identification and documentation of adult malnutrition (undernutrition). *JPEN J Parenter Enteral Nutr.* 2012;36(3):275-283.
11. Jensen GL, Mirtallo J, Compher C, et al. Adult starvation and disease-related malnutrition: a proposal for etiology-based diagnosis in the clinical practice setting from the international consensus guideline committee. *JPEN J Parenter Enteral Nutr.* 2010;34(2):156-159.
12. Jensen GL, Compher C, Sullivan DH, Mullin GE. Recognizing malnutrition in adults: definitions, characteristics, screening, assessment, and team approach. *JPEN J Parenter Enteral Nutr.* 2013;37(6):802-807.
13. Jensen GL, Wheeler D. A new approach to defining and diagnosing malnutrition in adult critical illness. *Curr Opin Crit Care.* 2012;18(2):206-211.
14. Jeejeebhoy KN. Nutrition assessment. *J Nutr.* 2000;16(7/8):585-590.
15. Cederholm T, Bosaeus I, Barazzoni R, et al. Diagnostic criteria for malnutrition—an ESPEN consensus statement. *Clin Nutr.* 2015;34(3):335-340.
16. Jensen GL, Hsiao PY, Wheeler D. Adult nutrition assessment tutorial. *JPEN J Parenter Enteral Nutr.* 2012;36(3):267-274.
17. Soeters PB, Schols AMWJ. Advances in understanding and assessing malnutrition. *Curr Opin Clin Nutr Metab Care.* 2009;12(5):487-494.
18. Alberda C, Graf A, McCargar L. Malnutrition: etiology, consequences, and assessment of a patient at risk. *Best Pract Res Clin Gastroenterol.* 2006;20(3):419-439.
19. Sabol VK. Nutrition assessment of the critically ill adult. *AACN Clin Issues.* 2004;15(4):595-606.
20. Kondrup J, Allison SP, Elia M, Vellas B, Plauth M. ESPEN guidelines for nutrition screening 2002. *Clin Nutr.* 2003;22(4):415-421.
21. Kondrup J, Rasmussen HH, Hamberg O, Stanga Z, an ad hoc ESPEN Working Group. Nutritional risk screening (NRS 2002): a new method based on an analysis of controlled clinical trials. *Clin Nutr.* 2003;22(3):321-336.
22. Hejazi N, Mazloom Z, Zand F, Rezaiazadeh A, Amini A. Nutrition assessment in critically ill patients. *Iran J Med Sci.* 2016;41(3):171-179.
23. Isabel M, Correia TD, Waitzberg DL. The impact of malnutrition on morbidity, mortality, length of hospital stay and costs evaluated through a multivariate model analysis. *Clin Nutr.* 2003;22(3):235-239.
24. Saunders J, Smith T, Stroud M. Malnutrition and undernutrition. *Medicine.* 2011;39(1):45-50.
25. Lim SL, Ong KCB, Chan YH, Loke WC, Ferguson M, Daniels L. Malnutrition and its impact on cost of hospitalization, length of stay, readmission and 3-year mortality. *Clin Nutr.* 2012;31(3):345-350.
26. Skipper A, Ferguson M, Thompson K, Castellanos VH, Porcari J. Nutrition screening tools: an analysis of the evidence. *JPEN J Parenter Enteral Nutr.* 2012;36(3):292-298.
27. Poulia KA, Klek S, Doundoulakis I, et al. The two most popular malnutrition screening tools in light of the new ESPEN consensus definition of the diagnostic criteria for malnutrition. *Clin Nutr.* 2017;36(4):1130-1135.
28. Phillips W, Zechariah S. Minimizing false-positive nutrition referrals generated from the malnutrition screening tool. *J Acad Nutr Diet.* 2017;117(5):665-669.
29. Patel V, Romano M, Corkins MR, et al. Nutrition screening and assessment in hospitalized patients: a survey of current practice in the united states. *Nutr Clin Pract.* 2014;29(4):483-490.
30. Anthony PS. Nutrition screening tools for hospitalized patients. *Nutr Clin Pract.* 2008;23(4):373-382.
31. van Bokhorst-de van der Schueren MA, Guaitoli PR, Iansma EP, de Vet HCW. Nutrition screening tools: Does one size fit all? A systematic review of screening tools for the hospital setting. *Clin Nutr.* 2014;33(1):39-58.
32. Rasmussen HH, Holst M, Kondrup J. Measuring nutritional risk in hospitals. *Clin Epidemiol.* 2010;21(2):209-216.
33. Gur AS, Atahan K, Aladag I, et al. The efficacy of nutrition risk screening-2002 (NRS-2002) to decide on the nutritional support in general surgery patients. *Bratisl Lek Listy.* 2009;110(5):290-292.
34. Mercadal-Orfila G, Lluch-Taltavull J, Campillo-Artero C, Torrent-Quetglas M. Association between nutritional risk based on the NRS-2002 test and hospital morbidity and mortality. *Nutr Hosp.* 2012;27(4):1248-1254.
35. Boban M, Laviano A, Persic V, Rotim A, Jovanovic Z, Vcev A. Characteristics of NRS-2002 nutritional risk screening in patients hospitalized for secondary cardiovascular prevention and rehabilitation. *J Am Coll Nutr.* 2014;33(6):466-473.
36. Orell-Kotikangas H, Österlund P, Saarilahti K, Ravasco P, Schwab U, Mäkitie AA. NRS-2002 for pre-treatment nutritional risk screening and

36. [continued] nutritional status assessment in head and neck cancer patients. *Support Care Cancer*. 2015;23(6):1496-1502.
37. Guo W, Ou G, Li X, Huang J, Liu J, Wei H. Screening of the nutritional risk of patients with gastric carcinoma before operation by NRS 2002 and its relationship with postoperative results. *J Gastroenterol Hepatol*. 2010;25(4):800-803.
38. Malnutrition Advisory Group. The 'MUST' report. Nutritional screening of adults: a multidisciplinary responsibility. Development and use of the malnutrition universal screening tool (MUST) for adults. BAPEN; 2003. https://www.health.gov.il/download/ng/N500-19.pdf
39. Stratton RJ, Hackston A, Longmore D, et al. Malnutriton in hospital outpatients and inpatients: Prevalence, concurrent validity, and ease of use of the 'malnutrition universal screening tool' ('MUST') for adults. *Br J Nutr*. 2004;92:799-808.
40. Stratton RJ, King CL, Stroud MA, Jackson AA, Elia M. 'Malnutrition universal screening tool' predicts mortality and length of hospital stay in acutely ill elderly. *Br J Nutr*. 2006;95:325-330.
41. Cooper PL, Raja R, Golder J, et al. Implementation of nutrition risk screening using the malnutrition universal screening tool across a large metropolitan health service. *J Hum Nutr Diet*. 2016;29(6):697-703.
42. Rahman A, Wu T, Bricknell R, Muqtadir Z, Armstrong D. Malnutrition matters in Canadian hospitalized patients: malnutrition risk in hospitalized patients in a tertiary care center using the malnutrition universal screening tool. *Nutr Clin Pract*. 2015;30(5):709-713.
43. Boléo-Tomé C, Monteiro-Grillo I, Camilo M, Ravasco P. Validation of the malnutrition universal screening tool (MUST) in cancer. *Br J Nutr*. 2012;108(2):343-348.
44. Dutch Malnutrition Steering Group. SNAQ tools in English. Fight Malnutrition Web site. www.fightmalnutrition.eu. Updated 2017. Accessed February 10, 2017.
45. Kruizenga HM, Seidell JC, de Vet H.C., Wierdsma NJ, van Bokhorst-de van der Schueren, M.A. Development and validation of a hospital screening tool for malnutrition: the short nutritional screening questionnaire (SNAQ©). *Clin Nutr*. 2005;24(1):75-82.
46. Kruizenga HM, de Jonge P, Seidell JC, et al. Are malnourished patients complex patients? Health status and care complexity of malnourished patients detected by the short nutritional assessment questionnaire (SNAQ). *Eur J Intern Med*. 2006;17(3):189-194.
47. Neelemaat F, Kruizenga HM, de Vet HC, Seidell JC, Butterman M, van Bokhorst-de van der Schueren, MA. Screening malnutrtion in hospital outpatients. Can the SNAQ malnutrition screening tool also be applied to this population? *Clin Nutr*. 2008;27(3):439-446.
48. van Venrooij LM, de Vos R, Borgmeijer-Hoelen AM, Kruizenga HM, Jonkers-Schuitema CF, de Mol BA. Quick-and-easy nutritional screening tools to detect disease-related undernutrition in hospital in- and outpatient settings: a systematic review of sensitivity and specificity. *e-SPEN Eur E J Clin Nutr Metab*. 2007;2:21-37.
49. Ferguson M, Capra S, Bauer J, Banks M. Development of a valid and reliable malnutrition screening tool for adult acute hospital patients. *Nutrition*. 1999;15(6):458-464.
50. Abbott Nutrition. Malnutrition screening tool (MST). Abbott Nutrition Web site. https://abbottnutrition.com/tools-for-patient-care/rd-toolkit. Updated 2017. Accessed October 29, 2017.
51. Isenring E, Cross G, Daniels L, Kellett E, Koczwara B. Validity of the malnutrition screening tool as an effective predictor of nutritonal risk in oncology outpatients receiving chemotherapy. *Support Care Cancer*. 2006;14(11):1152-1156.
52. Ferguson ML, Bauer J, Gallagher B, Capra S, Christie DR, Mason BR. Validation of a malnutrition screening tool for patients receiving radiotherapy. *Australas Radiol*. 1999;43(3):325-327.
53. Raslan M, Gonzalez MC, Dias MC, et al. Comparison of nutritinal risk screening tools for predicting clinical outcomes in hospitalized patients. *Nutrition*. 2010;26(7-8):721-726.
54. Kyle UG, Kossovsky MP, Karsegard VL, Richard C. Comparison of tools for nutritional assessment and screening at hospital admission: a population study. *Clin Nutr*. 2006;25(3):409-417.
55. Neelemaat F, Meijers J, Kruizenga H, van Ballegooijen H, van Bokhorst-de van der Schueren, M. Comparison of five malnutrition screening tools in one hospital inpatient sample. *J Clin Nurs*. 2011;20(15-16):2144-2152.
56. Pogatshnik C, Hamilton C. Nutrition-focused physical examination: skin, nails, hair, eyes, and oral cavity. *Support Line*. 2011;33(2):7-13.
57. Gorstein J, Akré J. The use of anthropometry to assess nutritional status. *World Health Stat Q*. 1988;41(2):48-58.
58. Shah B, Sucher K, Hollenbeck CB. Comparison of ideal body weight equations and published height-weight tables with body mass index tables for healthy adults in the United States. *Nutr Clin Pract*. 2006;21(3):312-319.
59. Madden AM, Smith S. Body composition and morphological assessment of nutritional status in adults: a review of anthropometric variables. *J Hum Nutr Diet*. 2016;29(1):7-25.
60. Beghetto MG, Fink J, Luft VC, de Mello ED. Estimates of body height in adult inpatients. *Clin Nutr*. 2006;25(3):438-443.
61. Cereda E, Bertoli S, Battezzati A. Height prediction formula for middle-aged (30-55 y) Caucasians. *Nutrition*. 2010;26(11-12):1075-1081.
62. Venkataraman R, Ranganathan L, Nirmal V, et al. Height measurement in the critically ill patient: a tall order in the critical care unit. *Indian J Crit Care Med*. 2015;19(11):665-668.
63. Centers for Disease Control and Prevention (CDC). National Health and Nutrition Examination survey (NHANES): Anthropometry procedures manual. https://www.cdc.gov/nchs/data/nhanes/nhanes_07_08/manual_an.pdf Updated January, 2007. Accessed October 29, 2017.
64. Hickson M, Frost G. A comparison of three methods for estimating height in the acutely ill erderly population. *J Hum Nutr Diet*. 2003;16(1):13-20.
65. Brown JK, Whittemore KT, Knapp TR. Is arm span an accurate measure of height in young and middle-age adults? *Clin Nurs Res*. 2000;9(1):84-94.
66. Brown JK, Feng J, Knapp TR. Is self-reported height or arm span a more accurate alternative measure of height? *Clin Nurs Res*. 2002;11(4):417-432.
67. Gorber SC, Tremblay M, Moher D, Gorber B. A comparison of direct vs. self-report measures for assessing height, weight, and body mass index: a systematic review. *Obes Rev*. 2007;8(4):307-326.
68. Berger MM, Cayeux M, Schaller M, Soguel L, Piazza G, Chioléro RL. Stature estimation using the knee height determination in critically ill patients. *e-SPEN Eur E J Clin Nutr Metab*. 2008;3(2):e84-e88.
69. Chumlea WC, Guo SS, Steinbaugh ML. Prediction of stature from knee height for black and white adults and children with application to mobility-impaired or handicapped persons. *J Am Diet Assoc*. 1994;94(12):1385-1388.
70. Hwang IC, Kim KK, Kang HC, Kang DR. Validity of stature-predicted equations using knee height for elderly and mobility impaired persons in koreans. *Epidemiol Health*. 2009;31:e20009004.
71. Chumlea WC, Guo SS, Wholihan K, Cockram D, Kuczmarski RJ, Johnson CL. Stature prediction equations for elderly non-hispanic white, non-hispanic black, and Mexican-American persons developed from NHANES III. *J Am Diet Assoc*. 1998;98(2):137-142.
72. Buchman AL. *Handbook of Nutritional Support*. Baltimore: Williams & Wilkins; 1997.
73. Pai MP, Paloucek FP. The origin of the "ideal" body weight equations. *Ann Pharmacother*. 2000;34(9):1066-1069.

74. Müller MJ. Ideal body weight or BMI: so, what's it to be? *Am J Clin Nutr*. 2016;103(5):1193-1194.

75. Peterson CM, Thomas DM, Blackburn GL, Heymsfield SB. Universal equation for estimating ideal body weight and body weight at any BMI. *Am J Clin Nutr*. 2016;103(5):1197-1203.

76. Hamwi GJ. Changing dietary concepts. In: Donowski TS, ed. *Diabetes mellitus: Diagnosis and treatment*. New York, NY: American Diabetes Association;1964:73-78.

77. Ireton-Jones C. Adjusted body weight, con: Why adjust body weight in energy-expenditure calculations? *Nutr Clin Pract*. 2005;20(4):474-479.

78. Kohn JB. Adjusted or ideal body weight for nutrition assessment? *J Acad Nutr Diet*. 2015;115(4):680.

79. Barak N, Wall-Alonso E, Sitrin MD. Evaluation of stress factors and body weight adjustments currently used to estimate energy expenditure in hospitalized patients. *JPEN J Parenter Enteral Nutr*. 2002;26(4):231-238.

80. Krenitsky J. Adjusted body weight, pro: Evidence to support the use of adjusted body weight in calculating calorie requirements. *Nutr Clin Pract*. 2005;20(4):468-473.

81. McClave SA, Taylor BE, Martindale RG, et al. Guidelines for the provision and assessment of nutrition support therapy in the adult critically ill patient: Society of Critical Care Medicine (SCCM) and American Society for Parenteral and Enteral Nutrition (A.S.P.E.N.). *JPEN J Parenter Enteral Nutr*. 2016;40(2):159-211.

82. Andrews AM, Pruziner AL. Guidelines for using adjusted versus unadjusted body weights when conducting clinical evaluations and making clinical recommendations. *J Acad Nutr Diet*. 2017;117(7):1011-1015.

83. Osterkamp LK. Perspective on assessment of human body proportions of relevance to amputees. *J Am Diet Assoc*. 1995;95(2):215-218.

84. Mozumdar A, Roy SK. Method for estimating body weight in persons with lower-limb amputation and its implication for their nutritonal assessment. *Am J Clin Nutr*. 2004;80(4):868-875.

85. Gunal A. How to determine 'dry weight'? *Kidney Int Suppl*. 2013;3(4):377-379.

86. Frankenfiled DC, Rowe WA, Cooney RN, Smith JS, Becker D. Limits of body mass index to detect obesity and predict body composition. *Nutrition*. 2001;17(1):26-30.

87. Flegal KM, Kit BK, Orpana H, Graubard BI. Association of all-cause mortality with overweight and obesity using standard body mass index categories. *JAMA*. 2013;309(1):71-82.

88. Zin T, Yusuff ASM, Myint T, Naing DKS, Htay K, Wynn AA. Body fat percentage, BMI and skinfold thickness among medical students in Sabah, Malaysia. *South East Asia J Public Health*. 2014;4(1):45-40.

89. Jensen TG, Dudrick SJ, Johnston DA. A comparison of triceps skinfold and upper arm circumference measurements taken in standard and supine positions. *JPEN J Parenter Enteral Nutr*. 1981;5(6):519-521.

90. Burden ST, Stoppard E, Shaffer J, Makin A, Todd C. Can we use mid upper arm anthropmetry to detect malnutrition in medical inpatients? A validation study. *J Hum Nutr Diet*. 2005;18(4):287-294.

91. Zuchinali P, Souza GC, Alves FD, et al. Triceps skinfold as a prognostic predictor in outpatient heart failure. *Arq Bras Cardiol*. 2013;101(5):434-441.

92. University of Colorado Denver. Waist circumference measurements in clinical research. http://www.ucdenver.edu/research/CCTSI/programs-services/ctrc/Nutrition/Documents/Waist%20Circumference%20Info%20for%20Web.pdf. Accessed March 14, 2017.

93. Jeyakumar A, Ghugre P, Gadhave S. Mid-upper-arm circumference (MUAC) as a simple measure to assess the nutritional status of adolescent girls as compared with BMI. *ICAN: Infant Child Adol Nutr*. 2013;5(1):22-25.

94. Cattermole GN, Graham CA, Rainer TH. Mid-arm circumference can be used to estimate weight of adult and adolescent patients. *Emerg Med J*. 2016;0:1-6.

95. Sultana T, Karim N, Ahmed T, Hossain I. Assessment of under nutrition of Bangladeshi adults using anthropometry: can body mass index be replaced by mid-upper-arm-circumference? *PLoS One*. 2015;10(4):1-8.

96. Powell NJ, Collier B. Nutrition and the open abdomen. *Nutr Clin Pract*. 2012;27(4):499-506.

97. Mei Z, Grummer-Strawn LM, de Onis M, Yip R. The development of a MUAC-for-height reference, including a comparison to other nutritional status screening indicators. *Bull World Health Organ*. 1997;75(4):333-341.

98. Powell-Tuck J, Hennessy EM. A comparison of mid upper arm circumference, body mass index and weight loss as indices of undernutrition in acutely hospitalized patients. *Clin Nutr*. 2003;22(3):307-312.

99. Tang AM, Dong K, Deitchler M, et al. Use of cutoffs for mid-upper arm circumference (MUAC) as indicator or predictor of nutritional and health-related outcomes in adolescents and adults: a systematic review. *Food and Nutrition Technical Assistance III Project (FANTA)*. 2013;FHI 360/FANTA.

100. Hymers R. The use of mid upper arm circumference in the nutritional assessment of the critically ill patient. Scottish Intensive Care Society Web site. Scottish Intensive Care Society. http://www.scottishintensivecare.org.uk/uploads/2014-05-28-23-52-56-TheuseofMidUpperArmCircum-59986.pdf. Updated 2009. Accessed March 10, 2017.

101. Tartari RF, Ulbrich-Kulczynski JM, Filho AF. Measurement of mid-arm muscle circumference and prognosis in stage IV non-small cell lung cancer patients. *Oncol Lett*. 2013;5(3):1063-1067.

102. Wang J, Thornton JC, Bari S, et al. Comparisons of waist circumferences measured at 4 sites. *Am J Clin Nutr*. 2003;77(2):379-384.

103. de Koning L, Merchant AT, Pogue J, Anand SS. Waist circumference and waist-to-hip ratio as predictors of cardiovascular events: meta-regression analysis of prospective studies. *Eur Heart J*. 2007;28(7):850-856.

104. Janssen I, Katzmarzyk PT, Ross R. Waist circumference and not body mass index explains obesity-related health risk. *Am J Clin Nutr*. 2004;79(3):379-384.

105. Vazquez G, Duval S, Jacobs Jr. DR, Silventoinen K. Comparison of body mass index, waist circumference, and waist/hip ratio in predicting incident diabetes: a meta-analysis. *Epidemiol Rev*. 2007;29:115-128.

106. Ma W, Yang C, Shih S, et al. Measurement of waist circumference: midabdominal or iliac crest? *Diabetes Care*. 2013;36(6):1660-1666.

107. Mason C, Katzmarzyk PT. Variability in waist circumference measurements according to anatomic measurement site. *Obesity (Silver Spring)*. 2009;17(9):1789-1795.

108. World Health Organization Expert Consultation. Waist circumference and waist-hip ratio. *Report of a WHO Expert Consultation*. http://www.who.int/nutrition/publications/obesity/WHO_report_waistcircumference_and_waisthip_ratio/en/ December,2008. Accessed October 29, 2017.

109. National Institutes of Health (NIH). According to waist circumference. Guidelines on Overweight and Obesity: Electronic Textbook Web site. https://www.nhlbi.nih.gov/health-pro/guidelines/current/obesity-guidelines/e_textbook/txgd/4142.htm Accessed March 14, 2017.

110. Cerhan JR, Moore SC, Jacobs EJ, et al. A pooled analysis of waist circumference and mortality in 650,000 adults. *Mayo Clin Proc*. 2014;89(3):335-345.

111. Britton KA, Massaro JM, Murabito JM, Kreger BE, Hoffmann U, Fox CS. Body fat distribution, incident cardiovascular disease, cancer, and all-cause mortality. *J Am Coll Cardiol*. 2013;62(10):921-925.

112. Price GM, Uauy R, Breeze E, Bulpitt CJ, Fletcher AE. Weight, shape, and mortality risk in older persons: Elevated waist-hip ratio, not high body mass index, is associated with a greater risk of death. *Am J Clin Nutr*. 2006;84(2):449-460.

113. Lear SA, James PT, Ko GT, Kumanyika S. Appropriateness of waist circumference and waist-to-hip ratio cutoffs for different ethnic groups. *Eur J Clin Nutr*. 2010;64:42-61.

114. Silver HJ, Welch EB, Avison MJ, Niswender KD. Imaging body composition in obesity and weight loss: challenges and opportunities. *Diabetes Metab Syndr Obes*. 2010;3:337-347.

115. Andreoli A, Scalzo G, Masala S, Tarantino U, Guglielmi G. Body composition assessment by dual-energy X-ray absorptiometry (DXA). *Radiol Med*. 2009;114:286-300.

116. Ross R, Goodpaster B, Kelley D, Boada F. Magnetic resonance imaging in human body composition research from quantitative to qualitative tissue measurement. *Ann N Y Acad Sci*. 2000;904:12-17.

117. Lee Y, Kwon O, Shin CS, Lee SM. Use of bioelectrical impedance analysis for the assessment of nutritional status in critically ill patients. *Clin Nutr Res*. 2015;4(1):32-40.

118. Kyle UG, Boseaus I, De Lorenzo AD, et al. Bioelectrical impedance analysis - part I: Review of principles and methods. Clin Nutr. 2004;23(5):1225-1243.

119. Kyle UG, Boseaus I, De Lorenzo AD, et al. Bioelectrical impedance analysis - part II: Utilization in clinical practice. *Clin Nutr*. 2004;23(5):1430-1453.

120. Walter-Kroker A, Kroker A, Mattiucci-Guehlke M, Glaab T. A practical guide to bioeletrical impedance analysis using the example of chronic obstructive pulmonary disease. *Nutr J*. 2011;10(35):1-8.

121. Savalle M, Gillaizeau F, Maruani G, et al. Assessment of body cell mass at bedside in critically ill patients. *Am J Physiol Endocrinol Metab*. 2012;303:E389-E396.

122. Chahar PS. Comparison of skinfold thickness measurement and bioelectrical impedance method for assessment of body fat. *World Appl Sci J*. 2013;28(8):1065-1069.

123. Andreoli A, Garaci F, Cafarelli FP, Guglielmi G. Body composition in clinical practice. *Eur J Radiol*. 2016;85(8):1461-1468.

124. Litchford M. Putting the nutrition focused physical assessment into practice in long-term care settings. *Ann Longterm Care*. 2013;21(11):38-41.

125. Radler DR, Lister T. Nutrient deficiencies associated with nutrition-focused physical findings of the oral cavity. *Nutr Clin Pract*. 2013;28(6):710-721.

126. Mordarski B. Nutrition-focused physical exam hands-on training workshop. *J Acad Nutr Diet*. 2016;116(5):868-869.

127. Fischer M, JeVenn A, Hipskind P. Evaluation of muscle and fat loss as diagnostic criteria for malnutrition. *Nutr Clin Pract*. 2015;30(2):239-248.

128. Esper DH. Utilization of nutrition-focused physical assessment in identifying micronutrient deficiencies. *Nutr Clin Pract*. 2015;30(2):194-202.

129. Russell MK. Functional assessment of nutrition status. *Nutr Clin Pract*. 2015;30(2):211-218.

130. Norman K, Stobäus N, Gonzalez MC, Schulzke J, Pirlich M. Hand grip strength: outcome predictor and marker of nutritional status. *Clin Nutr*. 2011;30(2):135-142.

131. Bohannon RW. Muscle strength: Clinical and prognostic value of hand-grip dynamometry. *Curr Opin Clin Nutr Metab Care*. 2015;18(5):465-470.

132. Wang AY, Sea MM, Ho ZS, Lui S, Li PK, Woo J. Evaluation of handgrip strength as a nutritional marker and prognostic indicator in peritoneal dialysis patients. *Am J Clin Nutr*. 2005;81(1):79-86.

133. Hillman TE, Nunes QM, Hornby ST, et al. A practical posture for hand grip dynamometry in the clinical setting. *Clin Nutr*. 2005;24(2):224-228.

134. Matos LC, Tavares MM, Amaral TF. Handgrip strength as a hospital admission nutritional risk screening method. *Eur J Clin Nutr*. 2007;61(9):1128-1135.

135. Jakobsen LH, Rask IK, Kondrup J. Validation of handgrip strength and endurance as a measure of physical function and quality of life in healthy subjects and patients. *Nutrition*. 2010;25(5):542-550.

136. Tufts University Nutrition Collaborative, Center for Drug Abuse and AIDS Research. Hand grip strength protocol. http://cdaar.tufts.edu/protocols/Handgrip.pdf. Updated September 2003. Accessed October 29, 2017.

137. Mendes J, Azevedo A, Amaral TF. Handgrip strength at admission and time to discharge in medical and surgical inpatients. *JPEN J Parenter Enteral Nutr*. 2014;38(4):481-488.

138. Flood A, Chung A, Parker H, Kearns V, O'Sullivan TA. The use of hand grip strength as a predictor of nutrition status in hospital patients. *Clin Nutr*. 2014;33(1):106-114.

139. Garcia MF, Meireles MS, Führ LM, Donini AB, Wazlawik E. Relationship between hand grip strength and nutritional assessment methods used of hospitalized patients. *Rev Nutr*. 2013;26(1):49-57.

140. Norman K, Stobäus N, Smoliner C, et al. Determinants of hand grip strength, knee extension strength and functional status in cancer patients. *Clin Nutr*. 2010;29(5):586-591.

141. Luna-Heredia E, Martín-Peña G, Ruiz-Galiana J. Handgrip dynamometry in healthy adults. *Clin Nutr*. 2005;24:250-258.

142. Jonnalagadda SS, Mitchell DC, Smiciklas-Wright H, et al. Accuracy of energy intake data estimated by a multiple-pass, 24-hour dietary recall technique. *J Am Diet Assoc*. 2000;100(3):303-308.

143. Kubena KS. Accuracy in dietary assessment: on the road to good science. *J Am Diet Assoc*. 2000;100(7):775-776.

144. Timon CM, van den Barg R, Blain RJ, et al. A review of the design and validation of web- and computer-based 24-h dietary recall tools. *Nutr Res Rev*. 2016;29(2):260-280.

145. Kirkpatrick SI, Collins CE. Assessment of nutrient intakes: introduction to the special issue. *Nutrients*. 2016;8(4):184-187.

146. Subar AF, Freedman LS, Tooze JA, et al. Addressing current criticism regarding the value of self-report dietary data. *J Nutr*. 2015;145(12):2639-2645.

147. Moshfegh AJ, Rhodes DG, Baer DJ, et al. The US Department of Agriculture automated multiple-pass method reduces bias in the collection of energy intakes. *Am J Clin Nutr*. 2008;88(2):324-332.

148. Blanton CA, Moshfegh AJ, Baer DJ, Kretsch MJ. The USDA automated multiple-pass method accurately estiamtes group total energy and nutrient intake. *J Nutr*. 2006;136(10):2594-2599.

149. Conway JM, Ingwersen LA, Moshfegh AJ. Accuracy of dietary recall using the USDA five-step multiple-pass method in men: an observational validation study. *J Am Diet Assoc*. 2004;104(4):595-603.

150. Chambers EI, McGuire B, Godwin S, McDowell M, Vecchio F. Quantifying portion sizes for selected snack foods and beverages in 24-hour dietary recalls. *Nutrition Research*. 2000;20(3):315-326.

151. Subar AF. Developing dietary assessment tools. *J Am Diet Assoc*. 2004;104(5):769-770.

152. National Cancer Institute. Usual dietary intakes: The NCI method. Epidemiology and Genomics Research Program Web site. https://epi.grants.cancer.gov/diet/usualintakes/method.html Updated July 17, 2015. Accessed October 29, 2017.

153. Sharp DB, Allman-Farinelli M. Feasibility and validity of mobile phones to assess dietary intake. *Nutrition*. 2014;30(11-12):1257-1266.

154. Bloomfield R, Steel E, MacLennan G, Noble DW. Accuracy of weight and height estimation in an intensive care unit: implications for clinical practice and research. *Crit Care Med*. 2006;34(8):2153-2157.

155. Heyland DK, Dhaliwal R, Jiang X, Day AG. Identifying critically ill patients who benefit the most from nutrition therapy: the

development and initial validation of a novel risk assessment tool. *Crit Care*. 2011;15(6):R268.

156. Rosa M, Heyland DK, Fernandes D, Rabito EL, Oliveira ML, Marcadenti A. Translation and adaptation of the NUTRIC score to identify critically ill patients who benefit the most from nutrition therapy. *Clin Nutr ESPEN*. 2016;14:31-36.

157. Kalaiselvan MS, Renuka MK, Arunkumar AS. Use of nutrition risk in critically ill (NUTRIC) score to assess nutritional risk in mechanically ventilated patients: a prospective observational study. *Indian J Crit Care Med*. 2017;21(5):253-256.

158. Rahman A, Hasan RM, Agarwala R, Martin C, Day AG, Heyland DK. Identifying critically-ill patients who will benefit most from nutritional therapy: further validation of the "modified NUTRIC" nutritional risk assessment tool. *Clin Nutr*. 2016;35(1):158-162.

Chapter 2

Biochemical Assessment

Katelyn Castro
Kelly Kane

Chapter Outline

Core Concepts
Introduction
Specimen Types
Assay Types
Routine Medical Laboratory Tests

CORE CONCEPTS

1. Biochemical assessment is an important component of the nutrition care process, which must be interpreted with other methods (i.e., physical findings, patient history, anthropometrics) for accuracy.

2. Nutrient concentrations in plasma do not reflect the amount of the substance stored in body pools and may be influenced by disease, inflammation, and recent dietary intake.

3. Refeeding syndrome can result in malnourished patients when carbohydrate feedings stimulate insulin, resulting in the intracellular shift of potassium, phosphorus, and magnesium, and fluid retention.

4. Fluid, electrolyte, and acid–base imbalances can lead to serious complications, ranging from metabolic and gastrointestinal problems to cardiovascular, respiratory, and neurological concerns, each requiring careful evaluation, monitoring, and treatment.

5. Visceral proteins can be altered by acute and chronic metabolic stress, making them more accurate indicators of inflammation than indicators of nutritional status.

6. Lipid profile results can be used to assess risk of cardiovascular (elevated low-density lipoprotein, decreased high-density/low-density lipoprotein ratio) and metabolic (elevated triglycerides) disorders, as well as risk of malnutrition (decreased cholesterol) in patients.

7. Deficiencies in iron, vitamin B_{12}, and folate, and toxicities of copper and zinc can all compromise red blood cell functioning and contribute to anemia.

Learning Objectives

1. Describe the role of biochemical assessment in the implementation of the nutrition care process.
2. Identify the causes and treatments of serum electrolyte and fluid imbalances.
3. State the metabolic changes that occur during refeeding syndrome.
4. Compare the causes and treatments of different metabolic and respiratory acid–base imbalances.
5. Specify two biomarkers used to assess each of the following: endocrine, renal, liver, and cardiovascular functioning.
6. Name two protein biomarkers used to assess nutritional status and the advantages and disadvantages of them.
7. Justify the need for careful interpretation of protein markers for malnutrition during inflammation.
8. Identify components of a hematological test and the role of each in diagnosis of anemias.

Introduction

Biochemical assessment is an essential component of nutrition assessment, the first step in implementing the Nutrition Care Process (NCP) in clinical practice. Laboratory tests of patients' blood, urine, feces, and tissue samples are important indicators of nutritional status and organ function. Because disease states, subsequent treatments, and hydration status can have a significant impact on biochemical indices, evaluation of laboratory values is critical in patients with both acute and chronic diseases. While patients with acute illness or injury may experience dramatic changes in laboratory results, patients with chronic illness may develop abnormal lab results more slowly. Comparing patients' laboratory results to reference values and interpreting discrepancies in the context of patients' clinical symptoms and medical history allows clinicians to prevent or diagnose diseases and develop appropriate nutrition interventions. Laboratory values are necessary to monitor effectiveness of medical treatment, evaluate NCP interventions, and adjust the plan of care appropriately. Unlike the other components of nutrition assessment, biochemical assessment is a carefully controlled process and considers only objective data used in the NCP. However, no single laboratory test or panel can be used to make diagnosis of nutritional status and needs.

> **CORE CONCEPT 1**
>
> Biochemical assessment is an important component of the nutrition care process, which must be interpreted with other methods (i.e., physical findings, patient history, anthropometrics) for accuracy.

Specimen Types

There are several types of specimens used for nutrient and nutrient-related analyses. Although the ideal specimens reflect the total body content of the nutrient being assessed, the optimal specimen is not always readily available. The most common specimens utilized for analysis in medical nutrition therapy include the following blood components:

- **Whole blood**: Contains red blood cells (RBCs), white blood cells (WBCs), and platelets suspended in plasma; collected with an anticoagulant when the entire content of the blood is evaluated and none of the elements are removed (**Figure 2.1**)
- **Serum**: Fluid remaining in blood after blood has been clotted and centrifuged to remove the clot and blood cells
- **Plasma**: Component of blood composed of water, blood proteins, organic electrolytes, and clotting factors
- **Blood cells**: Measurement of cellular components, separated from anticoagulated whole blood

In addition to blood, other specimens can also be used for analysis:

- **Urine**: Contains a concentrate of excreted metabolites from random samples or timed collection
- **Feces**: Determines composition of gut flora and presence or absence of adequate nutrient absorption, from random samples or timed collection
- **Hair and nails**: Stable, easy to collect, and noninvasive media which determines exposure to toxic metals and is a helpful indicator of levels of trace elements (zinc, copper, chromium, and manganese)
- **Saliva**: Noninvasive medium with high turnover used to evaluate functional adrenal stress and hormone levels
- **Breath tests**: Performed on the air generated from exhalation; less common and less invasive tool to assess nutrient metabolism, use, and malabsorption, particularly of sugars

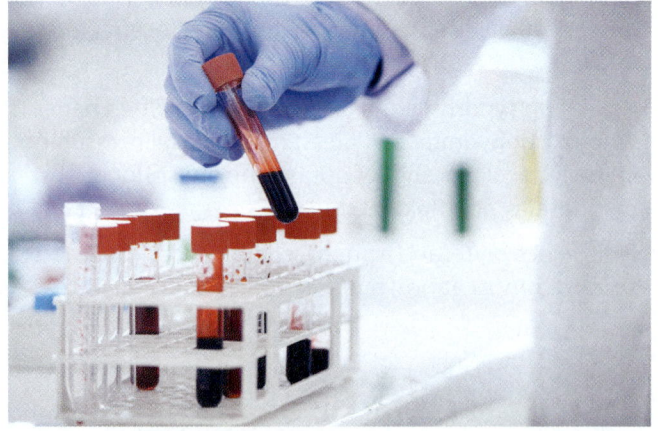

FIGURE 2.1 Example of Specimens Collected in Laboratory for Biochemical Assessment
© PeopleImages/Getty Images.

CASE STUDY INTRODUCTION

Adam is a 68-year-old male admitted to the hospital with a 1-month history of nausea, vomiting, and diarrhea resulting in weight loss and fatigue. He presents tachycardic with abdominal pain, fever, and chills. Adam is a retired engineer and lives at home with his wife.

Anthropometric Data:
Height: 165 cm (65")
Weight: 75 kg (165 lbs)
BMI: 27.5 kg/m²
Weight History
Usual body weight: 82 kg (180 lbs) 1 year ago

Biochemical Data:

Sodium 129 (135-145 mEq/L)
Potassium 3.2 (3.6-5.0 mEq/L)
Chloride 90 (98-110 mEq/L)
Carbon dioxide 43 (20-30 mEq/L)
Blood urea nitrogen 30 (6-24 mg/dL)
Creatinine 0.5 (0.4-1.3 mg/dL)
Glucose 166 (70-139 mg/dL)
Magnesium 1.3 (1.3-2.1 mg/dL)
Calcium 8.0 (8.5-10.5 mEq/L)
Phosphorus 2.7 (2.7-4.5 mg/dL)
Serum osmolality 250 (275-295 mOsm/kg)
Albumin 2.6 (3.5-5.0 g/dL)

Total cholesterol 233 (Desirable <200 mg/dL)
Low-density lipoprotein 41 (Desirable <100 mg/dL)
High-density lipoprotein 52 (Desirable ≥40 mg/dL)
Triglycerides 40 (Desirable <150 mg/dL)
Hemoglobin 11.1 (13.5-17.5 mg/dL)
Hematocrit 36.4 (42%-52%)
White blood cells 6×10^9 ($5\text{-}10 \times 10^9$/L)
Mean corpuscular volume 89 (80-99 fL)
Mean corpuscular hemoglobin concentration 32 (32-36 g/dL)
Red cell distribution width 50 (39-36 fL)

Clinical Data:
Past Medical History: Hypertension, hypercholesterolemia, hypertriglyceridemia, gastroesophageal reflux disease
Medications: Lipitor, Captopril, aspirin, imodium, omeprazole
Vital Signs: Blood pressure 110/50 mm Hg, Temperature 99.6° F, Heart rate 115 beats/min, tachycardic
Nutrition-focused Physical Exam: Patient noted to be pale with dry skin and poor skin turgor. Temporal muscles mildly wasted. Upper arm and lower extremity fat loss evident. Abdomen appears slightly distended. Oral exam notable for a dry tongue and good dentition. No wounds observed and no edema noted. No shortness of breath evident.

Dietary Data:
Dietary History: Normal appetite. Adam reveals he has avoided high-fat foods for the past year, and limits his sodium intake. He reports that he has had minimal intake for 3 to 4 days prior to admission.
Usual Diet Recall:
Breakfast: 8 oz orange juice, hard-boiled egg, ½ bagel with 2 oz cream cheese
Lunch: Sandwich with 3-4 oz turkey or ham and mustard on white bread, canned soup, 1 oz potato chips, 1% milk, apple
Dinner: 4 oz baked chicken, 2/3 cup rice, ½ cup cooked green beans
Diet Prescription: NPO (nil per os or nothing by mouth)

Questions

1. Describe the possible pathophysiologic etiology associated with Adam's electrolyte abnormalities.
2. What are Adam's nutritional risk factors?
3. What additional information and labs would you like to obtain?
4. What are your priorities for this patient?

Assay Types

Two types of laboratory assays are available to measure nutrient levels in specimens. A **static assay** is used to measure the actual level of a nutrient in the specimen. This type of assay is specific to the nutrient of interest. Unfortunately the concentration of the nutrient within the specimen does not always reflect its amount stored in body pools and tissues. Serum levels may be influenced by the status of their protein carriers, which may be altered by inflammation. The amount of nutrient found in serum, plasma, or another fluid or tissue is influenced by recent dietary intake in static assays. To address this limitation, overnight (8-12 hour) fasting is recommended when collecting some specimens.[1] Examples of static assays include serum iron and white blood cell ascorbic acid.

In contrast, a **functional assay** measures the specific biochemical or physiological functioning of a nutrient, rather than just the quantity of the nutrient. Usually a functional assay is sensitive for a nutrient at its functional site. Functional assays are not always specific for one nutrient of interest because many physiological and biochemical functions rely on several biological factors beyond the specific nutrient. One example of a functional assay is serum ferritin, which represents the functioning of iron present in the cellular storage pool.[2]

> ### CORE CONCEPT 2
> Nutrient concentrations in plasma do not reflect the amount of the substance stored in body pools and may be influenced by disease, inflammation, and recent dietary intake.

> ### PRACTICE POINT
> Biochemical assessment values in patients with hemodilution and hemoconcentration must be cautiously interpreted and treated.

Decreased red blood cell concentrations and increased plasma levels (**hemodilution**) and increased red blood cell concentrations and decreased plasma levels (**hemoconcentration**) can result from a gain or loss of plasma volume, respectively. As with abnormalities in fluid volume, an imbalance of plasma volume can contribute to an imbalance in **electrolytes**, or substances that dissolve into ions in solution, and lead to poor interpretation of biochemical assessment tests. For instance, during pregnancy, an increase in total cell and plasma volume can cause hemodilution and create artificial anemia also known as "physiologic anemia of pregnancy." Another example may occur when a patient has extreme edema. Hemodilution may decrease serum sodium levels, providing a false hyponatremia, requiring different treatment than a patient with true hyponatremia.

Routine Medical Laboratory Tests

Most laboratory tests can be ordered as a panel, a grouping of tests, or as individual tests. The most commonly ordered groups of tests include the **basic metabolic panel** (glucose, sodium, potassium, carbon dioxide, chloride, blood urea nitrogen [BUN], and creatinine) and **comprehensive metabolic panel** (all of the above measures plus albumin, total protein, alkaline phosphatase, alanine transaminase, aspartate transaminase, and bilirubin). A **complete blood count** (CBC) provides a count of the cells in the blood and description of red blood cells, while a **differential count** is a CBC for white blood cells. Stool tests can also be performed to assess the presence of blood, pathogens, and gut flora, especially among adults older than 50 years and individuals with unexplained anemia. Stool culture testing may also be ordered for patients with prolonged diarrhea, suspected food-borne illness, chronic gastrointestinal (GI) symptoms, or unexplained weight loss. Several chemical tests in a urinalysis are also commonly performed, including specific gravity, pH, protein, glucose, ketones, blood, and bilirubin. A urine specific gravity test compares the density of urine to the density of water, which can help to determine how efficiently kidneys can dilute urine.

Laboratory values must be used with other assessment data, such as clinical history and physical examination, to confirm diagnosis or monitor effectiveness of treatment. Specific biomarkers used to estimate nutrition availability in biological fluids and tissues often detect deficiencies before clinical or anthropometric changes are recognized. Understanding how to interpret biomarkers and laboratory values for nutrition diagnoses is a critical part of the NCP to provide the most effective and appropriate care for patients. This chapter will focus on interpreting biochemical laboratory values of electrolytes, glucose measures, proteins, enzymes, lipids, hematological tests, and iron studies, and their significance in identifying fluid and electrolyte imbalances, organ dysfunction, and nutritional abnormalities in clinical practice.

> ### PRACTICE POINT
> Interpreting changes in laboratory value trends has more clinical significance than simply comparing laboratory values within the established absolute reference ranges.

Fluid and Electrolytes

Bodily fluids can vary greatly in the amount of dissolved substances and their distribution in the body. To maintain an environment necessary for normal cell functioning, different regulatory mechanisms work simultaneously to achieve appropriate electrolyte and fluid balance, regardless of changes in intake. Cells also need acid–base homeostasis because hydrogen ion concentration plays an important role in nearly all biochemical reactions. The presence of both acute injury and chronic illness can alter fluid and electrolyte levels and requirements. Evaluation and treatment of fluids, electrolytes, and acid–base imbalance is critical in practice because disruption in normal levels of these substances can have a significant physiological impact on many organ systems.

Fluid Distribution

Water constitutes approximately 50% to 60% of body weight, with a higher percentage among infants and children and a lower percentage among women, the elderly, and obese individuals. Those with more body fat have proportionally less water because adipose tissue contains less water than lean body mass. As a consequence, total body water is a function of weight, age, sex, and lean body mass. Total body water is divided into three main compartments: intracellular fluid (ICF), extracellular fluid (ECF), and transcellular fluid compartments. Approximately two-thirds of the total body water is found within cells (ICF) and most of the remaining one-third is found outside cells. Only about 1% of total body water accounts for transcellular fluid, which includes specialized fluids such as cerebrospinal fluid, the aqueous of the eye, and secretions of the GI tract. Table 2.1 provides the ionic composition of intracellular and extracellular fluid.

ECF is the most clinically important fluid compartment because it contains interstitial fluids (surrounding cells) and intravascular fluid (within blood). The distribution of water between each fluid compartment (**Figure 2.2**) is primarily determined by **osmotic pressure**, defined as the pressure needed to maintain equilibrium with no net movement of solvent. Each compartment has one major active solute that determines its osmotic pressure and holds water within the compartment. Sodium is the dominant extracellular osmole, potassium is the main intracellular osmole, and plasma proteins are the primary substances in intravascular space. Under normal conditions, the sodium-potassium-adenosine triphosphate (Na^+-K^+-ATPase) pumps maintain the solute compositions of ECF and ICF and play an important role in fluid balance. Serum osmolality is used to express osmotic pressure by calculating the number of osmoles acting to hold fluid within the ECF. Serum osmolality (in mOsm/kg) can be calculated using the following equation:

$$S_{osm} = (2 \times \text{Sodium mEq/L}) + (\text{Glucose mg/dL})/18 + (\text{BUN mg/dL})/2.8$$

Sample Calculation: Sodium 135 mEq/L, Glucose 105 mg/dL, BUN 33 mg/dL

$$S_{osm} = (2 \times 135) + 105/18 + 33/2.8$$
$$S_{osm} = 270 + 5.8 + 11.8$$
$$S_{osm} = 288 \text{ mOsm/kg}$$

Normal serum osmolality ranges from 275 to 295 mOsm/kg.[3] Osmolalities of ECF and ICF are assumed

TABLE 2.1 IONIC COMPOSITION OF INTRACELLULAR AND EXTRACELLULAR FLUID

Electrolytes	Extracellular* fluid concentration meq/L	Intracellular† fluid concentration meq/L
Cations		
Sodium (Na^+)	140	13
Potassium (K^+)	5	140
Calcium (Ca^{2+})	5	Minimal
Magnesium (Mg^{2+})	2	7
Total	151	160
Anions		
Chloride (Cl^-)	104	3
Bicarbonate (HCO_3^-)	24	10
Sulfate (SO_4^{2-})	1	—
Phosphate (HPO_4^{2-})	2	107
Proteins	15	40
Organic anions	5	—
Total	151	160

*Values are for plasma. Interstitial fluid concentration varies slightly (about 4%).
†Values are for cell water in muscle.
Modified from Shils ME, Shike M, Ross AC, et al., eds. *Modern Nutrition in Health and Disease*. 10th ed. Philadelphia: Lippincott Williams & Wilkins; 2005:149–193.

to be equal (**isotonic**) under normal conditions. When cells are exposed to solutions that have an osmolality greater than that of blood (**hypertonic**), fluids move out of cells in an attempt to establish equilibrium and results in cellular dehydration. In contrast, when cells are exposed to solutions with osmolality less than that of blood (**hypotonic**) fluid moves into cells and causes cell swelling. **Figure 2.3** illustrates the red blood cell responses to solutions of varying tonicities.

To better understand the mechanisms of water distribution to ECF and ICF, consider the composition of commonly used intravenous (IV) fluids administered in practice. For example, when 1,000 mL of 5% dextrose (hypotonic, solute-free water) is infused, the dextrose is metabolized and the free water distributes evenly

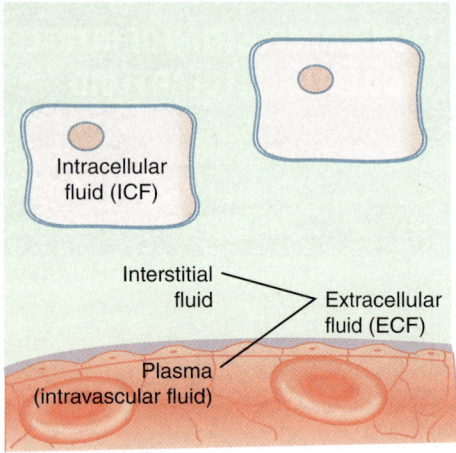

FIGURE 2.2 Intracellular Fluid is Found Within Cells Extracellular fluid includes interstitial fluid and intravasular fluid and is found outside of cells.

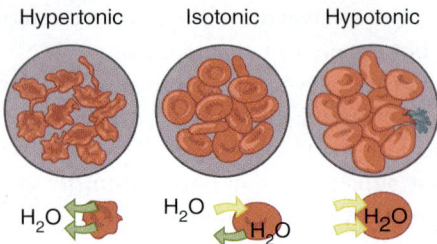

FIGURE 2.3 Fluid Distribution Based on Tonicity: Red blood Cells in Hypertonic, Isotonic, and Hypotonic Solution

across all compartments. That is, two-thirds (667 mL) of the solution goes to the ICF, where water enters the cell, and approximately one-third (333 mL) goes to the ECF. Alternatively, if 1,000 mL of 0.9% sodium chloride (normal saline) is administered, the water is distributed completely to the ECF because sodium is found mainly in the ECF. Approximately 25% (250 mL) will go to intravascular space and 75% (750 mL) will go to interstitial space. In contrast, administration of 3% sodium chloride (hypertonic saline) causes water to move out of cells and into ECF until osmotic equilibrium is reached. The addition of sodium chloride to ECF and the loss of water to ICF eventually would lead to increased osmolalities of both compartments, with the change in volume proportional to the degree of increase in ECF osmolality. **Table 2.2** outlines the composition of commonly used intravenous fluids.

While osmotic pressure determines the distribution of fluid between ECF and ICF, plasma oncotic and hydrostatic pressures influence the movement of fluid between the plasma and interstitial fluid. Under normal conditions these compartments are maintained in a steady state and the pressures are generally balanced, despite large fluid exchanges between compartments.

When disruption in oncotic and/or hydrostatic pressure favors fluid movement from intravascular to interstitial fluid, **third spacing** occurs. Third spacing is the accumulation of fluid in the interstices (edema) or in the potential fluid spaces (effusion) between body cavities. An example of edema can be seen in **Figure 2.4**. Third spacing is common during critical illness when capillary permeability increases, causing albumin to leak into interstitial space leading to a decrease in plasma oncotic pressure. Although over a period of days fluid will be absorbed back into extracellular compartments, the acute drop in blood volume can cause severe volume depletion so fluid intake and output should be monitored carefully.

Fluid and Electrolyte Disorders

Disorders in fluid and electrolyte balance can be classified by disturbances of volume, concentration, or

TABLE 2.2 COMPOSITION OF COMMONLY USED INTRAVENOUS FLUIDS

Commonly Used Intravenous Solutions	Dextrose (g/L)	Sodium (mEq/L)	Tonicity	Free Water
D5W (5% Dextrose)	50	0	Hypotonic	1,000 mL
0.45% NaCl (1/2 Normal Saline)	0	77	Hypotonic	500 mL
0.9% NaCl (Normal Saline)	0	154	Isotonic	0 mL
3% NaCl (hypertonic saline)	0	513	Hypertonic	Negative (Loss of free water)

Modified from Langley, G., & Tajchman, S. (2012). A.S.P.E.N. Adult Nutrition Support Core Curriculum Chapter 7: Fluids, Electrolytes, and Acid-Base Disorders (2nd ed., p.100). Washington DC: American Society for Parenteral & Enteral Nutrition.

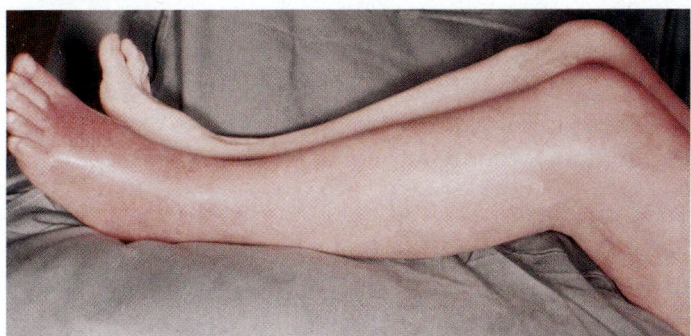

FIGURE 2.4 Localized Edema

composition, which often occur concurrently in clinical practice. Volume overload (**hypervolemia**) and volume depletion (**hypovolemia**) occur when there is a gain or loss in fluid (both water and solute) that alters extracellular fluid volume. The loss of extracellular fluid volume described in circumstances of volume depletion can result from vomiting, diarrhea, diuresis, or GI hemorrhage. Disorders of fluid balance can occur simultaneously with imbalance of electrolytes including sodium, potassium, magnesium, calcium, phosphate, chloride, bicarbonate, or hydrogen ions. For example, a change in sodium concentration leading to a change in plasma osmolality contributes to gain or loss of water (overhydration or dehydration, respectively). Excessive losses from the GI tract and abnormalities in kidney function are often found to be the primary contributors to electrolyte imbalances. Understanding the composition of specific body fluids can be helpful in the management of fluid and electrolyte disorders because many causes of water loss also lead to significant losses of electrolytes.

Management of Electrolyte Disorders

Safe and effective treatment of electrolyte imbalance requires careful assessment of the etiology of the electrolyte imbalance. If laboratory results are inconsistent with the patient's clinical condition, no treatment should be considered before validating the accuracy of the specimen sample. This is a critical step to prevent improper treatment of electrolyte values that may be based on errors in sample collection or handling. Only after laboratory results are validated should clinicians develop a treatment plan.

Generally, when electrolyte levels are above the normal range, removal of exogenous sources or facilitation of elimination of electrolyte is recommended. The severity of the electrolyte disorder and presence or absence of symptoms will determine the most appropriate treatment approach. Treatment may include removal of electrolyte supplementation from IV fluids or parenteral/enteral nutrition, discontinuing medications that may contribute to electrolyte disorder, and/or inducing renal or GI elimination of the electrolyte(s).

When electrolyte levels are below the normal range, electrolyte replacement through oral or IV replacement is appropriate based on patient-specific factors. Intravenous electrolyte replacement is considered optimal for patients with critically low electrolyte levels who are NPO ("nil per os," meaning nothing by mouth) or who have impaired GI functioning or difficulty swallowing. Patients with impaired renal function should receive conservative electrolyte replacement, unless actively receiving renal replacement therapy. Patients with volume overload should receive volume-restricted electrolyte replacement or oral therapy when possible. Identifying peripheral or central venous access is also important because peripheral administration may limit the volume and rate of administration. Tissue damage and potential harm can result from exceeding these limits in patients with peripheral access.

Because patients often have more than one electrolyte abnormality, all electrolyte values should be reviewed. The presence of concurrent electrolyte abnormalities requires clinicians to consider optimizing and minimizing replacement. For example, optimizing treatment should be considered if a patient has both hypomagnesemia and hypokalemia. Because potassium repletion can rarely occur if magnesium is deficient, magnesium should be corrected before potassium to optimize replacement.[3] Minimizing replacement can occur when patients have conditions, such as hypokalemia and hypophosphatemia, where potassium phosphate can be used to correct both of these imbalances simultaneously. Clinicians should also be aware of product availability and shortages to determine whether conservation or alternate therapy may be required.

Sodium

Sodium (Na^+) is the principal cation in the ECF, with a normal serum concentration of sodium range of 135 to 145 mEq/L. Sodium is the major osmotic determinant regulating volume and water distribution in the body, under the direct influence of the kidneys and central nervous system. Maintaining sodium levels requires a careful balance between sodium and water through the renin-angiotensin-aldosterone system, ECF volume, and renal function. Sodium also assists in acid–base balance; activation of enzyme reactions; nerve impulse conduction; and contraction of myocardial, skeletal, and smooth muscles.

Hyponatremia Hyponatremia, or low serum sodium, is the most common electrolyte disorder seen in medical care facilities, occurring in about 25% of hospitalized patients.[4]

Signs and Symptoms Evaluation of symptoms, rate of onset, and etiology can help clinicians determine the most effective treatment. Most patients with chronic hyponatremia have values in the range of

> ## CASE STUDY REVISITED
>
> Adam requires treatment for his hyponatremia (Na⁺ 129 mEq/L; normal: 135-145 mEq/L). The medical team asks for possible means of correcting his sodium through nutritional modifications of his diet.
>
> ### Questions
> 1. What are the possible causes of Adam's hyponatremia?
> 2. What labs might help you determine its cause?
> 3. How would you recommend his hyponatremia be treated?
> 4. Explain your rationale.

125 to 135 mEq/L and are asymptomatic or have mild symptoms (nausea, malaise, vomiting, and disorientation). Headaches, lethargy, agitation, confusion, and altered mental status are common symptoms for patients with lower sodium levels in the range of 115 to 125 mEq/L. More severe symptoms, including seizures, coma, respiratory distress, and death, are typically present when serum sodium values are less than 115 mEq/L due to the sodium's inability to maintain blood pressure and support nerves and muscles, which are critical for respiratory and cardiac functioning.

By determining the rate of onset of hyponatremia and assessing medical history and patient symptom information, clinicians can more effectively correct the disorder at a rate similar to that at which it was developed. Acute hyponatremia (developing in <48 hours) is more likely to result in cerebral edema, herniation of the brain, and cardiopulmonary arrest. These rapid adaptations to decreased intracellular osmolality can increase risk of developing **osmotic demyelination syndrome (ODS)** or widespread brain demyelination, which can also develop in patients with chronic hyponatremia when sodium correction is too rapid. Regardless of the severity of symptoms associated with hyponatremia, sodium correction rate should not exceed the target range of 5 to 10 mEq/L per day in order to prevent ODS.[5]

Etiology and Treatment After initial identification of hyponatremia, clinicians should assess serum osmolality to determine etiology and appropriate treatment of hyponatremia. Calculated serum osmolality should be compared to measured serum osmolality. Hyponatremia can occur with high plasma osmolality (hypertonicity), normal osmolality (isotonicity), and low plasma osmolality (hypotonicity). *Hypertonic hyponatremia* (>295 mOsm/kg H₂O) is caused by the presence of other osmotically active substances in the ECF, in addition to sodium. This is most commonly caused by severe hyperglycemia with dehydration or retention of hypertonic infusions of mannitol. To estimate the correction of serum sodium due to hyperglycemia, the following equation can be used:

$$\text{Corrected Sodium} = \text{Serum Sodium (mEq/L)} + 0.016\,[\text{Serum Glucose (mg/dL)} - 100]$$

Sample Calculation: Sodium 125 mEq/L, Glucose 350 mg/dL

$$\text{Corrected Sodium} = 125 + 0.016\,[350 - 100]$$
$$\text{Corrected Sodium} = 125 + 4$$
$$\text{Corrected Sodium} = 129 \text{ mEq/L}$$

The constants in this equation (0.016 and 100) reflect that serum sodium concentration falls approximately 1.6 mEq/L for every 100 mg/dL increment in elevated glucose. For a patient with a serum glucose of 350 mg/dL, the corrected sodium would be 129 mEq/L.

Isotonic hyponatremia (within normal serum osmolality values) occurs when there is a smaller fraction of serum that is composed of water, often resulting from excess plasma proteins or lipids. Normally, serum is 93% water, and the remaining 7% is made up of lipid and proteins. Because there is a larger non-aqueous phase occupied by lipids and proteins, and a smaller aqueous component (and sodium is restricted to the aqueous or water component), the resulting value from laboratory analysis of serum for sodium is low. This condition also called pseudohyponatremia may be caused by hyperlipidemia, hyperproteinemia, infusion of hypertonic solutions, or mannitol, resulting in a larger non-aqueous component to the plasma. Pseudohyponatremia does not reflect true hyponatremia because the concentration of sodium in plasma is normal. Once other laboratory values are corrected, sodium levels return to normal. With laboratory analysis advancing, pseudohyponatremia is less frequently observed in practice.[6] For practical purposes, hyponatremia in the presence of normal serum osmolality is usually attributed to pseudohyponatremia.

Hypotonic hyponatremia (<275 mOsm/kg H₂O) is the most common form of hyponatremia. Once this determination is made, a more detailed assessment of volume status must be done. Hypovolemic (lower than normal ECF volume), hypervolemic (higher than normal ECF volume) and euvolemic (normal ECF volume) hyponatremia each require different treatments.

Hypovolemic hypotonic hyponatremia (low volume, low osmolality) occurs when patients lose more sodium in relation to water. Urine osmolality in these patients is usually greater than 450 mOsm/L because excess sodium in relation to water is excreted in the body's attempt to retain fluid. Common signs of hypovolemia include decreased blood pressure, tachycardia, dry tongue, flattened neck veins, sunken eyeballs, increased body temperature, and acute weight loss. Determining the source of fluid loss is critical. Renal losses are identified by a urine sodium >20 mmol/L and are usually caused by diuretic excess, osmosis diuresis, mineralocorticoid deficiency, salt-wasting nephritis, pseudohypoalderonism, bicarbonaturia, renal tubular acidosis, or ketonuria. Extrarenal losses are commonly associated with a urine sodium <20 mmol/L and can be due to vomiting, diarrhea, fistula output, excess sweating, burns, open wounds, or fluid drains.

Isotonic saline is most often the recommended treatment for most patients with this condition to replenish sodium and water and to increase ECF volume. To calculate sodium deficits in patients, the following equation can be used:

$$\text{Sodium Deficit (mEq)} = [\text{Desired Sodium (mEq/L)} - \text{Actual Sodium (mEq/L)}] \times \text{Weight (kg)} \times 0.6$$

Sample Calculation: Desired Sodium: 135 mEq/L, Actual Sodium 129 mEq/L, Weight 70 kg

$$\text{Sodium Deficit (mEq)} = (135 - 129) \times 70 \times 0.6$$

$$\text{Sodium Deficit} = 252 \text{ mEq}$$

A 70-kg patient with hyponatremia (sodium 129 mEq/L), would require a gradual administration of 252 mEq of sodium (sodium deficit) to obtain the desired serum sodium of 135 mEq/L.

The constant in this equation is 0.6 to reflect the fact that approximately 60% of body weight is water. Note that due to variations of body water with age and sex, some formulas will adjust this constant for females, children, and the elderly. This formula can be used to determine the amount of sodium needed to reach appropriate serum sodium levels. With 154 mEq/L of sodium, isotonic or normal saline increases sodium gradually at approximately 1 mEq/L for each liter administered. Clinicians should be cautious not to replenish sodium too quickly because this can lead to fluid shifts in the brain and cause adverse effects of the central nervous system (CNS). If patients are receiving nutrition support, clinicians should consider changes to fluids or sodium content of formulas.

Sodium can be increased by using a formula with higher sodium content, administering sodium chloride tablets, or replacing water flushes with saline solution. For patients receiving parenteral nutrition (PN), changing the formula can increase both fluid and sodium levels. If diuretics are the cause of hypovolemia, clinicians should consider possible medication changes as part of treatment. Potassium supplementation should be considered in estimating sodium deficit because potassium can increase plasma sodium and osmolality in hyponatremic patients. The following equation can be used to calculate this effect:

$$\Delta \text{ Plasma [Sodium]} = [\text{Infusate Sodium} + \text{Infusate Potassium} - \text{Plasma Sodium}]/(\text{Body Weight} \times 0.6 + 1)$$

Sample Calculation: Infusate Sodium 154 mEq, Infusate Potassium 30 mEq,

Plasma Sodium 129 mEq/L, Body Weight 70 kg

$$\Delta \text{ Plasma [Sodium]} = [154 + 30 - 129] / (70 \times 0.6 + 1)$$

$$\Delta \text{ Plasma [Sodium]} = 55 / 43$$

$$\Delta \text{ Plasma [Sodium]} = 1.3$$

For a 70-kg patient with hyponatremia (sodium 129 mEq/L), infusing 1 L of normal saline (containing 154 mEq sodium) and 30 mEq potassium will raise the plasma sodium by 1.3 units (to approximately 130 mEq/L).

Euvolemic hypotonic hyponatremia (normal volume and low osmolality) often occurs in patients with syndrome of inappropriate antidiuretic hormone (SIADH), which causes excessive release of antidiuretic hormone (ADH). These patients have stable sodium intake and output but retain large amounts of water due to excess ADH. SIADH can be caused by brain or CNS malignancies, head trauma, lung malignancies, or pneumonia. Urine osmolality >100 mOsm/L and urine sodium >20 mEq/L indicate that kidneys are concentrating urine efficiently. Fluid restriction of 500 to 1,000 mL/day and administration of exogenous salt is the primary treatment for SIADH.[7] Pharmacological therapy with vasopressin-2 receptor antagonists may be required for SIADH refractory to conventional therapy. Other causes of euvolemic hypotonic hyponatremia include psychogenic polydipsia (ingestion of large amounts of water), hypothyroidism, hypopituitarism, medications, and reset osmostat, a condition that occurs when the kidneys adequately concentrate and dilute urine but the threshold for ADH secretion is reset downward. For these conditions, treatment should involve correcting the underlying disorder and fluid restriction.

Hypervolemic hypotonic hyponatremia (high volume and low osmolality) is often present in patients with renal failure, cardiac failure, hepatic cirrhosis, or nephritic syndrome because these conditions result in fluid retention or third spacing. To address water retention and edema, which is a common symptom, the recommendation for medical nutrition therapy is to restrict sodium and water from oral intake, enteral nutrition (EN), or PN. Administration of diuretics may be recommended and vasopressin receptor antagonists may also help to increase serum sodium in cirrhosis and cardiac failure. **Figure 2.5** provides an algorithm to define hyponatremia.

Hypernatremia Hypernatremia, or increased serum sodium, occurs in approximately 2% of hospitalized patients, with values >160 mEq/L associated with increased mortality.[8]

Signs and Symptoms Clinical manifestations of hypernatremia are similar to hyponatremia, including

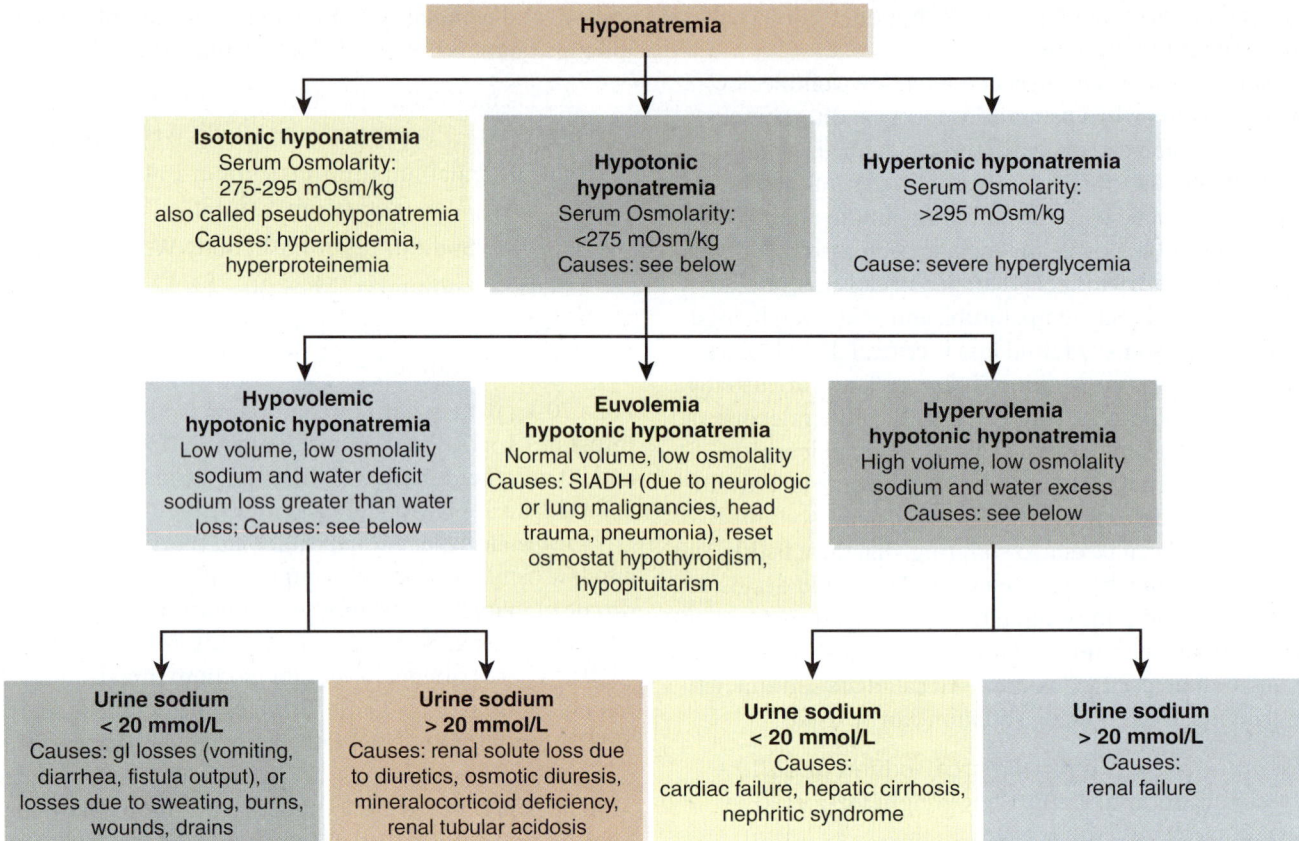

FIGURE 2.5 Algorithm to Define Hyponatremia
Data from Douglas I. Hyponatremia: Why it matters, how it presents, how we can manage it. *Cleve Clin J Med*. 2006;73(3):S5.

neurologic problems ranging from headaches and dizziness to more severe symptoms of seizures, coma, or death. Similar to hyponatremia, assessment of volume status is the first step in diagnosing hypernatremia.

Etiology and Treatment

Hypovolemic hypernatremia occurs when patients have higher sodium levels relative to fluid volumes. Renal losses due to diuretic use, solute diuresis, or acute tubular necrosis are common causes. Extrarenal losses, such as diarrhea and excessive sweating, are also causes of hypovolemia hypernatremia. Initially, patients need salt and water replacement to perfuse vital organs, which is typically administered via enteral or parenteral routes. Hypertonic solutions are only considered appropriate once volume status is corrected.

Euvolemic hypernatremia occurs when patients have water losses that exceed sodium losses. This is commonly caused by thermal injury, fever, or diabetes insipidus (DI). Central DI, which occurs when there is impairment of ADH secretion, and nephritic DI, which occurs when there is inability of the kidneys to respond to ADH circulating in the serum, lead to excessive water loss via urine. While treatment differs depending on the etiology, all require replacement of water via diet, enteral, or parenteral routes.

Hypervolemic hypernatremia occurs when there is an excess of sodium that is greater than the excess of water. This can be iatrogenic (excess administration of isotonic or hypertonic sodium) or caused by mineralocorticoid excess (exogenous administration, Cushing's syndrome, or adrenal malignancy). Treatment involves correcting the underlying disorder, minimizing fluids, eliminating sodium, and in some cases administering diuretics. To evaluate and treat hypernatremia, free water deficit should be calculated with the following equation where 140 refers to a desired sodium of 140 mEq/L:

$$\text{Free Water Deficit (L)} = \text{Total Body Weight (kg)} \times 0.6 \times ([\text{Serum Sodium mEq/L}/140] - 1)$$

Sample Calculation: Weight 70 kg, Sodium 153 mEq/L

$$\text{Free Water Deficit (L)} = 70 \times 0.6 \times ([153/140] - 1)$$
$$\text{Free Water Deficit (L)} = 42 \times (1.09 - 1)$$
$$\text{Free Water Deficit (L)} = 42 \times 0.09$$
$$\text{Free Water Deficit (L)} = 3.8 \text{ L}$$

A 70-kg patient with hypernatremia (sodium 153 mEq/L) has a fluid deficit of 3.8 L. A gradual infusion of this 3.8-L deficit would be required in order to decrease the serum sodium to normal range of 140 mEq/L sodium.

As with hyponatremia, sodium correction should not exceed 10 mEq/L per day, due to risk of cerebral edema and neurological impairment. Specifically, to prevent cerebral edema and convulsions, the maximal rate to reduce serum sodium levels is 0.5 mEq/L/hour for hypernatremia treatment. Hypotonic saline (1/4 normal saline or 38 mEq Na$^+$/L), free water, and water replacements with diuretics may be recommended depending on the etiology and patients' condition.

> **PRACTICE POINT**
>
> Sodium is considered as a critical electrolyte because high and low serum sodium can lead to serious, irreversible complications. Careful assessment and monitoring of sodium is critical, especially in the acute care setting.

Potassium

Potassium (K$^+$) is the major intracellular cation, with 98% of total body potassium located within cells. Normal serum concentration of potassium is 3.5 to 5.0 mEq/L and daily requirements range from 0.5 to 1.5 mEq/kg per day.[9] The most important factors regulating potassium balance include the Na$^+$-K$^+$-ATPase pump and the plasma potassium concentration. Extracellular pH, cellular breakdown, exercise, or hormonal secretions (insulin and catecholamines) can also affect potassium distribution indirectly by regulating the activity of the Na$^+$-K$^+$-ATPase pump. Potassium plays an important role in cell metabolism, transportation of glucose into the cell, and protein and glycogen synthesis. Although only a small amount of potassium is found in ECF, the ratio of serum potassium levels in ICF and ECF is crucial for neurotransmission and muscle contraction function due to potassium's role in maintaining resting membrane potential. The body strives to maintain potassium levels within a very narrow range because movement of only 1.5% to 2% of cellular potassium to ECF can be fatal.[10]

Hypokalemia

Signs and Symptoms Hypokalemia, or low serum potassium, is found in approximately 20% of hospitalized patients.[11] When this disorder is mild (3.0-3.5 mEq/L), patients are typically asymptomatic but may present with nonspecific symptoms including generalized weakness, lethargy, muscle cramping, anorexia, and constipation. Symptoms in more severe cases are muscle necrosis, ascending paralysis, arrhythmias, and possible death.

Etiology Abnormal potassium loss via urine is one of the most common causes of hypokalemia. Loop diuretics, such as furosemide, increase urine excretion and can contribute to potassium loss. Natural licorice and chewing tobacco, if swallowed, stimulate urinary potassium excretion because they contain an aldosterone compound. Hypokalemia may also result from GI losses, due to vomiting, nasogastric suction, or diarrhea. The compensatory actions in acid–base balance contribute to hypokalemia secondary to GI losses. For example, the loss of gastric acid from vomiting can lead to metabolic alkalosis, which results in sodium retention and potassium excretion. An increase in insulin or catecholamines (epinephrine) can also cause a transcellular shift of potassium from ECF to ICF, decreasing serum potassium levels. Inadequate dietary intake of potassium, common in eating disorders, and certain medications including loop and thiazide diuretics, insulin, corticosteroids, lithium, foscarnet, aminoglycosides, amphotericin B, cisplatin, and laxatives can also contribute to hypokalemia. Cellular shifts due to insulin, metabolic alkalosis, and refeeding syndrome are additional causes of hypokalemia.

Treatment The goals of treatment for hypokalemia include resolving the underlying cause, managing symptoms, restoring serum potassium concentrations, and preventing hyperkalemia. Oral correction of hypokalemia is often preferred due to its safety and the reduced risk of overcorrection and rebound hyperkalemia. Oral supplements of potassium chloride are available as a capsule, tablet, or liquid, although liquid forms may be poorly tolerated, sometimes contributing to nausea, vomiting, and diarrhea, and can also have an unpleasant taste. Clinicians are recommended to administer oral dosages of 40 to 100 mEq/day, divided into two to four doses, to correct deficiency.[12] Diet or oral supplements of potassium are recommended for mild or moderate depletion.

Only patients with severe hypokalemia or GI disturbances require IV potassium supplementation, with doses varying by severity and renal function. Intravenous potassium supplements include chloride, acetate, and phosphate salts. In the presence of metabolic acidosis, potassium acetate is recommended in place of potassium chloride. In general, with every 10 mEq of IV potassium administered, there is an increase in 0.1 mEq/L of serum potassium levels in patients with normal renal function. In most cases, infusion rates should not exceed 10 to 20 mEq/hour, although infusion rates of 40 mEq/hour have been reported and used in emergent cases or severely symptomatic patients.[12] Continuous cardiac monitoring is recommended if infusion rates exceed 10 mEq/hour to detect potential signs of hyperkalemia. A central venous catheter is the preferred administration route to minimize phlebitis and burning. It is recommended that clinicians not administer more than 40 to 100 mEq/day of total daily potassium supplementation. Some patients with severe potassium wasting, however, may require 200 mEq/day or higher, with careful cardiac monitoring.[13] **Table 2.3** provides guidelines for hypokalemia treatment through IV replacement.

To avoid worsening hypokalemia, clinicians should use saline as the diluent instead of dextrose, because dextrose can promote an intracellular shift of potassium due to increased insulin release. In addition, magnesium

TABLE 2.3 EMPIRICAL TREATMENT OF HYPOKALEMIA

Serum Potassium Concentration (mEq/L)	Intravenous Potassium Dose (mEq)
3–3.4	20–40
2.5–2.9	40–80
<2.5	80–120

Data from Kraft MD, Btaiche IF, Sacks GS, Kudsk KA. Treatment of electrolyte disorders in adult patients in the intensive care unit. Am J Health Syst Pharm. 2005;62(16):1663.

deficiency should be corrected if present. Treatment of hypomagnesemia is critical because magnesium deficiency can result in refractory hypokalemia due to increased potassium loss or impairment of Na^+-K^+-ATPase pump activity.

Hyperkalemia

Hyperkalemia, or increased serum potassium, rarely occurs in healthy individuals due to the body's efficient regulatory mechanisms. Individuals are often asymptomatic until serum potassium concentration exceeds 5.5 mEq/L.[14]

Signs and Symptoms Signs and symptoms of hyperkalemia are related to changes in neuromuscular and cardiac functions, including muscle twitching, cramping, weakness, ascending paralysis, electrocardiogram changes, and arrhythmias. These clinical manifestations are due to inactivation of electrical transmissions across the membrane. Other electrolyte imbalances, such as hypocalcemia or hyponatremia, or acid–base imbalance, can enhance the adverse effects of hyperkalemia.

Etiology The most common cause of hyperkalemia is inadequate potassium excretion due to renal insufficiency or severe burns. Excessive use of potassium-sparing diuretics, often used to treat hypertension, can also result in inadequate potassium excretion.

A shift in potassium from ICF to ECF can also result in hyperkalemia. This can be due to metabolic acidosis, tissue catabolism, and pseudohyperkalemia. Metabolic acidosis occurs when extracellular potassium shifts to maintain electroneutrality when some of the excess hydrogen atoms are buffered intracellularly. In general, potassium increases by 0.6 mEq/L for every 0.1 change in pH. Cellular shifts can also result from insulin deficiency and hyperosmolality. Tissue catabolism and strenuous exercise can also cause hyperkalemia due to the release of intracellular potassium into the ECF. Pseudohyperkalemia can occur when there is an artificial increase in serum potassium resulting from a release of intracellular potassium during or after blood sampling. Trauma during venipuncture is most commonly associated with pseudohyperkalemia, but a blood sample contaminated with infused potassium or that have been hydrolyzed can also cause pseudohyperkalemia. Hemolysis can also lead to falsely elevated serum potassium. If an elevated hyperkalemia is not commonly seen in a patient, a repeat potassium level should be obtained to confirm hyperkalemia diagnosis. Leukocytosis (increased white blood cells) or thrombosis may also increase potassium in ECF when there is increased hemolysis of red blood cells. Drugs including captopril, cyclosporin, digitalis, lithium, propanolol, and spironolactone also increase serum potassium levels.

Although rare, excessive ingestion from consumption of potassium-containing salt substitutes (KCl) can also result in hyperkalemia, especially if patients have renal insufficiency. While a large decrease in total body potassium is required to cause a slight decrease in serum potassium, only a small excess of total body potassium is needed for a significant increase in serum potassium. It should be noted that serum potassium does not always reflect total body potassium. Typically changes in serum potassium are the result of cellular shifting as opposed to changes in total body potassium. Consumption of potassium-containing salt substitutes should be evaluated, especially in renal patients, to prevent or treat hyperkalemia. Blood transfusions and excessive administration of potassium in IV solutions can also cause hyperkalemia.

Treatment Treatment goals differ based on the degree of hyperkalemia and the severity of symptoms. As with other electrolyte disorders, treating the underlying cause is crucial. If patients experience severe cardiac symptoms of hyperkalemia in short-term emergency situations, IV calcium gluconate is recommended to decrease abnormalities in cardiac cells that could lead to cardiac arrest and to restore membrane excitability. If excess exogenous potassium or other medications may have contributed to hyperkalemia, these should be discontinued or decreased if feasible. If a shift in ICF to ECF was the primary etiology, then insulin, dextrose, sodium bicarbonate and alpha$_2$-adreneric agonists can cause potassium to move intracellularly. Diuretics and cation-exchange resins (sodium polystyrene sulfonate) can also be administered to increase potassium excretion. For patients with renal insufficiency, dialysis and a potassium-restricted diet are recommended for long-term treatment. If patients have mild hyperkalemia, 2 g potassium/day dietary restriction is recommended.

Serum potassium levels should be monitored frequently in symptomatic patients during treatment because acute hyperkalemia can cause potassium to be redistributed within the body, without it being removed. After symptom removal, serum potassium should continue to be monitored until potassium levels have returned to normal.

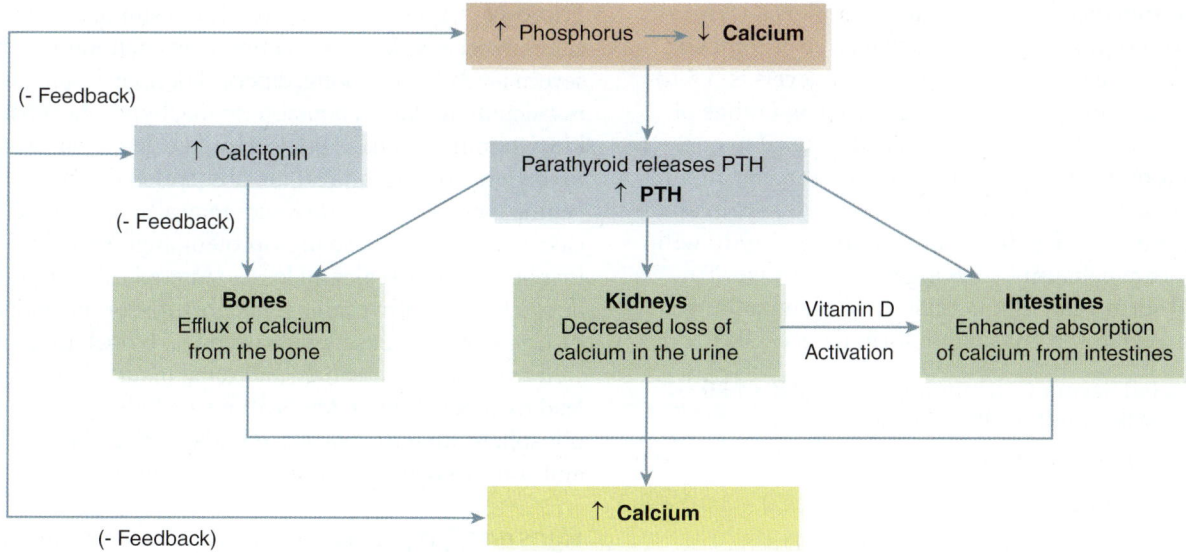

FIGURE 2.6 Mechanisms Involved in Phosphorus and Calcium Homeostasis
Data from Kraft MD. Phosphorus and calcium: A review for the adult nutrition support clinician. *Nutr Clin Pract*. 2015;30(1):21-33.

Phosphorus and Calcium

Phosphorus (P^{3-}) and calcium (Ca^{2+}) are closely interrelated in the body. Phosphorus and calcium homeostasis can be affected by many factors including disease states, clinical conditions, severity of illness, and medications. Homeostasis of phosphorus and calcium is primarily maintained by the regulation of serum phosphorus levels and ionized calcium levels, and the actions of parathyroid hormone (PTH), vitamin D, and calcitonin. An increase in serum phosphorus levels can lead to a decrease in serum ionized calcium levels, which stimulates release of PTH. The function of PTH is to increase calcium resorption and phosphorus excretion via kidneys, stimulate vitamin D activation in the kidneys, and increase absorption of phosphorus and calcium in the intestine. Vitamin D then upregulates intestinal absorption of phosphorus and calcium, stimulates calcium and phosphorus release from bone, and increases renal calcium resorption and urinary phosphorus excretion. The increase in serum ionized calcium levels and vitamin D will suppress PTH release, decreasing vitamin D activation. The increase in ionized calcium levels will also stimulate release of calcitonin, which inhibits bone resorption and decreases ionized calcium levels as a result. **Figure 2.6** demonstrates the processes involved in phosphorus and calcium homeostasis. Magnesium can also affect calcium homeostasis because it has been found to impair the synthesis and/or release of PTH. Clinicians must understand the relationship between serum phosphorous and serum ionized calcium in order to take measures needed to appropriately prevent and/or correct disorders when they occur, especially in patients who are acutely ill and patients receiving PN and/or EN.

Calcium

Calcium (Ca^{2+}) is the most abundant divalent cation in the body and plays a key role in bone structure, blood coagulation, platelet adhesion, endocrine and exocrine secretory functions, neuromuscular activity, and cardiac and smooth muscle functioning. **Figure 2.7** describes the essential functions of calcium. Calcium is closely regulated by the endocrine system, more specifically PTH, calcitonin, and calcitriol. Most of the body's calcium is located in bones and teeth, while the remaining 1% of calcium is found in body fluids. In serum, 40% of calcium is bound

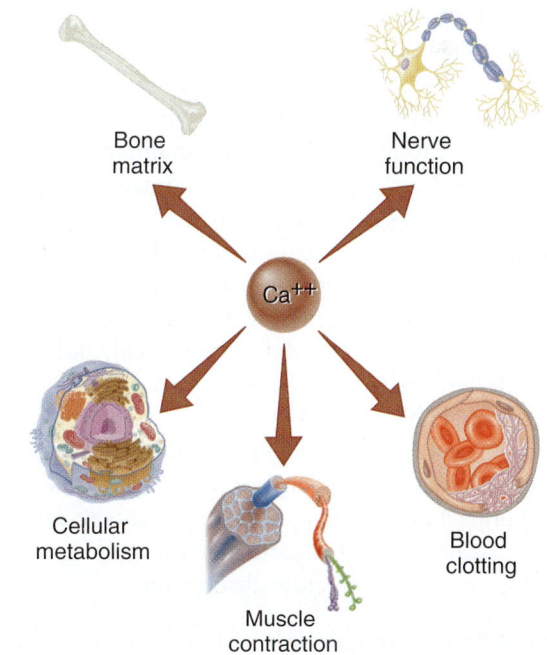

FIGURE 2.7 Essential Functions of Calcium

to proteins (mostly albumin), 13% is complexed (typically with citrate and phosphate), and 47% is free or ionized. The normal range for total serum calcium levels is 8.5 to 10.5 mg/dL, and ionized calcium has a normal range of 1.12 to 1.30 mmol/L.[15] An equation can be used to correct serum calcium due to hypoalbuminemia. Serum calcium levels must be corrected if a patient has a low serum albumin because a decrease in serum albumin by 1 g/dL will decrease serum calcium by 0.8 mg/dL, on average. To assess total serum calcium in relation to serum albumin levels, a corrected serum calcium formula is used:

$$\text{Corrected Serum Calcium (mg/dL)} = (0.8 \times [4.0 - \text{Albumin Level}]) + \text{Serum Calcium}$$

Sample Calculation: Calcium 8.0 mg/dL, Albumin 3.0 g/dL

$$\text{Corrected Serum Calcium (mg/dL)} = (0.8 \times [4.0 - 3.0]) + 8.0$$
$$\text{Corrected Serum Calcium} = (0.8 \times 1) + 8.0$$
$$\text{Corrected Serum Calcium} = 8.8 \text{ mg/dL}$$

A patient who has an albumin level of 3.0 g/dL, has a corrected serum calcium that is 8.8 instead of 8.0 mg/dL.

The 0.8 in the equation takes into account the 0.8 mg/dL that total calcium concentration decreases with every 1 g/dL reduction in serum albumin concentration while the 4.0 refers to a normal albumin level. Hypoalbuminemia causes a decrease in total serum calcium, but has less of an impact on ionized calcium. Therefore, ionized calcium is considered a better indicator of the functional status of calcium metabolism than serum calcium. In particular, there is a poor correlation between ionized calcium and total calcium in those with hypoalbuminemia, acid–base disorders, and critical illness, resulting in ionized calcium being the preferred indicator of calcium status in these populations.

The recommended adequate intake for calcium is approximately 1,000 to 1,200 mg/day for healthy adults, depending on age and sex. Most EN formulas contain approximately 700 to 1,200 mg/L (~17-30 mmol) of calcium and most adult patients with normal renal function require a dose of 10 to 15 mEq/day for maintenance with PN admixtures. Calcium doses can be adjusted by approximately 20% to 50%, depending on the daily calcium dose, serum calcium levels, responses to dose changes, and underlying clinical conditions. Absorption of calcium from diet and supplements ranges from 25% to 35%, influenced by source, salt form, presence of stomach acid, and whether or not it is taken with food. The recommended individual dose for optimal absorption is ≤500 mg.[16] Calcium citrate is also recommended in place of calcium carbonate because it appears to have better absorption. Calcium citrate is the preferred oral calcium supplement for patients receiving acid-suppression therapy or patients with achlorhydria, who may have reduced calcium absorption.

Hypocalcemia Hypocalcemia, or low serum calcium or low ionized calcium, has been observed in approximately 15% to 88% of hospitalized patients, and has been reported in 21% of critically ill trauma patients.[17]

Etiology Hypocalcemia is rarely a result of low intake of calcium because bone resorption helps maintain normal serum levels for a prolonged period of time despite variation in calcium intake. Hypomagnesemia, hyperphosphatemia, low vitamin D intake, and decreased calcium absorption due to phytate, oxalate, and fat malabsorption can cause hypocalcemia. Increased calcium losses may also contribute to hypocalcemia as a result of a high-protein, high-sodium diet, which increases urinary calcium losses. Altered calcium regulation due to hypoparathyroidism, pancreatitis, or metabolic bone disease can also cause hypocalcemia. Hypoalbuminemia, as well as sepsis, pancreatitis, and renal insufficiency can also lead to hypocalcemia. Medications including loop diuretics, phosphate, dilantin, corticosteroids, citrated blood, fluoride, and contrast dye can also cause hypocalcemia.

Signs and Symptoms Tetany (intermittent muscle spasms) is the most common sign of severe acute hypocalcemia (<7 mg/dL). Mild-moderate hypocalcemia may present other neuromuscular, cardiovascular, and central nervous symptom symptoms, including muscle cramps, paresthesias (tingling, numbness of extremities), seizures, ventricular arrythmias, prolonged QT interval, heart block, and ventricular fibrillation. Patients with chronic hypocalcemia may experience dermatologic manifestations including dermatitis; eczema; brittle, grooved nails; and hair loss.

Treatment

Hypocalcemia treatment involves removing the underlying cause, correcting hypomagnesemia (if present), and taking appropriate calcium supplementation. Because magnesium deficiency may impair release of PTH and/or PTH activity and contribute to hypocalcemia, magnesium supplements can be used to correct deficiency if it is concurrent with calcium deficiency. Phosphate binders may also be recommended if hyperphosphatemia is the underlying cause. Fixed IV doses of calcium gluconate are determined by symptoms and ionized calcium levels, rather than weight-based doses. If ionized calcium is not available, empirical treatment with 1 to 2 g calcium gluconate may be recommended followed by measurement of ionized calcium levels.[11] Calcium gluconate is recommended as the preferred calcium salt for routine calcium maintenance dosing and supplementation, while calcium chloride is recommended for use in urgent and emergency situations only. Severe, symptomatic hypocalcemia (i.e., seizures, tetany, arrhythmias, or refractory hypotension) should be corrected promptly with IV calcium administration over 10 minutes to control symptoms. Calcium gluconate is the preferred salt for peripheral venous administration to avoid extravasation (leakage of liquid into surrounding tissue) and tissue necrosis from calcium chloride. **Figure 2.8** shows an example of extravasation. Clinicians must be careful to prevent dosing errors from confusion about calcium salts and calcium dose, as well as the manner calcium is ordered. Calcium chloride provides three times more elemental calcium than an equivalent of calcium gluconate.[18] To prevent dosing errors, orders should contain dose of calcium, calcium salt, and dose in grams, milligrams, or

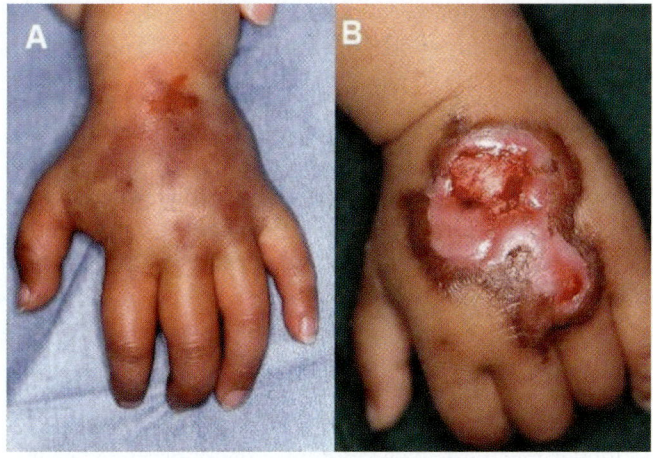

FIGURE 2.8 Extravasation or Leakage of Fluid into Surrounding Tissue
Reproduced from Cutaneous Necrosis Induced by Extravasation of Arginine Monohydrochloride. Hiroo Amano, DOI: 10.2340/00015555-0420.

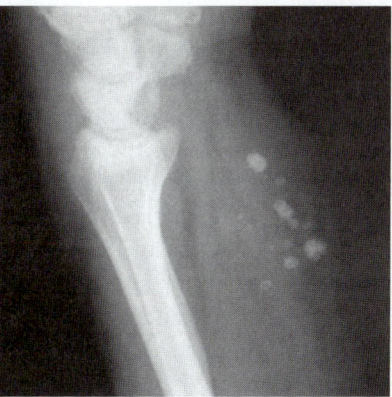

FIGURE 2.9 Tissue Calcification Due to Severe Hypercalcemia and Hyperphosphatemia
Published with permission from LearningRadiology.com.

milliequivalents. Clinicians must also be sure not to infuse calcium in the same IV line as solutions containing phosphate due to the risk of calcium-phosphorus precipitation.

In patients with mild-moderate hypocalcemia who are receiving EN or can tolerate oral medication, oral calcium supplements (calcium gluconate, calcium acetate, calcium citrate, or calcium carbonate) may be considered. Vitamin D status and evaluation of PTH may need to be considered prior to oral administration. If patients are receiving PN, adjustments of daily calcium maintenance doses in PN formulations or daily oral supplements may be recommended depending on patient's clinical condition and underlying cause of hypocalcemia.

As discussed earlier, hypoalbuminemia can produce a falsely low serum calcium (pseudohypocalcemia). If a patient has asymptomatic hypocalcemia due to hypoalbuminemia with normal ionized calcium levels, then no treatment is needed to correct hypocalcemia. Although there is debate over the need to correct asymptomatic hypocalcemia, most clinicians treat hypocalcemia to avoid the potential negative consequences of severe hypocalcemia, especially in critically ill patients.

Hypercalcemia Hypercalcemia is increased serum calcium or increased ionized calcium.

Etiology Hypercalcemia most frequently results from increased resorption from bone in malignancies with bone metastases (predominantly breast cancer, lung cancer, and multiple myeloma), and from decreased urinary excretion in patients with primary hyperparathyroidism.[15] Other causes include vitamin A or D toxicity, chronic ingestion of milk and/or calcium carbonate–containing antacids in patients with renal insufficiency (milk-alkali syndrome), or adrenal insufficiency. Immobilization, tuberculosis, Paget's disease, rhabdomyolysis, and medications including thiazide diuretics, estrogens, tamoxifen, and aluminum intoxication are other potential causes of hypercalcemia.

Early signs and symptoms of hypercalcemia are nonspecific and include fatigue, nausea, vomiting, constipation, anorexia, and confusion. Chronic hypercalcemia may lead to calcium-phosphate precipitation, metastatic calcification, and renal failure. Patients with severe cases can experience cardiac manifestations such as bradycardia (slow heart rate) or arrhythmias with electrocardiograph changes. Immediate treatment is required for severe hypercalcemia because acute kidney injury, ventricular arrhythmias, obtundation, coma, and death are potential consequences. Prolonged hypercalcemia can lead to tissue calcification (**Figure 2.9**), which can be irreversible.

As with other electrolyte disorders, treatment of hypercalcemia must include treatment or removal of the underlying cause if possible. Mild hypercalcemia (total serum calcium of 10.5-12.9 mg/dL or ionized calcium of 1.31-1.49 mmol/L) does not require immediate therapy; hydration and ambulation are typically effective treatments. Patients receiving PN may benefit from temporary reduction or removal of calcium from the PN prescription, based on the underlying cause and severity of hypercalcemia. Severe hypercalcemia (total serum calcium ≥13 mg/dL or ionized calcium ≥1.5 mmol/L) should be treated immediately with IV hydration to reverse the IV volume depletion caused by hypercalcemia. After hydration is restored, furosemide (40-100 mg) is recommended to enhance renal calcium excretion; however, careful monitoring is necessary to avoid further IV volume depletion.[19] Within the first 48 hours of treatment, saline hydration and furosemide have been found to reduce serum calcium by 2 to 3 mg/dL.[20] Calcitonin inhibits bone resorption and increases renal calcium elimination. This may also be used to treat acute hypercalcemia, although tachyphylaxis (diminishing response of successive doses) limits its effectiveness. In addition, biphosphonates are potential inhibitors of bone resorption and are often recommended for treatment of hypercalcemia in patients with malignancies or critical illness who have accelerated bone breakdown and associated metabolic bone disease. Serum or ionized calcium levels should be monitored every 4 to 8 hours during active treatment of severe hypercalcemia and every 24 to 48 hours after hypercalcemia is treated. Cardiac monitoring is critical for patients receiving treatment of hypercalcemia.

Phosphorus Phosphorus (P^{3-}) is the primary intracellular anion in the body, existing mainly as phosphate (PO_4) in the serum. Phosphate is the key form of phosphorus as it relates to medical nutrition therapy because it is also the primary form ingested in the diet and in exogenous administration of phosphorus. Only a small percentage of total body phosphorus is found in extracellular fluid, with the remaining 99% located in bones and soft tissues.

Phosphorus has many important functions in the body, including bone and cell membrane composition (phospholipids) and maintenance of normal pH. Phosphorus also provides the energy-bonds in the form of adenosine triphosphate (ATP), which supplies energy needed for many cellular processes and functions. Phosphorus is a key component of 2,3-diphosphoglycerate (2,3-DPG), which is essential for oxygen release from hemoglobin and delivery to tissues. Total body phosphorus is necessary for glucose use and glycolysis, protein synthesis, neurological function, and muscular function.

Serum phosphorus concentration is determined by the amount of intestinal absorption, renal excretion, hormonally regulated bone resorption and deposition, and distribution within intracellular and extracellular compartments. Intracellular shifts in phosphorus may be a result of insulin administration, catecholamines, and alkalosis while extracellular shifts may occur from cellular destruction and acidosis. Normal serum phosphorus concentration ranges from 2.7 to 4.5 mg/dL; however, serum phosphorus levels may not correlate well with total body phosphorus as serum phosphorus is only a small percentage of total phosphorus. As a result, clinicians must take a complete assessment of patient and consider factors that may affect serum levels and total body homeostasis of phosphorus including chronic kidney disease, severe malnutrition, and certain medications.

Hypophosphatemia Hypophosphatemia, or low serum phosphorus, has been found to occur in approximately 2% to 3% of hospitalized patients, but is reported in 28% to 80% of critically ill patients.[21]

Etiology Potential causes of hypophosphatemia include decreased intake (diet, PN, IV fluid), malnutrition, vomiting, or diarrhea. Decreased GI absorption due to antacids, vitamin deficiency, malabsorption, and chronic alcoholism or alcohol withdrawal may also cause hypophosphatemia. Many acutely ill and critically ill patients have underlying conditions or receive medications that predispose them to developing hypophosphatemia. Medications that increase urine phosphorus losses include antacids, phosphate binders, sucralfate, insulin, and corticosteroids. Low serum magnesium or phosphorus, osmotic diuresis, hyperparathyroidism, and renal tubular defects can also increase urine losses and cause phosphorus imbalance. Cellular shifts from respiratory and metabolic alkalosis (following treatment of diabetic ketoacidosis) can also result in hypophosphatemia due to decreased hydrogen ion secretion. Many clinicians have reported hypophosphatemia associated with initiation of nutrition support, including oral nutrition, EN, and PN. Hypophosphatemia can be a result of metabolic consequences of refeeding syndrome due to increased phosphorus needs during increased glucose utilization.

Signs and Symptoms Hypophosphatemia can cause a variety of adverse effects on respiratory, neurological, neuromuscular, and cardiopulmonary functions. Severe hypophosphatemia (serum phosphorus concentration <2 mg/dL) has been associated with impaired contractibility of diaphragm, acute respiratory failure, tissue hypoxia, decreased myocardial contractibility, paresthesia, confusion, disorientation, encephalopathy, areflexic paralysis, seizures, coma, and death. Some studies have found that hypophosphatemia is associated with higher mortality, longer hospitalization, and longer mechanical ventilation. Low phosphate levels can also result in mobilization of calcium and phosphorus in bone, contributing to osteomalacia and rickets.

Treatment The magnitude of the abnormality and presence of symptoms must be considered in treatment of hypophosphatemia. Treatment should focus on treating the underlying cause of phosphate abnormality (medically induced, malabsorption, inadequate maintenance dose, etc.). Patients with asymptomatic mild hypophosphatemia can be treated with oral phosphorus supplement if the GI tract is functioning, although absorption may vary among patients and diarrhea may result.

Patients with moderate–severe hypophosphatemia who are symptomatic and cannot tolerate oral supplements can be treated with IV phosphorus supplementation. A fixed IV dose of phosphorus is considered appropriate for patients with normal renal function based on serum phosphorus levels. Estimating doses is largely empirical because serum phosphorus levels may not correlate with total body stores of phosphorus. Patients with persistent hypophosphatemia may require a daily phosphorus supplement, IV supplementation, or increased maintenance phosphorus dose in PN admixtures. The recommended IV phosphorus dose should be provided over 4 to 6 hours to reduce risk of $Ca-PO_4$ precipitation and minimize infusion-related adverse effects, such as thrombophlebitis.

Hyperphosphatemia

Etiology Hyperphosphatemia, or increased serum phosphorus concentration, is most commonly caused by acute or chronic renal insufficiency, especially in hospitalized and critically ill patients. Decreased urinary phosphorus excretion can also result in patients with hypoparathyroidism and vitamin D toxicity. Excessive IV and/or oral administration of phosphorus could also cause hyperphosphatemia, which would be more likely found in patients with impaired renal function. Cellular shifts resulting from dehydration, hemolysis, rhabdomyolysis, and tumor lysis are also causes of hyperphosphatemia. Metabolic and respiratory acidosis are other potential causes of hyperphosphatemia. Oral and rectal administration of phosphorus-containing laxatives has also been reported to cause hyperphosphatemia. In addition, medications including enemas, salts, diuretics, biphosphonates, and lipid emulsions can lead to hyperphosphatemia.

Signs and Symptoms Many of the signs of hyperphosphatemia are concurrent with signs of hypocalcemia. Flaccid paralysis, mental confusion, hypertension, cardiac arrhythmias, and tissue calcification are common symptoms in patients with prolonged phosphorus toxicity. Due to the risk of calcium-phosphate precipitation, hyperphosphatemia can lead to hypocalcemia, further leading to its clinical manifestations such as altered nerve transmission and tetany. Calcium-phosphorus crystals can also cause further organ damage, particularly in the lungs, myocardium, and blood vessels, and can deposit on soft tissue. Evaluation of individual serum levels of calcium and phosphorus is recommended to guide treatment plans and prevent these complications.

Treatment A complete assessment of the patient is required for appropriate treatment of hyperphosphatemia. Identifying and correcting the underlying cause of this condition should be the first approach, followed by adjustment or restriction of phosphorus intake (reduced daily doses of PN prescription or initiating a renal EN formula). Volume deficit should be corrected if the cause is dehydration. Oral phosphorus binders are also recommended with meals and snacks to control high serum phosphorus levels by binding dietary phosphate. Common phosphate binders include calcium-, aluminum-, and magnesium-containing antacids. Individuals with hyperphosphatemia due to renal failure on renal replacement therapy may require different therapies for hyperphosphatemia treatment because various forms of renal replacement therapy, such as continuous renal replacement therapy, peritoneal dialysis, or intermittent hemodialysis, vary in their ability to remove phosphorus.

Magnesium

Magnesium (Mg^{2+}) is an abundant mineral in the ICF, with approximately 50% to 60% of magnesium located in bones and most of the remaining found within in cardiac muscle, skeletal muscle, and other soft tissues. Magnesium is an important cofactor in more than 300 biochemical processes in the body, including glucose metabolism, fatty acid synthesis, and DNA and protein metabolism. Magnesium also plays an important role in maintenance of the Na^+-K^+-ATPase, which is necessary for nerve impulse conduction, muscle contraction, and normal heart rhythm. Magnesium also is required for the synthesis of glutathione, and is a factor in PTH synthesis, and vasomotor tone.

As an important structural component of bone, magnesium also plays a role in maintaining intracellular potassium and calcium levels. The GI system, kidneys, and bones tightly regulate cellular and extracellular magnesium concentrations. Healthy individuals absorb about 30% to 40% of dietary magnesium; this occurs primarily in the distal jejunum and ileum. Normally about one-third of absorbed magnesium is excreted, but absorption varies with intake to maintain normal serum concentrations. Normal serum magnesium levels ranges from 1.3 to 2.1 mEq/L, but these serum levels do not accurately assess total body magnesium because less than 1% of total magnesium is found in serum. As the majority of magnesium is bound to albumin, hypoalbuminemia can cause a falsely low serum magnesium level.

Hypomagnesemia Hypomagnesemia, or low serum magnesium, has been found in up to 47% of hospitalized patients and in up to 65% of critical care patients.[22]

Etiology Decreased intake or absorption or excessive losses and redistribution into ICF are possible causes of hypomagnesemia. Protein-calorie malnutrition and prolonged administration of magnesium-free IV fluids or PN contribute to decreased intake. Chronic alcoholism or withdrawal of alcohol, malabsorption syndromes, short bowel syndrome, and intestinal bypass surgeries can lead to reduced magnesium absorption and GI losses. Renal losses of magnesium also occur in patients with acute tubular necrosis, renal tubular acidosis, Bartter syndrome, and hyperaldosteronism. Certain medications including cyclosporine, thiazide, loop diuretics, laxatives, cisplatin, amphotericin B, amino-glycosides can also cause hypomagnesemia. In addition, pancreatitis, low serum phosphorus, refeeding syndrome, diabetic ketoacidosis, hyperthyroidism, and myocardial infarction can also cause intracellular shifts of magnesium, decreasing serum magnesium levels.

Signs and Symptoms The primary symptom of magnesium deficiency is neuromuscular hyperexcitability. Latent tetany, muscular weakness, convulsions, and seizures may also occur. Cardiac complications, including electrocardiogram changes, arrhythmias, and increased sensitivity to cardiac glycosides, such as digoxin, are also common with magnesium deficiency. General symptoms may include depression, anorexia, nausea, vomiting, and ileus. Many of the signs and symptoms of hypomagnesemia are difficult to differentiate from those of hypokalemia and hypocalcemia, both of which are refractory to treatment in the presence of hypomagnesemia. Reports indicate that approximately 38% to 61% of patients with hypokalemia and 22% to 28% of patients with hypocalcemia also present with hypomagnesemia.[23]

Treatment Serum levels may not correlate with intracellular concentrations of magnesium or total body magnesium. As a result, hypomagnesemia treatment goals are largely empirical. Treatment should focus on addressing the underlying cause and correcting coexisting electrolyte imbalances following magnesium repletion. Oral salts are recommended for mild to moderate depletion, although they should be used with caution because they may cause diarrhea. For severe depletion or GI impairment, such as short bowel syndrome, IV administration of $MgSO_4$ is often preferred. The slow onset of action and GI intolerance limit the effectiveness oral administration, especially in severe cases of hypomagnesemia. For asymptomatic patients, clinicians should not exceed 1 g/L/hour of magnesium infusion because high levels of magnesium can cause cardiac arrest. In addition, patients with renal impairment should be administered 50% or less of recommended empirical doses to reduce risk of overcompensating and causing hypermagnesemia.

CASE STUDY REVISITED

On hospital day (HD) 3, you visit Adam and learn that he has been NPO since admission due to his medical GI evaluation. Because Adam is feeling better and his GI symptoms have resolved, the medical team has just advanced Adam to a regular diet. Adam reports an excellent appetite and is looking forward to eating.

Anthropometric Data:
Weight: 73 kg (161 lbs)
Last weight: 75 kg (165 lbs) at admission

Biochemical Data: (HD 3)
Sodium 134 (135-145 mEq/L)
Potassium 3.3 (3.6-5.0 mEq/L)
Blood Urea Nitrogen 22 (6-24 mg/dL)
Creatinine 0.2 (0.4-1.3 mg/dL)
Glucose 95 (70-139 mg/dL)
Phosphorus 2.9 (2.7-4.5 mg/dL)
Magnesium 1.4 (1.3-2.1 mEq/L)

Clinical Data:
Medications: protonix, lipitor, captopril

Dietary Data:
Diet Prescription: Regular

Questions
1. Is Adam at risk for refeeding syndrome? Explain.
2. What biochemical indices should be monitored with refeeding syndrome?
3. What factors mediate the refeeding process?
4. Do you have any recommendations for interventions for Adam?

Hypermagnesemia Hypermagnesemia, or high serum magnesium, is uncommon, occurring primarily in patients with renal insufficiency.

Etiology
In addition to renal insufficiency, medications interfering with magnesium excretion, such as lithium and spironolactone, and excessive supplementation of magnesium-containing antacids or laxatives (such as Milk of Magnesia) can also contribute to hypermagnesemia.

Signs and Symptoms Dehydration, nausea, vomiting, diaphoresis (excessive sweating), flushing, sensation of heat, drowsiness, depressed mental status, hypotension, and bradycardia are common symptoms of mild–moderate hypermagnesemia. Neuromuscular functions can also be impaired, leading to decreased reflexes, muscle weakness, and paralysis. Severe cases of hypermagnesemia may also cause respiratory paralysis, cardiac arrest, liver dysfunction, coma, and possibly death.

Treatment In mild cases, where medications or supplementation were the cause of hypermagnesemia, discontinuation of medications containing magnesium or supplementation of antacids or laxatives can treat the abnormality. Rehydration is recommended for those with symptoms of dehydration. In patients with asymptomatic hypermagnesemia, the recommended treatment is to remove or restrict other exogenous sources from PN or IV fluids. Patients with more severe symptomatic hypermagnesemia may need to be treated with IV calcium gluconate to alleviate neuromuscular and cardiovascular symptoms. Elimination of magnesium from IV fluids and PN are the preferred treatment; however, clinicians must consider the potential for ECF to ICF shifts when decreasing magnesium in PN. For patients with renal failure, hemodialysis may be recommended. Clinicians may also consider administering diuretics to increase magnesium excretion.

Refeeding Syndrome

Refeeding syndrome is a condition that can occur in malnourished patients during the initiation of concentrated calorie delivery, characterized by several metabolic complications due to derangements in phosphorus, potassium, magnesium, and glucose control. Together, the effects of depletion, repletion, and compartmental shifts in electrolytes, fluids, and other substrates in response to excessive nutritional resuscitation define refeeding syndrome. Patients with malnutrition, history of long-term inadequate intake, and those with minimal intake for several days are considered at risk for refeeding syndrome.

Reintroduction of carbohydrates (oral, enteral, or parenteral) after starvation induces a shift from ketones as the primary energy source to glucose. During this shift to anabolism particularly with the introduction of insulin, phosphorus, potassium, and magnesium shift intracellularly leading to low serum levels. The carbohydrate delivery also suddenly enables massive phosphorylation of ADP to ATP, leading to a rapid depletion of marginal phosphorus stores as well as thiamin. In addition, sodium and water is retained, leading to the potential for fluid overload. **Figure 2.10** outlines the metabolic changes associated with refeeding syndrome. According to case reports, refeeding syndrome can continue up to 5 days after initiation of feedings.[24]

Electrolyte abnormalities in refeeding syndrome can lead to neurologic, respiratory, and cardiac abnormalities, while vitamin deficiencies can cause severe encephalopathy and sodium retention can contribute to pulmonary edema and cardiac decompensation. Many strategies have been suggested to prevent the adverse effects of refeeding syndrome. Any electrolyte abnormalities should be addressed prior to initiating feedings, and sodium and fluids should be closely monitored in severely malnourished patients during the first days of nutrition repletion. By initiating feedings more slowly or at a lower level, clinicians can help prevent or reduce the metabolic effects of refeeding syndrome from occurring in patients. Starting energy intake at 15 to 20 kcal/kg/day, 1,000 kcal/day, or 50% of estimated needs are common recommendations, with a gradual increase to goal over 5 to 7 days.[25] Clinicians must recognize the risks of refeeding syndrome for severely malnourished patients and the dynamic process requiring continual monitoring and modification according to metabolic needs to maintain stability and promote nutritional repletion.

> **CORE CONCEPT 3**
>
> Refeeding syndrome can result in malnourished patients when carbohydrate feedings induce insulin, resulting in the intracellular shift of potassium, phosphorus, and magnesium, and fluid retention.

> **PRACTICE POINT**
>
> Screening patients for malnutrition (i.e., evaluating anthropometrics, functional assessment, diet history) prior to initiating feeds is critical to prevent and reduce the adverse effects of refeeding syndrome. Slow advancement of feeds to 30% to 50% of caloric requirement is recommended.

Chloride

Chloride (Cl^-) is the most abundant anion in the ECF, with approximately 88% found in ECF and only 12% located intracellularly.[26] Normal serum chloride levels range from 98 to 110 mEq/L, with serum chloride levels closely regulated by the kidneys. Chloride is most commonly found in the body as sodium chloride (NaCl) and hydrochloric acid (HCl). With a negative charge, chloride is usually associated with positively charged sodium and is typically regulated in the same proportion of sodium in extracellular fluid. As a result, chloride works closely with sodium to maintain cell membrane integrity via regulation of fluid balance and serum osmolality. The formation of hydrochloric acid also plays a crucial role in digestion and in acid–base balance. High serum chloride results in metabolic acidosis and low serum chloride can lead to metabolic alkalosis. As a large component of gastric

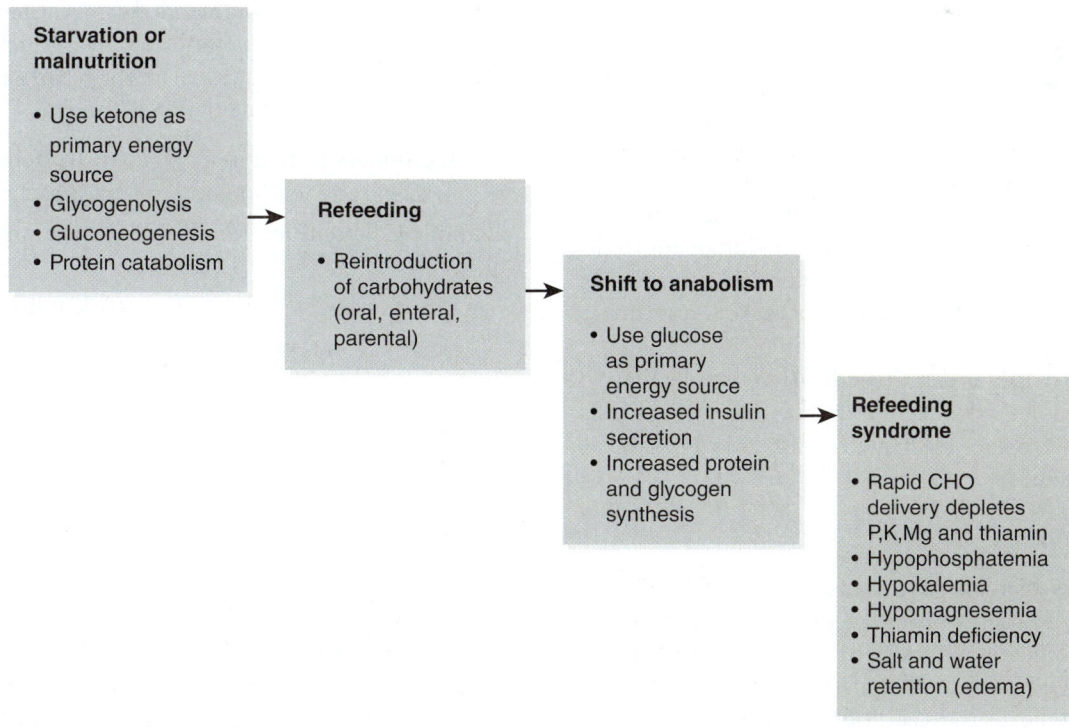

FIGURE 2.10 Metabolic Changes Occuring During Refeeding Syndrome

juice, HCl also alters the pH of the stomach, assists in protein digestion, and activates other digestive enzymes.

Hypochloremia

Etiology Hypochloremia, or low serum chloride, can occur from vomiting, diarrhea, nasogastric suction, GI fistulae, renal failure with salt restriction, and excessive sweating. Chronic respiratory acidosis, metabolic alkalosis, diabetic ketoacidosis, SIADH, adrenal insufficiency, and hyperaldosteronism may cause hypochloremia. Chronic use of laxatives, bicarbonate, corticosteroids, and diuretics may also lead to hypochloremia.

Signs and Symptoms Many people with hypochloremia are asymptomatic, with symptoms only present at extremely low levels. Common symptoms may include dehydration, hyperirritability, tetany, slowed respirations, and hypotension resulting from fluid loss.

Treatment Treatment of hypochloremia must initially address the underlying cause. Assessment of hydration status, severity of hypochloremia, and presence of concurrent electrolyte disorders (hypokalemia, hyponatremia) and metabolic alkalosis is critical. In acute hypochloremia, if the patient is in shock, isotonic fluid, preferably saline, should be administered. Clinicians should treat chronic hypochloremia more slowly because rapid treatment can lead to more serious complications. Intravenous administration of isotonic sodium chloride and potassium chloride is recommended, with doses determined by patients' serum chloride levels. To calculate chloride deficit, the following equation is used:

$$\text{Chloride Deficit in mEq} = (0.27)(\text{Weight in kg})(100 - \text{Chloride level})$$

Sample Calculation: Weight 70 kg, Chloride 92 mEq/L

$$\text{Chloride Deficit in mEq} = (0.27)(70)(100 - 92)$$

$$\text{Chloride Deficit} = 151 \text{ mEq}$$

The 100 in the equation refers to a desired chloride level and the 0.27 refers to the chloride distribution in the body. A 70-kg patient with hypochloremia (chloride 92 mEq/L) has a chloride deficit of 151 mEq if a chloride level of 100 mEq is desired. Furthermore, an infusion of approximately 1 L normal saline (which contains 154 mEq NaCl) would correct this deficit in order to increase the serum chloride to normal range.

If the abnormality is due to medication use, decrease or remove medication if possible. For hypochloremic acidosis, clinicians should replace electrolytes with chloride salts as primary treatment.

Hyperchloremia

Etiology Hyperchloremia, or increased serum chloride, can also result from a variety of health conditions. Renal failure, nephritic syndrome, renal tubular acidosis, dehydration, overtreatment with saline, and hyperparathyroidism are the most common causes. In addition, diabetes insipidus, metabolic acidosis from diarrhea, respiratory alkalosis, and hyperadrenocorticism can also result in hyperchloremia. Certain drugs including acetozolamide, androgens, hydrochlorothiazide, and salicylates can also cause hyperchloremia.

Signs and Symptoms The most common symptoms of hyperchloremia are weakness and lethargy, with more serious symptoms including unconsciousness and Kussmaul respirations, which are deep and labored breaths often associated with diabetic ketoacidosis or kidney failure.

Treatment Treatment of hyperchloremia varies based on the etiology. If excessive intake or inadequate excretion of chloride causes hyperchloremic acidosis, clinicians should substitute acetate, citrate, or phosphate salts for chloride salts in infusions. To treat GI causes of hyperchloremia, clinicians are recommended to administer saline solutions to treat volume losses and to administer potassium. Acidosis should be treated with bicarbonate-containing solutions with potassium replacement due to the potential consequences of rapid introduction of potassium into cells (cardiac arrhythmias and muscular paralysis). If chronic acidosis is present with hyperchloremia due to diarrhea, long-term therapy with sodium and potassium citrate solutions may be recommended.

Bicarbonate

Bicarbonate is a compound in the blood that works closely with chloride to maintain acid–base balance in the body. Bicarbonate usually refers to HCO_3 or carbon dioxide (CO_2), with normal serum levels ranging from 20 to 30 mEq/L. High serum bicarbonate results in metabolic alkalosis, while low serum bicarbonate causes metabolic acidosis. Treatment for metabolic acidosis is typically sodium bicarbonate ($NaHCO_3$) via IV administration. Due to the instability of bicarbonate in patients receiving PN, acetate, the biological precursor of bicarbonate, is recommended for treatment in these patients, assuming they have normal liver function to convert acetate to bicarbonate. To calculate the bicarbonate deficit in patients, the following calculation is used:

$$\text{Bicarbonate Deficit in mEq} = (0.50)(\text{Weight in kg})(\text{Desired Bicarbonate} - \text{Serum Bicarbonate})$$

Sample Calculation: Weight 70 kg, Serum Bicarbonate 17 mEq/L

$$\text{Bicarbonate Deficit in mEq} = (0.50)(70)(24 - 17)$$

$$\text{Bicarbonate Deficit} = 245 \text{ mEq}$$

The value of 0.50 is used in this equation to calculate the bicarbonate deficit because the bicarbonate volume of distribution is usually 50% of body weight under normal conditions. A 70-kg patient with a serum bicarbonate of 17 has a bicarbonate deficit of 254 mEq if a bicarbonate level of 24 mEq is desired.

Acid–Base Physiology

An acid is any substance that releases hydrogen ions (H^+) in solution, whereas a base is a substance that accepts or combines with H^+. The free hydrogen ion concentration, represented by the pH, determines the acidity of body

CASE STUDY REVISITED

On HD 6, Adam undergoes an urgent laparotomy for a severe gastric ulcer with perforation. On postoperative (postop) day 1/HD 7, you visit Adam for reassessment. He is currently in the ICU on mechanical ventilation with increased drainage from a nasogastric tube.

Anthropometric Data:
Weight: 77 kg (169 lbs) on HD 7
Last weight: 73 kg (161 lbs) on HD 3

Biochemical Data: (postop day 1/HD 7):

Sodium 143 (135-145 mEq/L)
Potassium 3.5 (3.6-5.0 mEq/L)
Chloride 88 (98-110 mEq/L)
Carbon Dioxide 41 (20-30 mEq/L)
Blood Urea Nitrogen 24 (6-24 mg/dL)

Creatinine 0.2 (0.4-1.3 mg/dL)
Glucose 139 (70-139 mg/dL)
Calcium 7.7 (8.5-10.5 mEq/L)
Phosphorus 3.0 (2.7-4.5 mg/dL)
Magnesium 1.4 (1.3-2.1 mEq/L)

Arterial Blood Gas:
pH 7.48 (7.35-7.45)
$PaCO_2$ 48 (35-45 mm Hg)
PaO_2 90 (80-100 mm Hg)
HCO_3 29 (22-26 mEq/L)

Dietary Data:
Diet Prescription: NPO

Questions

1. Describe Adam's acid–base status.
2. What specific acid–base disorder does he have?
3. What interventions would you recommend to manage this acid–base imbalance?

---

fluids. Because the pH varies inversely with the hydrogen ion concentration, a decrease in hydrogen ion concentration raises the pH and an increase in hydrogen ion concentration lowers the pH. In arterial blood, the pH is normally maintained within the narrow range of 7.35 to 7.45. An increased concentration of hydrogen ion concentration in the blood reflected by a blood pH below 7.35 is called **acidemia**, while a decreased concentration of hydrogen ion concentration in the blood reflected by blood pH above 7.45 is called **alkalemia**. **Acidosis** is the condition of increased hydrogen ion concentration and **alkalosis** is the condition of decreased hydrogen ion concentration. These terms are important to understand when evaluating acid–base disorders in patients because both acidotic and alkalotic processes can coexist. **Figure 2.11** illustrates the pH scale and hydrogen ion concentration range.

As with fluid and electrolyte balance, acid–base balance is critical for many physiologic functions and biochemical reactions. Serum chloride and bicarbonate levels are the most common electrolytes associated with acid–base imbalance. In a healthy individual, the kidneys, lungs, and buffering systems tightly regulate the pH level within the body, despite changes in acidity from diet and tissue metabolism. Metabolic and respiratory disorders can disrupt acid–base balance, resulting in alkalosis and acidosis. Adverse consequences of acid–base imbalance can be life threatening in severe cases. Clinicians must

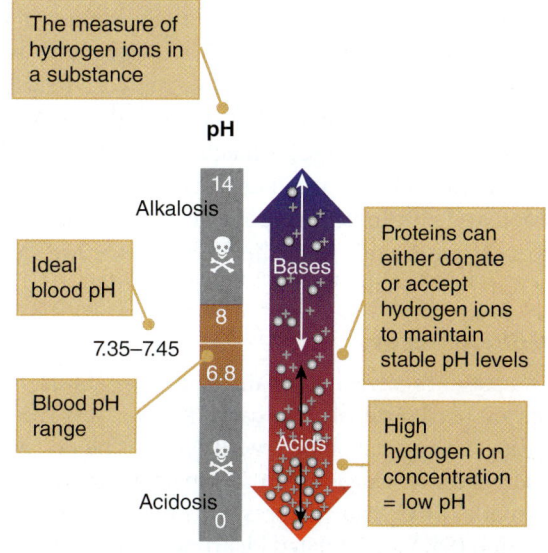

FIGURE 2.11 pH Scale in Relation to Hydrogen Ion Concentration

understand the underlying physiological processes and/or exogenous causes that occur in acid–base disorders to accurately diagnose and determine therapy regarding fluids, PN, and electrolyte managements.

Most hydrogen ions originate as a byproduct or end product of cellular metabolism, although a small amount of acidic substances enter the body via ingested food. Together, carbohydrates and fats produce approximately 15,000 mmol of CO_2, which forms carbonic acid when combined with water. Also, protein metabolism produces 50 to 100 mEq/day of noncarbonic acid.[27] Without tight regulation, progressive accumulation of acids can be detrimental. Hydrogen ion regulation within the body involves three steps: (1) chemical buffering via intracellular and extracellular mechanisms; (2) control of partial pressure of carbon dioxide in blood by changes in rate of alveolar ventilation; and (3) control of plasma bicarbonate concentration by alterations in renal H^+ excretion.

Chemical Buffers (1): Buffering systems prevent large changes in hydrogen ion concentration and are the first line of defense, occurring immediately to resist changes in pH. In general, the buffering systems consist of weak acid and base pairs that can take up or release hydrogen ions to minimize changes in free concentration. The carbonic acid/bicarbonate (H_2CO_3/HCO_3^-) system is the principal buffer system in the body, while the others (proteins, phosphate, and hemoglobin) also contribute to maintain a normal pH.

Lungs (2): The primary role of the lungs in maintaining acid–base balance is to control the pressure exerted by dissolved CO_2 gas in the blood. Among all chemicals impacting respiration, CO_2 is considered the most powerful respiratory stimulant. The rate and depth of ventilation can both be changed to allow diet and cellular metabolism to generate CO_2. Within minutes of acid–base disturbances, the rate and depth of ventilation begins to be compensated. As a result, any condition that impairs respiratory system functioning can lead to acid–base imbalances.

Kidneys (3): Alterations in renal hydrogen ion excretion is the last and slowest mechanism used to maintain acid–base balance within the body. Both the reabsorption of filtered bicarbonate and the excretion of hydrogen ions, which is produced daily from protein metabolism, work to achieve this balance. The acid–base regulatory mechanism of the kidneys is unique from the prior mechanisms because the kidneys have the ability to regulate alkaline substances in the blood and eliminate metabolic acids (organic acids, other than carbonic acid) from the body. **Figure 2.12** outlines the renal and respiratory acid–base regulation.

Arterial Blood Gases

To assess a patient's oxygenation and acid–base status, blood gas values are used. **Arterial blood gases (ABGs)** assess the lung's ability to oxygenate blood, while venous blood gases (VBGs) reflect tissue oxygenation. The partial pressure of carbon dioxide (PCO_2), partial pressure of oxygen (PO_2), oxygen saturation (SaO_2), calculated bicarbonate, pH, and base excess are the most common blood gas measurements used.

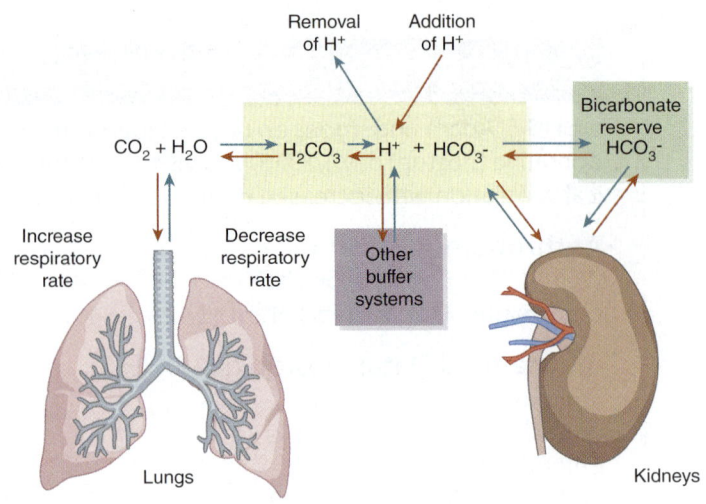

FIGURE 2.12 Renal and Respiratory Acid-Base Regulation

Normal values are listed in the **Table 2.4**. The normal ranges of these measurements differ for ABGs and VBGs, and evaluations also differ in aspects of ventilation and perfusion.

The $PaCO_2$ reflects the lung's ability to excrete carbon dioxide. Changes in $PaCO_2$ are associated with respiratory processes that can cause acid–base disorders. Because $PaCO_2$ is the acid component of the carbonic acid/bicarbonate buffer system, an increase in $PaCO_2$ reflects an acidosis and a decrease in $PaCO_2$ reflects an alkalosis. PaO_2 reflects hemoglobin's ability to carry oxygen, and is directly related to hemoglobin saturated with oxygen (SaO_2). When the partial pressure of oxygen is high, oxygen saturation of the blood is also high, and vice versa.

Changes in bicarbonate are associated with metabolic processes that can lead to acid–base disorders. Either calculated bicarbonate reported in blood gas or serum bicarbonate can be used to evaluate acid–base status. Because

TABLE 2.4 REFERENCE RANGE FOR BLOOD GAS VALUES

Blood Gas Values for Acid–Base Balance		
Laboratory Test	Normal Arterial	Normal Mixed Venous
pH	7.35-7.45	7.33-7.43
PCO_2	35-45 mm Hg	41-51 mm Hg
PO_2	80-100 mm Hg	35-40 mm Hg
HCO_3^-	22-26 mEq/L	24-28 mEq/L
O_2 saturation	>95%	70-75%
Base excess	−2 to +2	0 to +4

bicarbonate is the base component of the carbonic acid/bicarbonate buffer system, an increase in serum or calculated bicarbonate reflects an alkalosis, and a decrease reflects an acidosis. Base excess is another value that can be calculated and estimates the metabolic component of acid–base disorder. An increase in base excess occurs a metabolic alkalosis, while base deficit occurs in metabolic acidosis.

Acid–base Disorders

Acid–base disorders can be assessed using a systematic approach to avoid misdiagnosis and inappropriate treatment. The following steps can be useful for adequate evaluation for clinicians:

1. Use pH value to determine whether patient is acidemic (pH <7.4) or alkalemic (pH >7.4). A pH of 7.4 should not be excluded from assessment because compensation or a mixed acid–base disorder could contribute to a normal pH range.
2. Assess $PaCO_2$ to determine respiratory status. Elevated $PaCO_2$ indicates respiratory acidosis, while low $PaCO_2$ indicates respiratory alkalosis. (**Table 2.5** highlights the characteristics of primary acid–base imbalances.)
3. Assess HCO_3^- to determine metabolic status. Elevated HCO_3^- indicates metabolic alkalosis, while low HCO_3^- indicates metabolic acidosis.
4. Calculate the anion gap to determine the presence of metabolic acidosis. The anion gap can be calculated using the equation below (normal range is 8-16 mEq/L). Calculating anion gap is critical to assess the etiology of acid–base and determine appropriate treatment:

$$\text{Anion gap} = Na^+ - (Cl^- + HCO_3^-)$$

5. Determine whether the acid–base disorder is an acute or chronic condition and assess whether the acid–base disorder is appropriately compensated. If appropriate compensation is not evident, a mixed acid–base disorder may be present.

Respiratory acidosis is characterized by a low pH, high $PaCO_2$, and a variable increase in plasma HCO_3^- concentration. This disorder is most commonly caused by decreased effective alveolar ventilation and not an increase in carbon dioxide production. When there is interference in the ventilation at any step, hypoventilation can occur. In patients with severely impaired CO_2 excretion and/or life-threatening hypoxemia, adequate oxygenation should be provided. The most common causes include central nervous system depression, neuromuscular disorders, chronic obstructive pulmonary disease, and interstitial pulmonary disease. The underlying cause should be treated accordingly (bronchodilators and steroids, adjustment of ventilation, etc.), with sodium bicarbonate reserved for treatment of severely acidotic patients (pH <7.15).

Respiratory alkalosis is characterized by a high pH, low $PaCO_2$, and a variable decrease in plasma HCO_3^- concentration. This often occurs with increased effective alveolar ventilation beyond the level needed to eliminate metabolically produced CO_2, leading to hyperventilation. Common causes of respiratory alkalosis include pulmonary disease, hypoxemia, and increased central stimulation of respiration. See **Table 2.6** for more a complete list of the

TABLE 2.5 CHARACTERISTICS OF PRIMARY ACID–BASE IMBALANCES

Disorder	pH	Primary Disturbance	Compensatory Response
Metabolic Acidosis	Low	Low HCO_3^-	Low $PaCO_2$
Metabolic Alkalosis	High	High HCO_3^-	High $PaCO_2$
Respiratory Acidosis	Low	High $PaCO_2$	High HCO_3^-
Respiratory Alkalosis	High	Low $PaCO_2$	Low HCO_3^-

Data from Charney P. Ch.7: Clinical: Water, Electrolytes, and Acid-Base Balance. In *Krause's Food & the Nutrition Care Process*. 13th ed. St. Louis, Missouri: Elsevier Saunders; 2012:188.

TABLE 2.6 CAUSES OF RESPIRATORY ACID–BASE DISORDERS

Respiratory Acidosis	Respiratory Alkalosis
• Acute respiratory distress syndrome (ARDS)	• Altitudes (high)
• Aspiration	• Anemia (severe)
• Asthma	• Anxiety
• Cardiac arrest	• Asthma
• Central depression of respiration	• Brain tumor
• Chronic obstructive pulmonary disease (COPD)	• Central stimulation of respiration
• Drugs (opioids, anesthetics, sedatives)	• Drugs (catecholamines, salicylates)
• Head injury	• Fever
• Hypoventilation	• Head trauma
• Hypoxemia	• Hyperventilation
• Multiple sclerosis	• Hypoxemia
• Perfusion abnormalities	• Pain
• Parenteral nutrition	• Peripheral stimulation of respiration
• Pulmonary abnormalities, such as pulmonary edema and severe pulmonary embolism	• Pregnancy
• Sleep apnea	• Pulmonary issues, such as pulmonary edema and pulmonary embolism
• Stroke	• Pneumonia
	• Vascular accident

Modified from Langley G, Tajchman S. *A.S.P.E.N. Adult Nutrition Support Core Curriculum Chapter 7: Fluids, Electrolytes, and Acid-Base Disorders*. 2nd ed. Washington DC: American Society for Parenteral and Enteral Nutrition; 2012:116.

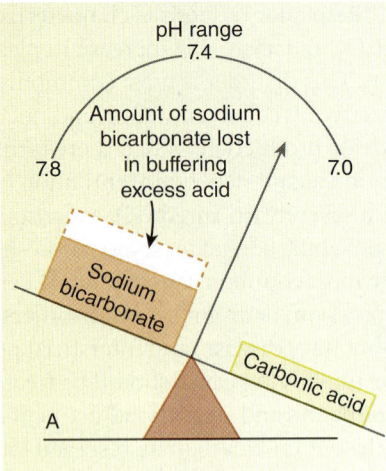 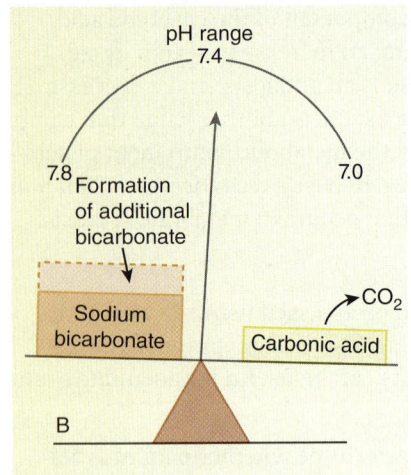

FIGURE 2.13 Metabolic Acidosis: Bicarbonate and Carbonic Acid Imbalance

causes of respiratory acid–base imbalances. For more information on respiratory disorders and nutritional therapy, please refer to Chapter 16, *Nutrition in Pulmonary Disease*.

Metabolic acidosis is characterized by a low pH, a low HCO_3^- concentration, and a compensatory hyperventilation that contributes to a decreased $PaCO_2$. **Figure 2.13** illustrates bicarbonate and carbonic acid imbalance in metabolic acidosis and compensation. This condition can result from either the inability of kidneys to excrete the dietary hydrogen ion load or an increase in hydrogen ion generation due to an addition of hydrogen ions or a loss of bicarbonate. Calculating the anion gap with the equation listed above can assist in the diagnosis of metabolic acidosis. The anion gap (approximately 8-16 mEq/L) represents the unmeasured serum ions including proteins, phosphate, sulfate, and organic ions.[28] In particular, albumin accounts for a large portion of unmeasured serum anions. For every decrease in 1 g/dL in serum albumin, the anion gap increases by approximately 2.5 mEq/L.[10] Calculating the anion gap allows clinicians to differentiate between normal anion gap acidosis or elevated anion gap acidosis.

Normal anion-gap acidosis (anion gap 8-16 mEq/L) occurs when there is milliequivalent-for-milliequivalent replacement of extracellular bicarbonate by chloride. As a result, there is a normal anion gap because the sum remains constant for the major measured anions. The most common causes of this disorder, also known as hyperchloremic metabolic acidosis, include increased GI or renal bicarbonate loss. *High anion-gap metabolic acidosis* (anion gap >25 mEq/L) is a result of metabolic acidosis associated with accumulation of unmeasured anions. This condition is most commonly caused by renal failure to excrete acid, diabetic ketoacidosis, and lactic acidosis from shock. Hypovolemia must be addressed with expansion of extracellular volume and IV insulin infusion should be administered to stop production of ketoacids. Once volume is replenished and insulin is administered, potassium should be replaced. **Table 2.7** outlines the causes of normal and increased anion gap metabolic acidosis.

Metabolic alkalosis is characterized by a high pH, a high bicarbonate concentration, and compensatory

TABLE 2.7 CAUSES OF METABOLIC ACIDOSIS

Normal Anion Gap	Increased Anion Gap
Gastrointestinal loss of HCO_3^- • Anion-exchange resins • Diarrhea • Ingestion of calcium or magnesium chloride • Obstructed ileal loop • Pancreatic fistula	Increased production of endogenous acid
Ingestions • Ammonium chloride • Parenteral nutrition (chloride salts) • Sulfur	Inborn errors of metabolism • Ketoacidosis • Lactic acidosis
Renal loss of HCO_3^- • Carbonic anhydrase inhibitors • Hypoaldosteronism • Hyperparathyroidism • Renal tubular acidosis	Failure to excrete acids • Ingestion of exogenous acid • Salicyclates, methanol, ethanol • Renal failure

Modified from Langley G, Tajchman S. *A.S.P.E.N. Adult Nutrition Support Core Curriculum Chapter 7: Fluids, Electrolytes, and Acid-Base Disorders*. 2nd ed. Washington DC: American Society for Parenteral and Enteral Nutrition; 2012:116.

hypoventilation that contribute to an increased $PaCO_2$. This disorder is reported in approximately 33% to 55% of hospitalized patients with acid–base disturbances.[29] The most common causes of this disorder include loss of gastric acid from vomiting or nasogastric suction and loss of intravascular volume and chloride from diuretic use. In the clinical setting, the most common cause is overtreatment of metabolic acidosis with bicarbonate or an excess of acetate in PN, which becomes metabolized to bicarbonate. Hypokalemia in patients can cause a transcellular shift of hydrogen ions, which can also contribute to the development of metabolic alkalosis. Normally, the kidneys can correct this disorder by excreting the excess bicarbonate in urine. Therefore, maintenance of metabolic alkalosis indicates that patients may have some degree of impairment in renal bicarbonate excretion. Urine chloride concentration can be used to classify metabolic alkalosis into volume mediated (saline responsive) and volume independent (saline resistant) and predict which patients will respond to volume replacement.

Saline-responsive metabolic alkalosis (urine chloride <10 mEq/L) is the most common metabolic alkalosis. To treat this disorder, administration of normal saline is recommended to reverse the increase in bicarbonate reabsorption that maintains alkalosis. While sufficient repletion of sodium chloride can typically normalize bicarbonate concentration, metabolic alkalosis will not be reversed if associated with hypokalemia. Potassium chloride is required to correct this underlying disorder. *Saline resistant metabolic alkalosis* (urine chloride >10 mEq/L) is most frequently associated with hyperaldosteronism. Treatment of this disorder requires first addressing the underlying cause of mineralocorticoid excess. When hypokalemia is present with this disorder in primary hyperaldosteronism, clinicians should treat this deficiency with aggressive potassium repletion. **Table 2.8** outlines common causes of saline-responsive and saline-resistant metabolic alkalosis.

Mixed acid–base disorders occur when patients have more than one acid–base disturbance occurring simultaneously. To diagnose a mixed acid–base disorder, clinicians must have an understanding of the extent of renal and respiratory compensations for each of the acid–base disturbances. When a set of blood gases does not fall within the range of expected responses for a simple acid–base disturbance, then clinicians should suspect that a mixed disorder exists. The most common mixed disorders include mixed respiratory acidosis and metabolic acidosis; mixed respiratory alkalosis and metabolic alkalosis; mixed metabolic acidosis and respiratory alkalosis; and mixed metabolic alkalosis and respiratory acidosis. If patients present with normal pH and alterations in pCO_2 and plasma bicarbonate, then clinicians should expect that a mixed acid–base disorder is present.

> **CORE CONCEPT 4**
>
> Fluid, electrolyte, and acid–base imbalances can lead to serious complications ranging from metabolic and gastrointestinal problems to cardiovascular, respiratory, and neurological concerns, each requiring careful evaluation, monitoring, and treatment.

Endocrine Function: Glucose and Glycosylated Hemoglobin

Glucose values are important in screening and diagnosing endocrine disorders and in monitoring patients with acute stress and critical illness. Evaluating trends in glucose measures is essential to determine glucose tolerance and to prevent adverse and potentially fatal consequences that may occur in patients experiencing abnormal glucose values.

Blood glucose, the measure of glucose in the plasma, is a short-term measure of glycemic response and glucose tolerance. Normal *fasting blood glucose* values range from 70 to 99 mg/dL or 3.9 to 5.5 mmol/L, while fasting blood glucose >100 mg/dL suggests impaired glucose metabolism. Diagnostic criteria for diabetes mellitus (DM) include the following: fasting plasma glucose ≥126 mg/dL (7.0 mmol/L), 2-hour postprandial plasma glucose ≥200 mg/dL (11.1 mmol/L), or classic symptoms of hyperglycemia or hyperglycemic crises with random plasma glucose ≥200 mg/dL.[30] Clinicians can use glucose testing to screen and diagnose patients, as well as to monitor patients receiving total PN. **Figure 2.14** illustrates the comparison of blood glucose levels in nondiabetic and diabetic individuals after a glucose tolerance test.

Urine glucose, although not a diagnostic criteria, is also abnormal in patients with DM. Normal urine glucose tests should be negative, while patients with DM may present with

TABLE 2.8 CAUSES OF METABOLIC ALKALOSIS

Saline-Responsive (Urine Chloride <10 mEq/L)	Saline-Resistant (Urine Chloride >10 mEq/L)
• Diuretic therapy • Excessive bicarbonate administration • Gastrointestinal loss • Nasogastric suction • Rapid correction of hypocapnia • Renal loss • Vomiting	• Cushing's syndrome • Excess mineralocorticoids • Excessive licorice ingestion • Hyperaldosteronism • Profound potassium depletion

Modified from Langley G, Tajchman S. *A.S.P.E.N. Adult Nutrition Support Core Curriculum Chapter 7: Fluids, Electrolytes, and Acid-Base Disorders.* 2nd ed. Washington DC: American Society for Parenteral and Enteral Nutrition; 2012:116.

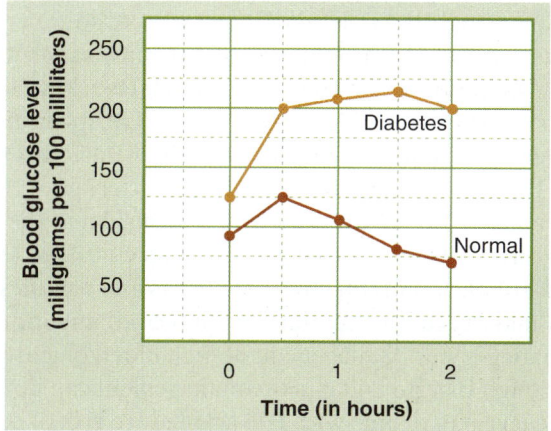

FIGURE 2.14 Comparison of Blood Glucose levels of a Non-Diabetic and Diabetic After a Glucose Tolerance Test

levels of 2 to 10 g/dL. A positive urine glucose result (glucosuria) is rarely found in benign conditions. Treatment includes managing DM and improving hydration status, due to the loss of water that follows when glucose is present in urine.

Urine ketones should be tested if glucose levels are elevated in patients during periods of illness or stress. For patients with DM, urine ketones should be tested if blood glucose is consistently greater than 300 mg/dL. In healthy nondiabetic patients, urine ketones should be negative. Uncontrolled DM is the most common cause of positive urine ketones. Other potential causes include fever, anorexia, certain GI disturbances, persistent vomiting, cachexia, fasting, and starvation. Positive urine ketones represent a condition that can lead to diabetic ketoacidosis, resulting in dehydration and electrolyte imbalances due to osmotic diuresis. Without immediate treatment of diabetic ketoacidosis, this condition can be fatal. Treatment includes assessment and treatment of severe hyperglycemia with IV fluids, insulin, and electrolytes. Doses of supplemental insulin are required until metabolic stability returns.

Glycosylated hemoglobin (HbA1c) is a measure of the percentage of glucose bound to hemoglobin in red blood cells. The subfraction of HbA1c in hemoglobin has a unique chemical structure that causes nonenzymatic glycation at the amino-terminal valines of the beta chains of hemoglobin A. As the lifespan of red blood cells is approximately 3 months, HbA1c is directly related to the average blood glucose levels during this length of time. A 1% change in HbA1c means a change in plasma glucose by approximately 35 mg/dL.[32] Unlike blood glucose levels, an HbA1c test does not reflect recent changes, making it a useful measure to differentiate between short-term hyperglycemia in individuals under stress or those with DM. HbA1c has been added to the diagnostic criteria for DM. In adults with normal blood glucose control, HbA1c values range from 4.3% to 5.8%.[33] **Table 2.9** correlates HbA1c with average blood glucose levels.

Diagnosis of DM is confirmed when an initial value is followed up with a repeat HbA1c ≥6.5% or plasma glucose ≥200 mg/dL. Because HbA1c is related to the lifespan of the erythrocyte, conditions that increase or decrease red blood cell turnover may alter results. For example, anemias which prolong erythrocyte turnover can lead to falsely elevated HbA1c levels. Conversely, conditions that increase erythrocyte production and turnover such as such as gestational diabetes can lead to falsely low HbA1c. Because of this, HbA1c is not a useful diagnostic indicator after the first few months of pregnancy. In addition to using HbA1c as a component of diagnostic criteria, HbA1c and trends in blood glucose levels are considered the best indicators of glycemic control in patients with DM. Clinicians can interpret trends in these levels and use these values to make recommendations for improved nutrition and DM management. Management of high blood glucose levels through insulin and glucose management can decrease HbA1c levels in people with DM and reduce risk of comorbidities associated with DM.

TABLE 2.9 HEMOGLOBIN A1C AND ESTIMATED EQUIVALENT AVERAGE BLOOD GLUCOSE[31]

Hemoglobin A1c	Mean Blood Glucose
6%	126 mg/dL
7%	154 mg/dL
8%	183 mg/dL
9%	212 mg/dL
10%	240 mg/dL
11%	269 mg/dL
12%	298 mg/dL

Data from Nathan DM, Kuenen J, Borg R, Zheng H, Schoenfeld D, Heine RJ. A1c-Derived Average Glucose Study Group. Translating the A1C assay into estimated average glucose values. *Diabetes Care*. 2008;31:1473–1478.

Hypoglycemia or low blood glucose can be caused by glycogen storage disease, liver disease, renal insufficiency, alcohol, abrupt PN cessation, cancer, or prolonged exercise. HbA1c is frequently used to assess for hypoglycemia, with values of 4.3% to 5.8% defining hypoglycemia for nondiabetic patients. Target HbA1c values for patients with DM range from 6.5% to 8% according to a patient's history of diabetes, hypoglycemia episodes, and diabetes-related health complications.[30]

Hyperglycemia is defined as blood glucose levels higher than the normal range. Mild hyperglycemia can result from uncontrolled diabetes, pancreatitis/pancreatic insufficiency, obesity, acute stress, or cirrhosis. Medications including thiazide and loop diuretics can cause mild hyperglycemia. Severe hyperglycemia (>400 mg/dL) is more commonly caused by diabetic ketoacidosis due to insulin deficiency and hyperosmolar hyperglycemic nonketotic dehydration. Common symptoms of severe hyperglycemia include increased urine output, glucosuria, hypernatremia, and headaches. Treatment of severe hyperglycemia requires replacement of fluids and electrolytes and insulin administration. See Chapter 9, *Nutrition in Diabetes Mellitus* for further discussion of blood glucose, HbA1c, and diabetes management.

Protein Assessment

Adequate protein in the body is essential for cellular growth and metabolism. Despite the large amount of protein in muscle and viscera, the body strives to protect it from being used as an energy source by drawing primarily

CASE STUDY REVISITED

It is now postoperative day 6/HD 12 and Adam remains in the ICU. He is currently receiving enteral nutrition support since postop day 3, which provides him with 1,700 calories and 100 g protein.

Anthropometric Data:
Weight: 76 kg (167 lbs)
Last Weight: 77 kg (169 lbs) postop day 1/HD 7
Admit weight 75 kg (165 lbs)

Biochemical Data:
Albumin 2.1 g/dL (3.5-5.0 g/dL)
Prealbumin 14 g/dL (17-36 g/dL)
Urine urea nitrogen (UUN) 10 g/24 hours

Questions

1. How do you interpret Adam's current albumin and prealbumin levels? What information does this provide to your assessment of Adam's nutritional status?
2. Calculate Adam's nitrogen balance. Is he in positive or negative nitrogen balance?
3. Based on this information, how would you assess Adam's current nutrition plan?
4. What biochemical indices can you monitor to further assess nutritional adequacy?

---

from fat and glycogen stores. When the body experiences acute or chronic metabolic stress, protein from muscle may be drawn to meet energy needs. Although no single laboratory value can determine the precise protein status of a patient, a combination of measures can provide a more complete picture of protein status, including anthropometric, dietary, physical, and biochemical findings. Clinicians must interpret these measures in combination to adequately assess protein status and monitor and treat patients according to the etiology and severity of illness. Biochemical assessment of protein focuses on evaluation from two compartments: visceral and somatic proteins. Visceral proteins consist of approximately 25% of total body protein and include non-muscular protein in organs, structural components, serum proteins, and blood cells. Somatic proteins make up the other 75% of total body protein within skeletal muscle.

Total serum protein measures the total amount of protein in the blood, including albumin and globulin (alpha-1, alpha-2, and beta) levels. Normal total serum protein levels range from 6.4 to 8.3 g/dL, while abnormalities are likely due to change in volume of plasma fluid or change in concentration of one or more plasma proteins. A low total serum protein level can result from decreased production or increased protein loss. Some common causes of hypoproteinemia include liver disorders, kidney disorders, and GI malabsorption disorders (such as celiac disease or inflammatory bowel disease). Low total protein levels are also found in patients with severe malnutrition, but clinicians must assess other possible factors contributing to low protein levels before determining appropriate treatment. In contrast, high total protein levels or hyperproteinemia can result from chronic inflammation or infection including viral hepatitis or human immunodeficiency virus (HIV). Bone marrow disorders such as multiple myeloma may cause hyperproteinemia. Medications, inflammation, infection, prolonged bed rest, chronic illness, and pregnancy can also impact total serum protein levels. If patients have abnormal total serum protein levels, clinicians must further assess serum globulin and serum albumin levels to evaluate etiology and determine appropriate nutrition therapy.

Visceral Proteins

Visceral protein indirectly measures protein stores by assessing the proteins made by the viscera, namely, organs (primarily the liver). Because serum protein is affected by the amount of amino acids needed for protein synthesis in the liver, a change in serum proteins is consistent with a change in visceral protein status. When acute illness or trauma causes inflammatory and/or metabolic stress, hormones and cell-mediated responses trigger muscle breakdown. In response to inflammation, **acute-phase proteins** respond by either increasing (positive acute-phase proteins) or decreasing (negative acute-phase proteins). As a result, protein status can be difficult to assess in acutely ill patients because these acute-phase proteins do not accurately reflect changes in protein status. Inflammation identified by serum visceral protein can contribute to several nutrition-related issues as inflammation contributes to net protein loss from catabolism and can induce anorexia. Clinicians must take into account the differences in specificity, sensitivity, and reliability of each visceral protein measurement when assessing and treating patients with acute, stress-related illnesses.

Positive acute-phase proteins such as C-reactive protein, ferritin, and ceruloplasmin increase during inflammation. *C-reactive protein (CRP)* is a nonspecific inflammatory biomarker and a normal serum CRP level is less than 1 mg/dL. CRP increases as transport protein levels (such as prealbumin and albumin) decrease. Although the exact function of CRP is unclear, it increases during the initial stage of acute hypermetabolic stress, which is usually within 4 to 6 hours of surgery or other trauma. Generally, a higher CRP indicates increased nutritional risk.

Negative acute-phase proteins include serum albumin, prealbumin, retinal binding protein, and transferrin. These **constitutive** (or constantly active) transport proteins are synthesized in the liver and decrease during acute-inflammatory stress, injury, or illness.

Albumin accounts for approximately 60% of total serum proteins, and is mostly found in skin, muscle, and organs. Normal serum albumin levels range from 3.5 to 5.0 g/dL. Albumin serves many important functions in the body, including transport and vascular fluid and electrolyte balance. Major blood constituents, hormones, enzymes, medications, minerals, ions, fatty acids, and metabolites are all transported via albumin. Maintenance of colloidal osmotic pressure also requires albumin, with albumin making up approximately 80% of colloidal osmotic pressure of the plasma. Serum albumin is a biomarker that has been widely used in hospital settings and is often correlated with outcomes and mortality.[34,35] However, albumin has been found to be a poor indicator of nutrition support adequacy because proteolysis occurs despite nutrition provision. The half-life of albumin is 18 to 21 days, which decreases albumin's sensitivity to short-term changes in protein status or short-term nutrition therapy to improve protein status.

Several non-dietary factors can alter serum albumin levels, with decreased levels commonly due to changes in fluid distribution, decreased synthesis, or increased degradation of albumin. Acute stress and inflammatory response decrease serum albumin levels by altering at least one of the factors listed above. Specifically, albumin loss occurs with trauma such as burn injuries, nephritic syndrome, protein-losing enteropathy, and cirrhosis. Hypoalbuminemia may also occur with surgery, infection, multiple myeloma, acute or chronic inflammation, rheumatoid arthritis, and aging. Liver disease, cancer, and malabsorption can also decrease albumin levels. Hydration status also affects serum albumin levels because water in the plasma shifts between the interstitial compartment if patients are overhydrated (leading to decreased albumin) or dehydrated (leading to increased albumin).

Albumin levels also vary according to the specific types of malnutrition, **kwashiorkor** or **marasmus**. In patients with marasmus, associated with severe caloric depletion, the body conserves visceral protein levels. In this condition, weight may be less than or equal to 80% of normal body weight, while albumin levels remain within reference range.[36] In contrast, in patients with kwashiorkor, which is associated with protein degradation with or without caloric deficit, visceral protein stores become depleted. As a result, low albumin levels may be present, but weight may be normal or elevated due to edema (**Figure 2.15**).

Increased albumin levels (hyperalbuminemia) can result from dehydration and exogenous albumin administration. Anabolic hormones and corticoid steroids can also raise albumin levels higher than normal. Clinicians must interpret changes in albumin level with caution, recognizing that low albumin is likely an indicator of stress or inflammation and not overall protein status.

Prealbumin (PAB), also called transthyretin, is a hepatic protein transported in the serum bound to retinol-binding protein and vitamin A. Normal PAB levels range from 17 to 36 g/dL (177-363 mg/L). Prealbumin is responsible for transporting the thyroid hormones (triiodothyronine and thyroxine) and T_4-binding globulin. It is synthesized in the liver and is renally excreted, although it is not influenced by hydration status. Because PAB has a relatively short half-life of 2 to 3 days, clinicians may use levels as a possible indicator of protein status. As with albumin, serum PAB levels decrease with illness, infection, trauma, burns, surgery, and metabolic stress. Liver disorders such as hepatitis or cirrhosis, malabsorption, and hyperthyroidism may also cause low PAB levels. Serum PAB also decreases in the presence of zinc

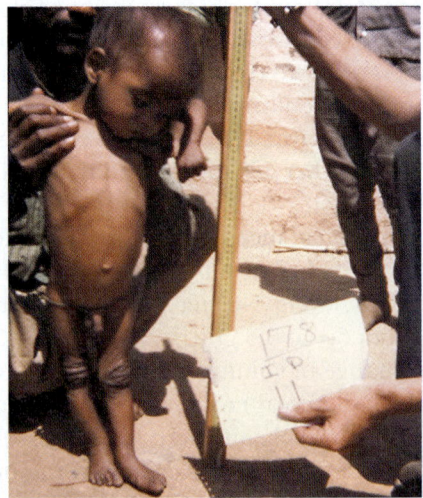

FIGURE 2.15 Kwashiorkor Extremity edema and a bloated abdomen are common in kwashiorkor.
Courtesy of CDC/Dr. Lyle Conrad.

deficiency because zinc is needed for synthesis and secretion of PAB in the liver. Clinicians must consider zinc status from diet intake and medical history and inflammation when interpreting low serum PAB levels.

PAB levels can be maintained in uncomplicated malnutrition and decreased in well-nourished individuals who have undergone recent stress or trauma. Also, when inflammatory stress causes a large drop in levels of PAB, its use as an indicator of nutritional status despite aggressive nutrition support is compromised. As a result, PAB may be assessed simultaneously with CRP. If CRP is also high, then PAB is not a reliable indicator of nutrition status. Other conditions can also increase PAB levels. Pregnancy may increase serum levels because changes in estrogen levels may stimulate PAB synthesis. Nephrotic syndrome can also increase PAB levels because proteinuria and hypoproteinemia may be present. With increased PAB synthesis, a disproportionate percentage of PAB exists in blood while other proteins take longer to produce. Hodgkin's disease and high doses of steroids can also increase serum PAB by stimulating PAB synthesis. Clinicians must take into account the etiology of PAB levels to assess and monitor the condition appropriately.

Retinol-binding protein (RBP) is an acute-phase protein produced in the liver whose main function is to transport vitamin A in the blood. RBP, whose normal levels range from 2.7 to 7.6 mg/dL, is considered one of the most sensitive indicators of protein status because of its short half-life (10-12 hours). RBP is a small protein that does not pass through the renal glomerulus because it circulates bound to PAB. Once RBP releases retinol in peripheral tissue, its affinity to PAB decreases and causes the PAB-RBP complex to dissociate. RBP is then filtered by the glomerulus and catabolized in the renal tubule.

As with the other negative acute-phase proteins, RBP decreases in the presence of inflammatory stress. Although a low RBP concentration is common in uncomplicated calorie malnutrition, RBP levels are not as affected by inflammatory stress as albumin, transferrin, or PAB in acutely stressed patients. Serum RBP is also low in patients with hyperthyroidism, liver failure, cystic fibrosis, vitamin A deficiency, and zinc deficiency. Therefore, when a patient has vitamin A deficiency, RBP cannot reliably assess protein status until the deficiency is addressed. Patients with renal failure are likely to have high serum RBP because it is not catabolized by the renal tubules. Therefore, RBP cannot accurately measure protein-energy status in patients with renal insufficiency.

Transferrin is a globulin protein that transports iron in blood to bone marrow for hemoglobin production. Normal serum transferrin levels range from 200 to 400 mg/dL. Serum transferrin can be measured directly or derived from total iron binding capacity (TIBC):

$$\text{Transferrin} = 0.8 \, (\text{TIBC}) - 43$$

Serum transferrin levels are most strongly affected by the size of the iron storage pool. Transferrin levels increase when iron stores are depleted to accommodate the need for increased levels of transport. High transferrin levels are common in iron-deficiency anemia and dehydration. In contrast, serum transferrin levels can decrease due to impaired synthesis, which is often caused by infection, fever, malignancies, collagen vascular disease, liver disease, cirrhosis, and malnutrition. Although transferrin has a shorter half-life (8-10 days) than albumin, it does not respond fast enough to changes in intake to be a useful indicator of protein status in acute care patients. Transferrin is therefore not a specific indicator for malnutrition and not a valid measure for iron-deficiency anemia in acute illness.

CORE CONCEPT 5

Visceral proteins can be altered by acute and chronic metabolic stress, making them more accurate indicators of inflammation than indicators of nutritional status.

PRACTICE POINT

During acute stress, exogenous protein alone will not attenuate loss of endogenous protein.

Somatic Proteins

Similar to assessment of visceral proteins, assessment of somatic proteins (in skeletal muscle) can provide clinicians with a more in-depth understanding of protein status and requirements, while recognizing how certain conditions may influence interpretation of these values.

Nitrogen balance occurs when nitrogen input (Nin) or intake (oral, enteral, or parenteral) is equal to nitrogen output (Nout) or excretion (urinary, fecal, or wound drainage). Because nitrogen is a key component of protein, its measure is used to assess protein status in patients. Urine urea nitrogen (UUN) is the primary biochemical measure used to calculate Nout. It is the end product of protein breakdown in the body and signifies protein catabolism. One gram (g) of nitrogen loss is thought to equal about 30 g of lean tissue loss. The extent of protein breakdown can be categorized into mild catabolism (5-10 g UUN), moderate catabolism (10-15 g UUN), and severe catabolism (>15 g UUN).[36] To calculate nitrogen balance (Nbal) a 24 hour urine collection is needed for analysis of UUN. Because urea nitrogen only represents 85% of total urine nitrogen (TUN), with ammonia being the other significant contributor of nitrogen in the urine, a correction factor of 0.85 is applied. In addition, a factor of 2-4 g of nitrogen is added to Nout to represent non-urinary nitrogen losses that occur in sweat, stool, and wound exudate, which can also vary based on the output of these variables. To calculate Nin, a 24-hour dietary intake of protein is determined.

Total protein intake is converted to g of nitrogen using a factor of 6.25 (1 g nitrogen = 6.25 g protein). The following equation is used to calculate Nbal:

$$Nbal = Nin - Nout$$

$$Nbal = \text{Dietary protein intake}/6.25 \text{ g Nitrogen} - [(UUN/0.85) + 2]$$

Sample Calculation: Protein intake = 94 g protein; UUN = 13 g/24 hours; Non-urinary nitrogen losses = 2 g/24 hours

$$Nbal = 94/6.25 - [(13/0.85) + 2]$$
$$Nbal = 15 - 17$$
$$Nbal = -2 \text{ g nitrogen}$$

For patients with a dietary intake of 94 g protein and a UUN of 13 g/24 hours, the Nbal would be negative by 2 g, meaning they are in negative nitrogen balance. Protein intake would have to be increased by 2 g nitrogen (or 12.5 g protein) to reach balance. Because the goal for anabolism requires the patient be positive by 2-4 g nitrogen an additional 12-25 g of protein may be added to their protein intake goal.

Nitrogen balance can be used for critically ill patients receiving nutrition support. If patients have a negative nitrogen balance, recommendations typically include increasing protein and caloric intake via diet, enteral, or parenteral nutrition. Nitrogen balance is imprecise as an indicator of protein status in acute care patients because it cannot accurately reflect protein anabolism and catabolism. True protein status can be better described by protein turnover or flux, which requires labeled protein (stable isotope) to measure protein synthesis and breakdown. This is done primarily as part of a research protocol as opposed to routine protein assessment. A valid 24-hour urine collection can be inconvenient and tedious to collect unless a patient has a catheter. Urine collection also fails to take into account nitrogen losses from wounds, burns, diarrhea, and vomiting. Equally confounding is the use of a factor of 0.85 to determine TUN from UUN, which is flawed in patients with variable excretion of ammonia, as is true during trauma, renal disease, and liver failure. If nitrogen balance is used to estimate protein status in critically ill patients or those with conditions that alter the nitrogen content of urine, clinicians must recognize the limitations of this UUN as a measure of nitrogen output. When possible, TUN should be measured; however, this is often not available in a clinical setting.

Creatinine is another value used to assess somatic protein status in patients. It is formed from muscle creatine phosphate at a constant daily rate. Creatine is formed from amino acids glycine and arginine with addition of a methyl group from the folate and vitamin B_{12}–dependent methionine-S-adenosylmethionine (SAM)-homocysteine cycle. Creatine phosphate, which is found almost exclusively in muscle, works as a high-energy phosphate buffer by providing a constant supply of ATP for muscle contractions. Through an irreversible, nonenzymatic reaction, some creatine phosphate is converted to creatinine during dephosphorylation. While creatinine is not stored in muscle and has no specific biologic function, it is continuously cleared from muscle and excreted by the kidneys. As a result, daily urine output of creatinine has been found to correlate with total muscle mass.

Although urinary creatinine can be effective in assessing somatic protein status in some patients, this indicator is confounded by many variables. First, dietary creatinine cannot be distinguished from endogenously produced creatinine in the body. As a result, the size of the somatic muscle protein pool is directly proportional to the amount of creatinine excreted only when a patient is following a meat-restricted diet. This factor accounts for the higher serum levels and larger amounts of creatinine excreted in men in comparison to women and among those with greater muscular development than those with less muscle.

Creatinine height index (CHI) is often calculated to take into account height and sex, by expressing creatinine excretion rate as a percentage of a standard value. A calculated CHI >80% is considered normal; 60% to 80% suggests mild skeletal muscle depletion; 40% to 60% suggests moderate skeletal muscle depletion; and <40% suggests severe skeletal muscle depletion.[37] CHI is calculated using the following equation:

$$CHI = \text{Actual 24-hour urine creatinine (mg)} / \text{Expected 24-hour urine creatinine (mg)}$$

where expected creatinine excretion is:

Female: 18 mg/kg

Male: 23 mg/kg

Sample Calculation: 66 kg female; 24-hour creatinine excretion: 890 mg

$$890 \text{ mg} / (18 \text{ mg/kg} \times 66 \text{ kg})$$
$$890/1188 \times 100 = 75\%$$

Therefore, a female weighing 66 kg with a 24 creatinine excretion of 890 mg/24 hours has CHI of 75% suggesting mild depletion.

CHI has limitations in measurement that clinicians must consider. As with UUN excretion, a test of urine creatinine excretion can be difficult to obtain. Furthermore, standards in the calculations for urinary creatinine do not account for variations in age, disease, physical training, body frame size, or weight status. Many conditions have been found to increase or decrease creatinine excretion. Sepsis, trauma, fever, strenuous exercise, and the second half of menstruation can also increase creatinine excretion. In contrast, renal function, low urine output, aging, and muscle atrophy unrelated to malnutrition can decrease creatinine excretion. Clinicians must account for these factors, beyond protein intake, that can alter urine creatinine laboratory values when evaluating and determining appropriate nutrition therapy.

While urinary creatinine has been used to assess somatic proteins status, *serum creatinine* is more commonly used in addition to BUN to assess renal function. Normal serum creatinine levels range from 0.4 to 1.3 mg/dL. Since serum creatinine is maintained within a relatively narrow range by the kidneys, elevated levels are most commonly a result of impaired renal function due to poor clearance of creatinine from the blood. In contrast, low serum creatinine levels can result from protein catabolism, which is common in patients with protein-energy malnutrition and muscular dystrophy, or in aging. Clinicians need to evaluate serum creatinine among other measures before determining etiology and treatment of abnormal values.

Blood urea nitrogen (BUN) is primarily used to assess renal function in addition to serum creatinine, but many other conditions can also alter BUN values. Normal BUN levels are 6 to 24 mg/dL. Urea is the metabolic byproduct of protein metabolism that is formed in the liver. Dietary protein is also broken down into amino acids, which are then catabolized to form free ammonia. Ammonia is then converted to urea and renally cleared. The kidneys filter urea out of the blood and into the urine, effectively eliminating excess nitrogen in the body. As a result, blood urea nitrogen consists of the normal waste products from endogenous protein metabolism and exogenous protein intake. In healthy individuals, there is usually a small amount of urea nitrogen in the blood, although many factors can alter BUN levels.

High BUN levels can often result from altered urea excretion rate due to renal insufficiency or dehydration. Altered protein metabolic rate from excessive protein intake, GI bleeding, and catabolism can also increase BUN levels. BUN should be interpreted in conjunction with creatinine to assess kidney function. In kidney and liver disease, BUN levels may rise and then return to normal. Clinicians should be careful in interpreting this drop because it does not suggest improved renal excretory function, but rather may reflect the inability of the liver to form urea. While BUN may remain normal or only slightly elevated, blood ammonia levels will increase as the liver continues to decline in these patients. Dehydration can also temporarily increase BUN levels and can be important in assessing hydration status in patients. Starvation, excessive protein intake, GI bleeding, and excessive protein catabolism (fever, burns, stress) can also increase BUN levels. Increased BUN levels is also common in patients with acute myocardial infarction because a decrease in cardiac function decreases renal blood flow, reducing renal excretion of BUN and consequently increasing serum BUN.

In contrast, low BUN levels are much less common and found in only a few conditions. Low BUN levels may result in patients with negative nitrogen balance, low protein intake, protein-energy malnutrition, increased protein synthesis (such as in pregnant women and in infancy), severe liver damage, impaired absorption, nephritic syndrome, and overhydration. However, low BUN levels are rarely used to diagnose or monitor the conditions described above.

A BUN:creatinine ratio can be used to help clinicians determine the etiology of abnormal BUN levels. A normal BUN:creatinine ratio ranges from 12 to 20, with most individuals ranging from 12 to 16. A normal BUN/high creatinine is usually indicative of muscle wasting, steroid administration, acute tubular necrosis, low protein intake, or severe liver disease. A high BUN/normal creatinine (BUN/creatinine >15:1) is common in dehydration, protein-energy malnutrition (catabolic state of tissue breakdown), excessive protein intake, GI bleeding, and catabolism. However, a ratio may be found to be normal in patients with renal insufficiency because both BUN and creatinine levels are higher than normal. Both BUN and BUN:creatinine values must be interpreted cautiously. Treatment of abnormal BUN levels will vary depending on the etiology and should take into account other protein assessment measures in addition to BUN.

Enzymes

A biochemical assessment of specific serum enzymes can provide clinicians with a more comprehensive evaluation of conditions affecting various organ systems. Aspartate transaminase, alanine transaminase, alkaline phosphatase, and lactate dehydrogenase are among the most common enzymes found within the blood in abnormal levels when patients have a variety of health conditions such as liver, kidney, cardiac, and bone disorders. Clinicians must evaluate these serum enzyme values in conjunction with the other serum proteins listed above to assess and treat patients according to the etiology and symptoms presented in patients.

Aspartate transaminase (AST) is an enzyme found primarily in the heart, liver, skeletal muscle cells, and to a lesser extent in the kidneys and pancreas. Normal serum AST values range from 10 to 35 IU/L. High serum AST values can be found in hepatocellular disease and coronary occlusive heart disease. An increase in AST is directly correlated to the number of cells affected by the disease or injury, with levels peaking about 8 hours after cell injury. In patients having a myocardial infarction, AST typically rises within 6 to 10 hours, peaking at 12 to 48 hours, and then returning to normal levels in 3 to 7 days unless another cardiac injury occurs.[39] Therefore, AST levels are often evaluated to estimate the time of myocardial infarction. Despite therapy, a second rise of AST may indicate additional cardiac injury. AST does not rise in angina, pericarditis, or rheumatic carditis. Liver damage also increases AST levels, peaking at up to 20 times the normal value then falling. As with myocardial infarction, the rise in AST is directly related to the degree of active inflammation. In chronic liver disease, high AST levels persist. Other conditions that may increase AST levels include hypothyroidism, acute pancreatitis, pulmonary emboli, Reye's syndrome, and skeletal muscle diseases.

Low serum AST is common in patients with vitamin B_6 deficiency, beriberi (thiamin deficiency), diabetic ketoacidosis, kidney disorders (acute, renal dialysis, uremia), chronic liver disease, and pregnancy. Treatment of abnormal AST values will vary based on the underlying cause. Monitoring AST levels and comparing values to other serum enzymes tests is important in determining etiology and appropriate treatment.

Alanine transaminase (ALT) is an enzyme found mostly in the liver and to a lesser extent in the kidneys, heart, and skeletal muscle. Normal serum ALT levels range from 4 to 36 units/L. High ALT levels are most commonly found in liver disorders (cholestasis, hepatitis, hepatic ischemia, cirrhosis or necrosis, liver cancer, obstructive jaundice). Very high ALT levels (10 times normal) are often due to acute hepatitis and may remain high for months before returning to normal. Drugs or other substances toxic to the liver and decreased blood flow to the liver (hepatic ischemia) also result in extremely high ALT levels (up to 100 times normal). In comparison, chronic hepatitis, cholestasis, cirrhosis, heart damage, alcohol abuse, and malignancies in the liver cause a more moderate increase in ALT levels (less than 4 times normal). Myocardial infarction, myositis, pancreatitis, infectious mononucleosis, severe burns, and shock may also cause elevated ALT levels. Strenuous exercise, medications injected into muscle tissue, and other medications including statins, antibiotics, aspirin, and chemotherapy can also increase ALT levels. Although ALT is more specific to the liver, AST:ALT ratio is frequently used to determine the etiology of abnormal ALT values and recognize heart or muscle injury in patients. In most types of liver diseases, ALT level is higher than AST (AST:ALT <1.0), with a few exceptions. An AST:ALT ratio >1.0 is commonly seen in patients with alcoholic hepatitis, cirrhosis, and heart or muscle injury for a few days after the onset of acute hepatitis.[39] Although AST and ALT are often referred to as "liver function tests," they are a better measure of hepatocellular damage instead of function, which makes the designation confusing. Note that certain proteins, such as albumin and clotting factors, which can reflect the liver's synthetic function, may be better indicators of actual liver function.

While low AST levels are not typically a concern, low ALT can be correlated to malnutrition and urinary tract infection. Treatment of abnormal ALT values will depend upon the underlying cause and severity. Clinicians must look to other markers for a comprehensive assessment and appropriate treatment.

Alkaline phosphatase (ALP) is an enzyme found in the liver and bones. Normal serum ALP values range from 30 to 120 units/L. High ALP levels are common in patients with liver disorders and can be useful in detecting blocked bile ducts and tumors (leukemia and lymphoma) if one or more bile ducts are obstructed. ALP levels are elevated as much as AST and ALT in hepatitis, while bile duct obstruction (gallstones, scars, surgery, previous gallstones, cancer) usually results in increased ALP more than AST or ALT. Because ALP is also present in bone, high levels of ALP can result from conditions affecting bone growth or increased activity of bone cells including osteomalacia, osteoblastic tumors, rickets, Paget's disease, and hyperparathyroidism. In cases of bone cancer or Paget's disease, where bones become enlarged and deformed, ALP levels will increase initially and then decrease, returning to normal over time in response to treatment. Moderately elevated ALP levels can also result from congestive heart failure, ulcerative colitis, and certain bacterial infections. ALP levels may also be temporarily elevated in women during pregnancy, in children and adolescents during large growth spurts, and with some medications such as anti-epileptics.

In contrast, ALP levels may decrease temporarily after blood transfusions or heart bypass surgery. Malnutrition, protein deficiency, zinc deficiency, vitamin B_{12} deficiency, hypothyroidism, hypophosphatemia, and Wilson's disease can also cause low ALP levels. Hypophosphatasia is a rare genetic disorder caused by a mutation in the gene producing ALP, while Wilson's disease is another genetic disorder causing copper to accumulate, leading to low ALP levels as a result of severe liver failure. Some medications including oral contraceptives and estrogen replacement therapy can also lower ALP levels. Treatment of abnormal ALP values varies based on the etiology and must address underlying cause and symptoms, such as vitamin D deficiency in bone disorders or zinc deficiency. Monitoring ALP can provide clinicians with important insight on progression and treatment of certain diseases.

Lactate dehydrogenase (LDH) is an enzyme present in the heart, liver, skeletal muscle, brain, red blood cells, and lung cells. LDH is released when a disease of injury affects cells and causes cell lysis. Normal serum LDH values range from 208 to 378 IU/L. LDH is not considered an indicator of any one disease affecting one organ. In contrast, five isoenzymes of LDH differentiate LDH among different organs: LDH-1 is mainly from the heart and blood vessels; LDH-2 is mostly from the reticuloendothelial system; LDH-3 is primarily from the lungs; LDH-4 is from the kidney, placenta, and pancreas; and LDH-5 is primarily from striated muscle and the liver.

In healthy individuals, LDH-2 is typically higher than the other isoenzymes. An elevated LDH-1 above LDH-2 (LDH flip) most often results from hemolytic anemia, megaloblastic anemia and/or sickle cell anemia. By assessing the time elapsed to peak values, clinicians can differentiate among these conditions. The LDH flip is also common in patients with myocardial infarction, although this is not the primary measure used for this diagnosis. An elevated LDH-5 in isolation most often suggests hepatocellular injury or disease, while elevated LDH-2 and LDH-3 suggest pulmonary injury or disease. When all LDH isoenzymes are high, the cause is likely multi-organ failure, advanced malignancy, or diffuse autoimmune inflammatory disease. Clinicians must treat abnormal LDH levels according to etiology. Patients with abnormal LDH levels should be monitored closely to monitor effectiveness of treatment and evaluate potential progression of certain diseases.

Troponin is a complex of three regulatory proteins—troponin C, troponin I, and troponin T—that are critical for muscle contraction in skeletal and cardiac muscle cells. A troponin test is most commonly performed to assess cardiac conditions because troponin is released into the blood when the heart muscle is damaged. In a healthy individual, troponin will not be detected in a blood sample. In contrast, a slight increase in troponin is often an indication of some damage to the heart, with very high levels most often indicating that a myocardial infarction has occurred. Typically patients who have had a myocardial infarction have raised troponin levels within 6 to 12 hours after the episode.[40] Other causes of high troponin levels include abnormally fast heartbeat, hypertension in lung arteries, congestive heart failure, long-term kidney disease, and cardiomyopathy. Medical nutrition therapy will vary according to the patient's cardiac condition and will require close monitoring to assess patient's needs.

Lipid Profile

As with proteins, lipids also serve many critical functions in the body. Triglycerides are an important source of stored energy in the body and cholesterol is the building block of hormones and cell membranes. When cholesterol is bound to protein (apolipoproteins) in the blood, it also plays an important role in transporting lipids throughout the body. Several health conditions can alter lipid metabolism, reflected in a lipid profile consisting of serum total cholesterol, very-low-density lipoprotein cholesterol (VLDL), low-density lipoprotein cholesterol (LDL), high-density lipoprotein cholesterol (HDL), and triglycerides. Both low and high lipid values are correlated to serious health conditions, impacting many organs in the body. The term *hyperlipidemia* or *dyslipidemia* is often used to refer to a condition of abnormal blood lipid levels, which may include total cholesterol, VLDL, LDL, HDL, and/or triglycerides. Clinicians must become skilled at interpreting abnormal blood lipid values as part of the nutrition care process because adequate medical nutrition therapy can play an important role in prevention, treatment, and symptom management of various disease states.

Lipoproteins transport endogenous lipids from the liver to the rest of the body and are characterized by their density. The density of lipoproteins varies according to the lipid-to-protein ratio and lipid composition (cholesterol, triglyceride, and phospholipids). VLDL cholesterol have the least amount of protein and the highest amount of triglycerides compared to LDL and HDL. VLDLs are produced in the liver and travel in the blood, converted to intermediate-density lipoprotein (IDL), and then to LDL as they lose triglycerides.

Currently, there is no simple way to measure VLDL cholesterol in the blood. However, this value can be estimated based on triglyceride values because VLDL cholesterol contains most of the circulating triglycerides and the composition of the different particles is relatively constant. To estimate VLDL cholesterol, divide fasting triglyceride value (in mg/dL) by five. This is not accurate for triglyceride levels higher than 400 mg/dL or in patients who have not fasted.

An elevated VLDL cholesterol level (>30 mg/dL) increases an individual's risk of heart disease and stroke because high VLDL cholesterol suggests that conversion to LDL cholesterol is slowed, causing an accumulation of intermediate particles in the blood and contributing to atherosclerosis and coronary heart disease. VLDL cholesterol levels must be assessed in conjunction with other lipid values before determining appropriate nutrition therapy. Low VLDL cholesterol levels are generally not of concern and do not require nutrition therapy.

LDL cholesterol which are higher in protein and cholesterol, are considered the end point of forward transport of lipids to tissues. LDL particles are removed from circulation and taken up by tissues in need of cholesterol for structural support. If there is too much LDL cholesterol in the blood, these particles can adhere to the walls of arteries, forming plaque. Plaque can narrow arteries, contribute to high blood pressure, and initiate the process of atherosclerosis, or the buildup of fatty deposits in artery walls. Oxidized LDL cholesterol is more likely to be taken up by atherosclerotic plaque and continue development of existing plaque, increasing risk for myocardial infarction and stroke. For these reasons, LDL cholesterol is commonly known as the "bad" cholesterol.

As with the other lipid values, patients ideally fast 12 hours for an accurate laboratory result. Elevated LDL cholesterol (>100 mg/dL) is the lipid biomarker most closely associated with increased risk of heart disease and is commonly found in patients with preexisting coronary heart disease.[41] There is strong evidence that dietary saturated fat and trans fat are positively associated with LDL cholesterol, while dietary cholesterol is not as strongly correlated with LDL levels or risk of cardiovascular disease.[42] The source of saturated fat may differ in its effect on LDL cholesterol and risk of cardiovascular disease. Genetics (family history of premature heart disease), age and sex (>45 years for men and >55 years for women), cigarette smoking, high blood pressure, diabetes mellitus, and pregnancy can also raise LDL cholesterol levels. Nutrition therapy will vary depending on the underlying cause. For instance, management of DM with carbohydrate control, blood pressure with sodium restriction, or cardiovascular risk factors with limited trans fat and saturated fat may be recommended. Depending on the severity and comorbidities, cholesterol-lowering medications may be prescribed in conjunction to a dietary intervention.

Low LDL cholesterol (<60 mg/dL) is rarely seen, but can occur in a few conditions. Acute illness, immediately following a myocardial infarction, and stress from surgery or trauma can lower LDL cholesterol temporarily.[43] In addition, malnutrition, cancer, infection, inflammation, hyperthyroidism, cirrhosis, and people with inherited lipid disorders may have low LDL cholesterol. Low LDL is not generally a concern and should be evaluated with other measures to determine effective nutrition therapy. Malnutrition should be further assessed with other protein biomarkers to determine etiology and treatment with continuous monitoring.

HDL cholesterol is involved in the reverse cholesterol transport, taking cholesterol from tissues and other lipoproteins and transporting it back to the liver. HDL cholesterol is considered the "good" or protective cholesterol because of its role in returning cholesterol to the liver reduces cholesterol in plaque, which is associated with cardiovascular problems. Normal blood HDL cholesterol levels range from 40 to 59 mg/dL, while patients with HDL cholesterol levels less than 40 mg/dL are at increased risk of heart disease, independent of other risk factors such as LDL cholesterol levels. As with LDL cholesterol, HDL cholesterol levels may also be altered during acute illness, immediately increasing after an myocardial infarction, during stress, and during pregnancy.[43] To address low HDL cholesterol, treatment should focus on addressing the underlying cause, with treatment ranging from smoking cessation and increasing physical activity to nutrition therapy, with similar recommendations to that of LDL cholesterol. **Figure 2.16** illustrates the composition of LDL and HDL cholesterol.

Total cholesterol is a calculated value representing the total amount of cholesterol found within the blood. It equals the sum of HDL cholesterol, LDL cholesterol, and 20% of triglycerides levels in mg/dL during 12 hours of fasting. Normal total cholesterol levels range from 140 to 200 mg/dL. Borderline high is considered in the range of 200 to 239 mg/dL, and high cholesterol or hypercholesterolemia is classified as greater than 240 mg/dL for adults and greater than 170 mg/dL for children and adolescents.[43] As with LDL and HDL cholesterol, several factors can increase total cholesterol levels including age, smoking, hypertension, family history, myocardial infarction, DM, obesity, and pregnancy. A diet high in saturated fat and trans fat is also directly correlated to high total cholesterol levels and increased risk of cardiovascular disease. Medications, including anabolic steroids, beta-blockers, epinephrine, oral contraceptives, and vitamin D, can also increase total cholesterol levels.

Low total cholesterol (<100 mg/dL) is commonly found in patients with malnutrition, liver disease, and cancer. Although there is no evidence that low cholesterol causes any of these issues, low total cholesterol values can be assessed with other protein biomarkers to determine underlying cause and appropriate treatment.

Total/HDL cholesterol is considered to be a more accurate measure of heart disease risk than total cholesterol and LDL cholesterol because this ratio takes into account HDL relative to total cholesterol. An optimal ratio of total cholesterol to HDL cholesterol is less than 3.5:1, while a ratio greater than 3.5:1 is associated with increased risk of heart disease.[43] Clinicians should treat elevated total/HDL ratio and elevated total cholesterol similar to elevated LDL cholesterol; restrict trans fats and limit saturated fats, depending on the underlying cause.

> **PRACTICE POINT**
>
> Interpreting LDL and HDL cholesterol levels in the context of total cholesterol provides more clinical significance than any one lipid value alone. A patient with an elevated HDL with an elevated total cholesterol will likely be at lower risk of health complications than a patient with both elevated LDL and elevated total cholesterol.

Triglycerides make up the largest percentage of fat in the body and are an important source of energy. As a component of lipoproteins, triglycerides are also important in transporting fat to cells. Normal triglyceride levels range from 40 to 150 mg/dL.[43] Borderline high triglyceride levels are 150 to 199 mg/dL and high triglyceride levels or hypertriglyceridemia are defined as values greater than 200 mg/dL. Hypertriglyceridemia is often found in patients who are overweight or obese, and those who have DM, kidney disease, and thyroid or liver disease. In addition, extremely high triglyceride levels greater than 1,000 mg/dL, known as severe hypertriglyceridemia, is associated with hypertriglyceridemic pancreatitis and cardiovascular disease.[44]

Dietary intake (high in refined grains, saturated fat, and trans fats), lack of exercise, smoking, and excess alcohol consumption can also increase triglyceride levels. Patients with hypertriglyceridemia combined with either low or high HDL are also considered at increased risk of atherosclerosis. Patients receiving PN who have combined hypertriglyceridemia are also at increased risk of glucose intolerance. Triglycerides levels should be closely monitored in patients at risk for these conditions. Nutrition therapy should focus on treating the underlying cause and reducing symptoms with a diet low in saturated fat, added sugar, refined grains, and alcohol.

> **CORE CONCEPT 6**
>
> Lipid profile results can be used to assess risk of cardiovascular (elevated low-density lipoprotein, decreased high-density/low-density lipoprotein ratio) and metabolic (elevated triglycerides) disorders, as well as risk of malnutrition (decreased cholesterol) in patients.

Hematology

A hematological assessment is another important component of biochemical assessment that is key to diagnosis and treatment for patients with all types of anemia and other blood disorders impacting nutrition needs. **Anemia** is defined as a reduction in erythrocytes per unit of blood

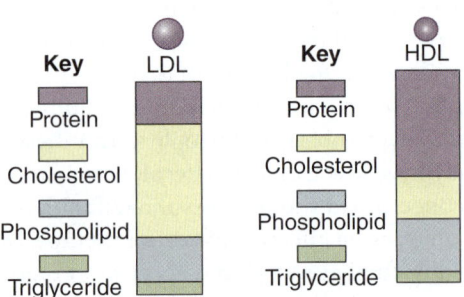

FIGURE 2.16 Composition of LDL and HDL Cholesterol

Clinical Roundtable

Topic: Use of LDL Cholesterol Particle Size in Assessing Cardiovascular Disease Risk

Background: An addition to the blood lipid test assessing the size and density of LDL particles has been studied but is not a standard measurement used in healthcare settings. Researchers are finding that the role of LDL cholesterol in cardiovascular disease risk may depend on the size and density of particles. As with other lipid values, composition of LDL particles, ranging from large, buoyant particles to small, dense particles, can be influenced by diet, genetics, and body weight.

Studies have found that high LDL particle size (LDL-P), which contains small, dense particles, may be associated with cardiovascular disease and metabolic syndrome more than low LDL-P, regardless of LDL cholesterol levels. High LDL-P can be seen with elevated LDL cholesterol levels as well as in individuals with normal and low LDL cholesterol levels.

Roundtable Discussion

1. How might these findings influence the way clinicians assess and diagnose risk of cardiovascular disease or metabolic syndrome?
2. Discuss whether you would use composition of LDL particle size to interpret a patient's risk of cardiovascular disease. Why or why not?

References

1. Kathiresan S, Otvos JD, Sullivan LM, et al. Increased small low-density lipoprotein particle number: A prominent feature of the metabolic syndrome in the Framingham heart study. *Circulation*. 2006;113(1):20-29.

2. Davidson MH, Ballantyne CM, Jacobson TA, et al. Clinical utility of inflammatory markers and advanced lipoprotein testing: Advice from an expert panel of lipid specialists. *J Clin Lipidol*. 2011;5(5):338-367.

CASE STUDY

It is now HD 15 and Adam is recovering well. He has been moved out of the ICU to the medical ward and is preparing for discharge home. His appetite and oral intake are improving. Based on his labs and symptom of fatigue, an iron supplement is ordered.

Biochemical Data (HD 15):
Hemoglobin 12.0 (13.5-17.5 g/dL)
Hematocrit 34 (42-52%)
Mean corpuscular volume 98 (80–100 fL)
Red cell distribution width (RDW-SD) 50 (39-46 fL)

Clinical Data:
Medications: iron, protonix, lipitor, captopril

Dietary Data:
Diet Prescription: Regular

Questions

1. Describe the abnormalities in Adam's biochemical data.
2. What type of anemia or anemias might Adam have? What are his risk factors?
3. What additional biochemical measures would be required to make a more accurate assessment?

volume or a decrease in hemoglobin of blood to below level of physiological needs. Although anemia is not a disease, it is a symptom of various conditions and the cause of anemia is usually multifactorial. Anemia can result from extensive blood loss (acute or chronic bleeding), excessive blood cell destruction (hemolytic anemia), or decreased red blood cell formation/production (bone marrow failure, micronutrient deficiency, erythropoietin deficiency). **Figure 2.17** compares healthy and anemic red blood cells. The causes of anemia are not mutually exclusive, as many patients have multiple causes leading to anemia. Anemia is observed in many hospitalized patients, varying in micro-

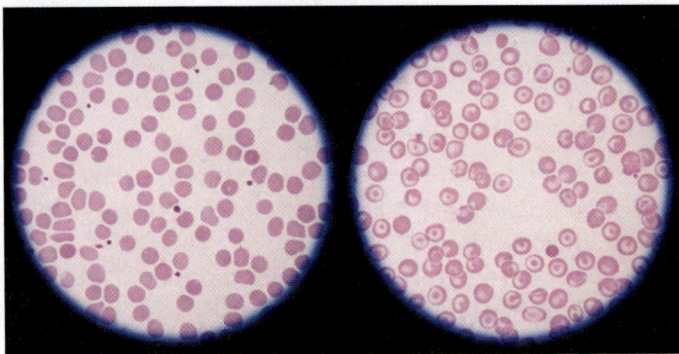

FIGURE 2.17 Comparison of a Image of a Healthy Red Blood Cell (left) and an Anemic Red Blood Cell (right)
© toeytoey2530/Getty Images.

nutrients involved (iron, folate, vitamin B_{12}, copper, zinc) and etiology (nutritional inadequacy, acute or chronic disease). See **Table 2.10** for a summary of the key roles of iron, folate, copper, vitamin B_{12}, and zinc in red blood cell synthesis. Malnourished patients; young children; pregnant women; older adults; and patients with kidney disease, uncontrolled chronic illness, cancer, and extensive GI surgeries are considered at higher risk of anemia. **Table 2.11** outlines the primary sites of GI absorption of macronutrients associated with anemia.

The size, shape, and color of erythrocytes (red blood cells) and a CBC can help clinicians evaluate etiology, severity, and appropriate treatment of these conditions. A CBC provides a count of cells in the blood and description of red blood cells including serum red blood cells, white blood cells, hemoglobin concentration, hematocrit, mean corpuscular volume, red cell distribution width, and mean corpuscular hemoglobin concentration. Laboratory assessment of several of these blood parameters should be evaluated to distinguish between nutrition adequacies and other factors contributing to anemia. Biochemical assessment in addition to clinical signs and symptoms (**Table 2.12**) and medical status should be used to help clinicians evaluate etiology, severity, and appropriate treatment of anemia and other blood-related conditions.

Hemoglobin (Hgb) concentration is a measure of the total amount of hemoglobin in peripheral blood. Hemoglobin is the protein in erythrocytes that delivers oxygen to cells and picks up CO_2 for expiration by the lungs. **Figure 2.18** depicts the structure of hemoglobin. Hgb concentration is considered the primary biochemical marker for diagnosis of anemia, defined as a hemoglobin concentration <95th percentile for healthy reference populations. According to World Health Organization recommendations, the cutoff of hemoglobin concentrations in defining anemia varies by age and sex: adult males (older than 15 years) <13.0 g/dL, adult females (older than 15 years) <12.0 g/dL, and pregnant adult females (older than 15 years) <11.0 g/dL.[44]

Low hemoglobin levels can be found in patients with four different types of nutritional anemias. However, Hgb concentration is not a sensitive or specific test for differentiating between nutritional anemias. Therefore, other laboratory values and a recent medical history need to be evaluated to determine appropriate nutrition therapy for patients with signs and symptoms of anemia. Hyperthyroidism,

TABLE 2.10 KEY MINERALS INVOLVED IN RED BLOOD CELL SYNTHESIS

Micronutrient	Major Physiological Role
Iron	Key component of hemoglobin
Vitamin B_{12}	Cofactor for amino acid synthesis and tricarboxylic acid cycle, facilitated in maturation and differentiation of erythroid lining
Folate	Key component of 1-carbon transfer system for protein and DNA synthesis and cell division
Copper	Key for regulation of iron transport from intestine and release into circulation
Zinc	Cofactor required for protein synthesis, and regulation for cell differentiation

Data from from Chan LN, Mike LA. The science and practice of micronutrient supplementations in nutritional anemia: An evidence-based review. *JPEN J Parenter Enteral Nutr*. 2014;38(6):656-672.

TABLE 2.11 PRIMARY GI ABSORPTION SITES OF MICRONUTRIENTS ASSOCIATED WITH ANEMIA

Micronutrient	Primary Site of Absorption
Non-heme iron	Duodenum (transporter also has affinity for lead, cobalt, manganese, copper, and zinc)
Heme iron	Duodenum and proximal jejunum
Vitamin B_{12}	Terminal ileum
Folate	Duodenum and proximal jejunum (transporter enhanced by vitamin D and inhibited by alcohol)
Copper	Most of small intestine
Zinc	Duodenum and jejunum

Modified from Chan LN, Mike LA. The science and practice of micronutrient supplementations in nutritional anemia: An evidence-based review. *JPEN J Parenter Enteral Nutr*. 2014;38(6):656-672.

TABLE 2.12 CLINICAL SIGNS AND SYMPTOMS OF ANEMIA

Fatigue, lethargy
Irritability
Difficulty concentrating, sleepiness
Pallor, pale sclera
Cold extremities
Muscle aches
GI distress (nausea, vomiting, diarrhea, cramping)
Reproductive dysfunction (amenorrhea, loss of libido)
Paresthesia
Cheilosis, glossitis
Spoon-shaped fingernails
Clubbing of joints in the digits
Cardiovascular sequelae (heart palpitation, tachycardia, dyspnea, angina)

Data from Pirker R. Symptoms of anemia. In: Recombinant Human Erythropoietin (rhEPO) in Clinical Oncology. New York, NY: Springer;2008:307-315

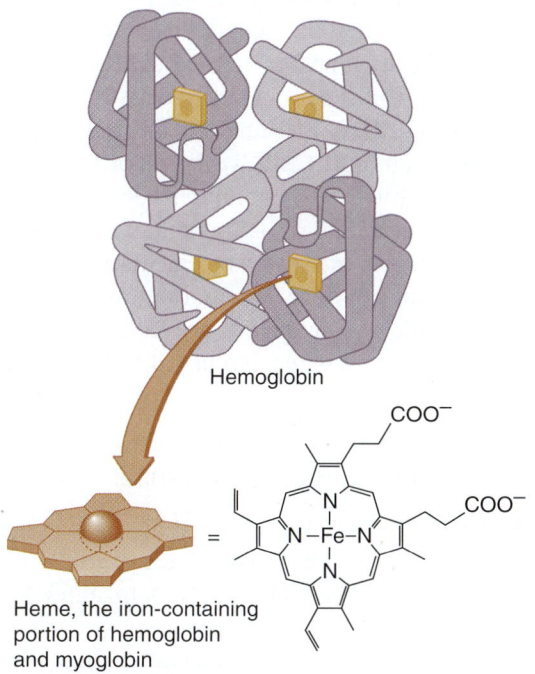

FIGURE 2.18 Structure of Hemoglobin

in femoliters (fL), which is one-quadrillionth of a liter. Red blood cells contain hemoglobin and make up the largest percentage of blood volume. They are regenerated approximately every 4 months with production, development, and function dependent on nutritional status, genetics, and environmental influences. Normal serum RBC values range from 4.7 to $6.1 \times 10^6/\mu L$ in males and 4.2 to $5.4 \times 10^6/\mu L$ in females. As with low hemoglobin concentrations, low RBC values may result from nutritional deficits or in patients with hemorrhage, hemolysis, genetic aberrations, marrow failure, renal disease, or consumption of certain medications. As with Hgb, RBC values are not sensitive to nutritional causes of anemia.

Hematocrit (Hct) percentage is also used with Hgb concentration to evaluate anemia. Hematocrit is the measure of the percentage of red blood cells in total blood volume and is often referred to as packed RBC volume. In healthy individuals, hematocrit percentage is typically three times the Hgb concentration in grams per deciliter. Normal serum Hct percentage values range from 42% to 52% in males, 35% to 47% in females, 33% in pregnant women, and 44% to 64% in newborns.[45] Hct percentage values are lower than normal under the same conditions that cause low Hgb and RBCs. Anemia, leukemia, hyperthyroidism, cirrhosis, massive blood loss, pregnancy, and poor iron intake can decrease Hct levels. On the other hand, high Hct levels may result from COPD, dehydration, or shock. As with Hgb, Hct is also not a sensitive or specific test for anemia. For example, Hct value is affected by an extremely high white blood cell count and hydration status. Also, high altitudes can increase Hct values during the first 72 hours in a high altitude because adaptations are made to lower arterial oxygen partial pressure due to diminished barometric pressure.[46] In addition, patients older than 50 years have slightly lower Hct values than younger adults, which can be caused by several factors including decreased production of intrinsic factor, physiological changes postmenarche, and chronic disease. As a result of the variation among individuals, other laboratory values and a recent medical history should be evaluated to determine appropriate nutrition therapy for patients with abnormal Hct values.

Mean corpuscular volume (MCV) or mean cell volume is the average size or volume of red blood cells. Normal serum MCV ranges from 80 to 99 fL in adults and 96 to 108 fL in newborns. MCV can be a helpful biomarker to characterize anemia by red blood cell size and can provide clinicians with a better understanding of the cause of dysregulation. High levels of MCV are associated with macrocytic anemia, pernicious anemia, and vitamin B_{12} (cyanocabalamin) and/or folate deficiency. In contrast, low MCV values are associated with microcytic anemia, iron-deficiency anemia, and anemia of chronic disease. **Microcytic anemia** (small cell size) is defined as MCV less than 80 fL, **macrocytic anemia** (large cell size) is MCV greater than 100 fL, and **normocytic anemia** (normal cell size) occurs when MCV is between 80 and 99 fL. This

cirrhosis, leukemia, chronic infection, hemolysis, marrow failure, and kidney disease can lower Hgb levels. Genetic aberrations, aging, lead poisoning, pregnancy, and overhydration can also cause low Hgb levels. In contrast, high Hgb concentration is found in patients with blood transfusions and in patients at higher altitudes.

Red blood cell (RBC) count is a component of the CBC that measures the volume of red blood cells in the blood

TABLE 2.13 DIETARY SOURCES OF IRON

Food Sources	Iron (mg)
Heme Iron:	
Clams (3 oz)	14
Beef (3 oz)	4
Sardines (3 oz)	3
Poultry (3 oz)	1
Nonheme Iron:	
Fortified cereal (1 cup)	9
Spinach (1 cup)	6
Kidney beans (1 cup)	5
Pumpkin seeds (1 oz)	3

Data from US Department of Agriculture, Agricultural Research Service, USDA Food Composition Databases. USDA National Nutrient Database for Standard Reference, Release 28. Version Current: September 2015. Internet: https://ndb.nal.usda.gov/ndb/nutrients/report/.

categorization can provide clinicians with a better understanding of the cause of dysregulation.

Microcytic anemia can result from impaired heme synthesis (inability to absorb, transport, store, or utilize iron) or impaired synthetic abilities (protein, iron, ascorbate, vitamin A, pyridoxine, copper, or manganese deficiency). The most common conditions associated with microcytic anemia are iron deficiency, thalassemia (genetic blood disorder), and inflammation from chronic disease. Copper, zinc, lead, cadmium, and other heavy metals can also impair heme synthesis. **Table 2.13** provides examples of common dietary sources of iron.

Macrocytic anemia results from the decreased ability of the red blood cell to divide appropriately or to synthesize new cells and DNA, leading to larger than normal red blood cells. Macrocytic anemia may be due to deficiency or impaired utilization of vitamin B_{12}, folate, thiamin, or pyroxidine. Dietary intake, genetic disorders in DNA synthesis, alcoholism, and liver disease are common causes of macrocytic anemia. Further evaluation of folate and vitamin B_{12} status is needed to determine etiology of anemia.

Normocytic anemia is associated with several chronic and inflammatory diseases including rheumatic disease, chronic heart failure, chronic infection, cancer, severe tissue injury, multiple fractures, and Hodgkin's disease. These conditions cannot be treated effectively with iron supplementation. MCV may appear within normal range if iron deficiency is concurrent with vitamin B_{12} and/or folate deficiency because the large size cell volume of the macrocytosis is masked by the small size cell volume of the microcytosis in the MCV value. MCV may also appear within normal range in the early stages of iron deficiency. In these cases, vitamin B_{12} and folate deficiency must be ruled out before iron-deficiency anemia is diagnosed and treated. Microcytosis and macrocytosis are not sensitive to marginal nutrient deficiencies. Additional laboratory values are needed to distinguish between various nutritional and non-nutritional causes of anemia and to determine appropriate treatment.

PRACTICE POINT

Evaluation of a patient's mean corpuscular volume (MCV) is an important in determining a patient's type of anemia (microcytic, macrocytic, normocytic) and developing appropriate nutrition therapy for the patient.

Mean corpuscular hemoglobin concentration (MCHC), or mean cellular hemoglobin concentration, is another one of the RBC indices that make up the CBC test. MCHC is the average concentration of hemoglobin within red blood cells presented as a ratio of hemoglobin mass to volume of red blood cells. It is calculated from the Hgb concentration and Hct using the following formula:

$$MCHC = Hgb\ (g/dL)/Hct\ (\%)$$

Normal serum MCHC levels range from 32 to 36 g/dL for children and adults and 32 to 33 g/dL for newborns. Abnormal MCHC values are evaluated similarly to MCV values; decreased MCHC is common in patients with iron deficiency and thalassemia trait. As with MCV, MCHC is not sensitive to marginal nutrient deficiencies.

Red cell distribution width (RDW) and MCV have become the most useful parameters in classifying anemias in clinical settings. RDW measures the degree of anisocytosis, or variation in RBC size variation or volume, as a coefficient of variation (CV) or standard deviation (SD). RDW-SD (fL) is the actual measurement of the width of RBC size distribution, measured by calculating the width at 20% height level of RBC size distribution range. Therefore, RDW-SD is not affected by the average RBC size (MCV). RDW-CV (%) is also used and can be calculated with the following equation:

$$RDW - CV = 1\ \text{standard deviation of}\ RBC\ \text{volume}/MCV \times 100\%$$

Unlike RDW-SD, RDW-CV is affected by the average RBC size (MCV). Normal serum RDW values in adults range from 39 to 46 fL for RDW-SD and 11.6% to 14.6% for RDW-CV.

Because RDW becomes elevated earlier than other blood measures, high RDW can be important in diagnosing early nutritional deficiencies, including iron, folate, or vitamin B_{12}. In addition, evaluation of RDW in conjunction with MCV can help clinicians determine the etiology of anemia by differentiating among microcytic, macrocytic, and normocytic anemia. Normal MCV and elevated RDW are common in patients with early iron, vitamin B_{12}, or folate deficiency; sickle cell disease; and chronic liver disease. Low MCV and normal RDW are associated with heterozygous thalassemia and anemia of inflammation and chronic disease, while low MCV and high RDW are associated with iron deficiency and sickle cell-β-thalassemia. In patients with high MCV and normal RDW, aplastic anemia, liver disease, chemotherapy, or alcohol is likely the cause. High MCV and high RDW is also associated with chronic liver disease, in addition to folate or vitamin B_{12} deficiency. If patients have normal RDW and normal MCV, anemia is likely associated with chronic disease, acute blood loss or hemolysis, or renal disease. While RDW and MCV values can further evaluate etiology of blood disorders, these measures must be assessed with other blood measures and clinical signs and symptoms before diagnosis and treatment of anemia or blood disorder. Treatment of blood disorders should focus on addressing the underlying causes and addressing protein and/or micronutrient deficiencies when appropriate.

White blood cell (WBC) count is another component of CBC that can help differentiate non-nutritional causes of anemia. White blood cells, also called leukocytes, are produced in bone marrow and play an important role in immune functioning, fighting infection or inflammation.

Normal serum WBC values are 5 to 10×10^9/L for adults, 6 to 17×10^9/L for children, and 9 to 30×10^9/L for newborns. Increased WBC count (leukocytosis) may be caused by infection, inflammation (rheumatoid arthritis, irritable bowel disease), leukemia, neoplasm, allergic response, or stress (trauma, burns, surgery). Decreased WBC count (leucopenia) may result from bone marrow damage or disorder, lymphoma or other cancer spreading to bone marrow, autoimmune disease, protein-energy malnutrition, overwhelming infection (e.g., sepsis), or effects chemotherapy or radiation therapy. Abnormal WBC values often require further assessment when symptoms are nonspecific and inflammatory autoimmune disease is expected. Reticulocyte (immature red blood cells) and platelet (components of red blood cells that function to clot blood) counts can help clinicians determine etiology and appropriate treatment of the underlying condition and anemia. Monitoring WBC levels can be useful for clinicians to assess whether the condition is generally worsening or improving if WBC counts are decreasing or increasing, respectively.

In addition to WBC count, differential WBC measures can be assessed to evaluate the levels of different types of leukocytes and related infections. These WBC measures include neutrophils (pyogenic infection), eosinophils (allergy and parasitic infection), basophils (parasitic infection), lymphocytes (viral infection), monocytes (severe infection), polymorphonuclear leukocytosis or PMNs (circulating mature cells), and bands (circulating immature cells).

Interpretation of Anemia

Iron Studies (Microcytic Anemia from Iron Deficiency)

Iron-deficiency anemia is the most prevalent of all types of anemia worldwide and one of the most common nutritional

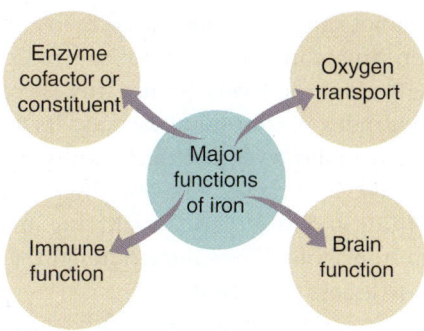

FIGURE 2.19 Major Functions of Iron

deficiencies. Suboptimal iron stores can have significant detrimental effects on biochemical processes of cellular metabolism including impaired growth and mental status in children, and depressed immune and cognitive function in adults. **Figure 2.19** shows the major functions of iron. In contrast, iron overload can lead to cell destruction, tissue injury, and organ failure. Clinicians must understand the etiology of iron-deficiency anemia and interpret lab values appropriately to determine effective nutrition therapy with careful monitoring.

Iron-deficiency anemia can result from blood loss, decreased iron intake or absorption, or increased iron requirements. Infants, young children, adolescents, women, and patients with renal insufficiency or undergoing gastric bypass surgery are at risk of iron-deficiency anemia. The most common symptoms are fatigue, anorexia, growth abnormalities, koilonychia (spoon-shaped nails), and glossitis. Typically, patients with iron-deficiency anemia have low Hgb, low Hct, and low MCV.

While these are the primary indicators of iron-deficiency anemia, folate and vitamin B_{12} deficiency can both mask iron deficiency by keeping MCV levels within a normal range. In addition, these tests are not sensitive to marginal deficiencies so they cannot detect early stages of anemia. If abnormal results are found with a CBC test, iron studies are often used to further assess presence of iron-deficiency anemia, including tests of serum iron, ferritin, transferrin, and total iron binding capacity. Clinical signs and symptoms should also be compared to results from iron studies to differentiate among iron-deficiency anemia, anemia of inflammation and chronic disease (described in detail below), and anemia of acute infection, because iron stores can be heavily influenced by many medical conditions causing inflammation and infection.

Serum iron measures the amount of circulating iron that is bound to transferrin, the iron transport protein in the blood. Normal serum iron levels range from 50 to 170 µg/dL. Levels less than 15 µg/dL reflect absent or reduced iron stores. Low serum iron levels are common in patients with gastric surgery due to peptic ulcer disease or obesity, GI bleed, malabsorption, leukemia, end-stage renal disease, and infection. Levels greater than 170 µg/dL may reflect iron overload, but can also be increased in liver disease, inflammation, and malignancies. Oral contraceptives may also increase serum iron levels. Serum iron is considered a relatively poor index of iron status because its value varies greatly from day to day, even in healthy individuals. In addition, diurnal variation occurs, with higher levels occurring midmorning and lower levels occurring in midafternoon. Serum iron should be evaluated in light of other iron study values to assess iron status.

Serum ferritin is a more accurate indicator of iron stores in patients. Normal ferritin levels are 20 to 500 ng/mL in males and 20 to 200 ng/mL in females. Ferritin is a storage protein that holds iron inside hepatocytes and other iron storage cells for later use. In healthy individuals, as iron supply increases, ferritin levels increase intracellularly to accommodate iron storage. Serum ferritin less than 12 to 15 ng/mL indicates that iron stores are depleted. Decreased serum ferritin can result from iron deficiency and malnutrition, with 1 ng/mL decrease of serum ferritin equal to approximately 8 mg decrease of stored iron.[47] During conditions of acute inflammation and some chronic diseases, serum ferritin is not an accurate indicator of serum ferritin status. Inflammatory disease, renal failure, malignancy, hepatitis, and iron overload can increase serum ferritin levels.

As a positive acute-phase protein, ferritin levels rise during stress and inflammation with increased synthesis and ferritin leakage from cells. Increased ferritin is often associated with acute inflammation, uremia, metastatic cancer, or alcohol-related liver disease, with elevated ferritin evident 1 to 2 days after onset of acute illness peaking at 3 to 5 days after injury or illness.[48] Under these conditions, other iron biomarkers must be used to evaluate the presence of iron deficiency.

Ferritin also fails to correlate with iron stores in **anemia of inflammation and chronic disease (AICD)**, a common form of anemia in hospitalized patients. In patients with AICD, cytokines such as interleukin-1 and tumor necrosis factor are released during inflammation due to inadequate mobilization of iron stores, which decreases red blood cell production. Low Hgb and Hct are the common indicators of AICD, and can occur in normocytic–hypochromic, microcytic-hypochromic, and normocytic-normochromic anemias due to failure of compensatory erythropoiesis.

AICD often occurs in patients with cancer or chronic inflammatory or infectious disorders, such as rheumatoid arthritis. Iron stores may also become depleted in arthritis from reduced absorption and in patients with regular use of nonsteroidal anti-inflammatory drugs or with GI blood loss. In patients with microcytic anemia, serum ferritin may remain normal or increase while serum iron levels are low. In this case, inflammatory mediators may also cause ferritin levels to remain normal, although iron stores can be depleted. Clinicians must distinguish the many forms of AICD from iron-deficiency anemia by comparing iron laboratory measures so that iron supplementation is not initiated when anemia is not caused by iron deficiency.

Transferrin is a globulin protein synthesized in the liver that transports iron to bone marrow for production of hemoglobin. The size of the iron storage pool controls the level of plasma transferrin. In healthy individuals, when iron stores are depleted, transferrin synthesis increases. Normal serum transferrin levels range from 170 to 370 mg/dL.[48] Increased transferrin levels are associated with iron-deficiency anemia, while low transferrin levels are common in liver disease, cirrhosis, malnutrition, infection, and fever. Like albumin, transferrin is a negative acute-phase protein, which means that decreased transferrin is found in patients with acute inflammation, malignancies, collagen vascular diseases, and liver diseases. Protein energy malnutrition and fluid overload can also decrease serum transferrin levels. As a result, low iron stores may not be reflected in transferrin measures when these conditions are present because transferrin levels may be falsely increased or remain within a normal range. Other iron biomarkers are needed to further assess the underlying cause of anemia and develop appropriate treatment. Clinicians may use transferrin as a measure of severity of illness and to monitor for progress if patients have these conditions.

Total iron binding capacity (TIBC) measures the saturation ability of transferrin, or the potential for plasma transferrin to bind to ferric acid (Fe^{3+}). Under normal conditions, approximately 30% of iron-binding sites on transferrin molecules are saturated. Each transferrin molecule binds to ferric ions at two or more binding sites and two bicarbonate ions at different sites. TIBC can be calculated using the following equation:

$$\text{Transferrin Saturation (\%)} = (\text{serum iron level} / \text{TIBC}) \times 100$$

Sample Calculation: serum iron 48 μg/dL; TIBC 352 μg/dL

$$\text{Transferrin Saturation \%} = (48/352) \times 100$$
$$\text{Transferrin Saturation \%} = 14\%$$

Therefore, an individual with a serum iron of 48 and TIBC of 352 has a total iron binding capacity of 14%, which suggests iron deficiency.

Under most conditions, as the body's requirements for iron and overall iron status changes, transferrin saturation changes in response. Normal TIBC values range from 300 to 360 μg/dL. Generally, decreased transferrin saturation and increased TIBC values are associated with iron-deficiency anemia. Increased TIBC can also result from hypoxia, pregnancy, and medications including oral contraceptives and estrogen replacement therapy. TIBC decreases in patients with malignancies, nephritis, hemolytic anemia, and iron overload. As with serum transferrin, TIBC will remain normal or decrease in response to chronic or acute

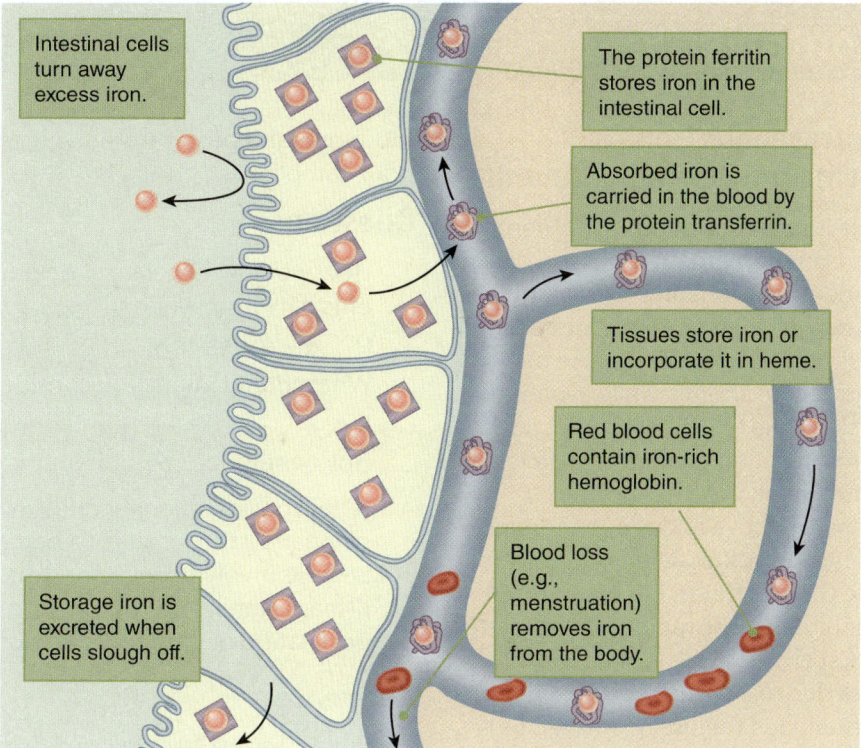

FIGURE 2.20 Iron Absorption in the Gastrointestinal Tract

inflammation. TIBC and transferrin saturation values persist until severe deficiency develops. Other biomarkers of iron status are necessary to accurately assess iron stores and detect early signs of anemia in patients.

Treatment of iron-deficiency anemia involves managing the underlying cause(s) of deficiency, restoring Hgb concentrations, and replenishing iron stores. Supplemental iron should increase serum reticulocyte count within a few days, although an increase in Hgb concentrations will not be evident for 2 to 3 weeks because iron utilization by bone marrow takes longer. Repletion of iron stores, measured by normalization of ferritin, will take even longer to improve. As a result, treatment duration should be at least 3 months to fully restore serum ferritin concentration. Iron supplementation can be administered orally (enterally) or intravenously. **Figure 2.20** illustrates iron absorption. Oral iron supplementation is preferred, as ferric salt, with amounts of elemental iron varying depending on salt form of product (ferrous calcium citrate, ferrous gluconate, ferrous ammonium citrate, ferrous dextran, and ferrous sucrose). After iron levels are restored, clinicians are recommended to recheck levels every 3 to 4 months for up to 1 year.[48]

Parenteral iron administration has historically been reserved for patients in whom oral iron therapy is ineffective or for those with malabsorptive disorders. Certain parenteral iron supplements such as iron dextran come with the risk of anaphylactic reactions. As a result, patients receiving iron dextran may benefit from a small test dose in a facility equipped for resuscitation with close monitoring for adverse reactions prior to receiving the full infusion. Other IV iron formulations such as iron sucrose have lower risk of anaphylaxis and may be better tolerated.

Macrocytic Anemias from B-Vitamin Deficiencies

Iron, vitamin B_{12}, and folate are the most important micronutrients for generation of erythrocytes. While iron deficiency alters production of hemoglobin, resulting in microcytic anemia, vitamin B_{12}, and folate deficiency impair synthesis of DNA and proteins and cell division, resulting in macrocytic anemia (large, nucleated red blood cells). Clinicians must assess patients further for vitamin B_{12} and folate deficiencies if abnormal CBC results (high MCV, low Hgb) indicate that macrocytic anemia may be present. Because MCV and Hgb are nonspecific measures and MCV value may be masked if iron deficiency is present, further assessment is needed to evaluate for vitamin B_{12} and folate deficiencies. As the clinical symptoms of vitamin B_{12} and folate deficiency are similar, a biochemical assessment of these vitamin levels is necessary to distinguish between B deficiencies. A static measurement of folate and vitamin B_{12} deficiency in the blood is used, testing the ability of a patient's blood specimen to support growth of microbes requiring folate or vitamin B_{12}.

Serum cobalamin was most commonly used to measure vitamin B_{12} status. Vitamin B_{12} is absorbed in the

> ## ⚠ Clinical Controversy
>
> ### Oral Iron versus Intravenous Iron Supplementation in Iron-Deficiency Anemia
>
> Iron-deficiency anemia is the most common nutrient deficiency worldwide. Iron supplementation is crucial in the treatment of iron-deficiency anemia, particularly in at-risk groups such as pregnant and postpartum women. Because anemia can be associated with adverse outcomes, adequate treatment of anemia while avoiding red blood cell transfusions due to increased infectious risk, possibility of allergic reactions, cost, and scarcity is critical. Use of oral iron in the treatment of iron-deficiency anemia is cost effective and easy to administer but can be limited by absorption as well as noncompliance due to adverse GI side effects. Intravenous (IV) iron may replete hemoglobin more rapidly, but concern exists with side effects such as allergic reactions and increased infection risk due to iron's pro-oxidant nature. Various studies have examined the use of oral versus IV iron to ascertain the preferred treatment route in pre- and postpartum women. Many studies have identified that IV iron is an effective mode of therapy over oral iron in the treatment of iron deficiency in pregnant and postpartum women. However, Litton et al. examined the use of IV iron through a meta-analysis of 75 randomized clinical trials (across many conditions and disease states) and found that IV iron administration was associated with increased hemoglobin and reduced risk of blood transfusion, but was also associated with an increased risk of infection when compared to oral or no iron supplementation. As oral iron is a common treatment for the prevention and treatment of iron deficiency in pregnant and postpartum women, IV iron may warrant consideration as an alternate iron delivery method for those pre- and post-partum women with anemia or poor compliance.
>
> ### Questions
>
> 1. How would you balance the potential risks and benefits of IV iron over oral iron in pregnant and post-partum women?
> 2. What criteria might you consider in recommending iron therapy treatment to this population?
> 3. How would you monitor for potential risks?
> 4. What considerations should you be mindful of when comparing the results of a heterogeneous meta-analysis involving wide range of conditions and disease states to clinical trails involving the target population of pregnant and post-partum women?
>
> ### References
>
> 1. Rudra S, Chandna A, Nath J. Comparison of intravenous iron sucrose with oral iron in pregnant women with iron deficiency anaemia. *Int J Reprod Contracept Obstet Gynecol*. 2016;5(3):747-751.
> 2. Neeru S, Sreekumaran Nair N, Rai L. Iron sucrose versus oral iron therapy in pregnancy anemia. *Indian J Community Med*. 2012; 37(4):214–218. doi: 10.4103/0970-0218.103467
> 3. Verma S, Inamdar SA, Malhotra N. Intravenous iron therapy versus oral iron in postpartum patients in rural area. *JSAFOG*. 2011;3(2):67-70.
> 4. Litton E, Xiao J, Ho KM. Safety and efficacy of intravenous iron therapy in reducing requirement for allogeneic blood transfusion: systematic review and meta-analysis of randomized clinical trials. *BMJ*. 2013;347:f4822. doi: https://doi.org/10.1136/bmj.f4822

ileum and stored in the liver and plays an important role in DNA synthesis and myelin synthesis. Normal values of serum cobalamin range from 200 to 900 pg/mL[49]. However, serum cobalamin has low sensitivity except in extremely deficient states, making its wide reference range for deficiency difficult to detect accurately. Serum levels may be elevated if patients receive IV minerals and vitamin infusions. Generally, low serum levels indicate macrocytosis and are associated with high MCV, high RDW, and low Hgb.

Vitamin B_{12} deficiency is now more accurately assessed using parameters in the metabolic pathways of *homocysteine (Hcy)* and *methylmalonic acid (MMA)*. This represents a functional assay as it describes the physiologic functioning of vitamin B_{12} as opposed to simply its quantity in the blood. Vitamin B_{12} plays a key role in converting homocysteine into methionine, one of the building blocks needed for protein synthesis. Vitamin B_{12} is a coenzyme in the reaction of MMA to succinyl coA. Therefore, high levels of serum MMA and Hcy are strongly associated with vitamin B_{12} deficiency. For patients with renal insufficiency, MMA is considered to be a more specific marker than Hcy because Hcy may be elevated due to decreased renal function, with or without the presence of vitamin B_{12} deficiency.

Subclinical vitamin B_{12} deficiency, defined as low serum vitamin B_{12} concentration and/or elevated MMA or Hcy that is responsive to vitamin B_{12} therapy, is commonly found in geriatric and vegan patients. Elderly patients and patients taking proton pump inhibitors are at higher risk of vitamin B_{12} deficiency due to decreased production of gastric acid, which is necessary for vitamin B_{12} absorption. For these patients, chronic supplementation of vitamin B_{12} may not be necessary. Oral cyanocobalamin, the synthetic form of vitamin B_{12}, is considered an effective treatment approach for vitamin B_{12} deficiency, but only if a significant portion of ileum is present and functional. For the first week, doses should range from 250 to 2,000 µg/day. This treatment should be followed by a maintenance period with at least 125 µg/day until symptoms have resolved in patients.[50] If treatment is taking several months for repletion of vitamin B_{12} stores and if clinical symptoms are not improving, a more intense therapy is needed. If neurological symptoms are present with deficiency, parenteral therapy is the preferred approach. Clinicians can use both MMA and Hcy to monitor progress and evaluate effectiveness of treatment.

Folate is absorbed in the small intestine and required for DNA synthesis. *Red blood cell folate (RBC folate)* is considered the most accurate measure of folate status in patients. Normal serum folate levels vary by age and are: 2-20 ng/mL in adults; and 5-21 ng/mL in children. In comparison to serum folate, RBC folate is more concentrated and more closely reflects tissue stores despite fluctuations in dietary intake. Normal RBC folate is 140-628 ng/mL in adults and >160 ng/mL in children. Low RBC folate is associated with folate deficiency and macrocytosis (high MCV, high RDW). Because folate is absorbed in the jejunum, folate deficiency may be caused by malabsorption in patients with celiac disease and those who have had bariatric surgery. Chronic alcohol consumption and long-term use of folate antagonists or antifolate medications including anticonvulsants and sulfasalazine can also cause folate deficiency. **Table 2.14** outlines common biochemical measures in iron-deficiency anemia, AICD, and folate and vitamin B_{12} deficiency anemias.

Before treating folate deficiency, vitamin B_{12} status must be assessed because treatment of folate deficiency can mask the symptoms of untreated vitamin B_{12} deficiency such as neuropathy. Once vitamin B_{12} status is sufficient or corrected, treatment of folate deficiency should focus on correcting anemia and replenishing folate stores as reflected by

TABLE 2.14 LABORATORY MEASURES IN IRON DEFICIENCY ANEMIA, ANEMIA OF INFLAMMATION AND CHRONIC DISEASE, FOLATE DEFICIENCY AND VITAMIN B_{12} DEFICIENCY

Laboratory Measure	IDA	AICD	Folate Deficiency	B_{12} Deficiency
Hemoglobin (Hgb)	↓	↓	↓	↓
Hematocrit (Hct)	↓	↓	↓	↓
Mean Corpuscular Volume (MCV)*	↓	↓	↑	↑
Red Cell Distribution Width (RDW)*	↑	WNL	↑	↑
Serum Ferritin	↓	WNL/↑	WNL	WNL
Serum Iron	↓	↓	WNL	WNL
Serum Transferrin	↑	↓/WNL	WNL	WNL
Transferrin Saturation	↓	↓	WNL	WNL
Red Blood Cell Folate	WNL	WNL	↓	WNL
Methylmalonic acid (MMA)	WNL	WNL	WNL	↑

*Expected levels may vary if more than one anemia or deficiency is present
↓ = reduced
↑ = increased
WNL = within normal limits
Modified from Clark, S. F. Iron deficiency anemia. *Nutr Clin Pract*. 2008; 23(2):128-141.

normal RBC folate concentration. Although the appropriate dose of folate to prevent anemia in nonpregnant individuals is not well established by clinical trials, current data suggest that oral folic acid supplementation of 5 to 10 mg/day is well tolerated.[51] Treatment duration should be at least 3 to 4 months depending on patients' RBC folate levels. If RBC folate levels remain low due to increased demand or malabsorptive disorders, a daily folic acid supplementation may be recommended to prevent recurrent anemia. In these circumstances, 500 to 800 µg daily may be a reasonable dose, although the most effective dose remains unclear.[52] **Table 2.15** differentiates microcytic and macrocytic anemia classifications.

Supplemental doses should take into account dietary intake of folate and RBC folate concentrations. Although folate-deficiency anemia can be prevented in most patients by optimizing diet intake, including foods fortified with folic acid, patients with suboptimal dietary folate intake may benefit from a weekly supplement of 500 µg of folic acid to prevent folate deficiency anemia. Because folate deficiency during pregnancy increases risk of neural tube defects, the U.S. Public Health Service and Centers for Disease Control and Prevention recommend that all women of childbearing age consume 400 µg of folic acid supplements before and during early pregnancy.[53] Women at high risk of neural tube defects are recommended to consume an extra 4 mg of synthetic folic acid supplements.[52] Unlike most supplement forms of vitamins and minerals, synthetic folic acid has been found to be more bioavailable than food sources of folate,[54] which supports the use of synthetic folic acid supplementation for primary treatment of folate deficiency. **Table 2.16** outlines the different types of anemias and associated nutrition deficiencies and toxicities.

TABLE 2.15 CLASSIFYING NUTRITIONAL ANEMIA (MICROCYTIC VERSUS MACROCYTIC)

Macrocytic	Deficiencies: • Vitamin B_{12}, folate, thiamin, pyridoxine
Microcytic	Deficiencies: • Protein, iron, ascorbate, vitamin A, pyridoxine, copper, manganese Toxicities: • Copper, zinc, lead, cadmium, other heavy metals

Data from Chulilla, J. A. M., Colás, M. S. R., & Martín, M. G. (2009). Classification of anemia for gastroenterologists. *World journal of gastroenterology: WJG*, 15(37), 4627.

TABLE 2.16 TYPES OF ANEMIAS AND RELATED NUTRITION DEFICIENCIES/TOXICITIES

Micronutrient Deficiency	Laboratory Values	Factors Affecting Laboratory Values
Iron	Low serum iron Low transferrin saturation or high TIBC Low ferritin Low MCV High Zinc protoporphyrin	Ferritin increases with inflammation (not accurate indicator in critically ill patient, or patients with acute inflammation) MCV may appear normal if concurrent deficiency in vitamin B_{12} and/or folate
Vitamin B_{12}	High MMA High serum homocysteine High MCV	Homocysteine can increase in presence of renal dysfunction (not an accurate indicator in these patients) MCV may appear normal if concurrent with iron deficiency
Folate	Low erythrocyte folate Low serum folate (fasting) High MCV	Serum folate can increase for up to 5 hours after meal, so measures made during fasting are most accurate MCV may appear normal if concurrent with iron deficiency
Copper	Low plasma copper Low ceruloplasmin	Plasma copper and ceruloplasmin increase with inflammation (not accurate indicators if inflammation present)
Zinc	Low 24-hour urine zinc excretion Low plasma/serum zinc	Plasma zinc decreases with inflammation (do not check in critically ill, consider checking C-reactive protein instead)

Modified from Chan LN, Mike LA. The science and practice of micronutrient supplementations in nutritional anemia: An evidence-based review. *JPEN J Parenter Enteral Nutr*. 2014;38(6):656-67.

> **CORE CONCEPT 7**
>
> Deficiencies in iron, vitamin B_{12}, and folate, and toxicities of copper and zinc, can all compromise red blood cell functioning and contribute to anemia.

Chapter Summary

Biochemical assessment is a critical component of the nutrition care process, providing important information regarding an individual's nutritional status as it relates to pertinent underlying health conditions. Interpreting trends in electrolyte, fluid, and acid–base levels can provide critical information about the progression or treatment of health conditions and about the most appropriate nutrition therapy plan. Consideration of these values in the context of other assessment measures (anthropometrics, functional assessment, and diet history) is crucial to accurately evaluate a patient's condition and nutritional needs. A collective evaluation of endocrine biomarkers, liver enzymes, lipid levels, and visceral proteins can help clinicians evaluate endocrine, liver, and cardiovascular function, as was a level of inflammatory stress, because these conditions can have a significant impact on a patient's nutritional status and needs. By assessing trends in these values, a clinician can determine whether a patient's health condition is progressing or improving, having important nutritional implications. Several biochemical values are also used to assess iron status and anemia and understanding how values can differentiate between types of anemia and treatment methods is critical. Prioritizing a patient's most severe and pertinent abnormal laboratory values in the context of nutritional status and needs is important in order for clinicians to provide the most effective nutrition therapy to patients.

Key Terms

static assay, functional assay, hemodilution, hemoconcentration, electrolytes, basic metabolic panel, comprehensive metabolic panel, complete blood count, differential count, osmotic pressure, isotonic, hypertonic, hypotonic, third spacing, hypervolemia, hypovolemia, hyponatremia, osmotic demyelination syndrome (ODS), hypernatremia, hypokalemia, hyperkalemia, hypocalcemia, hypercalcemia, hypophosphatemia, hyperphosphatemia, hypomagnesemia, hypermagnesemia, refeeding syndrome, hypochloremia, hyperchloremia, acidemia, alkalemia, acidosis, alkalosis, arterial blood gases (ABGs), respiratory acidosis, respiratory alkalosis, metabolic acidosis, metabolic alkalosis, hypoglycemia, hyperglycemia, visceral protein, acute-phase proteins, positive acute-phase proteins, negative acute-phase proteins, constitutive, marasmus, kwashiorkor, nitrogen balance, creatinine height index (CHI), anemia, microcytic anemia, macrocytic anemia, normocytic anemia, iron-deficiency anemia, anemia of inflammation and chronic disease (AICD)

References

1. Litchford MD. *Laboratory Assessment of Nutritional Status: Bridging Theory and Practice*. Greensboro, NC: CASE Software; 2010.
2. Oh MS: Evaluation of renal function, water, electrolyte and acid-base balance. In: McPherson RA, Pincus MR, eds. *Henry's Clinical Diagnosis and Management by Laboratory Methods*. 22nd ed. Philadelphia: W.B. Saunders; 2011:169-192.
3. Holcombe B. Parenteral nutrition product shortages. Impact on safety. *JPEN J Parenter Enteral Nutr*. 2012;36(2 suppl):44S-47S.
4. Hawkins RC. Age and gender as risk factors for hyponatremia and hypernatremia. *Clinica Chimica Acta*. 2003;337(1):169-172.
5. Verbalis JG, Goldsmith SR, Greenberg A, et al. Diagnosis, evaluation, and treatment of hyponatremia: expert panel recommendations. *Am J Med*. 2013;126(10):S1-S42.
6. Elhassan EA, Schrier RW. Hyponatremia: Diagnosis, complications, and management including V2 receptor antagonists. *Curr Opin Nephrol Hypertens*. 2011;20(2):161-168.
7. Sterns RH, Nigwekar SU, Hix JK. The treatment of hyponatremia. *Semin Nephrol*. 2009;29(3):282-299.
8. Snyder NA, Feigal DW, Arief AI. Hypernatremia in elderly patients: a heterogeneous, morbid, and iatrogenic entity. *Ann Intern Med*. 1987;107(3):309-319.
9. Burton D, Theodore P. *Clinical Physiology of Acid-Base and Electrolyte Disorders*. 5th ed. New York: McGraw-Hill; 2001.
10. Rose BD. *Clinical Physiology of Acid-Base and Electrolyte Disorders*. New York: McGraw-Hill; 1977.
11. Paice BJ, Paterson KR, Onyanga-Omara F, Donnelly T, Gray JM, Lawson DH. Record linkage study of hypokalaemia in hospitalized patients. *Postgrad Med J*. 1986;62(725):187-191.
12. Kraft MD, Btaiche IF, Sacks GS, Kudsk KA. Treatment of electrolyte disorders in adult patients in the intensive care unit. *AJHP*. 2005;62(16):1663.
13. Kruse JA, Clark VL, Carlson RW, Geheb MA. Concentrated potassium chloride infusions in critically ill patients with hypokalemia. *J Pharmacol Clin Toxicol*. 1994;34(11):1077-1082.
14. Mandal AK. Hypokalemia and hyperkalemia. *Med Clin North Am*. 1997;81(3):611-639.
15. Bushinsky DA, Monk RD. Calcium. *The Lancet*. 1998;352(9124):306-311.
16. Hanzlik RP, Fowler SC, Fisher DH. Relative bioavailability of calcium from calcium formate, calcium citrate, and calcium carbonate. *J Pharmacol Exp Ther*. 2005;313(3):1217-1222.
17. French S, Subauste J, Geraci S. Calcium abnormalities in hospitalized patients. *South Med J*. 2012;105:231-237.
18. Semple P, Both C. Calcium chloride: a reminder. *Anaesthesia*. 1996;51(1):93-93.
19. Davis KD, Attie MF. Management of severe hypercalcemia. *Crit Care Clin*. 1991;7(1):175-190.
20. Mundy GR, Guise TA. Hypercalcemia of malignancy. *Am J Med*. 1997;103(2):134-145.
21. Brunelli SM, Goldfarb S. Hypophosphatemia: clinical consequences and management. *J Am Soc Nephrol*. 2007;18(7):1999-2003.
22. Rude RK. Magnesium metabolism and deficiency. *Endocrinol Metab Clin North Am*. 1993;22(2):377-395
23. Whang R, Oei TO, Aikawa JK, et al. Predictors of clinical hypomagnesemia: hypokalemia, hypophosphatemia, hyponatremia, and hypocalcemia. *Arch Intern Med*. 1984;144(9):1794-1796.
24. Skipper A. Refeeding syndrome or refeeding hypophosphatemia: a systematic review of cases. *Nutr Clin Pract*. 2012;27(1):34-40.

25. Mehanna HM, Moledina J, Travis J. Refeeding syndrome: what it is, and how to prevent and treat it. *BMJ*. 2008;336(7659):1495-1498.

26. Sherwood L. *Human Physiology: From Cells to Systems*. 8th ed. Boston, MA: Cengage Learning; 2015.

27. Kurtz I, Maher T, Hulter HN, Schambelan M, Sebastian A. Effect of diet on plasma acid-base composition in normal humans. *Kidney Int*. 1983;24(5):670-680.

28. Winter SD, Pearson JR, Gabow PA, Schultz AL, Lepoff RB. The fall of the serum anion gap. *Arch Intern Med*. 1990;150(2):311-313.

29. Hodgkin JE, Soeprono FF, Chan DM. Incidence of metabolic alkalemia in hospitalized patients. *Crit Care Med*. 1980;8(12):725-728.

30. American Diabetes Association. Standards of medical care in Diabetes—2018. *Diabetes Care*. 2018;41(1):S1–S159.

31. Nathan, DM, Kuenen J, Borg R, Zheng H, Schoenfeld D, Heine RJ. Translating the A1C assay into estimated average glucose values. *Diabetes Care*. 2008; 31(8):1473-1478.

32. Rahbar S. The discovery of glycated hemoglobin: a major event in the study of nonenzymatic chemistry in biological systems. *Ann N Y Acad Sci*. 2005;1043(1):9-19.

33. American Diabetes Association. (6) glycemic targets. *Diabetes Care*. 2015;38(suppl):S33-40.

34. Keys A. Caloric undernutrition and starvation, with notes on protein deficiency. *J Am Med Assoc*. 1948;138(7):500-511.

35. Jensen GL, Bistrian B, Roubenoff R, Heimburger DC. Malnutrition syndromes: a conundrum vs continuum. *JPEN J Parenter Enteral Nutr*. 2009;33(6):710-716.

36. Dickerson RN, Tidwell AC, Minard G, Croce MA, Brown RO. Predicting total urinary nitrogen excretion from urinary urea nitrogen excretion in multiple-trauma patients receiving specialized nutritional support. *Nutrition*. 2005;21(3):332-338.

37. Blackburn GL, Bistrian BR, Maini BS, Schlamm HT, Smith MF. Nutritional and metabolic assessment of the hospitalized patient. *JPEN J Parenter Enteral Nutr*. 1977;1(1):11-22.

38. Fuhrman MP, Charney P, Mueller CM. Hepatic proteins and nutrition assessment. *J Am Diet Assoc*. 2004;104(8):1258-1264.

39. Chalasani N, Younossi Z, Lavine JE, et al. The diagnosis and management of non-alcoholic fatty liver disease: practice guideline by the American Association for the Study of Liver Diseases, American College of Gastroenterology, and the American Gastroenterological Association. *Hepatology*. 2012;55(6):2005-2023.

40. Patil H, Vaidya O, Bogart D. A review of causes and systemic approach to cardiac troponin elevation. *Clin Cardiol*. 2011;34(12):723-728.

41. Sharrett AR, Ballantyne CM, Coady SA, et al. Coronary heart disease prediction from lipoprotein cholesterol levels, triglycerides, lipoprotein(a), apolipoproteins A-I and B, and HDL density subfractions: the atherosclerosis risk in communities (ARIC) study. *Circulation*. 2001;104(10):1108-1113.

42. Wilson PW, D'Agostino RB, Levy D, Belanger AM, Silbershatz H, Kannel WB. Prediction of coronary heart disease using risk factor categories. *Circulation*. 1998;97(18):1837-1847.

43. Ewald PDN, Kloer H. Treatment options for severe hypertriglyceridemia (SHTG): the role of apheresis. *Clin Res Cardiol Suppl*. 2012;7(1):31-35.

44. World Health Organization. Haemoglobin concentrations for the diagnosis of anaemia and assessment of severity. Vitamin and Mineral Nutrition Information System. Geneva, 2011 (WHO/NMH/NHD/MNM/11.1) http://www.who.int/vmnis/indicators/haemoglobin.pdf Accessed November 5, 2017.

45. Clark SF. Iron deficiency anemia. *Nutr Clin Pract*. 2008;23(2):128-141.

46. Zubieta-Calleja G, Paulev P, Zubieta-Calleja L, Zubieta-Castillo G. Altitude adaptation through hematocrit changes. *J Physiol Pharmacol*. 2007;58(5):811-818.

47. Chan LN, Mike LA. The science and practice of micronutrient supplementations in nutritional anemia: an evidence-based review. *JPEN J Parenter Enteral Nutr*. 2014;38(6):656-672.

48. Taylor P. Martinez-Torres C, Leets I, Ramirez J, Garcia-Casal MN, Layrisse M. Relationships among Iron Absorption, percent saturation of plasma transferrin and serum ferritin concentration in humans. *J Nutr*. 1988;118:1110-1115.

49. Stabler SP. Vitamin B_{12} deficiency. *N Engl J Med*. 2013;368(2):149-160.

50. Solomon LR. Disorders of cobalamin (vitamin B_{12}) metabolism: emerging concepts in pathophysiology, diagnosis, and treatment. *Blood Rev*. 2007;21(3):113-130.

51. Butterworth CE Jr, Tamura T. Folic acid safety and toxicity: a brief review. *Am J Clin Nutr*. 1989;50(2):353-358.

52. Joseph B, Ramesh N. Weekly dose of iron-folate supplementation with vitamin-C in the workplace can prevent anaemia in women employees. *Pak J Med Sci*. 2013;29(1):47-52.

53. Folic acid recommendations. Centers for Disease Control and Prevention website. https://www.cdc.gov/ncbddd/folicacid/recommendations.html Updated December 28, 2016. Accessed November 9, 2017.

54. Suitor CW, Bailey LB. Dietary folate equivalents: interpretation and application. *J Am Diet Assoc*. 2000;100(1):88-94.

Chapter 3

Enteral Nutrition

Nusheen Orandi
Kathy Prelack

Chapter Outline

Core Concepts
Introduction
The Evolution of Enteral Nutrition
Determining the Route of Enteral Nutrition
Types of Enteral Tubes
Gastric Versus Small-Bowel Feeding
Formula Delivery Methods
Enteral Formula Compositions
Disease-Specific Formulas
Developing an EN Feeding Plan
Complication Monitoring
Early Enteral Nutrition
Immunonutrition

CORE CONCEPTS

1. Enteral nutrition includes food, oral supplements, and formulas created specifically to prevent malnutrition and accommodate nutrient needs in various disease states.
2. A patient's specific disease state and anticipated length of feeding time determine the route of enteral nutrition.
3. Gastric feeding more closely mimics how the gastrointestinal tract functions physiologically, which offers a metabolic and lifestyle benefit.
4. Small-bowel feedings are recommended for patients with gastric complications, gastroparesis, or increased aspiration risk.
5. The feeding–fasting environment associated with bolus feeding induces a favorable hormonal and nutrient response that promotes protein synthesis and anabolism.
6. Enteral nutrition formulas include carbohydrates, fat, protein, vitamins and minerals, and fiber, and are nutritionally complete.
7. Disease specific formulas that deviate from standard formulations can be used in many disease states to aid patients in meeting their nutritional needs.
8. Patients must be monitored closely for complications related to enteral feeding or side effects to medical treatment. Feeding method and formula should be adjusted as needed.

Learning Objectives

1. Explain the evolution of today's enteral nutrition.
2. Identify a patient's enteral nutrition route based on the current disease state and anticipated length of feeding time.
3. Explore the various short-term and long-term tube placements.
4. Describe the types of tubes and devices available for tube feeding.
5. State the advantages and disadvantages of gastric versus small-bowel feeding.
6. Identify three different formula delivery methods.
7. Describe the standard composition of enteral formulas.
8. Explain characteristics of specialty formulas and indications for their use.
9. Recognize complications associated with enteral nutrition and strategies to manage them.

Introduction

Enteral nutrition (EN) refers to the delivery of nutrients into the gastrointestinal tract either by mouth or through a feeding tube. EN includes food, oral supplements, and formulas created specifically to prevent malnutrition and accommodate nutrient needs in various disease states.[1-2] The development of EN has transformed nutritional care in a hospital setting, where the inability to receive adequate nutrition by normal means is common. Obstacles to oral intake have many causes, including gastrointestinal disease, swallowing inabilities, or increased nutrient needs related to critical illness or wound healing.[3] The use of EN to target specific immune-related and physiologic processes and alter the course of disease is an exciting aspect of enteral nutrition support that is supported by a robust research platform.

The Evolution of Enteral Nutrition

Enteral nutrition has a long history that dates back to the early 20th century. The first nasoduodenal tube was placed in 1910 and had a formula of raw egg, milk, and lactose.[4] In 1918, the first reported jejunal feeding took place using a formula of peptonized milk, dextrose, and whiskey.[4] It was not until the 1950s that the first commercial formulas were used.[4] It was at this time that flexible polyethylene tubes were developed as well. The 1970s brought increased food technology, including the formulation of more synthetic tube feeds (TFs). Low-residue and lactose-free TFs were developed, as well as TFs with a range of osmolalities.

In the 1980s, EN resurged and became more clinically formalized to support nutrition and digestion, aid wound healing, help the immune system, and support the critically ill.[5] Around this time, the first **percutaneous endoscopic gastrostomy (PEG) tube** was placed.[6,7] Tube placement capabilities became more advanced and TF products proliferated. Formula began to be fortified with fiber, predigested to include di- and tri-peptides, and enhanced to be more calorically dense. Product developers soon began to create more specialized formulas specific to certain diseases.

EN technology continued to advance in the 1990s. The potential pharmacologic role of micronutrients in modulating cellular and systemic physiology demonstrated a clear connection among disease, inflammation, and nutrient metabolism. The era of **immunonutrition**, marked by the predominance of specialty formulas enhanced with glutamine, arginine, and omega-3 fatty acids, had arrived. Research on the safety and efficacy of these formulas in altering the progression of disease, at times lagging industrial gains, continues to help guide the appropriate use of these immune-enhancing enteral products.

> **CORE CONCEPT 1**
>
> Enteral nutrition includes food, oral supplements, and formulas created specifically to prevent malnutrition and accommodate nutrient needs in various disease states.

Determining the Route of Enteral Nutrition

Determination of the site and route of EN should consider an individual's anticipated length of feeding time; their medical condition or disease state, including anatomical barriers within the gastrointestinal tract; and the surgical options for that individual (**Figure 3.1**).

The timing of enteral delivery is determined according to several considerations. First is the anticipated duration of enteral support. If a person is expected to require short-term tube feeding, generally 4 weeks or fewer, then a **nasoenteric** or **oroenteric** tube may be used.[1,8] Nasoenteric or oroenteric feeds require that a tube be placed in the nose or mouth and advanced into the stomach or past the pylorus. Nasoenteric tubes are used more often than oroenteric tubes for short-term feeding because they are better tolerated by the patient. If a person is in need of long-term nutrition care, or nutrition care lasting for longer than 4 weeks, then a more permanent gastrostomy or jejunostomy method is used.[2,8,9] A patient's specific needs or gastrointestinal function determines the specific enteral route, as seen in **Figure 3.2**.

> **CORE CONCEPT 2**
>
> A patient's specific disease state and anticipated length of feeding time determine the route of enteral nutrition.

> **PRACTICE POINT**
>
> If a patient requires tube feeding for 4 weeks or fewer, utilize a nasoenteric tube. If a patient requires significantly more than 4 weeks of nutrition care, a gastric or postpyloric percutaneous tube placement can be considered.

CASE STUDY INTRODUCTION

Laura is a 58-year-old female admitted to the hospital due to severe epigastric distress. She has not been able to eat in the last 48 hours due to pain. A medical work up has identified a large lesion in the distal portion of her stomach. Laura now awaits gastric surgery for removal of the tumor. She will be unable to eat for the next 2 weeks. After surgery, she will require a 12-week course of radiation and chemotherapy. Laura lives alone at home. She has two adult children. Her oldest daughter is a nurse and lives nearby.

Anthropometric Data:
Height: 152 cm (60")
Weight: 74 kg (163 lb)
Body mass index: 32 kg/m^2
Weight History
Usual Weight: 79 kg (167 lb)

Biochemical Data:
Sodium 147 (135-145 mEq/L)
Potassium 4.7 (3.6-5.0 mEq/L)
Chloride 101 (98-110 mEq/L)
Carbon dioxide 23 (20-30 mEq/L)
Blood urea nitrogen 28 (6-24 mg/dL)
Creatinine 0.5 (0.4-1.3 mg/dL)
Glucose 101 (70-139 mg/dL)
Hemoglobin 11.1 (12.0-15.5 g/dL)
Hematocrit 30 (35%-42%)

Calcium 8.7 (8.5-10.5 mEq/L)
Phosphorus 4.7 (2.7-4.5 mg/dL)
Magnesium 1.6 (1.3-2.1 mEq/L)
Total protein 6.0 (6.4-8.3 g/dL)
Albumin 3.2 (3.5-5.0 g/dL)

Clinical Data:
Past Medical History: Hyperlipidemia, gastric reflux, migraines
Medications: Avorostatin, Prevacid
Vital Signs: Blood pressure 155/77 mm Hg; temperature 99.0°C; heart rate 98 beats/min
Nutrition-focused Physical Exam: Patient appears pale and tired. Abdominal exam reveals a distended, nontender abdomen. Skin, hair, nail and oral exam appear normal. Patient noted to have adequate fat and muscle stores. No edema noted.

Dietary Data:
Dietary History: Laura typically has a good appetite. "I tend to eat healthy, but for the last 2 days, I have had pain when eating foods, and have only had broth and water or cranberry juice."
24-hour Diet Recall:
Breakfast: Coffee (cream and sugar), oatmeal with honey, or fruit with yogurt
Lunch: Turkey on whole grain bread with mustard, chocolate chip cookies, diet soda
Dinner: Salmon, rice pilaf, garden salad, glass of wine
Diet Prescription: NPO (nothing by mouth) for surgery. Nutrition consult is placed for suggestion for enteral tube feeding recommendation.

Questions
1. What are Laura's nutritional risk factors?
2. What labs are concerning? What additional labs might you ask for?
3. What type of enteral tube feeding placement do you recommend? Explain your rationale.
4. Provide recommendations for enteral feeding type and method of delivery.

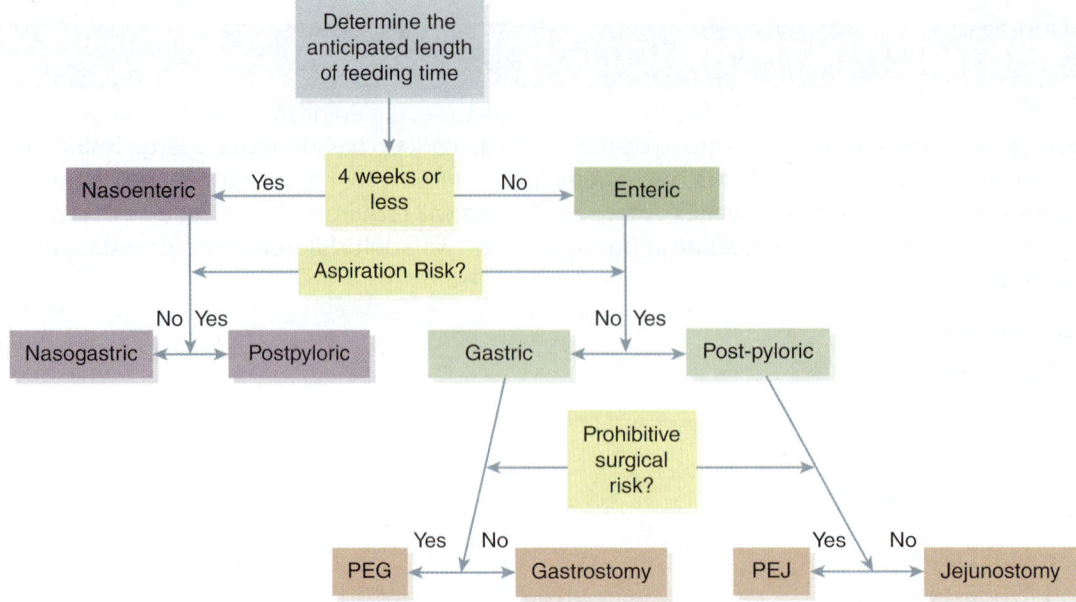

FIGURE 3.1 Algorithm for Selection of Feeding Tube Placement

Data from Gorman RC, Morris JB: Minimally invasive access to the gastrointestinal tract. In Rombeau JL, Rolandelli RH, eds. *Clinical nutrition: enteral and tube feeding.* 3rd ed. Philadelphia: WB Saunders; 1997.

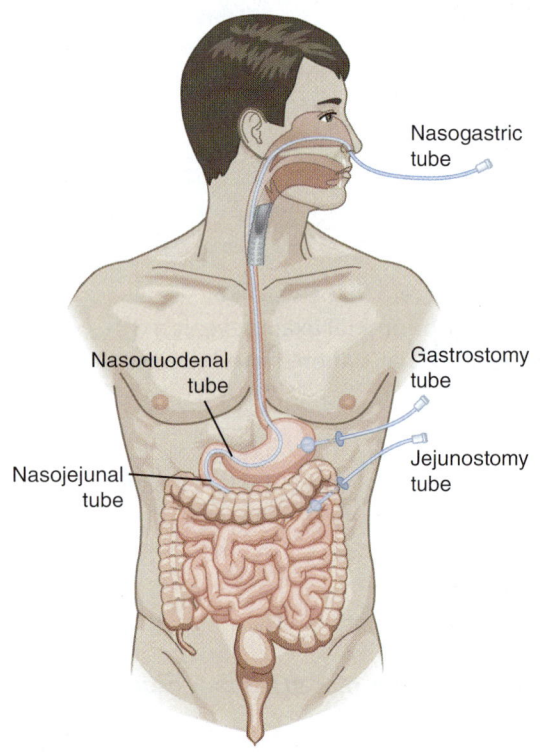

FIGURE 3.2 Basic Tube Placement Options

Short-term Placement

As mentioned, for patients who need short-term feeding, a nasoenteric or oroenteric method is used.[1,8,10-12] Nasoenteric tubes can be placed at the bedside, endoscopically, or fluoroscopically. **Nasogastric tube** placement is appropriate for patients who have normal gastric function. A tube is entered through the nose or mouth and is placed directly into the stomach. Postpyloric placement of nasoenteric tubes is used if a patient has gastric complications or aspiration risk but otherwise normal small intestine function.

Nasoduodenal tube feeding requires the tube be placed from the nose, through the stomach, to the duodenum of the small intestine, and **nasojejunal tube** feedings require that the tube is placed from the nose and advanced to the jejunum of the small intestine. While nasogastric tubes can usually be placed at the bedside, nasojejunal tubes are better placed with endoscopic or fluoroscopic methods.[10,11]

Bedside Nasoenteral Technique

The bedside nasogastric tube placement begins by obtaining a small-bore tube, about 8 to 12 French (1 French [Fr] is equal to 0.33 mm in diameter).[13] A large-bore tube can also be used and is thought to prevent clogging; however, the small-bore tube can be more comfortable for the patient.[15] The length of the tube is determined by first measuring the distance from the patient's nose to the earlobe, and then from the earlobe to the xiphoid.[14] The patient lies on his or her right side and, as air is insufflated, the tube is bent and slowly enters through the patient's nose (**Figure 3.3**).[15,16] **Prokinetics**, which are medications that promote motility

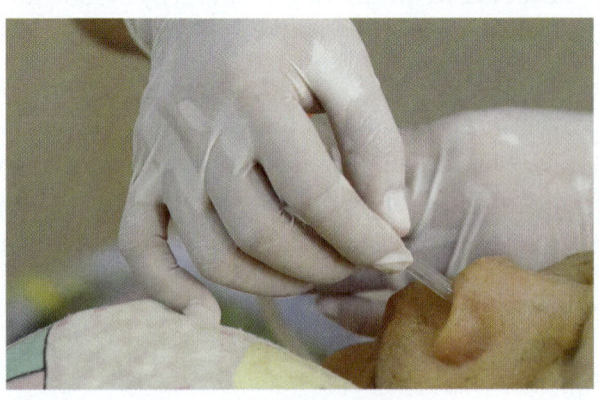

FIGURE 3.3 Insertion of Nasoenteric Feeding Tube

© Anukool Manoton/Shutterstock.

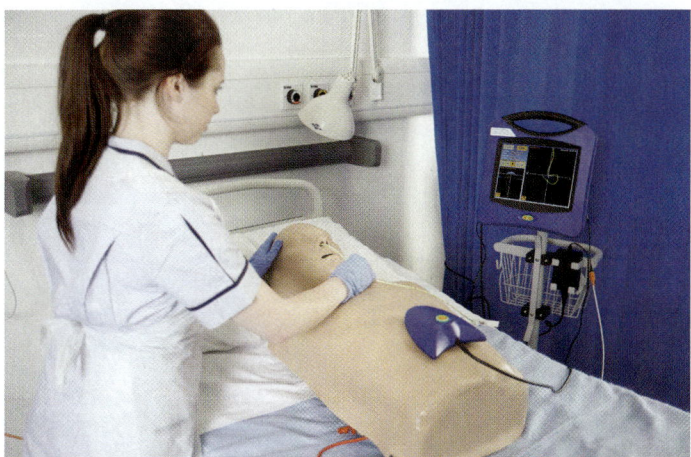

FIGURE 3.4 Use of an Electromagnetically Guided Tube Placement Allows for Feedings to be Initiated Sooner and Without the Need for X-Ray
Reproduced with permission Adam, Rouilly Limited.

by increasing small intestine contractions (such as metoclopramide and erythromycin) are often used to facilitate this technique.[14,16,17] Certain technologies are also used to ensure that the nasogastric tube is placed correctly; these include radiographs, typically a chest x-ray, as well as magnetically guided feeding tubes and electromagnetic imaging systems.[14,16,18-20] Electromagnetically guided feeding tubes have the advantage of being able to immediately confirm tube placement or identify tube misplacement so that the tube can be adjusted during placement. Not only does this alleviate the need for an additional chest x-ray, it also allows for feedings to be initiated sooner (**Figure 3.4**).[20]

Endoscopic Nasoenteral Technique

Nasoduodenal and nasojejunal tube placements are most easily done by endoscopic insertion.[16] A drag and pull technique is often utilized, where a suture is placed at the end of the nasoenteric tube and pushed with the tube from the patient's nostril to the stomach.[14,20] Meanwhile, an endoscope, with forceps, is advanced orally to the stomach.[16] In the stomach, the endoscopic forceps takes hold of the nasoenteric tube and suture, and the entire unit then enters the duodenum, or even the jejunum if possible.[14,16] In the small intestine, the forceps release the tube and the endoscope retracts.[14] Many studies suggest that there is greater placement success if the tube is placed after the ligament of Treitz.[11,14,16] With endoscopic aid, the nasoenteral tube is now properly placed in the small intestine.

Another endoscopic nasoenteral technique involves pushing an endoscope all the way to the small intestine with a guidewire to allow tube entry.[11,14,17] The guidewire is pushed through the transnasal channel with the endoscope and then remains in the small intestine while the endoscope is removed. The feeding tube is advanced over the guidewire to ultimately be placed in the small intestine through the same passage.

Fluoroscopic Nasoenteric Technique

Fluoroscopic nasoenteric tube placement involves using x-ray imaging as a guide when placing the feeding tube from the nose to the stomach or small intestine.[21] While there is success with this technique, it is not used as often as the bedside or endoscopic techniques because of radiation exposure or if the patient requires bedside attention due to critical illness.[11,17,21]

> **PRACTICE POINT**
>
> Nasogastric tube placement is commonly done on the patient at bedside. Nasoduodenal and nasojejunal tubes are more easily placed using endoscopic, and less commonly fluoroscopic, methods.

Long-term Placement

Percutaneous Endoscopic Gastrostomy Technique

Percutaneous endoscopic gastrostomy is the most common long-term tube placement method and can be performed at the bedside.[6,8,16,22,23] In what is called the pull technique, an endoscope is placed into the abdomen (**Figure 3.5**). Air is insufflated into the abdomen through the endoscope. The abdomen is then transilluminated to find the optimal spot for the tube placement and an indentation is placed on that spot.[16,23] After a small incision is made, a needle is placed through the abdominal wall and into the stomach so that a guidewire can be placed through the needle. An endoscopic snare is attached to the needle. The endoscope, needle, and snare are pulled back through the mouth, and the feeding tube is attached to the guidewire or placed over the guidewire.[20] The guidewire and tube are then pulled back through the esophagus and to the stomach. The tube is internally held in place by a bumper. An external bumper also ensures secure gastronomic placement.[16]

Percutaneous Endoscopic Jejunostomy Technique

If the patient has gastric complications, a **percutaneous endoscopic jejunostomy (PEJ)** can be performed. If there is an existing gastrostomy tube, a transpyloric feeding tube can be placed through the previously placed PEG tube and placed endoscopically into the jejunum.[16]

Another way of performing this procedure is to place the tube directly into the small bowel. The technique is similar to the PEG method, except the guidewire and tube are placed endoscopically into the jejunum.[6,16,22,24]

Surgical Methods

If a patient is in a traumatic condition or is undergoing surgery, a surgical means of tube placement may be used. This can be done in an open tube procedure or with laparoscopy under general anesthesia.[16,25] In **laparoscopy**, small ports are placed on the abdominal wall so that the peritoneal cavity can be accessed.[16] Once a camera and second port are placed, the stomach is attached to

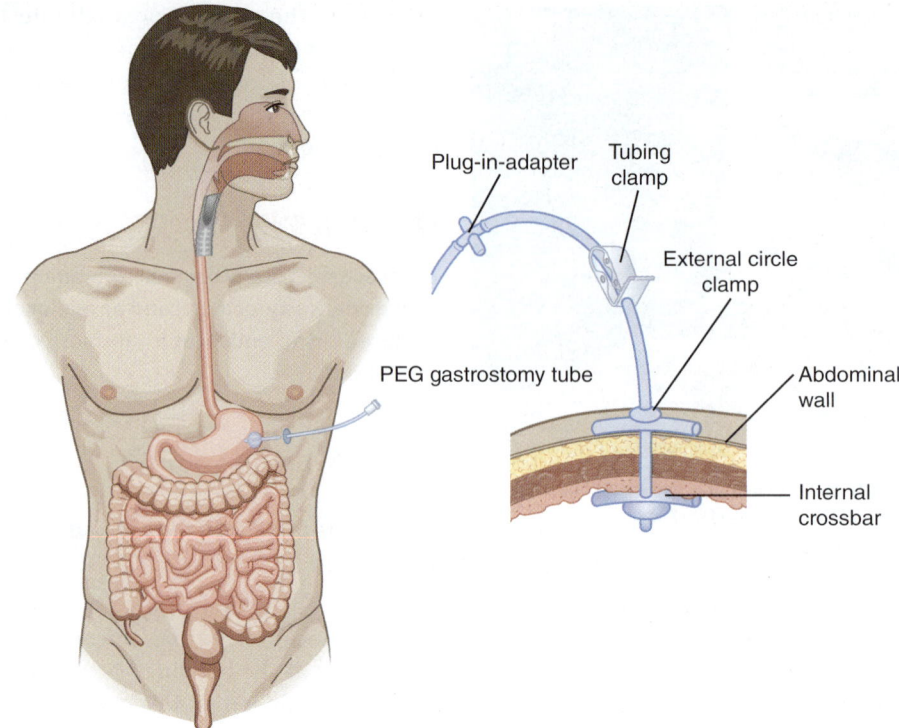

FIGURE 3.5 Percutaneous Endoscopic Gastrostomy is the Most Common Long Term Tube Placement Method and can be Performed Bedside

the abdominal wall by use of small structures called T-fasteners.[16,25] A needle and wire can then be placed into the stomach lumen so that a gastrostomy tube can finally be placed.

In the **open tube placement** technique, a small incision is made on the abdomen so that the gastrostomy tube can enter.[15,24] Sutures are placed to fasten the stomach around the feeding tube, as well as to fasten the stomach to the top of the abdomen wall.[15] Jejunostomy tubes can also be entered via open and laparoscopic techniques. A similar procedure is used in order to access the small bowel.

Types of Enteral Tubes

Feeding tubes have developed over time to become more comfortable for the patient and experience less clogging and other malfunctions. Nasogastric tubes made of polyvinyl chloride are more rigid and allow simple access. They can also be used for gastric suctioning and administering medications. Currently, most nasoenteric tubes are made out of polyurethane or silicone.[16,26,27,28] Polyurethane tubes are more pliable than polyvinyl chloride tubes and cause less nasopharyngeal erosion, which gives greater comfort to the patient. The structure of these tubes also makes it more difficult for a patient to aspirate, mitigating feeding complications. Silicone tubes are also flexible, more so than polyurethane, and therefore more comfortable to the patient. Nasoenteric tubes are generally sized 8 to 12 Fr.[16,27] For PEG tube placements, polyurethane and silicone tubes can be used, although silicone tubes tend to be used more often.[16] PEG tubes are generally sized 15 to 28 Fr in diameter.[27]

Gastric Versus Small-Bowel Feeding

There are certain indications that might prompt a clinician to initiate gastric versus postpyloric feeding in a patient. Both types have advantages and disadvantages that will be discussed further in this section.

Gastric Feeding

If normal gastric function is presumed, then gastric feedings are generally used. One advantage of gastric feedings is that they are more physiologic. The stomach acts as a natural reservoir for nutrients, so gastric placement of the feeding tube more closely mimics how the body receives nutrients.[12] It also allows for intermittent and bolus feeds, which have both metabolic and lifestyle benefits. Bolus intragastric feeding more closely resembles how the gastrointestinal tract functions physiologically, allowing contents to slowly empty into the small bowel.[12] The hydrochloric acid in the stomach also acts as bactericidal agent, providing less risk from any contaminants in the tube feeding. Also, certain nutrients require this acidification for proper absorption. Large-bore gastric tubes have less clogging than the small-bore tubes used in small-bowel feeding.[29,30] In addition, there is more ease to gastric tube placement; there are usually fewer attempts to place the tube correctly, and it can be done at bedside.[29,30] This usually makes gastric feeding more cost-effective than small-bowel feeding.[30] Lastly, the ease of bolus feedings has considerable lifestyle benefit. Incorporating bolus feedings on a routine schedule limits the amount of time the patient needs to be connected to a feeding pump, allowing more flexibility for the patient.

Clinical Roundtable

Background: One challenge to enteral feeding in a critical care setting is the need for interruption due to clinical interventions and procedures such as operating room visits, high-risk dressing changes, and extubation from a ventilator. Various strategies are employed to compensate for the energy and nutrient deficits associated with these procedures. Included among these are use of postpyloric feedings through the procedures, intermittent parenteral feedings during NPO phases, and volume-based feedings that increase the volume of feeding prior to and after procedures to assure adequate amount of feedings. Each of these strategies is associated with some degree of risk related to intolerance of feedings, aspiration, infection (in the case of PN), or hyperglycemia.

Roundtable Discussion

Discuss the pros and cons of these approaches. Are there certain patient populations that might benefit more from one approach or another? How does placement of feeding tube and central venous catheter access effect your decision?

References

1. McClave SA, Saad MA, Esterl M, et al. Volume-based feeding in the critically ill patient. *J Parenter Enteral Nutr.* 2015;39(6):707-712.
2. Varon DE, Freitas G, Goel N, et al. Intraoperative feeding improves calorie and protein delivery in acute burn patients. *J Burn Care Res.* 2017;38(5):299-303. doi: 10.1097/BCR.0000000000000514

Certain disadvantages also exist for gastric feeding. There can be several procedure-related feeding interruptions or other forms of intolerance.[29] A commonly cited risk is **aspiration**, or the movement of liquid into the patient's lungs.[29-31] Aspiration risk with continuous nasogastric feeding can lead to nosocomial (hospital-acquired) pneumonia.[12,29-31] Those who are at risk of aspiration include patients who are neurologically impaired, have experienced severe trauma, had a surgical operation, are heavily sedated, or have **gastroparesis** (delayed gastric emptying) due to a metabolic condition or operation.[29] In these cases, it may be more suitable to utilize small-bowel feeding.[29,30]

> **CORE CONCEPT 3**
>
> Gastric feeding more closely mimics how the gastrointestinal tract physiologically functions, which offers a metabolic and lifestyle benefit.

Small-bowel Feeding

Duodenal or jejunal feeding may be preferred if a patient has gastroparesis or reflux, or is diagnosed with aspiration risk.[29,31] It may also accommodate early satiety problems.

Small-bowel feedings afford an important advantage for patients who may have gastric complications or gastroparesis[29]. They decrease the risk of microaspiration, as well as of aspiration pneumonia.[29-31] Some studies demonstrate that small-bowel feedings allow patients to achieve a goal rate of infusion that may have not been attained with gastric feedings, providing a means of adequate nutrition.[29] It has also been shown that small-bowel feedings lead to decreased commencement of parenteral nutrition (PN). The benefit of being able to provide small-bowel feedings through clinical procedures has contributed to this decreased reliance on PN. Postpyloric feedings are now often continued during clinical interventions requiring anesthesia, either at the bedside or in the operating room. Major advancements in practice have led in some cases to intraoperative feedings, where EN is continuously provided throughout an operation. This practice has proven to be safe and effective in minimizing the energy and protein deficits that normally take place during planned surgeries.[32]

There is an increased cost associated with using small-bowel feedings, especially when using x-rays in fluoroscopy. Often, multiple attempts are needed to place the feeding tube correctly due to dislodgment of the feeding tube, and this can also be costly. Because it lacks holding capacity, the small intestine tends to be more sensitive to volume and osmotic load, so small-bowel feedings can lead to symptoms similar to **dumping syndrome**, a condition that causes rapid gastric emptying.[12] In this condition, food and liquid move from the stomach to the small intestine too quickly, causing abdominal pain and diarrhea shortly after a meal or feeding. Another disadvantage to small-bowel feedings is that bolus or large volume intermittent feeding cannot be provided.

> **CORE CONCEPT 4**
>
> Small-bowel feedings are recommended for patients with gastric complications, gastroparesis, or increased aspiration risk.

Formula Delivery Methods

There are several ways of delivering formula to make sure the patient is receiving adequate nutrition. Whether continuous, intermittent, or bolus feedings are used depends on the location of the feeding tube, the patient's gastrointestinal function and history of tolerance, and lifestyle considerations. Formula can be delivered to a patient via two systems. In a **closed tube feeding system**, a ready-to-use container or bag of formula is connected to the patient's feeding access.[26,33] In an **open tube feeding system**, formula from a can or package is poured into a separate container that is then attached to the patient's feeding access point.[26,33] A closed system product can safely be at room temperature for 24 to 48 hours, whereas an open system product should be at room temperature for 4 to 8 hours, depending upon the formula hanging.[26,33] This is known as the **hang time**. Reconstituted formulas should hang for no more than 4 hours while sterile decanted formula has an 8 hour hang time (except for neonates).[26,33] Clinicians may also wish to limit hang time for certain high risk populations, such as patients with burns or those who are immunocompromised. While closed tube feeding systems are preferred from an infection-control standpoint, at times open tube feeding systems are used when modular components are needed to enhance protein or calories specific to the patient's requirements.

Continuous

Continuous feeding is a common delivery method used for hospital patients. This method provides a slow infusion of feedings into the stomach or small intestine on an hourly basis. Using this method decreases risk for aspiration and gastric distention.[1] It tends to be the most easily tolerated because of its gradual delivery of feeding, and it allows for greater nutrient uptake in patients who may have marginal absorptive capacity. It also reduces the effect of thermogenesis. Most importantly, continuous feeding may be preferred for those patients with gastrointestinal complications or severe trauma because it has less risk of diarrhea and has been shown to reach nutrition goals more often.[34-36]

Despite a lack of evidence-based protocols for tube feeding advancement, conventional therapy consists of a moderate-to-low volume at initiation, followed by gradual advancement while continuously monitoring patient tolerance. Typically, continuous feeds begin at 20 to 55 mL/hour for adults and 0.5 to 1 mL/kg for children (depending on age). Once the patient can tolerate the tube feeding, the feeding rate advances incrementally. For adults, this rate increases by about 10 to 25 mL/hour every 4 to 24 hours until the goal rate is achieved. For children, this rate increases by 0.5 to 1 mL every 4 to 8 hours until the goal rate is achieved.

Intermittent

With **intermittent feeding**, feeding is delivered over a 20- to 60-minute interval, 4 to 6 times per day.[1] The duration and timing of intervals depend on the patient's formula need to attain adequate nutrition. Intermittent feeding can be administered using an infusion pump or by using the gravity drip method. Intermittent feeding provides the benefit of cyclic elevation of insulin levels. The rise in insulin in response to feeding creates an anabolic environment that promotes protein synthesis and improved protein nutritional status.[34]

Bolus Feedings

In **bolus feedings**, a specific volume of feeding is delivered over a short period of time a certain number of times per day.[1] An example feeding regimen would be rapid delivery of 200 to 400 mL of TF over approximately 5 to 20 minutes, 3 to 6 times per day.[1] Bolus feedings provide the benefit of mimicking normal eating.[1,12] Hormonal response to a feeding-fasting regimen is more anabolic than that seen with continuous feedings, resulting in increased amino acid and insulin levels and ultimately improved protein synthesis.[34] Often, a bolus regimen is preferable for stable patients because it does not rely on pumps and devices as much as the other methods, giving the patient an easier lifestyle.[1] While bolus feedings are less commonly used due to presumed risk of aspiration pneumonia and issues with tolerance, studies do not consistently support this notion, even in high-risk patients. This method of feeding, when compared to continuous feeding in critically ill adult patients, is shown to be equally well tolerated with no difference in gastroesophageal reflux, aspiration, aspiration pneumonia, glycemic variability, or time to reach calorie goal.[35-37]

> **CORE CONCEPT 5**
>
> The feeding–fasting environment associated with bolus feeding induces a favorable hormonal and nutrient response that promotes protein synthesis and anabolism.

CASE STUDY REVISITED

A percutaneous jejunostomy was successfully placed for enteral feedings. Laura is to remain NPO for 2 days. A nutrition consult is written for initiation of enteral feedings in 48 hours.
Her estimated energy and protein requirements based on your nutrition standard of care for surgical patients with mild stress/trauma are below:

Energy: 2,220 kcals per day (30 kcal/kg)

Protein: 111 g protein per day (1.5 g/kg)

Questions

1. What general type of enteral feeding do you recommend (intact, semi-elemental, elemental)?
2. Do you recommend a standard or disease-specific enteral type of feeding?
3. Provide a recommendation for EN, including EN type, goal volume, method of delivery, and guidelines for initiation and advancement.

Enteral Formula Compositions

A clinician must determine a formula that will meet a patient's nutrient needs. Many different standard formulas exist that are strategic compilations of carbohydrates, fat, protein, fiber, prebiotics and probiotics, vitamins, minerals, and water. Formulas for individuals with impaired digestion, also known as predigested; semi-elemental; or elemental formulas are available as well. Additionally, certain EN feedings are created for patients with specific diseases and conditions, such as diabetes; severe wounds; or complications with renal, pulmonary, or liver function. Lastly, immune-enhancing feedings are available for the critically ill and patients with altered metabolism. Table 3.1 shows various EN products categorized by composition and indication for use.

TABLE 3.1 TYPES OF TUBE FEEDING FORMULAS FOR ADULTS

Formula	Indication	Examples
Standard	Normal gastrointestinal function and fluid needs, feeding well-tolerated	Osmolite Promote Nutren Replete
Standard with Fiber	Long-term need for tube feeding; diarrhea and/or constipation	Jevity Promote with fiber Nutren with fiber Replete with fiber
Standard-Nutrient Dense (high nitrogen or high calorie)	Increased wound healing	Osmolite 1.2, 1.5 Jevity 1.2, 1.5 Isosource 1.5 Nutren 1.5
Fluid-Restricted	Restricted fluid allowance	Two Cal HN Nutren 2.0
Peptide-Based (partially hydrolyzed whey protein)	Impaired digestion	Peptamen, Peptamen 1.5 w/Prebio Vital Vital 1.5
Amino Acid Based (100% free amino acids)	Impaired digestion	Vivonex T.E.N
Immune-Enhanced	State of stress or trauma	Impact, Oxepa, Pivot
Renal	Kidney dysfunction and restrictions of potassium, phosphorus, and fluid	Nepro, Suplena Novosource Renal
Diabetes	Moderate carbohydrate, fiber enhanced	Glucerna Glytrol Diabetisource
Pulmonary	Moderate to low carbohydrate, higher fat content	Pulmocare Nutren Pulmonary
Hepatic	High branched-chain amino acids, low aromatic amino acids	Nutrihep

Tables **3.2** and **3.3** provide the nutrient composition of standard polymeric formulas and products used for patients with impaired digestion. The general nutritional content of these is similar; however, for those with impaired digestion, simpler or easier to digest forms of carbohydrate, protein, and fat are provided.

Carbohydrates

Carbohydrates are the primary energy source of enteral formula. They generally comprise 40%–90% of the formula.[38] Carbohydrate sources include monosaccharides such as glucose or fructose, and disaccharides including sucrose and maltose. Lactose is often omitted from enteral feeding products because it requires lactase, which is insufficient in some patients, leading to poor tolerance and symptoms of cramping, bloating and diarrhea.[38]

Other types of carbohydrates incorporated into formula include oligosaccharides and polysaccharides. Oligosaccharides are made of 2 to 10 glucose units. The most common oligosaccharide used in formula is maltodextrin, which is

TABLE 3.2 NUTRIENT COMPOSITION OF STANDARD ADULT POLYMERIC ENTERAL FORMULATIONS

Formula Name	Jevity Jevity 1.2 Jevity 1.5	Osmolite Osmolite 1.2 Osmolite 1.5	Promote Promote with Fiber	Replete Replete with Fiber	Nutren 1.0 Nutren 1.0 with Fiber Nutren 1.5	Two Cal HN Nutren 2.0
Concentration (kcal/mL)	1.06 1.2 1.5	1.06 1.2 1.5	1.0 1.0	1.0 1.0	1.0 1.0 1.5	2.0 2.0
Protein g/1,000 mL (% kcal)	44.3 (16.7) 55.5 (18.5) 63.8 (17)	44.3 (16.7) 55.5 (18.5) 62.7 (16.7)	62.5 (25) 62.5 (25)	64 (25) 64 (25)	40 (16) 40 (16) 68 (18)	83.5 (16.7) 48 (16)
Carbohydrate g/1,000 mL (% kcal)	154.7 (58.3) 169.4 (56.4) 215.7 (57.5)	143.9 (54.3) 157.5 (52.5) 203.6 (54.3)	130 (52) 138.3 (55)	112 (45) 124 (45)	136 (54) 148 (54) 176 (47)	218.5 (43.2) 216 (43)
Fat g/1,000 mL (% kcal)	34.7 (29) 39.3 (29) 49.8 (30)	34.7 (29) 39.3 (29) 49.1 (29)	26 (23) 28.2 (25)	34 (30) 34 (30)	34 (30) 34 (30) 60 (35)	90.5 (40.1) 92 (41)
Sodium/ Potassium (mg/1000 mL)	930/1570 1,350/1850 1,400/2150	930/1570 1,340/1810 1,400/800	1,000/1,980 1,300/2,100	880/1,600 880/1,600	880/1,600 880/1,600 1,300/2,400	1,450/2,440 1,500/2,100
Calcium/ Phosphorus (mg/1000 mL)	910/760 1,200/1,200 1,200/1,200	760/760 1,200/1,200 1,000/1,000	1,200/1,200 1,200/1,200	800/800 800/800	800/800 800/800 1,200/1,200	1,050/1,050 1,600/1,400
Vitamin D (IU/1000 mL)	305 400 400	305 400 400	400 400	400 400	400 400 640	415 800
Zinc/Copper (mg/1000 mL)	18/1.6 23/2.0 23/2.0	18/1.6 23/2.0 23/2.0	24/2 24/2	16/1.6 16/1.6	14/1.6 14/1.6 20/2	24/2.1 24/2.4
Selenium (mcg/ 1000 mL)	54 70 70	54 70 70	70 70	60 60	60 60 80	74 100

TABLE 3.3 NUTRIENT COMPOSITION OF HYDROLYZED AND MONOMERIC ENTERAL FORMULATIONS

Formula Name	Vivonex TEN	Vital	Peptamen	Peptamen 1.5 with Prebio
Concentration (kcal/mL)	1.0	1.0	1.0	1.5
Protein g/1,000 mL (% kcal)	38.3 (14)	40 (16)	40 (16)	68 (18)
Carbohydrate g/1,000 mL (% kcal)	206 (83)	130 (52)	128 (51)	184 (48)
Fat g/1,000 mL (% kcal)	3 (3)	38.1 (34)	39.2 (33)	56 (34)
Sodium/Potassium (mg/1,000 mL)	617/937	1,050/1,400	560/1,500	1,020/1,860
Calcium/Phosphorus (mg/1,000 mL)	500/500	705/705	800/700	1,000/1,000
Vitamin D (IU/1,000 mL)	403	280	13.2 (mcg)	20 (mcg)
Zinc/Copper (mg/1,000 mL)	11/1.0	21/1.4	24/2.0	36/3.0
Selenium (mcg/1,000 mL)	37	56	50	76

more soluble than starch and contributes less to the osmolality of the formula than glucose alone. Polysaccharides are made of more than 10 glucose units and include corn syrup solids and cornstarch.

Fats

Fats, or triglycerides, are composed of glycerol and fatty acids. They consist of chains of carbons with a carboxyl group at the end. The chain length influences the feeding tolerance, and the type of chain (such as monounsaturated fatty acids, saturated fatty acids, or polyunsaturated fatty acids) influences a patient's physiology.[38] Lipids are a secondary energy source in formula composition. Common sources of lipids in formula include corn oil, safflower oil, and coconut oil.[38] In addition to providing energy, lipids are an important component of enteral formulas because they carry fat-soluble vitamins and essential fatty acids that are important for physiologic function. Lipids are also isotonic, which helps lower the osmolality of the formula.

Often, a mixture of long-chain and medium-chain fatty acids are used in enteral formulations. Long-chain fatty acids are carbon chains of 14 to 24 units. These are cleared slowly from the bloodstream and are preferentially re-esterified and stored as triglycerides. Long-chain fatty acids require carnitine, which aids in the transport of long-chain fatty acids across the mitochondrial membrane for energy production. Long-chain fatty acids are also a source of essential fatty acids, such as linoleic and linolenic fatty acids.

For patients with impaired digestion, absorption, and transport of fats, medium-chain fatty acids can be added to the formula.[35] Medium-chain fatty acids are carbon chains of 6 to 12 units. Common sources include palm kernel oil and coconut oil. Medium-chain fatty acids are easier to digest because they absorbed directly into portal circulation and are not re-esterified to triglycerides. They do not require pancreatic enzymes or bile salts for absorption. They also do not require carnitine for transport across the mitochondrial membrane. Therefore, medium-chain fatty acids are a rapid energy source. However, because medium-chain fatty acids do not provide any essential fatty acids, some long-chain fatty acids are usually concurrently added to make sure the patient meets nutrient needs.[35]

> **PRACTICE POINT**
>
> Medium-chain fatty acids are absorbed directly into the portal system and are easier to digest; however, they do not provide essential fatty acids and so long-chain fatty acids should be provided as well.

Protein

Protein in enteral formulas can come in different forms, depending on what is indicated by the patient's need and medical condition. These forms of protein include intact proteins, hydrolyzed protein, or free amino acids.[38] Intact proteins are large in size and have limited impact on the osmolality of a formula. They are the original, natural form of the protein, called an **isolate**.[38] Examples of intact proteins include soy isolates, casein or whey protein from milk, and the albumen from egg white. Intact proteins require normal levels of pancreatic enzymes for adequate digestion. For patients with gastrointestinal dysfunction or malabsorption issues, semi-elemental or elemental formulations may be used. These include hydrolyzed proteins such as di-peptides, tri-peptides, and free amino acids. These types of proteins are enzymatically broken down to smaller particles and increase the osmolality of the formula. The intestine can digest both smaller peptides and free amino acids because they use separate transport systems. Formulas may prefer smaller peptides because they are thought to more efficiently absorb nitrogen, but free amino acids and di- and tri-peptides cause less trophic stimulation on the bowel than intact protein.

Vitamins and Minerals

Vitamins and minerals are vital components in enteral formula. These micronutrients play an important role in the body as essential cofactors and coenzymes that are needed for metabolism and other physiologic functions. Formulas generally have 100% of the recommended dietary allowance (RDA) of each vitamin and mineral at specific volumes. Different metabolic stresses and disease states may require a higher or lower amount of certain micronutrients.

Fiber

Dietary fiber comes in soluble and insoluble forms and is added to some enteral formulas. Fiber is a plant polysaccharide that is indigestible by human digestive enzymes. The formulas that include fiber generally have about 4 to 14 g/L of total fiber.

Soluble fiber is viscous and found in legumes, oat bran, pectins, and gums. Anaerobic bacteria in the cecum rapidly ferment soluble fiber into short-chain fatty acids. Short-chain fatty acids offer the health benefits of maintaining colonic structure and function. This includes lowering the colonic pH to balance intestinal flora. It also enhances fluid and electrolyte absorption, which may help with diarrhea. Soluble fiber intake is also linked to lower serum cholesterol, as well as improved glucose tolerance. Soluble fiber is important to include in enteral formulas of patients who have glucose intolerance, have had bowel surgery, or are undergoing antibiotic therapy.

Insoluble fiber is nonviscous and found in the cellulose of plant foods. Insoluble fiber is beneficial because it holds water. This increases bulk in fecal mass and allows softer stools, which helps prevent constipation and is recommended for those undergoing long-term feeding. Insoluble fiber may also be beneficial for patients with diverticulosis, which is when pouches accumulate in the colon.

Pre- and Probiotics

Some formulas also include prebiotics and probiotics to promote gut health; however, the benefit of these additions is still under debate. Because outcomes differ per patient and condition, it is currently difficult to make any broad recommendation for prebiotics and probiotics in formula.

Prebiotics are energy sources for the beneficial bacteria in the colon, commonly provided in EN formulas as fiber, fructo-oligosaccharides, and inulin. Food sources include artichokes, banana, onions, garlic, and soy. Prebiotics are generally included with probiotics so that the microorganisms can flourish. **Probiotics** are ingested microorganisms thought to promote beneficial gut microflora and gastrointestinal function, as well as compete against pathogenic bacteria. A common form used in formula is lactic acid bacteria. Research suggests that prebiotics and probiotics in preterm infant formula have had successful outcomes, helping gut microbiota and gastrointestinal function, as well as decreasing mortality risk.[39,40] Use of probiotics also has been shown to reduce the risk of necrotizing enterocolitis in preterm infants, a condition in which damaged intestinal tissue cause bloating, diarrhea, inflammation, and infection.[39]

Because critical illness and its management alter the microflora, resulting in a loss of commensal flora and abundance of pathogenic flora, considerable interest in probiotic therapy exists.[41-43] Meta-analyses show a reduction in antibiotic-associated diarrhea with probiotic use, but the heterogeneity of the pooled data makes it difficult to draw conclusions to specific populations.[42] While favorable, the data have not been consistent with respect to risk and benefit of probiotics. Systematic reviews reveal no improvement in mortality, pneumonia, or length of intensive care unit stay with use of probiotics. Furthermore, safety concerns have been raised due to increased gut ischemia in probiotic treatment groups.[41,44] The risk of translocation and improper administration of probiotics, resulting in blood infection, has caused the U.S. Food and Drug Administration to issue a black box warning for probiotic use in hospitalized patients. Prebiotics and probiotics are not generally included in standard formula because evidence is still inconclusive on their health benefits for mortality risk or infectious complications. Research is also needed to clarify which strands are most beneficial to humans, especially because the microbiota in the gastrointestinal tract are so complex.

> **PRACTICE POINT**
>
> Enteral feedings can provide a mixture of soluble and insoluble fiber. Advancement of fiber-containing feeds should take into consideration the total amount of fiber provided based on EN goal rate as well as history of gastrointestinal function to assure adequate tolerance.

> **CORE CONCEPT 6**
>
> Enteral nutrition formulas include carbohydrates, fat, protein, vitamins and minerals, and fiber adequate for meeting full nutrient requirements in most patients.

Disease-Specific Formulas

Certain health conditions require specific enteral formulations to ensure a patient meets their nutrient needs. Selection of enteral formula takes into account a patient's fluid limitations, electrolyte imbalances, increased nutrient requirement, decreased ability to receive nutrients due to disease or condition, and ease of digestion (Table 3.4).

Renal Dysfunction

Patients with renal dysfunction may require a formula that is more calorically dense and lower in phosphorus and potassium than standard polymeric TFs. Renal formulas should also assure protein of high biological value to include proportionately more essential amino acids. Patients who have stage 3 or 4 chronic kidney disease and are not yet on dialysis may need less protein in their formula. Amounts of potassium, phosphorus, and sodium are also reduced. When on dialysis or renal replacement therapy, formula composition is higher in protein to reflect increased protein losses associated with these therapies. Supplementation with enteral feedings designed for renal patients or essential amino acids is associated with improved markers of nutritional status (as evidenced by body mass index, hand grip strength, and mid-arm circumference) as well as serum albumin and prealbumin.[45]

TABLE 3.4 DISEASE-SPECIFIC ENTERAL FORMULATIONS

Formula Name	Nutrihep	Nepro	Glucerna	Pulmocare
Concentration (kcal/mL)	1.5	1.8	1.0	1.5
Protein g/1,000 mL (% kcal)	40 (11)	81 (18)	41.8 (17)	62.6 (17)
Carbohydrate g/1,000 mL (% kcal)	290 (77)	161 (36)	95.6 (38)	105.7 (28)
Fat g/1,000 mL (% kcal)	21.2 (13)	96 (48)	54.4 (49)	93.3 (56)
Sodium/Potassium (mg/1,000 mL)	160/1,320	1,060/1,060	930/1,570	1,310/1,960
Calcium/Phosphorus (mg/1,000 mL)	956/1,000	1,060/720	705/705	1,060/1,060
Vitamin D (IU/1,000 mL)	400	85	285	425
Zinc/Copper (mg/1,000 mL)	15.2/2.0	27/2.1	16/1.5	24/2.2
Selenium (mcg/1,000 mL)	NA	74	50	74

Pulmonary Dysfunction

Formulas for patients with pulmonary dysfunction have a modified carbohydrate-to-fat ratio to decrease carbohydrate intake. Oxidation of carbohydrate results in greater carbon dioxide (CO_2) production than fat oxidation. This is considered especially useful in patients with **hypercapnia** (CO_2 retention). Clinically, use of high-fat, low-carbohydrate TF in patients with chronic obstructive pulmonary disease may improve pulmonary function (forced expiratory volume in 1 second, minute ventilation, oxygen consumption, and CO_2 production) as well as arterial blood gases.[46,47] Many formulas for pulmonary patients also incorporate immune-enhancing nutrients such as omega-3 fatty acids and antioxidants. Omega-3 fatty acids are anti-inflammatory and signal pathways that complement therapeutic efforts to maximize lung function. Use of omega-3 fatty acids in patients with acute respiratory distress is associated with improved lung injury scores, fewer days on mechanical ventilation, and reduced stays on the intensive care unit.[48] The role of antioxidants in fighting free radicals and reducing lung cell injury remains a primary research interest.

Liver Dysfunction

Patients with advanced liver disease often have ascites, or fluid accumulation in the abdomen, which may cause them to not utilize nutrients efficiently. Because of this condition, formulas for these patients are often calorically dense, providing a high calorie-to-nitrogen ratio. Protein composition in formulations designed for patients with liver failure include a higher proportion of branched chain amino acids (BCAA) with lesser amounts of aromatic amino acids in attempt to minimize hepatic encephalopathy (a condition that is associated with liver disease). Levels of BCAA are often low in patients with liver disease due to their increased uptake in skeletal muscle to help detoxify and reduce ammonia.[49] While there is a lack of compelling evidence that nutritional support (enteral, parenteral, or oral) improves clinical outcomes in liver failure overall, use of BCAA-enhanced formulas during hepatic encephalopathy may be considered.[50]

Diabetes

Most patients with diabetes can be treated with standard polymeric TFs. Fiber-containing TFs by slowing gastric emptying and digestion of carbohydrates, can improve glycemic control. For better glycemic control, diabetes-specific feedings, which are higher in fructose and monounsaturated fatty acids, can be used.[51] These formulas generally have a carbohydrate content of about 35% to 40% of calories, approximately 10 to 15 g/L of soluble fiber, and fat (40%-50% of calories). In critically ill patients, where hyperglycemia can be exacerbated, diabetes-specific formulas improve glycemic control, lower insulin requirements, and decrease risk of acquired infections.[52] Because gastroparesis is common among diabetics, diabetes-specific formulas, given their higher fat and soluble fiber, may be poorly tolerated; postpyloric feedings can be used in these instances.

Trauma/Wound Healing

Specialty formulations are available for use in patients with trauma or increased wound healing requirements. EN solutions that are high in protein and include arginine and glutamine, as well as micronutrients zinc and vitamin C, should enhance the process of wound healing due to their effects on protein anabolism (arginine and glutamine) and collagen synthesis (zinc and vitamin C). Pressure injury healing time has been shown to decrease with use of these formulations.[53] Use of immune-enhancing formulas to promote wound healing in critically ill patients continues to be explored. These will be described in more detail in the immunonutrition section of this chapter.

> **CORE CONCEPT 7**
>
> Disease specific formulas that deviate from standard formulations can be used in many disease states to aid patients in meeting their nutritional needs.

Developing an EN Feeding Plan

Table 3.5 provides a step-wise procedure for developing an EN feeding plan for a patient. The first step is selection of EN type. Based on the plethora of EN products, a clinician must evaluate what formula to select based on a patient's nutrient requirements; clinical status, including fluid restrictions and electrolyte requirements; degree of metabolic stress; wound healing requirements; gastrointestinal function; cost; and supporting evidence of benefit and risk of specific nutrient components provided, particularly in disease-specific and immune-enhancing feeds. Figure 3.6 shows a mechanism for determining an optimal TF type.

Complication Monitoring

Patients who are receiving TF must be monitored routinely, because complications can arise. Clinicians must check for signs of nausea and vomiting, make note of the **gastric residuals** (volume of liquid that remains in stomach during enteral feeding), obtain a baseline of the abdominal girth with routine subsequent monitoring, and keep track of stool patterns. Certain complications can be associated with enteral feeding, as well as illness or treatment side effects that a patient may be experiencing. These include nausea and vomiting, aspiration, abdominal distention, delayed gastric emptying, constipation, and diarrhea.[54,55]

Aspiration

Aspiration is a common complication associated with tube feeding. It occurs when a patient inhales a substance, such as water or tube feed, into the airway, which causes dyspnea and coughing. Prolonged aspiration is dangerous because it can lead to pneumonia.[54]

TABLE 3.5 STEP-WISE PROCESS FOR DETERMINATION OF TUBE FEEDING VOLUME AND DELIVERY

Step	Description	Example
Step 1	Choose the EN formula type based on condition. Examples: Standard, Condition (Impaired Digestion, Stress/Trauma), Disease-Specific	Example: 58-year-old male with head injury due to motorcycle accident with a nasogastric feeding tube EN Formula: Replete
Step 2	Determine the amount of EN volume needed to meet the calorie goal.* 24-hour Calorie Goal/Formula Concentration (kcal/mL) = Total volume of EN needed over 24 hours *Consider: Stress level, malnourished vs. well nourished; clinical factors (intubated, sedated, sepsis); physical activity	Energy Goal: 2,000 kcal Protein Goal: 130 g protein Replete (1.0 kcal/mL) = 2,000 mL
Step 3	Calculate protein intake at that EN volume to assure protein is in range of patient's goal (Total EN volume/1000) × protein (g/L) = g protein/day OR (Total calorie intake at EN goal rate × % calories as protein)/4 = g protein/day	Replete has 62.5 g protein per 1,000 mL. 2,000/1000 = 2.000 × 62.5 g = 125 g protein on this regimen Protein intake is sufficient
Step 4	If both calorie and protein needs are met, determine hourly rate: EN volume/24 = hourly rate * Rounding numbers is preferred to make daily calculations of input/output and order writing simplified If protein needs are not met, consider a nutrient-dense feeding with higher nitrogen or adding modular protein	Hourly EN = ~2,000 mL/24 = 83.3 mL/hr Round up to 85 mL/hr
Step 5	Provide your TF type and hourly goal rate.	Full-strength Replete @ 85 mL/hr
Step 6	Document what the TF will actually provide. Note: This may be a little different from your initially established goal, due to rounding and fine-tuning	This regimen provides 2,040 kcal/128 g protein

CASE STUDY REVISITED

Laura was seen today in the clinic after completion of her first 6 weeks of chemotherapy. Treatment is going well for Laura; however, despite previously good tolerance, she is now experiencing diarrhea. It is unclear whether this is due to her treatment or the TF she is receiving.

Questions
1. What factors might be contributing to her diarrhea?
2. How might you resolve antibiotic-induced diarrhea?

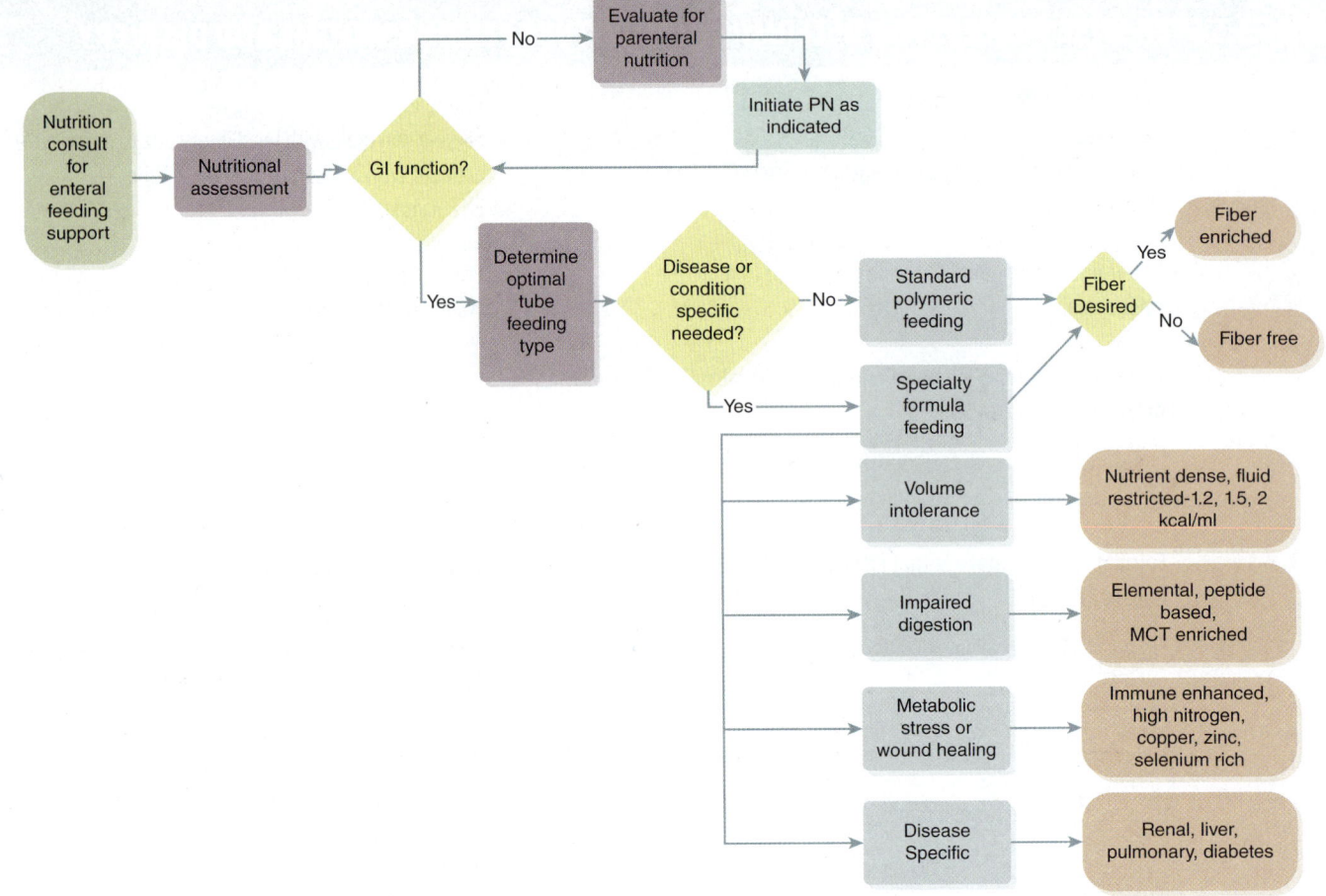

FIGURE 3.6 Algorithm for Determining Tube Feeding Type

Nausea/Vomiting

Nausea and vomiting are common complications to enteral feeding and increase the risk of aspiration and pneumonia.[54] There are many possible causes of nausea or vomiting. Both gastric retention and rapid infusion of hyperosmolar formula can cause nausea/vomiting. In these cases, a clinician must reduce the rate of feeding, but if the patient is vomiting, feedings should be held. The fat content of feeds also affects a patient's tolerance, with feedings that are lower in fat being generally better tolerated. The smell of the formula can affect the patient. Elemental formulas usually have a more unpleasant odor than polymeric formulas.

Abdominal Distention

Abdominal distention is the accumulation of air or liquid in a patient's abdomen and can cause major discomfort to the patient. Abdominal distention can be diagnosed by observing an increase in abdominal girth (about 8-10 cm) and/or palpating the abdomen.[54] A patient's report of symptoms such as bloating and cramping can also indicate abdominal distention.[54] Rapid bolus or intermittent feeds of cold formula can cause abdominal distention. Using continuous and room-temperature feeds can treat this. Abdominal distention can also be caused by nutrient malabsorption, delayed gastric emptying, or the onset of a septic episode.

> **PRACTICE POINT**
>
> Baseline and daily measurement of abdominal girth is useful for monitoring feeding tolerance and onset of sepsis. Sudden increases in abdominal girth may indicate the onset of a septic episode.

Gastroparesis (Delayed Gastric Emptying)

Many factors can delay the emptying of gastric contents into the small bowel. Gastroparesis can be induced by trauma or be caused by certain medications, such as opiates or paralytics. In order to mitigate the risk of gastroparesis, a clinician may check gastric residual volume (GRV) before initiating tube feeding, as well as every 4 hours after tube feeding. When monitoring gastric residuals, gastric fluid is suctioned. The amount of fluid collected is measured over 24 hours. Normal GRVs range from 250 to 500 mL.[56,57] Anything greater than 600 mL may indicate delayed gastric emptying, which puts a patient at risk for aspiration. Feeding tolerance, feeding administration rate, and duodeno-gastric reflux may also contribute to delayed gastric emptying and aspiration risk; therefore, certain adjustments may be instituted.[57] Continuous feeds may be preferred over intermittent or bolus feeds to normalize gastric emptying. A formula free of fiber and low in fat can also help. Prokinetic agents, such as metoclopramide and erythromycin, can mitigate delayed gastric emptying by increasing gastric motility.[14,16,17] Controversy exists about whether checking gastric residuals is truly necessary.[56,57] However, despite this controversy, it remains a common practice for patients in critical care.[57]

Constipation

Certain medications can cause constipation. It is therefore important to have a proactive bowel regime. Dehydration and lack of fiber are also frequent causes of constipation. Adding additional fluid to the formula in addition to fiber can prevent waste buildup.[45] Fecal impaction or obstruction is a type of stool accumulation that can be diagnosed by a rectal exam. Fecal implantation can be alleviated by rectal exam if it is close to the rectum, but surgical or endoscopic methods may have to be used if the impaction is higher in the colon.[45]

Diarrhea

Diarrhea is higher stool frequency, volume, and water content.[54] Most causes of diarrhea are not incidental to tube feeding. Certain medications, especially those containing magnesium, phosphorus, and sorbitol, can be hyperosmolar, causing diarrhea. Diarrhea can also be due to bacterial growth.[54] Prolonged antibiotic use creates an imbalance in gut microflora, resulting in antibiotic associated diarrhea. Despite the fact that *Clostridium difficile*, a bacteria that causes diarrhea, is only one of the possible causes, a stool culture is often done to confirm antibiotic-induced diarrhea. Use of pre- and probiotics promotes proliferation and can restore the patient's microbiota to resolve diarrhea associated with harmful bacterial overgrowth.[41,42]

Diarrhea can also be caused by aspects directly related to tube feeding. Included among these are rapid feed infusion, hyperosmolar formula, carbohydrate malabsorption, or intolerance to lactose in the formula. Additionally, patients can be exposed to bacterial growth on the tubing itself, leading to diarrhea. To prevent this, a closed tube feeding system can be used every 24 to 48 hours. Tubing should be changed every 24 hours. In an open system, formula hang time should be limited to 4 to 8 hours.[26,33] Tube feeding containers and tubing should be flushed frequently. Sterile water must always be used for reconstitution.

> **CORE CONCEPT 8**
>
> Patients must be monitored closely for complications related to enteral feeding or side effects to medical treatment. Feeding method and formula should be adjusted as needed.

Early Enteral Nutrition

Early enteral nutrition (EEN) generally refers to the initiation of EN within 48 hours of illness or a traumatic event. There are numerous proposed benefits to EEN, particularly in patients with systemic inflammation as is associated with multiple trauma, large burn injury, and acute pancreatitis. However, certain risks and complications associated with EEN mean that its use is controversial.[58-65] Evidence suggests that EEN reduces all-cause mortality,[59-62] shortens time needed to meet caloric and protein needs, and decreases hospital length of stay.[61,63,64] EEN also reduces cost of hospital-related expenses.[62] Many disease-related complications, including infections, are minimized with EEN.[61,63,64,66] There may be some benefit of EEN attenuating the postsurgical or trauma stress response.[64,67]

Although it is intuitive that enteral nutrition maintains gut integrity, EEN does so through increased **postprandial hyperemic response**.[68,69] With many diseases, blood flow to the intestine is diminished to accommodate other vital organs, complicating gastrointestinal function. However, enteral nutrients increase perfusion to the gastrointestinal tract; when cautiously delivered, EEN can be beneficial to gut integrity and prevention of ischemia.[70]

Although many benefits with EEN have been presented, EEN may not be indicated in certain scenarios. There are insufficient data to support whether EEN could be beneficial to respiratory-compromised or unstable hyperemic patients.[69-71] Because feedings can increase gut oxygen needs beyond what can be met, as well as induce gut ischemia or worsen an existing ischemic condition, EEN may be contraindicated. These findings underscore the delicate balance between promoting perfusion with judicious EEN and inducing gut ischemia through excessive nutrient provision.[70] Aspiration pneumonia is another concern because a patient may not be able to handle a substantial feeding load so early in treatment, depending on the disease or complication.[70] There are also inconsistencies in data supporting EEN reducing length of stay and infections.[70] Some studies also suggest that EEN alone may not be sufficient for a patient to meet nutritional needs.[70,71] These findings are a reminder that provision of EEN should be in conjunction with standardized criteria and close monitoring (**Table 3.6**).[59,71]

TABLE 3.6 CONTRAINDICATIONS FOR EARLY ENTERAL FEEDING[60]
Hemodynamically unstable; uncontrolled shock
Uncontrolled hypoxemia, hypercapnia, or acidosis
Overt bowel ischemia
High-output fistula if EEN cannot be safely provided distal to fistula
Abdominal compartment syndrome
Upper gastrointestinal bleed
Large gastrointestinal aspirates (>500 mL/24 hours)

Data from Reintam Blaser A, Starkopf J, Alhazzani W, et al. Early enteral nutrition in critically ill patients: ESICM clinical practice guidelines. *Intensive Care Medicine*. 2017;43(3):380-398. doi: 10.1007/s00134-016-4665-0.

Immunonutrition

Immunonutrition refers to the use of nutrients to alter or attenuate the inflammatory or immune response. This differs from conventional nutrition support therapy, where provision of nutrients is aimed at preventing deficiency or meeting requirements for increased utilization or losses. Nutrients such as the conditionally essential amino acids glutamine and arginine, omega-3 fatty acids, and antioxidants are considered to be beneficial in modulating inflammation and the course of disease. Today, numerous enteral formulations exist with these nutrients, either alone or in combination. These products often are used in critically ill patients in an attempt to counteract the inflammatory response to stress, both at the systemic and cellular levels. Research into the role of these select nutrients is ongoing and inconclusive despite the plethora of immune-enhancing specialty formulas. Scientific evidence of the potential benefit of these products, as well as possible harm, is ongoing.

Gastrointestinal Tract as an Immune Organ

Traditionally the gastrointestinal tract is viewed for its primary role in digestion and absorption (**Figure 3.7**). However, a better understanding of its morphology, structure, and mediatory response to stress clearly establishes the gut as having immunologic functions. First and foremost, the gut acts as a barrier to invasive organisms, preventing the spread of bacteria and toxins to other organs. This is accomplished through microbial, immunologic, and mechanical aspects of the gut. Increasing evidence confirms the role of the microbiome in immunology and health. Bacteria that are part of the normal intestinal flora inhibit colonization of invading bacteria, most basically by limiting the amount of space for bacteria to exist

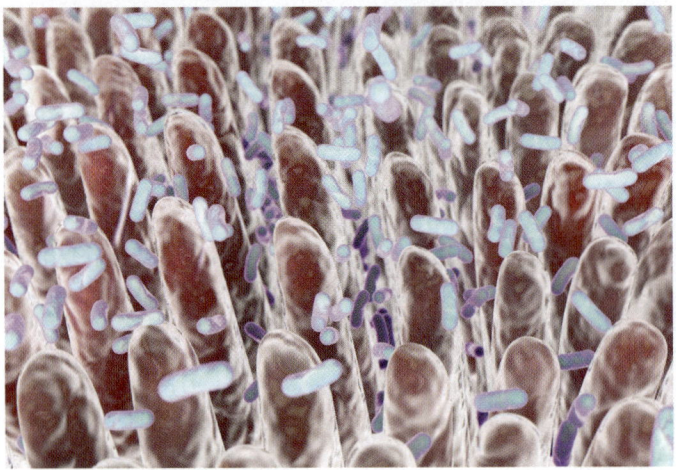

FIGURE 3.8 The Intestine is Home to the Microbiome
© Kateryna Kon/Shutterstock.

(**Figure 3.8**). Simply by virtue of their numbers, the normal gut bacteria can reduce the potential for bacterial invasion. In addition to space, the existing microbiome competes with foreign bacteria for nutrients, limiting the ability of pathogens to survive in the gut. This bacterial antagonism is essential for gut health and organ protection. Secondarily, the gut also contains immunologic factors, such as immunoglobulins that fight off foreign particles. Combined with the gut-associated lymphoid tissue (GALT), the gut is very effective at capturing and destroying invading bodies.[72]

From a mechanical perspective, the gut has a mucous gel layer, which prevents bacterial adhesion. Additionally, peristalsis protects against prolonged stasis, hindering the ability for bacteria to grow and multiply. The epithelial cell layer also plays a role in immunity by creating tight junctions and rearranging or shifting during -desquamation,

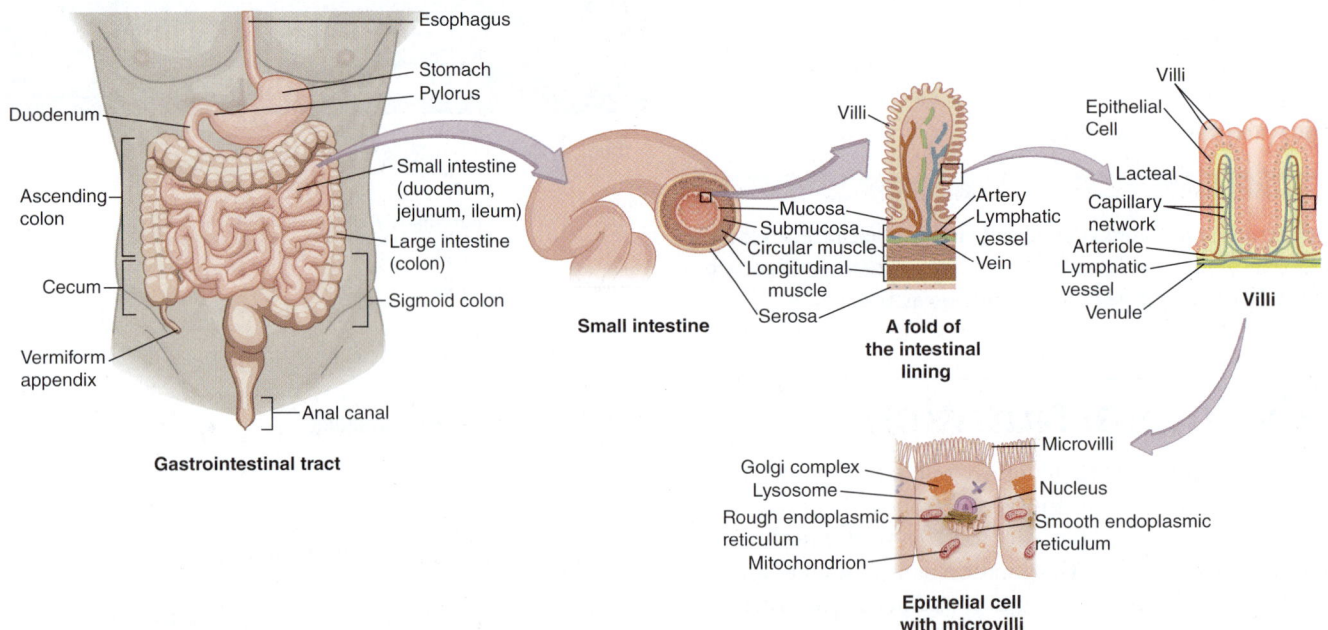

FIGURE 3.7 Morphology of the Intestinal Tract

making it difficult for foreign bacteria to enter from the lumen. Rearrangement of tight junctions prevents intestinal permeability. This aspect of the gut, combined with GALT, may explain why bacterial translocation in humans rarely progresses to the blood stream and other organs. Furthermore, the epithelial cells secrete cytokines that promote the synthesis of lymphocytes and immunity. By maintaining the epithelial layer and microbiome, EN facilitates the gut's immune function capacity.[72,73]

The Gut and Systemic Inflammatory Response System

The interaction between the gut and immunologic nutrients can be best seen in the context of the systemic inflammatory response. In systemic inflammatory response syndrome (SIRS), the intestine becomes a cytokine-generating organ due to ischemia (versus infection) as a result of certain conditions such as trauma, burns, obstructive gastrointestinal injury, hemorrhagic shock, or sepsis. Select nutrients can serve as substrates that mediate this cytokine-induced response. As shown in **Figure 3.9**, various nutritional substrates can induce immune activity both at the cellular and systemic level. For example, omega-3 fatty acids act as a substrate that systemically promotes anti-inflammatory eicosanoids and cytokines, as well as modulates smooth vascular muscle tone. The result is increased dilation of the vessels, improved platelet function, and reduction of bronchoconstriction. Similarly, the amino acids glutamine and arginine participate in macrophage activity at the cell-mediated immunity level.[74-76] The optimal dose and route of provision of these nutrients remain unknown, yet are imperative to achieving the beneficial aspects of these nutrients without posing harm. **Table 3.7** provides examples of immune-enhancing EN formulas.

Conditionally Essential Amino Acids

Stress-induced depletion of glutamine and arginine in blood and tissue pools has earned these amino acids the title of conditionally essential amino acids. While they can be synthesized within the body, during stress, synthesis does not meet their requirement.

Glutamine

Glutamine is a gluconeogenic amino acid that is synthesized in all tissues, with skeletal muscle as the major site. It is an important fuel source for rapidly dividing cells such as the gut epithelium, macrophages, lymphocytes, and fibroblasts. It contains two amine groups, making it a useful nitrogen shuttle to other organs. Glutamine also donates nitrogen to purines and pyrimidines for DNA synthesis. Because it is a precursor to glutathione, a potent antioxidant, glutamine helps protect cells from free radical damage.[75] Due to its properties, glutamine is used therapeutically in patients with gastrointestinal disease and in patients with immune function disorders. It is also widely used among patients with metabolic stress, such as burn and trauma patients.

Arginine

Arginine plays a fundamental role in protein metabolism. As a precursor to insulin and growth hormone, it can play

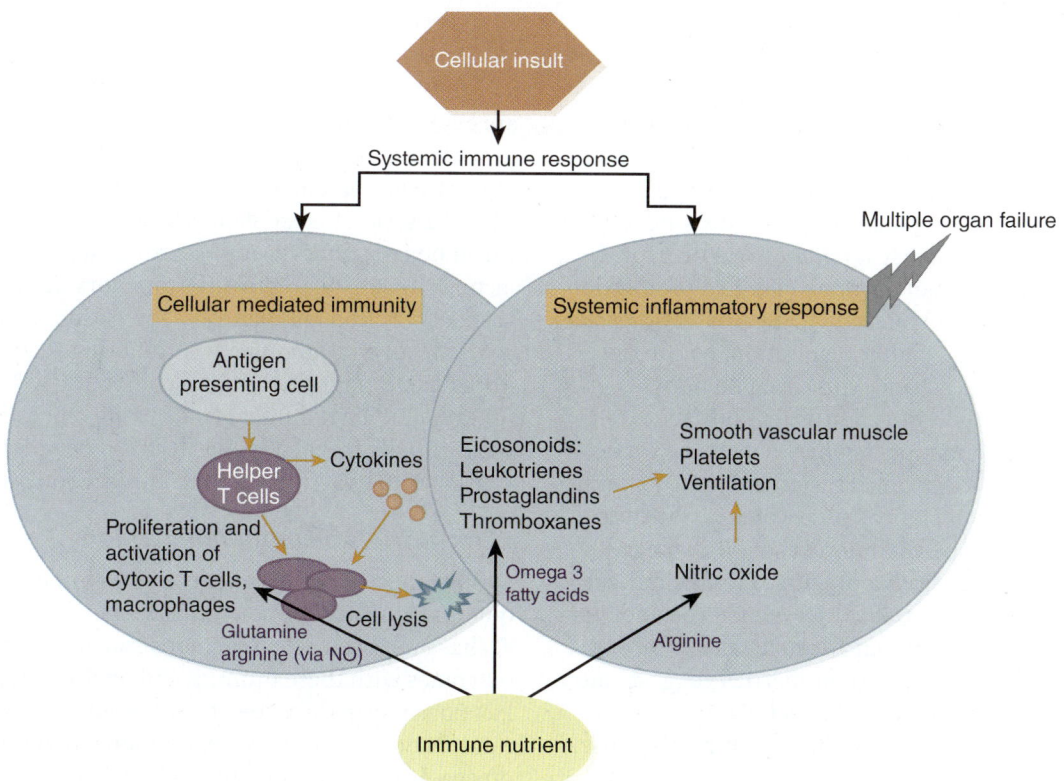

FIGURE 3.9 Immune Modulating Nutrients Act at Both the Cellular and Systemic Level

Data from Krauss H, Jablecka A, Sosnowski P, Bogdanski P. Influence of L-arginine on the nitric oxide concentration and level of oxidative stress during ischemia-reperfusion injury in a rat model. *J Clin Pharmacol Ther*. 2009 Aug;47(8):533-8; and 76. Gadek JE, DeMichele SJ, Karlstad MD. Enteral nutrition in ARDS study group. Effect of enteral feeding with eicosapentaenoic acid, gamma linolenic acid, and antioxidants in patients with acute respiratory distress syndrome. *Critical Care Medicine*. 1999; 27(8):1409-1420.

TABLE 3.7 NUTRIENT COMPOSITION OF IMMUNE-ENHANCING ENTERAL FORMULATIONS

Formula Name	Impact	Perative	Pivot 1.5	Oxepa
Concentration (kcal/mL)	1.0	1.3	1.5	1.5
Protein g/1,000 mL (% kcal)	56 (22)	66.7 (20.5)	93.8 (25)	62.7 (16.7)
Carbohydrate g/1,000 mL (% kcal)	132 (53)	180.3 (53)	172.4 (46)	105.3 (28)
Fat g/1,000 mL (% kcal)	28 (25)	35.2 (24)	50.8 (30)	93.8 (56)
Sodium/Potassium (mg/1,000 mL)	960/1,600	980/1,640	1,400/2,000	1,310/1,960
Calcium/Phosphorus (mg/1,000 mL)	800/800	840/840	1,000/1,000	1,060/1,060
Vitamin D (IU/1,000 mL)	13.2 (mcg)	332	400	425
Zinc/Copper (mg/1,000 mL)	15.2/1.7	18.8/1.68	25/2.0	24/2.2
Selenium (mcg/1,000 mL)	100	60	70	74

a major role in wound healing. Arginine is also a precursor to nitric oxide (NO), which provides cellular defense through the stimulus of increased lymphocyte activity, macrophage activation, and phagocytosis. NO is beneficial for tissue oxygenation because it reduces vascular tone, acting as a vasodilator.[74] Notably, uncontrolled production of NO can be damaging. Increased NO results in excessive inflammation, impaired cellular respiration, cytotoxicity, coagulation abnormalities, and worsening hemodynamic instability. NO is also a significant contributor in the ischemia reperfusion model, where a lack of oxygen and blood flow, followed by reperfusion of blood, generates powerful free radical substances such as perioxynitrate that can later cause tissue and microvascular damage.[77-79] Because NO can serve as both a precursor to free radical substances as well as a free radical scavenger, the need for the appropriate balance between adequate and excessive NO cannot be understated. These properties suggest caution when providing arginine in the diet. **Figure 3.10** outlines the impact of NO in the systemic immune response.

Omega-3 Fatty Acids

Many specialty products will now provide information on their omega-6 to omega-3 fatty acid ratio. While both are essential fatty acids, they have unique and contrasting properties due to the physiologic pathways they undergo. Omega-6 is a precursor to arachidonic acid and the eicosanoid 2 series, and substances such as prostaglandin 2, thromboxanes, and series 4 leukotrienes (**Figure 3.11**). These factors participate in pro-inflammatory activities such as vasoconstriction and platelet aggregation. Omega-3 fatty acids are anti-inflammatory, promoting vasodilation, inhibiting platelet aggregation, and competing with omega-6 production. Early clinical trials using omega-3 fatty acids were initially promising, with shown benefit to decreasing ventilator days and improving clinical outcome.[76, 80,81]

Clinical Trials on Immunonutrition

Despite the mechanistic benefit of arginine, glutamine, omega-3 fatty acids, and antioxidants, recent clinical trials have not been able to demonstrate improved clinical outcomes with these immune-enhancing formulas, and in fact have raised the issue of adverse consequences.[82,83] One randomized trial providing immune-enhanced (glutamine, omega-3 fatty acid, and antioxidants), high-nitrogen formulas versus a simple high-nitrogen feeding failed to show a benefit with respect to infection rate and duration or length of stay. In fact, 6-month mortality was increased in the

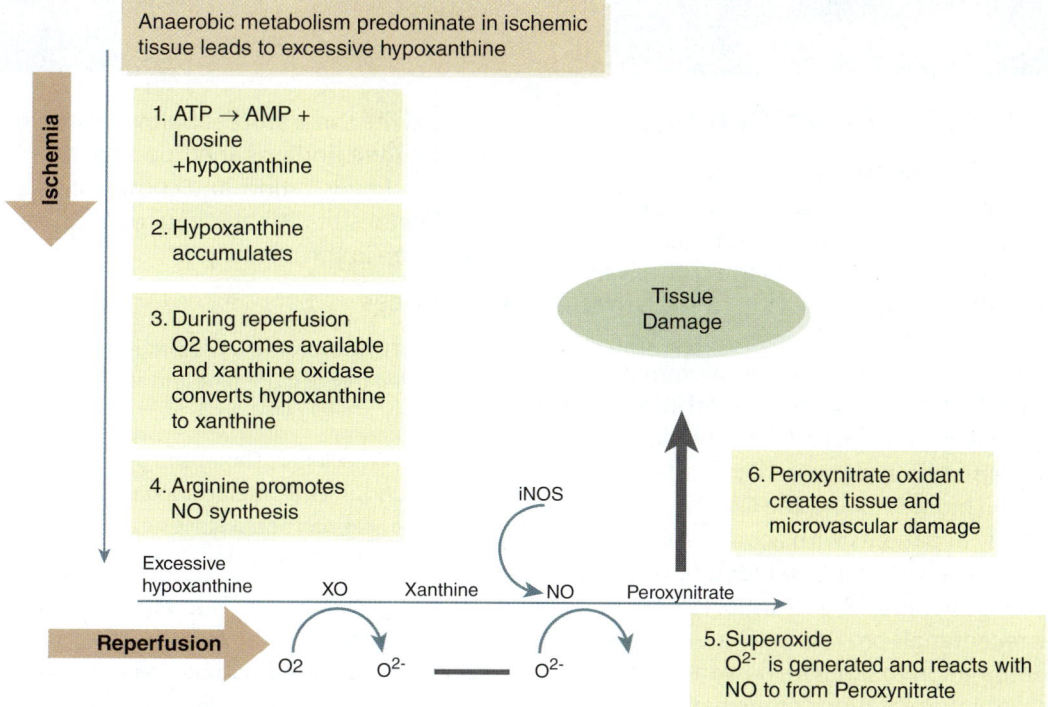

FIGURE 3.10 Nitric Oxide and the Ischemia-Reperfusion Model

Data from Yapca OE, Borekci B, Suleyman H. Ischemia-Reperfusion Damage. *The Eurasian Journal of Medicine*. 2013;45(2):126-127. doi: 0.5152/eajm.2013.24; and Beckman JS, Koppenol WH. Nitric oxide, superoxide, and peroxynitrite: the good, the bad, and ugly. *Am J Physiol*. 1996;271(5):C1424-C1437.

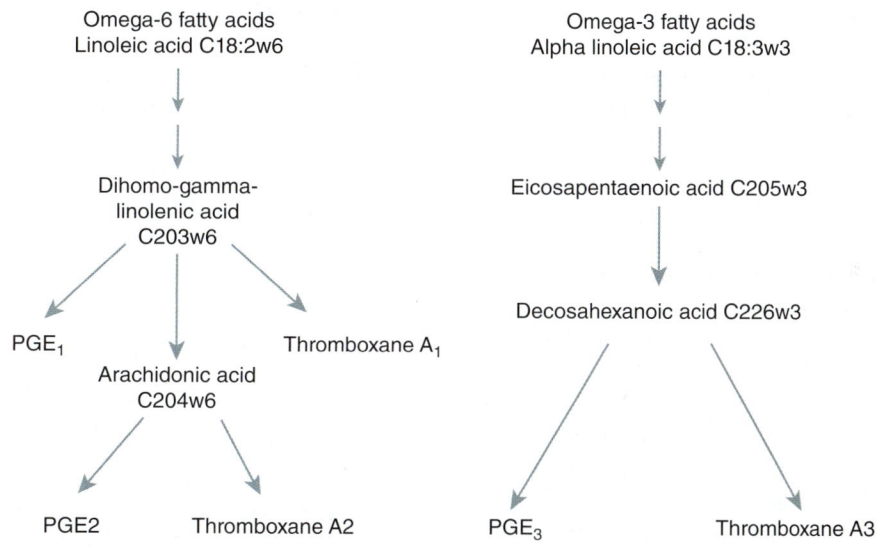

FIGURE 3.11 Omega-3 Versus 6 Fatty Acid Pathways

Data from Singer P, Theilla M, Fischer H, Gibstein L. Grozovski E, Cohen J. Benefit of an enteral diet enriched with eicosapentaenoic acid and gamma-linolenic acid in ventilated patients with acute lung injury. *Critical Care Medicine*. 2006;34(4):1033-1038.

immune-enhanced group by a hazard ratio of 1.57 (95% CI, 1.03 – 2.39; P = .04).[82] Meta-analysis of similar trials with glutamine showed no benefit in infectious complications or mortality.[83] Route of administration is considered particularly important in establishing glutamine as a beneficial immune nutrient. Unlike traditional practice and belief of enteral nutrient provision as superior, in the case of glutamine, parenteral delivery may be more advantageous in promoting protein synthesis during critical illness.[84] Intravenous glutamine results in a uniform uptake of glutamine in the splanchic region, which is more physiologic and typical of endogenous glutamine synthesis. This permits a more even distribution of glutamine throughout the body. Conversely, enteral glutamine undergoes a first-pass elimination at the gut level. Here, glutamine uptake by the enterocytes is substantial, reducing the amount of glutamine that enters the circulation.[85] Currently, IV glutamine is advocated over enteral for patients in the intensive care unit.[84] Finally, although initial studies with omega-3 fatty acids were promising, subsequent studies on omega-3 fatty acid–enriched diets with antioxidants added demonstrated no clinical benefit in ventilator-free days or ICU days.[86,87]

⚠ Clinical Controversy

Immunonutrition and Clinical Outcome

While meta-analyses demonstrate that immune-enhancing nutrients improve clinical outcomes, more recent clinical trials have raised questions regarding the general use of immunonutrition in the critically ill. The REDOX study (Reducing Deaths Due to Oxidative Stress) used selenium and found higher mortality in patients receiving enteral and parenteral glutamine. The detrimental effects were most profound in patients with multi-organ failure, and given that enteral and parenteral glutamine provision were used, overall dosing may have been too high. Similarly, the OMEGA found increased mortality in patients with acute respiratory distress syndrome. The study diet included omega-3 fatty acids, alpha-linolenic acid, and antioxidants. Notably, some recent trials provide immune-enhancing nutrients in combination to simulate how they interact in vivo. This makes interpretation somewhat obscured.

Read the three studies below on immunonutrition. Consider their findings and how study design, dosing, route of administration, and combination of nutrients may affect results. What is your opinion on use of immunonutrition in the critically ill?

References

1. Heyland D, Muscedere J, Wischmeyer PE, et al. A randomized controlled trial of glutamine and antioxidants in the critically ill patient. *N Engl J Med.* 2013;368(16):1489-1497.
2. Rice TW, Wheeler AP, Thompson BT, deBoiseblane BP, Steingrub J, Rock P. Enteral omega-3 fatty acid, gamma-linolenic acid, and antioxidant supplementation in acute lung injury. *JAMA.* 2011;306(14):1574-1582.
3. van Zanten AR, Sztark F, Kaisers UX, et al. High-protein enteral nutrition enriched with immune-modulating nutrients vs standard high-protein enteral nutrition and nosocomial infections in the ICU: a randomized clinical trial. *JAMA.* 2014;312(5):514-524.

Chapter Summary

Enteral nutrition is the preferred mode of feeding for most patients requiring nutrition support. Optimal outcome, however, depends on proper selection of feeding site, mode of delivery, and formula. Enteral feeding tube placement should take into consideration length of required support, gastric function, aspiration risk, and lifestyle needs of the patient. Formula selection is based on clinical and disease-related requirements of the patients. Over the past several decades, an abundance of specialized feeding products has become available. Choosing an appropriate formula can help support metabolic and disease-related needs in many patients. Disease- and condition-specific formulas are recognized for their unique nutrient characteristics, which can enhance provision of nitrogen and wound-healing nutrients. Differences in composition related to fiber, fluid, macronutrients, and micronutrients provide options to coincide with the medical management of the patient.

Key Terms

enteral nutrition (EN), percutaneous endoscopic gastrostomy (PEG) tube, immunonutrition, nasogastric tube, nasoenteric, oroenteric, nasoduodenal tube, nasojejunal tube, prokinetics, fluoroscopic tube placement, percutaneous endoscopic jejunostomy (PEJ), laparoscopy, open tube placement, aspiration, gastroparesis, dumping syndrome, closed tube feeding system, open tube feeding system, hang time, continuous feeding, intermittent feeding, bolus feeding, isolate, prebiotics, probiotics, hypercapnia, gastric residuals, early enteral nutrition (EEN), postprandial hyperemic response

References

1. Brantley S, Mills M. Overview of enteral nutrition. In: Mueller C, ed. *The A.S.P.E.N. Adult Nutrition Support Core Curriculum.* 2nd ed. Silver Spring, MD: American Society for Parenteral and Enteral Nutrition; 2012:170-184.
2. Volkert D, Berner YN, Berry E, et al. E.S.P.E.N guideline on enteral nutrition: geriatrics. *J Clin Nutr.* 2006;25(2):330-60.
3. White J, Guenter P, Jenson G, Malone A, Schofield M. Consensus Statement of the Academy of Nutrition and Dietetics/American Society for Parenteral and Enteral Nutrition: Characteristics Recommended for the Identification and Documentation of Adult Malnutrition (Undernutrition). *J Acad Nutr Diet.* 2012;112(5):730-738.
4. Harkness L. The history of enteral nutrition therapy: from raw eggs and nasal tubes to purified amino acids and early postoperative jejunal delivery. *J Am Diet Assoc.* 2002;102(3):399-404.
5. Bechtold ML, Mir FA, Boumitri C, et al. Long-term nutrition: a clinician's guide to successful long-term enteral access in adults. *Nutr Clin Pract.* 2016. [Epub ahead of print.] doi: 10.1177/0884533616670103
6. Dwolatzky T, Berezovski S, Friedmann R, et al. A prospective comparison of the use of nasogastric and percutaneous endoscopic gastrostomy tubes for long-term enteral feeding in older people. *Clin Nutr.* 2001;20(6):535-540.
7. Gauderer MW. Percutaneous endoscopic gastrostomy and the evolution of contemporary long-term enteral access. *Clin Nutr.* 2002;21(2):103-110.
8. Gopalan S, Khanna S. Enteral nutrition delivery technique. *Curr Opin Clin Nutr Metab Care.* 2003;6(3):313-317.
9. Nunes G, Santos CA, Santos C, Fonseca J. Percutaneous endoscopic gastrostomy for nutritional support in dementia patients. *Aging Clin Exp Res.* 2016;28(5):983-989.
10. Shastri YM, Shirodkar M, Mallath MK. Endoscopic feeding tube placement in patients with cancer: a prospective clinical audit of 2055 procedures in 1866 patients. *Aliment Pharmacol Ther.* 2008;27(8):649-658.

11. Fang JC, Hilden K, Holubkov R, Disario JA. Transnasal endoscopy vs. fluoroscopy for the placement of nasoenteric feeding tubes in critically ill patients. *Gastrointest Endosc*. 2005;62(5):661-666.

12. Jabbar A, McClave SA. Pre-pyloric versus post-pyloric feeding. *Clin Nutr*. 2005;24(5):719-726.

13. Nelms M, Sucher KP, Lacey K, Roth SL. *Nutrition therapy and pathophysiology*. 2nd ed. Boston, MA: Cengage Learning; 2010.

14. Vanek VW. Ins and outs of enteral access. Part 1: short-term enteral access. *Nutr Clin Pract*. 2002;17(5):275-283.

15. Haslam D, Fang J. Enteral access for nutrition in the intensive care unit. *Curr Opin Clin Nutr Metab Care*. 2006;9(2):155-159.

16. Fang John C, Bankhead R, and Kinikini M. Enteral access devices. In: Mueller C, Ed. *The A.S.P.E.N. Adult Nutrition Support Core Curriculum*. 2nd ed. Silver Spring, MD: American Society for Parenteral and Enteral Nutrition; 2012:206-217.

17. Niv E, Fireman Z, Vaisman N. Post-pyloric feeding. *World J Gastroenterol*. 2009;15(11):1281-1288.

18. Roberts S, Echeverria P, Gabriel SA. Devices and techniques for bedside enteral feeding tube placement. *Nutr Clin Pract*. 2007;22(4):412-420.

19. Disario JA. Endoscopic approaches to enteral nutritional support. *Best Pract Res Clin Gastroenterol*. 2006;20(3):605-630.

20. Bear DE, Champion A, Lei K, Smith J, Beale J, Camporota L, Barrett NA. Use of an electromagnetic device compared with chest x-ray to confirm nasogastric feeding tube position in critical care. *J Parenter Enteral Nutr*. 2016;40:581-586.

21. Kozin ED, Remenschneider AK, Cunnane ME, Deschler DG. Otolaryngologist-assisted fluoroscopic-guided nasogastric tube placement in the postoperative laryngectomy patient. *Laryngoscope*. 2014;124(4):916-920.

22. Ponsky JL. Percutaneous endoscopic gastrostomy. *J Gastrointest Surg*. 2004;8(7):901-904

23. Schrag SP, Sharma R, Jaik NP, et al. Complications related to percutaneous endoscopic gastrostomy (PEG) tubes. A comprehensive clinical review. *J Gastrointestin Liver Dis*. 2007;16(4):407-418.

24. Löser C, Aschl G, Hébuterne X, et al. ESPEN guidelines on artificial enteral nutrition-percutaneous endoscopic gastrostomy (PEG). *Clin Nutr*. 2005;24(5):848-861.

25. Bankhead RR, Fisher CA, Rolandelli RH. Gastrostomy tube placement outcomes: comparison of surgical, endoscopic, and laparoscopic methods. *Nutr Clin Pract*. 2005;20(6):607-612.

26. Bankhead R, Boullata J, Brantley S, et al. Enteral nutrition practice recommendations. *J Parenter Enteral Nutr*. 2009;33(2):122-167.

27. Kwon RS, Banerjee S, Desilets D, et al. Enteral nutrition access devices. *Gastrointest Endosc*. 2010;72(2):236-248.

28. Metheny NA, Titler MG. Assessing placement of feeding tubes. *Am J Nurs*. 2001;101(5):36-45.

29. Schlein K. Gastric versus small bowel feeding in critically ill adults. *Nutr Clin Pract*. 2016;31(4):514-522.

30. Marik PE, Zaloga GP. Gastric versus post-pyloric feeding: a systematic review. *Crit Care*. 2003;7(3):R46-51.

31. Jiyong J, Tiancha H, Huiqin W, Jingfen F. Effect of gastric versus post-pyloric feeding on the incidence of pneumonia in critically ill patients: observations from traditional and Bayesian random-effects meta-analysis. *Clin Nutr*. 2013;32(1):8-15.

32. Varon DE1, Freitas G, Goel N, et al. Intraoperative feeding improves calorie and protein delivery in acute burn patients. *J Burn Care Res*. 2017;38(5):299-303. doi: 10.1097/BCR.0000000000000514

33. Silva SMR, Silva de Assis MC, Rosane de Moraes Silveira C, Gomes M, Daniel de Mello E. Open versus closed enteral nutrition systems for critically ill adults: is there a difference? *Revista da Associação Médica Brasileira* (English Edition) 2012; 58(2): 229-233.

34. Davis TA, Fiorotto ML, Suryawan A. Bolus versus continuous feeding to optimize anabolism in neonates. *Curr Opin Clin Nutr Metab Care*. 2015;18(1):102-108.doi: 10.1097/MCO.0000000000000128

35. Bowling TE, Cliff B, Wright JW, Blackshaw PE, Perkins AC, Lobo DN. The effects of bolus and continuous nasogastric feeding on gastro-oesophageal reflux and gastric emptying in healthy volunteers: a randomised three-way crossover pilot study. *Clin Nutr*. 2008;27(4):608-613.

36. Evans DC, Forbes R, Jones C, et al. Continuous versus bolus tube feeds: Does the modality affect glycemic variability, tube feeding volume, caloric intake, or insulin utilization? *Int J Crit Illn Inj Sci*. 2016;6(1):9-15.

37. Kadamani I, Itani M, Zahran E, Taha N. Incidence of aspiration and gastrointestinal complications in critically ill patients using continuous versus bolus infusion of enteral nutrition: a pseudo-randomised controlled trial. *Aust Crit Care*. 2014;27(4):188-193. doi: 10.1016/j.aucc.2013.12.001.

38. Cresci G, Lefton J, Esper DH. Enteral formulations. In: Mueller C, ed. *The A.S.P.E.N. Adult Nutrition Support Core Curriculum*. 2nd ed. Silver Spring, MD: American Society for Parenteral and Enteral Nutrition; 2012:186-203.

39. Athalye-jape G, Deshpande G, Rao S, Patole S. Benefits of probiotics on enteral nutrition in preterm neonates: a systematic review. *Am J Clin Nutr*. 2014;100(6):1508-1519.

40. Dang S, Shook L, Garlitz K, Hanna M, Desai N. Nutritional outcomes with implementation of probiotics in preterm infants. *J Perinatol*. 2015;35(6):447-450.

41. Preiser J-C, van Zanten AR, Berger MM, et al. Metabolic and nutritional support of critically ill patients: consensus and controversies. *Crit Care*. 2015;19(1):35. doi: 10.1186/s13054-015-0737-8.

42. Hempel S, Newberry SJ, Maher AR, et al. Probiotics for the prevention and treatment of antibiotic-associated diarrhea: A systematic review and meta-analysis. *JAMA*. 2012;307 (18):1959-1969. doi: 10.1001/jama.2012.3507.

43. Barraud D, Bollaert PE, Gibot S. Impact of the administration of probiotics on mortality in critically ill adult patients: a meta-analysis of randomized controlled trials. *Chest*. 2013;143(3):646-655.

44. Besselink MG, van Santvoort HC, Buskens E, Boermeester MA, van Goor H, Timmerman HM, et al. Probiotic prophylaxis in predicted severe acute pancreatitis: a randomised, double-blind, placebo-controlled trial. *Lancet*. 2008;371:651-659.

45. Kalantar-Zadeh K, Cano NJ, Budde K, et al. Diets and enteral supplements for improving outcomes in chronic kidney disease. *Nature Rev Nephrol*. 2011;7(7):10.1038/nrneph.2011.60. doi: 10.1038/nrneph.2011.60.

46. Cai B1, Zhu Y, Ma Yi, et al. Effect of supplementing a high-fat, low-carbohydrate enteral formula in COPD patients. *Nutrition*. 2003;19(3):229-232.

47. Elamin EM, Miller AC, Ziad S. Immune enteral nutrition can improve outcomes in medical-surgical patients with ARDS: A prospective randomized controlled trial. *J Nutr Disord Ther*. 2012;2:109. doi: 10.4172/2161-0509.1000109.

48. Hsieh MJ, Yang TM, Tsai YH. Nutritional supplementation in patients with chronic obstructive pulmonary disease. *J Formos Med Assoc*. 2016;115(8):595-601. doi: 10.1016/j.jfma.2015.10.008.

49. Koretz RL, Avenell A, Lipman TO. Nutrition support for liver disease. *Cochrane Database Syst Rev*. 2012;(5):CD008344. doi: 10.1002/14651858.CD008344.pub2. Review.

50. Plauth M, Cabré E, Riggio O, et al. ESPEN Guidelines on enteral nutrition: liver disease. *Clin Nutr*. 2006;25(2):285-294.

51. Ojo O, Brooke J. Evaluation of the role of enteral nutrition in managing patients with diabetes: A systematic review. *Nutrients*. 2014;6(11):5142-5152. doi: 10.3390/nu6115142.

52. Mesejo A, Montejo-González JC, Vaquerizo-Alonso C, et al. Diabetes-specific enteral nutrition formula in hyperglycemic, mechanically ventilated, critically ill patients: a prospective, open-label, blind-randomized, multicenter study. *Crit Care*. 2015;19:390. doi: 10.1186/s13054-015-1108-1.

53. Ellinger S. Micronutrients, arginine, and glutamine: Does supplementation provide an efficient tool for prevention and treatment of different kinds of wounds? *Adv Wound Care*. 2014;3(11):691-707. doi: 10.1089/wound.2013.0482.

54. Malone A, Seres D, Lord L. Complications of enteral nutrition. In: Mueller C, ed. *The A.S.P.E.N. Adult Nutrition Support Core Curriculum*. 2nd ed. Silver Spring, MD: American Society for Parenteral and Enteral Nutrition; 2012:219-231.

55. Pancorbo-hidalgo PL, García-fernandez FP, Ramírez-Pérez C. Complications associated with enteral nutrition by nasogastric tube in an internal medicine unit. *J Clin Nurs*. 2001;10(4):482-90.

56. Montejo JC, Minambres E, Bordeje L, et al. Gastric residual volume during enteral nutrition in ICU patients: the REGANE study. *Intensive Care Med*. 2010;36(8):1386-1393.

57. Arabi YM, Casaer MP, Chapman M, et al. The intensive care medicine research agenda in nutrition and metabolism. *Intensive Care Med*. 2017. doi: 10.1007/s00134-017-4711-6.

58. Bistrian BR. The who, what, where, when, why, and how of early enteral feeding. *Am J Clin Nutr*. 2012;95(6):1303-1304.

59. Doig GS, Heighes PT, Simpson F, Sweetman EA. Early enteral nutrition reduces mortality in trauma patients requiring intensive care: a meta-analysis of randomized controlled trials. *Injury*. 2011;42:50-56.

60. Reintam Blaser A, Starkopf J, Alhazzani W, et al. Early enteral nutrition in critically ill patients: ESICM clinical practice guidelines. *Intensive Care Med*. 2017;43(3):380-398. doi: 10.1007/s00134-016-4665-0.

61. Li JY, Yu T, Chen GC, et al. Enteral nutrition within 48 hours of admission improves clinical outcomes of acute pancreatitis by reducing complications: a meta-analysis. *PLoS ONE*. 2013;8(6):e64926.

62. Mikhailov TA, Kuhn EM, Manzi J, et al. Early enteral nutrition is associated with lower mortality in critically ill children. *JPEN J Parenter Enteral Nutr*. 2014;38(4):459-466.

63. Szabo FK, Fei L, Cruz LA, Abu-el-haija M. Early enteral nutrition and aggressive fluid resuscitation are associated with improved clinical outcomes in acute pancreatitis. *J Pediatr*. 2015;167(2): 397-402.e1.

64. Liu J, Kong K, Tao Y, Cai W. Optimal timing for introducing enteral nutrition in the neonatal intensive care unit. *Asia Pac J Clin Nutr*. 2015;24(2):219-226.

65. Melis M, Fichera A, Ferguson MK. Bowel necrosis associated with early jejunal feeding: A complication of postoperative enteral nutrition. *Arch Surg*. 2006;141:701-704.

66. Bakiner O, Bozkirli E, Giray S, et al. Impact of early versus late enteral nutrition on cell mediated immunity and its relationship with glucagon like peptide-1 in intensive care unit patients: a prospective study. *Crit Care*. 2013;17(3):R123.

67. Chen W, Zhang Z, Xiong M, et al. Early enteral nutrition after total gastrectomy for gastric cancer. *Asia Pac J Clin Nutr*. 2014;23(4):607-611.

68. Martindale RG, Warren M. Should enteral nutrition be started in the first week of critical illness? *Curr Opin Clin Nutr Metab Care*. 2015;18(2):202-206.

69. Ibrahim EH, Mehringer L, Prentice D, et al. Early versus late enteral feeding of mechanically ventilated patients: results of a clinical trial. *JPEN J Parenter Enteral Nutr*. 2002;26(3):174-181.

70. Khalid I, Doshi P, Digiovine B. Early enteral nutrition and outcomes of critically ill patients treated with vasopressors and mechanical ventilation. *Am J Crit Care*. 2010;19(3):261-268.

71. Flordelís lasierra JL, Pérez-vela JL, Umezawa makikado LD, et al. Early enteral nutrition in patients with hemodynamic failure following cardiac surgery. *JPEN J Parenter Enteral Nutr*. 2015;39(2):154-162.

72. Hegazi RA, DeWitt T. Enteral nutrition and immune modulation of acute pancreatitis. *World J Gastroenterol*. 2014;20(43):16101-16105.

73. O'Hara AM, Shanahan F. The gut flora as a forgotten organ. *EMBO Reports*. 2006;7(7):688-693. doi: 10.1038/sj.embor.740073

74. Krauss H, Jablecka A, Sosnowski P, Bogdanski P. Influence of L-arginine on the nitric oxide concentration and level of oxidative stress during ischemia-reperfusion injury in a rat model. *Int J Clin Pharmacol Ther*. 2009;47(8):533-538.

75. Smith RJ. Glutamine metabolism and its physiologic importance. *JPEN J Parenter Enteral Nutr*. 1990;14(4 Suppl):40S-44S.

76. Gadek, JE, DeMichele SJ, Karlstad MD. Enteral nutrition in ARDS study group. Effect of enteral feeding with eicosapentaenoic acid, gamma linolenic acid, and antioxidants in patients with acute respiratory distress syndrome. *Crit Care Med*. 1999;27(8):1409-1420.

77. Grootjans J, Lenaerts K, Derikx JPM, et al. Human intestinal ischemia-reperfusion–induced inflammation characterized: Experiences from a new translational model. *Am J Pathol*. 2010;176(5):2283-2291. doi: 10.2353/ajpath.2010.091069.

78. Yapca OE, Borekci B, Suleyman H. Ischemia-reperfusion damage. *Eurasian J Med*. 2013;45(2):126-127. doi: 10.5152/eajm.2013.24.

79. Beckman JS, Koppenol WH. Nitric oxide, superoxide, and peroxynitrite: the good, the bad, and ugly. *Am J Physiol*. 1996;271(5):C1424-C1437.

80. Singer P, Theilla M, Fischer H, Gibstein L, Grozovski E, Cohen J. Benefit of an enteral diet enriched with eicosapentaenoic acid and gamma-linolenic acid in ventilated patients with acute lung injury. *Crit Care Med*. 2006;34(4):1033-1038.

81. Pontes-Arruda A, Aragao AM, Albequerque JD. Effects of enteral feeding with eicosapentaenoic acid, gamma-linolenic acid and antioxidants in mechanically ventilated patients with severe sepsis and septic shock. *Crit Care Med*. 2006;34(9):2325-2333.

82. van Zanten AR, Sztark F, Kaisers UX, et al. High-protein enteral nutrition enriched with immune-modulating nutrients vs standard high-protein enteral nutrition and nosocomial infections in the ICU: a randomized clinical trial. *JAMA*. 2014;6;312(5):514-24.

83. van Zanten ARH, Dhaliwal R, Garrel D, Heyland DH. Enteral glutamine supplementation in critically ill patients: A systematic review and meta-analysis. *Crit Care*. 2015;19:294-310.

84. Rodas PC, Rooyackers O, Hebert C, Norberg Å, Wernerman J. Glutamine and glutathione at ICU admission in relation to outcome. *Clin Sci*. 2012;122(Pt 12):591-597. doi: 10.1042/CS20110520.

85. Wernerman J. Glutamine supplementation. *Ann Intensive Care*. 2011;1:25. doi: 10.1186/2110-5820-1-25.

86. Li C, Bo L, Liu W, Lu X, Jin F. Enteral immunomodulatory diet (omega-3 fatty acid, gamma-linolenic acid and antioxidant supplementation) for acute lung injury and acute respiratory distress syndrome: An updated systematic review and analysis. *Nutrients*. 2015;7:5572-5585.

87. Rice TW, Wheeler AP, Thompson BT, deBoiseblane BP, Steingrub J, Rock P. Enteral omega-3 fatty acid, gamma-linolenic acid, and antioxidant supplementation in acute lung injury. *JAMA*. 2011;306(14):1574-1582.

Chapter 4

Parenteral Nutrition Therapy

Katie Fort
Grace Ling
Kathy Prelack
Kelly Kane

Chapter Outline

Core Concepts
Introduction
Brief History of Parenteral Nutrition
Parenteral Nutrition Administration
Parenteral Nutrition Formulation
Initiation and Progression of Parenteral Nutrition
Parenteral Nutrition Monitoring
Central Venous Access Complications and Their Management
Metabolic Complications
Home Parenteral Nutrition

CORE CONCEPTS

1. Parenteral nutrition is a low-volume, high-risk form of nutrition therapy that should only be used when clinically indicated. Enteral nutrition, if tolerated, is preferable to parenteral nutrition in patients who require nutrition support.

2. Venous access for parenteral nutrition is based on duration of therapy, desired concentration and solution type, and disease state/condition of the patient.

3. Candidates for parenteral nutrition must be fully evaluated for nutritional risk and nutritional status with adherence to standardized protocols for initiation of parenteral nutrition.

4. Parenteral nutrition is a hypertonic solution made up of, but not limited to, carbohydrate in the form of dextrose, crystalline amino acids, lipid emulsions, vitamins, minerals, and sterile water.

5. Many lipid emulsions are composed of primarily omega-6 fatty acids and should be provided judiciously given their role in inflammation.

6. Prescription of parenteral nutrition is based on energy and protein requirements with consideration of fluid specifications and substrate utilization of macronutrients.

7. Carbohydrate infusion from parenteral nutrition should not exceed 5 mg/kg/min in adults and children over the age of 2 years.

8. Parenteral nutrition formulations are customizable to the specific needs of each patient or patient population.

9. Monitoring of anthropometric, clinical, and biochemical indices such as electrolytes, acid–base balance, serum glucose, and liver function tests are critical to ensure the safety of the patient.

10. Parenteral nutrition may be a long-term or even life-long therapy for some patients.

Learning Objectives

1. Understand the history of parenteral nutrition therapy and its importance as a form of nutrition support therapy.
2. Identify the various methods of central and peripheral venous access.
3. Assess whether a patient is a candidate for parenteral nutrition by critically evaluating their disease state and biochemical parameters.
4. Identify the nutrition components and additions that commonly comprise parenteral nutrition.
5. Calculate a sample parenteral nutrition prescription/order.
6. Identify the anthropometric, biochemical, and physical examination components that constitute effective monitoring of parenteral nutrition patients.
7. Describe the potential mechanical and metabolic complications of parenteral nutrition and strategies to prevent and/or resolve them.

Introduction

Parenteral nutrition (PN) is a type of nutrition support that relies on the intravenous administration of nutrients to patients who are unable or unwilling to take adequate nutrition orally or enterally. PN may be used as an addition to an oral diet or enteral nutrition (EN) in order to meet needs, as the sole source of nutrition during recovery from illness or injury of the gastrointestinal (GI) tract, or as a long-term life-sustaining therapy for patients who have compromised ability to enterally absorb nutrients.

A **hypertonic** solution is a solution with increased osmotic pressure as compared to bodily fluid. It is administered intravenously and is customizable to the individual needs of the patient and may contain carbohydrates, amino acids, lipids, vitamins, minerals, and sterile water. There are potentially serious metabolic and mechanical dangers associated with PN. For this reason, PN is only utilized when nutrition support is necessary and enteral nutrition is inadequate and/or contraindicated.[1]

> **CORE CONCEPT 1**
>
> Parenteral nutrition is a low-volume, high-risk form of nutrition therapy that should only be used when clinically indicated. Enteral nutrition, if tolerated, is preferable to parenteral nutrition in patients who require nutrition support.

Brief History of Parenteral Nutrition

Since the 17th century, intravenous nutrition has been of interest to the medical and nutrition communities as a means to improve nutrition status; however, it was not until the 1960s that it was successfully utilized in a human model.[2] The pioneers of parenteral nutrition, Dr. George Blackburn, Dr. Stanley Dudrick, Dr. Harry Vars, and Dr. Douglas Wilmore, were most interested in treating protein-energy malnutrition in patients who were either unable to use the gastrointestinal tract or were experiencing failure to thrive despite sufficient oral consumption.[3]

Dudrick and his colleagues began their studies on the feasibility, efficacy, and safety of parenteral nutrition with a laboratory study. Six pedigreed beagle puppies were fed with parenteral nutrition for either 72, 100, 235, or 256 days after weaning from their mother at 8 weeks of age. The weight gain, skeletal growth, development, and activity of these puppies were compared to their orally fed littermates. At the end of the study period, the researchers found that each of the six intravenously fed puppies surpassed their controls in weight gain and matched them in skeletal growth, development, and activity. There were no significant differences between growth rates or weight gain between the experimental puppies.

The success of parenteral feeding with the beagles was encouraging for the researchers and prompted a clinical study in 30 human patients with chronic complicated gastrointestinal disease. The parenteral solution provided to these patients was customized by a clinician daily to meet individual needs and compounded by a pharmacist with 20% glucose, 5% fibrin hydrolysate, electrolytes, trace minerals, and vitamins. The infusion was administered through a central catheter placed percutaneously into the superior vena cava for 10 to 200 days, depending on the patient. In this clinical study, positive nitrogen balance was achieved in all patients. As a result, patients experienced improvements in wound healing, fistula closure, weight gain, and strength and activity.[4] These findings were groundbreaking, as the general consensus within the medical and nutrition communities during the 1960s was that feeding entirely by vein was not possible, practical, or affordable.

Despite its success in improving nutrition status of recipients, the research team encountered problems related to the preparation and administration of parenteral nutrition. Major challenges included formulating complete parenteral nutrient solutions, which did not exist at the time; concentrating hypertonic substrate components without precipitation; demonstrating utility and safety of long-term central venous catheterization; demonstrating efficacy and safety of long-term infusion of hypertonic nutrient solutions; maintaining **asepsis**, or the absence of bacteria throughout solution preparation and delivery; and anticipating, avoiding, and correcting metabolic imbalances or derangements.[2] Despite advances in medicine, many of these issues continue to be of concern with the preparation and administration of PN.

Parenteral Nutrition Administration

Venous Access

Depending on the type of venous access selected, PN may be referred to as **central parenteral nutrition** or

CASE STUDY INTRODUCTION

Alex is a 43-year-old male with a history of adenocarcinoma of the ileum and which has been in remission for 3 years. He now presents with intermittent abdominal cramping, abdominal distension, constipation, and loss of appetite and has not eaten for the past 4 days. The physician suspects that Alex's cancer treatment, including intensive radiation and two prior surgeries, has led to a small bowel obstruction. She orders a computerized tomography (CT) scan, which confirms that several intestinal adhesions have formed in the distal ileum, resulting in a complete bowel obstruction. Alex is scheduled for surgery in 5 days and is admitted to the hospital for management of his small bowel obstruction. Alex lives with his wife and 6-year-old daughter and works from home as a graphic designer.

Anthropometric Data:
Current weight: 64 kg (141 lbs)
Usual body weight (UBW): 70 kg (155 lbs)
Height: 175 cm (69 in)
Body mass index (BMI): 21 kg/m^2

Biochemical Data:
Sodium 133 (135-145 mEq/L)
Potassium 3.5 (3.6-5.0 mEq/L)
Chloride 109 (98-110 mEq/L)
Carbon dioxide 20 (20-30 mEq/L)
Blood urea nitrogen 5 (6-24 mg/dL)
Creatinine 0.6 (0.4-1.3 mg/dL)
Glucose 88 (70-139 mg/dL)
Glomerular filtration rate 99 mL/min/1.73 m^2

Calcium 8.7 (8.5-10.5 mEq/L)
Phosphorus 2.9 (2.7-4.5 mg/dL)
Magnesium 1.5 (1.3-2.1 mEq/L)
Albumin 3.5 (3.5-5.0 g/dL)
Hemoglobin 12.7 (13.5-17.5 g/dL)
Hematocrit 35% (42%-52%)

Clinical Data:
Past Medical History: None
Medications: Imodium
Vitals: Blood pressure 110/77 mm Hg, Temperature 98.6°F
Nutrition-focused Physical Exam: Patient appears pale with decreased muscle tone and skin turgor. Abdomen is distended with minimal bowel sounds.

Dietary Data:
Dietary History: Alex states that he has experienced intermittent abdominal cramping and poor appetite for the past several weeks. As a result, he has been skipping meals or eating half-sized portions of his usual intake. He has not eaten for the past 4 days due to worsening cramping.
Diet Prescription: NPO

Questions

1. How would you assess Alex's preoperative nutritional status?
2. Would you suggest initiating parenteral nutrition support to the medical team? Justify your answer. If you believe that parenteral nutrition support should be initiated prior to surgery, what type of venous access would you recommend?

---

peripheral parenteral nutrition. In central PN, venous access is acquired in a central vessel, namely the superior or inferior vena cava or the right atrium.[5] In peripheral PN, access is obtained in a peripheral vessel, such as the vessels of the hand or forearm. Because catheters, also known as vascular access devices (VADs), may be advanced some distance through the vasculature, the distinction between central and peripheral PN is based solely on the location of the catheter tip. The location of the tip does not necessarily correspond with the site of **venipuncture** (the point where the catheter enters the vasculature) or the **exit site** (where the catheter exits the body).[5]

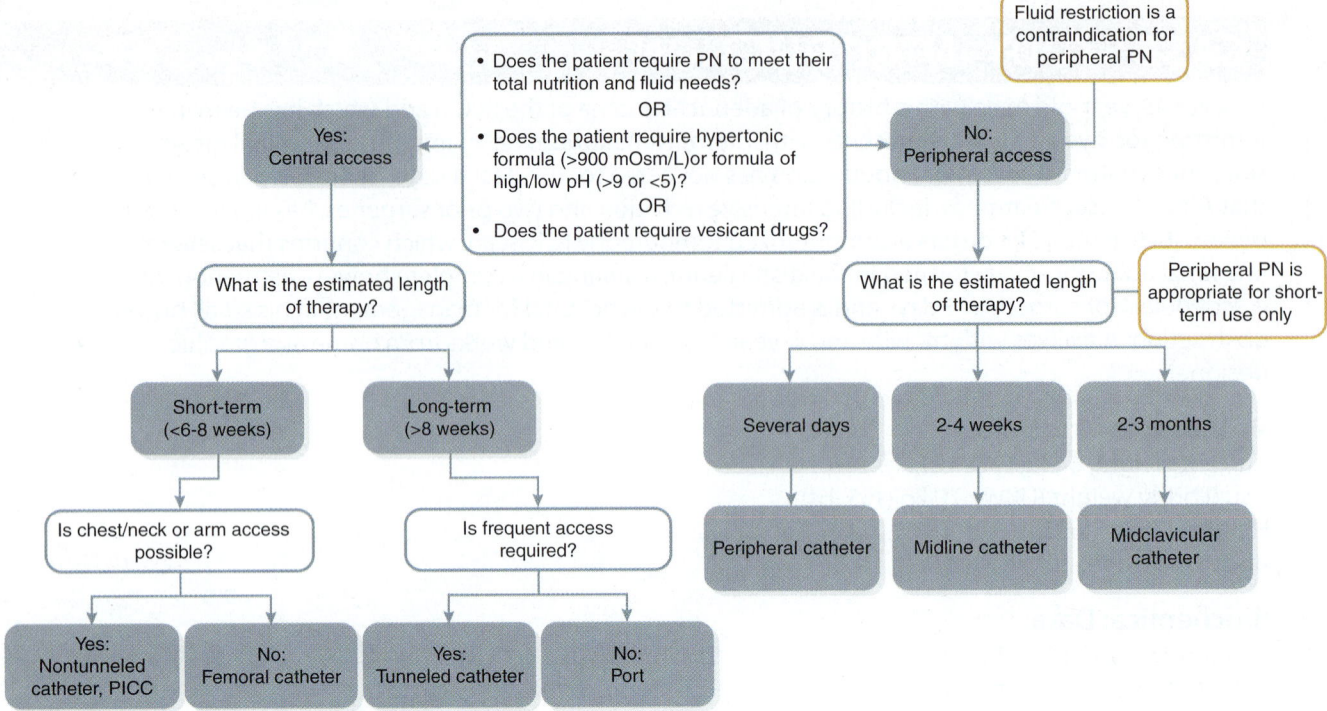

FIGURE 4.1 Determining Type of Intravenous Access

CORE CONCEPT 2

Several factors influence the decision to infuse centrally or peripherally, notably the type of PN formula. Because PN formulas are hypertonic to body fluids, the type of administration must be carefully considered to avoid complications.[3] Other considerations include the expected length of therapy; frequency of infusions; and patient characteristics such as medical history, preferences, and ability to care for the device.[6]

Figure 4.1 provides a basic algorithm for determining which form of access is appropriate for the patient.

Central Parenteral Nutrition

In central PN, the catheter tip is located in a large, high-flow vessel, typically the junction of the superior vena cava and right atrium. The vena cava and right atrium are sites of high blood flow that can quickly disperse PN solutions that might otherwise cause complications such as **thrombophlebitis**, or inflammation of a vein caused by a blood clot, and **extravasation**, or inadvertent administration or leakage of the PN into surrounding tissues instead of a vein.[5,7] The ideal tip location is the lower third of the superior vena cava or at the atrio-caval junction, as these locations are associated with the fewest mechanical and thrombotic complications.[7] However, the catheter tip should not be placed any deeper than this, as the risk of thrombotic complications increases when the catheter is inserted near the tricuspid valve or deeper.

The VAD may be centrally inserted and the location of the catheter tip is advanced from the site of venipuncture and threaded through the vasculature until the tip reaches the vena cava and/or right atrium.[5] There are two main types of central access: short-term and long-term **central venous catheters (CVCs)**. Short-term CVCs, often referred to as non-tunneled catheters, vary by insertion site and may be inserted in the subclavian, internal or external jugular, or femoral veins. Catheter insertion into the femoral vein is associated with a higher risk of infection and thrombosis, and is therefore not typically recommended for PN.[7] Alternately, short-term CVCs may be inserted in the arm via the cephalic or basilic vein. This form of access is considered a **peripherally inserted central catheter (PICC)** (**Figures 4.2** and **4.3**).[7]

Long-term central access seeks to separate the skin from the venous entry site in order to reduce infection risk. Long-term CVCs are often referred to as tunneled catheters (**Figures 4.4** and **4.5**) as they are tunneled under the skin to the venous site although the catheter exits through the

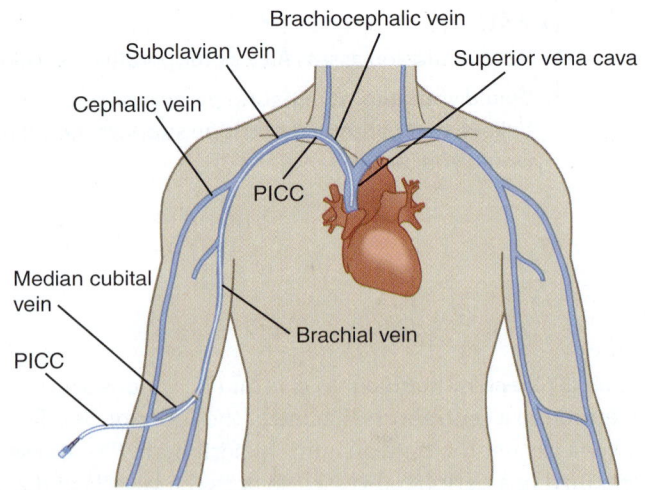

FIGURE 4.2 Peripherally Inserted Central Catheter (PICC) Placement

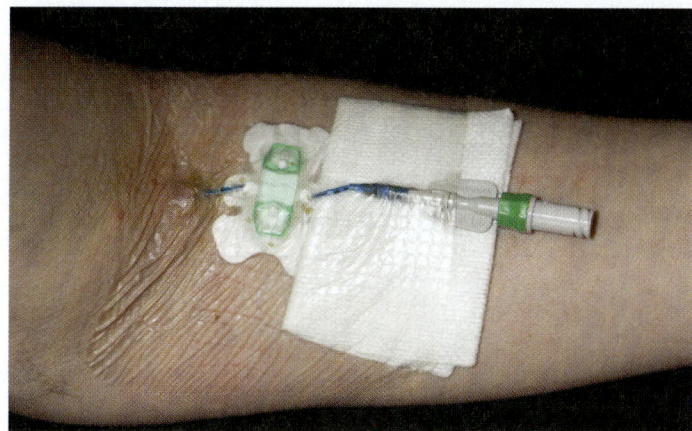

FIGURE 4.3 Patient with a PICC Line
© St Bartholomew's Hospital/Science Source.

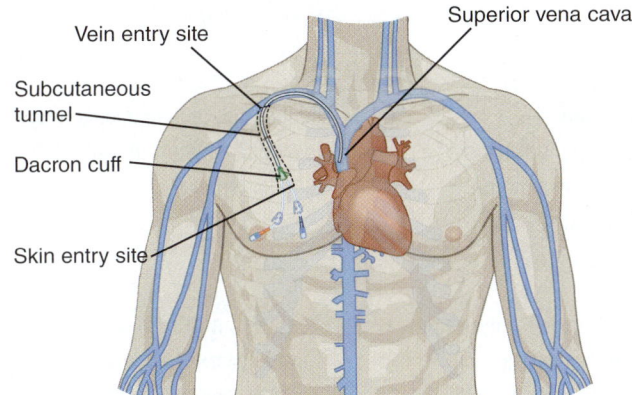

FIGURE 4.4 Tunneled Catheter Placement

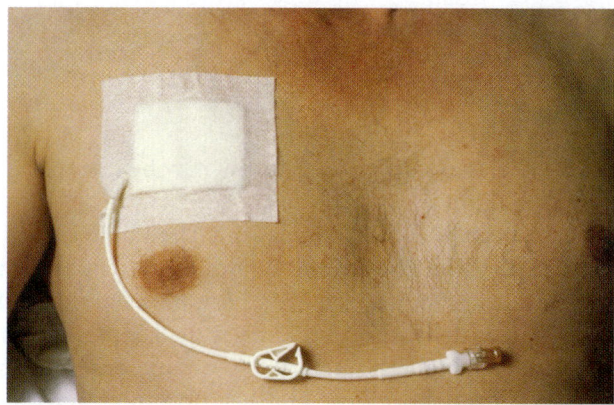

FIGURE 4.5 Patient with a Tunneled Catheter
© Dr P. Marazzi/Science Source.

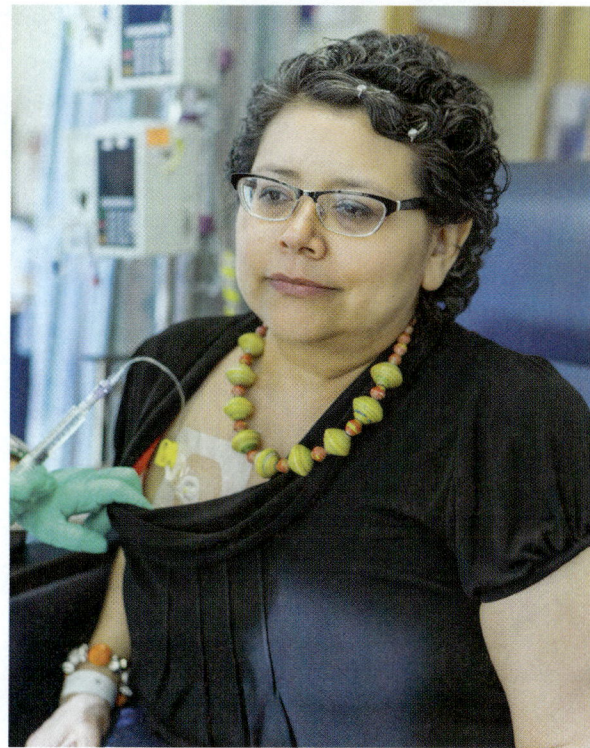

FIGURE 4.6 Patient Receiving an Infusion Through Central Venous Port
© Emerald Raindrops/Shutterstock.

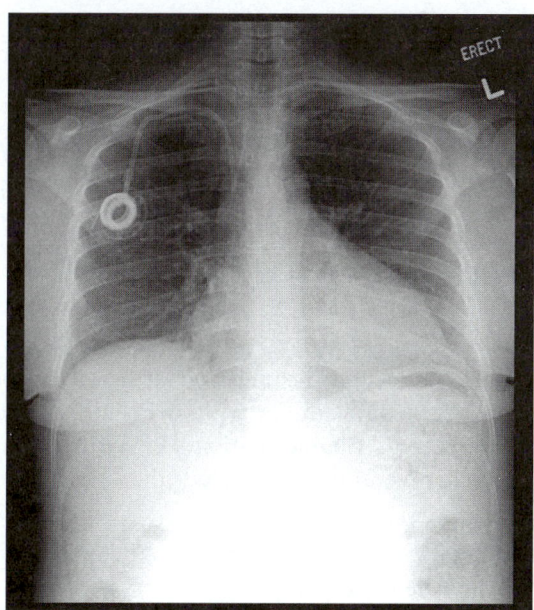

FIGURE 4.7 X-Ray Indicating Placement of Central Venous Port
© Living Art Enterprises / Science Source / Getty Images.

skin. Subcutaneously implanted ports are another form of long-term CVC where an entrance port is a device that exists under the skin with a catheter connecting the device to the vein. Implantable ports are different from tunneled catheters in that there is no catheter exiting the skin and access to the port requires puncturing the skin (**Figure 4.6**). Regardless of the entry site, the position of the tip should always be confirmed, whether through fluoroscopy or ultrasound during the procedure or through radiologic visualization after the procedure (**Figure 4.7**).[7]

There are advantages and disadvantages to both short-term and long-term CVCs. Short-term CVCs can typically be placed at the hospital bedside while long-term CVCs require surgical placement. Short-term CVCs, particularly those that are inserted through the subclavian, internal or external jugular, or femoral arteries, are more difficult to maintain sterile. Long-term CVCs are associated with lower infection risk and are preferred for use greater than 3 months.[7] **Table 4.1** describes various types of CVCs and their advantages and disadvantages.

TABLE 4.1 SUMMARY OF CENTRAL VENOUS CATHETERS[5]

Type of Central Venous Catheter	Description	Advantages	Disadvantages
Percutaneous non-tunneled catheter	Typically used for short durations (days to weeks) in the acute care setting	• Less costly to place • Easy to remove • Can be exchanged over a guidewire	• High risk of catheter-related infection • Self-care can be difficult • Requires sutures to secure in place • Repair kits not readily available if catheter breaks
Peripherally inserted central catheter (PICC)	A type of percutaneous nontunneled catheter. Venipuncture occurs in a peripheral vein (e.g., basilic, cephalic, or brachial), but the tip is located in the vena cava. Can be used for weeks to months, including short term home PN.	• Low risk of placement-related complications • Can be placed at bedside or radiology suite	• Self-care can be difficult if placed in forearm • Repair kits not readily available • Cannot necessarily be used to sample blood
Tunneled catheter	The venipuncture site is removed from the catheter exit site, theoretically reducing the risk of infection. Appropriate for long-term use (months to years), including home PN.	• Easier for self-care • Dressings and sutures can be removed after 1 month • Repair kits are available	• Requires placement in operating room and a minor surgical procedure for removal
Implanted catheter	A subcutaneous port, usually placed in the chest. The port can be accessed 1000 to 2000 times and is ideal for patients who need infrequent IV therapy. Appropriate for long-term use, including home PN.	• Easier to care for (only requires care when accessed and a monthly heparin flush) • Is discrete, thus preserving body image • Difficult to break • Lowest rates of infection of all central venous access devices	• Requires a needle to access • Must be placed in operating room • Requires surgical procedure for removal

Central PN is usually the preferred form of access because it allows greater flexibility in the types of PN infusions that can be administered.[5] Characteristics of PN formulas that would necessitate central access include the following:

- Hyperosmolarity (≥10% glucose or ≥5% amino acids, or 900 mOsm/L)[7,8]
- High (>9) or low (<5) pH[7]
- Infusions containing vesicant drugs (can cause the vessels to become leaky)[5]

Peripheral Parenteral Nutrition

In peripheral access, the catheter tip is located outside of a central vessel[7] Although central access is ideal, peripheral PN may be selected because it is a safer and easier way to access the vasculature, particularly for short-term use.[5] Peripheral PN is typically used for a maximum of 2 to 6 weeks at a time, as the risk of dislocation and complications (e.g., **phlebitis** or inflammation of the vein) is more common than in central PN and the risk increases as dwell time increases.[5,7] An advantage of peripheral PN is that there is evidence that it is associated with a lower risk of catheter-related infections, but this may be due to the shorter dwell time.[5]

Because peripheral PN infuses into the smaller veins of the extremities, the PN formula cannot be as hypertonic as those formulas used in central PN. Formulas should be of low osmolarity, defined as <900 mOsm/L. There is evidence that formulas of higher osmolarity do not increase the risk of phlebitis in the short term, but these formulas may cause a burning sensation.[7,8]

Indications and Contraindications

When evaluating whether a patient is eligible for PN, consider that PN carries a high risk of serious complications. It is also a costly therapy, due to the expense of vascular access devices, monitoring laboratory values, and treating potential complications.[3] While PN has been shown to improve markers of nutritional status, it does not consistently improve clinical outcomes.[3] PN is only clearly indicated for a narrow range of disease states and circumstances and should not be considered a first line of therapy in nutrition support. For these reasons, the expected benefits of PN therapy should outweigh the risks.

The benefits of enteral feeding are significant and every attempt should be made to trial enteral nutrition (EN) therapy before PN is considered.[3] It has been shown that when compared with PN, EN is associated with reduced risk of infection (e.g., pneumonia and central catheter infections) and reduced length of stay in intensive care unit (ICU) patients.[9] EN promotes blood flow to the gut and the maintenance of tight junctions, thereby preventing the gut from becoming leaky and reducing the risk of systemic infection and stress ulcers. EN is also key in maintaining the gut-associated lymphoid tissue, which is important in regulating the systemic immune response.[9] If EN has been attempted but has failed, PN could then be considered.

Despite the preference for EN from a clinical perspective, there are circumstances in which PN would be indicated:

1. EN has been attempted (including trialing different tube placements) but has failed.[3]
2. EN is contraindicated due to a dysfunctional GI tract. Causes of a dysfunctional GI tract include a paralytic ileus, mesenteric ischemia, small-bowel obstruction, a GI fistula distal to the feeding tube tip, and a GI fistula with outputs of greater than 200 mL/day.[3]

The patient's preference should always be considered. Some patients who are prescribed EN may refuse to have a tube placed and prefer to be fed via the parenteral route.[10] A discussion of the risks and benefits of enteral versus parenteral nutrition should occur so that a patient can make an informed decision.

Determining whether a patient is a candidate for PN requires a thorough nutrition assessment, the first step of the nutrition care process (NCP). If a patient cannot meet their nutritional needs through oral intake or EN alone, and is either at risk of malnutrition or is already malnourished, they may be a candidate for PN.[3] The American Society of Parenteral and Enteral Nutrition (A.S.P.E.N.) defines "nutritional risk" as a Nutrition Risk Screening (NRS) 2002 score of ≥5 or a Nutrition Risk in Critically Ill (NUTRIC) score of ≥5.[9] However, the exact length of time that a patient can remain either NPO or without adequate nutrition before negatively impacting clinical outcome is not clearly defined.[3]

> **Box 4.1**
>
> **Guidelines for PN in Critical Illness**
>
> While PN is clearly indicated when the gut is nonfunctional, indications for PN in critical illness are less well established. Critically ill patients usually experience a catabolic state and systemic inflammation and may experience increased infectious morbidity, multiple organ dysfunction, prolonged hospitalization, and high risk of mortality.[11] Early nutrition support in the form of EN is recommended to reduce disease severity, reduce the risk of complications, and decrease ICU length of stay.[11] Enteral access should be attempted within 24 to 48 hours of ICU admission if the patient cannot maintain oral intake.[11]
>
> There are, however, cases that necessitate PN as a last resort. PN may be indicated for patients in whom enteral access cannot be obtained or EN is not tolerated, although the timing of PN administration depends on nutrition status.[11]

> The 2016 A.S.P.E.N. guidelines on nutrition support of critically ill adults specify that if a patient is at low nutrition risk (e.g., NRS 2002 score of ≤3 or NUTRIC score of ≤5), early PN is associated with minimal benefit or even harm. In these patients, exclusive PN should be withheld for the first 7 days after ICU admission.[11] However, if the patient is at high nutrition risk (e.g., NRS 2002 score of ≥5 or NUTRIC score of ≥5), initiation of PN as soon as possible is associated with improved outcome. Regardless of nutritional risk status, if a patient cannot meet at least 60% of their energy and protein needs through the enteral route, supplemental PN should be considered after 7 to 10 days.[11]

> **Box 4.2**
>
> **Conditions in which PN should be used with caution**
>
> - Hemodynamic instability
> - Hyperglycemia: Glucose >300 mg/dL
> - Azotemia: BUN >100 mg/dL
> - Hyperosmolality: Serum osmolality >350 mOsm/kg
> - Hypernatremia: Na >150 mEq/L
> - Hypokalemia: K <3 mEq/L
> - Hyperchloremic metabolic acidosis: Cl >115 mEq/L
> - Hypophosphatemia: Phos <2 mg/dL
> - Hypochloremic metabolic alkalosis: Cl <85 mEq/L

In addition to assessing tolerance of EN, GI function, and disease state, it is also essential to assess whether the patient could tolerate PN. Patients must meet certain criteria in clinical status, including the ability to tolerate the quantities of fluid, carbohydrate, and protein required. PN should be used with caution in patients with fluid and metabolic imbalances. These conditions are outlined in Box 4.2.[3]

PRACTICE POINT

Severe hyperglycemia, azotemia, encephalopathy, and hyperosmolality, along with severe fluid and electrolyte imbalances, are associated with poor tolerance of any type of nutrition support, whether it be EN or PN. These abnormalities should be corrected prior to starting nutrition support therapy.[3]

⚠ Clinical Controversy

Early versus Late Parenteral Nutrition

A.S.P.E.N. currently recommends delaying administration of PN for 7 to 10 days in critically ill adult patients where enteral nutrition is not feasible, unless they are severely malnourished or at high nutritional risk. Similarly, their recommendations state that in both low- and high-risk patients who are unable to meet greater than 60% of their goal by EN, supplemental PN should be delayed 7 to 10 days. These guidelines are based on evidence that despite an increase in energy and protein intake, there is a lack of clinical benefit associated with early parenteral supplementation. Studies such as that by Heyland confirm the risk of PN use by demonstrating increased infection rates and intensive care unit length of stay as well as cost.

However studies have shown that PN can be used safely. In their study, Doig and colleagues demonstrated that PN use can be safe and also decrease number of days on ventilation, although length of intensive care and hospital stay were not improved. When providing nutrition support therapy, critical review of a patient's nutritional risk and status as well as clinical condition must accompany guidelines for PN use, particularly given that evidence does exist to support a benefit.

Based on the two studies referenced, provide how you might apply evidence-based findings and professional guidelines when providing nutrition support, and when you might determine that early supplemental PN may be indicated. What are the strengths and weaknesses of each study in terms of their design and rigor? How might study population or clinical status impact your conclusion based on these studies?

References

1. Doig GS, Simpson F; Early PN Trial Investigators Group. Early parenteral nutrition in critically ill patients with short term relative contraindications to early enteral nutrition. *JAMA*. 2013;309(20):2130-2138.

2. Heyland DK. Early supplemental parenteral nutrition in critically ill adults increased infections, ICU length of stay and cost. *Evid Based Med*. 2012;17(3):86-87.

If PN is to be used, the next step is determining the venous access site and type of venous access device. Central PN is appropriate when PN is required for longer term use (>2 weeks), peripheral venous access is inadequate, the patient has significant nutrient needs, or the patient is fluid restricted.[3] Peripheral PN may be considered if nutrition support is only needed for a short time frame (up to 2 weeks) if the patient is not a candidate for central PN.[3] Peripheral PN can provide partial or total nutrition, but because the peripheral PN solution is less concentrated, a higher volume must be administered to provide total nutrition. For this reason, a patient who requires fluid restriction (e.g., due to renal disease) would not be a candidate for peripheral PN.[3] In general, patients receiving peripheral PN should be able to tolerate 2 L to 3 L of fluid per day.

■ CORE CONCEPT 3

Candidates for parenteral nutrition must be fully evaluated for nutritional risk and nutritional status with adherence to standardized protocols for initiation of parenteral nutrition.

Parenteral Nutrition Formulation

Although there are standard PN formulas, PN solutions in the inpatient setting may be compounded daily and are customizable to the individual needs of the patient (**Figure 4.8**).

The components that can be included in the solution are carbohydrate, amino acids, lipids, vitamins, electrolytes, trace minerals, and a number of other specific additives.

Given in the appropriate amounts, the intravenous administration of these components can maintain nutrition status and support life-long term without use of the gastrointestinal tract.

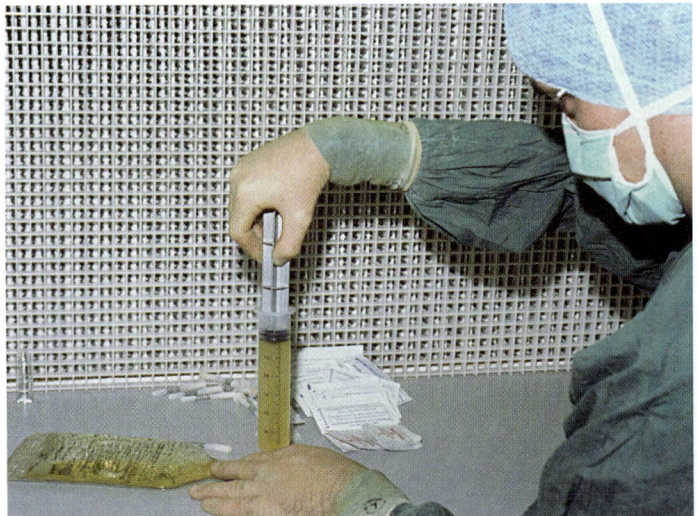

FIGURE 4.8 Sterile Preparation of Parenteral Nutrition Formula
© Eamonn McNulty/Science Source.

■ CORE CONCEPT 4

Parenteral nutrition is a hypertonic solution made up of, but not limited to, carbohydrate in the form of dextrose, crystalline amino acids, lipid emulsions, vitamins, minerals, and sterile water.

Carbohydrate

As the primary energy source for the body, the carbohydrate component of PN is critical. It is especially important during times of metabolic stress, when proteins can be catabolized as an energy source at an increased rate, causing negative nitrogen balance.[12] Carbohydrate should always be included in PN because of its protein-sparing effect.[13]

The most commonly used carbohydrate substrate used in PN formulas is dextrose monohydrate, the dextrorotatory form of glucose. In its hydrated form, dextrose provides 3.4 kcal per gram, not 4 kcal per gram like dietary carbohydrates.[1,14]

Commercially, dextrose is available in multiple concentrations ranging from 5% to 70%.[1] Because dextrose is an acidic molecule, the higher concentration solutions are more acidic. According to the United States Pharmacopoeia (USP), dextrose solutions range from pH 3.5 to 6.5. Dextrose solutions greater than 10% concentration are typically reserved for central venous administration because the hypertonicity and acidity of the solution has the potential to cause thrombophlebitis in peripheral veins.[14]

Dextrose infusion can be challenging due to its effect on blood sugar. Infusing dextrose directly into the bloodstream directly raises serum glucose, which commonly leads to hyperglycemia.[1] Appropriate monitoring of serum glucose and intervention of highs and lows beyond acceptable limits must be implemented to avoid more serious complications.

The most common dextrose solution used in parenteral nutrition is 50% dextrose in water (D50W). This concentration supplies 500 grams of dextrose per liter and 1700 kcal per liter. The mathematical process used to equate the grams of dextrose supplied per liter and the calories supplied per liter is shown as follows:

$$50\% \text{ dextrose} = \frac{50 \text{ grams dextrose}}{100 \text{ mL}} \times \frac{1000 \text{ mL}}{\text{L}}$$

$$= \frac{500 \text{ grams dextrose}}{\text{L}} \times 3.4 \frac{\text{kcal}}{\text{grams dextrose}}$$

$$= 1700 \text{ kcal}$$

In fluid-restricted patients, more concentrated PN is indicated. A more-concentrated dextrose solution like D60W or D70W is often used in compounding because less volume is required to meet carbohydrate requirements.[14] As an example, if a patient had a daily carbohydrate requirement of 400 grams, the PN formula would require 800 mL of D50W to meet that requirement. In contrast, the PN formula would only require 571 mL of D70W to meet the daily requirement of 400 grams of carbohydrate. This difference of 229 mL could be significant in a fluid-restricted patient.

How many mL of 70% dextrose is needed to provide 400 g dextrose?

$$70\% \text{ dextrose} = \frac{70 \text{ grams dextrose}}{100 \text{ mL}} \times \frac{1000 \text{ mL}}{\text{L}}$$

$$\frac{700 \text{ grams dextrose}}{1000 \text{ mL}} = \frac{400 \text{ grams}}{x \text{ mL}}$$

$$x = 571 \text{ mL}$$

Table 4.2 shows different dextrose solutions available for use in parenteral nutrition, grams of dextrose per liter, kcal per liter, and peripheral versus central access requirement.

Amino Acids

A variety of illnesses and catabolic conditions can disturb the blood amino acid profile, promote a decrease in lean

TABLE 4.2 DEXTROSE SOLUTIONS

Solution	Grams of Dextrose per Liter (g/L)	Kilocalories per Liter (Kcal/L)	Peripheral versus Central Administration
5% dextrose in water (D5W)	50	170	Peripheral or central
10% dextrose in water (D10W)	100	340	Peripheral or central
20% dextrose in water (D20W)	200	680	Central
30% dextrose in water (D30W)	300	1020	Central
40% dextrose in water (D40W)	400	1360	Central
50% dextrose in water (D50W)	500	1700	Central
60% dextrose in water (D60W)	600	2040	Central
70% dextrose in water (D70W)	700	2380	Central

body mass, and increase body protein requirements. Mixed amino acid formulations that provide both essential and nonessential amino acids are a standard component of complete PN prescriptions to support cell, organ, skeletal, and cardiac, and respiratory muscle functions, as well as wound healing.[15]

Amino acids are supplied through PN in their crystalline form. If oxidized for energy, crystalline amino acids supply 4 kcal per gram. As with other PN components, amino acid solutions are available in different concentrations ranging from 3% to 20%.[14] All commercially available amino acid solutions for PN contain all nine essential amino acids in varying amounts between 38% and 57% of total amino acids. Standard solutions also provide some nonessential amino acids at about 43% to 62% of total amino acids. Nitrogen content varies depending on the concentration of the solution and the amino acid profile.[15]

Specialty amino acid formulations are commercially available for use in certain disease states like renal failure, hepatic encephalopathy, metabolic stress, trauma, thermal injury, and hypercatabolic states. These products are generally more costly than standard formulas and should only be used in patients who meet the intended indications and who are expected to benefit clinically from the specialty amino acid formula.[14] A.S.P.E.N. has published guidelines for the use of these products in clinical practice.[16] **Table 4.3**

TABLE 4.3 COMMERCIALLY AVAILABLE CRYSTALLINE AMINO ACID SOLUTIONS

Brand Name, Manufacturer	Type/Indication	Stock Concentrations	Composition
Travasol, Baxter	Standard	3.5%, 4.25%, 5.5%, 8.5%, 10%	Essential amino acids + alanine, glycine, arginine, proline, serine, and tyrosine[15]
Clinisol, Baxter	Standard/fluid restriction	15%	Essential amino acids + alanine, glycine, arginine, proline, glutamic acid, serine, aspartic acid, and tyrosine[17]
ProSol, Baxter	Standard/fluid restriction	20%	Essential amino acids + alanine, glycine, arginine, proline, glutamic acid, serine, aspartic acid, and tyrosine[15]
Aminosyn II, Abbott	Standard	3.5%, 4.25%, 5%, 7%, 8.5%, 10%, 15%	Essential amino acids + alanine, glycine, arginine, proline, glutamic acid, serine, aspartic acid, tyrosine, and histidine[18]
FreAmine III, B.Braun	Standard	8.5%, 10%	Essential amino acids + alanine, glycine, arginine, proline, serine, histidine, and cysteine[19]
HepatAmine, B.Braun	Hepatic failure	8%	Essential amino acids + alanine, glycine, arginine, proline, serine, and histidine[19]
Hepatasol, Baxter	Hepatic failure	8%	Essential amino acids + alanine, glycine, arginine, proline, serine, histidine, and cysteine[17]
FreAmine HBC, B.Braun	Metabolic stress	6.9%	Essential amino acids + alanine, glycine, arginine, proline, serine, and histidine[19]
Aminosyn HBC, Abbott	Metabolic stress	7%	Essential amino acids + alanine, glycine, arginine, proline, serine, tyrosine, and histidine[19]
BranchAmin, Baxter	Metabolic stress	4%	Contains branched chain amino acids only (leucine, isoleucine, and valine)[14]
NephrAmine, B.Braun	Renal failure	5.4%	Contains essential amino acids only[14]
Aminosyn RF, Abbott	Renal failure	5.2%	Contains essential amino acids + arginine[14]
TrophAmine, B.Braun	Infants and young children	6%, 10%	Essential amino acids + alanine, glycine, arginine, proline, glutamic acid, serine, aspartic acid, tyrosine, taurine, and cysteine[15]

provides more information on some of the standard and specialty crystalline amino acid solutions available for use in PN.

Lipids

Energy deficit is a common and serious problem in intensive care unit patients and is associated with increased rates of complications, length of stay, and mortality.[20]

The infusion of lipid injectable emulsions (ILEs) provides a high energy supply, contributes to the prevention of high glucose infusion rates, and is indispensable for supplying the body with essential fatty acids (EFAs).[21]

In the United States, ILE components include an oil source, egg yolk phospholipid as an emulsifier, glycerin to render the formulation isotonic, and sodium hydroxide to adjust the final pH to a range of 6 to 9 (**Table 4.4**). Historically, the most common oil sources used in ILEs have been soybean oil and safflower oil, which contain long chain triglycerides (LCTs).[14] These oils were used because they are relatively inexpensive, abundant on the market, and effectively deliver nonglucose energy to the body. A disadvantage of soybean and safflower oils is their high levels of omega-6 fatty acid and low levels of omega-3 fatty acid, a ratio that is known to promote systemic inflammation. In an effort to address concerns associated with the soybean oil–based lipid emulsions, alternative sources of fatty acids were and continue to be investigated.[20]

In 2016, the Food and Drug Administration approved SMOFlipid™, which is comprised of four different oils: 30% soybean, 30% medium-chain triglycerides derived from coconut oil, 25% olive oil, and 15% fish oil. SMOFlipid, and others like it, have an improved omega-3:omega-6 ratio that may reduce the risk of harmful changes to the liver, such as **parenteral nutrition associated liver disease (PNALD)** and **hepatic steatosis**, and may preserve antioxidant capacity in critically ill patients. Ideally, this can contribute to better health outcomes such as shorter ICU stays.[22]

ILEs are commercially available in 10% (1.1 kcal per milliliter), 20% (2 kcal per milliliter), and 30% concentrations (2.9 to 3 kcal per milliliter, depending on the manufacturer); however, 30% ILE is not approved for direct intravenous administration. This high concentration is only approved for the compounding of a **total nutrient admixture** (TNA).

A 3 in 1 TNA is a PN formulation that contains 3 macronutrients (dextrose, amino acids, and lipid) in one solution. In addition, PN can be prepared as a 2 in 1 formulation containing 2 macronutrients (dextrose and amino acids) in one solution. When ILEs are infused as separate preparations from dextrose and amino acids as with a 2 in 1 formulation, there is enhanced microbial growth potential because the pH of the lipid emulsion is biologically compatible with bacteria. For this reason, the Centers for Disease Control and Prevention recommends a 12-hour hang time limit for ILE.[23] In contrast, a 3 in 1 TNA containing dextrose, amino acids, and ILE in the same container may be administered over 24 hours because the solution has a pH of 5.6 to 6, which is more likely to inhibit bacterial growth, and the increased total osmolarity with the combination of all three substrates in one container delays/inhibits microbial growth.[14,23]

In practice, lipid is not always given in PN. Although institutions may have their own criteria, it is common to hold lipid when a patient is receiving propofol, which is a short-acting hypnotic sedative provided in a 10% lipid emulsion. Lipids should also be withheld in patients who have an egg or soy allergy, or when they have hypertriglyceridemia prior to the initiation of lipid. According to A.S.P.E.N. guidelines, soybean oil–based ILE should be withheld from or limited in critically ill patients during the first week following initiation of parenteral nutrition to a maximum of 100 grams per week if there is concern for essential fatty acid deficiency. This provision is often divided into two doses of 50 grams or less per week. Alternative ILEs like SMOFlipid may provide outcome benefit over soy-based ILEs.[11]

TABLE 4.4 COMPOSITION OF PARENTERAL LIPID EMULSIONS

ILE, Manufacturer	Soybean Oil (%)	Safflower Oil (%)	Coconut Oil (%)	Olive Oil (%)	Fish Oil (%)
Intralipid, Fresenius Kabi	100	0	0	0	0
Liposyn II, Hospira	50	50	0	0	0
Lipofundin, B. Braun	50	0	50	0	0
SMOF Lipid™, Fresenius Kabi	30	0	30	25	15
ClinOleic, Baxter	20	0	0	80	0
Omegaven, Fresenius Kabi	0	0	0	0	100

> **CORE CONCEPT 5**
>
> Many lipid emulsions are composed of primarily omega-6 fatty acids and should be provided judiciously given their role in inflammation.

> **PRACTICE POINT**
>
> Most intravenous lipid emulsions contain egg yolk phospholipids as an emulsifying agent and soybean oil as the primary lipid source. For this reason, egg and soy allergies are contraindications of intravenous lipid infusion.

Electrolytes

Parenteral solutions represent a significant portion, if not all, of total daily fluid and electrolyte intake.[1] Maintenance or therapeutic amounts of various electrolytes are added to PN formulations depending on the patient's individual requirements. Acetate and chloride do not have specific ranges for intake; rather, they are adjusted as needed to maintain acid–base balance.[24] Other electrolytes are available in various salt forms as outlined in **Table 4.5**. For administration in PN, calcium gluconate and magnesium sulfate are the preferred forms of these electrolytes compared to calcium chloride, calcium glucaptate, and magnesium chloride because they are less likely to produce **physicochemical incompatibilities**, which are physical or chemical changes that can occur in PN leading to precipitation, color changes, or chemical degradation that can compromise the solution.[14]

> **PRACTICE POINT**
>
> Parenteral nutrition formulas that are high in amino acids can contribute to an increase in blood pH. To balance this effect, electrolytes in this situation can be provided as acetate.

Electrolytes are commercially available as individual salts and as combination products for ease in admixing. They are also pre-added to certain stock amino acid solutions or premixed PN formulations.[14]

Multivitamins

In addition to macronutrients and electrolytes, patients receiving PN require vitamins to prevent deficiency and promote optimal health. Clinical practice guidelines include the justification, dosage, and the route of delivery for inclusion of vitamins in patients receiving PN. Guideline adherence ensures optimum nutrition care and improves patient outcomes.

Commercially available vitamin products for parenteral nutrition supplementation include both single and multivitamin infusion products. In 2000, the Food and Drug Administration issued parenteral multivitamin dosing requirements.[14] In accordance with these requirements, parenteral multivitamins include vitamin A, vitamin D, vitamin E, vitamin K, vitamin B1, vitamin B2, vitamin B6, vitamin B12, niacin, folic acid, pantothenic acid, biotin, and vitamin C. One parenteral multivitamin product is available without vitamin K for patients on warfarin anticoagulant therapy.[25] Composition of the standard parenteral multivitamin products available in the United States is included in **Table 4.6**.

Single vitamins are used when a patient requires more of a vitamin than a parenteral multivitamin provides. Currently, there are no single vitamin products available for biotin, pantothenic acid, riboflavin, vitamin A, vitamin D, or vitamin E.[14]

Trace Elements

The need for trace elements in long-term parenteral nutrition was realized when patients began to develop deficiency symptoms that were alleviated through trace element supplementation. Some of the deficiencies that developed were copper, zinc, manganese, selenium, chromium, and molybdenum.[27] Of these, copper, zinc, manganese, selenium, and chromium are the most commonly supplemented trace elements in PN formulations. These trace minerals are available in both individual form and various trace element combinations at concentrations safe for use in neonates, pediatrics, and adults.[14] The American Medical Association and A.S.P.E.N. have published recommendations for daily parenteral dose of selenium, zinc, copper, manganese, and chromium, as seen in **Table 4.7**.

Other trace elements that are less commonly used in PN but are still available are molybdenum, iodine, and iron. Iron dextran is the only iron product approved for addition to PN. This product should only be added to 2 in 1 dextrose-amino acid formulations as opposed to PN formulas that contain lipid, like a 3 in 1 TNA, because ILEs are disrupted by iron.[14] If iron dextran is administered, strict protocol should be followed and the patient should be closely monitored as anaphylaxis is a potential side effect.[28] Nonetheless, iron is still an essential part of most long-term PN regimens and necessary in order to prevent deficiency.[29]

TABLE 4.5 COMMERCIALLY AVAILABLE PARENTERAL ELECTROLYTE SALTS

	Chloride	Acetate	Phosphate	Sulfate	Gluconate	Gluceptate
Sodium	X	X	X	–	–	–
Potassium	X	X	X	–	–	–
Calcium	X	–	–	–	X	X
Magnesium	X	–	–	X	–	–

TABLE 4.6 COMPOSITION OF ADULT PARENTERAL MULTIVITAMIN PRODUCTS AVAILABLE IN THE UNITED STATES[1,26]

Vitamin/Mineral	FDA requirement	MVI-12	MVI-13
Vitamin C (ascorbic acid)	200 mg	200 mg	200 mg
Niacin (niacinamide)	40 mg	40 mg	40 mg
Pantothenic acid (dexpanthenol)	15 mg	15 mg	15 mg
Vitamin E (dl-α-Tocopherol acetate)	10 mg (10 USP units)	10 mg (10 USP units)	10 mg (10 USP units)
Vitamin B6 (pyridoxine)	6 mg	6 mg	6 mg
Vitamin B1 (thiamin)	6 mg	6 mg	6 mg
Vitamin B2 (riboflavin)	3.6 mg	3.6 mg	3.6 mg
Vitamin A (retinol)	1 mg (3300 USP units)	1 mg (3300 USP units)	1 mg (3300 USP units)
Folic acid	600 mcg	600 mcg	600 mcg
Vitamin K (phylloquinone)	150 mcg	0	150 mcg
Biotin	60 mcg	60 mcg	60 mcg
Vitamin D (ergocalciferol)	5 mcg (200 USP units)	5 mcg (200 USP units)	5 mcg (200 USP units)
Vitamin B12 (cyanocobalamin)	5 mcg	5 mcg	5 mcg

TABLE 4.7 TRACE ELEMENT DEFICIENCIES ASSOCIATED WITH LONG-TERM PARENTERAL NUTRITION[24,27]

Deficiency	Symptoms	A.S.P.E.N. Recommendation
Copper	- Sensory ataxia - Lower extremity spasticity - Paresthesias in extremities - Hypochromic microcytic anemia - Leukopenia - Neutropenia - Hypercholesterolemia - Decreased ceruloplasmin and erythrocyte Cu/Zn - Increased erythrocyte turnover - Abnormal electrocardiographic patterns - Myeloneuropathy	0.3-0.5 mg/day
Zinc	- Inadequate growth - Acrodermatitis - Hypogonadism - Impaired night vision	2.5-5 mg/day

(continues)

TABLE 4.7 TRACE ELEMENT DEFICIENCIES ASSOCIATED WITH LONG-TERM PARENTERAL NUTRITION[24,27] *(Continued)*

Deficiency	Symptoms	A.S.P.E.N. Recommendation
Zinc (continued)	• Anorexia • Diarrhea • Alterations in taste and smell • Alopecia • Impaired epithelialization and wound healing • Impaired immune function	
Manganese	• Poor reproductive performance • Congenital abnormalities in offspring • Abnormal bone/cartilage formation • Ataxia • Growth retardation • Defects in lipid/carbohydrate metabolism	60-100 mcg/day
Selenium	• Oxidative injury • Increased susceptibility to mercury poisoning • Altered thyroid hormone metabolism • Increased plasma glutathione levels • Keshan disease	20-60 mcg/day
Chromium	• Weight loss • Hyperglycemia refractory to insulin • Glycosuria • Elevated plasma free fatty acids • Peripheral neuropathy • Hyperlipidemia	10-15 mcg/day
Molybdenum	• Tachycardia • Tachypnea • Visual/mental changes • Elevated methionine • Headache • Lethargy • Nausea • Vomiting	
Iron	• Microcytic hypochromic anemia • Tachycardia • Poor capillary refilling • Fatigue • Sleepiness • Headache • Anorexia • Nausea • Pallor • Impaired ability to maintain body temperature in cold environments • Increased lead absorption • Koilonychia • Glossitis	

Other Additives

Insulin

The development of hyperglycemia during inpatient parenteral nutrition therapy has been independently associated with higher rates of mortality and hospital complications. These observations indicate that prevention and correction of hyperglycemia through modification of nutrient composition or by insulin administration should be strongly considered during PN therapy.[30] Insulin can be administered through sliding scale coverage, subcutaneous injection of long-acting insulin, an intravenous insulin infusion, insulin mixed into the PN formula, or any combination of these. The most common initial regimen for insulin in PN is 1 unit of regular insulin per 10 grams of dextrose. In hyperglycemic patients (glucose >150 mg/dL), the regimen may increase to 1.5 units of regular insulin per 10 grams of dextrose.[31] It is critical to use hospital- or unit-specific protocols for insulin infusions that include careful monitoring blood glucose to allow for proper intervention of both high and low levels.

Medications

Addition of certain medications into PN solutions is generally not advised due to potential for the formation of precipitates, adverse reactions, and disturbances in acid–base balance.[14,31] Medication compatibility with PN often depends on the hydrophilicity or hydrophobicity of the drug/medication and the formulation of the PN solution. Lipid-based (hydrophobic) medications are more likely to be compatible with ILE or

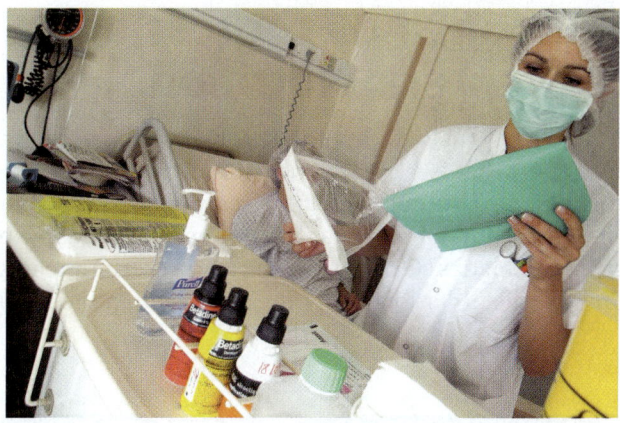

FIGURE 4.9 Clinician Preparing to Infuse Patient with Parenteral Nutrition
© Look at Sciences/Science Source.

TNA, while water-based medications (hydrophilic) are more likely to be compatible with a 2 in 1 dextrose-amino acid solutions.[14] Under current practice standards, pharmacists can admix certain medications into PN solutions; however, medication should never be added after the solution leaves the pharmacy or compounding center (**Figure 4.9**).[32]

> **PRACTICE POINT**
>
> When in doubt about compatibility or safety of a medication or parenteral nutrition additive, seek evidence in existing literature and contact the pharmacist responsible for admixing parenteral solutions at your institution.

Clinical Roundtable

Topic: PN Component Shortages: An Ethical Challenge

Background: PN component shortages have been consistently impacting hospitals and home infusion companies since spring 2010.[33] Since then, every parenteral nutrition component has been in short supply, including ILE, amino acids, vitamins, electrolyte additives, and sterile water.[34] Shortages arise due to issues in the manufacturing process. Because producing PN components and other drugs is a highly controlled process for safety and sterility, there are a limited number of production lines that can meet these requirements. When a problem arises at one of these locations, pharmaceutical companies are responsible for notifying the Food and Drug Administration if a decrease in supply is projected.

Currently, there is no mandatory timeframe to resolve the manufacturing issue. Because the PN drug market is not a particularly profitable one, there is little incentive for pharmaceutical companies to resolve shortages quickly.[35] These shortages pose a significant risk for patients who rely on PN as their sole source of nutrition. If a component is in short supply, clinicians are forced to administer a lower dose, prioritize which patients receive the component, or omit the component entirely. Various deficiencies have been reported as a result of this ongoing issue.[34]

In response to ongoing drug shortages, A.S.P.E.N. created the Parenteral Nutrition Product Shortage Committee as a subcommittee of the Clinical Practice Committee. This group continually disseminates information on current and expected component and drug shortages.[34] They have also developed and published a set of recommendations for managing shortages. The recommendations provide strategies for rationing and conserving products so that drugs and PN components are available for the most critical patients.[33-35]

Roundtable Discussion

Consider a scenario in which there was a PN component shortage at your institution.

1. How would you prioritize which patients would continue to receive PN and which patients would not?
2. What strategies could you use to ensure that as many patients as possible receive adequate nutrition despite the shortage?

Initiation and Progression of Parenteral Nutrition

As stated previously in this chapter, PN is a type of nutrition support that is typically individualized to the needs of the patient. This customization requires knowledge of each of the component parts that compose PN and use of basic mathematics. Calculating the PN prescription and filling out the order form appropriately is often the most intimidating aspect of PN for clinical trainees and novice clinicians. **Table 4.8** provides a commonly used method to calculate a PN prescription. An example of this method is provided in **Table 4.9**.

> **CORE CONCEPT 6**
>
> Prescription of parenteral nutrition is based on energy and protein requirements with consideration of fluid specifications and substrate utilization of macronutrients.

TABLE 4.8 PARENTERAL NUTRITION FORMULA CALCULATION METHOD

For steps where there is more than one way to determine needs, the most commonly used formulas are highlighted in gray.

Determine energy requirements	• Use the standard method utilized by your institution including but not limited to:
	  – Indirect calorimetry
	  – Harris–Benedict equation
	  – Mifflin–St. Jeor predictive equation
	  – Penn State predictive equation
	  – Estimation using kcal/kg

Determine protein requirements and calories from protein	Protein stress factor based on disease state or severity of disease $\times$ weight in kg = protein requirement (grams) $\text{protein (gram)} \times 4 \, \frac{\text{kcal}}{\text{gram}} = \text{kcal from protein}$

Determine ILE requirements	Does the patient need to receive lipids?
	No:
	  – If patient is receiving propofol **or**
	  – If patient has hypertriglyceridemia (TG >300 mg/dL) **or**
	  – If patient has egg or soy allergy **or**
	  – If the patient is critically ill and has received PN for fewer than 7 days
	Yes:
	If above conditions do not apply and/or if the patient has essential fatty acid deficiency
	If yes:
	total energy requirement (kcal) $\times$ x% energy from lipid = lipid requirement (kcal)
	*energy from lipid is typically 30% or less and should not exceed 60% kcal from lipid

Calculate kcal remaining for dextrose	Total energy requirement − [(protein kcal) + (lipid kcal)] = dextrose kcal protein kcal = grams protein $\times$ 4 kcals/gram protein
Calculate grams of dextrose	$\text{Dextrose (kcal)} \div 3.4 \, \frac{\text{kcal}}{\text{gram}} = \text{dextrose (g)}$
Determine desired total volume	Is the patient fluid restricted? If yes: Aim for 1 L volume of PN or less per day If no: Use predictive equation for fluid, typical PN volumes are 1.2 to 2 per day: $\text{X fluid} \left(\frac{\text{mL}}{\text{kg}}\right) \times \text{weight (kg)} = \text{fluid requirement (mL)}$

Chapter 4 Parenteral Nutrition Therapy

TABLE 4.8 PARENTERAL NUTRITION FORMULA CALCULATION METHOD (Continued)

	x is the factor being used to calculate fluid. Typical factors for maintenance fluid needs are listed below: If fluid losses are expected or the nutrition care plan includes home PN, be sure to provide at least maintenance fluid needs. • Young adults: 35 mL/kg body weight • Adults: 30 mL/kg body weight • Older Adults: 25 mL/kg body weight
Calculate component concentration/ volume	Protein (concentration): protein requirement (g) ÷ desired volume of parental nutrition (mL) × 1000 $\frac{mL}{L}$ = concentration of amino acid solution $\frac{grams\ AA}{L}$ grams AA/L ÷ 100 → percent AA% Round to the nearest available amino acid concentration Lipid (volume and gram): lipid requirement (kcal) ÷ ILE concentration $\frac{kcal}{mL}$ = lipid requirement (mL) lipid volume (mL) × ILE concentration $\frac{kcal}{mL}$ × $\frac{1g\ ILE}{10\ kcal}$ = lipid grams (g) ILE volume is considered anhydrous and some may prefer to exclude ILE volume from total fluid volume when providing maintenance fluid requirements. Dextrose (concentration): dextrose requirement (g) ÷ desired volume of parental nutrition (mL) × 1000 $\frac{mL}{L}$ = concentration of dextrose solution $\frac{grams}{L}$ grams dextrose/L ÷ 100 → percent dextrose% Round to the nearest available dextrose concentration
Determine goal rate	Total volume (mL) ÷ 24 $\frac{hours}{day}$ = goal rate $\frac{mL}{hour}$
Final answer	The PN prescription can be ordered per day or per liter. Per day: Total grams of dextrose per day, total grams of amino acids per day, and total grams of lipid per day = _____ kcal/day, _____ g protein/day Per liter: D(percent concentration of dextrose)AA(percent concentration of amino acid) with (concentration of ILE) ILE at (goal rate) mL/hour = _____ kcal/day, _____ grams protein/day

TABLE 4.9 PARENTERAL NUTRITION FORMULA CALCULATION METHOD: A SAMPLE CALCULATION

40-year-old male
178 cm, 91 kg
Trauma, hypermetabolic, intubated, sedated, 8 days NPO
All labs within normal limits
Propofol: 20 mL/hour, Maintenance fluid requirement: 114 mL/hour
The hospital utilizes 2 in 1 PN formulations and 20% ILE

Determine energy requirements	Penn State Equation = 2650 kcal per day
Determine protein requirements and calories from protein	Protein stress factor based on disease state or severity of illness × weight in kg = protein requirement $\frac{g}{kg}$ $$\left(1.4 \frac{g}{kg}\right) \times 91 \text{ kg} = 127 \text{ grams protein/day}$$ Protein requirement = 127 grams per day $$127 \text{ Protein (gram)} \times 4 \frac{kcal}{gram} = 508 \text{ kcal from Protein}$$
Determine ILE requirements	Does the patient need to receive IV lipids? No: <ul><li>If patient is receiving propofol **or**</li><li>If patient has hypertriglyceridemia (TG >300 mg/dL) **or**</li><li>If patient has egg or soy allergy **or**</li><li>If the patient is critically ill and has received PN for fewer than 7 days</li></ul> Yes: If above conditions do not apply and/or if the patient has essential fatty acid deficiency No, the patient is receiving propofol at 20 mL/hour. To calculate calories from propofol which is based in 10% ILE: $$20 \frac{mL}{hr} \times 24 \frac{hours}{day} = 480 \frac{mL}{day}$$ $$480 \text{ mL} \times 1.1 \frac{kcal}{mL} = 528 \text{ kcal}$$ This is supplying the patient with 528 kcal/day from lipid. If the patient was not receiving propofol, triglycerides were within normal limits, and his goal was set at 20% of total calories, his requirement would be 530 kcal. This is calculated with the following equation: $$\text{total energy requirement (kcal)} \times x\% \text{ energy from lipid} = \text{lipid requirement (kcal)}$$ $$2650 \text{ kcal} \times 20\% \text{ energy from lipid} = 530 \text{ (kcal)}$$ After 14 days of NPO status, if no other lipid source provided, the patient should be given essential fatty acids at a minimum of 2% to 4% of total kcals to prevent essential fatty acid deficiency.
Calculate kcal remaining for dextrose	Total energy requirement (kcal) − (protein (kcal) + lipid (kcal)) = dextrose (kcal) 2650 kcal − (508 kcal + 528 kcal) = 1614 kcal Kcal remaining for dextrose = 1614
Calculate grams of dextrose	$$\text{Dextrose (kcal)} \div 3.4 \frac{kcal}{gram} = \text{dextrose (g)}$$ $$1614 \text{ kcal} \div 3.4 \frac{kcal}{gram} = 475 \text{ grams}$$ 475 grams of dextrose/day

TABLE 4.9 PARENTERAL NUTRITION FORMULA CALCULATION METHOD: A SAMPLE CALCULATION *(Continued)*

Determine desired total volume	X fluid $\left(\frac{mL}{kg}\right) \times$ weight (kg) = fluid requirement (mL) $30 \left(\frac{mL}{kg}\right) \times 91$ (kg) = 2730 mL/day This patient is not on a fluid restriction, so the predictive equation for adults was used. The desired volume of both the patient's maintenance fluid and parenteral nutrition is 2730 mL per day.
Calculate component concentrations/volume	Protein (concentration): (Protein requirement (g) ÷ desired volume of parental nutrition (mL)) × 1000 $\frac{mL}{L}$ = concentration of amino acid solution $\frac{grams}{L}$ (127 (g) ÷ 2730 (mL)) × 1000 = 46.5 g/L → 4.7% amino acid (rounded) Lipid (volume): No ILE required. Sufficient lipid coming from propofol at 20 mL/hour. If the patient was not receiving propofol and required 530 kcal from ILE, the volume of 20% ILE needed to meet his lipid requirement would be calculated as follows: 530 kcal ÷ 2 $\frac{kcal}{mL\ ILE}$ = 265 mL ILE at 20% concentration 265 mL × 2 $\frac{kcal}{mL} \times \frac{1g\ ILE}{10\ kcal}$ = 53 g lipid Dextrose (concentration): (dextrose requirement (g) ÷ desired volume of parental nutrition (mL)) × 1000 $\frac{mL}{L}$ = concentration of dextrose solution $\frac{grams}{L}$ (475 (g) ÷ 2730 (mL)) × 1000 = 174 $\frac{g}{L}$ = 17.4% → 17% dextrose (rounded)
Determine goal rate	total volume (mL) ÷ 24 $\frac{hours}{day}$ = goal rate $\frac{mL}{hour}$ 2730 (mL) ÷ 24 $\frac{hours}{day}$ = 114 $\frac{mL}{hour}$
Final answer	Per day: 475 g dextrose/day, 127 g AA/day with propofol at 20 ml/hr = 2603 kcal/day, 127 grams protein/day Per liter: D17AA4.7 at 114 mL/hour with propofol at 20 mL/hour = 2623 kcal/day, 129 g protein/day Note that when ordering per liter, numbers tend to be rounded leading to slight difference in calculated calories and protein.

Safety Check of Macronutrient Infusion Rates

Due to risk for complications, there are maximum infusion rates set for both lipid and carbohydrate. The maximum lipid infusion rate is 1.7 mg/kg/min, the maximum rate of lipid oxidation.[21]

The maximum glucose infusion rate, also based on glucose oxidation rate in metabolically stressed adult patients, is 5 mg/kg/min.[36]

In order to calculate the glucose infusion rate, convert carbohydrate requirement in grams to milligrams by multiplying by 1000. Then, divide the requirement in milligrams by the weight of the patient in kilograms. Lastly, divide this number by 1440 minutes per day to give the infusion rate of milligrams per kilogram of body weight per minute (**Table 4.10**). If the glucose infusion rate is calculated to be greater than the maximum infusion rate, it is highly recommended that the PN formula be adjusted.

CORE CONCEPT 7

Carbohydrate infusion from parenteral nutrition should not exceed 5 mg/kg/min in adults and children over the age of 2 years.

Electrolyte Requirements

It is common that electrolytes are ordered in milliequivalents instead of milliliters in PN solutions. The standard daily electrolyte requirements in milliequivalents are listed in **Table 4.11**, although electrolyte levels should be monitored regularly and adjusted as needed. Each component of PN solution contributes to its osmolarity, which ultimately determines into which type of vein (central versus peripheral) the solution can be infused. Refer to **Table 4.12** for the method to calculate osmolarity.

Vitamin and Trace Element Requirements

Typically, the adult dose of multivitamin given per day is 10 mL. If a patient has needs beyond what is provided in MVI-12 or MVI-13, additional may be provided in single-vitamin form. This may add to the total volume of parenteral nutrition provided.[14]

The standard adult dose of the multiple trace elements solution given per day is 5 mL.

When the parenteral nutrition prescription is complete and safety checks have been made in regard to safe infusion rates, an order form must be completed and provided to the pharmacy. Most institutions have their own standard PN order form. It is crucial that the information input into the order form is specific and easily understood so that the formulation is made correctly.

CORE CONCEPT 8

Parenteral nutrition formulations are customizable to the specific needs of each patient or patient population.

TABLE 4.10 CALCULATING GLUCOSE INFUSION RATE

$$\text{Carbohydrate requirement (g)} \times 1000 \frac{mg}{g} = \text{requirement (mg)}$$

$$\text{requirement (mg)} \div \text{weight (kg)} = \text{infusion} \frac{mg}{kg\ body\ weight}$$

$$\text{infusion} \frac{mg}{kg\ body\ weight} \div 1440 \frac{minute}{day} = \text{infusion rate} \frac{\frac{mg}{kg\ body\ weight}}{minute}$$

TABLE 4.11 DAILY ELECTROLYTE REQUIREMENTS[24]

Electrolyte	Daily Parenteral Requirement
Sodium	1-2 mEq/kg
Potassium	1-2 mEq/kg
Chloride	As needed to maintain acid–base balance
Acetate	As needed to maintain acid–base balance
Calcium	10-15 mEq
Magnesium	8-20 mEq
Phosphate	20-40 mmol

TABLE 4.12 OSMOLARITY CALCULATION

1. Multiply grams of dextrose per liter by 5
2. Multiply grams of amino acids per liter by 8.8
3. Multiply mEq of sodium per liter by 2
4. Multiply mEq of potassium per liter by 2
5. Multiply mEq of calcium per liter by 1.5
6. Multiply mEq of magnesium per liter by 1
7. Add numbers 1-7 to calculate total osmolarity in mOsm/L

CASE STUDY REVISITED

You determine that PN is justified for Alex and are asked to provide Alex's PN prescription.

Questions

1. Is the provision of lipid as a component of Alex's PN indicated? Justify your answer.
2. Calculate a PN prescription for Alex assuming Alex requires 1920 kcal and 85 g protein
3. Calculate the glucose infusion rate of your prescription. Does the glucose infusion rate of your prescription follow safe protocol?

Progression of PN

Before initiating PN, ensure that the patient has stable vital signs and normal fluid and electrolyte balance. Box 4.2 details clinical scenarios in which PN should be used with caution. Any imbalances should be corrected and addressed either prior to PN initiation or in the PN formula.[3] Shortly after the initiation of PN is a common time for patients to experience fluid and electrolyte disturbances. It is critical for the clinician to monitor the patient closely during this time to reduce the risk of complications and/or slowing the advancement of the PN.

For patients previously on insulin or hypoglycemic agents, or fasting glucose ≥200 mg/dL, dextrose should be limited to approximately 100 g on the first day of PN.[31] However, if a patient's blood glucose exceeds 300 mg/dL, PN should be withheld until glycemic control improves.

Infusion may begin at a low rate (approximately half of energy needs) and gradually advance over 2 to 3 days to minimize the risk of refeeding syndrome, hyperglycemia, and hypervolemia.[3,36,37] Patients at risk of refeeding syndrome should progress at a slower rate over 3 to 4 days.[9] Aim for a glucose infusion rate of no more than 4 to 5 mg/kg/min to minimize the risk of hyperglycemia.[37] In the ICU, glucose infusion rate is typically initially held to 3 to 4 mg/kg/min. Blood glucose should be well controlled before advancing to the goal rate.[3]

Critically ill patients require special considerations for advancement of PN as they are at greater risk for hyperglycemia and insulin resistance. In addition, among some critically ill patients, excessive energy intake is associated with greater risk of infectious morbidity, increased duration of mechanical ventilation, and increased length of stay.[9] Permissive underfeeding (80% of target calorie intake) may be considered. Among obese critically ill patients, permissive underfeeding may be as low as 65% to 70% of target calories.[11] However, as the patient stabilizes, feeding may be advanced to 100% of goal.

Administration of PN may be through **continuous infusion** (over 24 hours) or **cyclical infusion** (10 to 12 hours per day). Hospitalized patients typically receive PN continuously, whereas those on long-term PN usually receive cyclical infusions in order to allow freedom from the pump.

Transitional Feeding

Use of the GI tract is ideal when possible, and so patients may be transitioned from PN to EN or oral intake under careful supervision. Among the critically ill, once a patient is stabilized on PN, EN should be periodically trialed. If transitioning to EN, begin at a slow rate of 30 to 40 mL/hour with a formula appropriate to the patient's needs to assess tolerance. As the volume of EN received increases, the amount of energy provided by PN should decrease accordingly to prevent overfeeding. However, PN should not be terminated until ≥60% of target calories are provided enterally.[9] As with initiating PN, terminating PN should be done gradually to prevent hypoglycemia.

Transitioning from PN to oral intake is a less-predictable process than transitioning from PN to EN due to variations in patients' appetite and motivation to eat. Patients may be introduced first to clear liquids followed by a low-fat, low-fiber, and lactose-free diet. Oral intake should account for approximately 75% of the patient's calorie needs before discontinuing PN. For patients who cannot meet this goal, PN may continue to provide supplementary nutrition.

Parenteral Nutrition Monitoring

Parenteral nutrition is a costly therapy that requires regular clinical monitoring and diligent care of the patient in order to support a good outcome. Nutritional monitoring is needed to determine efficiency of the solution being administered, to discover and prevent complications, and to document changes in the clinical course. Monitoring should preferably be carried out by a nutrition support team, which monitors efficiency and sufficiency of PN with regards to specific endpoints defined by the patient's underlying illness, clinical status, the facilities available in the institution caring for the patient, and patient requests.[11,38]

> **CORE CONCEPT 9**
>
> Parenteral nutrition formulations are customizable to the specific needs of each patient or patient population.

Anthropometrics

Weight monitoring of parenteral nutrition patients is important. Steep, short-term increases and decreases in body weight may indicate changes in fluid status such as dehydration or edema. Intake and output can give further insight to suspected changes in fluid status.

Vital Signs

Vital signs include temperature, blood pressure, pulse, and respiration rate. Temperature is important to monitor in PN patients because fever is an indicator of infection and increases energy requirements. This may change the course of clinical care and PN requirements.

Blood pressure is important to monitor because it reflects hemodynamic stability or instability. If a patient is hemodynamically unstable, he or she may not be able to tolerate PN and require a medical intervention in order to correct the issue.

Heart rate is important to monitor because many electrolyte imbalances, a common occurrence in patients receiving PN, present with changes in pulse and arrhythmias when severe enough.

In PN patients, respiratory quotient is more useful information than respiration rate. The respiratory quotient is the ratio of carbon dioxide eliminated to oxygen consumed. Measurement of respiratory quotient in patients receiving PN is important in the prevention of fat accumulation in the liver and alleviation of potential respiratory distress secondary to excess glucose. Respiratory quotient should ideally be maintained between 0.7 and 1.0 to avoid metabolic disturbances.[39]

Biochemistry

Biochemical monitoring of electrolyte balance, blood glucose, renal function, iron studies, liver function, vitamin and trace element levels is important for both acute and long-term PN. Biochemical markers should be measured and analyzed on a defined, regular basis since attention to and adjustment of biochemical trends can reveal and prevent complications related to parenteral nutrition. Table 4.13 contains a sample monitoring schedule for anthropometric measurements, vital signs, and biochemical markers.

TABLE 4.13 SUGGESTED PARENTERAL NUTRITION MONITORING SCHEDULE (*MAY VARY BETWEEN INSTITUTIONS*)

Parameter	Initiation Period	Stable Period	Long-term
Vital signs	3-4x/day	Daily	As needed
Weight	Daily	2x/week	Weekly
Intake and output	Daily	Daily	
Blood glucose	Every 6 hours	Daily	Monthly
Sodium	Daily	Weekly	Monthly
Potassium	Daily	Weekly	Monthly
Chloride	Daily	Weekly	Monthly
Bicarbonate	Daily	Weekly	Monthly
Blood urea nitrogen	Daily	Weekly	Monthly
Creatinine	Daily	Weekly	Monthly
Calcium	Daily	Weekly	Monthly
Magnesium	Daily	Weekly	Monthly
Phosphorus	Daily	Weekly	Monthly
Complete blood count with differential	Weekly	Weekly	Monthly
Liver function tests (ALT and AST)	Weekly	Weekly	Monthly
Triglycerides	Weekly	Weekly	Monthly
Prothrombin time	Weekly	Monthly	4x/year
Prealbumin	Weekly	Monthly	4x/year
Trace element levels	N/A	N/A	4x/year

TABLE 4.14 NUTRITION-FOCUSED PHYSICAL EXAM IN MONITORING PATIENTS ON PARENTERAL NUTRITION

Physical Sign	Etiology	Parenteral Nutrition Implication
"Tenting" of skin Dry mucosa Poor skin turgor Sunken eyes Decreased urine output	Dehydration	Increase fluid provided through PN if not on restriction
Edema (pitting or abdominal) Dilution per laboratory values Weight gain	Overhydration	Decrease fluid provided through PN by transitioning to more-concentrated solution
Inflammation at the catheter site (swollen, red, or hot to the touch)	Potential infection	Appropriate medical intervention and patient education on proper catheter-site care if applicable
Signs of nutrient deficiency in sites with high cell turnover (hair, skin, mouth, tongue)	Nutrient deficiency	Test to confirm and add to PN prescription to compensate
Changes in clinical status such as intubation/sedation		May require changes to PN prescription

Nutrition-Focused Physical Exam

Nutrition-focused physical exam (NFPE) of patients on PN is a necessary component of monitoring. Physical signs to evaluate in an NFPE, their etiology, and PN implications are further described in **Table 4.14**.

Central Venous Access Complications and Their Management

Patients receiving PN are at risk for a wide variety of **catheter-related complications (CRCs)**, beginning at the time of catheter placement. These complications may be mechanical (infectious or noninfectious) or metabolic in nature. Risk of CRCs is impacted by the type of catheter used, the team's procedural experience, the duration of PN therapy, the quality of catheter care, and the patient's underlying disease state.[40] Some complications may be relatively manageable, while others are more serious. For these reasons, careful monitoring by a skilled team is essential. The prevention of many CRCs is possible with strict adherence to evidence-based protocols.[41]

Mechanical Complications

Catheter-related Mechanical Complications

Mechanical complications are related to the insertion of and care for the catheter and can be classified as either infectious or noninfectious. Some complications may develop at the time of catheterization or soon after (e.g., pneumothorax, arterial puncture, air embolism), while others develop over time (e.g., occlusion, infection).[42]

Certain types of venous access devices and their method of securement (e.g., sutures versus suture-less) are associated with more or less frequent occurrence of complications. PICCs and implantable ports are associated with a particularly low rate of mechanical complications, whereas nontunneled catheters are associated with a higher rate of bloodstream infections and symptomatic venous thrombosis.[41] The method of catheter placement also impacts risk of complications. Using ultrasound-guided catheterization can significantly reduce complications such as pneumothorax and catheter-related thrombosis compared to "blind" catheterization that relies on anatomical landmarks.[41,43]

Noninfectious Mechanical Complications

Noninfectious mechanical complications include pneumothorax, arterial puncture, embolism, occlusion, and venous thrombosis. In general, these complications are rare, occurring in 1% to 4% of central catheter placements when access is established by an experienced operator, and potential complications can be identified early on by radiologic and clinical exam.[40]

Pneumothorax   Catheterization carries the risk of **pneumothorax**, a puncture in the pleura of the lung leading to air accumulation in the pleural space, resulting in a collapsed lung.[44] Depending on the severity of the pneumothorax, the patient may require a chest tube while the air leak seals. PICCs carry a lower risk of pneumothorax, although they are more likely to be malpositioned.[40]

Arterial puncture In general, the veins used for PN are large and easy for an experienced operator to access. Accidental arterial puncture can occur resulting in complications such as temporary occlusion, pseudoaneurysm, and hematoma. Factors that contribute to the risk of arterial puncture include darkly pigmented skin and anatomical variations such as thoracic outlet syndrome.[45]

Occlusion A **catheter occlusion** is the most common type of noninfectious mechanical complication and is defined as the inability to infuse, flush, and/or aspirate on the venous access device.[5,46] Occlusions can be caused by the precipitation of minerals, medications, and lipids, which then obstruct the catheter. Symptoms include neck vein distension, edema, tingling/pain in the arm and neck, a tight feeling in the throat, and prominent veins of the anterior chest.[5] Occlusions may be cleared via repeated saline flushes.[40] Failing this, flushing with other solutions such as thrombolytics, sodium bicarbonate, hydrochloric acid, and sodium hydroxide can be used. If the catheter cannot be cleared, it may need to be replaced.

Catheter-related venous thrombosis (CRVT) may occur when catheterization damages the vessel wall, activating the coagulation of platelets and fibrin and resulting in a thrombus.[5] This process can begin within minutes of catheter placement. The risk of thrombus development is influenced by the catheter tip location, catheter material, type of PN formula, and length of catheter duration. The major risks of venous thrombosis are the potential for **thrombotic occlusion** (the cannulated vessel is blocked) and **thromboembolism** (the thrombus breaks free and blocks an artery).[5,40] The symptoms of thrombotic occlusion are similar to a catheter occlusion (edema, neck vein distension, tingling of the arm and neck). If the catheter is still functional (i.e., not fully occluded), there is evidence that the catheter should be left in situ rather than removed. Removing the catheter could dislodge any thromboses in contact with the catheter and result in thromboembolism.[46] Thrombolytics injected into the catheter may be used to treat this complication. Currently, there is no universally accepted strategy to prevent CRVT. Commonly used strategies include the use of heparin and heparin-bonded catheters.[40]

Embolism Embolisms are a rare occurrence in which material becomes lodged in an artery, resulting in significant morbidity and mortality.[47] In PN, various types of embolism are possible, including thromboembolism, **catheter embolism**, and **air embolism**.[40] Catheter embolisms can occur if the catheter becomes damaged and a piece of the equipment breaks free. Air embolisms can occur when there is a connection between the air and the cannulated vessel.[47] The pressure gradient drives air into the bloodstream, halting blood flow. Depending on the location of the blockage, embolisms may affect the cardiovascular, pulmonary, and neurological systems.

Phlebitis Phlebitis, or inflammation of the vein, is a relatively common complication in PN and is more common in PICC lines than other forms of access.[40] Inflammation at the exit site often raises suspicion of a bloodstream infection. However, in phlebitis, the inflammation is due to physical or chemical irritation from the catheter as opposed to infection.[40] Unless the exit site is overtly inflamed, and particularly if the patient has a fever, the appearance of the site is not a reliable indicator of catheter-related bloodstream infection.[48]

Infectious Complications

Catheter-related infections may be local or systemic. Local infections include infections of the exit site, tunnel, and port-pocket. They are usually treated by removing the catheter or port and administering a course of systemic antibiotics.[44] An exit-site infection in a tunneled catheter may not necessitate removal of the catheter—rather, frequent dressing changes coupled with a course of antibiotics should be provided.

Conversely, **catheter-related bloodstream infection (CRBSI)**, also called **central line–associated bloodstream infection (CLABSI)**, is a systemic infection and is one of the most serious complications of PN. Not only does it contribute to increased costs per patient, but CRBSI also increases length of stay by approximately 3 weeks and increases mortality by 14% to 40%.[49] CRBSI may lead to **sepsis**, a condition in which the body's normal inflammatory response to infection is amplified.[50] Sepsis can lead to organ dysfunction, hypotension, and death. While it has been understood since the 1970s that PN contributes to the risk of bloodstream infection, PN has recently been identified as an independent risk factor for infection.[51] A proposed mechanism is that the highly concentrated dextrose content of PN increases blood glucose concentrations, which increases the risk of infection, particularly among critically ill patients. The catheter itself also provides a surface on which bacteria can colonize, forming a **biofilm**. Biofilms are particularly resistant to antibiotics, antibodies, and phagocytes because bacteria are protected by a polysaccharide matrix.

CRBSI is characterized by fever, chills, and increased white blood cell count, and the diagnosis is confirmed through positive blood cultures drawn from the catheter lumen(s) and peripherally.[44] Increased bacterial growth in blood drawn from the catheter indicates CRBSI. CRBSI is commonly caused by *Candida* or yeast species, gram-positive bacteria (including *Staphylococcus aureus*, *Staphylococcus epidermis*, and *Enterococcus*), and gram-negative bacteria (including *Pseudomonas*, *Serratia marcescens*, *Klebsiella pneumoniae*, and *Escherichia coli*).[44]

CRBSI is first treated by administering broad-spectrum antibiotics through the catheter in order to avoid catheter removal.[44] However, it is necessary to remove the infected catheter if the patient continues to deteriorate or if blood cultures remain positive.[40,44] Prevention of CRBSI requires following strict guidelines at every point from choosing the appropriate venous access device to caring for the exit site. **Table 4.15** contains evidence-based strategies for preventing CRBSI.

TABLE 4.15 POINTS AT WHICH CATHETER-RELATED BLOODSTREAM INFECTION CAN BE PREVENTED[7,5,44]

Time Point	Strategies to Prevent CRBSI
Device selection	• For long-term PN, use tunneled and implanted catheters • Antimicrobial coated catheters are effective for short-term PN • Use single-lumen catheters unless the patient requires multiple ports • If using multiple lumens, one lumen should be reserved exclusively for PN
Catheterization procedure	• Use ultrasound-guided venipuncture • Take maximal barrier precautions during insertion: cap, mask, disposable gown, gloves, and large drape
PN administration and site care	• Enforce a strict hand washing policy • Use 2% chlorhexidine as skin antiseptic • Appropriately dress the exit site • Disinfect hubs, stopcocks, and needle-free connectors • Regularly change administration sets • Use antibiotic-lock or ethanol-lock: catheter lumen is filled with antibiotic solution or ethanol when not in use

CASE STUDY REVISITED

Alex has been on PN for 2 weeks. Below are his weight and his most recent metabolic panel:

Anthropometric Data:
Weight: 68 kg (150 lbs)
Admission weight: 64 kg (141 lbs)

Biochemical Data:

Sodium 133 (135-145 mEq/L)
Potassium 3.7 (3.6-5.0 mEq/L)
Chloride 99 (98-110 mEq/L)
Carbon dioxide 22 (20-30 mEq/L)
Blood urea nitrogen 8 (6-24 mg/dL)
Creatinine 0.4 (0.4-1.3 mg/dL)
Glucose 180 (70-139 mg/dL)
Aspartate transaminase (AST) 110 (10-35 IU/L)
Alanine tranaminase (ALT) 99 (4-36 units/L)
Alkaline phosphatase (ALP) 130 (30-120 units/L)
Direct (conjugated) bilirubin 3.0 (0-0.3 mg/dL)
Total bilirubin 1.9 (0.3-0.9 mg/dL)

Calcium 9 (8.5-10.5 mEq/L)
Phosphorus 3.4 (2.7-4.5 mg/dL)
Magnesium 1.5 (1.3-2.1 mEq/L)
Albumin 3.0 (3.5-5.0 g/dL)

Questions
1. What is your interpretation of Alex's weight?
2. What biochemical labs are concerning?
3. How might you alter the PN composition or prescription? Provide specific changes to the initial PN prescription if necessary.
4. Are there other options you might consider for feeding Alex?

Metabolic Complications

Hyper- and Hypoglycemia
It is normal for blood glucose to rise after initiating PN. However, endogenous insulin secretion should bring glucose back to a normal range. Hyperglycemia is the most common metabolic complication of PN. Prolonged, uncontrolled hyperglycemia can lead to nonketotic dehydration, coma, and death.[37] It is usually caused by excessive dextrose infusion, although it can also be a result of the stress response in acutely ill or septic patients. These patients are known to develop insulin resistance, suppressed insulin secretion, and increased gluconeogenesis and glycogenolysis.[37] Patients with diabetes, acute pancreatitis, or on corticosteroid medication are also at risk of hyperglycemia. To prevent hyperglycemia, ensure that dextrose is infused at no higher than 5 mg/kg/min. In addition, identify other potential sources of dextrose or changes in medications (e.g., corticosteroids).[52] Hyperglycemia is treated with insulin, which can be administered subcutaneously, intravenously, or added to the PN formula itself.[37]

Patients receiving PN are typically secreting higher-than-normal levels of insulin due to the high concentration of dextrose in the formula. Abruptly stopping PN infusion can therefore result in reactive hypoglycemia within 15 to 60 minutes.[42] A blood glucose level <70 mg/dL would suggest hypoglycemia.[53] This complication can be prevented by slowly tapering PN over 1 to 2 hours or by infusing 10% dextrose immediately after PN cessation.[42] The safest way to provide and manage insulin therapy is through standardized protocols.

Electrolyte Abnormalities
As discussed in Parenteral Nutrition Formulation, the electrolyte content added to PN is customizable to the patient's needs. Biochemical monitoring should be performed regularly to assess whether a patient requires more or less of particular electrolytes.

When initiating PN, however, severe electrolyte disturbances may be indicative of refeeding syndrome, especially in malnourished patients. Refeeding syndrome is characterized by hypophosphatemia, hypokalemia, and hypomagnesemia in addition to disturbances in glucose metabolism and fluid and sodium balance.[52] Advancing PN gradually over several days and supplementing electrolytes can help to prevent refeeding syndrome.[42]

Electrolyte abnormalities may also result in acid–base disturbances. Arterial blood normally has a pH range of 7.35 to 7.45, and this range should be closely monitored to ensure optimal organ function.[54] Many factors can contribute to disturbances in a patient's acid–base balance, including components of the PN formula. Treatment of acid–base disturbances should address the underlying cause. Acidosis (arterial pH <7.35) may be corrected by decreasing the amount of chloride provided or by providing bicarbonate in the form of acetate (a bicarbonate precursor).[54] Bicarbonate itself should not be added to the PN formula, as it is unstable. Alkalosis (arterial pH >7.45) may be corrected by decreasing the amount of acetate salts provided or replacing any potassium and magnesium deficits.[54]

Hyper- and Hypovolemia
Patients may receive all of their fluid intake from PN alone, but some may also be consuming fluids orally.[55] For these patients, assess whether there have been any changes in oral intake. Hypervolemia, or fluid overload, is likely due to excessive PN or intravenous fluid infusion.[55] Symptoms include weight gain, edema, and shortness of breath. Manage hypervolemia by maintaining or decreasing PN volume, unless fluid overload is severe, in which case PN may need to be discontinued temporarily.[52]

Hypovolemia, or a deficit in the extracellular fluid, can occur in a variety of ways, including ostomy output, diarrhea, fistulae, fever, or diuresis.[55,56] Symptoms include weight loss, decreased urine output, decreased urinary sodium concentration (<15 mEq/L), low blood pressure, muscle cramps, weakness, dizziness, thirst, and dry mouth.[55,56] Hypovolemia may or may not be accompanied by an electrolyte deficit. Repletion with intravenous fluids should take into consideration whether any electrolytes must also be repleted.[56]

Overfeeding
Dr. Jonathan Rhoads, one of the founders of PN, originally described this form of nutrition support as "hyperalimentation" (overfeeding).[57] It was initially believed that malnourished or hypermetabolic patients should be fed much more than their required nutrient needs in order to stimulate an anabolic response. However, it is now recognized that overfeeding increases the risk of complications, particularly bloodstream infections.[58] Overfeeding is more common in the ICU setting because critically ill and septic patients do not metabolize glucose and lipids normally, excess glucose and lipids increase metabolic stress and exacerbate the storage impairments associated with insulin resistance.[59]

Essential Fatty Acid Deficiency
Linoleic acid, an omega-6 fatty acid, and α-linolenic acid, an omega-3 fatty acid, are considered EFAs because they cannot be synthesized by humans.[60] EFA deficiency can develop in infants and children receiving fat-free PN within a few days, and in adults receiving fat-free PN within 2 weeks.[61,62] Clinical signs of essential fatty acid deficiency include hepatomegaly; thrombocytopenia; impaired wound healing; hair loss; and dry, desquamated skin.[60] In order to prevent EFA deficiency in patients receiving fat-free PN, linoleic acid must be administered.[61,62] **Table 4.16** contains more information on the amount of EFA required to prevent deficiency.

TABLE 4.16 AMOUNT OF LINOLEIC ACID REQUIRED TO PREVENT ESSENTIAL FATTY ACID DEFICIENCY DURING DIFFERENT STAGES OF THE LIFE CYCLE[61,62]

Preterm infants	0.25 g/kg/day
Term infants and older children	0.1 g/kg/day
Adults	2%-4% of total calorie intake

Hepatobiliary Complications

There are essentially three types of hepatobiliary disorders associated with PN therapy: **hepatic steatosis**, **cholestasis**, and **cholelithiasis**.[63] These complications can happen without the use of parenteral nutrition; however, when attributable to the usage of PN, these complications are referred to as PN-associated liver disease (PNALD). It is estimated that PNALD develops in 40% to 60% of infants on long-term PN and 15% to 40% of adults on home PN for intestinal failure.[64]

Hepatic steatosis is the accumulation of fat in the liver. Although the development of hepatic steatosis is thought to be multifactorial, the use of soybean lipid emulsions is thought to be one of the largest contributing factors. Although the lipid particles in parenteral soybean oil emulsion mimic the size and structure of chylomicrons, they primarily contain omega-6 fatty acids and triglycerides and are devoid of cholesterol or protein. With reduced cholesterol, lipolysis is limited and the liver is prone to the accumulation of lipid particles. Although steatosis is reversible, it can advance to more serious stages of liver disease, and eventually to cirrhosis, if not appropriately managed.[65]

Cholestasis is a condition of reduced bile flow. This can be caused by any impairment between hepatocytes, which produce bile, and the duodenum, the site where bile is incorporated into the gastrointestinal tract. When bile flow is stopped, the pigment bilirubin escapes into the bloodstream and accumulates. For this reason, the primary indicator of cholestasis is a serum conjugated bilirubin >2 mg/dL. PNALD is initially characterized by cholestasis but can progress to fibrosis and cirrhosis with continued exposure to PN.[66,67]

Cholelithiasis is the presence of gallstones or gallbladder sludge. Gallstones can develop in patients receiving PN due to gallbladder stasis, or inactivity of the gallbladder. When the gallbladder is not stimulated to secrete stored bile, the bile begins to form sludge, which turns into gallstones.[68]

When a patient receiving PN develops hepatobiliary complications, it is necessary to rule out all treatable causes and minimize other risk factors. All potential hepatotoxic medications and herbal supplements should be eliminated. Modifications to the PN regimen that may be helpful include reduction of calories, reduction of ILE dose to <1 g/kg/day, replacement of an omega-6 lipid source with an omega-3 containing lipid source, supplementation of taurine in the infant, and use of cyclic infusion. Initiation of even small amounts of EN and use of ursodiol may be beneficial in stimulating bile flow. In the long-term PN patient with severe and progressive liver disease, intestinal or liver transplantation may be the only remaining treatment option.[63]

CASE STUDY REVISITED

Shortly after surgery, Alex remains on PN, but you believe that he is ready for trial oral feeding. A liquid diet is ordered, which he appears to tolerate well, and his PN is tapered. Two days later, Alex develops a fever, abdominal distention, and diarrhea. A CT scan reveals an enterocolonic fistula between the distal ileum and ascending colon. The surgeon determines that Alex will require further surgery to repair the fistula but advises waiting 3 to 6 months to allow the densest peritoneal adhesions to resolve. Until then, Alex will need to remain NPO and continue receiving PN. After another week in the hospital, Alex's fever, distention, and diarrhea have resolved and he is ready to be discharged on home PN.

Questions

1. What questions would you ask to determine whether Alex would be able to independently manage home PN?
2. Describe three common complications associated with long-term PN. What symptoms and lab values would you monitor?

Home Parenteral Nutrition

Indications and Access

Home parenteral nutrition (HPN) is becoming an increasingly common therapy. It is estimated that approximately 300 patients are placed on HPN in the United States each year.[69] The indications for HPN are similar to those for hospitalized patients. These patients have long-term (≥2 weeks) intestinal failure, cannot meet their nutritional needs through the enteral route alone, and can be treated outside of the acute care setting.[3,70] However, HPN is not recommended for terminally ill patients with a short life expectancy.[71] A.S.P.E.N. provides guidelines related to the ethical issues of nutrition support in end of life.[72]

Because hospitalization is no longer necessary, indications for HPN involve further considerations. Is the patient, family, or caregiver capable of administering PN? Is the home environment safe for PN? Will the patient's insurance cover HPN-related costs?

> **PRACTICE POINT**
>
> In the United States, the federal-level health insurance program Medicare will only cover HPN-related costs if it is documented that the patient's GI tract is nonfunctional, the condition is "permanent" (i.e., at least 90 days of therapy are needed), and the patient cannot tolerate EN.

In terms of type of venous access indicated for HPN, current guidelines recommend tunneled catheters or implanted ports.[69,70] As discussed earlier in this chapter, CRBSIs are one of the most common complications associated with catheters. PICCs have been shown to carry a lower risk of CRBSI in the hospital setting, but this has not yet been shown definitively in the home setting.[69] In addition, placement of PICCs do not have the potential for some of the serious mechanical complications associated with tunneled catheters, including pneumothorax and accidental arterial puncture.[73] Recent studies have assessed the feasibility of PICCs for HPN and have found that, overall, PICCs are associated with the same incidence of complications as traditional forms of access.

HPN is usually administered on a cyclic schedule. The infusion rate is controlled by an automatic pump that gradually increases the rate over the first 30 minutes, administers the total volume over 12 to 15 hours, then gradually tapers over the last 30 minutes.[70] Many patients choose to infuse overnight in order to allow freedom from the pump for daytime activities. The downside of nighttime infusion is frequent urination, so some patients may choose daytime infusion to ensure a better night's sleep.[74]

Once it has been established that a patient will return home on PN, it is essential to involve a interprofessional team to assist in the transition. This team may include a doctor, specialized nurse, dietitian, and pharmacist.[70] In reality, however, few HPN patients in the United States receive care from interprofessional nutrition support teams due to healthcare-cost restraints.[71] A psychologist and/or social worker may also be needed, depending on how HPN affects the patient's personal and social life. The primary goals of patient/caregiver education are to promote the patient's independence, improve their quality of life, and make living with HPN as normal as possible.[75]

HPN is a complex therapy that requires intensive education and training. Patients/caregivers must learn how to administer the PN formula, care for the IV site, and identify and address complications. Several factors can affect a patient's level of success in managing HPN. These include health literacy (performing basic reading and math skills in a healthcare environment), socioeconomic status, knowledge of the English language (or dominant language), and age (older than 65 years is associated with poorer health literacy).[75]

It can be difficult to assess HPN a patient's quality of life as it is affected both by HPN itself and the underlying disease state. Quality of life (QOL) is defined as "enjoying life" and "being able to do what you want to do when you want to do it."[76] Assessments of HPN patients' QOL have found that the poorest QOL is experienced during the first year, particularly if the patient was previously well.[55] QOL tends to improve with time. Strong self-esteem, spousal and family support, and financial security are associated with improved quality of life.[55,76]

Factors that negatively contribute to quality of life include frequent catheter-related infections; the inability to work and loss of income (although some patients can continue to work); decreased social interactions; lack of energy and stamina; the inconvenience of the catheter, tubing, and pump; and the rigidity of the infusion schedule.[55,76]

Transitioning to HPN can be an intense, stressful experience. Patients will have different attitudes in how they approach this new phase of their life. The infusion schedule can be particularly challenging. Some patients may be able to maintain a relatively spontaneous lifestyle and learn to adjust their infusion schedule accordingly, while others may feel burdened by a strict infusion schedule. Successful patients will acknowledge that their lives have changed, but will learn to redefine their "new normal." It can be helpful for patients to focus on what they can still do while on HPN, rather than what they cannot do.[76]

Prognosis of HPN

Retrospective cohort studies have found that the 5-year survival rate for patients on HPN range from 58% to 83%.[77] Because there are a wide variety of conditions that may necessitate HPN, the most influential and variable effect on survival rate is the underlying disease state.[55] For example, patients with cancer may have an expected survival of several months, whereas patients with Crohn's disease can expect to measure survival in decades. In the overwhelming majority of cases, death of a patient on HPN is due to the underlying disease and not a complication of HPN, particularly for patients on HPN for <1 year. As the length of HPN use increases, so does the risk of serious complications such as sepsis, liver failure, and thrombosis. Among long-term HPN patients, complications account for 15% to 20% of deaths.[55,77] Additional factors that influence prognosis of patients on HPN include the following:[55]

- Age (better prognosis amongst younger patients)
- Experience of supervising clinician
- Use of narcotics (associated with increased incidence of sepsis)
- Peer-support and education programs (associated with decreased incidence of sepsis)

While some patients will remain on life-long HPN, others may be able to transition off of HPN to an oral diet. Depending on the length and type of bowel that remains intact, patients with short-bowel syndrome may undergo a process known as adaptation. If the colon remains intact, absorption improves over 1 to 3 years, and with dietary counseling, patients may be able to reduce PN or transition off of PN entirely.[78] Recent studies have found that adaptation may even occur up to 5 years after onset of intestinal failure[77]

CORE CONCEPT 10

Parenteral nutrition may be a long-term or even life-long therapy for some patients.

Chapter Summary

Parenteral nutrition is a life-sustaining therapy for individuals with a nonfunctional GI tract who cannot consume nutrition through oral intake or enteral nutrition. It may be used to sustain patients before they are able to resume oral or enteral intake, whereas for those who have permanent GI dysfunction, it may be used for decades. PN is a highly complex therapy that requires careful calculation of nutrient needs, strict hygienic practices when administering PN and caring for the catheter site, and constant monitoring for complications. An experienced, interprofessional team is ideal for managing PN.

Key Terms

parenteral nutrition (PN), hypertonic, asepsis, central parenteral nutrition, peripheral parenteral nutrition, venipuncture, exit site, thrombophlebitis, extravasation, central venous catheter (CVC), peripherally inserted central catheter (PICC), phlebitis, parenteral nutrition associated liver disease (PNALD), hepatic steatosis, total nutrient admixture (TNA), physicochemical incompatibility, continuous infusion, cyclical infusion, catheter-related complication (CRC), pneumothorax, catheter occlusion, catheter-related venous thrombosis (CRVT), thrombotic occlusion, thromboembolism, catheter embolism, air embolism, catheter-related bloodstream infection (CRBSI), central line associated bloodstream infection (CLABSI), sepsis, biofilm, cholestasis, cholelithiasis.

References

1. Mahan KL E-SS, Raymond JL, Krause MV. *Krause's Food & the Nutrition Care Process*. 13th ed. St. Louis, MO.: Elsevier/Saunders; 2012.
2. Dudrick SJ. History of parenteral nutrition. *J Am Coll Nutr.* 2009;28(3):243-251.
3. Mirtallo JM, Patel M. Overview of parenteral nutrition. In: Mueller CM, ed. *The A.S.P.E.N. Adult Nutrition Support Core Curriculum*. 2nd ed. Silver Spring, MD: American Society for Parenteral and Enteral Nutrition; 2012:232-244.
4. Dudrick SJ, Wilmore DW, Vars HM, Rhoads JE. Long-term total parenteral nutrition with growth, development, and positive nitrogen balance. *Surgery*. 1968;64(1):134-142.
5. Krzywda EA, Andris DA, Edmiston CE. Parenteral access devices. In: Mueller CM, ed. *The A.S.P.E.N. Adult Nutrition Support Core Curriculum*. 2nd ed. Silver Spring, MD: American Society for Parenteral and Enteral Nutrition; 2012:265-283.
6. Derenski K, Catlin J, Allen L. Parenteral nutrition basics for the clinician caring for the adult patient. *Nutr Clin Pract*. 2016;31(5):578-595.
7. Pittiruti M, Hamilton H, Biffi R, MacFie J, Pertkiewicz M, ESPEN. ESPEN Guidelines on Parenteral Nutrition: Central venous catheters (access, care, diagnosis and therapy of complications). *Clin Nutr*. 2009;28(4):365-377.
8. Boullata JI, Gilbert K, Sacks G, et al. A.S.P.E.N. clinical guidelines: parenteral nutrition ordering, order review, compounding, labeling, and dispensing. *JPEN J Parenter Enteral Nutr*. 2014;38(3):334-377.
9. McClave SA, Martindale R, Taylor B, Gramlich L. Appropriate use of parenteral nutrition through the perioperative period. *J Parenter Enteral Nutr*. 2013;37(5 Suppl):73S-82S.
10. Muscaritoli M, Molfino A, Laviano A, Rasio D, Rossi Fanelli F. Parenteral nutrition in advanced cancer patients. *Crit Rev Oncol Hematol*. 2012;84(1):26-36.
11. McClave SA, Taylor BE, Martindale RG, et al. Guidelines for the provision and assessment of nutrition support therapy in the adult critically ill patient: Society of Critical Care Medicine (SCCM) and American Society for Parenteral and Enteral Nutrition (A.S.P.E.N.). *JPEN J Parenter Enteral Nutr*. 2016;40(2):159-211.
12. Şimşek T, Şimşek HU, Cantürk NZ. Response to trauma and metabolic changes: posttraumatic metabolism. *Turk J Surg*. 2014;30(3):153-159.
13. Bolder U, Ebener C, Hauner H, et al. Carbohydrates – Guidelines on Parenteral Nutrition, Chapter 5. *Ger Med Sci*. Vol 72009.
14. Barber JR, Sacks GS. Parenteral nutrition formulations. In: Mueller CM, ed. *The A.S.P.E.N. Adult Nutrition Support Core Curriculum*. 2nd ed. Silver Spring, MD: The American Society for Parenteral and Enteral Nutrition; 2012:245-264.
15. Yarandi SS, Zhao VM, Hebbar G, Ziegler TR. Amino acid composition in parenteral nutrition: what is the evidence? *Curr Opin Clin Nutr Metab Care*. 2011;14(1):75-82.
16. A.S.P.E.N. Board of Directors and the Clinical Guidelines Task Force. Guidelines for the use of parenteral and enteral nutrition in adult and pediatric patients. *JPEN J Parenter Enteral Nutr*. 2002;26(1 Suppl):1sa-138sa.
17. 15% Clinisol [package insert]. Deerfield, IL: Baxter Healthcare Corporation; 2006. https://dailymed.nlm.nih.gov/dailymed/archives/fdaDrugInfo.cfm?archiveid=2629.

18. Aminosyn II with Electrolytes [package insert]. Lake Forest, IL: Hospira, Inc.; 2004. https://www.accessdata.fda.gov/drugsatfda_docs/label/2005/019683s027lbl.pdf.
19. Friedman M. *Absorption and utilization of amino acids.* Vol 2. Boca Raton, FL: CRC Press; 1989.
20. Calder PC, Jensen GL, Koletzko BV, Singer P, Wanten GJ. Lipid emulsions in parenteral nutrition of intensive care patients: current thinking and future directions. *Intensive Care Med.* 2010;36(5):735-749.
21. Adolph M, Heller AR, Koch T, et al. Lipid emulsions – Guidelines on Parenteral Nutrition, Chapter 6. *Ger Med Sci.* 2009;7.
22. Antebi H, Mansoor O, Ferrier C, et al. Liver function and plasma antioxidant status in intensive care unit patients requiring total parenteral nutrition: comparison of 2 fat emulsions. *JPEN J Parenter Enteral Nutr.* 2004;28(3):142-148.
23. O'Grady NP, Alexander M, Burns LA, et al. Guidelines for the Prevention of Intravascular Catheter-related Infections. Clinical Infectious Diseases: An Official Publication of the Infectious Diseases Society of America. 2011;52(9):e162-e193.
24. Mirtallo J, Canada T, Johnson D, et al. Safe practices for parenteral nutrition. *JPEN J Parenter Enteral Nutr.* 2004;28(6):S39-70.
25. Clark SF. Vitamins and trace elements. In: Mueller CM, ed. *The A.S.P.E.N. Adult Nutrition Support Core Curriculum.* 2nd ed. Silver Spring, MD: The American Society for Parenteral and Enteral Nutrition; 2012:121-151.
26. M.V.I.-12 [package insert]. Westborough, MA: AstraZeneca; 2004.
27. Itokawa Y. Trace elements in long-term total parenteral nutrition. *Nihon Rinsho Jpn J Clin Med.* 1996;54(1): 172-178.
28. Rampton D, Folkersen J, Fishbane S, et al. Hypersensitivity reactions to intravenous iron: guidance for risk minimization and management. *Haematologica.* 2014;99(11):1671-1676.
29. Forbes A. Iron and parenteral nutrition. *Gastroenterology.* 2009;137 (5 Suppl):S47-54.
30. Gosmanov AR, Umpierrez GE. Management of hyperglycemia during enteral and parenteral nutrition therapy. *Curr Diab Rep.* 2013;13(1): 155-162.
31. Mirtallo J, Canada T, Johnson D, et al. Safe practices for parenteral nutrition. *JPEN J Parenter Enteral Nutr.* 2004;28(6): S39-70.
32. Hadaway LC. Administering parenteral nutrition with other I.V. drugs. *Nursing.* 2005;35(2):26.
33. Drug Shortages Update. A.S.P.E.N. website. https://www.nutritioncare.org/News/Product_Shortages/Drug_Shortages_Update/. Accessed January 31, 2017.
34. Mirtallo JM. The drug shortage crisis. *JPEN J Parenter Enteral Nutr.* 2011;35(4):433.
35. Product Shortages. A.S.P.E.N.website. http://www.nutritioncare.org/public-policy/product-shortages/. Accessed January 31, 2017.
36. Burke JF, Wolfe RR, Mullany CJ, Mathews DE, Bier DM. Glucose requirements following burn injury. parameters of optimal glucose infusion and possible hepatic and respiratory abnormalities following excessive glucose intake. *Ann Surg.* 1979;190(3):274-285
37. Kumpf VJ, Gervasio J. Complications of parenteral nutrition. In: Mueller CM, ed. *The A.S.P.E.N. Adult Nutrition Support Core Curriculum.* 2nd ed. Silver Spring, MD: The American Society for Parenteral and Enteral Nutrition; 2012; 284-297.
38. Hartl WH, Jauch KW, Parhofer K, Rittler P. Complications and Monitoring – Guidelines on Parenteral Nutrition, Chapter 11. *Ger Med Sci.* Vol 72009.
39. Hematology ASo. Sickle Cell Anemia. http://www.hematology.org/Patients/Anemia/Sickle-Cell.aspx. Accessed May 4, 2017.
40. Ghabril MS, Aranda-Michel J, Scolapio JS. Metabolic and Catheter Complications of Parenteral Nutrition. *Curr Gastroenteroly Rep.* 2004;6:327-334.
41. Cotogni P, Barbero C, Garrino C, et al. Peripherally inserted central catheters in non-hospitalized cancer patients: 5-year results of a prospective study. *Support Care Cancer.* 2015;23(2):403-409.
42. Ukleja A, Romano MM. Complications of parenteral nutrition. *Gastroenterol Clin N A.* 2007;36:23-46.
43. Cavanna, L, Civardi, G, Vallisa D, et al. Ultrasound-guided central venous catheterization in cancer patients improves the success rate of cannulation and reduces mechanical complications: A prospective observational study of 1,978 consecutive catheterizations. *World J Surg Oncol.* 2010;8(91).
44. Hamilton C. Vascular access. In: Charney P, Malone AM, eds. *ADA Pocket Guide to Parenteral Nutrition*: Chicago, IL: Academy of Nutrition and Dietetics; 2007:33-51.
45. Lirk P, Keller C, Colvin J, et al. Unintentional arterial puncture during cephalic vein cannulation: case report and anatomical study. *Br J Anaesth.* 2004;92(5):740-742.
46. Brandt CF, Tribler S, Hvistendahl M, et al. Home parenteral nutrition in adult patients with chronic intestinal failure: catheter-related complications over 4 decades at the main Danish Tertiary Referral Center. *JPEN J Parenter Enteral Nutr.* 2017;41(7):1178-1187
47. McCarthy CJ, Behravesh S, Naidu SG, Oklu R. Air embolism: Practical tips for prevention and treatment. *J Clin Med.* 2016;5(11).
48. Safdar N, Maki DG. Inflammation at the insertion site is not predictive of catheter-related bloodstream infection with short-term, noncuffed central venous catheters. *Crit Care Med.* 2002;30(12):2632-2635.
49. Fonseca G, Burgermaster M, Larson E, Seres DS. The relationship between parenteral nutrition and central line–associated bloodstream infections: 2009–2014. *JPEN J Parenter Enteral Nutr.* 2017:1-5.
50. Prasad, P, ed. Sepsis in adults. Dynamed website. http://www.dynamed.com/topics/dmp~AN~T115805/Sepsis-in-adults. Updated July 28, 2017. Accessed October 2, 2017.
51. Beghetto MG, Victorino J, Teixeira L, de Azevedo MJ. Parenteral nutrition as a risk factor for central venous catheter–related infection. *JPEN J Parenter Enteral Nutr.* 2005;29(5):367-373.
52. Roberts S. Initiation, advancement, and acute complications. In: Charney P, Malone AM, eds. *ADA Pocket Guide to Parenteral Nutrition*: Chicago, IL: Academy of Nutrition and Dietetics; 2007:76-102.
53. Olveira G, Tapia MJ, Ocon J, et al. Hypoglycemia in noncritically ill patients receiving total parenteral nutrition: a multicenter study. (Study group on the problem of hyperglycemia in parenteral nutrition; Nutrition area of the Spanish Society of Endocrinology and Nutrition). *Nutrition.* 2015;31(1):58-63.
54. Ayers P, Warrington L. Diagnosis and treatment of simple acid-base disorders. *Nutr Clin Prac.* 2008;23(2):122-127.
55. Howard L. Home Parenteral nutrition: Survival, cost, and quality of life. *Gastroenterology.* 2006;130(2):S52-S59.
56. Rhoda KM, Porter MJ, Quintini C. Fluid and electrolyte management. *JPEN J Parenter Enteral Nutr.* 2011;35(6):675-685.
57. Vinnars E WD. History of parenteral nutrition. *JPEN J Parenter Enteral Nutr.* 2003;27(3):225-231.
58. Jeejeebhoy KN. Total parenteral nutrition: potion or poison? *Am J Clin Nutr.* 2001;74:160-163.
59. Griffiths RD. Too much of a good thing: the curse of overfeeding. *Crit Care.* 2007;11(6):176.
60. Jeppesen PB, Hoy CE, Mortensen PB. Essential fatty acid deficiency in patients receiving home parenteral nutrition. *Am J Clin Nutr.* 1998;68(1):126-133.

61. ESPEN. Guidelines of Pediatric Parenteral Nutrition 4. Lipids. *J Ped Gastroenterol Nutr.* 2005;41(2):S19-S27.
62. Morlion B. Update on Parenteral Lipids: Therapeutic Goals. www.espen.org/presfile/Morlion-2-010902-web.doc. Updated September 14, 2017. Accessed October 2, 2017.
63. Kumpf VJ. Parenteral nutrition-associated liver disease in adult and pediatric patients. *Nutr Clin Pract.* 2006;21(3):279-290.
64. Xu ZW, Li YS. Pathogenesis and treatment of parenteral nutrition-associated liver disease. *Hepatobiliary Pancreat Dis Int.* 2012;11(6):586-593.
65. Nandivada P, Carlson SJ, Chang MI, Cowan E, Gura KM, Puder M. Treatment of parenteral nutrition-associated liver disease: the role of lipid emulsions. *Adv Nutr.* 2013;4:711-717.
66. Cholestasis. Merckmanuals.com. http://www.merckmanuals.com/home/liver-and-gallbladder-disorders/manifestations-of-liver-disease/cholestasis. Accessed September 30, 2017.
67. Guglielmi FW, Regano N, Mazzuoli S, et al. Cholestasis induced by total parenteral nutrition. *Clin Liver Dis.* 2008;12(1):97-110, viii.
68. Cholelithiasis. Merckmanuals.com. http://www.merckmanuals.com/professional/hepatic-and-biliary-disorders/gallbladder-and-bile-duct-disorders/cholelithiasis. Published August 2016. Accessed September 30, 2017.
69. Botella-Carretero JI, Carrero C, Guerra E, et al. Role of peripherally inserted central catheters in home parenteral nutrition: a 5-year prospective study. *JPEN J Parenter Enteral Nutr.* 2013;37(4):544-549.
70. Wanten G, Calder PC, Forbes A. Managing adult patients who need home parenteral nutrition. *BMJ.* 2011;342:d1447.
71. Kumpf VJ, Tillman EM. Home parenteral nutrition: Safe transition from hospital to home. *Nutr Clin Prac.* 2012;27(6):749-757.
72. Barrocas A, Geppert C, Durfee SM, et al. A.S.P.E.N. Ethics Position Paper. *Nutr Clin Prac.* 2010;25(6):672-679.
73. Christensen LD, Rasmussen HH, Vinter-Jensen L. Peripherally inserted central catheter for use in home parenteral nutrition: a 4-year follow-up study. *JPEN J Parenter Enteral Nutr.* 2014;38(8):1003-1006.
74. Hamilton C, Austin T. Home parenteral nutrition. In: Charney P, Malone AM, eds. *ADA Pocket Guide to Parenteral Nutrition.* Chicago, IL: Academy of Nutrition and Dietetics; 2007:118-146.
75. Gifford H, DeLegge M, Epperson LA. Education methods and techniques for training home parenteral nutrition patients. *Nutr Clin Prac.* 2010;25(5):443-450.
76. Winkler MF, Hagan E, Wetle T, Smith C, O'Sullivan Maillet J, Touger-Decker R. An exploration of quality of life and the experience of living with home parenteral nutrition. *JPEN J Parenter Enteral Nutr.* 2010;34(4):395-407.
77. Dibb M, Soop M, Teubner A, et al. Survival and nutritional dependence on home parenteral nutrition: Three decades of experience from a single referral centre. *Clin Nutr.* 2017;36(2):570-576.
78. Van Gossum A, Cabre E, Hebuterne X, et al. ESPEN Guidelines on Parenteral Nutrition: gastroenterology. In: Mueller CM, ed. *The A.S.P.E.N. Adult Nutrition Support Core Curriculum.* 2nd ed. Silver Spring, MD: American Society for Parenteral and Enteral Nutrition; 2012:415-437.

Chapter 5

Energy Expenditure and Body Composition in Metabolic Stress

Kathy Prelack

Chapter Outline

Core Concepts
Introduction
Characteristics of the Inflammatory Response
Ebb and Flow Phase
Alterations in Metabolism Associated with the Inflammatory Response
Determination of Energy Expenditure During Normal and Stressed Conditions
Estimating Total Energy Expenditure
Measuring Energy Expenditure—Direct and Indirect Calorimetry
Determination of Body Composition and Its Components During Metabolic Stress
Multi-Compartmental Models
Metabolic Support Aimed at Preserving Body Cell Mass

CORE CONCEPTS

1. The inflammatory response transgresses through phases known as the ebb and flow phases, each distinct in physiologic characteristics and clinical management.
2. Metabolic effects of the inflammatory response manifest as increased energy expenditure related to gluconeogenesis, protein synthesis and breakdown, and altered substrate utilization.
3. Stress hyperglycemia is common during the inflammatory response, as a result of increased gluconeogenesis, increased glucagon-to-insulin ratio and predominance of other counter-regulatory hormones, and insulin resistance.
4. Protein catabolism occurs in an effort to make acute-phase proteins and glucose. Muscle is the primary source of endogenous amino acids released in the body during stress for this use.
5. During inflammatory stress, adipose tissue is metabolically active, as evidenced by increased serum lipolysis and fatty acid levels, although fatty acid oxidation can be impaired.
6. Basal metabolic rate is primarily determined by body cell mass, the metabolically active component of the body.
7. Total energy expenditure is composed primarily of basal metabolic rate, energy cost of physical activity, and diet-induced thermogenesis.
8. During the inflammatory response, resting energy expenditure incorporates the energy cost associated with the physiologic and metabolic stress of disease and clinical interventions.
9. Expansion in extracellular water during illness confounds interpretation of weight, lean body cell mass, and erosion of body cell mass.
10. Metabolic Support of the inflammatory response should aim at preservation of the BCM.

Learning Objectives

1. Understand the components of energy expenditure and body composition and their changes during health and metabolic stress.
2. Describe the inflammatory response and its trajectory in the days to weeks following cell injury with respect to physiologic, endocrine, and metabolic changes.
3. Determine factors both metabolic and clinical that impact total energy expenditure and its components.
4. Distinguish the metabolic differences between stress and starvation and the impact on nutritional status.
5. Describe methods for determining estimates based on energy expenditure-including empirical equation, indirect calorimetry, and experimental models.
6. Identify the effects of the inflammatory response on body composition and its measurement.
7. Identify techniques that may be used to assess body composition in a clinical setting, their advantages, and their limitations.
8. Determine appropriate goals for nutrition support using information related to energy expenditure, protein turnover, and substrate utilization during metabolic stress.

Introduction

The goals of medical nutrition therapy are to support the metabolic demands of a specific disease state, uphold nutritional status, and improve clinical outcome. Differences in cell energetics arise based on the physiology of any given condition, preexisting nutritional status, degree of inflammation, and nutritional intake. Understanding the impact that pathophysiologic conditions have on nutrient metabolism and body composition is key to providing optimal nutrition support. This is particularly true in situations where a sustained inflammatory response and its accompanying array of metabolic alterations is found. When such a state ensues, nutrition therapy must be aggressive to counter the catabolic nature of this response, yet judicious given the many inefficiencies in substrate metabolism that exist. The case study underscores the alterations in substrate metabolism that occur during metabolic stress and the clinical implications of increased energy expenditure, hyperglycemia, protein catabolism, and lipolysis when planning nutrition support.

Characteristics of the Inflammatory Response

The inflammatory response is a complex series of metabolic and physiologic changes that take place following major trauma, disease, sepsis, or surgery. It occurs when there is significant insult or injury to the cell. Extreme physiologic changes are seen at every major organ level, including cardiac, respiratory, and gastrointestinal. Regardless of the initial cause, the ensuing response is universally the same, driven by an inflated systemic immune response with macrophage activation and the subsequent release of pro-inflammatory mediators. These mediators upregulate acute-phase reactants with concomitant down-regulation of visceral proteins. Endocrine changes lead to an accelerated catabolic state with major changes in energy, protein, and substrate metabolism. Nutrition support is required to alleviate severe lean body mass (LBM) wasting.[1]

Ebb and Flow Phases

The inflammatory response occurs in two unique phases each with distinct characteristics (**Figure 5.1**). The ebb phase, sometimes referred to as the shock phase, immediately follows injury or physical stress. During the ebb phase, there is a redistribution of fluid that, when in conjunction with losses due to trauma, leads to hypovolemia. Extracellular water shifts primary from plasma to interstitial space, placing vital organs at risk due to inadequate blood flow. Tissue hypoxia due to diminished perfusion and decreased cardiac output follow, with the primary focus of care being fluid resuscitation to restore plasma volume. Decreased oxygen consumption and body temperature contribute to this pathophysiologic picture, which essentially renders a hypometabolic state. Historically, this phase lasts 24 to 72 hours while attempts are made to reestablish homeostasis.[2,3]

Subsequently, increased substrate mobilization and oxygen transport take place and the system enters the flow, or hypermetabolic, phase. This phase, which can last for several months postinjury as recovery takes place, comprises the majority of the inflammatory response. This response is considered a necessary mechanism for survival. Unfortunately, severe catabolism results, with profound wasting when the response is prolonged. Nutritional status deteriorates as the body shifts from normal homeostasis and anabolism to instead produce necessary proteins for tissue repair and immunity. Preserving

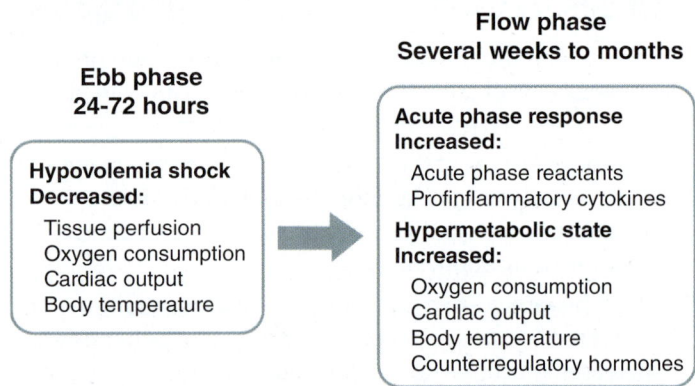

FIGURE 5.1 The Ebb and Flow Phase of the Inflammatory Response The ebb and flow phases are universal in their pattern of initial hypovolemia and decreased vital processes, followed by a hypermetabolic state which may be long lasting.

Chapter 5 Energy Expenditure and Body Composition in Metabolic Stress

CASE STUDY INTRODUCTION

Justin is a 35-year-old male who suffered major trauma following a motor vehicle accident on his way home from dinner. He is admitted into the emergency room with multiple long bone fractures and a crushing abdominal injury. He is accompanied by his wife and 2-year-old child, who were uninjured in the accident. Upon arrival to the intensive care unit, his vital signs and biochemical indices indicate he is hemodynamically unstable and in septic shock. Given his obesity, the team plans to hold off on nutrition support for now.

Anthropometric Data:
Height: 170 cm (67 in)
Weight: 96 kg (211 lbs)
Body mass index (BMI): 33.2 kg/m^2

Biochemical Data:
Sodium 135 (135-145 mEq/L)
Potassium 4.6 (3.6-5.0 mEq/L)
Chloride 99 (98-110 mEq/L)
Carbon dioxide 28 (20-30 mEq/L)
Blood urea nitrogen 17 (6-24 mg/dL)
Creatinine 1.3 (0.4-1.3 mg/dL)
Glucose 310 (70-139 mg/dL)

Calcium 7.2 (8.5-10.5 mEq/L)
Phosphorus 2.2 (2.7-4.5 mg/dL)
Magnesium 1.1 (1.3-2.1 mEq/L)
Albumin 1.4 (3.5-5.0 g/dL)

Clinical Data:
Past Medical History: None
Prior Medications: None

Vital Signs:
Blood pressure 87/52 mm Hg, Temperature 97°F, Mean arterial pressure 64 mm Hg, Pulse 58 beats beat/min

Nutrition-focused Physical Exam:
Obese appearing with abdominal and peripheral edema and poor capillary refill

Dietary Data:
Diet History: Unknown
Diet Prescription: NPO

Questions

1. How will Justin's physiology and metabolism change over the next 24 to 48 hours? How will it change over the next several weeks?
2. What is the impact of metabolic stress on energy expenditure and metabolism?
3. What laboratory values are of concern? How might they be explained? Which are a priority to address?
4. How might you describe his nutritional status? How might you describe his nutritional risk?

---

critical organs at the expense of skeletal muscle mass takes precedence. During this time, in addition to oxygen consumption, cardiac output and body temperature increase, pro-inflammatory cytokines, such as interleukin-1 (IL-1) and tumor necrosis factor (TNF), are released by the immune cells to regulate the host response to infection, inflammation, and trauma, acting on both at the endocrine and organ levels. A surge in counter-regulatory hormones to glucose and insulin, such as glucagon, cortisol, and growth hormone, stimulate gluconeogenesis and glycogen breakdown. Catecholamines such as epinephrine and norepinephrine are increased and mediate the aberrations seen in cell function and physiology.[3,4] **Figure 5.2** shows this cascade of events, which has considerable effects on energy and protein metabolism.

> **CORE CONCEPT 1**
>
> The inflammatory response transpires in two unique phases—the ebb and flow phases—each with distinct vital and physiologic characteristics.

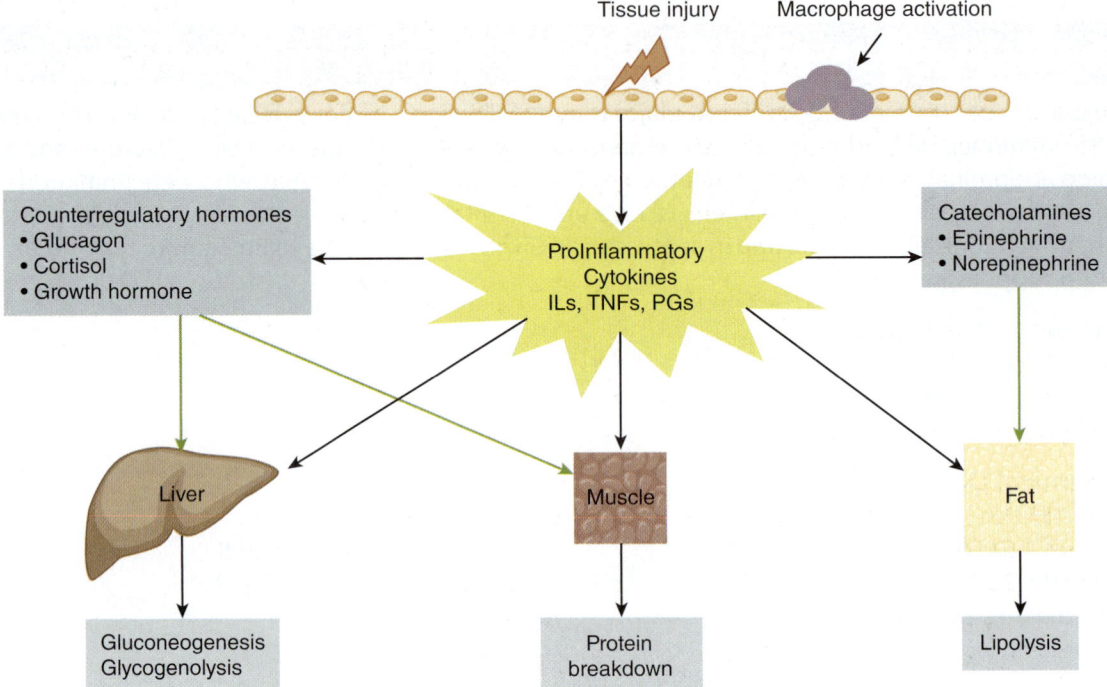

FIGURE 5.2 The Inflammatory Response to Cell Injury and Its Metabolic Sequalae Following injury, release of proinflammatory cytokines leads to a cascade of hormonal and neurologically driven metabolic pathways including gluconeogenesis, lipolysis and protein breakdown.

Alterations in Metabolism Associated with the Inflammatory Response

Energy Cost Associated with Altered Metabolism

Table 5.1 shows the energy cost associated with increased reliance on biochemical pathways including lipolysis, gluconeogenesis, and muscle protein breakdown. The cost of inefficient substrate recycling contributes to a 21% increase in energy expenditure above that of healthy individuals. Without consideration to other requirements such as wound healing and immunity, energy expenditure at baseline simply due to altered metabolism is greater than 50% above normal. The preponderance of counter-regulatory hormones and cytokines that stimulate increased reliance on these ATP-consuming biochemical pathways can be seen in **Table 5.2**. Glucagon, cortisol, and the catecholamines (epinephrine and norepinephrine) synergistically act to increase gluconeogenesis. Concurrently they promote insulin and growth hormone resistance, ensuring available amino acids and glucose for tissue and wound repair. Additional breakdown of endogenous adipose stores, mediated primarily by epinephrine and norepinephrine, complete the picture of this autocatabolism that favors injury repair and survival.[3,5,6]

> **CORE CONCEPT 2**
>
> Metabolic effects of the inflammatory response manifest as increased energy expenditure related to gluconeogenesis, protein synthesis and breakdown, and altered substrate utilization.

Hormonal and Metabolic Response to Stress Versus Starvation

Comparing stress to starvation essentially represents the difference between a state of adaptation, which occurs in starvation, and autocatabolism, which occurs in stress (**Figure 5.3**). In the later stages of starvation, after glycogen

TABLE 5.1 CONTRIBUTION OF ATP REQUIRING METABOLIC PATHWAYS TO INCREASED ENERGY EXPENDITURE

Biochemical pathway	Percentage Increase from Healthy
Protein synthesis	22
Urea synthesis	3
Gluconeogenesis	11
Substrate cycling Fat recycling Glycolytic-gluconeogenic	17 4
Total percent increase in energy expenditure	**57**

Modified from Yu YM, Tompkins RG, Ryan CM, Young VR. The metabolic basis of the increase of the increase in energy expenditure in severely burned patients. *JPEN J Parenter Enteral Nutr.* 1999;23(3):160-168.

TABLE 5.2 STRESS-INDUCED MEDIATORS OF CATABOLIC PATHWAYS FOR GLUCOSE, PROTEIN, AND FAT SUBSTRATE METABOLISM[6]

Hormone or Mediator	Mechanism
Glucagon	• Increased gluconeogenesis • Increased glycolysis
Cortisol	• Insulin resistance of skeletal muscle • Increased gluconeogenesis
Epinephrine	• Increased gluconeogenesis • Insulin resistance of skeletal muscle • Suppression of insulin secretion • Increased lipolysis • Increased free fatty acid release
Norepinephrine	• Increased gluconeogenesis • Increased lipolysis
Tumor necrosis factor	• Increased hepatic and skeletal muscle insulin resistance

stores have been depleted, gluconeogenesis provides necessary glucose for the brain and obligate users such as red blood cells and renal medulla. Energy expenditure is decreased to minimize loss of body stores, primarily LBM. Lipolysis increases with accompanying ketone production. Beta-hydroxybuterate is the ketone that becomes the primary fuel source for the brain. Muscle provides alanine as a source of glucose, but ultimately these biochemical pathways are kept to a minimum. Insulin levels are decreased due to the ultimate lack of substrate, and glucagon is increased to promote the gluconeogenesis and glycolysis that is needed.[7]

During stress, the body goes into a state of autocatabolism. Energy expenditure is increased, with glucose, amino acids, and fat all serving as primary fuel sources. Fat is broken down but rather than contributing to large ketone production, it is oxidized to support energy cost of gluconeogenesis. Much of the hydrolyzed fat enters a recycling process to ultimately be re-synthesized to triglyceride. Glucose production is increased. In the metabolically stressed state, insulin and glucagon are both increased. Insulin increases as the body tries to accommodate the increased hyperglycemia, but is ineffective. Protein breakdown is substantial. In addition to alanine, other amino acids that are likely needed during times of stress, such as glutamine, branched chain amino acids, and arginine, are released, leading further to the erosion of LBM.[8,9]

Glucose Metabolism and Stress Hyperglycemia

Abnormalities in glucose metabolism pose major obstacles in the clinical and nutritional management of patients undergoing metabolic stress. As described above, rates of gluconeogenesis are increased over normal states. This is accompanied by increased rates of glucose uptake and oxidation in the cell. However, the rate of glucose uptake relative to glucose production is impaired. This is due to an inability of insulin to suppress hepatic glucose production, as well as a blunting of insulin-mediated glucose uptake in peripheral tissues.[10,11]

CASE STUDY REVISITED

Due to his NPO status, Justin has essentially been in a fasting state for 5 days. Despite lack of nutritional intake, his blood sugars remain high. The medical student, suspecting Justin has an unknown history of prediabetes and metabolic syndrome, orders a serum triglyceride and cholesterol and a hemoglobin A1c. The results are as follows:

Biochemical Data:
Glucose 338 mg/dL (70-139 mg/dL)
Triglyceride 327 mg/dL (Desirable < 150 mg/dL)
Total Cholesterol 173 mg/dL (Desirable<200 mg/dL)
HDL Cholesterol 30 mg/dL (Desirable ≥40 mg/dL)

Hemoglobin A1C 5.8 (4.3-5.8%)
LDL Cholesterol 99 mg/dL (Desirable < 100 mg/dL)

Questions
1. Explain the disparity between Justin's blood sugar and HbA1c. Does Justin have prediabetes?
2. What is contributing to Justin's increased triglycerides?
3. Although Justin could be considered to be entering a semi-starvation state due to fasting, how does his metabolism differ due to metabolic stress?

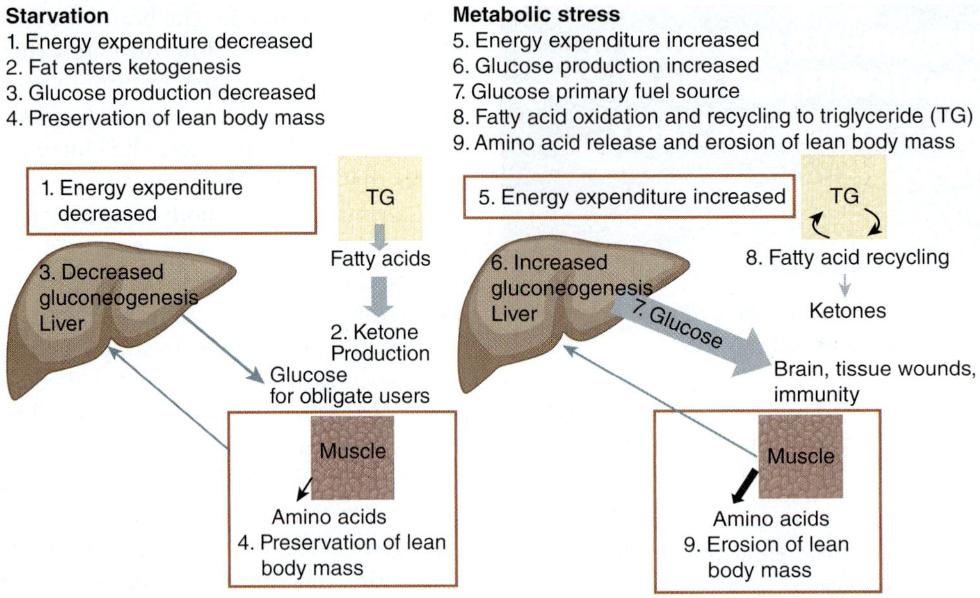

FIGURE 5.3 Metabolic Changes in Starvation Versus Stress Decreased energy expenditure and minimized gluconeogenesis help to preserve muscle mass while ketones provide glucose for obligate users. This process is reversed in stress, where energy expenditure and oxidation of substrate result in loss of muscle mass.

Starvation
1. Energy expenditure decreased
2. Fat enters ketogenesis
3. Glucose production decreased
4. Preservation of lean body mass

Metabolic stress
5. Energy expenditure increased
6. Glucose production increased
7. Glucose primary fuel source
8. Fatty acid oxidation and recycling to triglyceride (TG)
9. Amino acid release and erosion of lean body mass

The consequence of diminished insulin efficacy, or insulin resistance, is hyperglycemia. Unlike diabetes, "stress hyperglycemia" is associated with increased insulin production, but there is a relative insulin insufficiency related to increased glucose production.[12,13] This allows for greater glucose uptake in insulin-independent tissue. Because glucose is a main fuel source for non-insulin dependent cells such as wound and immune cells, this diversion of glucose through peripheral insulin resistance appears to be an inherent survival mechanism. As the proportion of hypoxic tissue and inflammatory cells such as macrophages and leukocytes increases, so does the rate of glucose production—hence the degree of **stress hyperglycemia** parallels the severity of injury.[3] Increases in glucose production up to 50% to 60% in septic patients and 100% in burn patients illustrate this concept. Use of insulin therapy can alleviate stress hyperglycemia. Once inside the cell, glucose utilization—as defined by glucose oxidation or the aerobic breakdown of glucose for the formation of ATP—is normal. Interestingly, despite increased glucose production, glucose oxidation in metabolic stress is similar to that in health. Stable isotope studies of glucose oxidation rates in metabolically stressed adult burn patients demonstrate that glucose oxidation is 5 mg carbohydrate/kg/min. Follow-up studies in critically ill children aged 2 to 18 years show a similar rate of glucose oxidation. Intakes of glucose beyond 5 mg carbohydrate/kg/min result in shunting of glucose to nonoxidative pathways, which may eventually lead to hepatic fat deposition.[10,11]

> **PRACTICE POINT**
>
> Glucose infusion rate during metabolic stress should rarely exceed 5 mg carbohydrate/kg/min.

> **CORE CONCEPT 3**
>
> Stress hyperglycemia is common during the inflammatory response, as a result of increased gluconeogenesis, increased glucagon-to-insulin ratio and predominance of other counter-regulatory hormones, and insulin resistance.

Protein Catabolic State

Many of the physiologic pathways that characterize the inflammatory response result in protein catabolism, or the release of amino acids for protein synthesis and glucose availability. The primary source of these amino acids is skeletal muscle.[14,15] During metabolic stress, rates of protein breakdown exceed rates of protein synthesis, resulting in a net negative protein balance.[16-18] Protein loss from skeletal muscle can be substantial, despite provision of nutrition, due to a regulated efflux of amino acids exceeding cellular influx.[19,20] Unfortunately, dietary protein alone cannot prevent protein catabolism. During critical illness, muscle wasting occurs quickly and if catabolism is prolonged, the extent of muscle loss is significant. Hormones such as insulin and insulin-like growth factor, growth hormone, oxandrolone, and propranolol serve as adjunctive therapy to nutritional support for reversal of net protein catabolism and muscle retention.[21-26]

> **CORE CONCEPT 4**
>
> Protein catabolism occurs in an effort to make acute-phase proteins and glucose. Muscle is the primary source of endogenous amino acids released in the body during stress for this use.

> **PRACTICE POINT**
>
> Serial measures of urinary urea nitrogen can help determine changes in protein catabolism and give an estimate of nitrogen balance.

Fat Metabolism and Lipolysis

Adipose tissue becomes metabolically active during the inflammatory response. Increased lipolysis (up to four times more than normal), mediated by stress hormones and inflammatory mediators, results in high levels of circulating triglycerides.[6] Triglycerides enter extrahepatic tissues and are hydrolyzed by lipoprotein lipase, releasing free fatty acids and glycerol. The increment in energy expenditure associated with free fatty acid turnover and oxidation is 130% of that in healthy individuals (as opposed to 33% and 41% above normal rates for glucose and protein oxidation, respectively).[6] **Table 5.3** shows the proportion of substrate oxidation to basal energy expenditure during health and stress. In healthy subjects, oxidation of glucose and protein combined contribute to 40% of energy expenditure, with fat making up the remaining 60%. Under stress conditions, fat metabolism accounts for up to 72% of total energy expenditure resulting in a relative decrease in the contribution of protein and carbohydrate. This table suggests that fat should be a predominant source

TABLE 5.3 RATE OF INCREASE IN SUBSTRATE OXIDATION AND CONTRIBUTION OF FAT, CARBOHYDRATE, AND PROTEIN TO TOTAL ENERGY EXPENDITURE

Substrate	Oxidation and turnover rate (percentage increase of health)	Percentage total energy expenditure (health)	Percentage total energy expenditure (stress)
Fat	132	60	72
Carbohydrate	33	25	17
Protein	41	15	11

CASE STUDY REVISITED

Seven days later, Justin is ready to begin nutrition support. You are consulted to provide an energy goal for Justin. He continues to be critically ill, septic, and metabolically stressed. His most recent weight (believed to be a dry weight) and labs are shown below.

Anthropometric Data:
Weight: 90 kg (198 lb)   Admission weight: 96 kg (211 lbs)
Height: 170 cm (67in)

Biochemical Data:
Sodium 136 mg/dL
Potassium 4.5 mg/dL
Blood urea nitrogen 10 mg/dL
Creatinine 1.1 mg/dL
Blood glucose 150 mg/dL

Calcium 8.2 mg/dL
Phosphorus 3.7 mg/dL
Magnesium 1.2 mg/dL

Clinical Data:
Key Medications: Oxandrolone, intravenous insulin infusion
Vitals: Blood pressure 160/64 mm Hg, Temperature 99°F, Mean arterial pressure 96 mm Hg
Pulse 75 beats per minute

Questions
1. What available methods exist to determine total energy expenditure in Justin?
2. What stress and activity factors are appropriate when using these methods?
3. Provide a goal for Justin's total energy requirement.
4. Indicate how each component of total energy expenditure is determined.

of energy provision in stressed individuals. However, although fatty acid oxidation is increased, the proportion of circulating fatty acids that are oxidized is blunted by the hyperinsulinemia and hyperglycemia that characterizes the stress response, resulting in significant recycling and deposition of fat in the liver.

Fat is poorly absorbed in metabolically stressed patients.[27] Other derangements include decreased synthesis of low-density and high-density lipoprotein fractions.[28] Increased triglyceride (TG) levels suggest that while fat stores are prone to lipolysis and free fatty acid release, they are not used to meet cellular energetics. This is further supported by carnitine deficiency and dysfunctional beta oxidation of fatty acids.[29] One theory is that hypertriglyceridemia may be protective because TG can neutralize and protect against the effects of endotoxins.[30]

CORE CONCEPT 5

During inflammatory stress, adipose tissue is metabolically active, as evidenced by increased serum lipolysis and fatty acid levels, although fatty acid oxidation can be impaired.

Determination of Energy Expenditure During Normal and Stressed Conditions

Total Energy Expenditure and Its Components

Total daily energy expenditure is comprised of three main components: basal metabolic rate, diet-induced thermogenesis, and activity energy expenditure (**Figure 5.4**). Basal metabolic rate (BMR) refers to energy expenditure associated with maintaining the metabolic activities of the body's cells and tissues.[31] These activities represent functions that are essential for life, such as cell function and replacement; hormone and protein synthesis; maintenance of body core temperature; and work associated with cardiac, respiratory, muscle, and brain function. BMR represents a postabsorptive state (for at least 12 to 14 hours) with the subjects lying supine, awake, in a thermoneutral environment. Measures of BMR should be at least 8 hours after physical activity and in the absence of mental or psychological stress. Once BMR is obtained, it can be expressed in kilocalories (kcal) per 24 hours, becoming then termed basal energy expenditure (BEE). Major determinants of BMR are age, gender, weight, and height. These indicators essentially serve as proxies for differences in body composition, primarily with respect to body cell mass (BCM), which encompasses all metabolically active tissue. BCM accounts for approximately 60% to 70% of BMR. Age-related differences can be appreciated throughout the lifecycle. A larger BMR per unit of body weight in neonates through infancy is attributable to a relatively larger brain, skin, and viscera than in older children and adults. Although skeletal mass is less during the infancy stages, deposition of LBM with rapid growth also contributes to increased BMR per unit of body weight. Thereafter, age-associated changes in BMR include decrease in BMR that is associated with a decline in LBM as a result of less activity. In older adults who are more active, BMR may be higher.[31]

CORE CONCEPT 6

Basal metabolic rate is primarily determined by body cell mass, the metabolically active component of the body.

Certain conditions in health can contribute to increases in BMR that are unrelated to BCM, such as deposition of tissue during growth, pregnancy, and lactation. During pregnancy, the energy required for growth of the fetus increases and maternal metabolism changes. Milk production during lactation also increases BMR. Thermoregulation can also contribute to energy expenditure. Usually this is minor, because humans can adjust clothing and environment to maintain ambient temperature, but in some conditions, such as burn injury, where extensive water losses result in evaporative cooling and a drop in body core temperature, energy associated with thermoregulation is more prominent.

Diet-induced thermogenesis (DIT), also referred to as the thermic effect of feeding, is the production of heat associated with the digestion and metabolism of food. This includes energy required for absorption, transport, cellular oxidation, and nutrient deposition. Although it is the smallest component of the three main contributing factors to TEE, DIT can be significant in the development of obesity. DIT is most often determined by measuring resting energy expenditure before and after a meal using indirect calorimetry. DIT can also be measured in a respiratory chamber, allowing for timing and duration of postprandial response. DIT increases TEE by 8% to 10% of BMR over a 24-hour period in a healthy individual eating a normal mixed diet. Diet composition differentially effects DIT, with protein and alcohol resulting in the largest increase in DIT and carbohydrate and fat contributing the least to DIT. Other factors that can alter DIT include weight gain (increase) or weight loss (decrease), intermittent versus continuous feeding (with DIT significantly reduced with continuous feeds), and ambient temperature.[31]

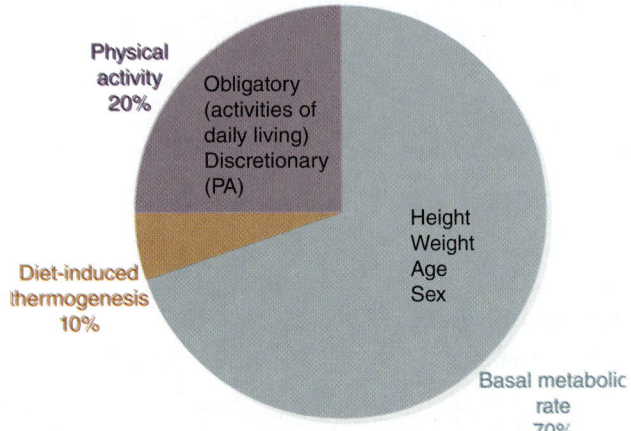

FIGURE 5.4 Components of Total Energy Expenditure Total energy expenditure is comprised of basal metabolic rate, diet-induced thermogenesis and physical activity.

Activity energy expenditure (AEE) is the energy expenditure associated with physical activity. In healthy individuals, this can be the second largest (after BMR), albeit most variable, component of TEE. AEE includes both obligatory physical activity and discretionary physical activity. Obligatory physical activity includes daily activities such as going to work or school, tending to children, household activities, and other demands an individual faces from their environment. Discretionary activities are not imposed on the individual, but rather are chosen for recreational or physical fitness. This component of AEE can vary dramatically based on the type, frequency, and intensity of activity.[32]

■ **CORE CONCEPT 7**

Total energy expenditure is composed primarily of basal metabolic rate, energy cost of physical activity, and diet-induced thermogenesis.

Estimating Total Energy Expenditure

Factorial Approach to Determining Energy Requirements Under Normal Conditions

Other than in research settings, total energy expenditure is typically estimated using a factorial approach. Here, a value for BMR can be obtained according to standard evidence-based references that incorporate weight, height, age, and gender. Table 5.4 shows equations for BEE throughout the lifespan. Additional factors are used to account primarily for physical activity. In normal, healthy individuals, energy cost associated with activities such as sleep, rest, work, leisure, and physical activity can be calculated to determine their physical activity ratio. For simplicity, physical activity levels (PALs) are assigned according to the general classification of light, moderate, or heavy. Table 5.5 shows the range of PALs within each lifestyle. Therefore, calculation of TEE in adults can be done easily using the equation BEE × PAL = TEE. For example, TEE for a female who is 52 years old, weighs 65 kg, and lives a sedentary lifestyle is 1372 (BMR) × 1.5 (PAL) = 2060 kcals/day. Although diet-induced thermogenesis is a component of total energy expen-

TABLE 5.5 PHYSICAL ACTIVITY LEVEL (PAL) BASED ON LIFESTYLE

Lifestyle	PAL Mean	PAL Range
Sedentary or light activity	1.25	1.0-1.30
Low Active	1.5	1.4-1.59
Active	1.75	1.6-1.89
Very Active	2.2	1.9-2.49

Modified from *Human energy requirements*. Report of the joint FAO/WHO/UNU Expert Consultation, Rome 17-24;October 2001.

TABLE 5.4 ESTIMATION OF BEE OR REE BY AGE AND GENDER IN HEALTHY INDIVIDUALS

Reference	Age (years)	Equation
Schofield[34]	0-3	M: 60.9W − 54 F: 61W − 51
	3-10	M: 22.7W + 495 F: 22.5W + 499
	10-18	M: 17.5W + 651 F: 12.2W + 746
	18-30	M: 15.3W + 679 F: 14.7W + 496
	30-60	M: 11.6W + 879.1 F: 8.7W + 829
	>60	M: 13.5W + 487.7 F: 10.5W + 596
Mifflin–St Jeor[35]	>18	M: 10(W) + 6.25 (H) − 5(A) + 5 W: 10(W) + 6.25 (H) − 5(A) − 16
Harris–Benedict[36]	>18	M: 66 + (13.7 W) + (5 H) − (6.8 A) F: 655 + (9.7 W) + (1.85H) − (4.7A)

Equations estimate basal energy expenditure except in the case of Mifflin-St Jeor which represents resting energy expenditure
Note: M= Male; F= Female; W = weight in kg; H = height in cm; A = age in years

diture, due to it's variability, it is often not incorporated into routine estimates of daily energy expenditure. In children, calculating energy requirements using this method does not incorporate energy cost associated with deposition of tissue and bone during growth. The Dietary Reference Intakes (DRIs) provide estimated energy requirements (EERs), which in children is the sum of TEE and energy deposition. An additional physical activity factor can be added for children 3 years and older (**Tables 5.6** and **5.7**).[31-36]

During critical illness, use of DRI for estimates of TEE is not recommended. Energy expenditure under these conditions does not parallel values obtained in healthy individuals. DRIs do not incorporate energy cost associated with metabolic stress and critical illness. Furthermore, DRIs incorporate increased needs for tissue building such as during growth and pregnancy and variations in activity level. These do not consistently apply in hospitalized, metabolically stressed, and often bedridden individuals. Energy devoted to activities such as growth and tissue deposition may be thwarted temporarily for the purpose of survival and recovery during illness. For example, growth in children who are physiologically stressed (such as in burn injury or congenital defects) is impeded until a later time with recovery.[37,38] For them, TEE is best estimated using BMR with stress factors associated with their condition until it is resolved or corrected.

Factorial Approach in Determining TEE in Hospitalized, Metabolically Stressed Patients

Achieving optimal conditions for true measure of BMR is difficult, particularly in a hospitalized setting; therefore, resting energy expenditure (REE) is most commonly described and used in these equations. REE represents the amount of calories required by the body at rest over a 24-hour period (Table 5.4). REE very closely represents BMR, and typically represents 60% to 70% of TEE.[31] Empirically derived estimates of REE poorly correlate with measured REE in stressed patients, a finding that has been consistent in the scientific literature. Prediction accuracy of most formulas rarely falls within 10% of measured REE.[39,40] This can be explained by the fact that in many disease states, particularly those associated with an inflammatory response, an additional component of TEE emerges representing increased energy requirement associated with metabolic stress. Actual measures of REE "capture" this additional component of stress, whereas when using the factorial approach, this component must be estimated and added on as a stress factor (**Table 5.8**). **Figure 5.5** illustrates the factors contributing to each component of TEE in a metabolically stressed, hospitalized individual.

As can be seen, while the stress component increases, AEE and DIT decrease. The decrease in AEE is primarily due to limited physical activity other than that associated with physical therapy and positioning.[41] Decline in DIT is most often attributed to a lower energy cost of nutrient storage and retrieval when administering nutrition continuously.[35] Although diet-induced thermogenesis is a component of total energy expenditure, due to it's variability, it is often not incorporated into routine estimates of daily energy expenditure.

Numerous predictive equations exist for energy assessment during critical illness (**Table 5.9**).[36,42-45] These equations vary based on the number of subjects used to develop them, as well as the subject's medical or clinical condition. The larger the study population, the greater likelihood of predictive accuracy of the equation. Similarly, it is useful to choose equations developed in the population type representative of the patient of interest. For example, equations such as the Penn State equation are best to use in critically ill, mechanically ventilated patients.

TABLE 5.6 ESTIMATED ENERGY REQUIREMENTS IN CHILDREN

Age	EER = TEE + Energy Deposition
0-3 months	(89W − 100) + 175
4-6 months	(89W − 100) + 56
7-12 months	(89W − 100) + 22
13-35 months	(89W − 100) + 20
3-8 years	M: 88.5 − (61.9 × A) + PA × (26.7 × W) + (903 × H) + 20 F: 135.3 − (30.8 × A) + PA × (10 × W) + (934 × H) + 20
9-18 years	M: 88.5 − (61.9 × A) + PA × (26.7 × W) + (903 × H) + 25 F: 135.3 − (30.8 × A) + PA × (10 × W) + (934 H) + 25

Note: M = Male; F = Female; W = weight in kg; H = height in cm; A = age in years
Modified from *Human energy requirements*. Report of the joint FAO/WHO/UNU Expert Consultation, Rome 17-24;October 2001.

TABLE 5.7 PHYSICAL ACTIVITY COEFFICIENTS IN CHILDREN AGED 3 TO 18 YEARS

Activity Level	Physical Activity Factor
Sedentary	M: 1.00 F: 1.00
Low	M: 1.13 F: 1.16
Active	M: 1.26 F: 1.31
Very Active	M: 1.42 F: 1.56

TABLE 5.8 STRESS AND ACTIVITY FACTORS FOR USE WITH PREDICTIVE EQUATIONS

Activity level	Factor
Bed rest	1-1.2 [hospitalized]
Ambulatory	1.3
Fever	12% increase in REE for every degree >37°C
Disease/condition	
Minor surgery	1.1-1.3
Mild/moderate stress	1.1-1.2
Infection	1.3
Long bone fracture	1.3
Major surgery	1.5
Major trauma	1.5-1.7
Sepsis	1.2-1.5
Burn injury	1.5-2.0
Closed head injury	1.3-1.5
Cardiac failure	1.0-1.3

When relying on standardized equations, prediction of REE, which is highly variable, is required, as well as factors associated metabolic stress of disease and AEE. Some of these equations regard clinical status by incorporating factors that would impact REE, such as temperature and ventilatory variables. However, during critical illness, clinical status is inconstant from day to day and patient to patient, and general stress factors may not capture these differences.[40,47] Measurement of energy expenditure to guide nutrition support in these patients is associated with reduced mortality.[48] Clinical conditions that can have changeable effects on energy expenditure are shown in **Table 5.10**. Clinical interventions targeting infection control, pain management, and anxiety reduce energy expenditure, while sepsis, fever, and respiratory effort increase energy expenditure.

> **PRACTICE POINT**
>
> Energy goals should be routinely reassessed to accommodate changes in the patient's clinical condition that may alter energy expenditure.

Measuring Energy Expenditure—Direct and Indirect Calorimetry

Use of calorimetry to determine energy expenditure is based on the construct that human metabolism involves the combustion of nutrients, a process that requires oxygen and produces carbon dioxide (which is eventually eliminated) and heat (which is used for cellular processes). Calorimetry relies on the first principle of thermodynamics, which states that energy cannot be created or destroyed, only transferred. A number of methods can be employed for determining TEE via calorimetry.

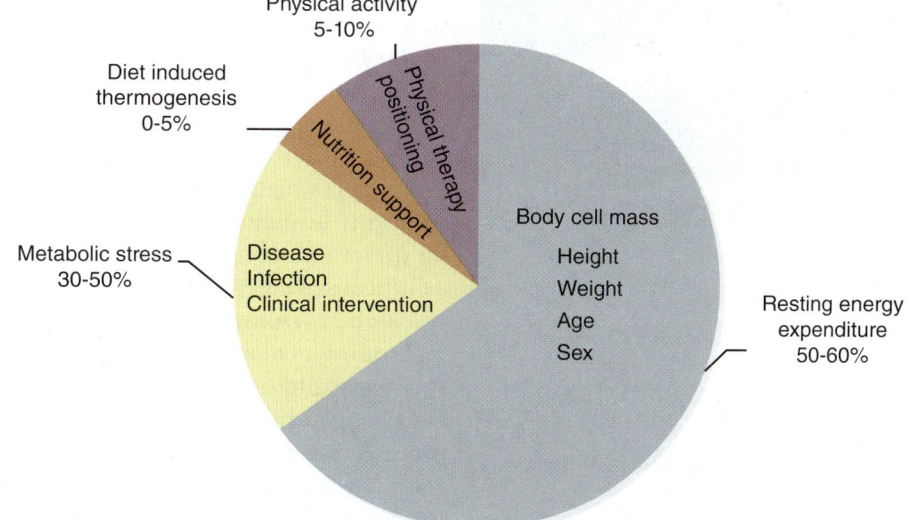

FIGURE 5.5 Components of Total Energy Expenditure During Metabolic Stress While the stress component increases, AEE and DIT decrease. The decrease in AEE is primarily due to limited physical activity other than that associated with physical therapy and positioning.[41] Decline in DIT is most often attributed to a lower energy cost of nutrient storage and retrieval when administering nutrition continuously.[35]

TABLE 5.9 PREDICTIVE EQUATIONS USED DURING CRITICAL ILLNESS AND METABOLIC STRESS

Source	Population	TEE Component Measured	Equation
Harris–Benedict[36]	N = 239 healthy subjects	BEE	M: 66 + (13.7 W) + (5 H) − (6.8 A) F: 655 + (9.7 W) + (1.85H) − (4.7A)
Revised Harris–Benedict[42]	N = 239 healthy subjects from original study plus additional 98 healthy subjects		M: 88 + (13.4W) + (5H) − (5.7A) F: 448 + (9.2W) + (3H) − (4.3A)
Mifflin–St Jeor[35]	N = 498 healthy subjects	REE	M: 10(W) + 6.25 (H) − 5(A) + 5 W: 10(W) + 6.25 (H) − 5(A) − 16
Penn State 2003b	N = 74 mechanically ventilated trauma/medical/surgical patients	REE, metabolic stress	Mifflin Equation (0.96) + Tmax (167) + VE (31) − 6212
Penn State 2010	N = 50 mechanically ventilated trauma/medical/surgical patients		Mifflin Equation (0.71) + VE (64) + TMax (85) − 3085
Swinamer[45]	N = 112 mechanically ventilated, critically ill trauma/medical/surgical patients	REE, metabolic stress	(945 BSA) − (6.4A) + (108T) = (24.2RR) + (817 Vt) − 4349
American College of Chest Physicians[46]	29 mechanically ventilated patients aged 16–79 years	TEE	25 W If BMI 16-25 use UBW If BMI >25 use IBW If BMI <16 use existing weight for 7-10 days, then use IBW

Note: M = Male; F = Female: W = weight in kg; H = height in cm; A = age in years; Tmax = maximum body temperature in the previous 24 hours (degrees Centigrade). Ve = minute ventilation recorded from ventilator in L per minute.; BSA = Body Surface Area

TABLE 5.10 CLINICAL FACTORS THAT CONTRIBUTE TO STRESS FACTOR IN ESTIMATING ENERGY EXPENDITURE

Decrease	Increase
Heated environment	Sepsis
Infection control	Fever
Pain control	Increased work of breathing
Sedation	Psychological stress/snxiety
Medications: Adrenergic blockade, muscle relaxants, opiates, barbituates, antipyretics	Medications: Epinephrine

One method, direct calorimetry, involves the direct measurement of heat produced or lost from this combustion reaction. Considered the gold standard, direct calorimetry assumes that metabolic rate is the sum of heat production and work of physical activity. In controlled circumstances, where the subject is not performing work of physical activity, the heat loss is considered to represent the subject's metabolic rate. Direct calorimetry requires the subject to be contained in a thermally controlled chamber for direct measure of heat produced. This is impractical in a clinical setting, making this tool more likely to exist in a research environment.[49]

Indirect calorimetry (IC) is the measure of respiratory gas exchange. In this process, volume of oxygen (VO_2) consumed and volume of carbon dioxide (VCO_2) produced is determined. These variables can be used to calculate both respiratory quotient and energy expenditure using calorimetric equations. Doubly labeled water (DLW) is a form of indirect calorimetry. It is based on the assumption of an exponential disappearance of hydrogen and oxygen isotopes from the body. Because oxygen

Clinical Roundtable

Topic: Predictive Equations: Which Weight Should be Used?

Background: Formulas for predicting energy requirements require inclusion of a patient's weight. Unfortunately, actual weight upon assessment may be unknown or skewed by edema or fluid overload. Many patients upon admission may have already experienced weight loss, which could be mild, moderate, or severe, designating some to a malnourished status in which weight gain is desired. In obese patients, using actual weight may lead to overestimation of energy requirements. The latter has prompted the use of adjusted body weight, which is the use of ideal body weight adjusted with a 25% increase to account for increased fat-free mass associated with obesity. Unfortunately, research evidence does not support the use of adjusted body weight, nor is it definitive as to which weight to use for estimating energy needs.

Roundtable Discussion:

Consider the use of actual, usual, ideal, and adjusted body weight when using predictive equations in critically ill patients.

1. When might you use each?
2. What are the risks or possible negative outcomes associated with your choices?
3. How might the weight you use alter the stress factor, if any, that you select?

atoms in exhaled carbon dioxide and body water are in isotopic equilibrium, the kinetics of water elimination and respiration are interdependent. Experimentally, a dose of water containing the combined stable isotopes deuterium oxide and oxygen 18 (hence doubly labeled water or D_2O^{18}) is consumed. Following equilibrium, DLW is eliminated from the body in the urine and breath. The H_2O^{18} is eliminated as both CO_2 and H_2O, while the D_2O is eliminated only as H_2O. Thus, the difference between these elimination rates is a measure of CO_2 flux, which can be related to energy expenditure using standard calorimetric equations (**Figure 5.6**).[50]

DLW is well validated for reproducibility and its ability to determine longitudinal changes in energy expenditure, intake, and body composition.[51] It serves as the gold standard by which other methods of determining TEE are compared. DLW provides an estimation of TEE over a period of 1 to 3 weeks, ideal for the study of energy

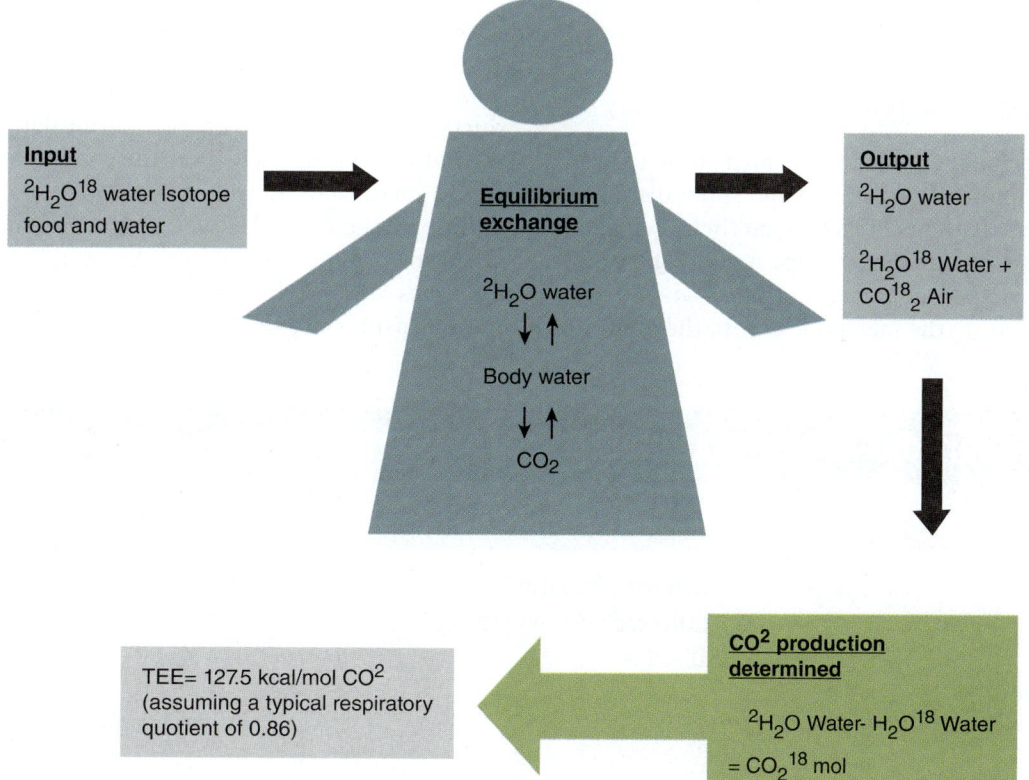

FIGURE 5.6 Doubly Labeled Water Method The doubly labeled water method measures elimination of CO_2 (in both air and water) and H_2O (water only) to determine, through subtraction, CO_2 production. CO_2 production is then used to calculate total energy expenditure.

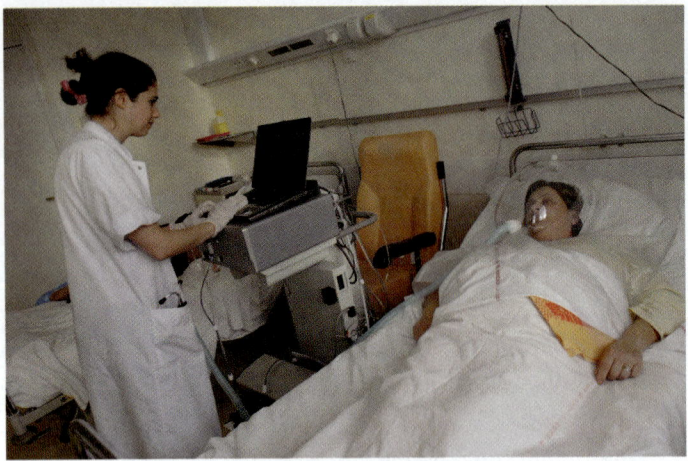

FIGURE 5.7 Indirect Calorimetry in Spontaneously Breathing Patient Using a Canopy Hood
© BSIP / Contributor/Getty Images.

metabolism in free-living individuals. The DLW method does rely on certain assumptions, including a constant rate of CO_2 production and a constant total body water pool. These assumptions can be confounded in patients with respiratory failure or significant evaporative water losses, as might be the case in patients with large wounds or burn injury. Combined with its expense and turnover time for results, it is not ideal in a clinical setting.

The more common form of IC in a hospital setting is the use of a portable "metabolic cart." In this form of IC, measures of VO_2 and VCO_2 in mL/min are obtained through breath analysis. These values are used to calculate REE using the Weir equation[52]:

Abbreviated Weir Equation:

REE (kcal/d) = 1.44 ([3.9 × VO_2] + [1.1 × VCO_2])

Indirect calorimetry can be performed at the bedside in both mechanically ventilated and spontaneously breathing patients. Patients breathing on their own can be measured using an attached canopy hood (**Figure 5.7**). Patients who are on a mechanical ventilator can be measured by attaching the metabolic cart to the expiratory port of a mechanical ventilator. Mechanically ventilated patients with a partial fraction of oxygen (FiO_2) greater than 60% should not be measured. Strategies for successful IC measurement are shown in **Table 5.11**. Breath-to-breath measures are captured and provided in minute-by-minute intervals. Ideally, measurements should be taken for a minimum of 30 minutes once a steady state has been achieved (as defined by less than a 10% minute-to-minute variability). Steady state measures, while important, are difficult to obtain in a clinical environment, which is a common frustration among clinicians. Studies looking at the validity of shorter measurements may offer ease and practicality in the future.[53]

Because measured REE (MREE) encompasses increases in REE due to inflammation and stress, it is greater than predicted REE (PREE). PREE requires an additional factor to account for these variables of stress that are not included in its estimate. The clear advantage of using MREE is the actual measurement of the stress associated with the disease as opposed to an estimated stress factor component that is prone to error. Usually, as a result, MREE in the metabolically stressed population represents up to 90% of TEE. **Figure 5.8** shows the elements captured by MREE. As components of metabolic stress, factors such as fever, pain, anxiety, and respiratory stress are measured. Additionally, if the patient is measured in a fed state (or during continuous feeding, which is customary), DIT is included in the measurement as well. By virtue of the fact that a larger component of TEE is actually measured versus estimated, indirect calorimetry provides greater accuracy than predictive equations.[54-56] However, while most of TEE is captured by indirect calorimetry, MREE represents a moment in time (as opposed to a 24-hour measurement). Changes that occur in the components of metabolic stress during the day (such as change in ventilator status, fever, or feeding regimen) will alter the validity of MREE. Therefore, a small factor must be incorporated to account for additional "activities" as well as changes that take place when the patient is not at rest. A common factor for this is 1.2 times MREE, which has been shown to compare well with measures of TEE.[57,58]

TABLE 5.11 CONDITIONS FOR OPTIMAL INDIRECT CALORIMETRY MEASUREMENT

Indirect Calorimetry Device	Patient Status	Environment
Precise calibration	• Stable respiratory status • Positive end expiratory pressure >12 • FiO_2 <60%	Thermoneutral
Adequate machine warm-up	Hemodynamically stable	Same setting for past 2 hours
Steady state achieved	No airway leaks, chest tubes	At least 24 hours postoperative

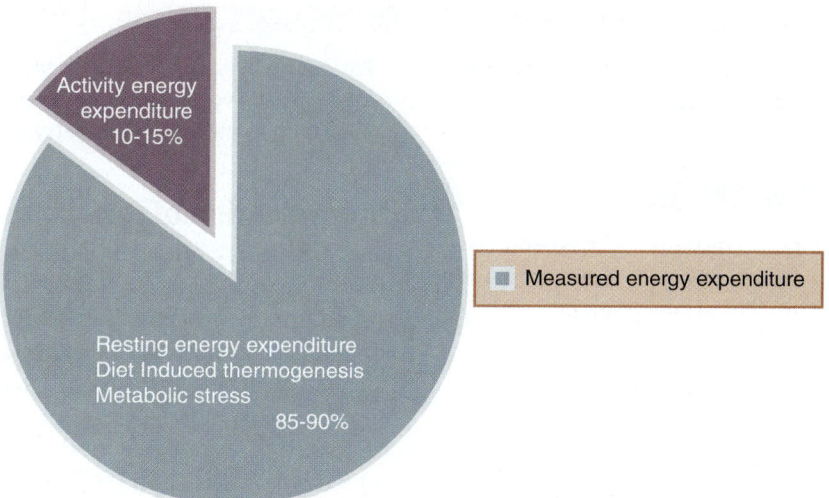

FIGURE 5.8 **Components of Energy Expenditure Captured by Indirect Calorimetry** Measures of resting energy expenditure (MREE) incorporate the stress of disease and diet induced thermogenesis. By capturing these elements, only physical activity must be estimated and included with MREE to determine total energy expenditure.

CASE STUDY REVISITED

Justin is established on a nutrition support regimen of enteral tube feedings per your recommendations. After 4 weeks of intensive care, the team is concerned because Justin's wounds are not healing well. The nurses measure his weight and he has lost 3 kg (6.6 lbs). The team consults you for a reassessment of energy requirements using indirect calorimetry. Your findings are below.

Anthropometric Data:
Weight: 87 kg (191 lbs)   Last weight: 90 kg (198 lbs)

Estimated Goals Upon Initial Assessment:
Energy goal = BEE of 1632 × 1.5 (stress factor) = 2448
Protein goal (based on 2.0 g/kg) =145 g/day

Nutrition Support Regimen:
Enteral tube feedings at goal rate = 2500 kcals/148 g protein
You perform indirect calorimetry and obtain the results below.

Indirect Calorimetry Results:
Patient was measured while on continuous tube feedings, rested, on a mechanical ventilator. Following achievement of a steady state, a 40-minute measurement was performed. Conditions for measurement are considered to be ideal; the results are presumed to be accurate.
MREE: 2500 kcals
Respiratory quotient (RQ): 0.75

Questions
1. What are the reasons for the difference in your MREE and your predicted BEE previously?
2. What information can you gain by your RQ? Are you under- or overfeeding your patient?
3. What stress factor if any will you use to adjust your IC measurement?
4. What is your new estimation for Justin's energy requirement?

> **PRACTICE POINT**
>
> A factor of 1.2 times MREE by indirect calorimetry may need to be used to accommodate for "physical activity."

> **CORE CONCEPT 8**
>
> During the inflammatory response, resting energy expenditure incorporates the energy cost associated with the physiologic and metabolic stress of disease and clinical interventions.

Use of Indirect Calorimetry to Prevent Over- and Underfeeding

Not surprisingly, studies show that predictive equations in critically ill, metabolically stressed patients are inaccurate. Because they both under- and overestimate measured REE, they contribute to morbidity risk factors such as hyperglycemia, hepatic steatosis, and difficulty weaning from the ventilator in the case of overfeeding. In the case of underfeeding, malnutrition, prolonged intensive care stay, impaired immune function, and delayed healing can occur. Nutrition support regimens guided by energy prescription according to IC measures of REE show improved mortality and outcomes.[49] Current guidelines suggest measurement of energy expenditure whenever possible.[59] It is understood that not all patient care settings have the resource or expertise for routine measurement of energy expenditure. Patients who benefit the most from measured energy expenditure include malnourished or obese, critically ill, and mechanically ventilated.

> **PRACTICE POINT**
>
> Patients who are malnourished, obese, or critically ill and mechanically ventilated should have their energy expenditure measured by indirect calorimetry when possible.

Interpretation of Respiratory Quotient

The respiratory quotient (RQ) is a measure of VCO_2/VO_2 and is useful for interpretation of both composition and adequacy of feeds. **Table 5.12** shows the physiologic range of RQs and their interpretation. RQ values for pure fat, protein, and carbohydrate oxidation are shown. When measuring a patient on a mixed diet, RQ values are usually in the range of 0.85 to 087; in fed patients, RQ values of less than 0.67 are considered nonphysiologic and suggest the need for a repeated measure. RQ values when fat oxidation is increased may represent a hypocaloric state leading to accelerated fat oxidation and ketogenesis. This clinical finding may warrant increase in caloric intake or a change in composition of the diet to include more carbohydrate as opposed to fat. Because lipogenesis results in increased CO_2 production, RQ is increased. When RQ values exceed 1.0, feedings may need to be decreased to avoid the consequences both of hepatic fat deposition and excessive CO_2 production on respiratory function.[60]

While interpretation of RQ is useful to determine dietary intake and substrate utilization, a number of nonnutritional factors influence the VCO_2 and therefore RQ. Among these are hyper- or hypoventilation and

---

⚠ Clinical Controversy

Hypocaloric versus Normocaloric Feeds in Critically Ill Patients

When rounding with the medical team on the ICU, the medical team questions the use of a hypocaloric feeding for a patient who is critically ill. Although you routinely use indirect calorimetry to determine feeding goals, you are asked whether the patient might have a better outcome when fed at 60% to 70% of energy goal. You let them know you will review the literature and return with your recommendation.

Optimal provision of calorie targets in metabolically stressed patients remains elusive. While consensus exists on the negative impact of overfeeding, eucaloric versus hypocaloric feeding continues to be debated. A study by Singer, et al. demonstrated the benefit of matching energy intakes with frequent, routine measures of indirect calorimetry on hospital mortality.

Conversely, Arabi et al. showed that hospital mortality was significantly lower in permissive underfeeding designed to provide 60% to 70% of calorie target. Using the two journal papers described, critically review study design, research findings, and conclusions. Based on the evidence, what is your recommendation for feeding your patient? Provide a persuasive argument and rationale for your decision.

References

1. Singer, P., Anbar, R., Cohen, J. et al. The tight calorie control study (TICACOS): a prospective, randomized, controlled pilot study of nutritional support in critically ill patients. *Intensive Care Med* (2011) 37: 601
2. Arabi, Y.M., Tamim, H.M., Dhar, G.S. et al. Permissive and Intensive Insulin Therapy in Critically Ill Patients. *Am J Clin Nutr* 2011;93:569-77

TABLE 5.12 RQ VALUES FOR AND INTERPRETATION FOR SUBSTRATE UTILIZATION

RQ value	Interpretation
<0.67	Nonphysiologic
0.7	Fat oxidation
0.8	Protein oxidation
0.85–0.87	Mixed diet
1.0	Carbohydrate Oxidation
>1.0	Lipogenesis

acid–base balance, where RQ is altered in response to shifts in associated respiratory dynamics and CO_2 elimination. Nutritional factors such as high carbohydrate feedings; inefficient substrate utilization; use of alternative, nonoxidative pathways; and defects in fat metabolism can also result in misinterpretation of the energy adequacy of feedings. Optimal interpretation of RQ requires a comprehensive look at all potential clinical and nutritional factors that may influence results as well as energy balance as indicated by daily intake and MREE.

Determination of Body Composition and Its Components During Metabolic Stress

Traditional Assessment of Nutritional Status

The systemic inflammatory response, when prolonged, can have devastating impact on nutritional status. While nutritional support of metabolically stressed patients is a priority in care planning, appropriate indicators for assessing nutritional adequacy are lacking. Among those most commonly used are measures of weight, energy, or nitrogen balance, and biochemical indices such as levels of visceral proteins. These indicators provide only crude estimates of nutritional status because they rely on many assumptions that are inaccurate in metabolically stressed patients. For example, measures of total body weight or weight changes as proxies for the adequacy of nutritional intake are usually confounded and complicated by derangements in fluid homeostasis. Overexpansion of fluid volume and weight gain may result even while tissue stores are being depleted. Protein nutritional status is also difficult to measure.

Hypoalbuminemia is the result of hemodilution, leakage from wound exudate, and marked protein catabolism, which includes enhanced albumin degradation. This is concurrent with diminished albumin synthesis due to the acute-phase response, making albumin a poor marker of protein nutritional status in stressed patients. Other

CASE STUDY REVISITED

After 3 weeks on his new regimen of increased feeds based on your IC measures, Justin still is not healing well. Along with a prealbumin, you order a 24-hour urine for urinary urea excretion (UUN) for calculation of nitrogen balance. The results are below.

Anthropometric:
Weight: 89 kg (196 lbs)   Last weight: 87 kg (191 lbs)

Biochemical:
Prealbumin 7 mg/dL
Nitrogen balance 1.3 g protein/kg/day

Questions

1. What are the limitations of each of these measures?
2. How do you explain the increase in weight despite the indices for protein status?
3. What is the most important component of body composition to maintain?
4. What tools are available to determine body composition and its change in a hospital versus a research setting?

serum proteins, such as retinol binding protein, transthyretin (prealbumin), sex hormone–binding globulin, fibronectin, and somatomedin C, have shorter half-lives and thus are more sensitive indicators of protein nutritional status. However, their production is also affected by the acute-phase response. Moreover, gains in these clinical markers do not necessarily correspond with improved clinical outcomes.[61]

Nitrogen balance studies are often flawed by overestimates of nitrogen intake and underestimation of nitrogen output, which lead to falsely positive results. Nitrogen balance is also a poor predictor of protein metabolic state as measured by isotope kinetics.[62] Isotopic amino acid kinetic studies have been used to determine rates of protein synthesis and breakdown during illness or in response to a specific dietary intervention. They provide valuable information about the alterations in metabolism that accompany the stress response. Comparisons of the relative rates of protein synthesis and breakdown only imply the extent of protein catabolism or anabolism that may be associated with nutritional therapy, but do not quantify changes in lean tissue.[63] Changes in body composition throughout the course of hospital stay are not routinely assessed in metabolically stressed patients, despite the common understanding that losses in LBM are associated with adverse clinical outcomes in other diseased populations.[64] A lack of reliable tools for measuring body composition at the beside is largely to blame. Given that most metabolically stressed patients are too ill to be transported to a lab for more sophisticated and accurate techniques, body composition and its change go unmeasured.

Models of Body Composition

Understanding the body's composition and its alterations during disease is fundamental for proper nutritional assessment and for gaging the efficacy of diet therapy. Various models for the analysis of body composition exist based on elemental, anatomical, or hydrational compartmentalization of the body.[65] While use of these sophisticated multicompartment methods of body composition analysis is predominately limited to a research environment, certain less-invasive techniques such as anthropometry, bioelectrical impedance, dual energy absorptiometry, stable isotope technology, and imaging techniques have been validated, enabling them to be applied in a clinical setting. When interpreted appropriately, they give the clinician tools for measuring patient progress and outcome.

Anthropometry

The simplest model, and one that is most commonly utilized in a clinical setting, is total body weight. A common misconception occurs when expansion of fluid volume results in weight gain, even while tissue stores are being depleted. Despite this, measures of total body weight remain clinically useful, particularly when taken routinely so that trends can be followed.

Body mass index (BMI), which is an index of weight proportional to height, does not measure body composition; however, it is used to screen for obesity, which is a measure of body fatness. BMI is imprecise as a measure of body composition due to differences in muscle mass, age, gender, and ethnicity. Muscle mass as a component of weight can vary dramatically among the individuals of the same height. In this context, BMI may falsely identify obesity among individuals with increased muscle mass. While BMI is useful in defining obesity in groups, it is inaccurate as a measure of body fat in the individual and varies significantly in response to age and gender.[66-68]

Anthropometric tools such as skinfold thickness and circumference measures continue to be used in clinical practice. Although as a means of body composition analysis they are criticized for their lack of precision and large interrater variability, they can be successfully applied as a screening tool, to evaluate change in nutritional status, and to diagnose malnutrition. Their advantages are simplicity, portability, and low cost. Combined measures of circumferences such as mid-upper arm circumference (MUAC) and skinfold thickness allow crude estimates of subcutaneous fat and muscle mass. Notably, skinfold thickness only measures fat under the skin, therefore provide little information on total body fat percentage. The use of many skinfold measures improves prediction of total body fat, but still does not provide a measure of visceral fat, which does not necessarily vary in the same fashion. Skinfold thickness is less accurate and there is also potential error in technique and interrater variability.[68,69]

Circumference measures are affected by edema and are not sensitive to acute changes in body composition, which are common in metabolically stressed patients. However, MUAC is resurfacing as a valid measure showing good sensitivity to change in nutritional status with treatment in children, correlating well with changes in weight during recovery from malnutrition. The World Health Organization recommends use of MUAC as a means of diagnosing malnutrition, making this measure useful in both initial assessment as well as an indicator of response to nutritional intervention.[70]

Two Compartment Model

The two compartment model divides the body into its fat and fat-free mass (FFM) as shown in **Figure 5.9**. FFM, while often used interchangeably with LBM, differs in that it does not include the fat that is contained within cell membrane structures. Measurement of the two compartment model relies on the assumption that these compartments are constant. This is important to recognize when applying these techniques during inflammation and illness, where derangements in fluid homeostasis confound interpretation of LBM and its change. A variety of techniques for measuring LBM exist and are applicable in the clinical setting, including bioelectrical impedance, isotope dilution estimates of total body water, and dual x-ray absorptiometry.

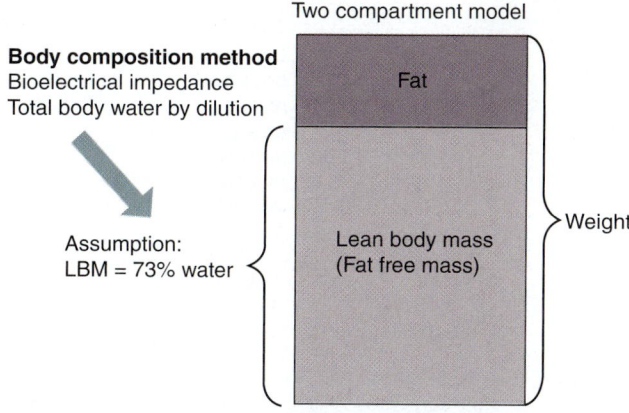

FIGURE 5.9 The Two Compartment Model for Assessing Fat and Fat-free Mass The two compartment model divides the body into fat and lean body mass (LBM). This method relies on the assumption of normal hydration of LBM (73%). Measures of total body water (TBW) can be divided by 0.73 to determine LBM. For example In a 70 kg male, whose TBW is 39 kg, LBM = 53 kg (39kg LBM/0.73 % water = 53kg LBM).

Methods Relying on Measures of Total Body Water

Bioelectrical Impedance

Because water comprises up to two-thirds of total body weight, models of body composition based on total body water and its properties are common. The assumption with this method is that neutral fat does not bind water or electrolytes, and therefore measurements of these compounds can be used to define the nonfat portion of the body. Bioelectrical impedance (BIA) has become an increasingly popular method of measuring total body water (TBW). It combines safety and noninvasiveness with the ease of portability. With BIA, a weak alternating electrical current is applied to the body, which can be visualized as resembling a series of conducing cylinders. Resistance to conduction of the electric current increases in proportion to body fatness because fat is a poor conductor. If the length and diameter of a cylinder are known, resistance can be used to determine the volume of the fluid within that cylinder (or segment of the body). Resistance measures taken across an arm or leg are felt to be representative of TBW. Impedance measures are well correlated with other measures of water space obtained by densitometry, anthropometry, computerized tomography (CT) scanning, and total body potassium in healthy populations, yielding daily coefficients of variation of approximately 2% in weight-stable patients. Unfortunately, the accuracy of this method in detecting fluid changes in hospitalized individuals has not yet been firmly established.[71]

Isotope Dilution Techniques

The isotope dilution technique is the classic method for measuring total body water. The main assumption involved in using this method is that isotopes of oxygen or hydrogen (either as deuterium or tritium) are exchanged in the body in a manner similar to water. Following ingestion of a known amount of tracer and allowing for an equilibration period, samples of blood, urine, or saliva can be used to determine the amount of TBW. The equation is $C_1V_1 = C_2V_2$, where C_1V_1 reflects the concentration of tracer ingested, C_2 reflects the concentration of tracer in sampling fluid, and V_1 represents TBW. When applying deuterium, adjustments must be made for nonaqueous exchange of hydrogen. The precision of this method is 3%.[72]

Labeled oxygen is more precise than deuterium, with a coefficient of variation of less than 1%. However, both methods for determining LBM, like all methods based on the two compartment model, are flawed by the presumption that the hydrational status of the fat-free body is constant at 73%. While this assumption is sufficiently precise to be acceptable in healthy populations, in diseased individuals, where derangements in fluid homeostasis are suspected, it is likely to be invalid.[73]

The Effect of Catabolic Disease on Body Composition

LBM is composed of extracellular mass and body cell mass (**Figure 5.10**). The extracellular mass consists of the structural proteins of the body, including skeleton, fascia, cartilage, dermis, and extracellular water (ECW). The extracellular solid mass remains relatively unchanged during acute injury, although the ECW can vary. The body cell mass (BCM) is the weight of the totality of all the cells (protoplasm, nucleus, cytoplasm, and cell membranes) in the body. It is within this component that all metabolic and synthetic processes are performed.

Figure 5.10 shows that significant changes in LBM and fat mass (FM) result from the prolonged hypermetabolic state that occurs in catabolic disease; this state may continue for several weeks. Fat represents a significant fuel source to aid in recovery from illness, and its losses account for approximately one-half of the weight loss experienced during severe catabolic injury. The remaining half of weight loss occurs within the LBM compartment, primarily within the soft tissue component. In this component there is a decrease in BCM accompanied by an expansion of ECW. While the etiology of this fluid expansion is not completely understood, it is thought that increased membrane permeability induced by shock of injury or sepsis allows the efflux of plasma proteins and cellular constituents, which is accompanied by the efflux of water into the interstitium. Increased levels of aldosterone and vasopressin occur following injury or starvation, suggesting that sodium and fluid retention are hormonally mediated as well. These alterations can mask the diminution of BCM that results from accelerated nitrogen losses. Not uncommonly, weight loss is marginal; however, the quality of LBM is diminished because its proportion of BCM to ECW is decreased.[73]

> **CORE CONCEPT 9**
>
> Expansion in extracellular water during illness confounds interpretation of weight, lean body cell mass, and erosion of body cell mass.

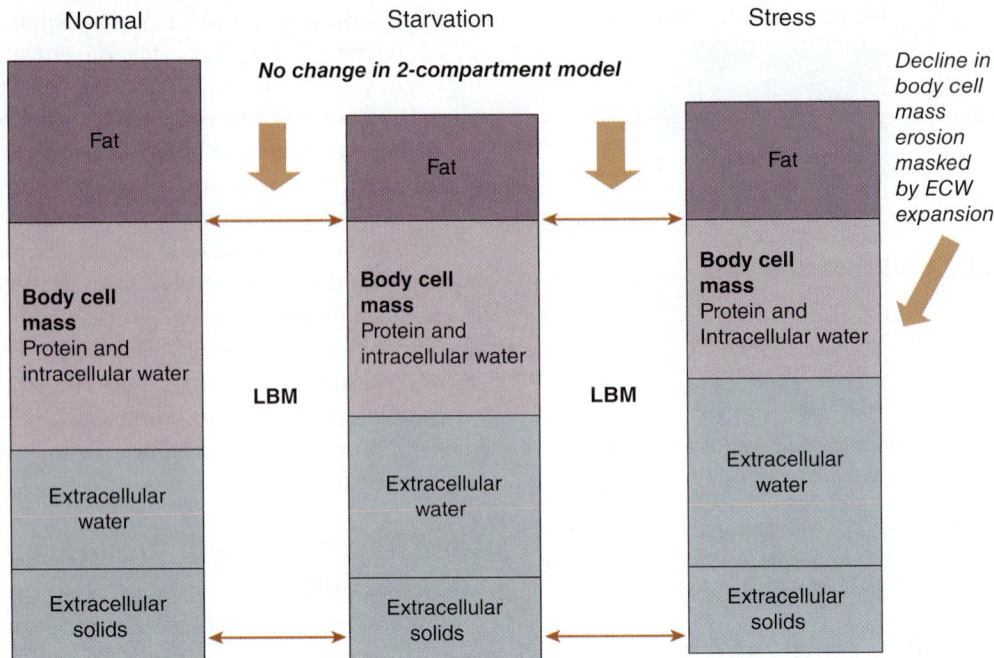

FIGURE 5.10 **The Effect of Starvation and Stress on Body Composition: The Two Compartment Model** Differences in metabolism between stress and starvation manifest in changes in body composition. While both demonstrate a decrease in fat mass from normal health, body cell mass (BCM) is diminished to a greater extent. When measuring lean body mass using the 2 compartment the loss in BCM cannot be appreciated due to the expansion of extracellular water.

Because significant depletion of the BCM has a direct, negative impact on immune competence, functional capacity, and, ultimately, survival, losses of BCM increase risks of adverse outcomes in metabolically stressed patients. The actual extent of BCM wasting is directly related to the degree and duration of the catabolic stimuli that are present. Therefore, individuals suffering from major trauma, burn injury, or sepsis can be expected to have greater losses than those with minor trauma. Measuring changes in various tissues and body compartments during stress can identify those patients at extremely high risk for BCM wasting, and may serve as a better compartment to assess response to nutritional therapy.

Multi-Compartmental Models

Combined Isotope Dilution Studies

An extension of the two compartment model is to use combined measurements of TBW and ECW to compensate for fluid alterations that are seen in the critically ill. In order to specifically measure ECW, a marker that exists exclusively (or nearly so) in the extracellular fluid component is needed. Bromide (Br) exchanges rapidly with chloride within the body and has essentially the same distribution as chloride, making it well suited for measuring ECW. Following the administration of a known quantity of Br and allowing for an equilibration period, corrected bromide space (CBS) is determined from the serum Br concentration. CBS can then be used to determine ECW. This technique has been successfully applied to measure ECW in hospitalized, acutely ill children.[74] The results of such studies have been useful in detecting abnormal states of hydration. Once measurements of both ECW and TBW are obtained, they can be used to estimate intracellular water (ICW), which is an indicator of the BCM. Monitoring of ICW as a marker of BCM and as a means of estimating nutritional adequacy has been used in hospitalized patients.[74-77]

Dual Energy X-ray Absorptiometry

Dual energy x-ray absorptiometry (DXA) has evolved as a well-accepted tool for measuring body composition. Traditionally used for measures of bone mineral density, the precision and accuracy of DXA has gained it distinction for estimating soft tissue as well such as LBM and fat mass(FM). Hence, DXA utilizes a three compartment model, where three components are measured: LBM, FM, and bone mineral density. This tool is shown to have good reliability for body composition measurement when compared with imaging studies of body fat by CT and magnetic resonance imaging (MRI), although its accuracy declines in more obese individuals.[79,80]

The DXA method involves use of x-ray beams at two photon energies to estimate body composition. As the energy from these beams passes through the bone or soft tissue, some of it is absorbed, while the rest passes through the body and is detected on the other side, providing information on the density of the bone or tissue. Although it is not portable, it is common in many clinical settings (**Figure 5.11**). Other advantages include providing a rapid measure (3-10 minutes for lumbar spine and whole body measures) with a minimal radiation dose. It also provides regional body composition. DXA measures are confounded by hydration status; therefore, standardization of timing, fasting state, and factors such as exercise or edema should be considered.[81]

Chapter 5 Energy Expenditure and Body Composition in Metabolic Stress

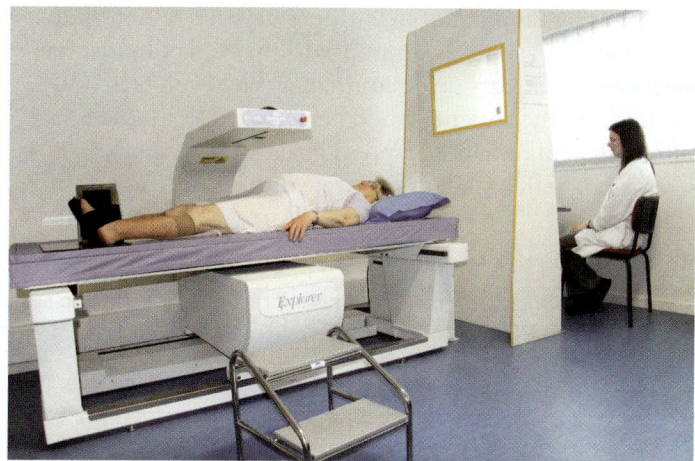

FIGURE 5.11 Measurement of Body Composition by Dual Energy X-ray Absorptiometry
© BSIP / Contributor/Getty Images.

Imaging Techniques

Development of imaging techniques such as MRI and CT have benefited body composition assessment as well as clinical medicine (**Figure 5.12**). Both of these methods assess body composition at the tissue level. Their use can provide information on skeletal muscle, visceral organs, bone, and the brain. Apart from their superior images and reliability, these techniques offer cross-sectional views. This is especially useful in evaluating visceral adipose tissue and its distribution. Another advantage is that these techniques are available in most medical centers. They are not influenced by hydration status. Lack of radiation exposure with the MRI allows it to be used longitudinally. Both are used to validate other anthropometric measures.[67,80-82]

Metabolic Support Aimed at Preserving Body Cell Mass

Metabolic support of the inflammatory response should aim at preservation of the BCM (**Figure 5.13**). In this context, nutrition support goals should be based on providing adequate energy and protein to minimize BCM wasting without exceeding the body's ability to utilize substrate. Energy requirements ideally are determined using indirect calorimetry given that large variability exists based on individual differences in physiologic stress, LBM composition, and the effect of clinical interventions. Typically, use of prediction equations results in overall goals ranging between 130% and 200% of BMR. Glucose infusion rates should match glucose oxidation rates 5-7 mg carbohydrate/kg/min. This is consistent with the maximum rate of glucose oxidation isotopically determined in both children and adults.[10,11]

Protein requirements depend on the degree of catabolism and potential sources of protein losses. In metabolically stressed patients 1.5 to 2.5 g/kg is recommended, with up to 4 g/kg in children.[83] The importance of calories versus protein is often debated in the scientific literature. While both are considered important, hypocaloric nutrition that is high in protein and micronutrient rich is advocated as an effective therapy for promoting positive outcomes, while avoiding complications.[82]

Lipid metabolism is altered during metabolic stress. Despite increased lipolysis, lipid oxidation is inefficient. Furthermore, endogenous fat lipolysis is often more than sufficient for providing necessary fatty acids for oxidation.

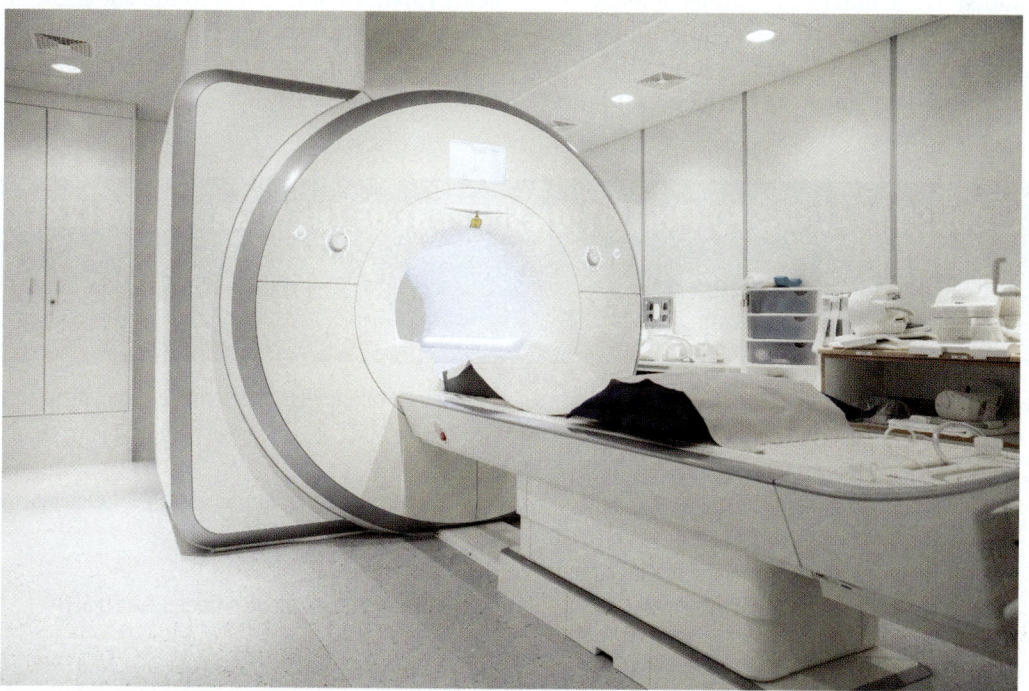

FIGURE 5.12 Body Composition can be Measured Using Imaging Techniques such as Magnetic Resonance Imaging
© Tyler Olson/Shutterstock.

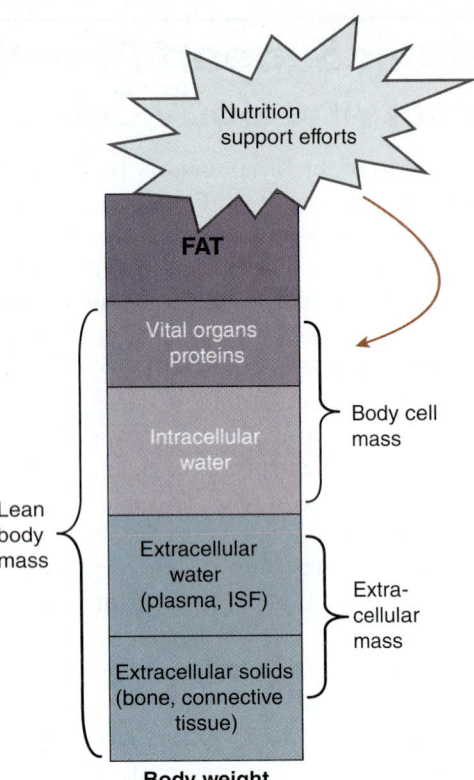

FIGURE 5.13 Metabolic Support of the Body Cell Mass Nutrition support should aim to minimize body cell mass wasting. This requires at minimum adequate energy and optimal protein provision. Losses in fat mass can be tolerated.

Complications such as hypertriglyceridemia can ultimately lead to fatty liver or pancreatitis. Withholding lipids during parenteral nutrition is common practice and currently recommended during the first week of parenteral nutrition infusion in the critically ill. Nevertheless, lipids should eventually be included in the nutrition support of metabolically stressed patients due to their role in cellular integrity, platelet metabolism, and absorption of fat-soluble vitamins. Essential fatty acid deficiency can develop in infants within 7 days and children within 2-5 weeks of lipid-free nutrition. Therefore, an appropriate quantity of lipids that meets essential fatty acid requirements and can be readily oxidized by the patient should be provided.[71,72] **Table 5.13** shows general nutrition support goals for the metabolically stressed patient based on substrate utilization.

> **CORE CONCEPT 10**
>
> Metabolic support of the inflammatory response should aim at preservation of the BCM.

Chapter Summary

The inflammatory response to traumatic injury represents a physiologic mechanism for survival that is mediated by a complex network of immune and neuroendocrine factors. Following injury, increased cellular production and release of cytokines lead to high circulating levels of TNF-1, IL-1, and interleukin 6. These cytokines activate the hypothalamic-pituitary-adrenal axis to produce glucagon, glucocorticoids, and catecholamines, which, in turn, have widespread effects on glucose, amino acid, and fatty acid metabolism.[1] Stimulation of gluconeogenesis concomitant with the development of insulin resistance results in increased glucose appearance, decreased glucose oxidation, and futile recycling of substrate. Enhanced lipolysis and impaired fat oxidation result in increased plasma free fatty acids and triglycerides. High cortisol levels have a permissive effect on muscle proteolysis and stimulate whole body protein turnover and protein breakdown. Net protein breakdown is most profound as the need to replenish diminished intracellular concentrations of specific amino acids further contributes to muscle protein catabolism. These aberrations in metabolism are clinically manifested by increased energy expenditure, impaired nutrient utilization, and LBM losses.

TABLE 5.13 CONSIDERATIONS FOR NUTRITION SUPPORT OF THE METABOLICALLY STRESSED PATIENT[84]

Substrate	Recommendation	General Guideline
Energy intake	• Avoid overfeeding • Consider limits to substrate utilization	• Indirect calorimetry to determine requirement on a weekly basis • Provide MREE × 1.2 to meet 24-hour energy requirement
Glucose	• Provide as primary fuel source	• 5 carbohydrate mg/kg/min glucose infusion rate
Protein	• Adequate protein for wound repair immunity and preservation of body cell mass	• 1.5-2.5 g/kg/day • High nonprotein calorie nitrogen ratio (85:1)
Fat	• Lipolysis of endogenous stores may suffice • Assure essential fatty acid intake is sufficient	• 3%-4% of energy intake as fat

Nutritional support cannot completely attenuate the inflammatory response. While aggressive feeding of protein and essential nutrients can enhance rates of protein synthesis, nutritional therapy does not abate protein breakdown. Metabolic support of these patients includes the provision of adequate protein and essential nutrients to enhance protein synthesis, optimize wound healing, support host immunological defenses, and at best, minimize losses of LBM.

Key Terms

inflammatory response, counter-regulatory hormones, pro-inflammatory cytokines, glucagon, cortisol, catecholamines, epinephrine, norepinephrine, protein catabolism, stress hyperglycemia, glucose oxidation, fat oxidation, basal metabolic rate, body cell mass, diet induced thermogenesis, activity energy expenditure, direct calorimetry, doubly labeled water, indirect calorimetry, resting energy expenditure, lean body mass, extracellular mass, dual x-ray absorptiometry

References

1. Williams, FN, Jeschke, MG, Chinkes, DL, Suman, OE, Branski, LK, Herndon, DN. Modulation of the hypermetabolic response to trauma: temperature, nutrition, and drugs. *J Am Coll Surg*. 2009;208(4):489-502.
2. Finnerty CC, Mabvuure NT, Ali A, Kozar RA, Herndon DN. The surgically induced stress response. *JPEN J Parenter Enteral Nutr*. 2013;37(5 Suppl):21S-9S.
3. Simsek T, Simsek HU, Canturk NZ. Response to trauma and metabolic changes: Posttraumatic metabolism. *Ulus Cerrahi Derg*. 2014;30(3):153-159.
4. Stahel PF, Flierl MA, Moore EE. "Metabolic staging" after major trauma: A guide for clinical decision making? *Scand J Trauma Resusc Emerg Med*. 2010;18:34.
5. Porter C, Tompkins RG, Finnerty CC, Sidossis LS, Suman OE, Herndon DN. The metabolic stress response to burn trauma: Current understanding and therapies. *Lancet*. 2016;388:1417-1426.
6. Yu YM, Tompkins RG, Ryan CM, Young VR. The metabolic basis of the increase of the increase in energy expenditure in severely burned patients. *JPEN J Parenter Enteral Nutr*. 1999;23(3):160-168.
7. Cahill GF. Fuel Metabolism in starvation. *Annu Rev Nutr*. 2006;26:1-22.
8. Weijs P, Cynober L, DeLegge M, Kreymann G, Wernerman J, Wolfe RR. Proteins and amino acids are fundamental to optimal nutrition support in critically ill patients. *Crit Care*. 2014;18:591-604.
9. Zhou M, Martindale RG. Arginine in the critical care setting. *J. Nutr*. 2007;137(6):1687S-1692S.
10. Sheridan RL, Yu YM, Prelack K, Young VR, Burke J, Tompkins RG. Maximal parenteral glucose oxidation in hypermetabolic young children: A stable isotope study. *JPEN*. 1998;22:212-216.
11. Burke JF, Wolfe RR, Mullany CJ, Mathews DE, Bier DM. Glucose requirements following burn injury. Parameters of optimal glucose infusion and possible hepatic and respiratory abnormalities following excessive glucose intake. *Ann Surg*. 1979;190(3):274-285.
12. Dungan KM, Braithewaite SS, Preiser JC. Stress hyperglycemia. *Lancet*. 2009;373:1798-1807.
13. Mizock BA. Alterations in fuel metabolism in critical illness: Hyperglycaemia. *Best Pract Res Clin Endocrinol Metab*. 2001;15(4):533-551.
14. Prelack K, Yu YM, Dylewski M, Lydon M, Sheridan RL, Tompkins RG. The contribution of muscle to whole-body protein turnover throughout the course of burn injury in children. *J Burn Care Res*. 2010;31(6):942-948.
15. Hart DW, Wolf SE, Chinkes DL, et al. Determinants of skeletal muscle catabolism after severe burn. *Ann Surg*. 2000;232(4):455-465.
16. Liebau F, Wernerman J, van Loon LJ, Rooyackers O. Effect of initiating enteral protein feeding on whole-body protein turnover in critically ill patients. *Am J Clin Nutr*. 2015;101(3):549-557.
17. Berg A, Rooyackers O, Bellander BM, Wernerman J. Whole body protein kinetics during hypocaloric and normocaloric feeding in critically ill patients. *Crit Care*. 2013;17:R158.
18. Kien CL, Young VR, Rohrbaugh DK, Burke JF. Increased rates of whole body protein synthesis and breakdown in children recovering from burns. *Ann Surg*. 1978;187(4):383-391.
19. Biolo G, Fleming RY, Maggi SP, Nguyen TT, Herndon DN, Wolfe RR. Inverse regulation of protein turnover and amino acid transport in skeletal muscle of hypercatabolic patients. *J Clin Endocrinol Metab*. 2002;87(7):3378-3384.
20. Tuvdendorj D, Chinkes DL, Zhang XJ, Sheffield-Moore M, Herndon DN. Skeletal muscle is anabolically unresponsive to an amino acid infusion in pediatric burn patients 6 months postinjury. *Ann Surg*. 2011;253(3):592-597.
21. Hart DW, Wolf SE, Ramzy PI, et al. Anabolic effects of oxandrolone after severe burn. *Ann Surg*. 2001;233(4):556-564.
22. Pham TN, Klein MB, Gibran NS, et al. Impact of oxandrolone treatment on acute outcomes after severe burn injury. *J Burn Care Res*. 2008;29(6):902-906.
23. Tuvdendorj D, Chinkes DL, Zhang XJ, et al. Long-term oxandrolone treatment increases muscle protein net deposition via improving amino acid utilization in pediatric patients 6 months after burn injury. *Surgery*. 2011;149(5):645-653.
24. Herndon DN, Rodriguez NA, Diaz EC, et al. Long-term propranolol use in severely burned pediatric patients: A randomized controlled study. *Ann Surg*. 2012;256(3):402-411.
25. Flores O, Stockton K, Roberts JA, Muller MJ, Paratz JD. The efficacy and safety of adrenergic blockade after burn injury: A systematic review and meta-analysis. *J Trauma Acute Care Surg*. 2016;80(1):146-155.
26. Nunez-Villaveiran T, Sanchez M, Millan P, Garcia-de-Lorenzo A. Systematic review of the effect of propanolol on hypermetabolism in burn injuries. *Med Intensiva*. 2015;39(2):101-113.
27. Abdelhamid YA, Cousins CE, Sim JA, et al. Effect of critical illness on triglyceride absorption. *J Parenter Enteral Nutr*. 2014;39:966-972.
28. Ilias I, Vassiliadi DA, Theodorakopoulou M, et al. Adipose tissue lipolysis and circulating lipids in acute and subacute critical illness: effects of shock and treatment. *J Crit Care*. 2014;29:1130; e5-1130.
29. Remaley AT, Norata GD, Catapano AL. Novel concepts in HDL pharmacology. *Cardiovasc Res* 2014;103:423-428.
30. Bonafé L, Berger M, Que YA, Mechanick JI. Carnitine deficiency in chronic critical illness. *Curr Opin Clin Nutr Metab Care*. 2014;179: 200-209.
31. *Human energy requirements*. Report of the joint FAO/WHO/UNU Expert Consultation, October 17-24, 2001; Rome, Italy.
32. Donahoo WT, Levine JA, Melanson EL. Variability in energy expenditure and its components. *Curr Opin Clin Nutr Metab Care*. 2004;7(6):599-605.
33. Institute of Medicine. *Dietary Reference Intakes for energy, carbohydrate, fiber, fat, fatty acids, cholesterol, protein, and amino acids*. Washington, DC: The National Academies Press; 2005.

34. Schofield WN. Predicting basal metabolic rate, new standards and review of previous work. *Hum Nutr Clin Nutr*. 1985;39c(1s):5-42.

35. Mifflin D, St Jeor ST, Hill, LA, Scott, B, Daugherty SA, Koh YO. A new predictive equation for resting energy expenditure in healthy individuals. *Am J Clin Nutr*. 1990;51:241-247.

36. Harris, JA, Benedict, FG. *A biometric study of basal metabolism in man*. Washington, DC: Carnegie Institution; 1919.

37. Prelack K, Dwyer J, Dallal GE, et al. Growth deceleration and restoration after serious burn injury. *J Burn Care Res*. 2007;28(2):262-268.

38. Rutan RL, Herndon DN. Growth delay in postburn pediatric patients. *Arch Surg*. 1990;125(3):392-395.

39. Walter RN, Heuberger RA. Predictive equations for energy needs in the critically ill. *Respiratory Care* 2009; 54(4):509-521.

40. De Waele E, Opsomer T, Honore PM, et al. Measured versus calculated resting energy expenditure in critically ill adult patients. do mathematics match the gold standard? *Minerva Anestesiol*. 2015;81(3):272-282.

41. Hickmann CE, Roeseler J, Castanares-Zapatero D, Herrera EI, Mongodin A, Laterre PF. Energy expenditure in the critically ill performing early physical therapy. *Intensive Care Med*. 2014; 40(4):548-555.

42. Roza AM, Shizgal HM. The Harris Benedict equation reevaluated: resting energy requirements and the body cell mass. *Am J Clin Nutr*. 1984;40(1):168-182..

43. Frankenfield D, Smith JS, Cooney RN. Validation of 2 approaches to predicting resting metabolic rate in critically ill patients. *JPEN*. 2004;28(4):259-264.

44. Frankenfield D. Validation of an equation for resting metabolic rate in older obese, critically ill patients. *JPEN*. 2011;35(2):264-269.

45. Swinamer DL, Grace MG, Hamilton SM, Jones RL, Roberts P. King G. Predictive equation for assessing energy expenditure in mechanically ventilated critically ill patients. *Crit Care Med*. 1990;18(6):657-661.

46. Cerra FB, Benitez BR, Blackburn GL, Irwin RS, Jeejeebhoy K, Katz DP. Applied nutrition in ICU patients: a consensus statement of the American College of Chest Physicians. *Chest*. 1997;111:769-778.

47. Prelack K, Dylewski M, Sheridan RL. Practical guidelines for nutritional management of burn injury and recovery. *Burns*. 2007;33(1):14-24.

48. Singer, P., Anbar, R., Cohen, J. et al. The tight calorie control study (TICACOS): a prospective, randomized, controlled pilot study of nutritional support in critically ill patients; *Intensive Care Med*. 2011;37:601.

49. Levine J. Measurement of energy expenditure. *Pub Health Nutr*. 2005;87(A):1123-1132.

50. Schoeller DA, Ravussin E, Schutz Y, et al. Energy expenditure by doubly labeled water: validation in humans and proposed calculation. *Am J Physiol*. 1986; 250:R823-R830.

51. Schoeller DA and Hnilicka J. Reliability of the doubly labeled water method for measurement of total daily energy expenditure in free-living subjects. *J Nutr*. 1996;126:348S-354S.

52. Weir JB de V. New methods for calculating metabolic rate with special reference to protein metabolism *J Physiol*. 1949;109(1-2):1-9.

53. Smallwood CD, Mehta NM. Accuracy of abbreviated indirect calorimetry protocols for energy expenditure measurement in critically ill children. *JPEN J Parenter Enteral Nutr*. 2012;36(6):693-699.

54. Frankenfield D, Roth-Yousey L, Compher C. Comparison of predictive equations for resting metabolic rate in healthy nonobese and obese adults: A systematic review. *J Am Diet Assoc*. 2005;105(5):775-789.

55. Mehta NM. Energy expenditure: How much does it matter in infant and pediatric chronic disorders? *Pediatr Res*. 2015;77(1-2):168-172.

56. Kross EK, Sena M, Schmidt K. A comparison of predictive equations and measured energy expenditure in critically ill patients. *J Crit Care*. 2012;27(3):321.e5-321.e12.

57. Goran MI, Peters EJ, Herndon DN, Wolfe RR. Total energy expenditure in burned children using the doubly labeled water technique. *Am J Physiol*. 1990;259(4 Pt 1):E576-E585.

58. Prelack K, Yu YM, Dylewski M, Lydon M, Keaney TJ, Sheridan RL. Measures of total energy expenditure and its components using the doubly labeled water method in rehabilitating burn children. *JPEN J Parenter Enteral Nutr*. 2017;41(3):470-480.

59. McClave SA, Taylor BE, Martindale RG, et al. Guidelines for the provision and assessment of nutrition support therapy in the adult critically ill patient: Society of Critical Care Medicine (SCCM) and American Society for Parenteral and Enteral Nutrition (A.S.P.E.N.). *JPEN J Parenter Enteral Nutr*. 2016;40(2):159-211. doi: 10.1177/0148607115621863 [doi].

60. McClave SA, Lowen CC, Kleber MJ, et al. Clinical use of respiratory quotient obtained from indirect calorimetry. *JPEN*. 2003;27(1):21-26.

61. Shields BA, Pidcoke HF, Chung KK, et al. Are visceral proteins valid markers for nutritional status in the burn intensive care unit? *J Burn Care Res*. 2015;36(3):375-380.

62. Prelack K, Dwyer J, Yu YM, Sheridan RL, Tompkins RG. Urinary urea nitrogen is imprecise as a predictor of protein balance in burned children. *JADA*. 1997;97:489-495.

63. Picou, D, Taylor-Roberts T. The measurement of total protein synthesis and catabolism and nitrogen turnover in infants in different nutritional states and receiving different amounts of dietary protein. *Clin. Sci Land*. 1969;36:283-301

64. Kotler DP. Nutritional considerations in AIDS. *Bol Asoc Med P R*. 1991;83(2):81-83.

65. Heymsfield SB, Ebbeling CB, Zheng J, et al. Multi-component molecular-level body composition reference methods: Evolving concepts and future directions. *Obes Rev*. 2015;16(4):282-294.

66. Adreoli A, Garaci F, Pio Cafarelli F, Guglielmi.G. Body composition in clinical practice. *Eur J Radiol*. 2016;85:1461-1468.

67. Ranasinghe C, Gamage P, Katulanda P, Andraweera N, Thilakarathne S, Tharanga P. Relationship between body mass index (BMI) and body fat percentage, estimated by bioelectrical impedance, in a group of sri lankan adults: A cross sectional study. *BMC Public Health*. 2013;13:797-2458-13-797.

68. Flegal KM, Shepherd JA, Looker AC, et al. Comparisons of percentage body fat, body mass index, waist circumference, and waist-stature ratio in adults. *Am J Clin Nutr*. 2009;89(2):500-508.

69. Wells JC, Fewtrell MS. Measuring body composition. *Arch Dis Child*. 2006;91(7):612-617.

70. Binns P, Dale N, Hoq M, Banda C, Myatt M. Relationship between mid upper arm circumference and weight changes in children aged 6-59 months. *Arch Public Health*. 2015;73:54-015-0103-y.

71. Langer RD, Borges JH, Pascoa MA, Cirolini VX, Guerra-Júnior G, Gonçalves EM. The Validity of bioelectrical impedance analysis to estimation fat-free mass in the army cadets *Nutrients*. 2016;8(3):121.

72. Schoeller DA, van Santen E, Peterson DW, Dietz W, Jaspan J, Klein PD. Total body water measurement in humans with 18O and 2H labeled water. *Am J Clin Nutr*. 1980;33(12):2686-2693.

73. Roubenoff R, Kehayias JJ. The meaning and measurement of lean body mass. *Nutr Rev*. 1991;49(6):163-175.

74. Prelack K, Sheridan R, Yu YM, et al. Sodium bromide by instrumental neutron activation analysis quantifies change in extracellular water space with wound closure in severely burned children. *Surgery*. 2003;133(4):396-403.

75. Prelack K, Dwyer J, Sheridan R, et al. Body water in children during recovery from severe burn injury using a combined tracer dilution method. *J Burn Care Rehabil*. 2005;26(1):67-74.

76. Monk DN, Plank LD, Franch-Arcas G, Finn PJ, Streat SJ, Hill GL. Sequential changes in the metabolic response in critically injured patients during the first 25 days after blunt trauma. *Ann Surg*. 1996;223(4): 395-405.

77. Plank LD, Hill GL. Sequential metabolic changes following induction of systemic inflammatory response in patients with severe sepsis or major blunt trauma. *World J Surg*. 2000;24(6):630-638.

78. Finn PJ, Plank LD, Clark MA, Connolly AB, Hill GL. Progressive cellular dehydration and proteolysis in critically ill patients. *Lancet*. 1996;347(9002):654-656.

79. Cheung AS, de Rooy C, Hoermann R, et al. Correlation of visceral adipose tissue measured by Lunar Prodigy dual X-ray absorptiometry with MRI and CT in older men. Int J Obesity. 2016;40(8):1325-1328.

80. Bredella M, Ghomi RH, Thomas BJ, et al. Comparison of DXA and CT in the assessment of body composition of premenopausal women with obesity and anorexia nervosa. *Obesity*. 2010;18(11):2227-2233.

81. Toomey CM, McCormack WG, Jakeman P. The effect of hydration status on the measurement of lean tissue mass by dual-energy X-ray absorptiometry. *Eur J Appl Physiol*. 2017;117:567-574.

82. Lacoste Jeanson A, Dupej J, Villa C, Brůžek J. Body composition estimation from selected slices: equations computed from a new semi-automatic thresholding method developed on whole-body CT scans. *PeerJ*. 2017;5:e3302.

83. Prelack K, Dylewski M, Sheridan RL. Practical guidelines for nutritional management of burn injury and recovery. *Burns*. 2007;33(1):14-24.

84. Hoffer AL, Bistrian BR. Energy deficit is clinically relevant for critically ill patients: No. *Intensive Care Med*. 2015;41:339-341.

Section 2

Nutrition in Disease States

Chapter 6   Nutrition in Critical Illness: A Burn Injury Model
Chapter 7   Nutrition in Wound Healing
Chapter 8   Nutritional Management of Obesity
Chapter 9   Nutritional Management of Diabetes Mellitus
Chapter 10   Nutrition in Cardiovascular Disease
Chapter 11   Nutrition in Oral Health
Chapter 12   Nutritional Management of Gastrointestinal Maldigestion
Chapter 13   Nutrition Management of Gastrointestinal Malabsorption
Chapter 14   Nutrition in Kidney Disease
Chapter 15   Nutrition in Liver Disease
Chapter 16   Nutrition in Pulmonary Disease
Chapter 17   Nutrition in Cystic Fibrosis
Chapter 18   Nutrition in Solid Organ Transplantation
Chapter 19   Nutrition in Oncology and Hematopoietic Stem Cell Transplant
Chapter 20   Nutrition in HIV/AIDS

Chapter 6

Nutrition in Critical Illness: A Burn Injury Model

Maggie Dylewski
Kathy Prelack

Chapter Outline

Core Concepts
Introduction
Pathophysiology of the Catabolic Response Following Acute Burn Injury
Medical Treatment/Clinical Course
Medical Treatment/Clinical Course Specific to Burn Patients
Nutritional Management
Chapter Summary

CORE CONCEPTS

1. The physiologic response to critical illness is characterized by hypermetabolism, protein catabolism, and hyperglycemia.
2. The SCCM and A.S.P.E.N. published evidence-based guidelines to assist with the nutritional assessment and treatment of critically ill patients.
3. Due to the catabolic characteristics of critical illness, malnutrition can develop quickly in the intensive care unit.
4. The Nutritional Risk Screening (NRS) and the Nutrition Risk in the Critically Ill (NUTRIC) are tools used to screen for malnutrition in critically ill patients.
5. Accurate height and weight measurements are needed to determine baseline and ongoing nutritional status.
6. Maintaining blood glucose levels between 70 and 149 mg/dL decreases morbidity and mortality.
7. Biochemical assessment of protein nutritional status is not accurate in critically ill patients.
8. The nutrition-focused physical exam assists with identifying signs of malnutrition, including muscle and fat wasting.
9. It is important to collect and analyze daily calorie and protein intake to ensure patients are receiving adequate energy and protein to support recovery.
10. Energy and protein requirements are increased during critical illness.
11. Enteral nutrition is the gold standard of nutrition support in the intensive care unit.

Learning Objectives

1. Describe the characteristics of the stress response associated with critical illness, including hypermetabolism, protein catabolism, and hyperglycemia.
2. Understand the pathophysiology specific to burn-injured patients.
3. List the elements included in a comprehensive nutritional assessment of a critically ill patient.
4. Calculate energy and protein needs of critically ill patients.
5. Establish an appropriate nutrition treatment plan for critically ill patients.
6. Determine the appropriate timing and route of nutrition support for critically ill patients.

Introduction

The term "critical illness" includes a variety of different disease states, such as trauma, burns, organ failure, sepsis, and acute pancreatitis. Although the severity of illness can vary, most critically ill patients present with catabolic stress and are at increased risk for significant morbidity and mortality. Optimal and appropriate nutrition support delivery is vital to the survival and outcome of critically ill patients. The following case study utilizes a burn injury model, the most severe and hypermetabolic category of critical illness.

Pathophysiology of the Catabolic Response Following Acute Burn Injury

The **catabolic stress response** associated with burn injury resembles that of any critically ill state, and is characterized by significant alterations in physiology, immune function, and metabolism. Propagated by inflammatory mediators, life-threatening changes in all of the major organ systems occur, often requiring intensive care management. Physiologic changes in cardiac function and circulatory hemodynamics are foremost in the response to injury, requiring fluid resuscitation and restoration of vascular integrity.[1] The inflammatory response that ensues calls upon a network of immune and endocrine mediators that work both locally and systemically to ultimately ensure survival. This comes at a metabolic cost, which includes increased energy expenditure, increased protein catabolism, and impaired glucose utilization. Increased resting energy expenditure, or **hypermetabolism**, persists throughout the disease process, necessitating the need for aggressive nutritional support.[2] The need for **acute-phase reactants** and proteins for wound healing draws upon the skeletal muscle for necessary amino acids. This leads to **catabolism** or breakdown of skeletal muscle. The extent of hypermetabolism and catabolism depends on the type and severity of illness. Burn injuries are among the most hypermetabolic disease states. The pathophysiology of the response to burn injury and its general management are shown in **Table 6.1**.

The shock (ebb) phase starts immediately after injury and continues for 24 to 72 hours.[1,2] During this time, capillary integrity is compromised, causing fluid to shift from the plasma into the interstitial space. This often results in edema, particularly in patients with severe trauma or burns. Additional fluid may be lost through wounds. The redistribution and loss of fluid leads to hypovolemia, hypotension, and reduced tissue perfusion. Inadequate blood flow to tissues may advance to organ failure. Aggressive fluid resuscitation, especially in burn patients, is required to replete plasma volume and reduce the risk of organ failure. The ebb phase is also characterized by a reduction in oxygen consumption, metabolic rate, and body temperature.[1,2]

The hyperdynamic or flow phase is characterized by a shift in cardiac dynamics, restoration of vascular fluid, and a full-blown systemic inflammatory response, which ultimately leads to hypermetabolism and muscle protein catabolism. This stage may persist for several months, depending on the degree of injury. Immune cells, in response to tissue injury, inflammation, or infection, release pro-inflammatory **cytokines**, such as interleukin-1, interleukin-6, and tumor necrosis factor.[2,3]

Throughout the flow stage, the body is working diligently to mobilize glucose and protein to support energy requirements, wound healing, and immune function. Oxygen consumption increases to support ATP-consuming metabolic pathways, including protein synthesis and hepatic gluconeogenesis. Burn injuries may increase metabolic rate by 40% to 80% and remain elevated for at least 1 year postinjury.[4-7]

Alterations in macronutrient metabolism mediated by **catecholamines** (epinephrine and norepinephrine), glucagon, and cortisol persist throughout the course of injury and result in muscle wasting and hyperglycemia (**Table 6.2**).[8-10]

Substrates required for gluconeogenesis, including glycerol, alanine, and lactate, are provided by adipose tissue lipolysis, hepatic glycogenolysis via the Cori Cycle, and gluconeogenesis via the alanine cycles[9,11-13] (**Figure 6.1**).

Glutamine is also released from muscle to provide fuel to the immune system and enterocytes. Although rates of lipolysis are increased, fatty acids are not efficiently utilized during critical illness, and thus are primarily re-esterified within adipose tissue.[14]

The catabolic nature of critical illness persists despite administration of nutrition, which, under normal physiologic conditions, would abate catabolic pathways such as proteolysis, lipolysis, and gluconeogenesis. Instead, these metabolic adaptations contribute to a state of hyperglycemia and muscle wasting. Stress hyperglycemia is further aggravated by insulin resistance, which is common during critical illness. In healthy individuals, glucose produced from gluconeogenesis or glycogenolysis is taken up by insulin-independent organs (such as the brain or red blood cells) or by insulin-dependent organs (such as muscle or liver) to be used for energy production. Among critically ill

CASE STUDY

Manuel is a 33-year-old male with a large burn from 1 day ago, involving 55% of his total body surface area. After admission to the Emergency Department, he was stabilized and transferred to the intensive care unit (ICU). He has a central venous catheter and a nasogastric tube.

Manuel is a lawyer at a local law firm and lives at home with his wife and two small children. A nutrition consult was initiated to assess Manuel and provide a treatment plan and nutrition support recommendations. The following clinical information was collected upon admission.

Anthropometric Data:
Weight: 81 kg (178 lbs)
Height: 173 cm (68″)
Body mass index (BMI): 27 kg/m^2
Weight history
Usual Weight: 81 kg (178 lb)

Biochemical Data:
Sodium 133 (135-145 mEq/L)
Potassium 5.2 (3.6-5.0 mEq/L)
Chloride 99 (98-110 mEq/L)
Carbon dioxide 28 (20-30 mEq/L)
Blood urea nitrogen 20 (6-24 mg/dL)
Creatinine 1.3 (0.4-1.3 mg/dL**)**
Blood glucose 190 mg/dL (70-139 mg/dL)

Calcium 7.0 (8.5-10.5 mEq/L)
Phosphorus 2.9 (2.7 to 4.5 mg/dL)
Magnesium 1.2 (1.3 to 2.1 mEq/L)
Albumin 1.3 (3.5 to 5.0 g/dL)

Clinical Data:
Past Medical History: None
Medications: None
Vital signs: Blood pressure 125/65 mm Hg
Nutrition-focused physical exam: Patient appears slightly edematous from fluid resuscitation. Otherwise appears well nourished. No apparent signs of muscle or fat wasting.
Disease severity scores:
APACHE II: 20
SOFA: 8

Dietary Data:
Dietary History: Follows a typical American diet. No food allergies or special diet.
Diet Prescription: NPO

Questions:
1. What will Manuel's trajectory be over the next few days with respect to the physiologic and metabolic response to this injury? What systems will be impacted?
2. What is Manuel's nutritional risk? Does Manuel's BMI decrease his risk for malnutrition while in the ICU?
3. Assess Manuel's biochemical data. What is concerning? How are his labs a reflection of his physical presentation and clinical data? What do his disease severity scores tell you?

---

patients, insulin resistance decreases glucose clearance and contributes to the hyperglycemia.[15,16]

Increased proteolysis, which provides alanine for gluconeogenesis, also depletes muscle protein and leads to muscle wasting. Burn patients are particularly susceptible to lean body mass depletion. Despite aggressive treatment strategies, a loss of up to 25% of total body mass may occur following a large burn injury.[17,18] Loss of lean body mass is highly correlated to morbidity and mortality (**Table 6.3**).[19,20]

Systemic inflammatory response syndrome and sepsis are potential complications of critical illness. **Systemic inflammatory response syndrome (SIRS)** describes an inflammatory response that occurs throughout the body in response to infection, inflammation, trauma, and

TABLE 6.1 CHARACTERISTICS OF THE PHYSIOLOGIC RESPONSE TO ACUTE BURN INJURY[1,2]

Primary Systems Effected	Etiology	Treatment Goals
Shock (Ebb) Phase		
Cardiac and Circulatory Tachycardia Decreased cardiac output	Myocardial depression	Fluid resuscitation/repletion of intravascular volume to maintain tissue perfusion and minimize ischemia
Hypovolemic Shock Loss of intravascular volume Hypotension Decreased tissue perfusion Oxygen consumption	Increased vascular permeability due to release of cytokines Increased systemic vascular resistance	Airway management and ventilatory support
Lungs/Pulmonary Pulmonary edema Bronchospasm Acute respiratory distress syndrome	Inhalation injury or increased vascular permeability and edema	Restore tissue perfusion
Kidneys Decreased urine output	Decreased glomerular filtration, elevated aldosterone and ADH	
Hyperdynamic, hypermetabolic (Flow) Phase		
Cardiac and Circulatory Tachycardia Increased oxygen saturation Increased oxygen consumption Increased carbon dioxide production	Cardiac dysfunction, metabolic stress, oxidative stress	Pharmacologic management including blockade of sympathetic nervous system
Lungs/Pulmonary Pulmonary edema Bronchospasm Acute respiratory distress syndrome	Resorption of edema Continued respiratory distress due to inhalation injury or inflammatory mediators released with cell damage	Supportive care, mechanical ventilation
Liver and Skeletal Muscle Altered metabolic function Fatty liver Fat recycling Increased gluconeogenesis Decreased coagulation Increased amino acid release Muscle wasting	Endocrine-mediated release of catabolic hormones: glucagon, cortisol, epinephrine, norepinephrine	Nutritional support and pharmacological modulation of increased energy expenditure and protein breakdown

Data from Bittner EA, Shank E, Woodson L, Martyn JAJ. Acute and Perioperative Care of the Burn-Injured Patient. Anesthesiology. 2015 February ; 122(2): 448-464. doi:10.1097/ALN.0000000000000559. 3. Simsek T, Simsek HU, Canturk NZ. Response to trauma and metabolic changes: Posttraumatic metabolism. Ulus Cerrahi Derg. 2014;30(3):153-159. doi: 10.5152/UCD.2014.2653 [doi].

burns. In general, **sepsis** is defined as a systemic infection that leads to the SIRS (**Table 6.4**)[21]. If organ failure is present, it is considered severe sepsis.

Most burn patients meet the SIRS criteria due to the nature of the burn injury, making these guidelines impractical for this population. The American Burn Association (ABA) suggested modified guidelines to diagnose sepsis among burn patients (**Table 6.5**).[22] In addition to these criteria, the ABA defines **septic shock** as consistent hypotension in the presence of adequate fluid resuscitation and/or lactate levels of 4 mmol (36 mg/dL) in patients with sepsis.

TABLE 6.2 ENDOCRINE AND METABOLIC RESPONSE TO BURN INJURY

Endocrine Response	Alterations in Macronutrient Metabolism	Metabolic Consequence
↑Epinephrine	Gluconeogenesis Lipolysis Insulin resistance	
↑Norepinephrine	Gluconeogensis Lipolysis Glycogenolysis	Hyperglycemia Muscle wasting
↑Glucagon	Gluconeogenesis Glycogenolysis	Poor lipid clearance
↑Cortisol	Gluconeogenesis Lipolysis Proteolysis	

TABLE 6.3 MORBIDITY AND MORTALITY ASSOCIATED WITH LEAN BODY MASS CATABOLISM

Loss of Lean Body Mass	Associated Morbidity	Associated Mortality Rate
10%	Reduced immune function Increased risk of infection	10%
20%	Decreased wound healing	30%
30%	Pressure sores	50%
40%	Increased risk for pneumonia	100%

Modified from Demling RH, Seigne P. Metabolic management of patients with severe burns. World J Surg. 2000;24(6):673-680. doi: 0.1007/s002689910109 [pii].

Sepsis imposes an additional metabolic demand that increases protein catabolism and energy expenditure by approximately 40%.[5] In addition, the hypotension and organ dysfunction during septic shock may interfere with the utility of the gastrointestinal tract. A substantial drop in blood pressure will reduce perfusion to the gut tissues and thus decreases peristalsis. Under these conditions, an ileus (lack of intestinal peristalsis) may develop, which may directly interfere with providing enteral nutrition (EN). Aggressively feeding a patient during septic shock, when blood flow to the gut is compromised, increases the risk for necrotic bowel.

> **PRACTICE POINT**
>
> In patients who are exhibiting signs of sepsis, provision of enteral feedings should be carefully evaluated. It may be necessary to hold feedings or delay initiation until the patient is hemodynamically stable.

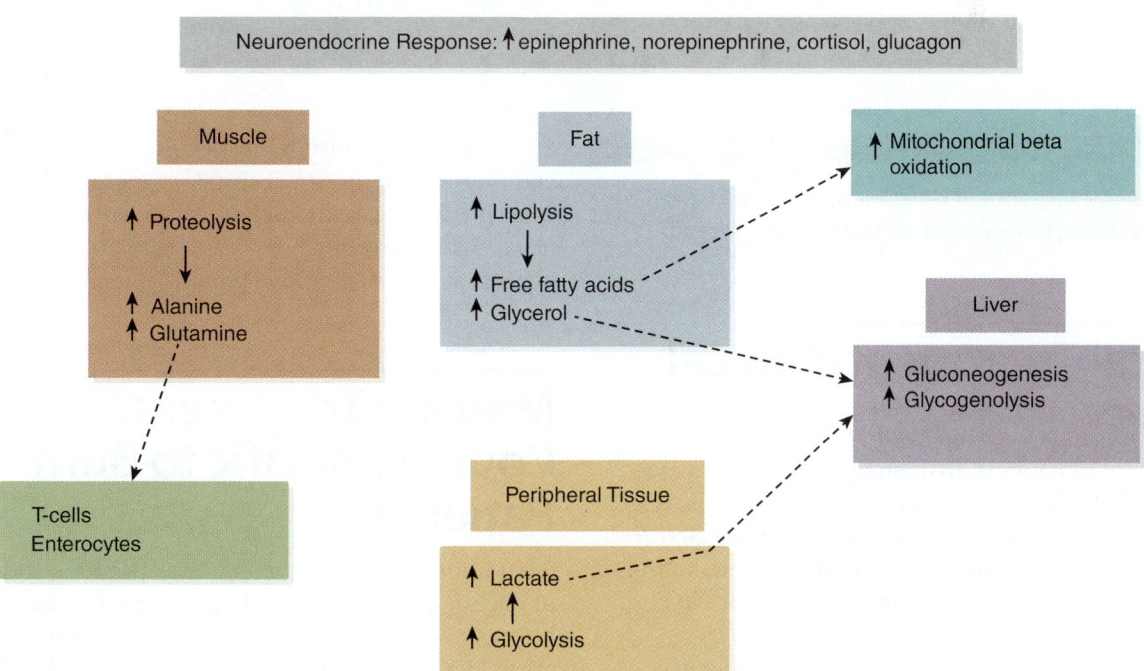

FIGURE 6.1 Inflammatory Mediated Alterations of Intermediary Metabolism Within the Muscle, Liver, and Adipose Tissue

TABLE 6.4 CRITERIA FOR DIAGNOSING SYSTEMIC INFLAMMATORY RESPONSE SYNDROME (SIRS)

A diagnosis of SIRS requires two or more of the following clinical outcomes:
- Heart rate: >90 beats/min
- Respiratory rate: >20 breaths/min
- Temperature: >38°C or <36°C
- White blood cell count: >12,000/mm^3, <4000/mm^3, or >10% bandemia

Data from Bone RC, Sprung CL, Sibbald WJ. Definitions for sepsis and organ failure. Crit Care Med. 1992;20(6):724-726.

TABLE 6.5 CRITERIA FOR DIAGNOSING SEPSIS IN ADULT BURN PATIENTS

A diagnosis of sepsis requires three or more of the following clinical outcomes

Clinical Outcome	Sepsis Diagnosis Criteria
Temperature	>39°C or <36.5°C
Progressive tachycardia	>110 beats/min
Progressive tachypnea	>25 breaths/min (not ventilated) Minute ventilation >12 L/min ventilated
Thrombocytopenia	<100,000/μL (not applicable until 3 days after initial resuscitation)
Hyperglycemia	Untreated plasma glucose >200 mg/dL Insulin resistance >7 units/hour insulin intravenous drip >25% increase in insulin requirements over 24 hours
Inability to continue enteral feed >24 hours	Abdominal distention Residual volume 2x feeding rate Diarrhea >2,500 mL/day

CORE CONCEPT 1

The physiologic response to critical illness is characterized by hypermetabolism, protein catabolism, and hyperglycemia.

Medical Treatment/Clinical Course

Most critically ill patients are managed in the intensive care unit (ICU). The heterogeneity of patients in the ICU is vast and may include those with or without mechanical ventilation, trauma, sepsis, obesity, malnutrition, and/or surgical requirements. Patients may be young or old and have a variety of comorbidities.

Thus, the clinical course depends on the diagnosis. The treatment of critical illness is highly interprofessional and includes input from physicians, nurses, occupational and physical therapists, respiratory therapists, dietitians, speech-language pathologists, social workers, and psychologists. Clinicians must work as a team to create treatment plans that support optimal patient outcomes.

Medical Treatment/Clinical Course Specific to Burn Patients

Burn injuries are classified by type (flame, scald, electrical, or chemical), size, and depth (**Figure 6.2**). The size of the burn is expressed as a percentage of the total body surface area (TBSA) and determined using the Lund and Browder chart (**Figure 6.3**).[23]

VARYING DEGREES OF BURN INJURIES

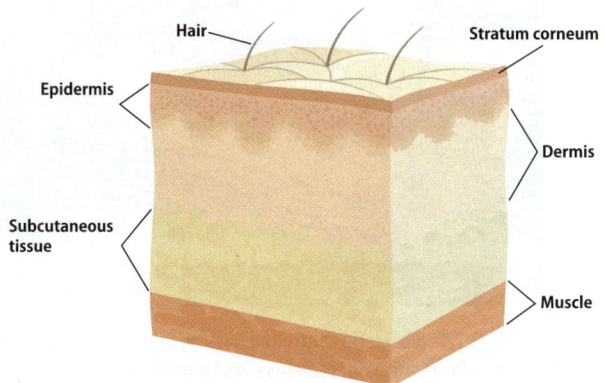

FIGURE 6.2 Varying Degrees of Burn Injuries
© logika600/Shutterstock.

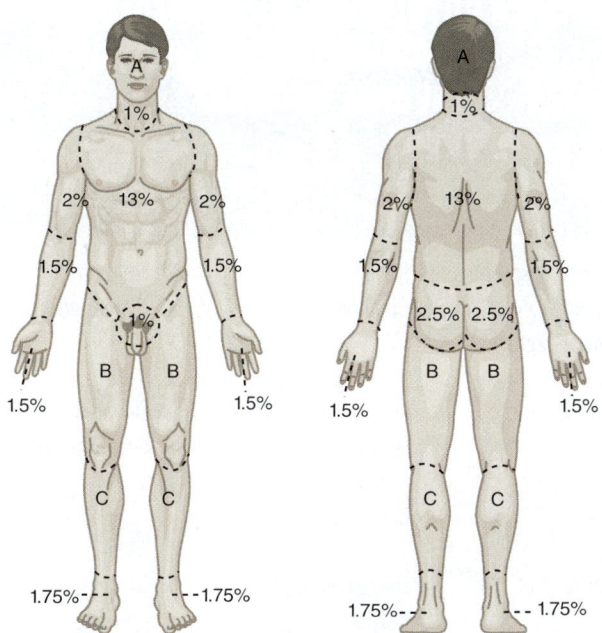

FIGURE 6.3 Lund and Browder Chart. This Chart is Used for Estimating the Extend of Body Surface Area that is Burned. Each Segment that is Burned is Given a Total Body Surface Area Burn
Modified from Lund, C.C., and Browder, N.C. Surg. Gynecol. Obstet. 1944;79:352-358.

The depth of the burn is classified as superficial, partial-thickness, or full thickness (**Table 6.6**). Previous terminology, such as first-, second-, and third-degree, is typically not used among burn clinicians. Of note, superficial burns are not included in the calculation of TBSA percentage.

A burn is considered to be large when it involves 30% or more TBSA. Regardless of size or depth, a burn injury greater

TABLE 6.6 CLASSIFICATION OF BURN DEPTH

Current Terminology	Old Terminology	Tissue Layer Affected
Superficial	First-degree	Epidermis
Partial-thickness	Second-degree	Epidermis and dermis
Full-thickness	Third-degree	Epidermis, dermis, and subcutaneous tissues

than or equal to 10% TBSA in children and 15% TBSA in adults often requires hospitalization for treatment.[24]

Once admitted to the burn unit, patients undergo fluid resuscitation to restore intravascular volume. The amount of fluid required is determined using age, weight, and burn size. The composition of the resuscitation formula typically includes a crystalloid component, such as lactated Ringer's, which contains sodium, chloride, calcium, potassium, and lactate. The addition of a colloid component, such as albumin or fresh frozen plasma, may also be utilized in larger burns.[25] Following the initial resuscitation period, fluid management should cover maintenance fluid needs and evaporative losses through the open wounds.

Early care of the burn patient focuses on reducing wound size, preventing infection, and blunting the hypermetabolic response. Subsequent total burn care also includes maintaining function and optimizing physical and psychological outcomes. The initial treatment plan must include a variety of surgical and supportive care strategies (**Table 6.7**).

Surgical interventions are the most effective way to reduce hypermetabolism, infection, and mortality.[5] Patients are routinely taken to the operating room for excising and grafting of wounds. Additionally, most patients will receive daily wound dressing changes.

Supportive strategies incorporate aggressive nutrition support, environmental manipulation, and pharmacological interventions. Continuous nutrition support must provide an optimal provision of protein to promote protein synthesis and reduce lean body mass catabolism.

Bacteria-controlled nursing units (BCNU) help to reduce infection, evaporative fluid loss, heat loss, and metabolic rate among patients with burns >30% TBSA (**Figure 6.4**). The four plastic walls of the BCNU maintain a warm, isolated environment. Temperatures range from 84°F to 88°F with 80% humidity, and a laminar airflow unit reduces bacterial cross-colonization.[26]

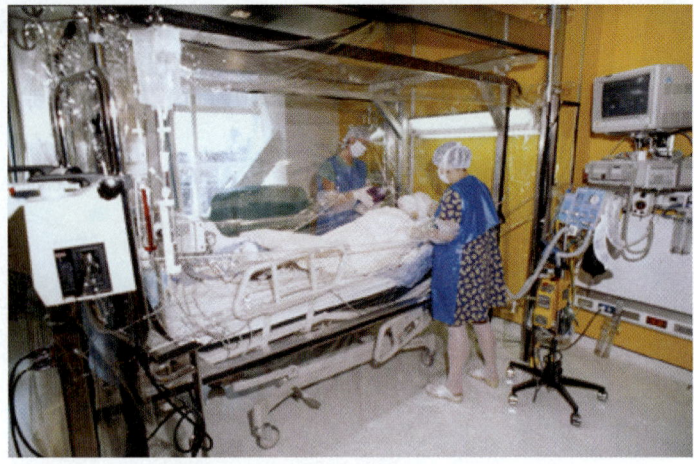

FIGURE 6.4 A bacteria Controlled Nursing Unit is Used to Maintain Infection and Temperature Control for Patients with Large Burn Injury

Pharmacological interventions include sedation, pain control, and antibiotics as needed. Adequate pain control decreases metabolic rate. Depending on the course of illness, a variety of other medications may be required to support the patient. For example, during septic episodes, vasopressor therapy may be used to manage hypotension. Pharmacotherapy, using oxandrolone or propranolol, may also be used to counteract the hypermetabolic response (**Table 6.8**).

Oxandrolone

Oxandrolone is an anabolic steroid that has been shown through kinetic studies to minimize lean body mass

TABLE 6.7 TREATMENT STRATEGIES FOR BURN PATIENTS

Surgical	• Early excision and wound closure
Nutrition Support	• Early initiation of nutrition support • High-protein diet
Pharmacologic	• Adequate sedation and pain control • Anabolic steroids • Beta-andrenergic medicationss
Environmental	• Infection control • Warm environment

TABLE 6.8 NUTRITIONAL PHARMACOLOGY IN MODULATING THE HORMONAL RESPONSE TO INJURY

Drug	Mechanisms of Action	Negative Side Effects
Growth hormone Insulin-like growth factor	Reduced protein breakdown	Fluid retention Hyperglycemia
Oxandrolone	Increased protein synthesis Reduced protein breakdown	Elevated liver function tests
Propranolol	Decreased cardiac output Decreased lipolysis Improved protein balance	Decreased blood pressure

wasting by increasing net protein balance in muscle in metabolically stressed patients.[27,28] Although a positive nitrogen balance is achieved using an aggressively high protein diet (>2.5 g protein/kg), a high-protein diet alone does not completely abate protein breakdown.[29] Oxandrolone can further improve protein net balance through the mechanism of enhancing muscle protein synthesis.[28]

Additional data indicate that oxandrolone use increases lean body mass, bone mineral content, and muscle strength after 6 months of therapy among pediatric burn patients.[30] This is relevant for metabolically stressed patients, particularly those with preexisting malnutrition, where prompt lean body mass accrual is desirable or in patients with prolonged hospital stays where large lean body mass losses can be profound over time.

Propranolol

As previously described, traumatic injury creates a hyperdynamic state, which includes elevated heart rate, increased cardiac output, and increased catecholamine production—all of which manifest in increased energy expenditure, protein breakdown, and muscle catabolism. Propranolol is a beta-adrenergic receptor antagonist that blocks catecholamine activity. Propranolol has been shown to decrease heart rate by 15% and lessen cardiac workload. Measures of resting energy expenditure are decreased, while protein breakdown and lean body mass losses are diminished.[31] Beta blockade has been effectively used in numerous populations of the critically ill, including adult and pediatric burn patients, as well as patients undergoing major elective surgeries.[31,32]

Nutritional Management

The nutritional management of critically ill patients is complex and dynamic. Assessment and treatment plans may differ among disease states, and the patient's past medical history must be carefully considered. The Academy of Nutrition and Dietetics (AND),[33] the Society of Critical Care Medicine (SCCM), and American Society for Parenteral and Enteral Nutrition (A.S.P.E.N.)[34] published specific recommendations to guide the nutritional management of critically ill patients. These tools provide the foundation for the nutrition assessment, diagnosis, treatment, and monitoring in the ICU.

> **CORE CONCEPT 2**
>
> The SCCM and A.S.P.E.N. published evidence-based guidelines to assist with the nutritional assessment and treatment of critically ill patients.

Malnutrition, both preexisting and hospital acquired, must routinely be assessed. Nutritional status can quickly deteriorate in the ICU due to the metabolic stress associated with critical illness coupled with potential intolerance to nutrition support or frequent cessation of nutrition support for medical procedures.[35-37] A joint statement from AND and A.S.P.E.N. provides recommendations for assessing and diagnosing malnutrition among critically ill patients.[38]

> **CORE CONCEPT 3**
>
> Due to the catabolic characteristics of critical illness, malnutrition can develop quickly in the intensive care unit.

> **PRACTICE POINT**
>
> Clinicians may use AND and A.S.P.E.N. guidelines coupled with current evidence-based recommendations and good clinical judgment to assess, diagnose, treat, and monitor nutritional status in the intensive care unit.

Assessment

Nutrition Screen

The Joint Commission mandates that all patients admitted to the hospital be screened for nutritional risk within 24 hours of admission.[39] Nutritional risk of ICU patients may be identified using a screening tool that captures characteristics of both nutritional status and disease severity. This combination allows for identification of current malnutrition and the risk of transitioning to a malnourished state while in the hospital.[40] It is particularly important to identify patients at risk for malnutrition so that the medical team can accurately prioritize nutrition support.

The Nutritional Risk Screening (NRS)[41] and the Nutrition Risk in the Critically Ill (NUTRIC)[42,43] score are both appropriate tools for assessing nutritional risk of the adult ICU patient and are supported by the 2016 SCCM/A.S.P.E.N. Guidelines.[34] Using the NRS (**Table 6.9**), risk is determined by adding the impaired nutritional status score to the severity of disease score (Risk = score >3; High risk = score ≥ 5). The NUTRIC tool (**Table 6.10**) was recently modified from its original version proposed in 2011[42] to increase the tool's clinical value.[43] High NUTRIC scores (≥5) indicate that the patient is at high nutritional risk.

> **CORE CONCEPT 4**
>
> The NRS and NUTRIC are tools used to screen for malnutrition in critically ill patients.

If a patient is identified as malnourished or at risk for malnutrition, the medical team should complete a full assessment and consider initiating aggressive nutrition support. Patients who are identified as well nourished should be routinely reassessed, as nutrition status may rapidly decline in the ICU.

Anthropometrics

Important anthropometric measurements in the ICU patient include height, weight, BMI, and weight history.[33] A patient's current BMI and recent weight change evaluate baseline nutritional status. Accurate height and weight

CASE STUDY REVISITED

1. According to the Nutritional Risk Screening and Nutrition Risk in the Critically Ill screening tools, what is Manuel's baseline nutritional risk?
2. At baseline, does Manuel meet the criteria for malnutrition?

TABLE 6.9 NUTRITIONAL RISK SCREENING TOOL (NRS)[41]

Impairment of Nutritional Status		Severity of Disease	
Absent Score 0	Normal nutritional status	Absent Score 0	Normal nutritional requirements
Mild Score 1	Weight loss >5% in 3 months OR Food intake below 50% to 75% of normal requirement in preceding week	Mild Score 1	• Hip fracture • Chronic illness patients, in particular those with acute complications (cirrhosis, chronic obstructive pulmonary disease) • Chronic hemodialysis, diabetes, or oncology patients
Moderate Score 2	Weight loss >5% in 2 months OR BMI 18.5 to 20.5 plus impaired general condition OR Food intake 25% to 50% of normal requirement in preceding week	Moderate Score 2	• Major abdominal surgery • Stroke • Severe pneumonia, hematologic malignancy
Severe Score 3	Weight loss >5% in 1 month (>15% in 3 months) OR BMI <18.5 plus impaired general condition OR Food intake 0% to 25% of normal requirement in preceding week	Severe Score 3	• Head injury • Bone marrow transplant • Intensive care patients (APACHE* >10)

Total Score (impaired nutritional status score + severity of disease score):
* Acute Physiology and Chronic Health Evaluation
Note: If age ≥ 70 years, add 1 to the total score
Reproduced from Kondrup J, Rasmussen HH, Hamberg O, Stanga Z, Ad Hoc ESPEN Working Group. Nutritional risk screening (NRS 2002): A new method based on an analysis of controlled clinical trials. *Clin Nutr*. 2003;22(3):321-336. doi: S0261561402002145 [pii].

measurements will also help the medical team determine energy requirements and appropriate rates for nutrition support and weight-based mediations.

Repeated measurements throughout the continuum of care are essential for diagnosing hospital-acquired malnutrition. Table 6.11 features characteristics associated with adult malnutrition according to the guidelines of AND/A.S.P.E.N.[38] Obtaining accurate height and weight measurements in the ICU may be difficult, as most patients are bed bound and sedated. Estimated height and weight may be inaccurate[44] and standardized evidence-based methods are not currently available. Clinicians may use bed scales and patient lifts to obtain weight and tape measures to determine recumbent height,[45] but should be mindful of possible measurement errors.[46] Frequent measurements will improve accuracy and confidence in the measurements.

Anthropometric measurements are often influenced by medical factors, such as hydration status. If a patient requires aggressive fluid resuscitation or has visual

TABLE 6.10 NUTRITION RISK IN THE CRITICALLY ILL (NUTRIC) SCREENING TOOL[43]

Variable	Criteria	Points
Age (years)	<50	0
	50-74	1
	≥75	2
APACHE II* score	<15	0
	15-19	1
	20-28	2
	≥28	3
SOFA† score	<6	0
	6-9	1
	≥10	2
Number of comorbidities	0-1	0
	≥2	1
Days from hospital to ICU admit	0-<1	0
	≥1	1

* Acute Physiology and Chronic Health Evaluation II
†Sequential Organ Failure Assessment
Reproduced from Rahman A, Hasan RM, Agarwala R, Martin C, Day AG, Heyland DK. Identifying critically-ill patients who will benefit most from nutritional therapy: Further validation of the "modified NUTRIC" nutritional risk assessment tool. *Clin Nutr.* 2016;35(1):158-162. doi: 10.1016/j.clnu.2015.01.015 [doi].

evidence of edema or ascites, clinicians should use a dry or usual body weight.[34] A dry weight is obtained in the absence of excess fluid and usual body weight may be collected from a knowledgeable family member.

> **CORE CONCEPT 5**
>
> Accurate height and weight measurements are needed to determine baseline and ongoing nutritional status.

Biochemical Assessment

Laboratory data, relevant to the nutritional care of the patient, varies among critical care diagnoses and may change throughout the hospital course. Monitoring glucose, electrolytes, acid–base balance, and liver and kidney function is often necessary.

Table 6.12 includes biochemical markers typically monitored during the acute phase of burn injury. Frequency of measurements may vary and is influenced by preexisting comorbidities and degree of injury. Hypophosphatemia and hypomagnesemia are common among burn patients and must be treated as needed.

> **PRACTICE POINT**
>
> Monitoring of electrolytes, including phosphorus and magnesium, before and during initiation of nutrition support is important, as initiation of feeds may result in cellular shifts. Low levels should be repleted despite advancement of feedings.

TABLE 6.11 INDICATORS OF MALNUTRITION DURING ACUTE ILLNESS

	Malnutrition*	
	Moderate	**Severe**
Energy intake	<75% of energy needs for >7 days	≤50% of energy needs for ≥5 days
Weight loss	1%-2% over 1 week 5% over 1 month 7.5% over 3 months	> 2% over 1 week > 5% over 1 month >7.5% over 3 months
Loss of subcutaneous fat	Mild	Moderate
Muscle loss	Mild	Moderate
Edema	Mild	Moderate/Severe
Reduced grip strength	N/A	Reduced

* Having two or more of these characteristics supports a malnutrition diagnosis.
Modified from White JV, Guenter P, Jensen G, et al. Consensus statement of the academy of nutrition and dietetics/american society for parenteral and enteral nutrition: Characteristics recommended for the identification and documentation of adult malnutrition (undernutrition). *J Acad Nutr Diet.* 2012;112(5):730-738. doi: 10.1016/j.jand.2012.03.012 [doi].

TABLE 6.12 BIOCHEMICAL MONITORING OF BURN PATIENTS

Biochemical Marker	Frequency
Electrolytes	2-4 times per day
Phosphorus	2-4 times per day
Magnesium	2-4 times per day
Glucose	2-4 times per day
Liver function tests	Weekly
Blood urea nitrogen/creatinine	Weekly
Triglycerides	Weekly
Serum lipase	Weekly
Urinary urea nitrogen	Weekly

Many ICU patients will have hyperglycemia, characterized by elevated blood glucose levels, due to the acute-phase response. Blood glucose control is critical in the ICU, as hyperglycemia among ICU patients increases mortality and infection rates.[47-49] Current guidelines from the SCCM recommend keeping blood glucose levels <150 mg/dL[47] (Table 6.13). Insulin protocols should maintain blood glucose levels below this threshold, while preventing episodes of hypoglycemia (blood glucose ≤70 mg/dL).[47]

> **PRACTICE POINT**
>
> Protocols or algorithms should be used when using insulin therapy for safety and efficacy.

TABLE 6.13 GENERAL GUIDELINES FOR BLOOD GLUCOSE MONITORING IN THE ICU[47]

- Maintain blood glucose between 70 mg/dL and 149 mg/dL
- Initiate IV insulin therapy for blood glucose ≥150 mg/dL
- For patients receiving intravenous (IV) insulin, blood glucose should be monitored every 1 to 2 hours
- Insulin is a high-risk medication. Standardized protocols are needed to reduce medication errors.

Data from Jacobi J, Bircher N, Krinsley J, et al. Guidelines for the use of an insulin infusion for the management of hyperglycemia in critically ill patients. *Crit Care Med*. 2012;40(12):3251-3276. doi: 10.1097/CCM.0b013e3182653269 [doi].

> **CORE CONCEPT 6**
>
> Hyperglycemia is common among ICU patients. Maintaining blood glucose levels between 70 and 149 mg/dL decreases morbidity and mortality.

Current SCCM/A.S.P.E.N. guidelines do not support the use of serum proteins (albumin, prealbumin, retinol-binding protein, transferrin) to assess protein status during critical illness.[34,53-55] Decreases in these acute-phase proteins most likely reflect reprioritization of protein synthesis in the liver and are not related to nutritional status.[34,56]

In some situations, obtaining a urinary urea nitrogen from a 24-hour urine collection and calculating nitrogen balance may be useful for assessing the adequacy of dietary protein intake.[57] Clinicians should aim for a nitrogen balance between –2 and +2 g/day. A considerably negative nitrogen balance indicates that dietary protein intake is insufficient to meet metabolic demands. Nitrogen balance studies may be unreliable if the patient has renal failure or significant protein losses via wounds, drains, or dialysate.[58,59]

Assessment of micronutrient status in the ICU may also be inaccurate due to potential alterations in absorption, transport, metabolism, and excretion.[60,61] Thus, interpretation of blood micronutrient levels among this population should be interpreted with caution.

> **PRACTICE POINT**
>
> Nitrogen balance is a useful way to determine protein adequacy. For burn patients, it is important to account for increased protein losses in the wound.

> **CORE CONCEPT 7**
>
> Biochemical assessment of protein nutritional status is not accurate in critically ill patients.

Nutrition-focused Physical Exam

A head-to-toe inspection of the patient will evaluate a variety of characteristics that are essential for the nutrition assessment of a critically ill patient. Elements of the nutrition-focused physical exam (NFPE) include the following:

- Overall appearance
- Skin (open wounds, decubitus ulcers, evidence of micronutrient deficiency)
- Muscle and fat wasting
- Fluid accumulation
- Assistive feeding devices (gastric tubes, enteric tubes)
- Peripheral and central catheters
- Ostomies

The NFPE is used, along with other assessment tools, to identify existing malnutrition or changes in nutritional status. If a patient is identified as having two or more of the criteria listed in Table 6.11, a diagnosis of malnutrition is indicated.[38]

⚠ Clinical Controversy

Stress Hyperglycemia

Stress hyperglycemia is a common occurrence in metabolically stressed intensive care patients. However, the optimal range for maintaining blood glucose levels remains controversial. In 2001, van den Berghe et al[50] demonstrated a significant reduction in mortality compared with a conventional insulin therapy, which lead to a paradigm shift in glucose management in an intensive care setting.[50] In 2009, The NICE-SUGAR Study Investigators[51] showed conflicting results, with an increasing mortality risk among adults in the ICU with tight glucose control. Furthermore, moderate blood glucose control resulted in lower mortality.

Questions

1. Review the articles cited below. Choose your position on glucose control for patients in the ICU and provide persuasive argument for your position, using evidence from the study described.

References

1. van den Berghe G, Wouters P, Weekers F, et al. Intensive insulin therapy in critically ill patients. *N Engl J Med*. 2001;345(19):1359-1367. doi: 10.1056/NEJMoa011300 [doi].
2. NICE-SUGAR Study Investigators, Finfer S, Chittock DR, et al. Intensive versus conventional glucose control in critically ill patients. *N Engl J Med*. 2009;360(13):1283-1297. doi: 10.1056/NEJMoa0810625 [doi].

Completing a NFPE may be challenging in patients who require extensive wound dressings, such as a multiple-trauma or burn patient. A thorough inspection of the patient should be completed when the dressings are removed, such as during daily dressing changes or during an operative procedure.

> **CORE CONCEPT 8**
>
> The NFPE assists with identifying signs of malnutrition, including muscle and fat wasting.

Dietary Assessment

In the absence of reliable biochemical markers, evaluation of dietary intake is one of the only methods to determine optimal energy and protein intake. If possible, a complete dietary history should be obtained upon admission either from the patient or a reliable family member.

Ongoing documentation of nutrient intake while in the ICU is critical to assessing adequate oral intake and/or provision of nutrition support. Daily calorie/protein counts are useful for documenting macronutrient deficits. It is important to remember that some medications contain calories (propofol, dextrose) and should be included in the dietary intake totals.

Sufficient protein intake is especially important for ICU patients, as it is the primary macronutrient responsible for wound healing, immune function, and lean body mass preservation.[34]

> **PRACTICE POINT**
>
> Dietary energy and protein deficits should be calculated daily and communicated with the medical team on a regular basis.

Specific micronutrient requirements during critical illness have not been established and most likely differ across diagnoses. It is important to ensure that all patients

🩺 Clinical Roundtable

Topic: Nutrition Assessment in Critical Illness

Background: Indicators to assess nutritional status and nutritional adequacy are lacking in the critically ill patient. Measures of weight are useful to trend, but shifts and expansion within the extracellular fluid compartment mask changes in dry weight or lean body mass. Down regulation of visceral proteins makes serum albumin and prealbumin insensitive to changes in nutritional status. Protein balance provides insight into protein breakdown as indicated by urinary urea nitrogen; nitrogen and protein losses through the wound are difficult to predict, however. Monitoring effectiveness of nutrition therapy is challenging and requires interpretation of a collection of indices. Frequent and critical analysis is needed to adjust nutrition support to the patient's responsiveness to therapy.

Roundtable Discussion

1. Compare and contrast the utility of nutrition assessment methods in critically ill versus non-critically ill patients.
2. How would you determine nutritional status without biochemical markers in the critical care setting?

are receiving at least the Dietary Reference Intake (DRI) for all essential micronutrients.

> **CORE CONCEPT 9**
>
> It is important to collect and analyze daily calorie and protein intake to ensure patients are receiving adequate energy and protein to support recovery.

Determining Energy Needs

The best way to estimate energy requirements in the ICU is by using indirect calorimetry (IC).[33,34] Measurements should be repeated in timely intervals to account for the dynamic features of critical illness including changes in metabolic stress, wound healing, medications, and treatment plans.[34,62]

Predictive equations are inaccurate and should only be used if IC is not available. These equations tend to be particularly erroneous among obese and underweight patients.[63-66] Several predictive equations are supported by professional organizations when IC is not available (**Table 6.14**). Some of these equations do not require additional activity or stress factors. The 2016 SCCM/A.S.P.E.N. Guidelines support a simple weight-based equation (25-30 kcal/kg/day).[34] Although not superior to others, it is easy to use and is just as accurate as the more complex equations.

> **PRACTICE POINT**
>
> Clinicians should be mindful of fluid accumulation when utilizing predictive equations. To prevent overestimation of energy requirements, equations should include the patient's dry weight.

Calculating Protein Needs

For all critically ill patients, adequate protein is required to maintain lean body mass and support immune function. In some subsets of critical illness, protein is also needed to support wound healing. Protein requirements typically range from 1.2 to 2.0 g/kg actual body weight[34] and may

CASE STUDY REVISITED

Manuel is stabilized and a consult is made for nutrition support. His information is as follows:

Anthropometric Data:
Current weight: 90 kg (200.8 lbs)
Admission weight: 81 kg (178 lb)
Height: 173 cm (68")

Biochemical Data:
Sodium 138 (135-145 mEq/L)
Potassium 4.2 (3.6-5.0 mEq/L)
Chloride 114 (98-110 mEq/L)
Carbon dioxide 19 (20-30 mEq/L)
Blood urea nitrogen 21 (6-24 mg/dL)
Creatinine 1.0 (0.4-1.3 mg/dL)
Blood glucose 200 mg/dL (70-139 mg/dL)

Calcium 7.0 (8.5-10.5 mEq/L)
Phosphorus 2.0 (2.7 to 4.5 mg/dL)
Magnesium 1.4 (1.3 to 2.1 mEq/L)
Albumin 1.5 (3.5 to 5.0 g/dL)

Clinical Data:
Past Medical History: None
Nutritionally Relevant Medications: Oxandrolone, insulin per protocol, neutraphos
Vital signs: Blood Pressure: 170/90 mm Hg; temperature: 101°F; heart rate: 101 beats/min
Nutrition-focused Physical Exams: Patient remains edematous.
Disease severity Scores: APACHE II: 20; SOFA: 8

Dietary Data:
Dietary History: NPO for 3 days since admission
Diet Prescription: Initiate enteral feedings per dietitian recommendation

Questions:
1. Explain the change in Manuel's anthropometric measurements, biochemical parameters, and clinical data.
2. Estimate Manuel's energy and protein requirements. What weight would you use?
3. What is the best feeding plan for Manuel?

TABLE 6.14 ESTIMATING ENERGY REQUIREMENTS FOR CRITICALLY ILL PATIENTS

	Equation	Reference
Nonobese, mechanically ventilated	PSU 2003b RMR = Mifflin(0.96) + VE(31) + Tmax(167) − 6212	AND EAL[33]
Obese, mechanically ventilated <60 years	PSU 2003b RMR = Mifflin(0.96) + VE(31) + Tmax(167) − 6212	AND EAL[33]
>60 years	PSU 2010 RMR = Mifflin(0.71) + VE(64) + Tmax(85) − 3085	
Nonobese	25-30 kcal/kg/day	SCCM/A.S.P.E.N.[34]
Obese BMI 30-50 kg/m²	11-14 kcal/kg/day (use actual body weight)	SCCM/A.S.P.E.N.[34]
BMI > 50 kg/m²	22-25 kcal/kg (use ideal body weight)	

PSU: Penn State University
RMR: Resting metabolic rate
Mifflin: Mifflin–St Jeor equation
RMR males = 10 x weight (kg) + 6.25 x height (cm) − 5 x age (years) + 5
RMR females = 10 x weight (kg) + 6.25 x height (cm) − 5 x age (years) − 161
VE: minute ventilation (L/min)
Tmax: maximum temperature in Celsius
Data from Academy of Nutrition and Dietetics. Critical illness guidelines. http://www.andeal.org/topic.cfm?menu=5302. Updated 2012; and McClave SA, Taylor BE, Martindale RG, et al. Guidelines for the provision and assessment of nutrition support therapy in the adult critically ill patient: Society of critical care medicine (SCCM) and american society for parenteral and enteral nutrition (A.S.P.E.N.). *JPEN J Parenter Enteral Nutr.* 2016;40(2):159-211. doi: 10.1177/0148607115621863 [doi].

be higher among patients with burns, trauma, or dialysis requirements[8] (Table 6.15). Of note, it is not recommended to restrict protein during renal insufficiency or hepatic failure.[34] For critically ill obese patients, a high-protein, hypocaloric diet will help maintain lean body mass and promote the breakdown of adipose tissue.[34] The protein requirement of burn patients is particularly high (1.5-2 g/kg/day) and may even exceed 2.5 g/kg/day to improve nitrogen balance. Wound healing and nitrogen balance studies should be followed closely and correlated with protein intake as appropriate.

> **CORE CONCEPT 10**
>
> Energy and protein requirements are increased during critical illness.

Vitamins/Minerals

All critically ill patients should receive at least the DRI for all essential micronutrients. This can easily be accomplished in patients receiving EN, as most commercial EN products provide 100% or more of the DRI for all essential micronutrients. If parenteral nutrition (PN) is required, clinicians should ensure that micronutrient provision is adequate.

Specific guidelines for micronutrient supplementation during critical illness are not well established. According to the 2016 SCCM/A.S.P.E.N. Guidelines, current evidence suggests that supplementation with antioxidant vitamins (vitamins E and C) and trace minerals (selenium, zinc, copper) may reduce mortality.[34] Dosing, route of administration, and specific micronutrient combinations differ among clinicians who specialize in critical illness, and micronutrient requirements most likely vary among disease

TABLE 6.15 DAILY PROTEIN REQUIREMENTS FOR CRITICALLY ILL PATIENTS[34]

Nonobese	1.2-2.0 g/kg
Obese BMI 30-40 kg/m² BMI > 40 kg/m²	2 g/kg using ideal body weight up to 2.5 g/kg ideal body weight
Hemodialysis or continuous renal replacement therapy	Up to 2.5 g/kg
Burns	1.5-2 g/kg

Data from McClave SA, Taylor BE, Martindale RG, et al. Guidelines for the provision and assessment of nutrition support therapy in the adult critically ill patient: Society of critical care medicine (SCCM) and american society for parenteral and enteral nutrition (A.S.P.E.N.). *JPEN J Parenter Enteral Nutr.* 2016;40(2):159-211. doi: 10.1177/0148607115621863 [doi].

states. Thus, provision of micronutrients should be individualized and closely monitored to prevent deficiency and toxicity.

Treatment

Treatment options should be individualized and established using the data collected during the nutrition assessment. Nutritional risk and severity of disease will be significant factors when determining the appropriate nutrition intervention. Adequate provision of nutrition support will impact patient outcomes including infection rates and length of stay.[67-69]

Enteral Nutrition Support

Most critically ill patients require EN and/or PN support to meet the metabolic demands of the illness. EN is the preferred method of nutrition support, as it maintains gut integrity and blunts the hypermetabolic response.[70-72]

Current SCCM/A.S.P.E.N. and AND guidelines advocate for the introduction of EN within 24 to 48 hours of admission to the ICU.[33,34] Patients who receive timely EN have lower mortality and infection rates compared to those who receive delayed EN.[34]

> **CORE CONCEPT 11**
>
> Enteral nutrition is the gold standard of nutrition support in the intensive care unit.

Hemodynamic instability, a condition associated with sepsis and characterized by hypotension, is a contraindication of EN.[34] Providing EN to patients with advanced hemodynamic instability may result in ischemia/reperfusion injuries and, in severe cases, the development of ischemic bowel. EN should be stopped if mean arterial blood pressure is <50 mm Hg or if the patient requires aggressive use of vasopressor medications (norepinephrine, phenylephrine, epinephrine, dopamine) to maintain blood pressure.[34]

In most cases, specialty formulas (disease-specific, organ-specific, immune-modulating, elemental, semi-elemental) are not indicated for ICU patients. A standard, high-protein, polymeric (whole protein), 1 to 1.5 kcal/mL EN formula is sufficient to meet macro- and micronutrient requirements.[34]

According to the 2016 SCCM/A.S.P.E.N. guidelines, formulas with immune-modulating components (eicosapentaenoic acid, docosahexaenoic acid, glutamine, nucleic acid) and anti-inflammatory lipids (omega-3 fish oils) do not provide additional benefit to ICU patients.[34] Thus, these specialty formulas, which are often more expensive than standard formulas, are not necessary for ICU patients. The few exceptions to this recommendation are listed in **Table 6.16**.

The addition of fermentable soluble fiber is recommended for all ICU patients who are hemodynamically stable, especially among patients with diarrhea.[34] Loose bowel movements that progress to diarrhea are common among patients who require aggressive antibiotic therapy or hypertonic medications, such as sodium chloride.

Soluble fiber supports bowel health by producing short chain fatty acids and functioning as a prebiotic. **Short chain fatty acids**, products of soluble fiber fermentation in the colon, are fuel for colonocytes and promote water and electrolyte absorption.[73] As a prebiotic, soluble fiber stimulates the growth of healthy bacteria, including *Bifidobacteria* and *Lactobacillus*, in the colon.[74] For patients with diarrhea, the enhanced water absorption via the colon

---

Clinical Roundtable

Topic Micronutrient Supplementation During Critically Ill

Background: Many aspects of critical illness, particularly burn injury, intuitively increase micronutrient requirements. Antioxidant nutrients may be useful in fighting free radicals. Selenium, zinc, and copper are important for wound healing and infection control. The acute-phase response associated with critical illness and catabolic stress alters micronutrient status. Many nutrients are lost through wounds and urine. In addition, certain nutrients such as zinc and selenium depend on specific protein carriers to be transported to organs and wound tissue. These protein carriers may be downregulated during stress. In addition, because nutrients work in systems and/or can be antagonistic to one another, single nutrient supplementation may affect the status of other nutrients. Specific recommendations for micronutrient supplementation during critical illness are not available.

Roundtable Discussion: How do you assess micronutrient status? How would you prevent deficiency and toxicity? Which nutrients, if any, would you recommend providing to patients in addition to the amount they receive via nutrition support? What might you monitor? How well do enteral feeding products meet micronutrient requirements during illness?

Reference

1. Prelack, K and Sheridan RL. Micronutrient supplementation in the critically ill patient: strategies for clinical practice. *J Trauma*. 2001;51:601-620.

> ## CASE STUDY REVISITED
>
> EN support via Manuel's nasogastric tube was initiated within the first 24 hours of admission and advanced to goal rate by 48 hours. On day 5 of admission, Manuel's condition worsened, and he became hemodynamically unstable. He begins to have abdominal distention and high gastric residuals. The team asks if the feeding tube should be positioned postpylorically.
>
> ### Questions
> 1. What are your feeding plan options at this point?
> 2. Which do you recommend?

TABLE 6.16 APPROPRIATE USE OF ENTERAL NUTRITION FORMULAS FOR ICU PATIENTS[34]

Condition	Suggested Formula Type
Most critically ill patients	High protein, polymeric
Acute respiratory failure	Fluid-restricted, energy dense (1.5-2 kcal/mL)
Renal failure	High protein, polymeric
	If needed, formula low in phosphorus, potassium
Traumatic brain injury	Immune-modulating (with arginine)
Postoperative surgical ICU patients	Immune-modulating
Critically ill patients with persistent diarrhea due to malabsorption	Semi-elemental

Data from McClave SA, Taylor BE, Martindale RG, et al. Guidelines for the provision and assessment of nutrition support therapy in the adult critically ill patient: Society of critical care medicine (SCCM) and american society for parenteral and enteral nutrition (A.S.P.E.N.). *JPEN J Parenter Enteral Nutr*. 2016;40(2):159-211. doi: 10.1177/0148607115621863 [doi].

is especially beneficial for decreasing loose stools. The SSCM/A.S.P.E.N. guidelines recommend providing a total of 10 to 20 g fiber/day to all ICU patients.[34,75] Ideally, this dose would be provided in intervals throughout the day or added to the EN to provide a continuous infusion.

Full-strength EN formulas may be started at 10 to 40 mL/hour and advanced as tolerated (typically 10 to 20 mL every 8 to 12 hours).[76] Volume-based feeding regimens may also be useful in the ICU, especially if patients require frequent breaks in EN due to medical procedures.

The goal of this type of feeding protocol is to meet the daily volume of EN (instead of focusing on a specific hourly rate), which often requires fluctuating the rate of EN to account for periods when EN was held.[34,77]

> **PRACTICE POINT**
>
> For patients who are frequently going to the operating room or who have their feedings held for medical procedures, feeding volume can be upwardly adjusted to compensate for interruption of feedings.

Parenteral Nutrition Support

If EN is not a realistic or safe option, due to intolerance or hemodynamic instability, PN should be considered in most ICU populations. Nutritional status guides the initiation of PN according to SCCM/A.S.P.E.N. guidelines.[34] PN should be started immediately among malnourished patients or those at high risk for malnutrition. Among well-nourished patients, if EN cannot be established within 7 days, PN may be initiated. Additionally, if a patient is only able to tolerate small volumes of EN and thus is meeting <60% of estimated energy and protein needs, PN should be introduced after 7 to 10 days.[34]

In any case, judicial utilization and monitoring of PN is critical to prevent overfeeding and hyperglycemia. The SCCM/A.S.P.E.N. guidelines support hypocaloric (≤20 kcal/kg/day or up to 80% of estimated kcal needs) PN regimens that supply adequate amounts of protein (≥1.2 g/kg/day) during the first week. PN may be increased thereafter, as tolerated by the patient.[34] Glucose infusion rates should not exceed glucose oxidation capacity (5 mg/kg/min)[78]. Hypocaloric PN may reduce the incidence of hyperglycemia and infection.[79,80]

Lipids are not a preferred source of energy during critical illness and the addition of intravenous lipids may increase infectious complications[79]. Therefore, intravenous lipid injectable emulsion (ILE) are not recommended during the first week of PN provision and subsequently should only be used to prevent essential fatty acid deficiency. If necessary, the SCCM/A.S.P.E.N. guidelines recommend limiting ILE to a maximum dose of 20 g per week.[34]

CASE STUDY REVISITED

On day 12 of admission, Manuel remains hemodynamically unstable and EN has not restarted. Manuel's current dry weight is 77 kg (172 lbs).

Questions

1. Does Manuel now meet the criteria for malnutrition?
2. Is it appropriate to start PN?

Chapter Summary

Patients with critical illness have heightened protein and energy requirements due to the hypermetabolic and catabolic physiologic response. Burn injuries are the most hypermetabolic disease state. Comprehensive, ongoing nutrition assessments are essential to identify patients at risk for malnutrition. An interdisciplinary team approach is required for the development and implementation of successful treatment plans to optimize recovery, survival, and outcome measures.

Key Terms

catabolic stress response, hypermetabolism, acute phase reactants, catabolism, catecholamines, cytokines, systemic inflammatory response syndrome, sepsis, septic shock, hemodynamic instability, short chain fatty acids

References

1. Nielson CB, Duethman NC, Howard JM, Moncure M, Wood, JG. Burns: Pathophysiology of systemic complications and current management. *J Burn Care Res*. 2017;38(1):e469-e489.
2. Bittner EA, Shank E, Woodson L, Martyn JAJ. Acute and Perioperative care of the burn-injured patient. *Anesthesiology*. 2015;122(2):448-464. doi:10.1097/ALN.0000000000000559.
3. Simsek T, Simsek HU, Canturk NZ. Response to trauma and metabolic changes: Posttraumatic metabolism. *Ulus Cerrahi Derg*. 2014;30(3):153-159. doi: 10.5152/UCD.2014.2653 [doi].
4. Finnerty CC, Mabvuure NT, Ali A, Kozar RA, Herndon DN. The surgically induced stress response. *JPEN J Parenter Enteral Nutr*. 2013;37(5 Suppl):21S-29S. doi: 10.1177/0148607113496117 [doi].
5. Hart DW, Wolf SE, Mlcak R, et al. Persistence of muscle catabolism after severe burn. *Surgery*. 2000;128(2):312-319. doi: S0039-6060(00)62693-4 [pii].
6. Jeschke MG, Gauglitz GG, Kulp GA, et al. Long-term persistence of the pathophysiologic response to severe burn injury. *PLoS One*. 2011;6(7):e21245. doi: 10.1371/journal.pone.0021245 [doi].
7. Porter C, Herndon DN, Borsheim E, et al. Uncoupled skeletal muscle mitochondria contribute to hypermetabolism in severely burned adults. *Am J Physiol Endocrinol Metab*. 2014;307(5):E462-467. doi: 10.1152/ajpendo.00206.2014 [doi].
8. Harrison T. Sixth national burn seminar. adrenaline and noradrenaline excretion following burns. *J Trauma*. 1967;7(1):137-140.
9. McCowen KC, Malhotra A, Bistrian BR. Stress-induced hyperglycemia. *Crit Care Clin*. 2001;17(1):107-124.
10. Jeschke MG, Chinkes DL, Finnerty CC, et al. Pathophysiologic response to severe burn injury. *Ann Surg*. 2008;248(3):387-401. doi: 10.1097/SLA.0b013e3181856241 [doi].
11. Robinson LE, van Soeren MH. Insulin resistance and hyperglycemia in critical illness: Role of insulin in glycemic control. *AACN Clin Issues*. 2004;15(1):45-62. doi: 00044067-200401000-00004 [pii].
12. Wilmore DW, Mason AD, Jr, Pruitt BA, Jr. Insulin response to glucose in hypermetabolic burn patients. *Ann Surg*. 1976;183(3):314-320.
13. Tredget EE, Yu YM. The metabolic effects of thermal injury. *World J Surg*. 1992;16(1):68-79.
14. Wolfe RR, Herndon DN, Peters EJ, Jahoor F, Desai MH, Holland OB. Regulation of lipolysis in severely burned children. *Ann Surg*. 1987;206(2):214-221.
15. Little RA, Henderson A, Frayn KN, Galasko CS, White RH. The disposal of intravenous glucose studied using glucose and insulin clamp techniques in sepsis and trauma in man. *Acta Anaesthesiol Belg*. 1987;38(4):275-279.
16. Black PR, Brooks DC, Bessey PQ, Wolfe RR, Wilmore DW. Mechanisms of insulin resistance following injury. *Ann Surg*. 1982;196(4):420-435.
17. Newsome TW, Mason AD,Jr, Pruitt BA,Jr. Weight loss following thermal injury. *Ann Surg*. 1973;178(2):215-217.
18. Porter C, Tompkins RG, Finnerty CC, Sidossis LS, Suman OE, Herndon DN. The metabolic stress response to burn trauma: Current understanding and therapies. *Lancet*. 2016;388(10052):1417-1426. doi: S0140-6736(16)31469-6 [pii].
19. Demling RH, Seigne P. Metabolic management of patients with severe burns. *World J Surg*. 2000;24(6):673-680. doi: 10.1007/s002689910109 [pii].
20. Pollack SV. Wound healing: A review. III. Nutritional factors affecting wound healing. *J Dermatol Surg Oncol*. 1979;5(8):615-619.
21. Bone RC, Sprung CL, Sibbald WJ. Definitions for sepsis and organ failure. *Crit Care Med*. 1992;20(6):724-726.
22. Greenhalgh DG, Saffle JR, Holmes JH, 4th, et al. American Burn Association consensus conference to define sepsis and infection in burns. *J Burn Care Res*. 2007;28(6):776-790. doi: 10.1097/BCR.0b013e3181599bc9 [doi].
23. Lund C, Browder N. The estimation of areas of burns. *Surg Gynecol Obstet*. 1944;79:352-358.
24. Sheridan RL. Management of burns. *Surg Clin North Am*. 2014;94(4):xv-xvi. doi: 10.1016/j.suc.2014.06.001 [doi].
25. Pham TN, Cancio LC, Gibran NS, American Burn Association. American Burn Association practice guidelines burn shock resuscitation. *J Burn Care Res*. 2008;29(1):257-266. doi: 10.1097/BCR.0b013e31815f3876 [doi].
26. Weber JM, Sheridan RL, Schulz JT, Tompkins RG, Ryan CM. Effectiveness of bacteria-controlled nursing units in preventing cross-colonization

27. Pham TN, Klein MB, Gibran NS, et al. Impact of oxandrolone treatment on acute outcomes after severe burn injury. *J Burn Care Res*. 2008;29(6):902-906. doi: 10.1097/BCR.0b013e31818ba14d [doi].

28. Tuvdendorj D, Chinkes DL, Zhang XJ, et al. Long-term oxandrolone treatment increases muscle protein net deposition via improving amino acid utilization in pediatric patients 6 months after burn injury. *Surgery*. 2011;149(5):645-653. doi: 10.1016/j.surg.2010.12.006 [doi].

29. Hart DW, Wolf SE, Ramzy PI, et al. Anabolic effects of oxandrolone after severe burn. *Ann Surg*. 2001;233(4):556-564.

30. Herndon DN, Rodriguez NA, Diaz EC, et al. Long-term propranolol use in severely burned pediatric patients: A randomized controlled study. *Ann Surg*. 2012;256(3):402-411. doi: 10.1097/SLA.0b013e318265427e [doi].

31. Flores O, Stockton K, Roberts JA, Muller MJ, Paratz JD. The efficacy and safety of adrenergic blockade after burn injury: A systematic review and meta-analysis. *J Trauma Acute Care Surg*. 2016;80(1):146-155. doi: 10.1097/TA.0000000000000887 [doi].

32. Nunez-Villaveiran T, Sanchez M, Millan P, Garcia-de-Lorenzo A. Systematic review of the effect of propanolol on hypermetabolism in burn injuries. *Med Intensiva*. 2015;39(2):101-113. doi: 10.1016/j.medin.2014.08.002 [doi].

33. Academy of Nutrition and Dietetics. Critical illness guidelines. http://www.andeal.org/topic.cfm?menu=5302. Updated 2012. Accessed November 25, 2017.

34. McClave SA, Taylor BE, Martindale RG, et al. Guidelines for the provision and assessment of nutrition support therapy in the adult critically ill patient: Society of Critical Care Medicine (SCCM) and American Society for Parenteral and Enteral Nutrition (A.S.P.E.N.). *JPEN J Parenter Enteral Nutr*. 2016;40(2):159-211. doi: 10.1177/0148607115621863 [doi].

35. Jensen GL, Bistrian B, Roubenoff R, Heimburger DC. Malnutrition syndromes: A conundrum vs continuum. *JPEN J Parenter Enteral Nutr*. 2009;33(6):710-716. doi: 10.1177/0148607109344724 [doi].

36. Jensen GL, Mirtallo J, Compher C, et al. Adult starvation and disease-related malnutrition: A proposal for etiology-based diagnosis in the clinical practice setting from the international consensus guideline committee. *JPEN J Parenter Enteral Nutr*. 2010;34(2):156-159. doi: 10.1177/0148607110361910 [doi].

37. Jensen GL, Wheeler D. A new approach to defining and diagnosing malnutrition in adult critical illness. *Curr Opin Crit Care*. 2012;18(2):206-211. doi: 10.1097/MCC.0b013e328351683a [doi].

38. White JV, Guenter P, Jensen G, et al. Consensus statement of the Academy of Nutrition and Dietetics/American Society for Parenteral and Enteral Nutrition: Characteristics recommended for the identification and documentation of adult malnutrition (undernutrition). *J Acad Nutr Diet*. 2012;112(5):730-738. doi: 10.1016/j.jand.2012.03.012 [doi].

39. Standard FAQ Detail. The Joint Commission. https://www.jointcommission.org/standards_information/jcfaqdetails.aspx?StandardsFaqId=872&ProgramId=46 Accessed November 25, 2017.

40. Kondrup J, Allison SP, Elia M, Vellas B, Plauth M, Educational and Clinical Practice Committee, European Society of Parenteral and Enteral Nutrition (ESPEN). ESPEN guidelines for nutrition screening 2002. *Clin Nutr*. 2003;22(4):415-421. doi: S0261561403000980 [pii].

41. Kondrup J, Rasmussen HH, Hamberg O, Stanga Z, Ad Hoc ESPEN Working Group. Nutritional risk screening (NRS 2002): A new method based on an analysis of controlled clinical trials. *Clin Nutr*. 2003;22(3):321-336. doi: S0261561402002145 [pii].

42. Heyland DK, Dhaliwal R, Jiang X, Day AG. Identifying critically ill patients who benefit the most from nutrition therapy: The development and initial validation of a novel risk assessment tool. *Crit Care*. 2011;15(6):R268. doi: 10.1186/cc10546 [doi].

43. Rahman A, Hasan RM, Agarwala R, Martin C, Day AG, Heyland DK. Identifying critically-ill patients who will benefit most from nutritional therapy: Further validation of the "modified NUTRIC" nutritional risk assessment tool. *Clin Nutr*. 2016;35(1):158-162. doi: 10.1016/j.clnu.2015.01.015 [doi].

44. Bloomfield R, Steel E, MacLennan G, Noble DW. Accuracy of weight and height estimation in an intensive care unit: Implications for clinical practice and research. *Crit Care Med*. 2006;34(8):2153-2157. doi: 10.1097/01.CCM.0000229145.04482.93 [doi].

45. Dennis DM, Hunt EE, Budgeon CA. Measuring height in recumbent critical care patients. *Am J Crit Care*. 2015;24(1):41-47. doi: 10.4037/ajcc2015761 [doi].

46. Freitag E, Edgecombe G, Baldwin I, Cottier B, Heland M. Determination of body weight and height measurement for critically ill patients admitted to the intensive care unit: A quality improvement project. *Aust Crit Care*. 2010;23(4):197-207. doi: 10.1016/j.aucc.2010.04.003 [doi].

47. Jacobi J, Bircher N, Krinsley J, et al. Guidelines for the use of an insulin infusion for the management of hyperglycemia in critically ill patients. *Crit Care Med*. 2012;40(12):3251-3276. doi: 10.1097/CCM.0b013e3182653269 [doi].

48. Falciglia M, Freyberg RW, Almenoff PL, D'Alessio DA, Render ML. Hyperglycemia-related mortality in critically ill patients varies with admission diagnosis. *Crit Care Med*. 2009;37(12):3001-3009. doi: 10.1097/CCM.0b013e3181b083f7 [doi].

49. Bagshaw SM, Egi M, George C, Bellomo R, Australia New Zealand Intensive Care Society Database Management Committee. Early blood glucose control and mortality in critically ill patients in Australia. *Crit Care Med*. 2009;37(2):463-470. doi: 10.1097/CCM.0b013e318194b097 [doi].

50. van den Berghe G, Wouters P, Weekers F, et al. Intensive insulin therapy in critically ill patients. *N Engl J Med*. 2001;345(19):1359-1367. doi: 10.1056/NEJMoa011300 [doi].

51. NICE-SUGAR Study Investigators, Finfer S, Chittock DR, et al. Intensive versus conventional glucose control in critically ill patients. *N Engl J Med*. 2009;360(13):1283-1297. doi: 10.1056/NEJMoa0810625 [doi].

52. NICE-SUGAR Study Investigators for the Australian and New Zealand Intensive Care Society Clinical Trials Group and the Canadian Critical Care Trials Group, Finfer S, Chittock D, et al. Intensive versus conventional glucose control in critically ill patients with traumatic brain injury: Long-term follow-up of a subgroup of patients from the NICE-SUGAR study. *Intensive Care Med*. 2015;41(6):1037-1047. doi: 10.1007/s00134-015-3757-6 [doi].

53. Raguso CA, Dupertuis YM, Pichard C. The role of visceral proteins in the nutritional assessment of intensive care unit patients. *Curr Opin Clin Nutr Metab Care*. 2003;6(2):211-216. doi: 10.1097/01.mco.0000058592.27240.95 [doi].

54. Stroud M. Protein and the critically ill; do we know what to give? *Proc Nutr Soc*. 2007;66(3):378-383. doi: S0029665107005642 [pii].

55. Academy of Nutrition and Dietetics. Does serum albumin correlate with weight loss in four models of prolonged protein-energy restriction: Anorexia nervosa, non-malabsorptive gastric partitioning bariatric surgery, calorie-restricted diets or starvation. http://www.andeal.org/topic.cfm?cat=4302&evidence_summary_id=251043&highlight=albumin&home=1. Accessed November 25, 2017.

56. Davis CJ, Sowa D, Keim KS, Kinnare K, Peterson S. The use of prealbumin and C-reactive protein for monitoring nutrition support in adult patients receiving enteral nutrition in an urban medical center. *JPEN J Parenter Enteral Nutr*. 2012;36(2):197-204. doi: 10.1177/0148607111413896 [doi].

57. Choban P, Dickerson R, Malone A, Worthington P, Compher C, American Society for Parenteral and Enteral Nutrition. A.S.P.E.N. clinical guidelines: Nutrition support of hospitalized adult patients with obesity. *JPEN J Parenter Enteral Nutr.* 2013;37(6):714-744. doi: 10.1177/0148607113499374 [doi].

58. Young L, Kearns L, Schoepfel S, Clark N. Protein. In: American Society for Parenteral and Enteral Nutrition, ed. *The A.S.P.E.N. Adult Nutrition Support Core Curriculum.* 2nd ed. Silver Spring, MD: American Society for Parenteral and Enteral Nutrition; 2012:83-97.

59. Collier BR, Cherry-Bukowiek JR, Mills ME. Trauma, surgery, and burns. In: *The A.S.P.E.N. adult nutriton support core curriculum.* 2nd ed. Silver Spring, MD: American Society for Parenteral and Enteral Nutrition; 2012:392-411.

60. Visser J, Labadarios D, Blaauw R. Micronutrient supplementation for critically ill adults: A systematic review and meta-analysis. *Nutrition.* 2011;27(7-8):745-758. doi: 10.1016/j.nut.2010.12.009 [doi].

61. Berger MM, Shenkin A. Update on clinical micronutrient supplementation studies in the critically ill. *Curr Opin Clin Nutr Metab Care.* 2006;9(6):711-716. doi: 10.1097/01.mco.0000247466.41661.ba [doi].

62. McClave SA, Martindale RG, Kiraly L. The use of indirect calorimetry in the intensive care unit. *Curr Opin Clin Nutr Metab Care.* 2013;16(2): 202-208. doi: 10.1097/MCO.0b013e32835dbc54 [doi].

63. Anderegg BA, Worrall C, Barbour E, Simpson KN, Delegge M. Comparison of resting energy expenditure prediction methods with measured resting energy expenditure in obese, hospitalized adults. *JPEN J Parenter Enteral Nutr.* 2009;33(2):168-175. doi: 10.1177/0148607108327192 [doi].

64. Frankenfield DC, Ashcraft CM, Galvan DA. Prediction of resting metabolic rate in critically ill patients at the extremes of body mass index. *JPEN J Parenter Enteral Nutr.* 2013;37(3):361-367. doi: 10.1177/0148607112457423 [doi].

65. Frankenfield DC, Ashcraft CM. Estimating energy needs in nutrition support patients. *JPEN J Parenter Enteral Nutr.* 2011;35(5):563-570. doi: 10.1177/0148607111415859 [doi].

66. Kross EK, Sena M, Schmidt K, Stapleton RD. A comparison of predictive equations of energy expenditure and measured energy expenditure in critically ill patients. *J Crit Care.* 2012;27(3):321.e5-321.12. doi: 10.1016/j.jcrc.2011.07.084 [doi].

67. Heyland DK, Schroter-Noppe D, Drover JW, et al. Nutrition support in the critical care setting: Current practice in Canadian ICUs--opportunities for improvement? *JPEN J Parenter Enteral Nutr.* 2003;27(1):74-83. doi: 10.1177/014860710302700174 [doi].

68. Kreymann KG, Berger MM, Deutz NE, et al. ESPEN guidelines on enteral nutrition: Intensive care. *Clin Nutr.* 2006;25(2):210-223. doi: S0261-5614(06)00041-0 [pii].

69. McClave SA, Heyland DK. The physiologic response and associated clinical benefits from provision of early enteral nutrition. *Nutr Clin Pract.* 2009;24(3):305-315. doi: 10.1177/0884533609335176 [doi].

70. Kang W, Kudsk KA. Is there evidence that the gut contributes to mucosal immunity in humans? *JPEN J Parenter Enteral Nutr.* 2007;31(3):246-258. doi: 31/3/246 [pii].

71. Windsor AC, Kanwar S, Li AG, et al. Compared with parenteral nutrition, enteral feeding attenuates the acute phase response and improves disease severity in acute pancreatitis. *Gut.* 1998;42(3): 431-435.

72. Ammori BJ. Importance of the early increase in intestinal permeability in critically ill patients. *Eur J Surg.* 2002;168(11):660-661; author reply 662.

73. Wong JM, de Souza R, Kendall CW, Emam A, Jenkins DJ. Colonic health: Fermentation and short chain fatty acids. *J Clin Gastroenterol.* 2006;40(3):235-243. doi: 00004836-200603000-00015 [pii].

74. Silk DB, Walters ER, Duncan HD, Green CJ. The effect of a polymeric enteral formula supplemented with a mixture of six fibres on normal human bowel function and colonic motility. *Clin Nutr.* 2001;20(1):49-58. doi: 10.1054/clnu.2000.0359 [doi].

75. Homann HH, Kemen M, Fuessenich C, Senkal M, Zumtobel V. Reduction in diarrhea incidence by soluble fiber in patients receiving total or supplemental enteral nutrition. *JPEN J Parenter Enteral Nutr.* 1994;18(6):486-490. doi: 10.1177/0148607194018006486 [doi].

76. Bankhead R, Boullata J, Brantley S, et al. Enteral nutrition practice recommendations. *JPEN J Parenter Enteral Nutr.* 2009;33(2):122-167. doi: 10.1177/0148607108330314 [doi].

77. Heyland DK, Murch L, Cahill N, et al. Enhanced protein-energy provision via the enteral route feeding protocol in critically ill patients: Results of a cluster randomized trial. *Crit Care Med.* 2013;41(12):2743-2753. doi: 10.1097/CCM.0b013e31829efef5 [doi].

78. Burke JF, Wolfe RR, Mullany CJ, Mathews DE, Bier DM. Glucose requirements following burn injury. parameters of optimal glucose infusion and possible hepatic and respiratory abnormalities following excessive glucose intake. *Ann Surg.* 1979;190(3):274-285.

79. McCowen KC, Friel C, Sternberg J, et al. Hypocaloric total parenteral nutrition: Effectiveness in prevention of hyperglycemia and infectious complications--a randomized clinical trial. *Crit Care Med.* 2000;28(11):3606-3611.

80. Ahrens CL, Barletta JF, Kanji S, et al. Effect of low-calorie parenteral nutrition on the incidence and severity of hyperglycemia in surgical patients: A randomized, controlled trial. *Crit Care Med.* 2005;33(11):2507-2512. doi: 00003246-200511000-00010 [pii].

Chapter 7

Nutrition in Wound Healing

Caitlin Wong

Chapter Outline

Core Concepts
Introduction
Pathophysiology of Wounds and Wound Healing
Chronic Wounds
Medical Treatment of Wounds
Medical Nutrition Therapy for Wound Healing

CORE CONCEPTS

1. Wounds are caused by local and systemic factors and are influenced by the individual's nutritional status.
2. Completion of all three stages of wound healing is essential, and a disruption in any stage leads to chronic inflammation and delayed wound healing.
3. Uncontrolled diabetes increases risk of the development of chronic foot ulcers and often leads to amputations.
4. Wound healing creates a catabolic state; preservation of lean body mass is prioritized over wound healing in malnourished patients.
5. Poor nutritional status is associated with increased risk of developing pressure injuries.

Learning Objectives

1. Explain the difference between an acute wound and a chronic wound.
2. Describe the pathophysiology of wound healing.
3. Compare the types of chronic wounds and their etiologies.
4. Determine the consequences of inadequate nutrition in wound healing.
5. Evaluate how wound healing is differentially affected by starvation and metabolic stress.
6. Outline the roles of specific nutrients in wound healing.
7. Determine nutrition recommendations and the need for amino acid or micronutrient supplementation for wound healing.

Introduction

The skin is the largest organ of the human body. It comprises several layers that act as a barrier to the environment and serves several purposes. The skin aids with temperature regulation; helps maintain hydration status; synthesizes vitamin D; and, most importantly, protects the underlying muscle, bone, tissue, and organs from pathogens and damage. Under normal circumstances, skin remains intact. Skin integrity may be compromised by external and internal factors, such as abrasions and chronic diseases, which lead to the development of wounds.

A **wound** is defined as damage to the structure and function of tissue and can be a minor cut in the epidermis, or outer layer of the skin, or more severe, causing damage to subcutaneous tissue, including muscles, tendons, and bone.[1] Skin wounds are prevalent in all settings, primarily in acute care, long-term care, and home care. Depending on the severity of the wound(s), it can have a major impact on the patient's quality of life because he or she may experience pain, impaired mobility, social isolation, emotional stress, depression, loss of self-image, and increased length of institutional stay.[2,3] In some cases, wounds can also contribute to premature mortality.[3]

The estimated cost of treatment for pressure injuries alone was approximately $9.2 to $15.6 billion dollars in 2008.[3] According to the Centers for Medicare and Medicaid Services, it costs $43,180 per hospital stay to treat pressure injury in an acute care setting as a secondary diagnosis.[3] In addition to the cost of treatment, wounds create an economic burden for the patient. Patients with complicated wounds may need to take time off from work; lose their jobs; be forced into early retirement; or require assistance with activities of daily living, such as bathing, cooking, grooming, and feeding, all of which come at a monetary cost.[2]

To decrease healthcare costs and improve patients' quality of life, the prevention and treatment of wounds needs to be addressed using an interprofessional approach. A clear association exists between nutritional status and the risk of developing wounds, as well as with the healing of wounds. An understanding of the pathophysiology of wound healing, its effects on specific nutritional needs, and the implications for medical nutrition therapy is important in wound management.

Pathophysiology of Wounds and Wound Healing

Wounds can develop secondary to external injury, such as surgery, trauma, and friction. Certain diseases that cause poor circulation, neuropathy, or ischemia, such as venous stasis and diabetes mellitus, also put patients at risk for developing ulcers. Risk factors for wound development and impaired wound healing include poor dietary intake, weight loss, immobility, fecal incontinence, suppressed immune function, corticosteroid use, advanced age, and dry skin.[4,5]

> **CORE CONCEPT 1**
> Wounds are caused by local and systemic factors and are influenced by the individual's nutritional status.

Wounds can be classified as either acute or chronic. **Acute wounds** are caused by external injury, such as trauma or surgery, and heal through a normal sequence of events, usually within 5 to 10 days, or at least within 30 days.[1,6] Chronic wounds are unable to heal in such a timely manner. **Chronic wounds** are those that persist longer than 6 weeks or frequently reoccur and are typically associated with underlying conditions that lead to tissue breakdown, inadequate tissue perfusion, and chronic inflammation.[6,7] Wound healing starts immediately after injury, which begins with coagulation, forming the extracellular matrix and fibrous tissue that eventually leads to wound contraction and closure. There are three phases of wound healing: inflammation, proliferation, and remodeling.

Inflammation
Inflammation is the body's initial response to injury and is characterized by redness, warmth, swelling, pain, and loss of function. The initial goal after injury is to prevent further blood loss through hemostasis, which involves coagulation and clot formation. Immediately after injury, mediators, such as thromboxane A2 and prostaglandin 2α (which are both derived from lipids), and adhesive proteins, such as fibrinogen and fibronectin, are released, resulting in platelet aggregation, reflex vasoconstriction, and coagulation.[7-9] Within seconds, a fibrin clot is formed, which is comprised of platelets, collagen, thrombin, and fibronectin.[8] Subsequently, cytokines and growth factors are released, which are involved in cell signaling and cellular growth and differentiation. These include transforming growth factor β (TGF-β), platelet-derived growth factor (PDGF), fibroblast growth factor (FGF), and endothelial growth factor (EGF).[5] The inflammatory response begins when neutrophils are sent to the wound site by the cytokines and growth factors.[8]

CASE STUDY INTRODUCTION

Sean is a 38-year-old wheelchair-bound male who presents to the hospital with fever and chills. Sean sustained a gunshot wound (GSW) to his back 5 years ago, leading to a spinal cord injury and subsequent paraplegia. His history is notable for pressure injuries on his sacrum and coccyx.

Anthropometric Data:
Height: 173 cm (68 in)
Weight: 100 kg (220 lbs)
BMI: 33.5 kg/m^2
Weight history
Stable weight. No weight change reported in past 3 years.

Biochemical Data:
Sodium 141 (135-145 mEq/L)
Potassium 4.3 (3.6-5.0 mEq/L)
Chloride 103 (98-110 mEq/L)
Carbon dioxide 25 (20-30 mEq/L)
Blood urea nitrogen 22 (6-24 mg/dL)
Creatinine 0.5 (0.4-1.3 mg/dL)

Glucose 157 (70-139 mg/dL)
Calcium 8.5 (8.5-10.5 mEq/L)
Magnesium 1.7 (1.4-2.1 mEq/L)
Phosphorus 3.1 (2.7-4.5 mg/dL)
White blood cells 13 (4-11 K/uL)

Clinical Data:
Past Medical History: GSW to back, spinal cord injury, paraplegia, neurogenic bladder, depression, stage II sacral ulcer, stage III coccyx ulcer
Medications: Lovenox, Seroquel, Baclofen, multivitamin, Colace, senna
Vital Signs: Blood pressure: 100/65 mm Hg; Temperature: 101°F
Nutrition-focused Physical Exam: Patient appears obese yet pale, with decreased muscle tone in lower extremities. Skin feels very warm to touch. No edema noted. Good dentition with normal mouth and tongue. Wounds noted but not examined due to intact wound dressings.

Description Previously Documented By Wound Care Nurse:
Sacral wound—stage II: Partial-thickness wound on sacrum; shallow open ulcer measuring 2.7 cm x 2.4 cm with pink/red wound bed; no slough or exudate noted.
Coccyx wound—stage III: Full-thickness wound on coccyx; open ulcer measuring 3.5 cm x 4 cm with beefy red tissue and moderate foul-smelling, purulent wound exudate. Area around the wound noted to be red, swollen, and tender to the touch.

Dietary Data:
Dietary History: Sean reports fair appetite and normal intake, consuming three meals and one bedtime snack via a regular unrestricted diet. He has been trying to increase protein intake due to wounds.
Nutrition Prescription: Regular diet

Questions
1. How would you describe Sean's nutritional status and nutritional risk factors?
2. What are the nutritional priorities for Sean?
3. How does Sean's wound status effect your assessment?
4. What additional information would you like to obtain?

Neutrophils are white blood cells that essentially clean the wound, removing pathogens and other debris to prevent infection. This process occurs within 24 to 48 hours after injury and may continue for up to 2 weeks.[8,9]

As previously mentioned, coagulation is the other component of hemostasis. Between 48 and 96 hours postinjury, monocytes aggregate at the wound site and mature into macrophages that further clear the site of bacteria and damaged tissue.[8] Macrophages also release enzymes and cytokines that contribute to inflammation. Macrophages become the predominant cell type in the later stages of the inflammatory phase.[9] Two cytokines, interleukin (IL) and tumor necrosis factor-alpha (TNF-α), facilitate **angiogenesis**, the formation of new blood vessels, and the migration of fibroblasts to synthesize collagen and the extracellular matrix. This is necessary for endothelial and epithelial cell migration and blood vessel formation, which are essential for tissue repair.[6] IL-1 is responsible for the migration of keratinocytes and collagen synthesis, IL-2 stimulates fibroblasts and other inflammatory cells to the wound site, and IL-6 promotes fibroblast proliferation.[5] Keratinocytes, which comprise the epidermis, are stimulated by TGF-β and migrate to the wound site to begin the re-epithelialization process. Growth factors are responsible for the foundation of the healing wound and attract cells to the wound to form the fibrin matrix.[8] At this point, a barrier is created to protect exposed tissue and newly formed blood vessels. A matrix is now ready for cell migration in the later phases of the wound healing process.

Proliferation

Following the inflammatory phase, **proliferation**, or the increase in the number of cells, begins around the fourth day after injury.[8] Fibroblasts are the dominant cell type during proliferation and aggregate to the wound bed early in this stage to synthesize proteins and granulation tissue for proper wound healing.[8,9] During the proliferation phase, angiogenesis, epithelialization, granulation, tissue formation, and collagen deposition occur. The matrix previously formed in the inflammatory phase is then replaced by a collagen-fortified extracellular matrix produced by fibroblasts and endothelial cells. New granulation tissue can then be formed by fibroblasts as well as growth factors. The development of granulation tissue occurs between 1 and 2 weeks after the wound is inflicted and is composed primarily of glycosaminoglycans, proteoglycans, and collagen.[7,8]

TGF-β stimulates fibroblasts to produce **collagen**, which is the most abundant protein in the human body.[5,8] Collagen is collected into fibers and organized into cross-linkages to form the extracellular matrix and, subsequently, connective tissue. Collagen is the primary component of the extracellular matrix and continues to be produced over the next 6 weeks of healing.[7] Collagen production is a vital part of wound healing because, as the amount of collagen increases, so does tensile strength.[8] In addition to collagen, the number of keratinocytes and endothelial cells also grows. These cells secrete growth factors and are necessary for angiogenesis so that adequate blood supply, oxygen, and nutrients can be taken to the wound site and granulation tissue can be formed.[7-9]

As the extracellular matrix develops, the fibrin clot created in the inflammatory phase begins to degrade. Granulation tissue, which is composed of ground substance, collagen, capillaries, and fibroblasts, is deposited and continues to grow until the wound is closed.[7] At the same time, epithelial cells move from the wound edge to the center to close the wound. Following this step, fibroblasts evolve into myofibroblasts that allow the wound to contract and reduce in size.[7] As the wound contracts, new tissue replaces damaged tissue, and fibroblasts begin to differentiate. The extent of contraction depends on the depth of the wound.[9] For example, contraction can reduce the size of a wound by up to 40% in full-thickness wounds, but contraction is less in partial-thickness wounds.[9]

Remodeling

Approximately 1 week after injury, the remodeling, or maturation, phase begins.[8] **Remodeling** is the final phase of wound healing, but it can last up to 1 year or longer.[8] During this phase, new epithelium and final scar tissue are formed. Fibronectin, a glycoprotein in the extracellular matrix, forms a network for collagen deposition in the granulation tissue, as well as for cell migration and cell growth.[8] It is during the remodeling phase that the collagen is fashioned into an organized structure with increased tensile strength.[7] About 3 to 4 weeks after injury, the tensile strength is approximately 20% to 40% that of uninjured skin.[8,9] One year after injury, even after the wound is healed, the new flesh is only about 70% to 80% as strong as it originally was.[7,8] Collagen is now the predominant cell type in the wound healing process, and its synthesis and degradation are regulated by collagenases.[8] Its purpose is to provide strength, structure, and stiffness to the new tissue. Once epithelialization and tissue development is complete, fibroblasts undergo apoptosis, or cell death, and the individual is left with a scar.[5]

Chronic Wounds

Most wounds will heal in a timely manner; however, some wounds may persist for longer than 6 weeks or frequently reoccur.[7] These wounds are considered chronic wounds. The majority (85%) of patients with chronic wounds are older than 65 years of age, and approximately 3 to 6 million people in the United States suffer from chronic wounds.[10]

There are various reasons why chronic wounds develop, such as atherosclerosis, lymphedema, burns, obesity, and some neoplastic diseases. The majority of chronic wounds are due to ischemia as a consequence of pressure, venostasis, or diabetes mellitus.[10,11] Several factors can impair healing, as described in **Table 7.1**. Thus, the wound cannot advance through all three stages of healing and remains in a state of constant inflammation, resulting in delayed or incomplete wound healing.

On a cellular level, collagen synthesis, and therefore healing, may be impaired if excessive levels of TNF-α are

TABLE 7.1 FACTORS THAT IMPAIR WOUND HEALING[5,7,10,12]

Internal Factors	External Factors
Advanced age	Incontinence
Alcohol consumption	Improper wound care
Autoimmune/immunocompromised and muscle-wasting diseases	Impaired mobility
Corticosteroid, NSAIDS, or immunosuppressive drug use (chemotherapy)	Pressure/trauma
Elevated cortisol levels due to psychosocial stress	
Infections	
Poor circulation/tissue perfusion	
Poor nutritional status/malnutrition	
Smoking	
Uncontrolled diabetes mellitus	

NSAIDS = nonsteroidal anti-inflammatory drugs.
Data from Hackman DJ, Ford, HR. Cellular, biochemical, and clinical aspects of wound healing. *Surg Infec*. 2002;3:S23-S35; Wild T, Rahbarnia A, Kellner M, Sobotka L, Eberlein T. Basics in nutrition and wound healing. *Nutrition*. 2010;26:862-866; Guo S, DiPietro LA. Factors Affecting Wound Healing. *J Dent Res*. 2010;89(3):219-229; Ebrect M, Hextall J, Kirtley LG, Taylor A, Dyson M, Weinman J. Perceived stress and cortisol levels predict speed of wound healing in healthy male adults. *Psychoneuroendocrinology*. 2004;29:798-809.

produced because it overstimulates immune cells, causing cell damage and reduced amounts of hydroxyproline, a collagen precursor.[5] Wounds may fail to heal in advanced age because proliferation is slowed, collagenase activity is increased, and inflammatory cell response is reduced.[5] Delayed healing may also be observed in older adults as their body composition changes with age and lower activity levels.[8] Individuals on corticosteroids may also experience impaired wound healing because of their anti-inflammatory effects.[10] These medications affect cytokine activity by blunting angiogenesis and epithelial cell migration.[5]

Because healing is delayed in the chronic wound, many complications can occur, including infection, thrombosis, cellulitis, abscess formation, osteomyelitis, and gangrene.[11,13] Chronic wounds may require surgical intervention, which comes with its own complications. Patients' functional abilities may then be impaired, leading to decreases in quality of life. Chronic ulcers are also associated with decreased serum levels of vitamin A, vitamin E, and zinc, which may necessitate nutrient supplementation.[4]

CORE CONCEPT 2

All three stages of wound healing are essential, and a disruption in any stage can lead to chronic inflammation and delayed wound healing.

Pathophysiology of the Chronic Wound

Chronic wounds fall into a perpetual cycle of inflammation, which may be caused by polymicrobial colonization, proteinase imbalance, oxygen metabolites in the wound, and/or recurring injury.[6,7,11] As previously mentioned, neutrophils are recruited to the wound bed during the inflammatory phase of wound healing. When the wound is in a state of chronic inflammation, neutrophils continue to be recruited to the site of injury.[8] Matrix metalloproteinases (MMPs) accumulate at abnormally high levels, causing the extracellular matrix to degrade and leading to further tissue damage.[8,10] Neutrophils also cause oxidative damage to the wound.[8] Increased levels of MMPs impair fibroblast and endothelial cell proliferation and interfere with their functions, suppressing cell growth.[8,11] There are more damaging enzymes than protective enzymes, and the wound cannot proceed through the healing process.

Chronic Venous Ulcers

Approximately 80% of nonhealing wounds are venous ulcers, and an estimated 500,000 to 600,000 people in the United States experience these types of ulcers.[2] The prevalence of chronic venous ulcers increases with age and risk of development is higher in females.[2] Venous ulcers primarily occur on the lower extremities secondary to insufficient circulation and venous hypertension.[2] Venous ulcers are typically shallow wounds. Signs of venous ulcers include edema, varicose veins, and skin changes such as eczema and hyperpigmentation.[2] They consist of fibrotic cuffs that wrap around capillary vessels, which lead to further degradation of tissue as these cuffs inhibit the transportation of oxygen and nutrients to the dermal layer.[2] Leukocytes become trapped and release cytokines and enzymes that damage endothelial tissue.

Diabetic Ulcers

About 15% of all patients with diabetes will experience chronic nonhealing diabetic foot ulcers, which contribute to a large percentage of lower limb amputations.[10] Diabetic ulcers are caused by peripheral neuropathy, ischemia, and/or trauma. Diabetic ulcers can develop from one of these factors alone or a cascade of all three, as one irregularity can easily lead to another.[13] Diabetes mellitus has both micro- and macrovascular effects that contribute to the development of ulcers, specifically on the lower limbs. Prolonged hypoxia occurs and tissue perfusion is not adequate; therefore, the transportation of nutrients and oxygen is insufficient.[10]

Impaired healing is multifactorial. Healing may be impaired by the same factors that cause the diabetic ulcer, such as wound infection, pressure on the wound site, and callus formation.[13] When the diabetic ulcer develops or is inflicted by trauma, there is a delayed inflammatory response and decreased fibroblast and endothelial cell activity.[8] The inflammatory response is also extended, delaying the latter phases of wound healing. In patients with diabetes, cytokine concentrations may be abnormal, and these wounds may have decreased levels of keratinocyte growth factor and insulin-like growth factor, as well as decreased nitric oxide production.[5] Hyperglycemia increases oxidative stress and hinders the transport of ascorbic acid, which is necessary for collagen synthesis, into leukocytes and fibroblasts.[8,10] Hyperglycemia affects neutrophil activity and cell proliferation; granulation tissue formation is decreased, disrupting the healing process.[14] In studies using rats with diabetes, proper management of blood glucose with insulin has been shown to increase tensile strength and collagen production.[5] For this reason, it is imperative that patients with diabetes learn how to manage their blood glucose.

> **CORE CONCEPT 3**
>
> Uncontrolled diabetes increases risk of the development of chronic foot ulcers and often leads to amputations.

Pressure Ulcers

According to the National Pressure Ulcer Advisory Panel (NPUAP), **pressure ulcers**, also called pressure injuries, are defined as localized injuries to the skin and/or underlying tissue caused by external factors, including compression, shear force, friction, moisture, or a combination, primarily occurring on bony prominences.[2,8,15] Continuous pressure can cause deep tissue injury secondary to low blood perfusion and ischemia. Common areas where pressure injuries develop include heels, sacrum, coccyx, elbow, shoulder, and back of head.[16,17] Risk factors for developing pressure injuries include age older than 65 years, impaired mobility, loss of nerve sensitivity such as in neuropathy, prolonged hospital stay, dehydration, and malnutrition.[2,18] Age is not an independent risk factor for developing pressure injuries, but problems associated with older age put these patients at increased risk of pressure injury development.[16] These include hip fracture, immobility, incontinence, dry or inelastic skin, systemic disease, and terminal illness.[16] Patients with spinal cord injuries are also highly susceptible to pressure injuries. While poor nutritional status is associated with pressure injury development and impaired wound healing, obesity also puts patients at risk for developing pressure injuries because of the added weight and possible muscle atrophy.[18]

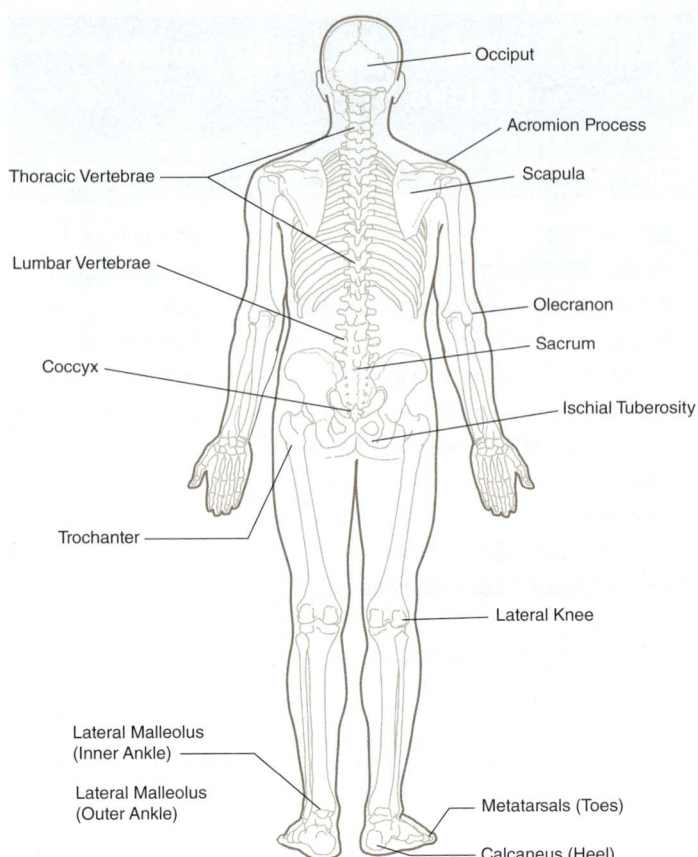

FIGURE 7.1 Common Locations for Chronic Wounds

Approximately 20% to 30% of people with spinal cord injuries will develop pressure injuries within 1 to 5 years after injury.[16] Pressure injuries are staged based on the gravity of the wound and range between small wounds to deep cavities with tissue necrosis and even damage to bone, as described in **Figure 7.1**, **Figure 7.2**, and **Table 7.2**.[2] Chronic pressure injuries exhibit decreased levels of fibronectin.[2] Wound healing is delayed as the formation of the fiber matrix for collagen and granulation tissue deposition is impaired.

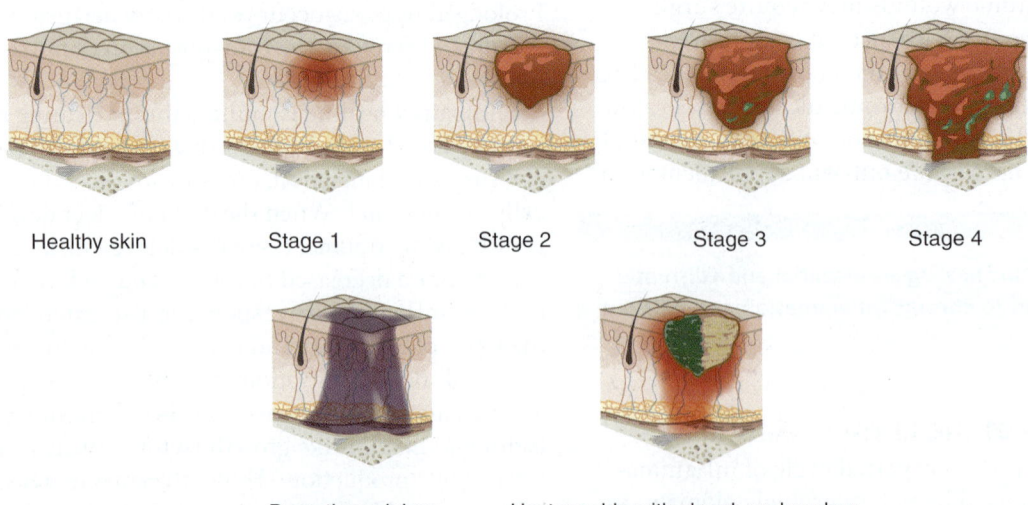

FIGURE 7.2 NPUAP Pressure Injury Staging Illustrations[15]

Reproduced from the National Pressure Ulcer Advisory Panel http://www.npuap.org/resources/educational-and-clinical-resources/pressure-injury-staging-illustrations/.

TABLE 7.2 NPUAP PRESSURE INJURY STAGES[15]

Stage 1 Pressure Injury: Nonblanchable erythema of intact skin	Intact skin with a localized area of nonblanchable erythema, which may appear differently in darkly pigmented skin. Presence of blanchable erythema or changes in sensation, temperature, or firmness may precede visual changes. Color changes do not include purple or maroon discoloration; these may indicate deep tissue pressure injury.
Stage 2 Pressure Injury: Partial-thickness skin loss with exposed dermis	Partial-thickness loss of skin with exposed dermis. The wound bed is viable, pink or red, and moist, and may also present as an intact or ruptured serum-filled blister. Adipose (fat) is not visible and deeper tissues are not visible. Granulation tissue, slough, and eschar are not present. These injuries commonly result from adverse microclimate and shear in the skin over the pelvis and shear in the heel. This stage should not be used to describe moisture-associated skin damage including incontinence-associated dermatitis, intertriginous dermatitis, medical adhesive–related skin injury, or traumatic wounds (skin tears, burns, abrasions).
Stage 3 Pressure Injury: Full-thickness skin loss	Full-thickness loss of skin, in which adipose (fat) is visible in the ulcer and granulation tissue and epibole (rolled wound edges) are often present. Slough and/or eschar may be visible. The depth of tissue damage varies by anatomical location; areas of significant adiposity can develop deep wounds. Undermining and tunneling may occur. Fascia, muscle, tendon, ligament, cartilage, and/or bone are not exposed. If slough or eschar obscures the extent of tissue loss, this is an Unstageable Pressure Injury.
Stage 4 Pressure Injury: Full-thickness skin and tissue loss	Full-thickness skin and tissue loss with exposed or directly palpable fascia, muscle, tendon, ligament, cartilage, or bone in the ulcer. Slough and/or eschar may be visible. Epibole (rolled edges), undermining, and/or tunneling often occur. Depth varies by anatomical location. If slough or eschar obscures the extent of tissue loss, this is an Unstageable Pressure Injury.
Unstageable Pressure Injury: Obscured full-thickness skin and tissue loss	Full-thickness skin and tissue loss in which the extent of tissue damage within the ulcer cannot be confirmed because it is obscured by slough or eschar. If slough or eschar is removed, a Stage 3 or Stage 4 pressure injury will be revealed. Stable eschar (i.e., dry, adherent, intact without erythema or fluctuance) on the heel or ischemic limb should not be softened or removed.
Deep Tissue Pressure Injury (DTPI): Persistent nonblanchable deep red, maroon, or purple discoloration	Intact or nonintact skin with localized area of persistent nonblanchable deep red, maroon, or purple discoloration or epidermal separation revealing a dark wound bed or blood-filled blister. Pain and temperature change often precede skin color changes. Discoloration may appear differently in darkly pigmented skin. This injury results from intense and/or prolonged pressure and shear forces at the bone–muscle interface. The wound may evolve rapidly to reveal the actual extent of tissue injury, or may resolve without tissue loss. If necrotic tissue, subcutaneous tissue, granulation tissue, fascia, muscle, or other underlying structures are visible, this indicates a full-thickness pressure injury (Unstageable, Stage 3, or Stage 4). Do not use DTPI to describe vascular, traumatic, neuropathic, or dermatologic conditions.
Additional Pressure Injury Definitions	
Medical Device–Related Pressure Injury: This describes an etiology	Medical device–related pressure injuries result from the use of devices designed and applied for diagnostic or therapeutic purposes. The resultant pressure injury generally conforms to the pattern or shape of the device. The injury should be staged using the staging system.
Mucosal Membrane Pressure Injury	Mucosal membrane pressure injury is found on mucous membranes with a history of a medical device in use at the location of the injury. Due to the anatomy of the tissue, these ulcers cannot be staged.

Used with permission of the National Pressure Ulcer Advisory Panel June 23, 2017. http://www.npuap.org/resources/educational-and-clinical-resources/npuap-pressure-injury-stages/.

Alterations in Physiological State and Metabolism During Wound Healing

In response to injury, the body undergoes various changes including increased catabolic hormones, decreased anabolic hormones, increased metabolic rate, increased cardiac output, increased body temperature, increased glucose needs, increased cellular protein turnover, and increased muscle breakdown.[19,20] Wounds and skin ulcers can result in a systemic inflammatory response, also known as the acute-phase response. The magnitude of

CASE STUDY REVISITED

Sean is admitted to the hospital with sepsis and begins intravenous antibiotics.

Questions
1. What are Sean's modifiable and nonmodifiable risk factors for wound development?
2. Would you address his modifiable risk factors? If so, how?

---

the acute phase response parallels the extent of wound injury and its associated trauma. Acute-phase response can also be induced by infection, trauma, surgery, neoplastic growth, or immunological disorders, and is thought to prevent microbial growth and to help restore homeostatis.[21] The acute-phase response is mediated by pro-inflammatory cytokines (TNF-α, IL-1, IL-6, transforming growth factor, and interferon), which lead to the activation of inflammatory tissue fibroblasts, endothelial cells, and macrophages; reduction in growth hormone secretion; and stimulation of protein catabolism.[21,22] TNF-α, IL-1β, and interferon gamma (IFNγ) are important to wound healing because they are needed to induce platelet-activating factor, prostaglandins, leukotrienes, and nitric oxide.[21] Pro-inflammatory cytokines also stimulate heat shock proteins and metallothionein synthesis, which decrease liver secretion of albumin, transferrin, and lactoferrin.[21] Because albumin transports zinc, serum zinc decreases, as well as iron, which is beneficial to the patient as iron is a key nutrient for microbial growth.[21] During the acute-phase response, other serum levels of nutrients fall, including calcium, vitamin A, and α-tocopherol.[21,22] Patients with pressure injuries can present with significant decreases in the concentration of ascorbic acid and α-tocopherol.[22]

Clinically, the acute-phase response is characterized by anorexia, fever, increased neutrophils and leukocytes, hyperglycemia, and anemia. Changes in the body are due to changes in acute-phase proteins as a result of changes in liver synthesis stimulated by the pro-inflammatory cytokines as described in **Table 7.3**.[21] Positive acute-phase proteins are released by hepatocytes and function to trap microorganisms and their products, activate the complement system, bind cellular remnants, neutralize enzymes, scavenge free hemoglobin and radicals, and modulate the host's immune response.[21] Other acute-phase proteins decrease in the acute-phase response and are called negative acute-phase proteins. Patients with pressure injuries and infections tend to have lower serum levels of total proteins, albumin, transferrin, and hemoglobin, and higher serum leukocytes and C-reactive protein.[22] Both positive and negative acute-phase proteins are used as markers of inflammation.

Metabolic stress and the acute-phase response put the body in an overall catabolic state, and there is a rapid loss of lean body mass (LBM) to provide energy and to synthesize new protein, particularly acute-phase proteins.[24] The loss of LBM is also dependent on the degree of metabolic stress and the body's response to injury. Healthy individuals in a fasting state may lose 60 to 70 g of protein per day (240-280 g muscle tissue).[7] In contrast, those with severe trauma or sepsis, such as with chronic wounds, may lose up to 250 g of protein daily (600-1,000 g muscle tissue).[7] Metabolic stress delays wound healing; in such a state, wound healing takes precedence and nutrients are allocated toward protein synthesis in the wound at the expense of LBM.[20] Adequate nutritional intake is important to meet the needs of the healing wound. Otherwise, LBM will continue to be broken down into amino acids for gluconeogenesis. Protein depletion and loss of LBM will continue until the wound has closed, the cause of metabolic stress has been resolved, and the body is no longer catabolic, which can take weeks to months.[20] At a certain point, if too much LBM is lost (30% or more), preserving LBM becomes the priority, and the wound will fail to heal until LBM is at least partially restored.[20]

Many patients with pressure injuries are malnourished. Malnutrition can occur as a preexisting condition

TABLE 7.3 ACUTE-PHASE PROTEINS[23]

Positive	Negative
α-1 antichymotrypsin	Albumin
α-1 antitrypsin	Retinol-binding protein
α-2 macroglobulin	Transcortin
Ceruloplasmin	Transferrin
Complement factors	Transthyretin (Prealbumin)
C-reactive protein	
D-dimer protein	
Factor VIII	
Ferritin	
Fibrinogen	
Haptoglobin	
Mannose-binding protein	
Plasminogen	
Prothrombin	
Serum amyloid A	
Serum amyloid P	
von-Willebrand factor	

Data from Jain S, Guatam V, Naseem S. Acute-phase proteins: As diagnostic tool. *J Pharm Bioallied Sci*. 2011;3(1):118-127.

TABLE 7.4 EFFECTS OF INADEQUATE NUTRITION ON WOUND HEALING[7,8,19,25]
Prolonged inflammatory and healing phase secondary to decreased: • Proliferation of fibroblasts • Angiogenesis • Collagen synthesis • Matrix protein deposition • Granulation tissue formation • Tensile strength
Increased risk of infection secondary to decreased: • B- and T-cell function • Phagocytic activity • Complement and antibody levels

Data from 7. Wild T, Rahbarnia A, Kellner M, Sobotka L, Eberlein T. Basics in nutrition and wound healing. *Nutrition*. 2010;26:862-866; Stechmiller JK. Understanding the Role of Nutrition and Wound Healing. *Nutr Clin Pract*. 2010;25:61-68;19. Arnold M, Barbul A. Nutrition and Wound Healing. *Plast Reconstr Surg*. 2006;117:42S-58S.25. Collins CE, Kershaw J, Brockington S. Effect of nutritional supplements on wound healing in home-nursed elderly: A randomized trial. *Nutrition*. 2005;21:147-155.

TABLE 7.5 TREATMENT METHODS FOR WOUNDS[1,5,6,13,26,27,28]
Dressings Fibrin glue Topical nitroglycerin, growth factors, antibiotics, antiseptics Irrigation and debridement Surgery (closure, skin grafting, skin flaps, musculocutaneous flaps) Vacuum-assisted closure (VAC; negative pressure therapy) Hyperbaric oxygen therapy

Data from Velnar T, Bailey T, Smrkolj V. The wound healing process: an overview of the cellular and molecular mechanisms. *Journal Int Med Res*. 2009;37:1528-1542; Hackman DJ, Ford, HR. Cellular, biochemical, and clinical aspects of wound healing. *Surg Infec*. 2002;3:S23-S35; Bowler PG. Wound pathophysiology, infection and therapeutic options. *Ann Med*. 2002;34:419-427.

or develop as a result of metabolic stress or injury.[19] In a state of unstressed starvation, metabolic rate and overall protein turnover decrease in an attempt to preserve LBM. As glycogen stores become exhausted within the first 24 hours after the onset of starvation, the body initially uses amino acids for gluconeogenesis, then begins to mobilize free fatty acids from adipose tissue for energy and muscle protein is catabolized at a slower rate.[8,19,20] The majority of energy is derived from fat and only 5% comes from protein.[20] Malnutrition can exacerbate already poorly healing wounds and can contribute to nonhealing wounds, but even mild protein-energy malnutrition or brief periods of starvation can impair wound healing (**Table 7.4**).[19] In malnourished patients, LBM preservation takes precedence over wound healing; thus, wound healing is delayed or halted until LBM is restored.[20] It is suggested that recent dietary intake may be more important than the patient's overall nutritional status when it comes to the healing wound.[19] Because starved patients who have wounds are also metabolically stressed, they may experience prolonged wound healing compared to those who are metabolically stressed yet adequately nourished.

> **CORE CONCEPT 4**
>
> Wound healing creates a catabolic state; preservation of lean body mass is prioritized over wound healing in malnourished patients.

Medical Treatment of Wounds

Some wounds will heal on their own, while others, such as chronic wounds, require medical treatment as described in **Table 7.5**. Wound care requires an interprofessional approach, and wound and ostomy care (WOC) clinicians, such as nurses and physicians, are an integral part of the wound healing process because they care directly for the wounds.

Wounds are cleaned with normal saline and, in some cases, antibiotics, to remove debris and bacteria.[26,27] If a wound contains eschar, or necrotic tissue, it may need to be debrided for healing to take place.[27] **Debridement** is the removal of dead or damaged tissue and can occur in four ways: (1) surgically (with a scalpel), (2) mechanically (such as wound irrigation), (3) enzymatically (with chemical debriding agents), and (4) autolytically (relying on the body's proteolytic enzymes to break down necrotic tissue).[27]

Once the wound has been cleaned, the WOC clinician may decide to use ointments or creams, such as antibiotics, to retain moisture within the wound and minimize bacterial growth.[27] Wounds can either be covered with dressings or left open to the air, depending on the severity of the wound. Both methods have advantages and disadvantages. For example, uncovered wounds are exposed to less friction from dressings.[27] On the other hand, the wound is also exposed to more environmental factors that may cause the scab to prematurely detach.[27] Uncovered wounds often take longer to heal because the wound is drier and epithelial cells need a moist, healthy wound bed to grow.[27] A possible disadvantage of covered wounds is the potential for bacterial overgrowth due to a dark, moist environment. If a dressing is applied with the proper technique, this risk is minimized. Regardless of the method, the goal of wound care is to keep the wound moist and the surrounding skin dry to prevent complications, such as infection, and promote healing.[6,27] Moisture from wound exudate and bodily fluids can damage the surrounding tissue and skin, so exudate is typically collected via gauze, wound drainage collector, or ostomy pouch.[27]

Newer medical treatments for wounds include fibrin glue, which essentially glues the epidermis together and allows the wound to close.[27] Another method is vacuum-assisted closure therapy (such as Wound VAC; **Figure 7.3**) and can be used for chronic, nonhealing wounds. The negative pressure that is created stimulates blood flow, allows cells to regenerate more quickly, and brings the cells closer together.[27] Hyperbaric oxygen therapy (HBOT; Figure 7.3) is also a promising treatment option for wound healing,

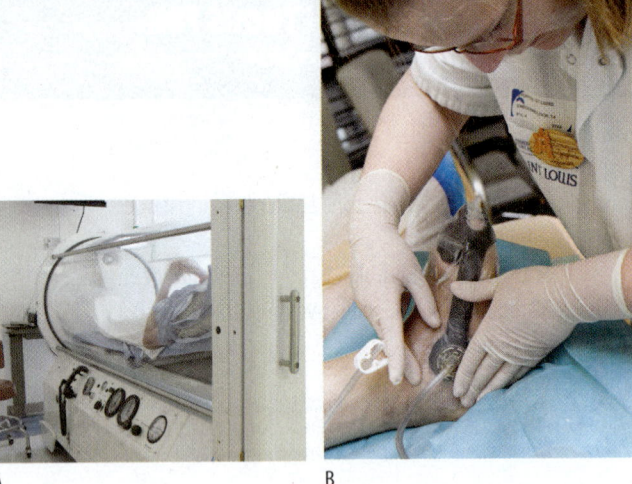

FIGURE 7.3 A. Hyperbaric Oxygen Therapy B. Vacuum-Assisted Closure (Wound VAC)
(A) © Dallas Events Inc/Shutterstock; (B) ©BSIP/UIG Via Getty Images.

particularly for those with diabetic foot ulcers.[6,27,28] Patients are placed in a chamber with 100% oxygen, which promotes angiogenesis, neovascularization, collagen and fibroblast synthesis, and epithelialization.[27] While HBOT has been found to beneficial in the short term, the same results are not seen long term, and more research is needed before this method can be used as widespread therapy.[28]

Medical Nutrition Therapy for Wound Healing

Screening

Given the correlation between wound healing and nutritional status, it is important to screen patients for malnutrition or risks for developing malnutrition. Approximately half of patients who are admitted to hospitals are malnourished, and about two-thirds of those patients will continue to worsen nutritionally.[29] In addition, an estimated one-third of patients who are not malnourished at time of arrival will become malnourished during their hospital stay.[29] Screening tools are useful to identify patients who have wounds or chronic ulcers, and also those at risk for developing wounds.

The **Braden Scale for Predicting Pressure Sore Risk** (Table 7.6) is used to predict the risk of injury development.[26,30] The Braden Scale is multifactorial and includes sensory perception, moisture, activity, mobility, friction and shear, and nutrition. Each factor is rated on a scale of 1 to 4 (with the exception of friction and shear, which is rated 1 to 3), for a total of 23 points. The total score indicates risk level as follows: 15 to 18 = mild risk, 13 to 14 = moderate risk, 10 to 12 = high risk, ≤9 = severe risk. The Braden Scale, including the nutrition section, is often completed by nursing staff, although it is important for the registered dietitian to complete a full nutrition assessment of the patient.

Assessment

The purpose of the nutrition assessment in wound healing is to identify any nutrition risks, ensure adequate nutrition intake to prevent further breakdown of the wound, promote anabolism, and prevent loss of LBM, especially in malnourished patients.[20,31] The number and stages of wounds should be assessed to help determine individualized protein and energy needs. However, there are no reliable or specific markers of malnutrition, and there are none specifically linked to wounds or pressure injuries.[29] Many patients with wounds have low albumin levels due to metabolic stress, inflammation, and infection, or related to comorbidities. Patients who have low BMI, recent weight loss, and poor intake are at risk for pressure injury development and impaired wound healing.[8] Malnourished patients are two to four times more likely to develop pressure injuries than normally nourished patients.[4,29,32] Hospitalized patients have an increased risk of developing pressure injuries secondary to loss of LBM during bed rest.[29] Wound healing is impaired with a loss of more than 15% of LBM, and greater than 30% loss of LBM significantly increases the risk of developing pressure injuries and wound dehiscence.[20] The goal of nutrition assessment is to detect and resolve any nutritional deficiencies as soon as possible because proper nutrition interventions can lead to improved quality of life, decreased length of hospital stay, and decreased risk of morbidity and mortality.[33]

> **CORE CONCEPT 5**
>
> Poor nutritional status is associated with increased risk of developing pressure injuries.

> **PRACTICE POINT**
>
> Patients with a low Braden Scale score (12 or lower) are considered high risk. Early screening and initiation of nutrition interventions can decrease the risk of developing skin ulcers.

Nutritional Requirements

There are currently no well-established, specific nutrient guidelines for wound healing, and it is unclear whether vitamin and mineral supplementation aids with the prevention and treatment of ulcers.[26,33] More research is needed to determine the optimal dosage of supplements. Various recommended intakes have been documented as described in **Table 7.7**.

> **PRACTICE POINT**
>
> The optimal nutrient needs for wound healing are still unknown, but adequate intakes of calories, protein, zinc, vitamin C, and vitamin A are essential for tissue growth and repair.

TABLE 7.6 BRADEN SCALE FOR PREDICTING PRESSURE SORE RISK[30]

Risk Factor	Score			
Sensory Perception Ability to respond meaningfully to pressure-related discomfort	**1—Completely Limited** Unresponsive (does not moan, flinch, or grasp) to painful stimuli, due to diminished level of consciousness or sedation; **OR** limited ability to feel pain over most of body.	**2—Very Limited** Responds only to painful stimuli. Cannot communicate discomfort except by moaning or restlessness; **OR** has a sensory impairment that limits the ability to feel pain or discomfort over one-half of body.	**3—Slightly Limited** Responds to verbal commands, but cannot always communicate discomfort or the need to be turned; **OR** has some sensory impairment that limits ability to feel pain or discomfort in one or two extremities.	**4—No impairment** Responds to verbal commands. Has no sensory deficit that would limit ability to feel or voice pain or discomfort.
Moisture Degree to which skin is exposed to moisture	**1—Constantly Moist** Skin is kept moist almost constantly by perspiration, urine, etc. Dampness is detected every time patient is moved or turned.	**2—Very Moist** Skin is often, but not always, moist. Linen must be changed at least once a shift.	**3—Occasionally Moist** Skin is occasionally moist, requiring an extra linen change approximately once a day.	**4—Rarely Moist** Skin is usually dry; linen only requires a changing at routine intervals.
Activity Degree of physical activity	**1—Bedfast** Confined to bed.	**2—Chairfast** Ability to walk severely limited or nonexistent. Cannot bear own weight and/or must be assisted into chair or wheelchair.	**3—Walks Occasionally** Walks occasionally during day, but for very short distances, with or without assistance. Spends majority of each shift in bed or chair.	**4—Walks Frequently** Walks outside the room at least twice a day and inside room at least once every 2 hours during waking hours.
Mobility Ability to change and control body position	**1—Completely Immobile** Does not make even slight changes in body or extremity position without assistance.	**2—Very Limited** Makes occasional slight changes in body or extremity position but unable to make frequent changes independently.	**3—Slightly Limited** Makes frequent though slight changes in body or extremity position independently.	**4—No limitations** Makes major and frequent changes in position without assistance.

(continues)

TABLE 7.6 BRADEN SCALE FOR PREDICTING PRESSURE SORE RISK[30] (continued)

Risk Factor	Score			
	1—Very Poor	2—Probably Inadequate	3—Adequate	4—Excellent
Nutrition Usual food intake pattern	Never eats a complete meal. Rarely eats more than one-third of any food offered. Eats two servings or less of protein (meat or dairy products) per day. Takes fluids poorly. Does not take a liquid dietary supplement; OR is NPO and/or maintained on clear liquids or IVs for more than 5 days.	Rarely eats a complete meal and generally eats only about one-half of any food offered. Protein intake includes only three servings of meat or dairy products per day. Occasionally will take a dietary supplement; OR receives less than optimum amount of liquid diet or tube feeding.	Eats over half of most meals. Eats a total of four servings of protein (meat, dairy products) per day. Occasionally will refuse a meal, but will usually take a supplement when offered; OR is on a tube feeding or TPN regimen, which probably meets most nutritional needs.	Eats most of every meal. Never refuses a meal. Usually eats a total of four or more servings of meat and dairy products. Occasionally eats between meals. Does not require supplementation.
	1—Problem	2—Potential Problem	3—No Apparent Problem	
Friction & Shear	Requires moderate to maximum assistance in moving. Complete lifting without sliding against sheets is impossible. Frequently slides down in bed or chair, requiring frequent repositioning with maximum assistance. Spasticity, contractures, or agitation leads to almost constant friction.	Moves feebly or requires minimum assistance. During a move, skin probably slides to some extent against sheets, chair, restraints, or other devices. Maintains relatively good position in chair or bed most of the time but occasionally slides down.	Moves in bed and chair independently and has sufficient muscle strength to lift up completely during move. Maintains good position in bed or chair.	
Total Score				

© Barbara Braden and Nancy Bergstrom, 1988. Reprinted with permission. All Rights Reserved.

Macronutrients

Energy Wound healing requires energy for anabolism, protein and collagen synthesis, cell proliferation, and enzyme activity. Calories can be utilized from carbohydrates, fat, and protein. Glucose is the primary source of energy in wound healing and for collagen synthesis.[8,25] Energy needs vary for each individual depending on age; sex; height; weight; activity and stress level; comorbidities; and number, size, and severity of wounds. In most settings, nutrition professionals use predictive equations or calories per kilogram as a starting point for estimating energy needs and make adjustments using clinical judgment. It is important for patients to meet their energy needs in order to spare protein as an energy source.[3] It is still unclear what the optimal calorie goal should be to promote wound healing. While wound healing does require energy, it has been suggested that additional calories alone do not improve healing, and that in older patients with ulcers, energy needs are not increased.[32,33,39]

> **PRACTICE POINT**
>
> Increased energy intake can be beneficial, especially in malnourished patients, to prevent the development of new wounds or further tissue damage, because an increase in body mass can provide a "cushion," especially on bony prominences.

TABLE 7.7 NUTRIENT RECOMMENDATIONS FOR WOUND HEALING

Nutrient	Wound Stage		
	Stages 1 & 2	Stages 3 & 4	Stage Not Specified (in the literature)
	Harris–Benedict × 1.2[34]	Harris–Benedict × 1.5[34]	30-35 kcal/kg[8] 30-40 kcal[34] 35-40 kcal/kg[7] 35-50 kcal/kg for those who are underweight or losing weight[8]
	For obese patients, consider using the Mifflin–St Jeor equation x stress factor or calculate energy needs based on adjusted body weight (using Harris–Benedict equation or kcal/kg ABW).[35-38]		
Protein	1.25-1.5 g/kg/day[8] 1.2-1.5 g/kg/day[34]	1.5-2 g/kg/day[8,34]	N/A
Arginine	No definitive guidelines for its safe and effective use have been established[34]		
Glutamine	Insufficient data to determine recommendations; glutamine should not be routinely used[34]		
Zinc	N/A	N/A	Up to 40 mg (176 mg zinc sulfate) for 10 days or 220 mg twice daily (25-50 mg elemental zinc) if deficiency present (no duration identified) for 2-3 weeks[8,34]
Vitamin C	100-200 mg/day[8,34]	1,000-2,000 mg/day[8,34]	N/A
Vitamin A	N/A	N/A	10,000-50,000 IU/day (oral)[8,34] or 10,000 IU intramuscularly for 10 days[8] 10,000 IU IV for 10 days for moderate to severely injured or malnourished patients[34]
Multivitamin + mineral	Daily[34]	Daily[34]	N/A

ABW = average body weight.

Data from Wild T, Rahbarnia A, Kellner M, Sobotka L, Eberlein T. Basics in nutrition and wound healing. *Nutrition*. 2010;26:862-866; Stechmiller JK. Understanding the Role of Nutrition and Wound Healing. *Nutr Clin Pract*. 2010;25:61-68; 34. Academy of Nutrition and Dietetics Evidence Analysis Library. Recommendations Summary: Spinal Cord Injury (SCI) Assessment of Nutritional Needs for Pressure Ulcers [Web page]. 2014. http://www.andeal.org/template.cfm?key=2378. Accessed May 28, 2017.

CASE STUDY REVISITED

Sean remains hospitalized due to sepsis. To address his wounds, a vacuum-assisted closure therapy is initiated. He continues to report good intake.

Anthropometric Data:
Weight: 99 kg (218 lbs)

Biochemical Data:
Sodium 138 (135-145 mEq/L)
Potassium 4.0 (3.6-5.0 mEq/L)
Blood urea nitrogen 18 (6-24 mg/dL)
Creatinine 0.5 (0.4-1.3 mg/dL)
Glucose 120 (70-139 mg/dL)
White blood cells 11.4 (4-11 K/uL)

Clinical Data:
Medications: Ciprofloxacin, Lovenox, Seroquel, Baclofen, multivitamin, Colace, senna
Vitals: Temperature: 99°F

Dietary Data:
Nutrition Prescription: Regular, high-protein diet with commercial supplement twice daily.

Questions
1. How would you assess Sean's energy needs? What factors are influencing his energy needs?
2. How would you assess Sean's protein needs? What factors are influencing his protein needs?
3. What specific nutrients, if any, or dietary supplements might you prescribe as part of Sean's diet prescription?

Protein Protein is an essential nutrient for repairing damaged tissue because it is needed for cell proliferation and tissue growth. The development of collagen, cytokines, growth factors, immune cells, and enzymes depends on adequate protein intake.[7] If protein intake is poor, these cells are not sufficiently synthesized to initiate a strong inflammatory response as soon as the wound is inflicted.[7] It may become more difficult for the wound to heal because there are not sufficient fibroblasts, and subsequently collagen, to fill the wound.[7] Because these cells are active in all stages of wound healing, protein is necessary in each stage as well.

Protein is lost through wound drainages, exudates, and negative pressure wound therapy; therefore, oral nutrition supplements are often prescribed to patients with multiple or severe wounds. Patients who consume increased amounts of protein may experience faster wound healing.[8] Protein intake is only beneficial if adequate calories are consumed as well. Otherwise, the protein will be used as an energy source rather than for tissue rebuilding.[3,8] Hydration status should be monitored when high-protein diets or formulas are administered because higher protein intake increases the risk for dehydration.[33]

Amino acids: Arginine Specific amino acids, including arginine, are important in wound healing. **Arginine** is a conditionally essential amino acid required for cell growth, protein synthesis, and collagen deposition. Arginine is necessary for maintenance of the immune system, aiding with T-cell reproduction, macrophage activity, and nitric oxide synthesis.[40,41] Citrulline, which is produced from proline, glutamate, and glutamine, is the major precursor for arginine synthesis. While arginine can be synthesized, it is primarily obtained from food and, on average, 3 to 6 g of arginine are consumed daily.[41,42] Approximately 50% to 60% of ingested arginine is taken up through the portal vein.[41,42] Under normal circumstances, arginine is synthesized in adequate amounts; if stress or injury occurs, arginine stores are depleted at a rapid rate. Malabsorption issues and uncontrolled diabetes can also lead to decreased serum arginine levels.[14,42] Arginine supplementation may be beneficial in wound healing, because it has been found to increase collagen accumulation in wounds in healthy rodents.[43] Hydroxyproline, a component of collagen, as well as total protein deposition and cell proliferation have also been found to be increased with arginine supplementation.[14,25] The mechanism by which arginine improves wound healing is still unknown.

In human subjects, arginine supplementation has been found to significantly reduce weight loss and nitrogen excretion.[43] In a small study, pressure ulcer healing rates were significantly improved in spinal cord injury patients who received 9 g of a commercial powdered arginine supplement (containing vitamins C and E) daily.[18] Standard oral and enteral formulas do not supply excess arginine, so arginine supplements may need to be given to see improvements in wound healing. Arginine supplementation may improve immune function; enhance tensile strength; and increase nitric oxide production, which regulates angiogenesis, collagen formation, and cell proliferation to close the wound.[5,8,41] Arginine can be metabolized into two byproducts: ornithine and nitric oxide. Ornithine is a precursor of collagen, and nitric oxide is important for wound healing because it affects the functions of macrophages, fibroblasts, and keratinocytes.[42] Low production of nitric oxide related to arginine-free diets is associated with impaired healing.[42,44] Patients who are malnourished, have diabetes, or are taking corticosteroids may have decreased nitric oxide production, which may explain the delayed healing process in many of these patients.[42] Witte and colleagues[14] found that arginine supplementation in diabetic rats restored nitric oxide levels and improved wound strength. While nitric oxide can be beneficial in wound healing, it can cause hemodynamic instability in critically ill patients.[8] Thus, arginine supplementation remains a controversial topic.

Amino acids: Glutamine Glutamine is the most abundant amino acid in the plasma.[8] It is also considered a conditionally essential amino acid because muscle and plasma stores of glutamine quickly decline after injury or trauma. Like arginine, glutamine is also necessary for protein synthesis as well as lymphocyte proliferation. Glutamine plays a significant role in wound healing because it is involved in nucleotide synthesis in the cells involved in the healing process: fibroblasts, macrophages, and epithelial cells.[8,25] Glutamine is particularly important in the inflammatory phase of wound healing because it is helps stimulate the inflammatory response.[8,19] Glutamine is utilized in gluconeogenesis as an energy and nitrogen source for cell proliferation.[8,25,45]

Although supplementation of glutamine has been shown to improve immune status and increase nitrogen balance after trauma, surgery, and sepsis, there is currently not enough evidence to determine guidelines for glutamine supplementation for wounds.[7,8,19] Glutamine supplementation may still be beneficial by improving protein synthesis and gut permeability, thereby decreasing hospital length of stay.[19]

β-hydroxy-β-methylbutyrate β-hydroxy-β-methylbutyrate (HMB) is a metabolite of leucine, an essential amino acid. Supplementation of HMB may prevent or delay muscle breakdown, increase cell proliferation and protein synthesis, and improve nitrogen balance.[43,46,47] HMB also stimulates LBM production, but the mechanism by which this occurs is unknown.[48] Dietary supplementation of HMB may also increase collagen deposition in wounds. A study conducted by Williams et al.[43] showed that supplementation with arginine, glutamine, and HMB significantly enhanced collagen synthesis in healthy adults ages 70 years or older. Sipahi and colleagues[46] found similar results in diabetic hemodialysis patients, ages 51 to 81 years.

HMB supplementation may be a safe and effective way to improve wound healing in patients with various diseases such as cancer, malnutrition, chronic obstructive pulmonary disease, HIV, and sepsis.[46]

Fat Lipids are an integral part of cell membranes and are necessary for eicosanoid synthesis, cell growth, and remodeling. People with essential fatty acid (EFA) deficiency will often exhibit dermatitis that resolves once the diet is supplemented with EFA. After injury, the need for essential fatty acids is increased.[8,19] Patients with chronic wounds may become deficient in linoleic and arachidonic acid, which are needed for prostaglandin synthesis for cell growth and inflammation.[8,19] This impairs wound healing because prostaglandins are critical for cellular metabolism and inflammation and phospholipids are integral parts of cell membranes.[19]

Omega-3 fatty acids (eicosapentaenoic acid and docosahexaenoic acid) may be beneficial in wound healing because of its possible actions on pro-inflammatory cytokine production (interleukin and TNF-α).[49] However, animals fed diets high in omega-3 fatty acids actually had weaker wounds.[19] Use of omega-3 fatty acids may help the wound healing process through improved immune function and reduced infections and complications, but there is currently not enough evidence to support the use of omega-3 fatty acids in clinical practice.[7,8,19]

Micronutrients

Zinc Zinc is the second most abundant trace element in the body.[50] It is responsible for catalyzing enzymatic reactions for the synthesis of RNA and DNA, as well as other proteins, and plays a role in immune function, glucose metabolism, and oxygen transport.[7,50] Zinc is particularly important in maintaining healthy skin, although the exact mechanism of how zinc impacts wound healing is not well understood.[51] Within epidermal and dermal tissue, zinc stabilizes cell membranes and is required for cell replication.[50] If zinc status is low, cells cannot reproduce enough for wound closure.[7] In patients who are zinc deficient, fibroblast proliferation and collagen synthesis are decreased, leading to impaired wound healing and decreased wound strength.[7,34,51] The wound may then enter a state of prolonged inflammation, and if the wound heals, the tensile strength may be decreased.[7,19]

Patients who have malnutrition, diarrhea, malabsorption, Crohn's disease, ulcerative colitis; are on long-term steroids; or are in catabolic states may exhibit zinc deficiency.[8,19,50] While zinc is necessary for all elements of wound healing, zinc supplementation is generally only beneficial when a patient is deficient in zinc.[7,8,50] Signs of zinc deficiency include loss of appetite, taste changes, lethargy, depression, dermatitis, and alopecia. Serum levels of zinc are not commonly measured but can be ordered to rule out zinc deficiency. It is important to be mindful that serum zinc levels can be increased or decreased by non-

⚠ Clinical Controversy

Do arginine, glutamine, and β-hydroxy-β-methylbutyrate enhance wound healing?

Wound healing success involves adequate provision of nutrient substrates and the specific amino acids and amino acid metabolites (arginine, glutamine, and β-hydroxy-β-methylbutyrate or HMB) have been identified to potentially improve the wound healing process.

Bozkirh et al. investigated the effect of glutamine, arginine, and HMB on 12 rats with two full-thickness wounds. The rats were randomized to a control or treatment group, and while both received standard rat food, the rats in the treatment group received extra glutamine, arginine, and HMB. Wound size was measured every 2 days for a total of 10 days. There was found to be no statistically significant difference in wound sizes or healing parameters for the two groups, which suggests that diets supplemented with the amino acid combination is not beneficial to healing in rats. The same research group also published a similar study. Gündoğdu et al. investigated the effect of glutamine, arginine, and HMB on 18 rats with two full-thickness ischemic wounds. Wound size was measured on days 0, 4, 10, and 14. This study found that the wound sizes of the rats in the treatment group were significantly smaller on days 10 and 14, which suggests that this amino acid combination seems to have a positive impact on the healing of *ischemic* wounds in rats. The finding in this study suggests that the efficacy of nutrient provision may depend upon wound type, which may be relevant since ischemia is commonly associated with chronic wounds.

The conflicting findings of these the studies by Bozkirh et al. and Gundoğdu at al. highlight that the amino acid mixture of arginine, glutamine, and HMB may influence healing differently in different types of wounds, although the mechanism by which this mixture imparts benefit is still unclear.

Questions

1. Are these findings derived from the rat model applicable to humans?
2. How do these conflicting results influence your decision to use or not use arginine, glutamine, and HMB when providing medical nutrition therapy to individuals with wounds?
3. How might it influence which selection criteria you use to determine which patients receive the amino acid combination?
4. What are the potential advantages and disadvantages of providing arginine, glutamine, and HMB to the wound population?

References

1. Bozkirh BO, Gündoğdu RH, Ersoy E, et al. Pilot experimental study on the effect of arginine, glutamine, and β-hydroxy-β-methylbutyrate on secondary wound healing. *JPEN J Parenter Enteral Nutr.* 2015;39:591-597.
2. Gundoğdu RH, Temel HT, Bozkirh BO, Ersoy E, Yazgan A, Yildirium Z. The mixture of arginine, glutamine, and β-hydroxy-β-methylbutyrate enhances the healing of ischemic wounds in rats. *JPEN J Parenter Enteral Nutr.* 2017; 41(6):1045-1050.

---

nutritional factors such as medications, inflammation, and metabolic stress.[52] In addition, serum zinc does not necessarily reflect the amount of zinc that is in tissue.[52] Clinical judgment is needed to determine the need for zinc supplementation.

Caution must be taken when supplementing zinc because zinc binds to iron and copper in the gut, which can lead to a deficiency in either of these minerals. Excess zinc intake can cause gastrointestinal issues, such as nausea, vomiting, diarrhea, and abdominal pain, increasing risk of poor oral intake and subsequent consequences of malnutrition. Zinc toxicity secondary to supplementation can also lead to delayed wound healing.[4] Lim and colleagues[51] found that high-dose zinc supplementation delays wound healing, possibly due to changes in the inflammatory response. Zinc supplementation that most accurately reflects the needs of the individual should be administered.

Vitamin C Vitamin C, or ascorbic acid, is necessary for collagen synthesis and the stabilization of the collagen structure. Specifically, vitamin C is required for the hydroxylation of proline and lysine, which are major components of collagen.[7] Vitamin C is essential during the inflammatory phase of wound healing. It aids with cell migration into the wound bed, capillary formation, neutrophil activity, and fibroblast proliferation.[7,8] Patients who eat a balanced diet or take daily supplements may not be deficient in vitamin C; however, those who smoke and consume alcohol frequently excrete more vitamin C.[8] A deficiency in vitamin C is correlated with delayed wound healing, and may lead to more severe wound infections due to impaired collagen synthesis and neutrophil activity.[19,34] Vitamin C supplementation is generally safe for patients with various wound stages, but may cause issues with patients with a history of kidney stones.[8,34]

CASE STUDY REVISITED

It is now hospital day (HD) 7 and Sean's infection is clearing and he is feeling better. His dietary intake remains good and he is meeting his calorie and protein goals with commercial supplements and high-protein snacks. The medical resident wants to initiate zinc, vitamin C, and vitamin A to aid in wound healing.

Anthropometric Data:
Weight: 100 kg (218 lbs)

Biochemical Data:
Glucose 105 (70-139 mg/dL)
White blood cells 9.1 (4-11 K/uL)

Clinical Data:
Medications: Ciprofloxacin, Lovenox, Seroquel, Baclofen, multivitamin, Colace, senna
Vital Signs: Temperature: 98.6°F

Description Documented By Wound Care Nurse On HD 7:
Sacral wound—stage II: Partial-thickness wound on sacrum, shallow open ulcer measuring 2.5 cm × 2.1 cm with pink wound bed; remains free of slough or exudate.
Coccyx wound—stage III: Full-thickness wound on coccyx, open ulcer measuring 3.3 cm × 3.9 cm with red tissue with light serosanguinous wound exudate; granulation tissue is present. Mild redness and swelling around wound noted. No odor or tenderness observed.

Dietary Data:
Diet Prescription: Regular, high-protein diet with commercial supplement twice daily

Questions

1. Do you agree with the initiation of zinc, vitamin C, and/or vitamin A? Why or why not?
2. How would you describe Sean's wound healing progress?
3. What dietary recommendations would you make to improve Sean's intake of micronutrients that aid in wound healing?
4. Are any adjustments to his nutrition prescription or energy and protein goals warranted? Why or why not?

Vitamin A Vitamin A is an antioxidant that is important for proper immune function and, like zinc and vitamin C, a deficiency is associated with impaired wound healing. During the inflammatory phase, vitamin A promotes the increase of macrophages and monocytes in the wound site.[8] It is also necessary for collagen deposition and epithelialization.[8,19] Vitamin A deficiency can be induced by stress or injury, and vitamin A requirements vary based on severity.[8] Patients on corticosteroids may also experience vitamin A loss, because high doses exhaust liver stores of vitamin A.[19] Vitamin A is not commonly used in clinical settings and, because it is a fat-soluble vitamin, excessive intake of vitamin A can cause toxicity. It has been reported that doses of vitamin A of 25,000 IU/day have been used without any serious side effects; however, any dose greater than this has not been found to be advantageous in wound healing.[19]

Fluids

Fluids are lost through wound exudates and wound treatment and therapy; therefore, fluid requirements are increased in wound healing. Patients with wounds may be receiving high amounts of protein, and adequate fluid intake is necessary to prevent dehydration.[8] Fluids maintain skin turgor and improve blood flow to wounded tissue. Adequate fluid intake can prevent further tissue breakdown. Daily fluid needs are estimated to be 1 to 1.5 mL/kcal consumed, or 30 mL/kg.[3,8] Some comorbidities, such as congestive heart failure and end-stage renal disease, may limit the amount of fluids an individual can ingest. Clinicians need to monitor changes in weight, urine output, electrolytes, respiratory status, and skin turgor.[3] Other issues that may increase fluid needs include excessive output from vomiting and/or diarrhea and elevated body temperature.[3]

Diet and Nutrition Intervention

Patients with wounds can benefit from a high-protein diet that incorporates a variety of foods rich in the essential nutrients, such as zinc, vitamin C, and vitamin A, at least to meet the Recommended Daily Allowance. Sources of these micronutrients can be found in **Table 7.8**. Patients should be encouraged to eat high-protein foods, including meat, poultry, fish, eggs, milk and other dairy products, nuts, beans, and legumes, at every meal and snack. Many high-protein foods are also high in zinc. Dietitians should also encourage patients to drink enough fluids, such as water, soup, juice, and milk, with and in between meals to maintain hydration balance. It is best to keep the patient on an unrestricted diet to allow for increased oral intake and to provide higher calorie foods. Diets should be individualized to meet the patient's protein and calorie needs, food preferences, swallowing abilities, and other comorbidities. Including portions of high-quality protein or other meal components may be helpful in providing for increased protein requirements. Extra food should be given before offering oral nutrition supplements, because this will likely improve patient satisfaction and compliance. If meal intake is inadequate, offer snacks and high-calorie beverages between meals that cater to the patient's likes/dislikes.

Many patients do not meet their energy and protein needs via oral intake and may become malnourished, especially in acute care settings. Patients may experience poor appetite and/or intake secondary to illness and gastrointestinal issues, difficulty chewing and swallowing, pain, and frequent NPO (*nil per os* or nothing by mouth) status that may lead to malnutrition. In a small study conducted by Raffoul et al.,[57] only two of nine patients were able to meet >90% of their energy needs through meals supplied at the hospital. Dietitians play a crucial role in identifying those at risk for malnutrition and preventing and treating skin ulcers through medical nutrition therapy. Even brief nutrition interventions can help prevent or overcome barriers to proper wound healing.[19] If a patient is not consuming adequate calories and protein from their diet, the first intervention would be to give oral nutrition supplements (ONS). ONS have been found to be an inexpensive, safe, and effective method to meet nutritional needs and may reduce healthcare costs.[32,57] Depending on the individual's cognitive and feeding abilities, enteral nutrition (EN) support may be another suitable option.

The administration of ONS may improve or accelerate wound healing and reduce complications associated with wounds.[25,58-61] Improved nutritional intake can prevent the development of pressure ulcers by repletion of nutrient deficiencies, improving skin condition, and increasing soft tissue to distribute pressure over bony prominences.[62] While ONS does contribute to improvements in nutritional status and dietary intake, it is unclear whether malnourished patients benefit more from nutrition interventions than well-nourished patients.[62] One study conducted by van Anholt and colleagues[32] showed that supplementation of high-protein, arginine- and micronutrient-enriched ONS

TABLE 7.8 DIETARY SOURCES OF MICRONUTRIENTS[53-56]

Micronutrient	Food Source	Amount per Serving
Zinc	Oysters, cooked	74 mg/ 3 oz
	Beef chuck roast, cooked	7 mg/ 3 oz
	Fortified breakfast cereal (fortified with 25% of the daily value for zinc)	3.8 mg/ ¾ cup
	Pork chop, cooked	2.9 mg/ 3 oz
	Yogurt, low fat	1.7 mg/ 8 oz
	Swiss cheese	1.2 mg/ 1 oz
	Milk	1 mg/ 1 cup
	Chicken breast, cooked	0.9 mg/ ½ breast
	Nuts	0.9-1.6 mg/ 1 oz
	Beans and peas	0.5-2.9 mg/ ½ cup
Vitamin C	Red peppers, sweet, raw	95 mg/ ½ cup
	Orange juice	93 mg/ ¾ cup
	Orange	70 mg/ 1 medium orange
	Green peppers	60 mg/ ½ cup
	Broccoli, cooked	51 mg/ ½ cup
	Broccoli, raw	39 mg/ ½ cup
	Strawberries	49 mg/ ½ cup
	Grapefruit	39 mg/ ½ medium grapefruit
	Cabbage, cooked	28 mg/ ½ cup
	Tomatoes	17 mg/ 1 medium tomato
	Spinach, cooked	9 mg/ ½ cup

TABLE 7.8 DIETARY SOURCES OF MICRONUTRIENTS[53-56] (continued)

Vitamin A	Beef liver	22,175 IU/ 3 oz
	Sweet potato, baked	21,909 IU/ 1 medium potato
	Spinach, cooked	11,458 IU/ ½ cup
	Carrots, raw	9,189 IU/ ½ cup
	Cantaloupe	2,706 IU/ ½ cup
	Red peppers, sweet	2,332 IU/ ½ cup
	Black-eyed peas, boiled	1,305 IU/ 1 cup
	Apricots, dried	1,261 IU/ 10 halves
	Egg, hard boiled	260 IU/ 1 large egg
	Summer squash, cooked	191 IU/ ½ cup

Data from Office of Dietary Supplements. Zinc: Fact Sheet for Health Professionals. National Institutes of Health. June 5, 2013. http://ods.od.nih.gov/factsheets/Zinc-HealthProfessional/. Accessed September 21, 2017; Office of Dietary Supplements. Vitamin C: Fact Sheet for Health Professionals. National Institutes of Health. June 5, 2013. https://ods.od.nih.gov/factsheets/VitaminC-HealthProfessional/. Accessed September 21, 2017; Office of Dietary Supplements. Vitamin A: Fact Sheet for Health Professionals National Institutes of Health. June 5, 2013. https://ods.od.nih.gov/factsheets/VitaminA-HealthProfessional/. Accessed September 21, 2017; US Department of Agriculture, Agricultural Research Service, Nutrient Data Laboratory. USDA National Nutrient Database for Standard Reference, Release 27. Version Current: May 2015. Internet: http://www.ars.usda.gov/ba/bhnrc/ndl

over a period of 8 weeks accelerated pressure ulcer healing and decreased wound severity in nonmalnourished patients. Well-nourished patients with wounds should not be overlooked by dietitians. Cereda et al.[33] showed that consumption of disease-specific formulas enriched with protein, arginine, zinc, and vitamin C over 12 weeks accelerated pressure ulcer healing, but more research is needed to confirm these beneficial effects. Desneves and colleagues[48,63] found similar results in just 3 weeks of using high-protein/energy supplements containing arginine, vitamin C, and zinc, which had a 2.5-fold greater improvement in pressure ulcer healing compared with a standard hospital diet and a standard diet plus high-protein/energy ONS. While many studies have demonstrated improvements in wound healing with ONS, results are mixed regarding the benefits of nutritional interventions on the prevention and treatment of pressure ulcers.[49,64]

> **PRACTICE POINT**
>
> Patients may benefit from specialized oral and enteral nutrition formulas to prevent and treat wounds.

If a patient is unable to meet their nutritional needs orally, partial (combined with oral intake) or total EN support may be warranted. EN support is always indicated over parenteral nutrition (PN) unless the gastrointestinal tract is not functional. Feeding through the gut stimulates the immune functions and promotes healing. EN support has been found to increase collagen deposition and tensile strength compared to total PN support, particularly in the early stage of wound healing.[19] While there is a clear connection between nutritional status and clinical outcomes,

Clinical Roundtable

Topic: Nutrition in Pressure Injury Prevention

Background: Although there is a strong epidemiological association between poor nutritional status and pressure injury development, there has been mixed evidence that nutrition interventions prevent pressure injury development. A common intervention for pressure injury prevention is to provide oral nutrition supplementation (ONS), a frequent practice in both the acute and long-term care setting. Many studies examining the practice of providing ONS to prevent pressure injuries tend to have small sample sizes and short durations, which may limit the power of the studies to detect clinical differences between the control and intervention groups.

Roundtable Discussion

1. Would you recommend using oral nutrition supplements for individuals at high risk of pressure injuries, such as older adults with compromised mobility or individuals who are bed or wheelchair bound?
2. What criteria would you consider when making this recommendation?
3. What are the advantages and disadvantages of providing or not providing oral nutrition supplements in this population?

References

1. Kennerly S, Batchelo-Murphy M, Yap TL. Clinical insights: understanding the link between nutrition and pressure ulcer prevention. *Geriatr Nurs*. 2015;36:477-481.
2. Thomas DR. Role of nutrition in the treatment and prevention of pressure ulcers. *Nutr Clin Pract*. 2014;29:466-472.

further research is needed to verify the effect of ONS or EN support on healing of pressure ulcers and mortality in malnourished patients.[4,8]

> **PRACTICE POINT**
>
> Nutrition therapy goals for patients receiving palliative care may be to prevent further tissue breakdown and to preserve quality of life, instead of wound healing.

Monitoring

Monitoring a patient's response to a nutritional intervention can be difficult, especially in an acute care setting, because many patients are discharged from the hospital before the wound is completely healed. Wound healing is not solely dependent on adequate nutrition. Other disciplines, such as nursing and physical therapy, also play vital roles in the wound healing process. While a patient's nutritional intake may be adequate, the wound may fail to heal due to other factors. In any setting, monitoring involves observing any changes to the wound stage. Dietitians may need to work with the interprofessional team to facilitate the timing of a nutrition-focused physical exam during wound dressing changes in order to evaluate and monitor wound healing. Photodocumentation and wound measurements by WOC clinicians can also be useful tools in monitoring wound healing. It is critical to communicate with all members of the interprofessional care team to provide optimal medical nutrition therapy.

Chapter Summary

wound healing is associated with each individual's nutritional status, but is also dependent on other factors, both local and systemic. further research is still needed to determine optimal nutrient recommendations for improved wound healing at each stage. patients should be encouraged to maintain adequate intake of energy and foods high in protein, zinc, vitamin a, and vitamin c to promote wound healing. current studies support the use of ons in both malnourished and well-nourished patients with chronic wounds. particularly, ons containing nutrients specific to wound healing (arginine, glutamine, zinc, and vitamin c) have been shown to improve rates of healing. larger, randomized controlled trials are needed to determine the true efficacy of nutrition supplementation. the impact of nutrition on wound healing is well-known and emphasizes the importance of clinical dietitians in the interprofessional approach to prevent and treat wounds.

Key Terms

wound, acute wound, chronic wound, inflammation, angiogenesis, proliferation, collagen, remodeling, pressure ulcer, debridement, Braden Scale for Predicting Pressure Sore Risk, arginine, glutamine, β-hydroxy-β-methylbutyrate (HMB)

References

1. Velnar T, Bailey T, Smrkolj V. The wound healing process: an overview of the cellular and molecular mechanisms. *Journal Int Med Res*. 2009;37:1528-1542.
2. Medina A, Scott PG, Ghahary A, Tredget EE. Pathophysiology of chronic nonhealing wounds. *J Burn Care Rehabil*. 2005;26(4):306-319.
3. Dorner B, Posthauer ME, Thomas, D. National Pressure Ulcer Advisory Panel. The Role of Nutrition in Pressure Ulcer Prevention and Treatment: National Pressure Ulcer Advisory Panel White Paper. NPUAP; 2009.
4. Mechanick JI. Practical aspects of nutritional support for wound-healing patients. *Am J Surgery*. 2004;188:52S-56S.
5. Hackman DJ, Ford, HR. Cellular, biochemical, and clinical aspects of wound healing. *Surg Infec*. 2002;3:S23-S35.
6. Bowler PG. Wound pathophysiology, infection and therapeutic options. *Ann Med*. 2002;34:419-427.
7. Wild T, Rahbarnia A, Kellner M, Sobotka L, Eberlein T. Basics in nutrition and wound healing. *Nutrition*. 2010;26:862-866.
8. Stechmiller JK. Understanding the role of nutrition and wound healing. *Nutr Clin Pract*. 2010;25:61-68.
9. Li J, Chen J, Kirsner R. Pathophysiology of acute wound healing. *Clinic Dermatol*. 2007;25:9-18.
10. Guo S, DiPietro LA. Factors affecting wound healing. *J Dent Res*. 2010;89(3):219-229.
11. Menke NB, Ward KR, Witten TM, Bonchev DG, Diegelmann RF. Impaired wound healing. *Clinic Dermatol*. 2007;25:19-25.
12. Ebrect M, Hextall J, Kirtley LG, Taylor A, Dyson M, Weinman J. Perceived stress and cortisiol levels predict speed of wound healing in healthy male adults. *Psychoneuroendocrinology*. 2004;29:798-809.
13. Falanga V. Wound healing and its impairment in the diabetic foot. *Lancet*. 2005;366:1736-1743.
14. Witte MB, Thornton FJ, Tantry U, Barbul A. L-arginine supplementation enhances diabetic wound healing: involvement of the nitric oxide synthase and arginase pathways. *Metabolism*. 2002;51(10):1269-1273.
15. National Pressure Ulcer Advisory Panel. Educational and Clinical Resources. http://www.npuap.org/resources/educational-and-clinical-resources/. Accessed June 23, 2017.
16. Grey JE, Enoch S, Harding KG. ABC of wound healing: Pressure ulcers. *BMJ*. 2006;332(7539):472-475.
17. Brown P. Assessment and Documentation for Wounds: A Step-by-Step Process. In: Brown P. *Quick reference to wound care: Palliative, home, and clinical practices*. 4th ed. Burlington, MA: Jones & Bartlett Learning; 2013:11-16.
18. Brewer S, Desneves K, Pearce L, et al. Effect of an arginine-containing nutritional supplement on pressure ulcer healing in community spinal patients. *J Wound Care*. 2010;19(7): 311-316.
19. Arnold M, Barbul A. Nutrition and wound healing. *Plast Reconstr Surg*. 2006;117:42S-58S.
20. Demling RH. Nutrition, anabolism, and the wound healing process: An overview. *ePlasty*. 2009;9:65-94.
21. Gruys E, Toussaint MJM, Niewold TA, Koopmans SJ. Acute phase reaction and acute phase proteins. *J Zhejiang Univ SCI*. 2005;6B(11): 1045-1056.
22. Cordiero MBC, Antonelli EJ, Ferreira da Cunha D, Jordao Jr. A, Rodrigues Jr. V, Vannucchi H. Oxidative stress and acute-phase response in patients with pressure sores. *Nutrition*. 2005;21:901-907.
23. Jain S, Guatam V, Naseem S. Acute-phase proteins: As diagnostic tool. *J Pharm Bioallied Sci*. 2011;3(1):118-127.

24. Desborough JP. The stress response to trauma and surgery. *Br J Anaesth*. 2000;85(1):109-117.
25. Collins CE, Kershaw J, Brockington S. Effect of nutritional supplements on wound healing in home-nursed elderly: A randomized trial. *Nutrition*. 2005;21:147-155.
26. Lyder CH. Pressure ulcer prevention and management. *JAMA*. 2003;289(2):223-226.
27. Harvey C. Wound healing. *Orthop Nurs*. 2005;24(2):143-157.
28. Kranke P, Bennett MH, Martyn-St James M, Schnabel A, Debus SE, Weibel S. Hyperbaric oxygen therapy for chronic wounds. *Cochrane Database Syst Rev*. 2015;6:1-72.
29. Tappenden KA, Quatrara B, Parkhurst ML, Malone AM, Fanjiang G, Ziegler TR. Critical role of nutrition in improving quality of care: An interdisciplinary call to action to address adult hospital malnutrition. *J Acad Nutr Diet*. 2013;113:1219-1237.
30. Braden B, Bergstrom N. Braden Scale for Predicting Pressure Sore Risk. 1988. http://bradenscale.com/images/bradenscale.pdf. Accessed August 17, 2017.
31. Mueller C, Compher C, Druyan, ME, American Society for Parenteral and Enteral Nutrition (A.S.P.E.N.) Board of Directors. A.S.P.E.N. Clinical Guidelines: Nutrition Screening, Assessment, and Intervention in Adults. *JPEN J Parenter Enteral Nutr*. 2011;35(1):16-24.
32. van Anholt RD, Sobotka L, Meijer EP, et al. Specific nutritional support accelerates pressure ulcer healing and reduces wound care intensity in non-malnourished patients. *Nutrition*. 2010;26:867-872.
33. Cereda E, Gini A, Pedrolli C, Vanottie A. Disease-specific, versus standard, nutritional support for the treatment of pressure ulcers in institutionalized older adults: A randomized control trial. *J Am Geriatr Soc*. 2009;57:1395-1402.
34. Academy of Nutrition and Dietetics Evidence Analysis Library. Recommendations Summary: Spinal Cord Injury (SCI) Assessment of Nutritional Needs for Pressure Ulcers [Web page]. 2014. http://www.andeal.org/template.cfm?key=2378. Accessed May 28, 2017.
35. Hasson RE, Howe CA, Jones BL, Freedson PS. Accuracy of four resting metabolic rate prediction equations: Effect of sex, body mass index, age, and race/ethnicity. *J Sci Med Sport*. 2011;14:344-351.
36. Kushner RF, Drover JW. Current strategies of critical care assessment and therapy of the obese patient (hypocaloric feeding): What are we doing and what do we need to do? *JPEN J Parenter Enteral Nutr*. 2011;35(1):36S-43S.
37. Anderegg BA, Worrall C, Barbour E, Simpson KN, DeLegge M. Comparison of resting energy expenditure prediction methods with measured resting energy expenditure in obese, hospitalized adults. *JPEN J Parenter Enteral Nutr*. 2009;33(2):168-175.
38. Kee AL, Isenring E, Hickman I, Vivanti A. Resting energy expenditure of morbidly obese patients using indirect calorimetry: a systematic review. *Obes Rev*. 2012;13:753-765.
39. Dambach B, Salle A, Marteau C, et al. Energy requirements are not greater in elderly patients suffering from pressure ulcers. *J Am Geriatr Soc*. 2005;53:478-482.
40. Bansal V, Ochoa JB. Arginine availability, arginase, and the immune response. *Curr Opin Clin Nutr Metab Care*. 2003;6:223-338.
41. Witte MB, Barbul A. Arginine physiology and its implication for wound healing. *Wound Rep Reg*. 2003;11:419-423.
42. Stechmiller JK, Childress B, Cowan L. Arginine supplementation and wound healing. *Nutr Clin Pract*. 2005;20:52-61.
43. Williams JZ, Abumrad N, Barbul A. Effect of a specialized amino acid mixture on human collagen deposition. *Ann Surg*. 2002;236(3):369-375.
44. Debats IB, Wolfs TG, Gotoh T, Cleutjens JP, Peutz-Kootstra CJ, van der Hulst RR. Role of arginine in superficial wound healing in man. *Nitric Oxide*. 2009;1-8.
45. Blass SC, Goost H, Tolba RH, et al. Time to wound closure in trauma patients with disorders in wound healing is shortened by supplements containing antioxidant micronutrients and glutamine: A PRCT. *Clin Nutr*. 2012;31:469-475.
46. Sipahi S, Gungor O, Gunduz M, Cilci M, Demirci MC, Tamer A. The effect of oral supplementation with a combination of beta-hydroxy-beta-methylbutyrate, arginine and glutamine on wound healing: a retrospective analysis of diabetic haemodialysis patients. *BMC Nephrology*. 2013;14(8):1-6.
47. Clements RH, Saraf N, Kakade M, Yellumahanthi K, White M, Hackett JA. Nutritional effect of oral supplement enriched in beta-hydroxy-beta-methylbutyrate, glutamine and arginine on resting metabolic rate after labaroscopic gastric bypass. *Surg Endosc*. 2011;25(5):1376-1382.
48. Eley HL, Russell ST, Baxter JH, Mukerji P, Tisdale MJ. Signaling pathways initiated by β-hydroxy-β-methylbutyrate to attenuate the depression of protein synthesis in skeletal muscle in response to cachectic stimuli. *Am J Physiol Endocrinol Metab*. 2007;293:E923-E931.
49. McDaniel JC, Belury M, Ahijevych K, Blakely W. ω-3 fatty acids effect on wound healing. *Wound Rep Reg*. 2008;16(3):337-345.
50. Lansdown ABG, Mirastschijski U, Stubbs N, Scanlon E, Agren MS. Zinc in wound healing: Theoretical, experimental, and clinical aspects. *Wound Rep Reg*. 2007;15:2-16.
51. Lim Y, Levy M, Bray TM. Dietary zinc alters early inflammation responses during cutaneous wound healing in weanling CD-1 mice. *J Nutr*. 2004;134:811-816.
52. Yanagisawa H. Zinc deficiency and clinical practice. *JMAJ*. 2004;129(5):613-616.
53. Office of Dietary Supplements. Zinc: Fact Sheet for Health Professionals. National Institutes of Health. http://ods.od.nih.gov/factsheets/Zinc-HealthProfessional/. Updated Accessed September 21, 2017.
54. Office of Dietary Supplements. Vitamin C: Fact Sheet for Health Professionals. National Institutes of Health. https://ods.od.nih.gov/factsheets/VitaminC-HealthProfessional/. Updated Accessed September 21, 2017.
55. Office of Dietary Supplements. Vitamin A: Fact Sheet for Health Professionals National Institutes of Health. https://ods.od.nih.gov/factsheets/VitaminA-HealthProfessional/. Updated June 5, 2013. Accessed September 21, 2017.
56. U.S. Department of Agriculture, Agricultural Research Service, Nutrient Data Laboratory. USDA National Nutrient Database for Standard Reference, Release 27. Version Current: May 2015. http://www.ars.usda.gov/ba/bhnrc/ndl. Accessed November 21, 2017.
57. Raffoul W, Far MS, Cayeux MC, Berger MM. Nutritional status and food intake in nine patients with chronic low-limb ulcers: importance of oral supplements. *Nutrition*. 2006;22:82-88.
58. Brown SA, Coimbra M, Coberly DM, Chao JJ, Rohrich RJ. Oral nutrition supplementation accelerates skin wound healing: A randomized, placebo-controlled, double-arm, crossover study. *Plast Reconstr Surg*. 2003;114:237-244.
59. Stratton RJ, Elia M. The skeleton in the closet: malnutrition in the community, Encouraging appropriate, evidence-based use of oral nutritional supplements. *Proc Nutr Soc*. 2010;69:477-487.
60. Chapman BR, Mills KJ, Pearce LM, Crow TC. Use of an arginine-enriched oral nutrition supplement in the healing of pressure ulcers in patients with spinal cord injuries: An observational study. *Nutr Diet*. 2011;68:208-213.

61. Cawood AL, Elia M, Stratton RJ. Systematic review and meta-analysis of the effects of high protein oral nutrition supplements. *Ageing Res Rev.* 2012;11:278-296.
62. Stratton RJ, Ek AC, Engfer M, et al. Enteral nutritional support in prevention and treatment of pressure ulcers: A systematic review and meta-analysis. *Ageing Res Rev.* 2005;4:422-450.
63. Desneves KJ, Todorovic BE, Cassar A, Crowe TC. Treatment with supplementary arginine, vitamin C and zinc in patients with pressure ulcers: A randomized controlled trial. *Clin Nutr.* 2005;24:979-987.
64. Langer G, Fink A. Nutritional interventions for preventing and treating pressure ulcers. *Cochrane Database of Syst Rev.* 2014;6:1-82.

Chapter 8

Nutritional Management of Obesity

Isadora Nogueira
Sonja Goedkoop
Jillian Reece

Chapter Outline

Core Concepts
Introduction
Prevalence
Classification of Obesity: Is Obesity a Disease?
Causes and Contributions to the Obesity Epidemic
Alterations in Body Composition in Obesity
Nutrition Assessment in Obesity
Biochemical Assessment

Clinical Assessment
Dietary Assessment
Other Considerations
Pathophysiology Associated with Obesity
Obesity Management
Micronutrient Concerns
Emerging Treatment Options

CORE CONCEPTS

1. Obesity is a risk factor for a variety of health conditions, including type 2 diabetes, hyperlipidemia, hypertension, heart disease, stroke, certain cancers, nonalcoholic fatty liver disease, sleep apnea, gallbladder disease, respiratory problems, arthritis, and depression.

2. The etiology of obesity is complex and includes many interacting factors, including genetics; environment; and social, biological, and developmental factors.

3. Body weight is regulated by a complex network of systems and signaling pathways that become overtaxed with obesity and chronic positive energy balance.

4. Body weight is regulated by metabolic, neuroendocrine, and autonomic systems in the body, including signals released from adipose, gastrointestinal, and endocrine tissues that are integrated by the liver and central nervous system.

5. Approaches to obesity management include individual and comprehensive lifestyle intervention, pharmacotherapy, and bariatric surgery.

Learning Objectives

1. Describe the magnitude and etiology of obesity.
2. Explain how obesity is defined and classified.
3. Identify the pathophysiology of obesity.
4. Assess nutritional status and develop a nutrition care plan for individuals with obesity.
5. Discuss the signaling pathways and hormones involved in body weight regulation.
6. Identify the disease states associated with obesity and their pathophysiology.
7. List the characteristics used to define metabolic syndrome.
8. Describe three nonsurgical nutrition interventions for weight loss.
9. Identify three types of medications used for treatment of weight management.
10. Classify the bariatric surgery procedure types.
11. List the recommended vitamin supplementation for a patient after having bariatric surgery.
12. Describe the diet progression following roux-en-Y gastric bypass or sleeve gastrectomy.

Introduction

Overweight and **obesity** are medical conditions in which an individual has excess body fat for a given height. The World Health Organization (WHO) uses **body mass index** (BMI; weight in kilograms divided by height in meters squared) to classify stages of overweight and obesity and the perceived health risk of an individual. A BMI of 25 to 29.9 is defined as overweight and a BMI ≥30 is defined as obese.[1] Childhood overweight and obesity is defined as the 85th to 95th percentiles and greater than the 95th percentile, respectively, using BMI-for-age scales.[2] Obesity is a risk factor for a variety of health conditions, including diabetes, hyperlipidemia, hypertension, heart disease, stroke, certain cancers, nonalcoholic fatty liver disease, sleep apnea, gallbladder disease, respiratory problems, arthritis, and depression.[3] Higher classes of obesity are associated with increased all-cause mortality, primarily from cardiovascular disease, diabetes, and certain cancers.[3] Additionally, obese individuals may experience social stigmatization and discrimination, and report a decreased quality of life.[4] Over the last decade, the estimated annual medical cost of obesity has increased, with current estimates ranging from $147 billion to $210 billion. Annual medical expenses for individuals with obesity are higher than those of normal weight by an estimated $1,429.[5] If current trends continue, obesity-related healthcare costs in the United States are expected to increase by $48 to $66 billion per year by the year 2030.[6] Nutrition interventions in the prevention and treatment of obesity are important initiatives in addressing this crisis.

CORE CONCEPT 1

Obesity is a risk factor for a variety of health conditions, including diabetes, hyperlipidemia, hypertension, heart disease, stroke, certain cancers, nonalcoholic fatty liver disease, sleep apnea, gallbladder disease, respiratory problems, arthritis, and depression.

Prevalence

According to the Centers for Disease Control and Prevention (CDC), more than one-third (37.9%) of adults and approximately 17% of children in the United States have obesity.[7] The most recent estimates of obesity prevalence in the United States are based on the 2013-2014 National Health and Nutrition Examination Survey.[8] While trends show that obesity prevalence increased over the last decades of the 20th century, rates have since slowed; there was minimal change among adults or children from 2007-2008 to 2011-2012.[9] Still, within these trends there are observed differences between age groups, sex, ethnicity, race, geographic location, and socioeconomic status (**Figures 8.1-8.3**). Women

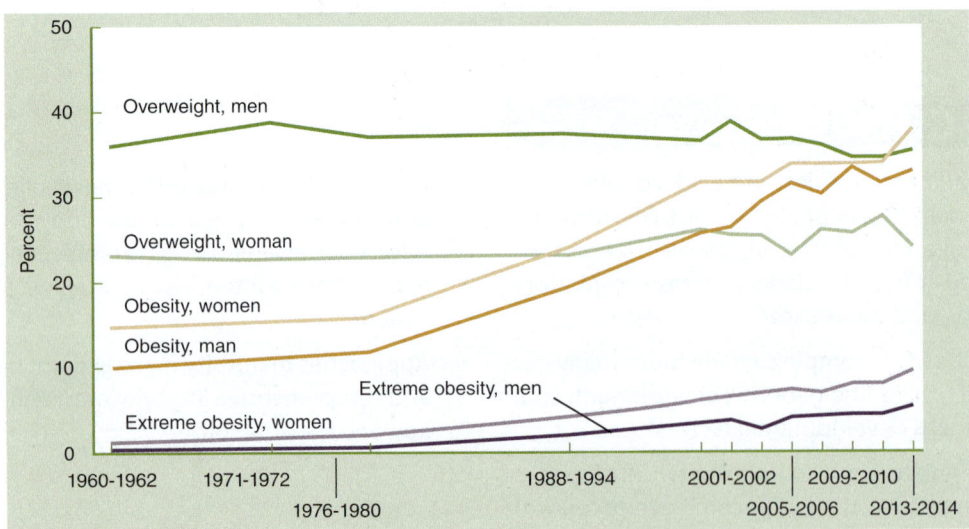

FIGURE 8.1 Overweight and Obesity Trends for Men and Women from 1960 to 2014

Reproduced from Fryar CD, Carroll, MD, et.al., Prevalence of Overweight, Obesity, and Extreme Obesity Among Adults Aged 20 and Over: United States, 1960–1962 Through 2013–2014. Hyattsville, MD: National Center for Health Statistics. 2016. Accessed at, https://www.cdc.gov/nchs/data/hestat/obesity_adult_13_14/obesity_adult_13_14.htm

CASE STUDY INTRODUCTION

Allison is a 30-year-old female presenting to nutrition clinic seeking weight loss and diabetes management. She had childhood-onset obesity and throughout her adult years gained weight due to chronic use of prednisone for asthma and insulin for her diabetes. She is single and works full time as an accountant.

Anthropometric Data:
Weight: 95 kg (208 lbs)
Height: 152 cm (62 in)
BMI: 38 kg/m^2
Weight History
Usual body weight: 95 kg (208 lbs)
Highest adult weight: 110 kg (220 lbs) 4 years ago
Lowest adult weight: 91 kg (200 lbs) 8 years ago

Biochemical Data:
Fasting blood glucose: 150 (70-99 mg/dL)
Hemoglobin A1c: 8.0% (4.3-5.8%)
Low-density lipoprotein (LDL-C): 119 (Desirable: <100 mg/dL)
High-density lipoprotein (HDL-C): 38 (Desirable: >40 mg/dL)
Triglycerides: 175 (Desirable: <150 mg/dL)
25 (OH) Vitamin D: 17 ng/mL (20-100 ng/mL)

Clinical Data:
Past medical history: Type 2 diabetes mellitus, obesity, asthma
Medications: Metformin 1000 mg with breakfast and dinner, glucotrol 10 mg with breakfast and dinner, glargine insulin 20 units at bedtime, prednisone 150 mg once per day
Vital signs: Blood pressure 119/78 mm Hg; Temperature 98.2°F; Heart rate 82 beats per minute
Nutrition-focused Physical Exam: Appears obese with notable central adiposity consistent with android body type. Mild ankle edema noted. Darkened skin consistent with acanthosis nigricans seen on back of neck.

Dietary Data:
Dietary History: Allison eats three meals/day and one to two snacks. Portions can be large, particularly at dinner. She tries to follow a balanced, lower carbohydrate meal plan with whole grains, fruits, and vegetables daily. Recently, she has been complaining of persistent hunger despite daily intake of around 1,800 calories/day. She is logging foods daily via a written journal.

Questions
1. What factors contributed to Allison's obesity?
2. What are the important considerations when determining the appropriate nutrition intervention? How would you evaluate her disease risk given her BMI?
3. What are your nutrition priorities for Allison?
4. How would you interpret Allison's labs?
5. What additional information would you like to obtain?

---

may be more likely to have obesity (40.4%) when compared to men (35%), and middle-aged adults rank the highest (age 41-59 years) compared to young adults (age 20-39) and older adults (age 60 and older).[9] Non-Hispanic blacks have the highest age-adjusted rates of obesity (48.4%) compared with Hispanics (42.6%), non-Hispanic whites, (36.4%) and non-Hispanic Asians (12.6%).[9] Geographically, U.S. obesity prevalence is currently highest in the South (31.2%), followed by the Midwest (30.7%), Northeast (26.4%), and the West (25.2%).[10] There are also varying rates of obesity based

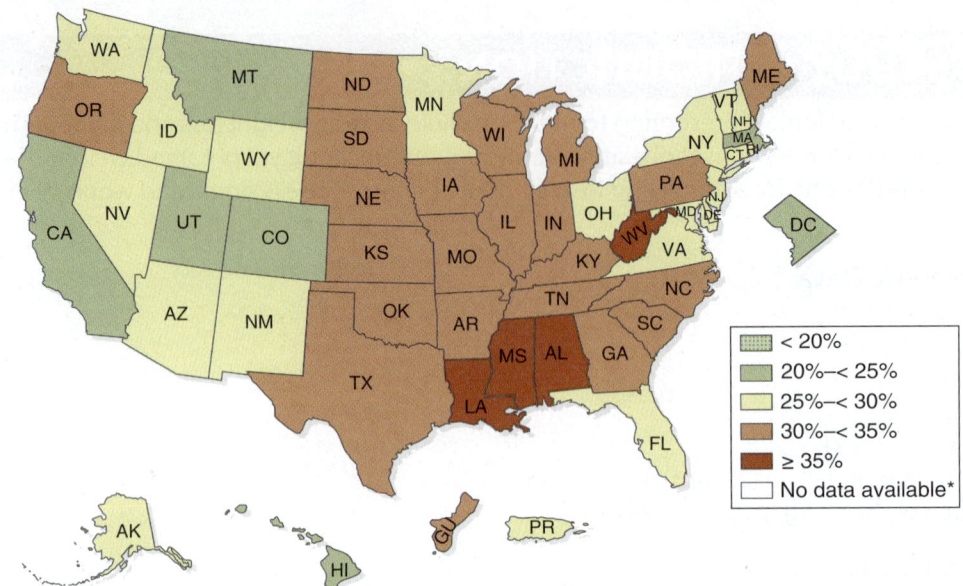

FIGURE 8.2 Prevalence of Self-Reported Obesity Among U.S. Adults by State and Territory, BRFSS, 2015

Reproduced from Centers for Disease Control and Prevention (CDC). Behavioral Risk Factor Surveillance System Survey Data. Atlanta, Georgia: U.S. Department of Health and Human Services, Centers for Disease Control and Prevention. Accessed at https://www.cdc.gov/obesity/data/prevalence-maps.html

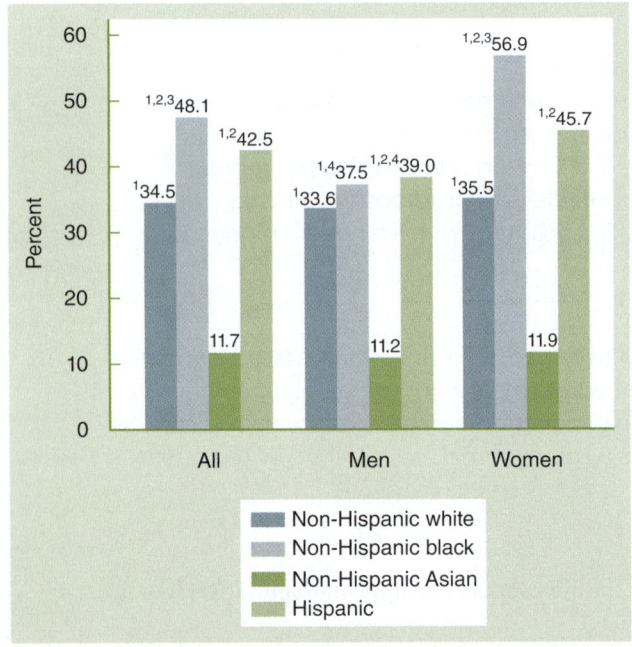

FIGURE 8.3 Prevalence of Obesity among Adults Aged 20 And Older, By Sex and Race And Hispanic Origin, in the United States, 2011 to 2014. [1]Significantly different from non-Hispanic Asian persons. [2]Significantly different from non-Hispanic white persons. [3]Significantly different from females of the same race and Hispanic origin. [4]Significantly different from non-Hispanic black persons

Reproduced from Ogden CL, Carroll MD, Fryar CD, Flegal KM. Prevalence of obesity among adults and youth: United States, 2011–2014. NCHS data brief, no 219. Hyattsville, MD: National Center for Health Statistics. 2015.

on education and socioeconomic status. Non-Hispanic black and Mexican American men with higher incomes are more likely to have obesity compared to those with lower income. Higher-income women are less likely to have obesity than low-income women. Education level does not appear to have an impact on obesity among men; however, women with college degrees are less likely to have obesity than those without college degrees.[11]

Classification of Obesity: Is Obesity a Disease?

In June 2013, the American Medical Association (AMA) adopted a policy that recognizes obesity as a disease requiring a range of medical interventions for treatment and prevention. BMI is used as a simple, noninvasive way to predict an individual's risk for disease; however, it does not directly measure body fat stores. As a result, some individuals may be classified as "obese" due to an elevated BMI without having excess body fat. Factors that contribute to disease risk but that cannot be captured by BMI measurements include body fat distribution, such as visceral versus subcutaneous fat; ethnicity; age; fitness level; and smoking status. The diagnosis of obesity must be individualized because health risks vary by ethnicity. For example, diabetes risk starts to increase at a BMI of 23 kg/m^2 for East Asian individuals (e.g., Japanese, Chinese), while disease risk may be lower in African Americans and whites with the same BMI. Despite the demonstrated shortcomings of BMI measurements, some studies suggest that it correlates well with morbidity and mortality for the general population.[12] **Table 8.1** lists the cutoff ranges used to determine overweight and obesity.

> **PRACTICE POINT**
>
> Body composition should be considered when using BMI to classify obesity in individuals who are very muscular.

TABLE 8.1 CLASSIFICATION OF OBESITY USING BODY MASS INDEX

BMI (kg/m²)	Classification
<18.5	Underweight
18.5 to 24.9	Healthy weight
25.0 to 29.9	Overweight
30.0 to 34.9	Obesity Class I
35.0 to 39.9	Obesity Class II
≥ 40.0	Obesity Class III, or Morbid/Extreme Obesity

Data from https://www.nhlbi.nih.gov/health/educational/lose_wt/BMI/bmi_dis.htm.

Causes and Contributions to the Obesity Epidemic

The etiology of obesity is complex and includes many interacting factors.[13]

Genetic Factors

Changes in the genotype of humans occur too slowly to explain the rapid rise in obesity over recent decades; however, the variation of weight regulation among individuals in the same environment suggests that genetics play a role. A systematic review of 12 studies, including 8,179 monozygotic and 9,977 dizygotic twin pairs in addition to individual participant data for 629 monozygotic and 594 dizygotic pairs from four twin registries, assessed the genetic influence of BMI.[14] Results suggest that the heritability of BMI ranged from 61% to 80% for both male and female subjects and was high across all age categories. The number of known markers and chromosome regions associated with obesity is greater than 250.[15] Numerous genes are involved in obesity, but there has been a major focus on two in particular: the ob gene and the β-adrenoreceptor gene. The ob gene produces leptin, a hormone involved in energy regulation, and the β-adrenoreceptor gene is one of many genes involved in regulation of resting metabolic rate (RMR) and fat oxidation in humans. It was thought that mutations of these genes were involved in weight gain, although one particular gene is not likely to be the major contributor of obesity, but rather several polygenic factors in combination with other determinants.[16] Although only a small number of rare, single genetic abnormalities that cause obesity have been identified, an area of research called epigenetics examines the relationship by which obesity-predisposing genes interact with the environment and may influence an individual's response to treatment.[17]

Environmental Factors

In addition to genetics, there are strong environmental influences on obesity. Food environment has shifted over the years to promote overeating through increased availability of inexpensive, calorie-dense foods, such as fast food restaurants, convenience stores, and vending machines. Not only has the availability of processed foods high in calories, fat, and sugar increased over time, but portion sizes have increased dramatically as well.[18] While fast-paced life in the United States may leave many individuals turning to high-calorie, convenience foods by choice, others may be limited by their geographical location. "Food deserts," described as areas where limited access to fresh and affordable foods exist, occur within the United States, making it difficult for certain individuals to eat an optimal diet for health and disease prevention.[19]

Decreased involvement in physical activity for both children and adults is another contributing factor to the obesity epidemic. According to a report by the CDC, only 1 in 5 individuals meet the 2008 Physical Activity Guidelines for Americans.[20] Generally, there has been a significant decrease in activities of daily of living over the past three or four decades due to many environmental factors.[13] The energy individuals used to spend in these activities has now been replaced by technology, such as purchasing groceries online from home instead of grocery shopping, remote controls, cell phones, drive-through restaurants, and computers.

Another contributing factor to weight gain and obesity is the use of weight-promoting medications. Many commonly used medications are associated with weight gain, including psychotropic medications, steroid hormones, contraceptives, diabetes medications, antihypertensives, antihistamines, and protease inhibitors (**Table 8.2**).[13] In some instances, alternative medications that do not have weight gain as a side effect may be available to treat the same condition. When visiting a primary physician or specialist who is prescribing medication, individuals should discuss in detail any potential side effects with its use.

Sleep deprivation may also be contributing to the rise in obesity. Americans now sleep less than they did a few decades ago. Mechanisms that may explain the relationship between sleep loss and obesity include both metabolic and endocrine changes within the body. These include a decrease in glucose tolerance and insulin sensitivity; increased concentrations of stress hormones such as cortisol, which occur later in the day; increased levels of ghrelin; and decreased levels of leptin. Cumulatively, these factors can contribute to increased appetite and hunger, which may result in overeating and weight gain in some individuals.[21]

Social Factors

Social determinants of health, defined by the WHO as conditions in which individuals are born, grow, live, work, and age, may also contribute to the obesity epidemic. Shaped by the distribution of money, power, and resources at national and local levels, this includes demographic characteristics, education level, socioeconomic status, and perceived social and

TABLE 8.2 MEDICATIONS THAT PROMOTE WEIGHT GAIN

Class	Drugs	Comments
Tricyclic antidepressants (TCAs)	Amitriptyline, nortriptyline, clomipramine, doxepin, imipramine, trimipramine, desipramine	Amytriptyline and imipramine have the greatest effect on weight gain; notriptyline and desimaprine have the smallest
Monoamine oxidase inhibitors (MAOIs)	Phenelzine	Weight gain is less intense than with TCAs
Selective serotonin reuptake inhibitors (SSRIs)	Paroxetine, citalopram	
Phenothiazines	Chlorpromazine	
Tetracyclic antidepressants	Mirtazapine	
Atypical antipsychotics	Clozapine, olanzapine, ripseridone	Clozapine may increase appetite
Antimanics	Lithium	
Anticonvulsants	Valproic acid, gabapentin, carbamazepine	Valproic acid and carbamazepine may increase appetite
Antidiabetic agents	Insulin; *meglitinides:* repaglinide, nateglinide; *sulfonylureas:* gluyburide; *thiazolidinediones:* rosiglitazone, ploglitazone	Insulin increases deposition of adipose tissue
Alpha-andrenergic blockers	Prazosin, doxazosin, terazosin	
Nonselective beta blockers	Propranolol	
Alpha-andrenergic agonists	Methyldopa, clonidine	
Anabolic steroids	Oxandrolone	
Corticosteroids	Hydrocortisone, prednisone	Indirectly promote weight gain by stimulating appetite; increase truncal fat (adipose) tissue deposits
Antihistamines	Meclizine, diphenhydramine	Indirectly promote weight gain by stimulating appetite
Antineoplastic agents	Megatrol	Indirectly promote weight gain by stimulating appetite

Data from Alexander Motylev, RPh, PhD. US Pharm. 2008;33(12):HS19-HS27. https://www.uspharmacist.com/article/the-operating-room-pharmacist-and-bariatric-surgery.

cultural norms.[22] Specifically, the interactions that individuals have with others, as described by their social network, can have a powerful influence on weight. A study examining 12,067 people from the Framingham Heart Study between 1971 and 2003 found that an individual's chance of developing obesity increased by 57% if a friend also had obesity. Additionally, among adult siblings, the risk of obesity increased by 40% if one sibling had obesity. Similar trends are observed with married couples: if one spouse has obesity, the likelihood that the other would become obese increased by 37%.[23]

Biological Factors

Recent research has examined the influence of intestinal microbiota on obesity, showing a potential link between alterations in the gut microbiome and weight gain. The human gastrointestinal tract is host to trillions of live bacteria that have metabolic interactions with each other and the human host, influencing human nutrition and metabolism.[24] Gut microbiota synthesize essential B vitamins and vitamin K, and harvest energy from the diet that is used to produce short-chain fatty acids that provide an energy source for cells in the colon and liver. The role of gut microbiota on body weight regulation originated from studies using mice models in which transplantation of intestinal microbiota from obese mice to lean mice led to 60% increase in body fat content and development of insulin resistance despite reduced food intake.[25] One mechanism by which obesity may be related to these changes in gut microbiota is the varying absorption of energy from dietary intake depending on the composition of the microbiota. Research suggests that obese mice absorb more energy (kilocalories) from dietary carbohydrate than conventional (nonobese) mice. While the data in humans are smaller, association studies indicate that obese humans have reduced microbial diversity and alterations in the genes involved in metabolic pathways compared to lean individuals. Similarly to mice, increased efficiency of energy absorption from food in obese compared to lean individuals is one possible mechanism explaining the link between gut microbiota and obesity.[24] The best current evidence supports the hypothesis that dietary factors induce changes in microbiota that support an obese phenotype through multiple mechanisms.

Developmental Factors

Early life determinants including in utero factors and the impact of breastfeeding have been studied. Research suggests that children with obesity are more likely to remain obese as adults; therefore, further studies involving this population are essential. While we still do not fully understand the direct causes of obesity, it is thought that breastfeeding may play a protective role early in life. A mother's breast milk is often lower in calories, fat, and proteins and contains satiety hormones such as leptin compared to infant formulas.[26] This balance may trigger less of an insulin response in the infant and protect against increased fat accumulation and weight gain.[27] Further studies examining the duration of breastfeeding during infancy and obesity suggest an inverse relationship; the longer an infant is breastfed, the lower the risk for overweight and obesity extending through childhood (<1 month compared to >6 months).[28] Despite the large number of studies in support of a inverse correlation between breastfeeding and obesity, further research is needed to examine its impact on weight and disease risk later in life.[29,30]

The numerous causes and influences of obesity continue to be a highly researched topic, and it is important for healthcare professionals to be aware of the complexity of this condition. Additional factors that may contribute to obesity not mentioned but worth considering include endocrine disruption due to environmental exposure, political influences on weight, changes in ethnicities and impact of increasing gravida age, infection, and inflammation.[13] The nutrition assessment for patients with obesity should include a thorough evaluation of each individual and, where possible, identify and evaluate the possible contributors in order to provide the best possible care.

> **CORE CONCEPT 2**
>
> The etiology of obesity is complex and includes many interacting factors including genetics; environment; and social, biological, and developmental factors.

Hormonal Factors

Body weight is regulated by metabolic, neuroendocrine, and autonomic systems as well as a complex network of signaling released from adipose, gastrointestinal, and endocrine tissues that are integrated by the liver and central nervous system (CNS). When the body experiences a slight change in energy intake or energy loss, these systems work together to maintain a state of weight equilibrium. As the systems become overtaxed, such as that with repeated overfeeding and a positive energy balance, weight gain can result. The term "adaptive thermogenesis" has been used to explain why individuals who have tried to achieve a state of negative energy balance tend to regain lost weight over time (with an 80% to 90% return rate to pre–weight loss levels of body fat). The effect is observed in both lean and obese individuals.[31] There is variability among individuals regarding the degree of weight gain when exposed to an adipogenic environment, which can be explained in part by genetic influences that reflect individual metabolic responses to increased energy intake or decreased expenditure.[31]

Understanding the interplay between gut hormones and the CNS and how these factors regulate appetite and food intake is essential to obesity management (**Figure 8.5**). The hypothalamus in the brain plays a central role in energy balance and weight regulation. It receives both peripheral signals (gastrointestinal tract, pancreas, adipocytes) and central signals that communicate how much energy from food is needed by the body in the short term and how much energy is available in the body for long-term use. The acruate nucleus region within the hypothalamus contains hormone receptors with two regions predominantly responsible for integrating these signals: the pro-opiomelanocortin (POMC) neurons, which aim to suppress appetite, and the neuropeptide Y (NPY) and agouti-related peptide (AgRP) neurons, which aim to stimulate appetite (**Figure 8.4**).[32] The hypothalamus manages input from the cortex and hedonic pathways, which are activated by the sight, smell, and social aspects of food. When these signals reach the regions in the hypothalamus, changes in their activity and the release of neuropeptides influence eating behavior, meal patterns, and energy expenditure (**Figure 8.5**).[33]

> **CORE CONCEPT 3**
>
> Body weight is regulated by a complex network of systems and signaling pathways that become overtaxed with obesity and chronic positive energy balance.

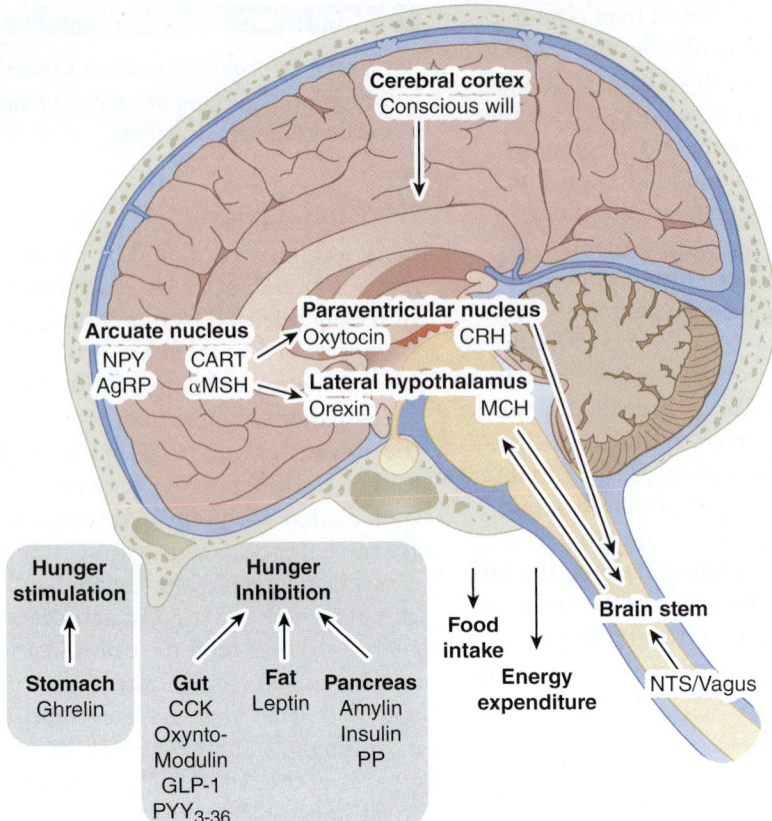

FIGURE 8.4 Selected Pathways Involved in Body Weight Regulation

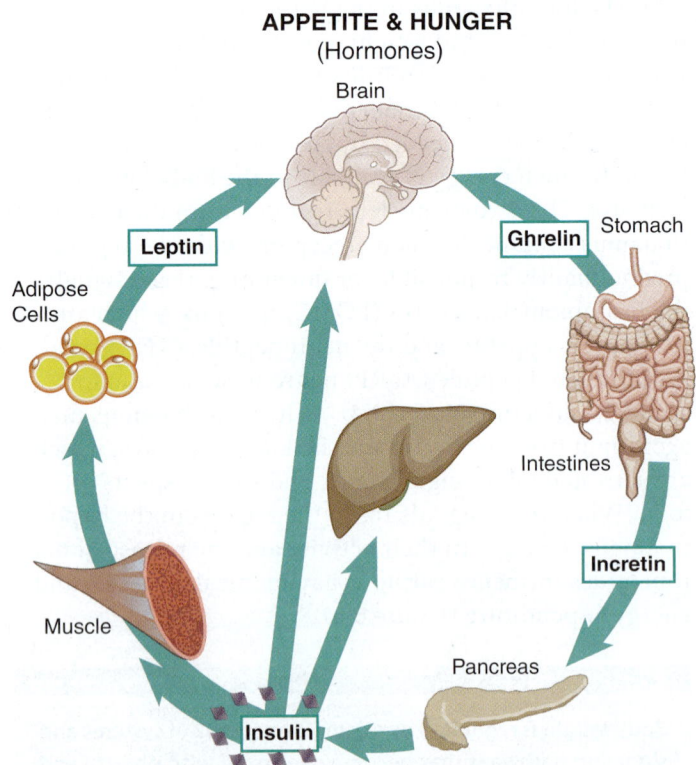

FIGURE 8.5 Hormones Involved in Appetite and Hunger in the Human Endocrine System: Incretin, Ghrelin, Leptin and Insulin

Orexigenic Hormones

Ghrelin

Ghrelin is the only **orexigenic**, or appetite-inducing, gastrointestinal hormone. It is short acting and secreted in the fundus of the stomach, in small quantities in other parts of the gastrointestinal tract, in the pancreas, and in ghrelin-neurons in the hypothalamus. Ghrelin levels are found to be at the highest preprandially to stimulate food intake and at the lowest postprandially to signal the end of eating. The release of ghrelin increases gastrointestinal motility and decreases insulin secretion. The exact mechanism of action of ghrelin remains unclear. Ghrelin may reach the hypothalamus via the bloodstream or inhibit activity of the vagus nerve and reduce activity of neurotransmitters in the brain, which then reduces the discharge of neurotransmitters. Afferent neurons contain ghrelin receptors. This may lead to the local release of ghrelin in the hypothalamus, which stimulates appetite by increasing activity of orexigenic neurons in the ACR. Ghrelin concentrations in the body appear to be inversely related with BMI and may be inadequately suppressed in obesity. Following a period of energy restriction or weight reduction, ghrelin levels will rise to stimulate appetite and assist the body in returning to its original weight. An exception to this relationship is observed with the sleeve gastrectomy, a bariatric surgical procedure that removes the fundus of the stomach and thus reduces ghrelin secretion.[34]

Anorexigenic Hormones

Leptin

Leptin is a hormone produced by white adipose tissue that relays the status of fat storage to the brain via the bloodstream and affects both energy intake and expenditure. Leptin inhibits appetite by decreasing the activity of orexigenic (NPY and AgRP) neurons and increasing the activity of the **anorexigenic** (POMC) neurons in the hypothalamus, leading to a loss of appetite; in a state of energy balance, leptin circulates at levels proportional to body fat. When an individual gains weight and adipose tissue increases, leptin levels will rise. Conversely, leptin will fall in a state of negative energy balance or weight loss. In individuals with obesity, there is suspected "leptin resistance," or impairment in the leptin signaling pathways that results in higher than expected leptin levels (for adipose tissue) and a reduced sense of satiety by the brain; this may lead to increased energy intake and weight gain. This concept is similar to that of insulin resistance observed in type 2 diabetes. When an individual with obesity attempts to lose weight and reduce adipose tissue, leptin levels will fall, although the body remains in a leptin-resistant state and will attempt to regain lost **adipose** or fat tissue over time. Impairments in this signaling pathway are partially responsible for why it is so difficult for many individuals with obesity to lose weight and keep it off.

The effects of white fat versus brown fat in the body is an ongoing and important area of obesity research. There is evidence to support that, in rodents, leptin increases energy expenditure through thermogenesis in brown adipose tissue due to increased sympathetic activation.[35] The loss of brown adipose tissue function in rodents is linked to metabolic dysfunction and obesity[36], and abnormalities in the sympathetic nervous system have been observed in leptin-deficient adults.[37] Much is still unknown about how brown adipose tissue behaves in adults; however, it is likely to play a major metabolic role in weight management.

Insulin

Insulin works in tandem with leptin and has an anorexigenic effect on the ACR in the hypothalamus. Insulin is produced and secreted by the beta cells of the pancreas in response to ingestion and breakdown of carbohydrate to glucose, and later absorption of glucose into the bloodstream. Insulin assists glucose into various cells in the body for energy, where it can be used or stored for later use. Individuals with obesity are at risk for insulin resistance, which occurs when cells such as those in muscle, fat, and the liver are no longer accepting glucose from the bloodstream. The beta cells in the pancreas continue to produce insulin to lower blood glucose levels and eventually are not able keep up with the body's demand, resulting in inflammation, development of type 2 diabetes, and other chronic health conditions.[38]

Islet Amyloid Polypeptide (Amylin)

Islet amyloid polypeptide or amylin is co-secreted with insulin by the beta cells of the pancreas and acts on receptors in the brain via the bloodstream. Amylin works to promote satiety by slowing gastric emptying, assisting with secretion of gastric acids, and preventing postprandial spikes in blood sugar. Amylin also enhances the effects of cholecystokinin.[39]

Cholecystokinin

Cholecystokinin (CCK) is secreted by cells in the intestine and stimulates bile production by the liver; influences release of bile from the gallbladder; stimulates release of enzyme from the pancreas; and, through the control of the gastric sphincter, decreases the rate of gastric emptying. CCK stimulates the vagus nerve, which affects the neurotransmitters in the brain and provides a message of satiety. CCK may also stimulate short-term satiety by influencing release of leptin.[40] When an individual with obesity attempts to lose weight, CCK levels will fall, resulting in decreased feelings of satiety.

Peptide YY (PYY)

Like CKK, peptide YY (PYY) acts as a satiety messenger and produces an anorexigenic effect via the ACR. It is stimulated by food entering in the gut; high-protein meals in particular may result in prolonged effects of PYY. PYY also delays gastric emptying and inhibits gastric acid secretion.[41] Levels of this hormone are decreased in obesity, leading to lower satiety.

Incretins (GLP-1 and GIP)

Glucagon-like peptide-1 (GLP-1) and glucose-dependent insulinotropic polypeptide (GIP) are two incretin hormones that are released by the intestine in response to carbohydrate and fat intake and stimulate release of insulin from the pancreatic beta cells. GLP-1 suppresses glucagon secretion from pancreatic alpha cells, which results in delaying gastric emptying and suppressing appetite, while GIP works with insulin to promote energy storage in adipose tissue. There is a decreased functionality of GLP-1 hormone resulting in a blunted effect on satiation.[42]

> **CORE CONCEPT 4**
>
> Body weight is regulated by metabolic, neuroendocrine, and autonomic systems in the body, including signals released from adipose, gastrointestinal and endocrine tissues that are integrated by the liver and central nervous system.

Alterations in Body Composition in Obesity

An individual's total body weight includes fat mass and fat-free mass (FFM). Fat mass includes fat from all the sources of the body, including adipose tissue, brain, and skeleton, while FFM is devoid of fat and includes water, protein, and mineral components. Individuals with obesity have a higher percentage of body fat compared with the normal-weight individual.[43]

Body fat is categorized as "essential" or "storage." Essential body fat is present in the nerve tissues, bone marrow, and organs, and is needed for normal physiological functioning. In men, 2% to 3% of body fat is considered essential compared to 5% to 12% for women, which is higher due to childbearing and hormonal functions. Lean body mass (LBM) is the FFM combined with the essential fat. Storage fat, or "nonessential" fat, represents an energy reserve in the subcutaneous adipose tissue or visceral fat. The optimal amount of total body fat, which includes essential plus storage fat, is 21% to 36% in females and 8% to 25% in males. These ranges vary depending on age and ethnicity.[44]

Adipocytes are connective tissue cells that can synthesize and store fat (**Figure 8.6**). The function of white adipocytes is to store energy, while the function of brown adipocytes is to dissipate energy in a heat-producing process called thermogenesis. Adipocytes play a role in maintaining proper energy balance by mobilizing sources of energy that are hormonally stimulated and storing calories in lipid form, as triacylglycerols. When fat stores are mobilized, non-esterified fatty acids are released into the bloodstream. Adipose tissue grows by two mechanisms: hyperplasia (cell number increase) and hypertrophy (cell size increase). Weight gain may result in hyperplasia, hypertrophy, or a combination. The enlargement of these adipocytes through increased fat storage may play a key role in weight gain in adults through the enlargement of the fat deposits. Genetics and diet may affect contributions of these two mechanisms to the growth of adipose tissue in obesity.[45] There has been evidence to support that adipocyte population growth starts at a young age; in people with early-onset obesity, this involves a more significant increase in adipocyte number, leading to a larger number of adipocytes when reaching adulthood. While the population of adipocytes increases throughout childhood and adolescence, it is tightly regulated during adulthood. Changes in fat mass in adults are likely the result of changes in adipocyte size as opposed to an increase in adipocyte number, and adipocyte populations are not influenced by energy balance.[46]

While total body fat is used to predict health risk, the distribution of fat in the body also plays a significant role.

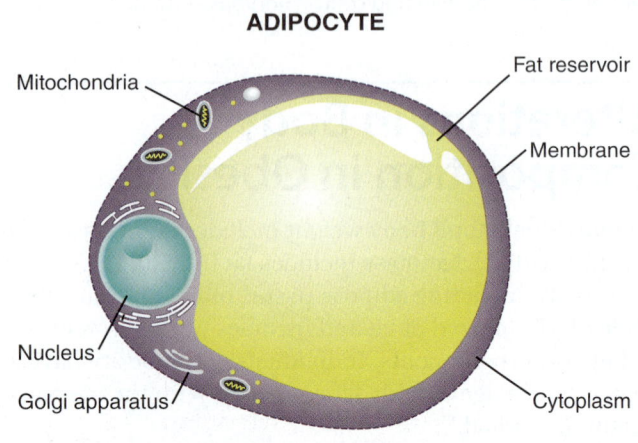

FIGURE 8.6 Adipocyte Structure

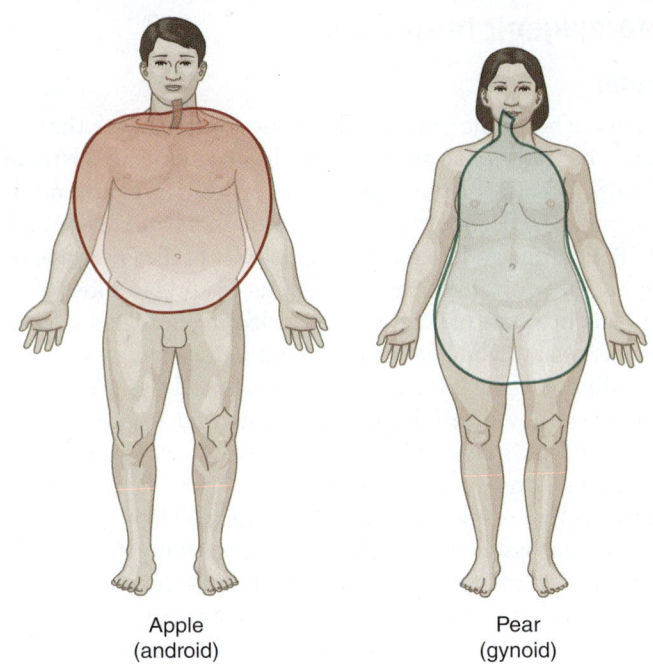

FIGURE 8.7 Apple versus Pear Body Shape

Higher waist circumference is associated with increased frequency of type 2 diabetes, dyslipidemia, hypertension, coronary heart disease, stroke, and early mortality.[4] An android distribution of fat (greater fat located around the abdomen, sometimes referred to as an "apple" figure) conveys greater risk of developing cardiovascular disease, hypertension, and type 2 diabetes. This type of fat distribution is more commonly seen in men. A gynecoid distribution of fat (greater fat located around the hips, also referred to as a "pear" figure) does not increase the risk of developing medical complications, and is more commonly seen among women (**Figure 8.7**).[4]

Nutrition Assessment in Obesity

A nutrition assessment completed by a registered dietitian nutritionist (RD or RDN) is a crucial component of the Nutrition Care Process and Model (NCPM) and the first step in evaluating a patient's current nutritional patterns and dietary history. The nutrition assessment is defined as a method for observing, obtaining, analyzing, and interpreting necessary data to identify nutrition-related problems and to develop a plan. Data are gathered from the medical record, patient/client interview, measurements, observation, and other healthcare providers involved in the patient's care. What follows are several areas for the dietitian to assess in order to evaluate for obesity and formulate an appropriate plan with the multidisciplinary team.

Anthropometric Assessment

Anthropometric assessment should include an accurate height and weight, BMI, waist-to-hip ratio and/or waist circumference, and body fat percentage if attainable.

Body Mass Index (BMI)
BMI is the most commonly used anthropometric measurement when assessing obesity status. As stated previously, a major limitation of BMI is that it fails to distinguish between lean and fat mass.[47] The current definition of obesity is based solely on body weight, although excess body fat has been linked with a variety of metabolic issues.[48] There have been numerous studies to measure the accuracy of BMI in determining body adiposity and metabolic risks, and the results significantly vary. Direct methods to accurately measure body fat such as dual energy x-ray absorptiometry, magnetic resonance imaging, and computed tomography analysis are rarely used in clinical practice due to high cost and impracticality. There are also indirect methods such as air-displacement plethysmography, bioelectrical impedance, hydrostatic weighing, skinfold thickness, waist circumference, and waist-to-hip ratio. Despite its limitations, BMI is used extensively in epidemiological studies and is incorporated regularly in clinical practice due to its practicality and simplicity. In addition to BMI, determination of individual energy needs through calculation of resting energy expenditure (REE) can help guide nutrition education.

Waist Circumference
Waist circumference should be measured annually in overweight and obese individuals.[3] Risk increases with a waist size that is greater than 35 inches for women or greater than 40 inches for men.

Waist-to-Hip Ratio
Waist-to-hip ratio is the comparison of waist circumference to that of the hips. There is evidence that shows increased health risk when the waist-to-hip ratio is above 1.0 for males and above 0.8 for females.[4] Data are lacking on appropriate cut-offs for waist-to-hip ratio for predicting risk of mortality in ethnic and population groups.[49]

Weight History
Weight history should include the highest and lowest adult weights, triggers, patterns of weight gain or loss throughout life, and family weight history.

Biochemical Assessment
Laboratory values are important to identify comorbidities related to lipid profile and hyperglycemia, as well as to evaluate for potential deficiencies, such as vitamin D, that are common with obesity.

Clinical Assessment
A clinical assessment is necessary in order to identify any medical or psychosocial issues, histories, or past or current therapies that may impact food and nutrient ingestion and absorption.

Medical and Psychosocial History
Medical and psychosocial history includes current and past medical conditions and obesity-related comorbidities, medications, past surgical history, and family medical history. For individuals who may qualify for weight loss surgery, a thorough evaluation by a mental health provider is required. Note that if a patient is in mental health treatment, asking permission from the patient to contact their provider may be of great value when considering medical nutrition therapy recommendations. Any history of eating disorders should be noted. A psychologist may evaluate history of binge eating, bulimia, or other specified feeding or eating disorders; current/past psychiatric diagnosis; alcohol/tobacco/drug use; self-care challenges; stress management; and coping mechanisms.

Nutrition-Focused Physical Exam
A nutrition-focused physical exam (NFPE) can also provide valuable information in obesity assessment by identifying fat, muscle, fluid, and micronutrient status as well as markers of inflammation, chronic disease, and nutrient deficiencies. An obesity-specific NFPE can include assessment of total and regional adiposity, hydration status, skin hyperpigmentation, numbness or tingling in extremities, and presence or absence of edema and/or wounds.

Dietary Assessment
Dietary assessment is important to identify nutrient intake, variety, and patterns in order to assess for inadequate, excessive, or imbalanced intake. It is possible for obese individuals to also be malnourished, so monitoring of both deficiencies and excesses is key.

Dietary History
A comprehensive nutrition evaluation for overweight and obesity should document previous weight loss attempts including medical programs, commercial programs, previous dietitian visits for weight loss, self-directed diets, weight loss medications, and weight loss surgery. Working with the patient to identify which method(s) were most effective may help to guide future recommendations for management.

Nutrition Patterns
Current intake (24-hour recall or food frequency questionnaire) of food/fluid, timing of meals and snacks, portion sizes, hunger and satiety levels, eating patterns, vitamin/mineral supplements, dietary supplements (i.e., protein supplements, fish oil, herbal supplements, etc.), and food allergies are important to assess and evaluate as a component of the comprehensive nutrition assessment.

Other Considerations
Physical Activity
Individuals should be evaluated for current activity level at work, time spent in sedentary activities, type and amount of time spent in planned activities, and barriers to activity. Address barriers that prevent exercise and determine which activities are most enjoyable. The goal of assessing physical activity is to determine activities of daily living, type and duration of structured exercise, and sedentary behaviors to aid the individual in creating realistic goals.

CASE STUDY REVISITED

Allison is eager to try to improve her weight and health through lifestyle management. She reports that she has a very sedentary lifestyle and spends most of her workdays at her desk. Her hobbies include reading and watching TV due to low energy and fatigue. You request more detailed information about her diet and she shares the following:

24-hour Diet Recall:
Breakfast (6 am): two 12-oz coffees with fat-free half and half and artificial sweetener
Lunch (11:30 am): Tuna sandwich on whole wheat bread, 2 cups strawberries, 1 can diet soda
Snack (3 pm): 1 cup grapes, 3 chocolate chip cookies, and a small coffee with half and half and artificial sweetener
Dinner at home (7 pm): Salad with romaine lettuce, carrots, tomatoes, and blue cheese salad dressing; baked chicken breast; 1 baked sweet potato with margarine and sour cream; water
Bedtime snack (10 pm): 6 crackers with peanut butter and 8 oz fat-free milk

Questions
1. What are Allison's energy needs?
2. What are your suggestions for Allison to address her diet? Her exercise regimen?
3. Given risk factors associated with obesity, what laboratories would you monitor?

Sleep Patterns

Hours of sleep, fatigue during the day, awakening at night, and symptoms of obstructive sleep apnea (OSA) may help to explain the sleep patterns of individuals. Assess whether the individual might be snoring, gasping for breath while sleeping, waking with a headache, or experiencing daytime somnolence, as these are possible symptoms of OSA. If the individual displays one of more of these symptoms, they may need referral to their primary care physician to assess for OSA.

Readiness/Motivation

Motivations/reasons for intervention; readiness to make behavioral changes; willingness to adhere to program; expected time, frequency, and duration of follow-up; and weight loss expectations should be included in the assessment.

Support System

The individual's support system, including friends, family, case workers, etc., and relationship to the individual should be evaluated. It is important to assess other individuals involved in the cooking, grocery shopping, and daily activities, because they may influence an individual's food choices or activity patterns.

Cultural and Socioeconomic Factors

Cultural factors include dietary restrictions, food/activity customs, and other cultural factors influencing eating behavior. Socioeconomic status and ability to purchase recommended foods and supplements should be evaluated.

Other

Assessment of obesity should also address any potential barriers to weight loss, including low literary skills, poor vision or hearing, language barriers, and/or learning disabilities.

> **PRACTICE POINT**
>
> The nutrition assessment of individuals with obesity should include collection of anthropometric measurements, past medical and psychosocial history, diet and weight history, nutrition, physical activity, sleep patterns, biochemical assessment, cultural factors, support systems, and readiness to change.

Assessment of Energy Requirement

Human energy requirements are estimated based on total energy expenditure (TEE), which is comprised of basal metabolic rate (BMR) or resting energy expenditure (REE), the thermic effect of food (TEF), and energy expended in physical activity.[50] BMR accounts for approximately 60% of TEE in sedentary individuals. This is the energy an individual expends at complete rest in the postabsorptive state measured in the morning and is highly predicted by lean body mass. TEF, or the energy required for digestion, absorption, and storage of food, accounts for approximately 10% of TEE. Lastly, energy expended by physical activity can be grouped into exercise-related activity and nonexercise-related activity thermogenesis (NEAT). Exercise-related activity ranges from 0% in sedentary individuals to about 10% of total energy expenditure in individuals who exercise regularly. NEAT accounts for activities of daily living (and other factors such as fidgeting and spontaneous muscle contraction) and the remainder of total energy expenditure.[50]

The different components of TEE can be measured through several methods, including direct and indirect calorimetry or through the use of validated predictive equations. Direct calorimetry techniques allow for direct determination of energy needs by measuring the rate of heat loss from an individual. Direct calorimetry has limited practical use due to extremely high cost and thus is generally only used in specialized research practice.

Indirect calorimetry methods involve measuring oxygen consumption and/or carbon dioxide production and using a formula to convert these measurements to energy expenditure. These methods include both stationary and portable systems with high levels of precision and pose moderate burden and cost to the individual. They are often performed with the use of an open-circuit system involving the use of hood, canopy, or mask-based equipment and yield accurate results with the use of standardized protocols and trained staff.[50]

The use of doubly labeled water (DLW) is considered the "gold standard" method of measuring energy expenditure in humans. In this method, an individual consumes an oral dose of water with a known amount of stable isotopes of hydrogen and oxygen. The isotopes mix with hydrogen and oxygen that are normally present in the body. When the body expends energy, carbon dioxide (CO_2) and water are produced and lost from the body. By measuring the difference in the rate of loss of the oxygen and hydrogen isotopes, the rate at which CO_2 is produced can be determined to estimate energy expenditure. To determine an even more reliable measure of energy expenditure, a ratio of CO_2 production to oxygen consumption (VO_2) can also be estimated using a variety of methods. The use of the DLW method to measure energy expenditure has shown usefulness in a variety of settings and individuals, including all age groups, hospitalized patients, obese individuals, and pregnant and lactating women. Despite the advantages to this method, the DLW method is also higher cost than many other methods of measuring energy expenditure.

There are also a number of questionnaire and physical activity recall methods that have been used to estimate energy expenditure in humans and have been validated against the DLW method. These methods include activity and recall questionnaires, the Baecke questionnaire, the Five-City questionnaire, and the Yale Physical Activity Survey.

Motion sensors, including basic pedometers and more highly advanced accelerometers, have also been tested as methods to estimate energy expenditure. In addition, there is a close relationship between energy expenditure and heart rate during physical activity, and thus measurements of heart rate have also been used to estimate energy expenditure. To account for the variation in fitness levels among individuals, simultaneous measurements of VO_2 must also be measured using indirect calorimetry. This type of measurement may have errors up to 30% in individuals, but for a group or population is likely to be within 10% of the true value.[51]

The most practical way to estimate RMR in the clinical setting is through the use of predictive equations using anthropometric data. These equations were developed from both indirect and direct calorimetry measures, although they still have varying margins of error. Of the most commonly used equations (Mifflin–St. Jeor, Harris–Benedict, Cunningham, Owen, and World Health Organization/Food and Agriculture Organization/United Nations University [WHO/FAO/UNU]), the Mifflin–St. Jeor has the least margin of error and is believed to estimate RMR within as little as 10% of normal-weight individuals and those with obesity.[52,53] Because there is no direct measurement of body stores, there are limitations when generalized to certain age and ethnic groups. In some cases, indirect calorimetry may be a more appropriate measure when the clinician deems that a predictive method fails in a clinically relevant way. The Mifflin–St. Jeor is the preferred equation to predict RMR for healthy individuals (Table 8.3); other equations may be more appropriate for various disease states.[52]

TABLE 8.3 ASSESSMENT OF RESTING ENERGY EXPENDITURE (REE)

Use the **Mifflin–St. Jeor** equation to estimate REE (kcal/day):
Women: RMR = (9.99 × actual weight) + (6.25 × height) − (4.92 × age) − 161
Men: RMR = (9.99 × actual weight) + (6.25 × height) − (4.92 × age) + 5
TEE = REE × AF (study or population-specific activity fact)
Multiply the REE by an activity factor of 1.3 for sedentary individuals.

> **PRACTICE POINT**
>
> The Mifflin–St. Jeor is the best predictive equation for estimating energy needs for healthy individuals and individuals with obesity.

Pathophysiology Associated with Obesity

Obesity meets standards of a medical disease, including a known etiology, recognized signs and symptoms, and a range of structural and functional changes that culminate in pathologic consequences. Excess adipose tissue produces excess free fatty acids, tumor necrosis factor-alpha (TNF-α), interleukin-6 (IL-6), leptin, and plasminogen activator inhibitor-1. This production is associated with hyperinsulinemia, hyperglycemia, insulin resistance, development of diabetes, endothelial damage, and the onset and progression of atherosclerotic lesions.[54]

Weight-Related Comorbidities

Obesity increases the risk of several conditions, including cardiovascular disease, type 2 diabetes, coronary heart disease, obstructive sleep apnea (OSA), gastroesophageal reflux disease (GERD), hypertension (HTN), arthritis, and certain cancers, among others (Figure 8.8).

Cardiovascular System

Obesity is strongly associated with HTN and cardiovascular conditions such as coronary heart disease, heart failure, atrial fibrillation, and sudden cardiac death.[55] Obesity-related HTN is caused by activation of the sympathetic nervous system and activation of the

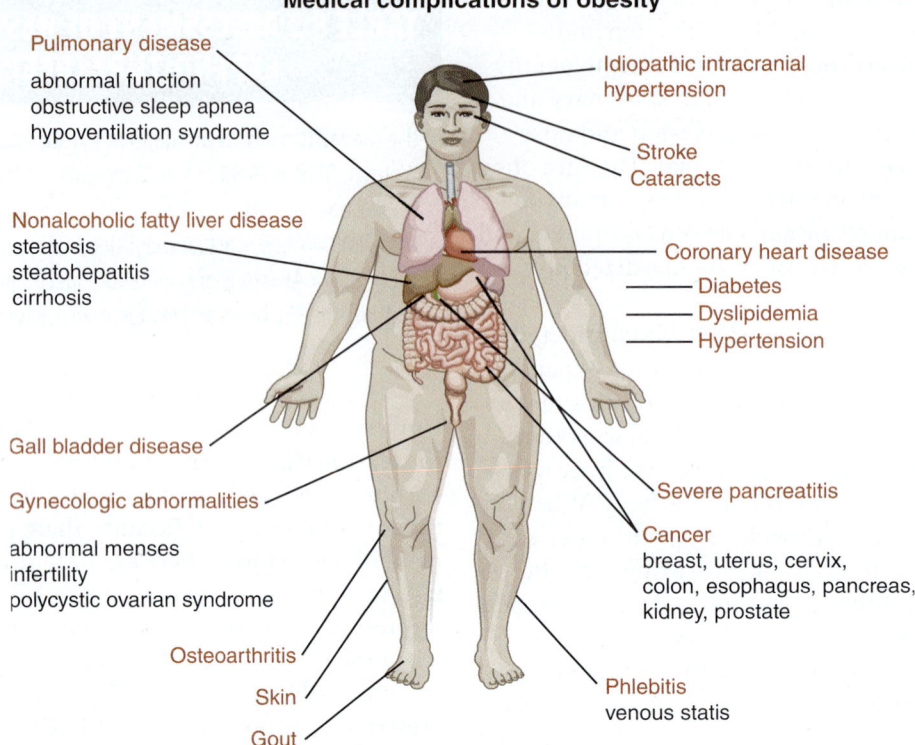

FIGURE 8.8 Medical Complications of Obesity

renin-angiotensin system, among other irregularities. Other factors considered to affect obesity-related HTN are hyperinsulinemia, structural changes in the kidney, and various adipokines (hormones) such as leptin.[56] These factors may contribute to sodium reabsorption and fluid retention contributing to HTN. Numerous studies suggest that obesity-related HTN is associated with an increased risk of renal insufficiency.[57]

Obesity may impact cardiovascular disease through its effect on its risk factors such as HTN, inflammatory markers, glucose intolerance, dyslipidemia, and other factors.[58] Increased levels of C-reactive protein (CRP) and leptin are associated with cardiovascular events.[59] In addition, several variations in cardiac function and structure may occur with excess adipose tissue, and individuals with obesity have higher cardiac workload and cardiac output.[60] Although obesity is associated with cardiovascular diseases, it is well documented that individuals with obesity who have heart disease have improved prognosis when compared to lean or underweight individuals.[55]

Metabolic/Endocrine System

Type 2 Diabetes Mellitus

Currently 11% of Americans (approximately 29 million people) are living with type 2 diabetes, an estimate that is up from 8.3% a few years ago. By 2050, diabetes prevalence is predicted to rise to 21%.[61] Type 2 diabetes accounts for 90% to 95% of all diabetes diagnoses in the United States.[62] The precursor to type 2 diabetes is insulin resistance, which results from gradual dysfunction of pancreatic islet beta-cells and the inability to effectively move glucose out of the bloodstream into various cells in the body. This eventually leads to low beta cell mass, impaired incretin response, and inadequate suppression of glucagon production. The lack of glucagon suppression leads to inadequate uptake, storage, and clearance of glucose, which is accompanied by elevated production of glucose by the liver and significant hyperglycemia. Once the body is no longer able to properly manage blood glucose levels effectively, type 2 diabetes results and can progress to an insulin-dependent state if not effectively treated.

Factors contributing to type 2 diabetes are both environmental and genetic. While the relationship of insulin resistance and pancreatic cell dysfunction is believed to be important in the development and progression of type 2 diabetes, the precise mechanisms are unclear. Adipose tissue likely plays an important role in the development of type 2 diabetes given that the majority of individuals with type 2 diabetes have excess central visceral (intra-abdominal) adiposity. Although corporal adipose tissue is associated with increased risk of type 2 diabetes, it is generally held that an accumulation of central visceral fat is an independent risk for type 2 diabetes, despite the level of obesity. Because not all obese individuals develop hyperglycemia, an underlying abnormality of the beta cell must coexist with excess adipose tissue to promote type 2 diabetes.[63]

Pro-inflammatory molecules produced by adipose tissue have been associated with the development of metabolic disease such as type 2 diabetes.[64] Excess adipose tissue releases higher amounts of glycerol, nonesterified fatty acids, hormones, pro-inflammatory cytokines, and other factors that are involved with the development of insulin resistance. Chronic increase in fatty acids reduces the usage of glucose as a source of energy, and also impairs beta cell function, acting in conjunction with insulin resistance to worsen hyperglycemia. Moderate weight reduction (7%-10%) can improve glycemic control and reduce diabetes risk.

Metabolic syndrome is a term used to define a combination of cardiovascular risk factors that may be present in individuals with obesity. These include dyslipidemia, hypertension, insulin resistance, abdominal adiposity, and a pro-inflammatory and prothrombotic state. Diagnostic criteria for metabolic syndrome differ by organization (Adult Treatment Panel III[65], WHO, American Association of Clinical Endocrinologists) due to differences among human populations, although the most common measures are included in Table 8.4. A diagnosis of metabolic syndrome is made when an individual exhibits three of the five qualifying characteristics.[66] Research suggests that there is strong evidence to support an association between metabolic syndrome and increased risk of developing type 2 diabetes and cardiovascular disease, so it should be monitored and treated appropriately.[3] While not used as diagnostic criteria, elevations in the pro-inflammatory marker CRP may be strong predictors of future cardiovascular disease events with or without a firm diagnosis of metabolic syndrome.[67]

Gastrointestinal System

Gastroesophageal Reflux Disease

Obesity has known effects on the gastrointestinal system and is associated with increased gastroesophageal reflux disease (GERD). GERD symptoms increase in severity with weight gain. Obesity is a risk factor for more serious conditions, including development of Barrett's esophagus and adenocarcinoma of the esophagus.[68] Research suggests that an increase in BMI is associated with increased acid exposure from the esophagus.[69] There are several mechanisms by which obesity may contribute to GERD, although the exact relationship is not clearly defined. One commonly described pathway is increased abdominal pressure associated with a higher waist circumference, which may cause the lower esophageal sphincter to relax and allow acidic gastric contents to come in contact with the esophageal mucosa. In addition to the suspected mechanical relationship, adipocytokines that are released from visceral fat, including IL-6 and TNF-α, may increase symptoms from GERD and play a role in consequent carcinogenesis.[70] Research suggests that weight loss decreases symptoms of GERD, though once erosions are present, it is unclear whether weight reduction would have beneficial effects. Improvement in GERD symptoms has been also observed in individuals following Roux-en-Y gastric bypass (RYGB) surgery with near-complete cessation of acid production.[68]

Steatohepatitis

Overweight and obesity is implicated as a primary cause in the development of nonalcoholic fatty liver disease (NAFLD), which describes a form of steatohepatitis in which excess fat builds up in the liver unrelated to alcohol consumption.[71] Liver cells, or hepatocytes, generally only contain small amounts of storage lipids. In NAFLD, these cells contain greater than normal amounts of triglycerides. Some individuals with NAFLD have liver cell injury and inflammation in addition to excessive fat, causing a more severe condition termed nonalcoholic steatohepatitis (NASH). NAFLD does not lead to increased short-term mortality or morbidity, although progression to NASH dramatically increases risk of cirrhosis, liver failure, and hepatocellular carcinoma (HCC).[72] The reported rates of disease progression from NAFLD to NASH and ultimately to cirrhosis, liver failure, and HCC vary greatly depending on disease definitions, populations studied, and the diagnostic methods used. Global guidelines from the World Gastroenterology Organization indicate that the prevalence of disease progression from NAFLD to NASH in the general population is 10% to 20%, while it is as high as 37% in high-risk individuals with higher classes of obesity.

The pathogenesis of NAFLD is not entirely understood and currently there are no evidence-based clinical therapeutic guidelines due to the lack of adequate prospective, double-blind controlled trials in this field.[72] Experts agree that NAFLD begins with overnutrition due to energy input that exceeds output mediated by important genetic and environmental factors. In particular, central obesity, glucose intolerance, type 2 diabetes, dyslipidemia, hypertension, and other features of metabolic syndrome are associated with NAFLD. Insulin resistance, oxidative stress, and cytokines are considered important contributing factors to

TABLE 8.4 ATP III CLINICAL IDENTIFICATION OF METABOLIC SYNDROME

Risk Factor Criteria	Level
Waist circumference: Men	≥102 cm (≥40 in)
Waist circumference: Women	≥88 cm (≥35 in)
HDL-C: Men	<40 mg/dL
HDL-C: Women	<50 mg/dL
Triglyceride	≥150 mg/dL
Blood pressure	≥130/85 mm Hg
Fasting blood sugar	≥110 mg/dL

Data from Om Murti Anil, Kathmandu, Nepal. http://www.jcpcarchives.org/userfiles/table-2-atp.jpg.

the pathogenesis of NAFLD.[71] These factors contribute to a pro-inflammatory cascade in the body that is mediated by various proteins and immune factors hypothesized to contribute to the development of NAFLD/NASH. States of hyperinsulinemia and hyperglycemia drive hepatic lipogenesis, which may cause insulin resistance in peripheral sites such as muscle and adipose tissue. This progression is mediated by inflammatory factors like TNF-α and IL-6, which also may arise from stressed and inflamed adipose tissue. Once insulin resistance is systemic, free fatty acids released from adipose tissue circulate continuously and likely cause the hepatic lipid accumulation and injury (lipotoxicity). Genetic factors that drive consumption of calorie-dense foods and those that affect lipid storage are likely to also play an important role in NAFLD/NASH pathogenesis. It is difficult to determine the relationship between steatosis and insulin resistance because both states can potentiate the other, and which arises first remains unclear.

Immune System

Cancer

Overweight and obesity are estimated to cause approximately 20% of all cancer cases.[73] A comprehensive systematic review of the evidence by the World Cancer Research Fund and American Institute for Cancer Research concluded that obesity is an established risk factor for several cancers, including those of the esophagus, pancreas, colon and rectum, endometrium, kidney, postmenopausal breast, and gallbladder.[74] The American Cancer Society also suggests that overweight and obesity are associated with increased mortality from liver cancer, pancreatic cancer, non-Hodgkin's lymphoma, and myeloma.[75] The mechanisms by which obesity increases cancer risk are still not fully understand and vary by type of cancer. Mechanisms that have been studied include the modulation of energy balance and calorie restriction, growth factors, multiple signaling pathways, and inflammatory processes that modulate cancer cell growth.[76]

Obesity and metabolic syndrome are associated with chronic low-grade inflammation, which is thought to be an important link between obesity and cancer. Individuals with a higher BMI show an elevated CRP level, which is a marker of inflammation and may be correlated with increased cancer risk.[77] Adipocytes release inflammatory markers that have been associated with poor prognosis from cancer.[73] Fat tissue also produces and releases hormones; adipokines; and cytokines such as leptin, adiponectin, TNF-α, and IL-6 that may play a role in cancer development. Leptin has been studied as a mediator in cancer development via its role in increasing inflammatory pathways, while adiponectin may have anticancer effects through decreasing inflammatory actions within the body.[76] Insulin and insulin-like growth factor-1 (IGF-1) may also be important factors contributing to cancer development. Observational studies have linked increased cancer mortality with type 2 diabetes and obesity, which may be due to increased insulin and/or elevated IGF-1 in these individuals.[78] Understanding the pathways that may link obesity with increased cancer risk is helpful in determining therapeutic targets; however, preventing overweight and obesity remains the number one priority.

Musculoskeletal System

Osteoarthritis

Obesity is associated with a number of musculoskeletal conditions, including osteoarthritis (OA), low back pain, diffuse idiopathic skeletal hyperostosis, gait disturbance, fibromyalgia, rheumatoid arthritis, osteoporosis, gout, and soft tissue conditions such as plantar fasciitis.[79] These conditions can lead to physical consequences including chronic pain, disability, and impaired quality of life, as well as the societal burden of increasing direct and indirect healthcare costs. According to the CDC, 31% of obese adults have arthritis compared to 16% of nonobese adults.[80] Researchers are beginning to identify potential mechanisms by which obesity increases musculoskeletal conditions, particularly for osteoarthritis. Studies suggest that weight loss is important for preventing and managing knee osteoarthritis because individuals with obesity and knee OA have elevated cartilage turnover biomarkers. Inflammatory cytokines released from adipose tissue may also play a role in the development of musculoskeletal conditions.[81] Other studies have shown that bariatric surgery reduces symptoms of OA and reduces pain in the spine, knee, and foot, though more research is needed in this area.[82]

Respiratory System

Obstructive Sleep Apnea

Obstructive sleep apnea (OSA) is a medical condition characterized by ongoing episodes of complete obstruction (apnea) or partial obstruction (hypopnea) of the upper airway. OSA leads to poor sleep and intermittent hypoxia during sleep.[83] It is estimated that 50% to 60% of individuals with obesity and metabolic syndrome have OSA.[84] Recent studies showed that individuals with OSA were 6 to 9 times more likely to have metabolic syndrome compared to subjects without OSA. Obesity is a significant risk factor for OSA as it may be associated with enlargement of soft tissue structures within and around the airway, resulting in pharyngeal airway narrowing. In addition, increased abdominal adipose tissue and recumbent posture may reduce lung volume. This can narrow the airway due to the decrease in pharyngeal wall tension and longitudinal tracheal traction forces.[85] There is evidence that markers of cardiovascular risk, such as systemic inflammation, sympathetic activation, and endothelial dysfunction, are increased in individuals with obesity with OSA compared to those with obesity without OSA. OSA may contribute to the pathogenesis of hypertension, CRP, and inflammation. Individuals with OSA have increased risk of hypertension, dysrhythmias, myocardial infarction, stroke, pulmonary hypertension, heart failure, and overall mortality.[86]

Continuous positive airway pressure treatment can undo pathophysiological changes associated with OSA, including lowering blood pressure and increasing insulin sensitivity. Modest weight loss will improve OSA as well as metabolic and cardiovascular risk.

Obesity Management

Successful weight management requires a lifelong commitment to healthy lifestyle behaviors, including sustainable eating patterns and daily physical activity.[87] Realistic weight loss goals should be set by the individual; sustained weight loss of even 3% to 5% is likely to lead to clinically significant health improvements, including reductions in triglycerides, blood glucose, HbA1c, and the risk of developing type 2 diabetes. Greater health improvements are seen as weight loss increases.[3]

Comprehensive Lifestyle Intervention

A widely recommended method for facilitating weight loss is through a comprehensive lifestyle program that includes diet, physical activity, and behavior modification lasting at least 6 months (**Figure 8.9**).[3] Individuals who enter a comprehensive lifestyle program should be ready to commit to behavioral changes such as monitoring food intake and physical activity, be free of any untreated major depressive symptoms, and enter at a stable juncture in their lives.[88] Intensive Behavior Programs (IBT), which include 14 or more sessions lead by a trained interventionist such as a dietitian, are often most effective.[3] Programs may be conducted in an individual or group setting, and in person or remotely (via Internet or phone). In some cases, electronic programs prove to be more convenient for the individual or the provider due to timing or location, although they may result in smaller weight loss than face-to-face programs (5-kg versus 8-kg weight loss at 6 months).[3]

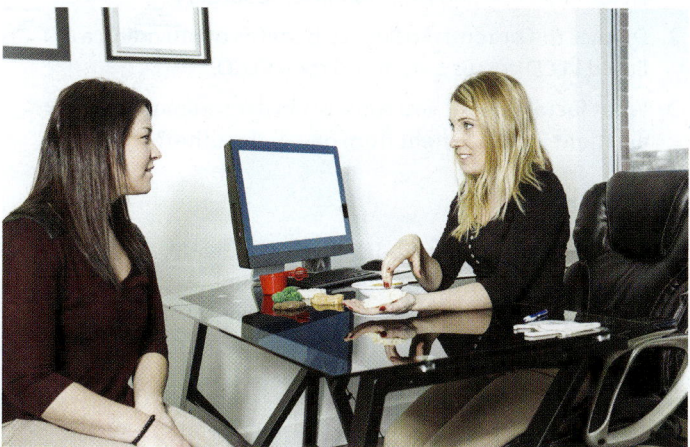

FIGURE 8.9 **Comprehensive Lifestyle Interventions Facilitated by a Dietitian Can Promote Weight Loss**

© Lopolo/Shutterstock.

Dietary

Nutrition prescriptions in a comprehensive lifestyle program should focus first on calorie reduction (versus macronutrient content, processing of foods, etc.), as this will initiate the greatest amount of weight change. This includes specific calorie prescriptions (usually 1,200 to 1,500 kcal/day for women and 1,500 to 1,800 kcal/day for men, adjusted based on body weight and physical activity), or a standard caloric reduction (500 to 1000 calories) taken from an individual's estimated energy needs using predictive equations.[3] A number of diets that restrict certain types of food or nutrients have been approved for weight loss when used in the setting of calorie reduction. These include the high-protein diet, low-fat and low carbohydrate diets, the DASH diet, and the Mediterranean-style diet, among others. Foods consumed on these diets are typically low in energy density (e.g., fruits, vegetables, whole grains, and lean protein) and aim to support an estimated weight loss of about 1 to 2 lb/week.[87] Federal guidelines further encourage balanced macronutrient intake for optimal health (<30% fat, <7% saturated fat, 15% protein, and the remainder from carbohydrate) and should be considered when formulating dietary prescriptions for an individual.

Within a reduced-calorie plan, few studies have examined the impact of specific dietary patterns on weight loss. The use of single-serve, portion-controlled meals; reduction in sugar sweetened–beverage intake; and consumption of more calories earlier in the day instead of at night may suggest a positive association with weight loss and should be discussed with the individual as part of a reduced-calorie eating plan.[89] While often encouraged, there is limited evidence to support that the sole consumption of breakfast and/or fruits and vegetables (specifically), reduction of fast-food intake, or increase in eating frequency will result in significant weight loss.[89] These patterns, combined with additional efforts aimed at weight loss (i.e., calorie reduction, behavioral changes, and physical activity), may have a cumulative positive effect. Further research is needed in these areas to determine the optimal dietary pattern for weight loss. Ultimately, the best prescription for the individual is one that is realistic and sustainable for their lifestyle.

Individuals looking for a more structured and specific meal prescription may benefit from the use of meal replacements. Meal replacements are typically defined as portion-controlled, vitamin and mineral–fortified entrees, shakes, and bars, and they provide an easy tool to reduce calories, manage portions, and simplify meal preparation (**Figure 8.10**). Research has shown that the use of meal replacements leads to greater weight loss than a prescribed diet with the same number of calories where individuals are left to select their own foods.[12] Meal replacements are often used as part of Low Calorie Diet (LCD) and Very Low Calorie Diet (VLCD) eating plans that prescribe very specific food choices and calorie levels. A LCD usually consists of 800 to 1600 calories per day and may offer a partial or full meal replacement plan, while a VLCD consists of <800 calories per day and usually consists of liquid shakes only.[89] Given

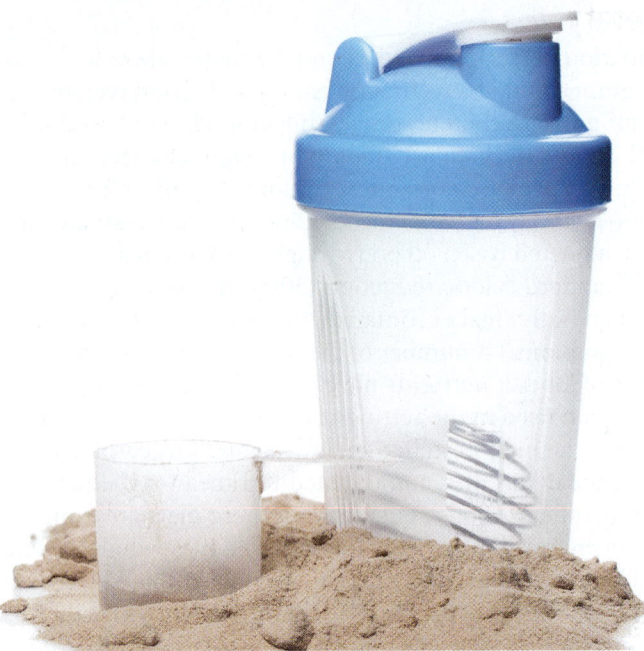

FIGURE 8.10 Meal Replacement Plans Often Include Protein Shakes
© Blackday/Shutterstock.

the aggressive calorie reduction of a VLCD plan, it is recommended only in limited circumstances and when delivered by a trained individual, because regular medical monitoring is required. This is due to rapid weight loss and the potential for health complications.[3] A VLCD will produce the greatest amount of weight loss, but research from randomized controlled trials (RCTs) suggests that both LCD and VLCD plans result in similar weight loss at 1 year later.[88,89]

Behavior

Behavior modification interventions should focus on habits that will encourage weight loss, including self-monitoring of food intake (paper or electronic records), physical activity (such as activity meters, step counters) and weight; goal setting and stress reduction techniques; stimulus control; and sustainable approaches to problem solving via cognitive restructuring. Self-monitoring in the form of food journals or records, for example, is associated with greater weight loss when compared to no self-monitoring.[90] Many new tools have emerged in recent years to track intake and physical activity, including online programs that allow individuals to search specific foods and track total calorie and nutrient intake. These programs have many advantages, although individuals should be aware that many programs have user-entered data that may not be entirely accurate regarding nutrient profiles.

Cognitive approaches involved in behavior change focus on building skills and habits that will promote long-term weight maintenance. Cognitive behavior therapy aims to help individuals examine the role that their thought process plays in behavior and can help to identify cognitive distortions such as "all-or-nothing thinking," which are commonly observed in humans and in weight-loss therapy.[91] Use of motivational interviewing techniques by the provider encourages collaboration with the individual rather than control and aims to enhance motivation and self-efficacy to ultimately drive behavior change.[89] Current research suggests that no one behavior change strategy is best for weight loss and that a combination can be used in effective treatment.[89]

Behavior interventions can be offered in a variety of settings, including clinical, community, commercial, and

⚠ Clinical Controversy

Methods of Weight Loss Before Bariatric Surgery

Patients undergoing bariatric surgery are often encouraged to lose weight prior to their procedure to help improve surgical outcomes such as operating times, re-operation rate, risk of infection, and overall safety for the patient. There is evidence to suggest that following a VLCD preoperatively can help to achieve this weight loss. There is much debate about what type of VLCD is best for the patient: liquid high-protein meal replacement shakes or a standard food diet. One group of researchers found that patients following a VLCD liquid diet preoperatively demonstrated greater weight loss and reduction in duration of surgical time. Conversely, in another study, it was demonstrated that patients following liquid diets and patients following standard food diets were both able to achieve comparable preoperative weight loss, although acceptance and tolerance of the standard food diet was better.

Questions

1. Based upon the two studies referenced, how might you apply evidence-based findings when recommending a weight loss method prior to bariatric surgery?
2. Discuss the potential risks and benefits of providing a liquid VLCD versus a standard food VLCD.
3. What factors might you consider in determining whether a patient would benefit from one or the other?

References

1. Faria SL, Faria OP, Almeida de Almeida Cardeal M, Ito MK. Effects of a very low calorie diet in the preoperative stage of bariatric surgery: a randomized trial. *Surg Obes Relat Dis*. 2015;11:230-237.
2. Schouten R, van der Kaaden I, van 't Hof G, Feskens PG. Comparison of preoperative diets before bariatric surgery: a randomized, single blinded, non-inferiority trial. *Obes Surg*. 2016: 26:1743-1749.

electronic. IBT programs are often offered in the academic and clinic settings and involve a medical team consisting of a physician, physician's assistant, behavioral provider, and RDN. While these programs can be very effective (i.e., Diabetes Prevention Program [DPP]), they may also be expensive and difficult for some individuals to access.[92] In one study where a version of the DPP was adopted at a YMCA community setting, participants lost 6% of their starting weight, compared to 2% in the control group, and paid a fraction of the cost of an IBT program.[92] Commercial weight loss programs such as Weight Watchers, Jenny Craig, and Nutrisystem are widely available and utilize a variety of behavior strategies such as prepackaged meals, dietary counseling, and group support self-monitoring. Emerging evidence also supports the use of electronically delivered interventions (such as telephone- or Internet-based) when in-person visits are not possible. These types of programs have been shown to be effective for weight loss, although the loss is less than that seen with in-person visits.[3]

Physical Activity

Regular physical activity can help individuals lose weight, maintain weight loss, and prevent weight regain after weight loss (**Figure 8.11**). Research suggests that caloric restriction is more effective at achieving weight loss than physical activity on its own, although increasing physical activity is an important part of weight management, and weight maintenance in particular.[12] When prescribed adjunct to a reduced calorie diet, exercise may result in an additional 1% to 3% of weight loss.[61] Individuals should be encouraged to participate in at least 150 minutes of moderately intense physical activity (e.g., walking) per week, with an additional 2 days of strength training to achieve health benefits and prevent weight gain.[93] More clinically significant weight loss is seen in individuals with overweight and obesity when a level of >250 minutes per week is achieved.[94] Individuals who are sedentary should be instructed to increase their physical activity gradually and begin with short episodes of activity.

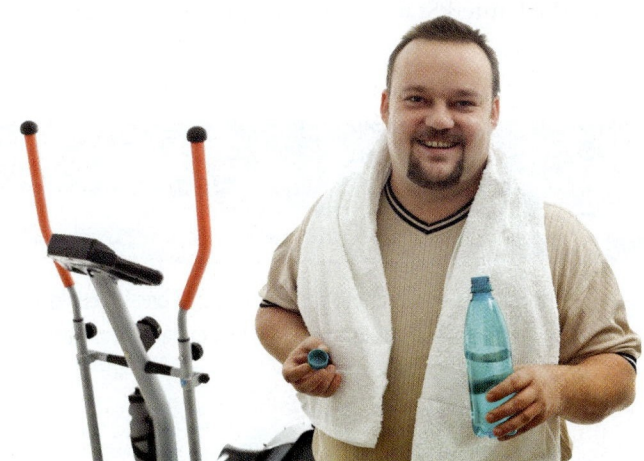

FIGURE 8.11 Regular Physical Activity Can Help Individuals Lose Weight, Maintain Weight Loss, and Prevent Weight Regain

© Nagy-Bagoly Arpa/Shutterstock.

Weight Maintenance

Results from the largest U.S. weight loss study (Look AHEAD study) show successful long-term weight loss maintenance following an intensive lifestyle intervention (>1 year comprehensive program).[95] This study, published in January 2014, found that participants in the lifestyle intervention program maintained more than half of their weight loss after 8 years and almost 40% of those who lost ≥10% of initial weight after the first year maintained the loss by the 8th year. This study shows meaningful results given its long duration and high retention rate, and participants likely achieved positive outcomes due to the intensive and comprehensive nature of the intervention.

Experts have proposed several recommendations for long-term weight loss maintenance. These include regular follow-up contact every other week (or monthly if biweekly is not possible) for 1 year with a trained interventionist (such as a dietitian) in either a group or individual setting.[12] Individuals should follow a reduced-calorie diet necessary to maintain their lower body weight. Physical activity, as mentioned previously, is also an essential component of long-term weight management. Individuals should be instructed to participate in 200 to 300 minutes per week of moderately vigorous aerobic activity. Occasional use of food records and/or activity monitoring tools may be beneficial. In addition, individuals should weigh themselves twice per week or daily and participate in a behavior change program that provides feedback on relapse prevention and problem solving.[12]

> **PRACTICE POINT**
>
> For health benefits, individuals should participate in at least 150 minutes per week of moderately vigorous physical activity with additional recommended strength training. For weight loss and maintenance, individuals should be instructed to participate in 200 to 300 minutes per week of moderately vigorous aerobic activity.

> **PRACTICE POINT**
>
> When creating a lifestyle program for weight management, aim for 14 or more sessions over a 6-month period led by a trained interventionist, such as a dietitian.

Pharmacotherapy

The use of medications to assist in weight loss is appropriate for those with a BMI ≥30 kg/m^2 or those with a BMI ≥27 kg/m^2 with a comorbid condition such as hypertension or type 2 diabetes (**Figure 8.12**). Any individual being treated with medications for weight loss should also participate in lifestyle modification through diet and exercise.[3] The FDA approved two new drugs for the treatment of obesity in 2012, lorcaserin and phentermine/topiramate, which were the first drugs approved for long-term weight management in 13 years.[96] Several other medications have been approved by the FDA for weight loss. Physicians may also prescribe medications, such as metformin, that result in weight loss as a side effect. The

CASE STUDY REVISITED

Allison has participated in a behavioral program for 6 months and this lifestyle intervention has not produced significant weight loss results.

Anthropometric Data:
Weight: 94 kg (207 lbs)
Height: 152 cm (62")
BMI: 38 kg/m^2

Biochemical Data:
Fasting blood glucose 152 (70-99 mg/dL)
Hemoglobin A1c 7.9% (4.3-5.8%)

Questions
1. What pharmacological approaches are available to Allison?
2. What are the advantages and disadvantages of these interventions?

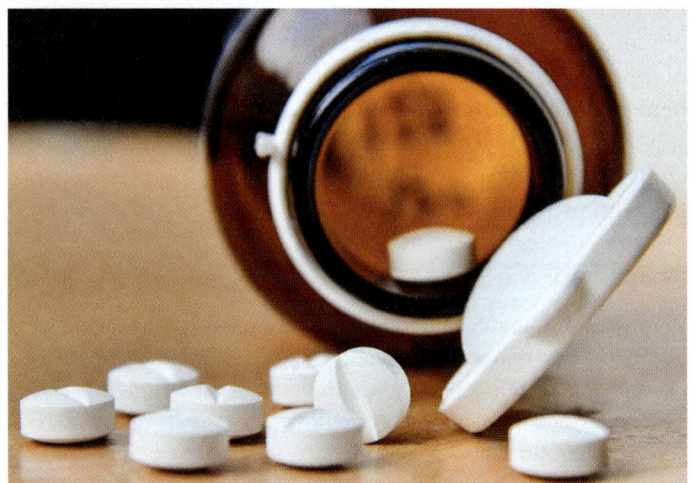

FIGURE 8.12 Pharmacotherapy for Weight Loss Can Be Used for Individuals with a BMI ≥30 or Those with a BMI ≥27 with a Comorbid Condition
©JJ IMAGE/Shutterstock.

use of medications in this way is deemed "off label" use. If a medication is effective, it is recommended for long-term use under medical supervision. A list of commonly prescribed weight loss medications (FDA approved and off label) are described in the **Table 8.5**.

> **CORE CONCEPT 5**
>
> Approaches to obesity management include individual and comprehensive lifestyle intervention, pharmacotherapy, and bariatric surgery.

Bariatric Surgery

This rise in individuals with obesity has led to an increased number of bariatric surgical procedures over the years. Close to half a million **bariatric surgery**, or weight loss surgery, operations were performed in 2013 worldwide; in the United States and Canada, 154,276 were

TABLE 8.5 FDA-APPROVED WEIGHT LOSS MEDICATIONS

Medication Name	Brand Name	Mechanism of Action	Contraindications
Phentermine	Adipex	Releases norepinephrine	Heart disease, uncontrolled HTN, pregnancy, breastfeeding, hyperthyroidism, drug abuse, use of monoamine oxidase inhibitors (MAOIs)
Diethylproprion	Tenuate	Releases norepinephrine	Same as phentermine
Phendimetrazine	Bontril	Releases norepinephrine	Same as phentermine

(continues)

TABLE 8.5 FDA-APPROVED WEIGHT LOSS MEDICATIONS (Continued)

Medication Name	Brand Name	Mechanism of Action	Contraindications
Benzphentamine	Didrex	Releases norepinephrine	Same as phentermine
Orlistat	Alli, Xenical	Inhibits pancreatic and gastric lipases	Pregnancy, breastfeeding, use of levothyroxine or warfarin, malabsorption syndrome, use of seizure drugs
Laceserin	Belviq	Activates serotonin receptor	Pregnancy, breastfeeding
Phentermine/Topiramate ER	Qsymia	Releases norepinephrine, modulates gamma-aminobutyric acid	Pregnancy, breastfeeding, hyperthyroidism, use of MAOIs, glaucoma
Naltrexone/bupropion (Contrave)	Contrave	Opioid antagonist; inhibits dopamine and norepinephrine uptake	Uncontrolled HTN, seizures, use of MAOIs, anorexia, bulimia, opioid/alcohol use
Liraglutide	Saxenda	Activates GLP-1	Medullary thyroid carcinoma history, multiple endocrine neoplasia type 2 history, pancreatitis history

Reproduced with permission of the American Association of Diabetes Educators. All rights reserved. May not be reproduced or distributed without the written approval of AADE.

CASE STUDY REVISITED

One year later, Allison is seeking the most effective intervention to improve her type 2 diabetes and does not want to take a medication for the rest of her life. Meal replacement and very low calorie diets have not yielded weight loss results, but rather Allison has continued to gain weight. After evaluation by a dietitian, physician, and psychologist, the multidisciplinary team recommends surgery for Allison as the best approach given her high BMI, comorbid conditions, and past failed weight loss attempts. She is referred for a surgical evaluation.

Anthropometric Data:
Weight: 104.5 kg (230 lbs)
Height: 152 cm (62 in)
BMI: 42 kg/m^2

Biochemical Data:
Fasting blood glucose 165 (70-99 mg/dL)
Hemoglobin A1C 9.4% (4.3-5.8%)

Clinical Data:
Allison has newly diagnosed obstructive sleep apnea.

Questions
1. What are Allison's options at this point?
2. How does Allison's anthropometric, clinical, and biochemical data guide this decision?
3. What are advantages and disadvantages of bariatric surgery?
4. Which surgery would have the greatest likelihood in improving Allison's type 2 diabetes?

performed.[97] The National Institutes of Health Consensus Development Conference on Gastrointestinal Surgery for Severe Obesity recommended that obesity surgery be considered for those with a BMI >35 kg/m² with significant comorbidities or for individuals with a BMI >40 kg/m² with or without comorbidities (Table 8.6).[98] Bariatric surgery is widely considered the most effective long-term treatment for obesity.

Procedure Type

There are several types of bariatric surgery procedures that support weight loss and work through different mechanisms. These include restrictive, malabsorptive, or both restrictive and malabsorptive procedures.

1. Restrictive procedures
   - **Laparoscopic adjustable gastric band (LAGB)**

TABLE 8.6 INCLUSION AND EXCLUSION CRITERIA FOR CONSIDERATION OF BARIATRIC SURGERY

Inclusion Criteria
- Body mass index ≥40 kg/m² or ≥35 kg/m² with comorbid conditions (HTN, type 2 diabetes, OSA)
- Absence of medical contraindications
- Failure of nonsurgical weight loss
- Well-informed, compliant, motivated patient

Exclusion Criteria
- Uncontrolled, severe psychiatric illness
- Reversible endocrine or other disorders that can cause obesity
- Current drug or alcohol abuse

Data from Gastrointestinal surgery for severe obesity: National Institutes of Health Consensus Development Conference Statement. Am J Clin Nutr. 1992 Feb; 55(2 Suppl):615S-619S.

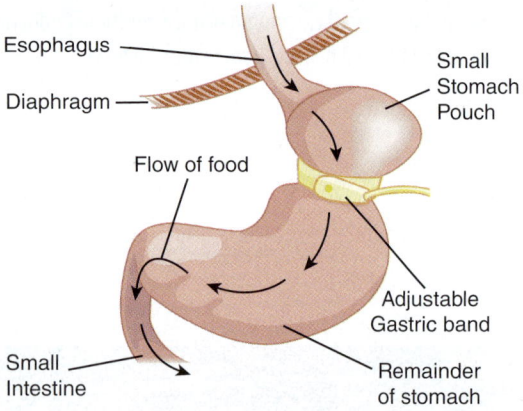

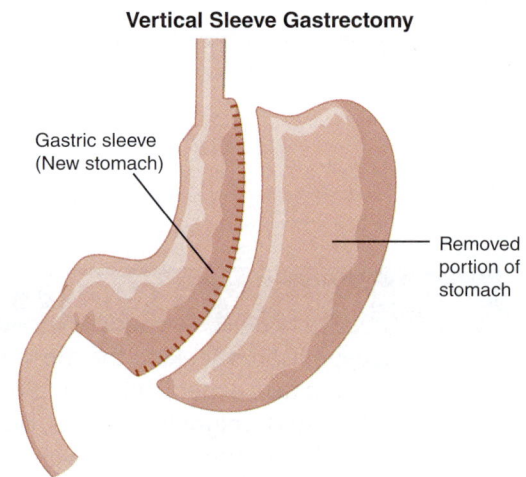

2. Restrictive and malabsorptive (combination):
   - **Sleeve gastrectomy (SG)** (mostly restrictive)
   - **Roux-en-Y gastric bypass (RYGB)**

3. Malabsorptive procedures:
   - Biliopancreatic diversion (BPD)
   - BPD with duodenal switch (BPD/DS)

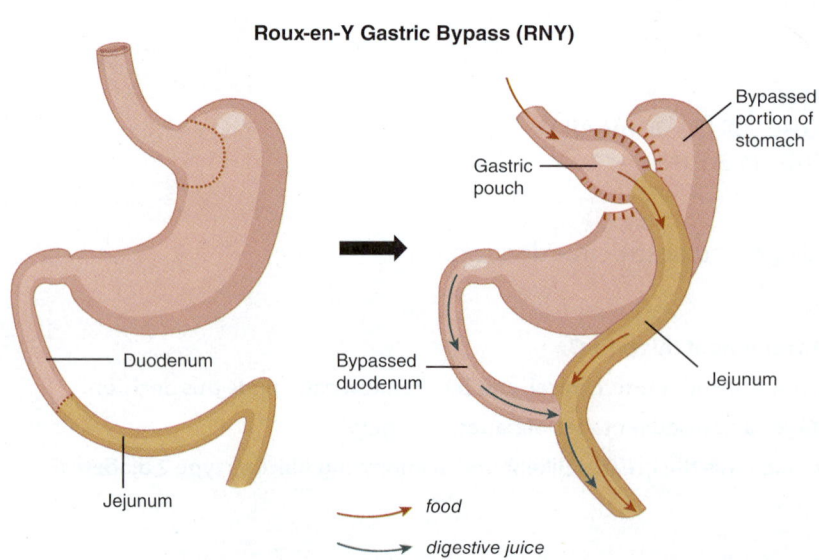

Restrictive Procedures

Laparoscopic Adjustable Gastric Banding (LAGB) The LAGB works by physically restricting the stomach, decreasing overall transit time of food and leading to early sense of satiety and decreased intake. It works primarily by restricting intake without neural or hormonal physiological influence. A small pouch is created by placing a hollow band around the stomach. The band is tethered to tubing connected to a port that is placed just underneath the skin. Approximately 6 weeks after placement, the band is inflated by injection of a small amount of saline into the port. These injections of saline are called "fills" or "adjustments" and are completed over a period of 6 to 8 weeks until the band is inflated enough to reduce the size of the individual's meal intake. The goal of the fill is to achieve just the right amount of restriction. The LAGB requires regular follow-up for band adjustment, at which time the individual should also participate in counseling sessions with the dietitian regarding mindful eating, avoidance of foods that can obstruct the outlet, and chewing food thoroughly. Individuals may find that soft, high-calorie foods and beverages (i.e., sodas, juices, ice cream, etc.) can easily pass through the restricted outlet, and therefore they will need to learn to limit or avoid these foods.

Many individuals are initially attracted to the LAGB because it is less invasive and potentially reversible, compared to other bariatric surgeries. In 2008, the LAGB accounted for over 90% of outpatient bariatric procedures in the United States, although numbers have since fallen dramatically.[99] The potential long-term complications associated with the band include band slippage, erosion, infection, and scar tissue formation, which have led to reports of a reoperation rate of up to 60%.[100] Inadequate weight loss is the most-reported basis for reoperation, with an average of 28% to 65% excess weight loss (EWL), where EWL is actual weight minus weight at a BMI at 2 years postoperatively.[3,101] Many surgeons are converting the LAGB to a SG or RYGB and, more recently, surgeons are choosing to perform the SG. Average weight loss with the band is approximately 20% of initial body weight 1 to 2 years after surgery and 14% 10 years postsurgery.[102] Long-term complications and/or dissatisfaction with weight loss has led to a failure rate approaching 80%.[103]

Combination Procedures

Sleeve Gastrectomy (SG) The SG was initially used as a first-step approach to the biliopancreatic diversion-duodenal switch (BPD/DS) procedure because individuals with severe obesity are at high risk for surgical complications. Once the individual lost weight after the SG procedure, the BPD/DS was performed. Because research demonstrated effective weight loss with SG, this became a standalone procedure. The SG involves a left partial gastrectomy, which removes about 80% of the stomach, including the fundus and greater curvature. The remaining gastric pouch resembles the shape of a banana. While the SG was initially thought to induce weight loss primarily due to restriction, there are data to support there are resulting gut hormonal changes and metabolic influences such as improvement in blood sugar control, increased satiety, and reduction in hunger.[104,105]

In 2013, the SG surpassed the RYGB as the number one procedure in the United States, and its numbers continue to climb. This is due to its substantial weight loss results with reduced postsurgical complications compared to RYGB.[105] In one study, individuals who had the SG showed a BMI reduction of 11.9 kg/m^2 compared to 7 kg/m^2 after LAGB and 15.3 kg/m^2 after RYGB.[106] The average EWL following the SG is >50% at 3 to 5 years postoperatively.[105] While there are limited long-term data on micronutrient deficiencies after SG, short-term studies have shown that there may be some risk involved. The current recommendations for vitamin and mineral supplementation are the same as those for RYGB (see below). Long-term (greater than 5-10 years) outcome data are needed to fully assess its efficacy.

Roux-en-Y Gastric Bypass (RYGB) The RYGB is considered a combination procedure involving both restriction and malabsorption and is widely accepted as the "gold standard" in bariatric surgery. Although all of the mechanisms by which the RYGB influences the weight regulatory system are not fully understood, there is strong evidence of changes in neural and hormonal pathways that favor durable and significant weight loss and improvement in obesity-related comorbid conditions. In the RYGB, a small gastric pouch is created in the upper portion of the stomach by dividing and reattaching the stomach and the distal jejunum. The remaining stomach, duodenum, and proximal jejunum are bypassed, and the remaining stomach aids in digestion by producing enzymes that will eventually mix with food in the jejunum. The accelerated passage of undigested nutrients directly into the jejunum activates chemoreceptors that decrease hunger and that stimulate satiety.[107] Changes in GLP-1 and PYY have been well studied. More recent data support that there may be specific effects of RYGB surgery on the microbiota that influence weight loss.[108] These combined factors may contribute to the long-term effectiveness of the RYGB and other combination procedures, with excess weight loss of 60% to 80%.[105] Improvement or remission of obesity-related comorbidities such as type 2 diabetes has been well documented, often occurring independent of weight loss and usually seen within days of surgery (see **Table 8.7**). Risks for complications (14.6%) include infection, bleeding, stricture, obstruction, and dehydration.[109] The mortality rate is relatively low, at around 0.1%.[109] Because major parts of the stomach, the entire duodenum, and proximal jejunum are bypassed, individuals are at risk for micronutrient deficiencies such as vitamin B12, iron, zinc, thiamine, calcium, and vitamin D, among others. Individuals need to consent to life-long vitamin and mineral supplementation to ensure optimal body functioning.

Comorbidity Outcomes

RYGB has the greatest documented improvement in comorbidities as compared to SG and LAGB. The 30-day postoperative complication rate is slightly higher (5.6 versus 5.9

TABLE 8.7 MORBIDITY OUTCOMES: PERCENTAGE OF PATIENTS WHO ACHIEVED COMORBIDITY REMISSION OR SIGNIFICANT IMPROVEMENT AT 1-YEAR POSTOP

Condition	Bariatric Surgery Type		
	Bypass	Sleeve	Band
Type 2 diabetes	83%	55%	44%
Hypertension	79%	68%	44%
Hyperlipidemia	66%	35%	33%
Sleep apnea	66%	62%	38%
Gastroesophageal reflux	70%	55%	64%

Data based on a longitudinal data collection system, 109 hospitals, 28,616 patients.
Modified from Hutter MH, Schirmer BD, Jones DB. Et al. Ann Surg. 2011;254(3);410-422.

for the RYGB compared to the SG, while weight loss and improvement of comorbidities is higher with the RYGB.[110] Reports of type 2 diabetes remission postsurgery vary significantly; in an RCT conducted by Shauer et al., there was 45% full remission at 1 year in RYGB patients.[111]

The changes that occur due to the manipulation of the stomach and/or digestive tract have been a field of investigation for the past decade, particularly related to gut hormones (Table 8.8). The mechanisms are not fully known, although the durability of weight loss is most likely due to changes in the physiological regulation of body weight.

The Swedish Obese Subjects study showed that patients who had bariatric surgery who maintained a loss of 15% to 25% of initial weight 10 years later had a 29% reduction in all-cause mortality when compared with a control group that was matched on 18 characteristics. The major reductions in mortality resulted from decreases in cardiovascular and cancer-related deaths. Due to its metabolic impact on the body and the durability of weight loss for most patients, bariatric surgery is considered one of the most effective therapies for obesity management.

Diet Progression for RYGB and SG

There is no standardization of diet stages, but the below diet advancement protocols provide adequate fluid, protein and fiber intake, as well as proper texture progression.

TABLE 8.8 GUT HORMONES AND MECHANISMS OF WEIGHT LOSS AFTER WEIGHT LOSS SURGERY

Gut Hormone/Mechanism	RYGB Postprandial	SG Postprandial	LAGB
GLP-1 • Slows gastric emptying • Inhibits glucagon secretion • Acts synergistically with PYY: satiety and inhibits food intake • Augments the insulin response to nutrients	Increased	Increased	No effect
PYY • Shown to induce satiety and reduce food intake • Inhibitory effect on gastrointestinal mobility	Increased	Increased	No effect
Ghrelin • Produced from the fundus of the stomach and the proximal intestine • Only known orexigenic gut hormone • Primary source is the gastric mucosa • Nutrient exposure to the small intestine is sufficient for food-induced ghrelin suppression in humans; therefore, gastric nutrient exposure is not necessary for suppression	Inconclusive	Decreased	Ghrelin has been shown to increase in response to caloric restriction after LAGB as seen in low-calorie dieting; this may be the reason for less weight loss and more hunger in patients post-LAGB

Data from Stefater MA, Wilson-Perez HE, Chambers AP, et al. Endo Rev, 2013, 33(4):595-622. ; Pournaras DJ, le Roux CW. World J Surg. 2009; 1983-1988. ;Ochner CN, Gibson C, Shanik N, et al. Int'l J Obes. 2011;36:153-166.

Clinical Roundtable

Topic: Estimating Energy Needs Post-bariatric Surgery

Background: The Mifflin–St. Jeor predictive equation for estimating energy needs has been found to have the least margin of error in estimating resting metabolic rate in healthy individuals with obesity and is a commonly used method of estimating energy needs in this population.[52,53] It is known that weight loss impacts total and resting energy expenditure because weight loss leads to loss of both fat mass and lean body mass. Although diet-induced weight loss's effect on energy expenditure has been studied, there is less information on the impact of bariatric surgery's effect on energy expenditure. It is not clear whether surgically induced weight loss, including the change in regulation of gut hormones that accompanies the procedures, modifies the various components of energy expenditure differently than diet-induced weight loss.

Roundtable Discussion

1. Can predictive equations used to estimate energy needs before bariatric surgery be applied post-operatively?
2. What factors would you consider in estimating energy needs in a post-bariatric surgery patient?
3. What methods might you utilize in your energy needs estimation?

References

1. Thivel D, Brakonieki K, Duche P, et al. Surgical weight loss: Impact on energy expenditure. *Obes Surg.* 2013;23(2):255-266.

Data from Thivel D, Brakonieki K, Duche P, et al. Surgical weight loss: impact on energy expenditure. Obes Surg. 2013;23(2):255-266.

CASE STUDY REVISITED

Immediately following Allison's surgery, you are consulted to educate Allison on her diet progression.

Questions

1. Describe your intervention.
2. What other concerns might you have regarding Allison's nutritional status?
3. What are her short-term nutrition goals?
4. What are her long-term nutrition goals?
5. Which biochemical parameters would you monitor postoperatively?

The same nutritional guidelines and diet advancements for post-RYGB are also recommended post-SG (**Table 8.9**). The protocol for diet staging following laparoscopic adjustable gastric banding (LAGB) is shown in **Table 8.10**.

Micronutrient Concerns

Following bariatric surgery, individuals need additional supplementation for vitamins and minerals compared to individuals who have not undergone surgery. There are several micronutrients that can become deficient based on the type of surgery performed. Across all procedures, the most common are vitamin B12, iron, zinc, folate, copper, thiamine, calcium, and vitamin D. Recommendations for dosages and frequency of vitamins and minerals are established by the American Society for Metabolic and Bariatric Surgery (ASMBS). Micronutrient deficiencies and recommendations for supplementation are described in the **Tables 8.11** and **8.12**.

> **PRACTICE POINT**
>
> Following bariatric surgery, individuals will need to take additional vitamin and mineral supplements in order to prevent deficiencies in vitamin B12, iron, zinc, folate, copper, thiamine, calcium, and vitamin D.

Emerging Treatment Options

Many new treatment options for severe obesity have emerged over the past several years due to the limited effectiveness of most current therapies and the need for less-invasive procedures/treatments. These include electrical stimulation systems such as the Maestro Rechargeable System, gastric emptying systems including the Aspire Assist, and a variety of gastric balloon systems. Specifically, the Orbera intragastric balloon was approved by the FDA

TABLE 8.9 DIET STAGE PROGRESSION FOR ROUX-EN-Y GASTRIC BYPASS AND SLEEVE GASTRECTOMY

RYGB and SG Diet Stage	Diet Initiation	Food/Fluid Stage	RYGB/SG Guidelines	Supplements
Stage I	Postop day 1 and 2	RYGB/SG clear liquids: noncarbonated, low calorie, low sugar, no caffeine	Postop RYGB day 1, patients may begin sips of water, ice chips, and low-calorie fluids; avoid carbonation.	
Stage II	Postop day 2 and 3 (discharge diet)	RYGB clear liquids: • Variety of low sugar liquids or artificially sweetened liquids • Salty fluids and solid liquids (sugar-free ice pops) encouraged Plus RYGB/SG full liquids: • Less than 25 g sugar per serving in full liquids • Protein rich liquids (limit 25 to 30 g protein per serving)	Minimum 48 to 64 oz total fluids per day: • 24 to 32 oz or more ounces RYGB clear liquids plus 24 to 32 oz any combination of full liquids: • Low-fat or fat-free milk mixed with: • Whey or soy protein powder (limit 20 g protein per serving) • Lactose-free milk or soy milk mix with soy protein powder • Light yogurt, blended • Plain yogurt	Begin supplementation: • Chewable multivitamin with minerals, 2x/day • Chewable or liquid 1200 to 1500mg/day calcium citrate with vitamin D
Stage III: Week 1	Postop day 10 to 14	Increase RYGB/SG clear liquids: Total liquids 48 to 64 oz or more per day and replace full liquids with soft, moist, diced, ground, or pureed protein sources as tolerated Stage III protein sources: • Eggs; ground meats and poultry; soft, moist fish; added gravy, bouillon, light mayo to moisten, cooked beans, hearty bean soups, cottage cheese, low-fat cheese, yogurt	• Protein food choices are encouraged for 3 to 6 small meals per day; patients may only be able to tolerate a couple of tablespoons at each meal/snack. • Mindful, slow, eating is essential. • Encourage patients not to drink with meals and to wait ~30 minutes after each meal before resuming fluids.	Daily supplements essential
Stage III: Week 2	4 weeks postop	Advance diet as tolerated; if protein foods are well tolerated, add well-cooked, soft vegetables and soft and/or peeled fruit. Always eat protein first.	Adequate hydration is essential and a priority for all patients during the rapid weight loss phase. Patient should be encouraged to add fruits/vegetables in a texture that is tolerated. Full liquids may be used for meal or snack replacement	Daily supplements essential

(continues)

TABLE 8.9 DIET STAGE PROGRESSION FOR ROUX-EN-Y GASTRIC BYPASS AND SLEEVE GASTRECTOMY (Continued)

RYGB and SG Diet Stage	Diet Initiation	Food/Fluid Stage	RYGB/SG Guidelines	Supplements
Stage III; Week 3	5 weeks postop	Continue to consume protein with some fruit or vegetable at each meal; some people tolerate salads 1 month to 6 weeks postop	**AVOID** rice, bread, and pasta until patient is comfortably consuming adequate protein per day and fruits/vegetables. **Consider diet a "nutrition prescription"** to meet nutritional needs during rapid weight loss and healing phase: Nutrition Prescription: 1. Adequate hydration 2. 1 to 2 oz protein sources 3 to 5 times a day with fruit and/or vegetables 3. Postsurgery supplementation As weight stabilizes, hunger increases, and patients are meeting the DRI for protein and consuming fruits and vegetables, grains can be introduced.	Daily supplements essential
Stage IV	As hunger increases and more food is tolerated	Healthy solid food diet	Healthy, balanced diet consisting of adequate protein, fruits, vegetables and whole grains. Calorie needs based on height, weight, age	Daily supplements essential. Nutritional labs should be drawn 3, 6, 12 months and annually indefinitely for RYGB and SG

*RYGB: Roux-en-Y gastric bypass; SG: sleeve gastrectomy
Table created with permission by Sue Cummings, MS, RD.

TABLE 8.10 DIET STAGE PROGRESSION FOR LAPAROSCOPIC ADJUSTABLE GASTRIC BANDING

LAGB Diet Stage	Diet Initiation	Fluids/Food Stage	LAGB Guidelines	Supplements
Stage I	Postop day 1 and 2	LAGB clear liquids: • Noncarbonated; low calorie, low sugar; no caffeine,	Postop LAGB day 1, patients may begin sips of water, ice chips, and low-calorie fluids; avoid carbonation.	
Stage II	Post-op day 2 and 3 (discharge diet)	LAGB clear liquids: • Variety of low-sugar liquids or artificially sweetened liquids Plus LAGB full liquids: • Less than 25 g sugar per serving, and no more than 3 g fat per serving of protein-rich liquids	Patients should consume a minimum of 48 to 64 oz of total fluids per day; 24 to 32 oz or more LAGB clear liquids; plus 24 to 32 ounces of any combination of full liquids: Low-fat or fat-free milk mixed with: • Whey or soy protein powder (limit 20 g protein per serving) • Lactose-free milk or soy milk mix with soy protein powder • Light yogurt, blended • Plain yogurt	Begin supplementation: • Chewable multivitamin with minerals, 2x/day • Chewable or liquid 1200 to 1500 mg/day calcium citrate with vitamin D

(continues)

TABLE 8.10 DIET STAGE PROGRESSION FOR LAPAROSCOPIC ADJUSTABLE GASTRIC BANDING (Continued)

LAGB Diet Stage	Diet Initiation	Fluids/Food Stage	LAGB Guidelines	Supplements
Stage III: Week 1	Postop day 10 to 14	Increase LAGB clear liquids (total liquids 48 to 64 oz per day) and replace full liquids with soft, moist, diced, ground, or pureed protein sources as tolerated: • Eggs; ground meats and poultry; soft, moist fish; added gravy; bouillon; light mayo to moisten; cooked beans; hearty bean soups; cottage cheese; low-fat cheese; yogurt	NOTE: Patients should be reassured that hunger is common and normal after LAGB. • Protein (moist, ground) choices are encouraged for 3 to 6 small meals per day to help with satiety, because hunger is common within a week or so after LAGB. • Mindful, slow eating is essential. • Encourage patients not to drink with meals and to wait ~30 minutes after each meal before resuming fluids	Vitamin and mineral supplementation daily
Stage III: Week 2	4 weeks postop	Advance diet as tolerated; if protein foods are well tolerated, add well-cooked, soft vegetables and soft and/or peeled fruit	Adequate hydration is essential and a priority for all patients during the rapid weight loss phase. Protein at every meal and snack, especially if increased hunger is noted prior to the initial fill or adjustment. Very well-cooked vegetables may also help to increase satiety.	Vitamin and mineral supplementation daily
Stage III: Week 3	5 weeks postop	Continue to consume protein with some fruit or vegetable at each meal; some patients tolerate salads 1 month to 6 weeks post-op	If patient is tolerating soft, moist, ground, diced, and/or pureed proteins with small amounts of fruits and vegetables, may add crackers (use with protein). AVOID rice, bread, and pasta	Vitamin and mineral supplementation daily
Stage IV	As hunger increases and more food is tolerated	Healthy solid food diet	Healthy, balanced diet consisting of adequate protein, fruits, vegetables and whole grains; Calorie needs based on height, weight, and age	Vitamin and mineral supplementation daily Nutritional labs should be drawn 3, 6, 9, 12 months and annually indefinitely; done density test at baseline and every 2 years

(continues)

TABLE 8.10 DIET STAGE PROGRESSION FOR LAPAROSCOPIC ADJUSTABLE GASTRIC BANDING (Continued)

LAGB Diet Stage	Diet Initiation	Fluids/Food Stage	LAGB Guidelines	Supplements
Post-LAGB fill/adjustment	~6 weeks postop LAGB, and possibly every 6 weeks until satiety/optimal adjustment reached	Full liquids for 2 days postfill; advance to Stage III, week 1 guidelines above, as tolerated for 4 to 5 days, then advance as above.	Same as Stage II liquids above for 48 hours (and/or as otherwise advised by surgeon). NOTE: When diet advances to soft solids, special attention to mindful eating and chewing until liquid is key, because more restriction may increase risk for food getting stuck above stoma of band if not properly chewed (e.g., if not chewed until liquid).	

Table created with permission by Sue Cummings, MS, RD.

TABLE 8.11 POTENTIAL VITAMIN/MINERAL DEFICIENCIES AFTER BARIATRIC SURGERY

Vitamin/Mineral	Markers	Deficiency Prevalence Postprocedure	Repletion
Iron	Fe Ferritin TIBC	3 months to 10 years 14% LAGB <18% SG 20% to 25% RYGB 13% to 62% BPD 8% to 50% DS	150 to 300 mg 2-3x/day iron infusion
Vitamin B12	Serum B12 (cobalamin) MMA	2 to 5 years <20% RYGB 4% to 20% SG	1,000 mcg orally/day 1,000 μ IM/month
Thiamine	Serum B1	<1% to 49%, depending on surgery May occur with IV hydration, vomiting	100 mg orally 2-3x/day 200 mg IV 3x/day 200 mg IM 1x/day
Folic acid	RBC folate	Reported in up to 65% patients	1,000 μg orally/day
Calcium	Serum Ca phosphorous Alk Phos PTH Bone density	N/A	1,500 to 2,000 mg/day for LAGB, SG, RYBP 1800 to 2400 mg/day for BPD/DS
Vitamin D	25-OH Vitamin D PTH Alk Phos	Up to 100% of patients	2,000 to 6,000 IU/day 50,000 IU D2 1-2x/week for 5 to 8 weeks, recheck

(continues)

TABLE 8.11 POTENTIAL VITAMIN/MINERAL DEFICIENCIES AFTER BARIATRIC SURGERY (Continued)

Vitamin/Mineral	Markers	Deficiency Prevalence Postprocedure	Repletion
Vitamin A Vitamin E Vitamin K	Plasma retinol Plasma alpha tocopherol Prothrombin time	Within 4 years 70% RYGB, BPD/DS Deficiencies uncommon	10,000 to 25,000 IU/day for 1 to 2 weeks 100 to 400 IU/day + 1 to 2 mg/day orally
Zinc	Plasma zinc	34% LAGB 19% SG 40% RYGB up to 70% BP/DS	Insufficient evidence to recommend dose
Copper	Serum copper Ceruloplasmin	As high as 10% to 20% RYBP 90% BPD/DS	3 to 8 mg/day oral copper gluconate or sulfate 2 to 4 mg/day IV copper for 6 days for severe deficiency

Data from J Parrot et al. American Society for Metabolic and Bariatric Surgery Integrated Health Nutritional Guidelines for the Surgical Weight Loss Patient 2016 Update: Micronutrients.

TABLE 8.12 CURRENT STANDARD FOR VITAMIN MINERAL SUPPLEMENTATION AFTER BARIATRIC SURGERY*

Supplement	Dosage
Multivitamin First month, chewable 2x/day	100% to 200% daily value
Calcium citrate with Vitamin D (Citrate preferred) Divided doses for maximum absorption	1,200 to 1,500 mg/day 400 to 800 IU of vitamin D
Vitamin D	3,000 IU daily
Elemental iron contained in multivitamin; additional as indicated (not to be taken with calcium)	18 to 27 mg/day elemental 40 to 65 mg/day for menstruating females
Vitamin B12	350 to 500 μg/day orally/—sublingual/nasal or 1,000 mcg IM

*Patients with preoperative or postoperative biochemical deficiency states are treated beyond these recommendations.
Modified from J Mechanick et al. Clinical Practice Guidelines for the Perioperative Nutritional, Metabolic, and Nonsurgical Support of the Bariatric Surgery Patient—2013 Update: Cosponsored by American Association of Clinical Endocrinologists, The Obesity Society, and American Society for Metabolic & Bariatric Surgery.

in August 2015 (**Figure 8.13**).[112] This device is a system that uses a gastric balloon to occupy space in the stomach. Once the balloon is in place, it is filled with 400 to 700 mL of saline to occupy the stomach and assist in reducing food intake. The balloon is only intended for temporary use and should be removed after 6 months. It is approved for adults with a BMI of 30 to 40 kg/m^2.

A meta-analysis of the Orbera intragastric balloon found an average EWL of 32.1% after 6 months with improvements in blood pressure, fasting glucose, and lipid profile.[113] Significant improvements in HbA1c have been seen among patients with diabetes who have used Orbera. However, more research is needed on long-term weight maintenance after the intragastric balloon. Nutrition guidelines following placement of the intragastric balloon have also not yet been established by the ASMBS. In general, the dietitian should work closely with patients to ensure they are following a nutrient-dense meal plan and meeting micronutrient needs. This procedure is not currently covered by insurance, and the cost may be

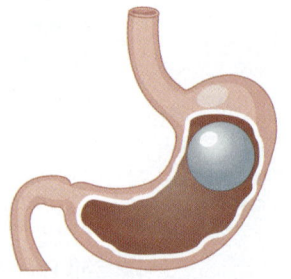

FIGURE 8.13 Intragastric Balloon

prohibitive for many individuals. Other endoscopic procedures are currently under investigation and aim to bridge the gap between medication and bariatric surgery by providing effective, but less-invasive, methods for weight loss.

Chapter Summary

Obesity is a multifactorial condition that involves genetic, environmental, social, biological, and developmental factors. Obesity is a risk factor for a variety of health conditions, including diabetes, hyperlipidemia, hypertension, heart disease, stroke, certain cancers, nonalcoholic fatty liver disease, sleep apnea, gallbladder disease, respiratory problems, arthritis, and depression and is currently an epidemic in the United States. Due to the complex nature of obesity, many approaches exist to address the condition. The cornerstone of obesity management is facilitating weight loss through a comprehensive lifestyle program that includes diet, physical activity, and behavior modification. All lifestyle interventions should be individualized. Additional approaches include pharmacological treatments, which can augment lifestyle programs, and bariatric surgery, which can elicit the greatest results. Because relapse is common, continued treatment and ongoing support are necessary to achieve and maintain desired results.

Key Terms

obesity, body mass index, ghrelin, leptin, orexigenic, anorexigenic, adipose, bariatric surgery, laparoscopic adjustable gastric band (LAGB), sleeve gastrectomy (SG), roux-en-Y gastric bypass (RYGB)

References

1. World Health Organization. Obesity and Overweight fact sheet. www.who.int/mediacentre/factsheets/fs311/en/index.html. Updated June 2016. Accessed September 30, 2017.
2. Centers for Disease Control and Prevention. Basics About Childhood Obesity. http://www.cdc.gov/obesity/childhood/basics.html. Updated October 20, 2016. Accessed September 30, 2017.
3. Jensen MD, Ryan DH, Apovian CM, et al. 2013 AHA/ACC/TOS Guideline for the Management of Overweight and Obesity in Adults: A Report of the American College of Cardiology/American Heart Association Task Force on Practice Guidelines and The Obesity Society. *J Am Coll Cardiol*. 2013;pii:S0735-1097(13)06030-0.
4. National Heart, Lung, and Blood Institute Obesity Education Initiative Expert Panel on the Identification, Evaluation, and Treatment of Obesity in Adults (US). Clinical Guidelines on the Identification, Evaluation, and Treatment of Overweight and Obesity in Adults: The Evidence Report. *Obes Res*. 1998; 6 Suppl 2:51S-209S.
5. Finkelstein EA, Trogdon JG, Cohen JW et al. Annual medical spending attributable to obesity: payer- and service-specific estimates. *Health Affairs*. 2009;28(5):w822-w831.
6. Wang LC, McPherson K, Marsh T, et al. Health and economic burden of expected of the expected obesity trends in the USA and UK. *Lancet*. 2011;78:815-825.
7. Centers for Disease Control and Prevention. Adult Obesity Facts. https://www.cdc.gov/nchs/data/hestat/obesity_adult_13_14/obesity_adult_13_14.htm. Updated July 20, 2016. Accessed September 30, 2017.
8. Centers for Disease Control and Prevention. Childhood Obesity Facts. http://www.cdc.gov/obesity/data/childhood.html. Updated April 20, 2017. Accessed June 3, 2017.
9. Flegal KM, Kruszon-Moran D, Carroll MD, et al. Trends in obesity among adults in the United States, 2005 to 2014. *JAMA*. 2016;315(21):284-2291.
10. Centers for Disease Control and Prevention. Obesity prevalence maps. https://www.cdc.gov/obesity/data/prevalence-maps.html. Updated August 29, 2017. Accessed September 30, 2017.
11. Centers for Disease Control and Prevention. Adult Obesity Trends. https://www.cdc.gov/obesity/data/adult.html. Updated August 31, 2017. Accessed September 30, 2017
12. Tsai AG, Wadden TA. In the Clinic Obesity. *Ann Intern Med*. 2013;159(5):ITC3-1.
13. Wright SM, Aronne LJ. Causes of obesity. *Abdom Imaging*. 2012;37(5):730-732.
14. Nan C, Guo B, Warner C, Zeegers M. Heritability of body mass index in pre-adolescence, young adulthood and late adulthood. *Eur J Epidemiol*. 2012;27(4):247-253.
15. Perusse L, Chagnon YC, Weisnagel SJ, Rankinen T, Snyder E, Sands J, et al. The human obesity gene map: the 2000 update. *Obes Res*. 2001;9:135-169.
16. Shuldiner AR, Sabra M. TRp64Arg 3-adrenoceptor; when does a candidate gene become a disease-susceptibility gene? *Obes Res*. 2001;9;806.
17. Choquet H, Meyre D. Molecular basis of obesity: current status and future prospects. *Curr Genomics*. 2011;12(3):154-168.
18. Ledikwe JH, Ello-Martin JA, Rolls BJ. Portion sizes and the obesity epidemic. *J Nutr*. 2005;135(4):905-909.
19. Beaulac J, Kristjansson E, Cummins S. A systematic review of food deserts, 1966-2007. *Prev Chronic Dis* 2009;6(3):A105.
20. Centers for Disease Control and Prevention. Facts about physical activity. https://www.cdc.gov/physicalactivity/data/facts.htm. Updated May 23, 2014. Accessed April 23, 2017.
21. Leproult R, Van Cauter E. Role of sleep and sleep loss in hormonal release and metabolism. *Endocr Dev*. 2010;17:11-21.
22. World Health Organization: Social determinants of health. http://www.who.int/social_determinants/sdh_definition/en/. Accessed April 23, 2017.
23. Christakis NA, Fowler JH. The spread of obesity in a large social network over 32 years. *N Engl J Med*. 2007;357(4):370-3379.
24. Ramakrishna BS. Role of the gut microbiota in human nutrition and metabolism. *J Gastroenterol Hepatol*. 2013;28 Suppl 4:9-17.
25. Bäckhed F, Ding H, Wang T, et al. The gut microbiota as an environmental factor that regulates fat storage. *Proc Natl Acad Sci U S A*. 2004;101(44):15718-15723.
26. Yan J, Liu L, Zhu Y, et al. The association between breastfeeding and childhood obesity: A meta-analysis. *BMC Public Health*. 2014;14:1267.
27. Hediger ML, Overpeck MD, Kuczmarski RJ, Ruan WJ. Association between infant breastfeeding and overweight in young children. *J Am Med Assoc*. 2001;285:2453-2460.
28. Wang L, Collins C, Ratliff M, et al. Breastfeeding reduces childhood obesity risks. *Childhood Obes*. 2017. DOI: 10.1089/chi.2016.0210.
29. Monasta L, Batty GD, Cattaneo A, et al. Early-life determinants of overweight and obesity: a review of systematic reviews. *Obes Rev*. 2010;11(10):695-708.

30. Casazza K, Fontaine KR, Astrup A, et al. Myths, presumptions, and facts about obesity. *N Engl J Med*. 2013;368(5):446-454.
31. Rosenbaum M, Leibel RL. Adaptive thermogenesis in humans. *Int J Obes*. 2010;34 Suppl 1:S47-55.
32. Sumithran P, Proietto J. The defence of body weight: a physiological basis for weight regain after weight loss. *Clin Sci (Lond)*. 2013 Feb;124(4):231-241.
33. Perry B, Wang Y. Appetite regulation and weight control: the role of gut hormones. *Nutr Diabetes*. 2012;2:e26.
34. Klok MD, Jakobsdottir S, Drent ML. The role of leptin and ghrelin in the regulation of food intake and body weight in humans: a review. *Obesity Rev*. 2007;8:21-34.
35. Rahmouni K Morgan DA. Hypothalamic arcuate nucleus mediates the sympathetic and arterial pressure responses to leptin. *Hypertension*. 2007;49:647-652.
36. Lowell BB, S-Susulic V, Hamann A, et al. Development of obesity in transgenic mice after genetic ablation of brown adipose tissue. *Nature*. 1993;366:740-742.
37. Ozata M, Ozdemir IC, Licinio J. Human leptin deficiency caused by a missense mutation: multiple endocrine defects, decreased sympathetic tone, and immune system dysfunction indicate new targets for leptin action, greater central than peripheral resistance to the effects of leptin, and spontaneous correction of leptin-mediated defects. *J Clin Endocrinol Meta*. 1999;84:3686-3695.
38. National Institute of Diabetes and Digestive and Kidney Diseases. Prediabetes and insulin resistance. https://www.niddk.nih.gov/health-information/diabetes/overview/what-is-diabetes/prediabetes-insulin-resistance. Accessed June 2, 2017.
39. Lutz, TA. The role of amylin in the control of energy homeostasis. *Am. J. Physiol Regul Integr Comp Physiol*. 2010;298(6):R1475-R1484.
40. Dockray GJ. Cholecystokinin and gut-brain signaling. *Regulatory Peptides*. 2009;155:6-10.
41. Parker SML, Balasubramanian A. Y2 receptors in health and disease. *Br J Pharmacol*. 2008;153:420-431.
42. Lean MEJ, Malkova D. Altered gut and adipose tissue hormones in overweight and obese individuals: cause or consequence? *Int J Obesity*. 2016;40(4):622-632.
43. Deurenberg P, Yap M. The assessment of obesity: methods for measuring body fat and global prevalence of obesity. *Baillieres Best Pract Res Clin Endocrinol Metab*. 1999;13(1):1-11.
44. Gallagher D, Heymsfield SB, Heo M, et al. Healthy percentage body fat ranges: an approach for developing guidelines based on body mass index. *Am J Clin Nutr*. 2000; 72(3):694-701.
45. Jo J, Gavrilova O, Pack S, et al. Hypertrophy and/or Hyperplasia: Dynamics of Adipose Tissue Growth. *PLoS Comput Biol*. 2009;5(3):e1000324.
46. Spalding, KL, Arner E, Westermark PO, et al. Dynamics of fat cell turnover in humans. *Nature*. 2008;453:783-787.
47. Kontogianni MD, Panagiotakos DB, Skopouli FN. Does body mass index reflect adequately the body fat content in perimenopausal women? *Maturitas*. 2005;51:307-313.
48. Romero-Corral A, Somers VK, Sierra-Johnson J, et al. Normal weight obesity: a risk factor for cardiometabolic dysregulation and cardiovascular mortality. *Eur Heart J*. 2010;31(6):737-746.
49. World Health Organization. Waist Circumference and Waist–Hip Ratio: Report of a WHO Expert Consultation. December 8-11, 2016; Geneva, Switzerland. whqlibdoc.who.int/publications/2011/9789241501491_eng.pdf. Accessed June 1, 2017.
50. Levine JA. Measurement of energy expenditure. *Public Health Nutr*. 2005;8(7A):1123-1132.
51. Ainslie P, Reilly T, Westerterp K. Estimating human energy expenditure: a review of techniques with particular reference to doubly labelled water. *Sports Med*. 2003;33(9):683-698.
52. Frankenfield D, Roth-Yousey L, Compher C. Comparison of predictive equations for resting metabolic rate in healthy nonobese and obese adults: a systematic review. *J Am Diet Assoc*. 2005;105(5):775-789.
53. Namazi N, Aliasgharzadeh S, Mahdavi R, et al. Accuracy of the common predictive equations for estimating resting energy expenditure among normal and overweight girl university students. *J Am Coll Nutr*. 2016;35(2):136-142.
54. Aronne LJ, Nelinson DS, Lillo J. Obesity as a disease state: a new paradigm for diagnosis and treatment. *Clin Cornerstone*. 2009;9(4):9-25.
55. Lavie CJ, Milani RV, Artham SM. The obesity paradox, weight loss, and coronary diasease. *Am J Med*. 2009;122(12):1106-1114se.
56. Ne R. Obesity-related Hypertension. *Ochsner J*. 2009;9(3):133-136.
57. Hall JE. Pathophysiology of obesity hypertension. *Curr Hypertens Rep*. 2000;2(2):139-147.
58. Poirier P, Giles T, Bray G, et al. Obesity and cardiovascular disease: pathophysiology, evaluation, and effect of weight loss. An Update of the 1997 American Heart Association Scientific Statement on Obesity and Heart Disease From the Obesity Committee of the Council on Nutrition, Physical Activity, and Metabolism. *Circulation*. 2006;113:898-918.
59. Romero-Corral A, Sierra-Johnson J, Lopez-Jimenez, et al. Relationships between leptin and C-reactive protein with cardiovascular disease in the adult general population. *Nat Clin Pract Cardiovasc Med*. 2008;5(7):418-425.
60. Poirier P, Martin J, Marceau P, et al. Impact of bariatric surgery on cardiac structure, function and clinical manifestations in morbid obesity. *Expert Rev Cardiovasc Ther*. 2004;2:193-201.
61. Garvey WT, Mechanick JI, Brett EM et al. American Association of Clinical Endocrinologists and American College of Endocrinology Comprehensive Clinical Practice Guidelines for Medical Care of Patients with Obesity. *Endocrine Prac*. 2016;22(Suppl 3):1-203.
62. Centers for Disease Control and Prevention. Diabetes at a Glance fact sheet. https://www.cdc.gov/chronicdisease/resources/publications/aag/diabetes.htm. Updated July 25, 2016. Accessed June 3, 2017.
63. Kahn SE, Hull RL, Utzschneider KM. Mechanisms linking obesity to insulin resistance and type 2 diabetes. *Nature*. 2006;444:840-846.
64. Hajer GR, van Haeften TW, Visseren FL. Adipose tissue dysfunction in obesity, diabetes, and vascular diseases. *Eur Heart J*. 2008;29:2959-2971.
65. Third report of the National Cholesterol Education Program (NCEP) expert panel on detection, evaluation, and treatment of high blood cholesterol in adults (Adult Treatment Panel III). Final report. *Circulation*. 2002;106:3143-3421.
66. Grundy SM, Brewer HB, Cleeman JI, et al. Definition of metabolic syndrome: Report of the National Heart, Lung, and Blood Institute/American Heart Association conference on scientific issues related to definition. *Circulation*. 2004;109(3):433-438.
67. Kaur, Jaspinder. A comprehensive review on metabolic syndrome. *Cardiol Res Prac*. 2014; 943162.
68. Anand G, Katz PO. Gastroesophageal reflux disease and obesity. *Gastroenterol Clin North Am*. 2010;39(1):39-46.
69. Ayazi S, Hagen JA, Chan LS. Obesity and gastroesophageal reflux: quantifying the association between body mass index, esophageal acid exposure, and lower esophageal sphincter status in a large series of patients with reflux symptoms. *J Gastrointest Surg*. 2009;13(8):1440-1447.

70. Emerenziani S, Rescio MP, Guarino MP, et al. Gastro-esophageal reflux disease and obesity, where is the link? *World J Gastroenterol.* 2013;19(39):6536-6539.
71. Fabbrini E, Sullivan S, Klein S. Obesity and nonalcoholic fatty liver disease: biochemical, metabolic, and clinical implications. *Hepatology.* 2010;51(2):679-689.
72. World Gastroenterology Organisation. Nonalcoholic fatty liver disease and nonalcoholic steatohepatitis. June 2012. http://www.worldgastroenterology.org/NAFLD-NASH.html. Accessed August 1, 2017.
73. Wolin KY, Carson K, Colditz GA. Obesity and cancer. *Oncologist.* 2010;15(6):556-565.
74. World Cancer Research Fund/American Institute for Cancer Research. food, nutrition, physical activity, and the prevention of cancer: a global perspective, 2007. http://www.dietandcancerreport.org/cancer_resource_center/downloads/Second_Expert_Report_full.pdf. Accessed February 2, 2014.
75. Calle EE, Rodriguez C, Walker-Thurmond K, et al. Overweight, obesity, and mortality from cancer in a prospectively studied cohort of U.S. adults. *N Engl J Med.* 2003;348:1625-1638.
76. Vucenik I, Stains JP. Obesity and cancer risk: evidence, mechanisms, and recommendations. *Ann NY Acad Sci.* 2012;1271:37-43.
77. van Kruijsdijk RC, van der Wall E, Visseren FL. Obesity and cancer: the role of dysfunctional adipose tissue. *Cancer Epidemiol Biomarkers Prev.* 2009;18(10):2569-2578.
78. Gallagher EJ, LeRoith D. Minireview: IGF, insulin, and cancer. *Endocrinology.* 2011;152(7):2546-2551.
79. Anandacoomarasamy A, Caterson I, Sambrook P, et al. The impact of obesity on the musculoskeletal system. *Int J Obes.* 2008:(32)211-222.
80. Centers for Disease Control and Prevention. Arthritis-related statistics. https://www.cdc.gov/arthritis/data_statistics/arthritis-related-stats.htm. Updated March 6, 2017. Accessed June 1, 2017.
81. Anandacoomarasamy A, Fransen M, March L. Obesity and the musculoskeletal system. *Curr Opin Rheumatol.* 2009;21(1):71-77.
82. Hooper MM, Stellato TA, Hallowell PT, et al. Musculoskeletal findings in obese subjects before and after weight loss following bariatric surgery. *Int J Obes.* 2007;31(1):114-120.
83. Sleep-related breathing disorders in adults: recommendations for syndrome definition and measurement techniques in clinical research. The Report of an American Academy of Sleep Medicine Task Force. *Sleep.* 1990;22;667-689.
84. Drager LF, Lopes HF, Maki-Nunes C, et al. The impact of obstructive sleep apnea on metabolic and inflammatory markers in consecutive patients with metabolic syndrome. *PLoS One.* 2010;5:12065.
85. Isono S. Obesity and obstructive sleep apnoea: mechanisms for increased collapsibility of the passive pharyngeal airway. *Respirology.* 2012;17:32-42.
86. Partinen M, Jamieson A, Guilleminault C. Long-term outcome for obstructive sleep apnea syndrome patients. Mortality. *Chest.* 1988;94:1200-1204.
87. Seagle HM, Strain GW, Makris A, et al. Position of the American Dietetic Association: weight management. *J Am Diet Assoc.* 2009;109(2):330-346.
88. Tsai AG, Wadden TA. The evolution of very-low-calorie diets: An update and meta-analysis. *Obesity.* 2006;14(8):1283-1293.
89. Raynor HA, Champagne, CM. Position of The Academy of Nutrition and Dietetics: Interventions for the Treatment of Overweight and Obesity in Adults. *J Acad Nutr Diet.* 2016;116 (2):339-340.
90. Kong A, Beresford SA, Alfano CM, et al. Self-monitoring and eating-related behaviors are associated with 12-month weight loss in postmenopausal overweight-to-obese women. *J Acad Nutr Diet.* 2012;112(9):1428-1435.
91. Fabricatore AN. Behavior therapy and cognitive-behavioral therapy of obesity: Is there a difference? *J Am Diet Assoc.* 2007;107(1):92-99.
92. Butryn ML, Webb V, Wadden TA. Behavior treatment of obesity. *Psychiatr Clin North Am.* 2011; 34(4):841-859.
93. Physical Activity Guidelines Advisory Committee. *Physical Activity Guidelines Advisory Committee Report, 2008.* Washington, DC: U.S. Department of Health and Human Services, 2008.
94. Donnelly JE, Blair SN, Jakicic JM, Manore MM, Rankin JW, Smith BK; American College of Sports Medicine. American College of Sports Medicine Position Stand: Appropriate physical activity intervention strategies for weight loss and prevention of weight regain in adults. *Med Sci Sports Exerc.* 2009;Feb 41(2):459-471. doi: 10.1249/MSS.0b013e3181949333.
95. Look AHEAD Research Group. Eight-year weight losses with an intensive lifestyle intervention: The look AHEAD study. *Obesity.* 2014;22(1):5-13.
96. U.S. Food and Drug Administration. Medications target long-term weight control. http://www.fda.gov/ForConsumers/ConsumerUpdates/ucm312380.htm. Updated March 19, 2017. Accessed August 1, 2017.
97. Angrisani L, Santonicola A, Iovino P, et al. Obesity worldwide 2013. *Obes Surg.* 2015;25:1822.
98. Gastrointestinal surgery for severe obesity: National Institutes of Health Consensus Development Conference Statement. *Am J Clin Nutr.* 1992;55(2):615S-619S.
99. Abraham A, Ikramuddin S, Jahansouz C, et al. Trends in bariatric surgery: Procedure selection, revisional surgeries, and readmissions. *Obes Surg.* 2016;26:1371.
100. Himpens J, Cadiere GB, Bazi M, et al. Long-term outcomes of laparoscopic adjustable gastric banding. *Arch Surg.* 2011;146(7):802-807.
101. American Society for Metabolic and Bariatric Surgery. Story of obesity surgery. https://asmbs.org/resources/story-of-obesity-surgery. Accessed May 19, 2017.
102. Sjöström L, Narbo K, Sjöström CD, et al. Effects of bariatric surgery on mortality in Swedish obese subjects. *N Engl J Med.* 2007;357(8):741-752.
103. Balsiger BM, Poggio JL, Mai J, et al. Ten and more years after vertical banded gastroplasty as primary operation for morbid obesity. *J Gastrointest Surg.* 2000;4:598-605.
104. Stefater MA, Wilson-Perez HE, Chambers AP, et al. All bariatric surgeries are not created equal: insights from mechanistic comparisons. *Endo Rev.* 2013;33(4):595-622.
105. American Society for Metabolic and Bariatric Surgery. Bariatric surgery procedures. https://asmbs.org/patients/bariatric-surgery-procedures. Accessed May 19, 2017.
106. American Society for Metabolic and Bariatric Surgery. Estimate of bariatric surgery numbers 2011-2015. https://asmbs.org/resources/estimate-of-bariatric-surgery-numbers. Accessed May 19, 2017.
107. Moran TH. Cholecystokinin and satiety: Current perspectives. *Nutrition.* 2000;16:858-865.
108. American Society for Metabolic and Bariatric Surgery. Metabolic and bariatric surgery. https://asmbs.org/resources/metabolic-and-bariatric-surgery. Accessed June 30, 2017.
109. Liou AP, Paziuk M, Luevano JM, et al. Conserved shifts in the gut microbiota due to gastric bypass reduce host weight and adiposity. *Sci Transl Med.* 2013;5(178):178ra41.
110. Hutter MH, Schirmer BD, Jones DB, et al. First report from the American College of Surgeons Bariatric Surgery Center Network,

Laparoscopic sleeve gastrectomy has morbidity and effectiveness positioned between the band and the bypass. *Ann Surg.* 2011;254(3);410-422.

111. Schauer PR, Kashyap SR, Wolski K, et al. Bariatric surgery versus intensive medical therapy in obese patients with diabetes. *N Engl J Med.* 2012;366(17):1567-1576.

112. U.S. Food and Drug Administration. ORBERA Intragastric Balloon System - P140008. 2015. http://www.fda.gov/MedicalDevices/ProductsandMedicalProcedures/DeviceApprovalsandClearances/Recently-ApprovedDevices/ucm457416.htm. Accessed June 3, 2015.

113. Imaz I, Martínez-Cervell C, García-Alvarez EE, et al. Safety and effectiveness of the intragastric balloon for obesity. A meta-analysis. *Obes Surg.* 2008;18:841-846.

Chapter 9

Nutritional Management of Diabetes Mellitus

Nora Saul

Chapter Outline

Core Concepts
Introduction: Incidence and Scope
Pathophysiology of Diabetes
Screening, Risk Factors, and Diagnosis of Diabetes
Nutritional Requirements in Diabetes
Medical Nutrition Therapy for Diabetes
Exercise
Glycemic Targets and Self-Monitoring of Blood Glucose
Acute and Chronic Complications of Diabetes
Medical Treatment of Diabetes
Surgical Treatment Options
Hospitalization and Illness in Patients with Diabetes

CORE CONCEPTS

1. Diabetes is a life-long, chronic disease in which patient self-management is key.

2. While relative or absolute insulin deficiency is the major defining characteristic of diabetes, diabetes is a host of metabolically differentiated diseases.

3. Type 1 diabetes is an autoimmune disease brought about by the interaction of genetics and environmental triggers, resulting in a near or complete beta cell failure.

4. Type 2 diabetes results from relative insulin deficiency triggered by insulin resistance at the cellular level, coupled with a reduction in insulin production in the beta cells.

5. Insulin resistance is exacerbated by obesity.

6. During exercise, in the presence of elevated circulating insulin, glycogenolysis is blunted and insulin-enhanced muscle glucose uptake augmented, leaving the individual at risk for hypoglycemia.

7. Improvements in glycemic control stimulated by physical activity are generally due to reductions in insulin resistance in skeletal muscle.

8. For every 1% drop in blood glucose levels, there is a corresponding reduction in risk of complications of approximately 40%.

9. Although diet and exercise remain the cornerstone of diabetes management, all people diagnosed with type 1 diabetes will require insulin as a life-long treatment modality.

10. The most common and serious side effect of insulin therapy is hypoglycemia.

Learning Objectives

1. Identify the magnitude and etiology of the diabetes epidemic today.
2. Describe the pathophysiology of the different types of diabetes.
3. Assess nutrition status and formulate a nutrition care plan for people with type 1 diabetes.
4. Describe three methods of meal planning for people with diabetes.
5. Identify nutrition interventions for nephropathy, neuropathy, and cardiovascular disease.
6. Specify the classes of diabetes medications and their mechanism of action.
7. State the benefits of exercise and the exercise recommendations for people with diabetes.
8. Determine best enteral and parenteral feeding practices for blood glucose control.

Introduction: Incidence and Scope

In ancient Greece, diabetes mellitus was known as the sweet urine disease because the taste of the urine of people with diabetes was honey tinged. Even then, "physicians" knew this sweetness was a sign of poor health. Today, we know that diabetes encompasses a large group of metabolic conditions, all stemming from the body's inability to produce or use sufficient insulin to transfer glucose in the bloodstream into cells to be converted into energy or stored as fat for later use. Alterations in insulin action affect the metabolism of protein and fat in addition to glucose and, if left untreated, can damage a wide range of organs from the heart to the oral mucosa to the kidneys.

In the United States today, 30.3 million people have diabetes and 84 million have prediabetes, a condition of abnormal blood glucose metabolism that is not as severe as diabetes.[1] Of those, at least 7 million are not aware they have it. The diabetes epidemic is expected to grow more ominous over the next several decades. By the year 2050, it is estimated that 1 out of 3 people will have diabetes. Diabetes is now a woldwide epidemic, with China and India leading in diabetes prevalence.

Diabetes is a major drain on economic resources. It is the seventh leading cause of death and a major cause of heart disease and stroke. In 2012, the United States spent over $245 billion in total costs related to diagnosed diabetes.[1] This includes medical costs associated with the diagnosis and treatment of the disease and its complications, but also indirect costs such as lost wages and missed days of work.

The face of diabetes has changed markedly over the past 20 years. No longer is type 2 diabetes a disease relegated to older adults. Type 2 diabetes now strikes at younger and younger ages in susceptible populations. There has been a 68% increase in the diagnosis of type 2 diabetes in American Indian and Alaskan native youth ages 15 to 19 years in the years 1994 to 2004.[2] Most youth diagnosed with type 2 diabetes are overweight, sedentary, and have a strong family history of diabetes.

Caring for patients with diabetes is a challenge in both outpatient and inpatient settings. Because diabetes is a life-long, chronic disease in which self-management by the patient is key, this chapter will focus on assessment and treatment options for the ambulatory patient, while reviewing key concepts for the management of glucose control in the inpatient setting.

> **CORE CONCEPT 1**
>
> Diabetes is a life-long, chronic disease in which patient self-management is key.

Pathophysiology of Diabetes

Although the major defining characteristics of relative or absolute insulin deficiency are commonalities, diabetes is not a single disease; rather, it is a host of metabolically differentiated diseases under one rubric. The majority of people diagnosed with diabetes have type 2 diabetes, which accounts for between 90% and 95% of all instances of diabetes.[1] Type 1 diabetes, gestational diabetes, latent autoimmune diabetes in adults (LADA), chemically or surgically induced diabetes, diabetes related to specific genetic variations, and maturity-onset diabetes of the young (MODY) account for the remaining cases.

> **CORE CONCEPT 2**
>
> While relative or absolute insulin deficiency is the major defining characteristics of diabetes, diabetes is a host of metabolically differentiated diseases.

Type 1 Diabetes

Type 1 diabetes is an autoimmune disease brought about by the interaction of genetics and environmental triggers. The Diamond Project reported that type 1 diabetes incidence rates rise from infancy and peak during puberty (ages 10-14 years).[3] The hallmark of type 1 diabetes is beta cell destruction in which antibodies to insulin attack the insulin-producing beta cells in the pancreas, destroying

CASE STUDY INTRODUCTION

Aubree is a 12-year-old female patient presenting to the emergency department with vomiting and abdominal pain. Her mom describes a 2-week history of polyuria and polydipsia, accompanied by an approximate 10-pound weight loss over the last 3 months and blurred vision.

Anthropometric Data:

Height: 155 cm (61")
Weight: 41 kg (90 lbs)
BMI: 17 kg/m²

Last Pediatrician Visit (3 months ago)
Height: 155 cm (61")
Weight: 45 kg (99 lbs)

Biochemical Data:

Sodium 131 (135-145 mEq/L)
Potassium 4.0 (3.6-5.0 mEq/L)
Chloride 100 (98-110 mEq/L)
Carbon dioxide 10 (20-30 mEq/L)
Blood urea nitrogen 30 (6-24 mg/dL)
Creatine 1.5 (0.4-1.3 mg/dL)
Glucose 466 (70-139 mg/dL)

Magnesium 1.1 (1.3-2.1 mEq/L)
Calcium 8.8 (8.5-10.5 mEq/L)
Phosphorus 3.7 (2.7-4.5 mg/dL)
Osmolarity 299 (275-295 mOsm/kg)
pH 7.29 (7.35-7.45)
beta-hydroxybuterate 3 mmol/L H (none)
Urine Acetone +2 H (none)

Clinical Data:
Past Medical History: None
Family History: Grandfather died of renal disease, age 35; no family history of type 1 diabetes
Medications: None
Vital Signs: Blood pressure 140/80 mm Hg
Nutrition-Focused Physical Exam: Patient appears pale, fatigued, and a fruity odor is present on her breath, Kussmaul breathing

Dietary Data:
Dietary History: Patient normally eats a regular diet. Typically has good appetite except for most recently with vomiting and abdominal cramping.

Questions
1. Describe what is happening based on symptoms and biochemical data.
2. What are the initial treatment priorities for this patient?
3. What are Aubree's nutritional risk factors?
4. Which laboratory values should be closely monitored?
5. Calculate the anion gap for this patient.

most or all insulin secreting capacity. When diagnosed in childhood or the teenage years, beta cell destruction usually occurs rapidly, while patients diagnosed as adults may have a much longer period of beta cell decline. Studies of 50-year medalists (people with type 1 diabetes who have lived with diabetes for 50 years) at Joslin Diabetes Center have shown preservation of some insulin-producing capacity in those people who have avoided many of the acute and chronic complications of the disease.[4] Although clinical symptoms usually have a rapid onset, autoantibodies to the islet cells are often present months to years before the onset of clinical indicators and are helpful in distinguishing among diabetes types. Ninety percent of people with type 1 diabetes have at least one islet cell or endogenous insulin autoantibody present at diagnosis. These include islet cell autoantibodies, glutamic acid decarboxylase autoantibodies, insulinoma-associated 2 autoantibodies, insulin autoantibodies, and zinc transporter autoantibodies.[5]

CORE CONCEPT 3

Type 1 diabetes is an autoimmune disease brought about by the interaction of genetics and environmental triggers, resulting in a near or complete beta cell failure.

Common presenting symptoms of type 1 diabetes include **polyphagia** (hunger), **polyuria** (frequent urination), **polydispia** (thirst), and weight loss. Severe insulin deficiency precipitates **hyperglycemia** (the increase of glucose in the blood) and cellular energy deprivation. Under circumstances of **euglycemia** (normal blood sugar levels), virtually 100% of glucose that is presented to the kidneys is reabsorbed in the proximal renal tubules.[6] When the renal threshold for glucose is exceeded, glucose is diverted into the urine. To maintain the required fluid volume to produce adequate urine for glucose excretion, the renin-aldosterone system is activated, stimulating the thirst mechanism and perpetuating the cycle of unquenchable thirst and urination. Inability to access glucose triggers both increased appetite and a shift to fat metabolism with production of the ketone bodies: **acetone**, **acetoacetic acid**, and **beta-hydroxybutyric acid**. Normally, the acidic hydrogen ions are buffered by bicarbonate. However, the large quantity of acid produced by metabolism of the ketone bodies soon depletes the supply of bicarbonate, and metabolic acidosis occurs. Left untreated, **diabetic ketoacidosis** (DKA) ensues, a condition where excessive ketone bodies cause the blood pH to drop to dangerous levels and can quickly lead to death. Patients often present with depleted sodium levels secondary to fluid shifts caused by severe hyperglycemia. Insulin deficiency and acidosis will cause potassium to shift to the extracellular space. DKA can develop in less than 24 hours.[7] Many patients in DKA present with nausea, vomiting, and a fruity odor to their breath from the ketone buildup. In severe DKA, patients may have **Kussmaul's respirations**, abnormally deep breathing associated with metabolic acidosis. Diagnostic criteria for DKA are listed in **Table 9.1**.

> **PRACTICE POINT**
>
> Common presenting symptoms of type 1 diabetes include polyphagia (hunger), polyuria (frequent urination), polydispia (thirst), and weight loss.

Initial treatment for ketoacidosis includes intravenous insulin administration, correction of the metabolic acidosis and electrolyte abnormalities, and repletion of fluids. When stable, patients are started on subcutaneous insulin. For many, the reduction of glucose levels and the correction of metabolic parameters temporarily restore glucose homeostasis. This period of limited exogenous insulin is known as the honeymoon phase. Lasting up to a year, the honeymoon phase eventually ends with an increasing need for exogenous insulin until complete insulin coverage is required for both basal requirements and prandial coverage. People with type 1 diabetes require life-long administration of both basal and bolus insulin either by injection or through an insulin pump. **Figures 9.1** and **9.2** show examples of an insulin pump and insulin injection, respectively.

Type 2 Diabetes

Unlike type 1 diabetes, in which complete or near complete beta cell failure occurs, type 2 diabetes results from relative insulin deficiency triggered by insulin resistance at the cellular level, coupled with a reduction in insulin production in the beta cells. Reduction in beta cell mass may be due to apoptosis (cell death) without compensatory regeneration. A number of causal factors, including prolonged exposure to elevated glucose levels (glucotoxicity) and fatty acid concentrations (lipotoxicity), infiltration of pro-inflammatory cytokines, and deposition of islet cell amyloid, have been postulated to explain the damage to the beta cells.[8]

TABLE 9.1 PARTIAL DIAGNOSTIC CRITERIA OF KETOACIDOSIS

	Mild DKA	Moderate DKA	Severe DKA
Plasma glucose (mg/dL)	> 250	> 250	> 250
Arterial pH	7.25-7.30	7.00-7.24	< 7.00
Serum bicarbonate (mEq/L)	15-18	10-< 15	< 10
Urine and serum ketones	Present	Present	Present
Beta-hydroxybutyrate	Elevated	Elevated	Elevated
Anion gap	> 10	> 12	> 12

Chart with diagnostic criteria of ketoacidosis Diagnostic Criteria for Diabetic Ketoacidosis and Hyperosmolar Hyperglycemic State Adapted from: http://www.aafp.org/afp/2005/0501/p1705.html

have it until a routine physical examination brings the condition to light. Initially, insulin resistance of the muscle and liver cells stimulates the pancreas to produce more insulin and normal glucose levels are maintained. In many cases, people in the early stages (prediagnostic) of type 2 diabetes will hypersecrete insulin in compensation for insulin resistance.[9]

Insulin resistance is often exacerbated by obesity. Metabolic defects contributing to hyperglycemia include excess hepatic glucose secretion mediated by the loss of insulin's effects on suppressing **glycogenolysis** (breakdown of glycogen stores for glucose) and **gluconeogenesis** (synthesis of glucose from noncarbohydrate sources, usually amino acids). High circulating levels of free fatty acids increase insulin resistance and further impair pancreatic insulin secretion in adults and children.[11,12]

> **CORE CONCEPT 5**
>
> Insulin resistance is exacerbated by obesity.

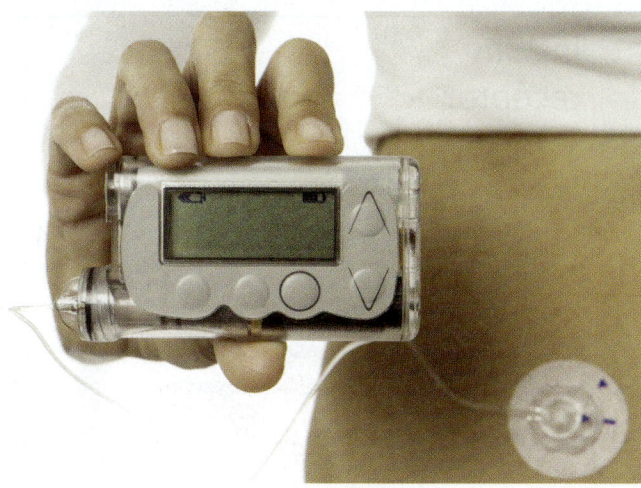

FIGURE 9.1 Example of an Insulin Pump Device
©Click and Photo/Shutterstock.

As the disease progresses, the pancreas's ability to meet the demand for insulin is overcome and diabetes ensues. The loss of postprandial euglycemia occurs, followed by the inability to maintain fasting glucose levels in target range. Insulin secretory capacity is diminished due the impairment of two incretin hormones, gastric inhibitory polypeptide (glucose-dependent insulinotropic polypeptide) and glucagon-like peptide 1 (GLP-1), which normally stimulate up to 50% of postprandial insulin secretion, as well as the loss of beta cell mass.[13]

By the time diabetes is diagnosed, islet cell function is reduced to approximately 50% of normal.[8] Insulin is secreted in two phases. After eating, there is an initial release of pre-formed insulin stored in granules in the beta cells. First phase insulin secretion occurs within 2 minutes of eating and lasts between 10 and 15 minutes. It is responsible for muscle cell glucose disposal, suppresses glucose production by the liver, and maintains normal blood glucose levels. The second phase, which may last 1 to 2 hours, is derived from newly formed insulin released in oscillating pulses. In type 2 diabetes, phase 1 response is destroyed and phase 2 is diminished, causing the insulin response time to a mixed meal to be delayed.[14]

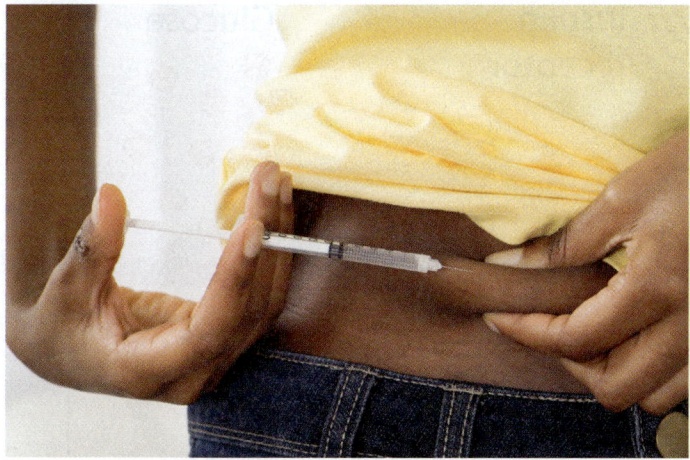

FIGURE 9.2 Injection of Insulin into the Abdominal Area
©Andrey_Popov/Shutterstock.

Insulin resistance is triggered by insulin receptor defects in target cells, with environmental factors such as obesity and lack of physical activity contributing to its development, as seen in **Figure 9.3**.[9]

Type 2 diabetes is not an autoimmune disease, but it has a large genetic component. Family history, in addition to lifestyle factors, plays a major role in its development. Risk factors include older age, family history, hypertension, dyslipidemia, obesity, lack of physical activity, ethnicity, polycystic ovary disease, and history of gestational diabetes.[10]

> **CORE CONCEPT 4**
>
> Type 2 diabetes results from relative insulin deficiency triggered by insulin resistance at the cellular level, coupled with a reduction in insulin production in the beta cells.

The onset of type 2 diabetes is usually insidious, occurring over a number of years. Many people are unaware they

> **PRACTICE POINT**
>
> By the time diabetes is diagnosed, islet cell function is reduced to approximately 50% of normal.

A third contributor to type 2 diabetes is the increase in hepatic glucose output due to greater gluconeogenesis driven by hepatic insulin resistance. The hormonal picture is one of high levels of glucagon and cortisol with even smaller amounts of insulin.

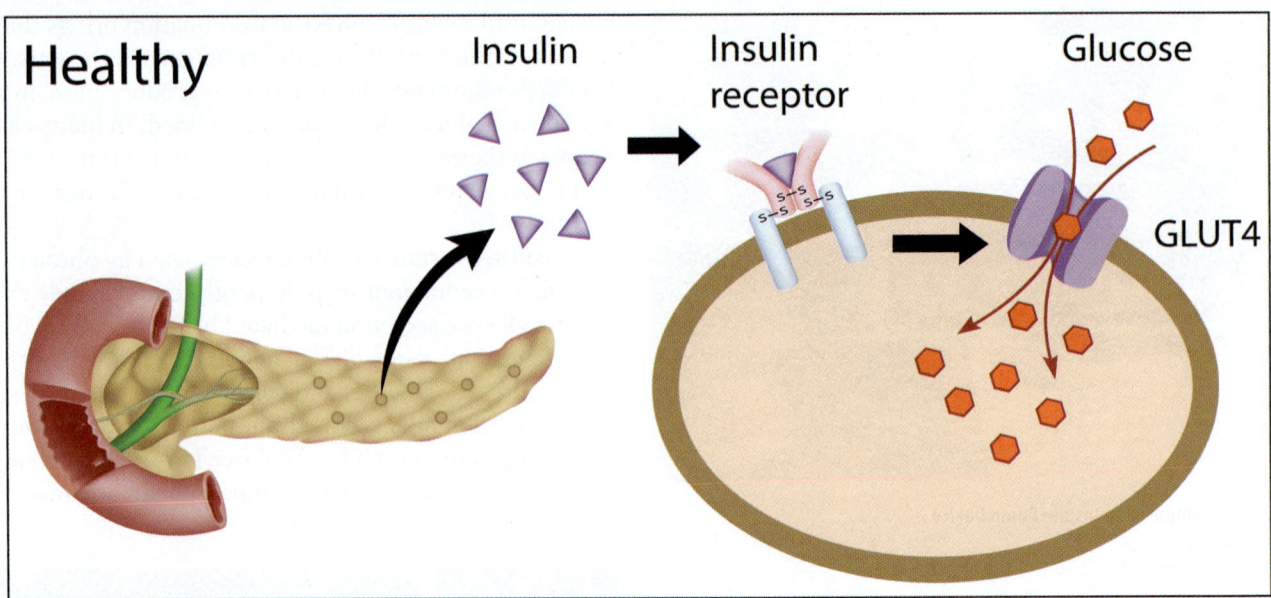
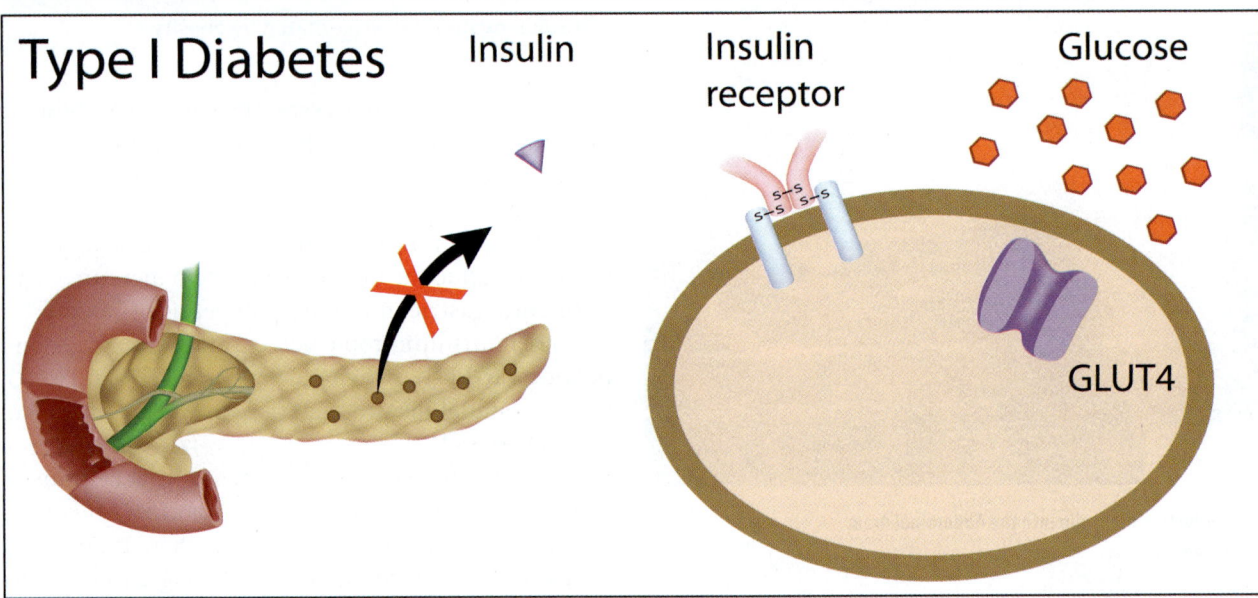
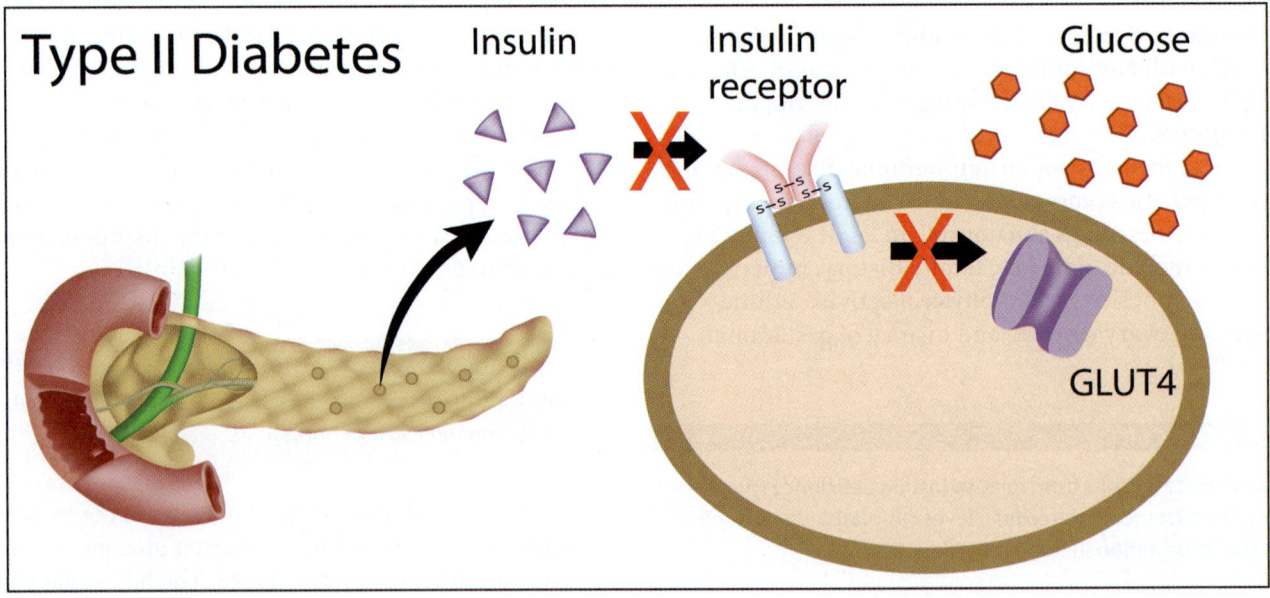

FIGURE 9.3 Insulin Receptor Defects
© Alila Medical Media/Shutterstock.

Treatment of type 2 diabetes focuses on its various metabolic defects and the degree of hyperglycemia present at the time of diagnosis. People may begin treatment with lifestyle measures and/or oral medications, but over time there is a diminution in beta cell mass, leading to the need for eventual insulin administration.

Gestational Diabetes

Gestational diabetes (GDM) is defined as any degree of abnormal glucose tolerance with first appearance or recognition during pregnancy.[15] Pregnancies complicated by glucose intolerance are on the rise due to the explosion of obesity and sedentary behavior in the United States, with higher rates among ethnic communities and those of limited economic resources. Current prevalence estimates vary widely, from between 2% and 10% of all pregnancies, depending on the groups surveyed.[16] Pregnancy distorts the normal hormonal milieu toward one of insulin resistance and decreased insulin output. During the first trimester, insulin secretion increases, fostering the accumulation of adipose tissue. In the later stages of pregnancy, insulin resistance and lipolysis develop. Late gestation is characterized by a several-fold increase in circulating postprandial free fatty acid levels, which further reduces insulin activity and stimulates liver glycogenolysis, increasing insulin resistance. Several pregnancy hormones facilitate this process. Human placental lactogen increases up to 30-fold throughout pregnancy and human placental growth hormone increases 6- to 8-fold during gestation, replacing normal pituitary growth hormone in the maternal circulation.[17]

Although glucose levels are usually not as elevated as those with overt diabetes, gestational diabetes carries significant risks for the mother and the fetus. GDM increases the mother's risk for preeclampsia and cesarean section. Infants born to mothers with uncontrolled gestational diabetes are at risk for excessive weight gain, shoulder dystocia, postdelivery hypoglycemia, and respiratory distress syndrome. Neonatal hypoglycemia, jaundice, polycythemia, and hypocalcaemia may complicate infant delivery. Women also face the possibility of developing obesity and type 2 diabetes later in life.[18] Any degree of maternal hyperglycemia is injurious to the fetus.[19] Alterations in glucose metabolism are a continuum, which has made choosing an ideal screening paradigm so difficult. The International Association of Diabetes and Pregnancy Study Groups published their recommendations on the Diagnosis and Classification of Hyperglycemia in Pregnancy in March 2010 after reviewing the results of the Hyperglycemia and Adverse Pregnancy Outcome study (HAPO).[20] They recommended a single method of screening for gestational diabetes. This method employs a 2-hour oral glucose tolerance test (OGTT) using a 75-g glucose solution. Blood glucose measurements are drawn fasting and at 1 hour and 2 hours after drinking a sweetened beverage. Diagnostic cutoffs for the diagnosis of GDM using both methods are listed in **Table 9.2**.

Some women with overt diabetes would be misdiagnosed following this guideline. Therefore, the American Diabetes Association recommends that women with risk

TABLE 9.2 SCREENING CRITERIA FOR GESTATIONAL DIABETES

Two-step approach	One-step approach
Prescreen with 50-g glucose challenge between 24 and 28 weeks' gestation. Screening threshold ≥140mg/dL	Screen with 2-hour OGTT using 75-g glucose between 24 and 28 weeks' gestation. One value exceeding the defined thresholds is diagnostic for GDM: • Fasting: ≥92 mg/dL (5.1 mmol/L) • 1 hour: ≥180 mg/dL (10.0 mmol/L) • 2 hours: ≥153 mg/dL (8.5 mmol/L)
3-hour OGTT using 100 g glucose	
Two values exceeding the defined threshold are diagnostic for GMD	
• Fasting: ≥95 mg/dL (5.3 mmol/L) • 1 hour: 180 mg/dL (10.0 mmol/L) • 2 hours: 155 mg/dL (8.6 mmol/L) • 3 hours: 140mg/dL (7.8 mmol/L)	

Data from Diabetes Care January 2003 vol. 26 no. suppl 1 s103-s105 and table 6 in Standards of Medical in Diabetes 2013.

factors for diabetes should be screened during their first prenatal visit.[21] However, the American College of Obstetricians and Gynecologists has voted to continue to use previous screening criteria involving a two-step approach, in which all women are screened using a 50-g glucose solution. Those whose blood levels exceed 140 mg/dL 1 hour after ingesting the beverage go on to take a 100-g OGTT O'Sullivan screening test.[22]

Screening, Risk Factors, and Diagnosis of Diabetes

Diabetes Screening and Risk Factors

In 2011, the Centers for Disease Control and Prevention undertook a study to determine when and if large-scale screenings for type 2 diabetes were warranted. They determined that the yield of diabetes diagnoses from community-based screenings is poor and did not represent a good use of resources, and that identification of persons with diabetes should be accomplished in the clinical setting. Currently it is recommended that screening for prediabetes and risk of future diabetes should be done for all individuals 45 years of age and older, asymptomatic adults who are overweight or obese with a body mass index (BMI) ≥25 (≥23 in Asian Americans), and adults having one or more risk factors as defined in **Table 9.3**.

Diagnostic Criteria and Staging

Diabetes is diagnosed by clinical presentation along with a causal glucose level above 200 mg/dL or with the variety of blood tests shown in **Table 9.4**. Fasting glucose and oral glucose tolerance tests have been used for many years. In 2010, the Hemoglobin A1C test (A1C), also known as HbA1c or glycohemoglobin test, was added to these other well-established methods of diagnosing diabetes. The A1C test is based on the attachment of glucose to hemoglobin, the protein in red blood cells. Since the average lifespan of a red blood cell is about 3 months, A1C reflects the 2-3 month average blood glucose level, reported as a percentage. The A1C is often the easiest test for patients to complete because it can be accomplished without fasting.

In type 1 diabetes, the progression of the disease that accompanies beta cell failure is well characterized. The American Diabetes Association provides staging for type 1 diabetes (**Table 9.5**). At least two autoimmune antibodies are persistently present well before the onset of symptoms or an increase in biochemical indices such as glucose and A1C, making these indices useful predictors of diabetes and hyperglycemia. During stage 1, despite the presence

TABLE 9.4 DIAGNOSTIC CRITERIA FOR DIABETES

Hemoglobin A1C ≥6.5

Fasting plasma glucose (FPG) ≥126 mg/dL (7.0 mmol/L)

Postprandial glucose (PPG) ≥200mg/dL

OGTT at 2 hours ≥200 mg/dL

A random plasma glucose ≥200 mg/dL in the presence of the classic clinical symptoms of diabetes

Data from American Diabetes Association. Classification and diagnosis of diabetes. Sec. 2. In Standards of Medical Care in Diabetes 2017. *Diabetes Care.* 2017;40(suppl 1):S11–S24.

TABLE 9.3 RISK FACTORS INDICATING THE NEED TO SCREEN FOR DIABETES AND PREDIABETES

Risk Factor Category	Indicators
Family history	First-degree relative with diabetes
Medical history	Cardiovascular disease, polycystic ovary syndrome, women diagnosed with gestational diabetes
Biochemical indices	HgA1c ≥ 5.7%, Impaired glucose tolerance (IGT)* or Impaired fasting glucose (IFG)**, High Density Lipoprotein cholesterol ≤ 35 mg/dL or Triglycerides ≥ 250 mg/dL
Clinical conditions	Hypertension (HTN): ≥140/90 mm Hg, factors associated with insulin resistance (acanthosis nigricans, severe obesity), physical inactivity
Ethnicity	High-risk ethnicity: African American, Latino, Native American, Asian American, Pacific Islander

*IGT is a higher than normal glucose level 2 hours after an oral glucose tolerance test (140-199 mg/dL). A result in that range is consistent with prediabetes.
**IFG is is a higher than normal fasting glucose level (100-125 mg/dL). A result in that range is consistent with prediabetes.
Data from American Diabetes Association. Classification and diagnosis of diabetes. Sec. 2. In: Standards of Medical Care in Diabetes 2017. *Diabetes Care.* 2017;40(suppl 1):S11–S24.

TABLE 9.5 CRITERIA FOR STAGING OF TYPE 1 DIABETES

Stages	Clinical Characteristics and Diagnostic Criteria	Laboratory Indices
1	Presence of autoimmunity Presymptomatic Euglycemia	Presence of two or more autoantibodies Normal FPG and PPG
2	Autoimmunity Dysglycemia (increased fasting glucose and impaired glucose tolerance) Presymptomatic	Presence of multiple autoantibodies FPG: 100-125 mg/dL PPG: 140-199 mg/dL HgA1c 5.7% to 6.4% or ≥10% increase in A1C
3	New-onset hyperglycemia Symptomatic	Meets standard diabetes screening criteria as described in Table 9.4

Data from American Diabetes Association. Classification and diagnosis of diabetes. Sec. 2. In Standards of Medical Care in Diabetes 2017. *Diabetes Care.* 2017;40(suppl 1):S11–S24.

of these antibodies, euglycemia exists. As beta cell failure progresses into stage 2, impaired glucose tolerance and fasting glucose levels becomes evident without clinical manifestations until the patient progresses into stage 3.

Nutritional Requirements in Diabetes

Nutritional requirements for people with diabetes are similar to those of the general healthy population. There is not one optimal macronutrient composition of the diet for people with diabetes. Studies have shown that a variety of dietary patterns can result in adequate glycemic control.[24] Low-fat and low-carbohydrate, omnivore and vegetarian diets have been demonstrated to be effective in promoting glycemic control and short-term weight loss. Low-carbohydrate diets have an advantage in producing a more favorable cardiac profile, improving triglyceride levels and diminishing the reduction in high-density lipoprotein levels that occur with weight loss.[25] Recently, research has determined that a Mediterranean-style eating pattern can be effective in achieving glycemic control and improving cardiovascular risk factors, including blood pressure and lipids, without the need for weight loss.[26,27]

Carbohydrate

The amount of carbohydrate consumed and the available insulin are the most important factors determining postmeal blood glucose levels.[28] Carbohydrate modification was the cornerstone of nutrition intervention prior to the discovery of insulin. An early treatment modality for diabetes was the near elimination of carbohydrate-containing foods from the diet. Although effective in lowering blood glucose levels, this approach ignored the role of carbohydrate as the body's main source of energy and needed vitamins, minerals, fiber, and phyto substances. Diets overly restricted in carbohydrate can cause ketosis and dehydration, which is a serious concern, particularly in the elderly. Low-carbohydrate diets are often constipating due to their lack of fiber and, because of what many perceive as a lack of palatability, can be difficult to follow long-term.

> **PRACTICE POINT**
>
> The amount of carbohydrate consumed and the available insulin are the most important factors determining postmeal blood glucose levels.

Neither the American Diabetes Association nor the Academy of Nutrition and Dietetics specify a particular amount of carbohydrate to be used in the diets of people with diabetes. Both organizations recommend that the percentage of carbohydrate in the diet be individualized to the needs and preferences of the individual with diabetes. Joslin Diabetes Center, in its Clinical Nutrition Guideline for Overweight and Obese Adults with Type 2 diabetes, Prediabetes, or a High Risk for Developing Type 2 Diabetes, recommends that carbohydrate be restricted to between 40% and 45% of calories as a means to reduce excess glycemic excursions.[29]

> **PRACTICE POINT**
>
> The percentage of carbohydrate in the diet should be individualized to the needs and preferences of the individual with diabetes.

Carbohydrate foods consist of grains, legumes, milk and yogurts, fruit, and starchy and nonstarchy vegetables. Nonstarchy vegetables, unless consumed in large quantities, provide little carbohydrate and in practical terms are often considered free foods in the diet. The brain and nervous system have an obligatory requirement for glucose, and the Institute of Medicine recommends a minimal intake of 130 g of carbohydrate per day to supply the brain, nervous system, and red blood cells with glucose without reliance on gluconeogenesis from other fuel sources.[30]

Glycemic Index

The type of carbohydrate consumed is secondary to the total quantity eaten in affecting glycemic response. However, the digestibility of different carbohydrate sources affects blood glucose excursions differently. The **glycemic index** (GI) describes the quantity and rate at which different carbohydrate foods influence blood glucose response.[31,32] Fifty grams of carbohydrate-containing foods are ranked according to how much they raise

⚠ Clinical Controversy

Although the superiority of low-carbohydrate diets for short-term improvements in metabolic parameters, such as fasting blood glucose and triglycerides, are well established, the distribution of nutrients that supplies the best strategy to achieve weight loss is still under consideration. Attaining and maintaining a 5% to 7% loss of body weight is considered a crucial element in the treatment of type 2 diabetes for those who are overweight or obese. There are various finding on this topic in the literature. Nordmann et al. found that low carbohydrate, non-energy restricted diets appear to be at least as effective as low fat, energy restricted diets for weight loss for up to 1 year. Sacks et al. report that reduced-calorie diets, regardless of the macronutrient emphasis, can result in meaningful weight loss. Hall et al. report that a fat restriction is more effective than a carbohydrate restriction in reducing body fat. Bazzano et al. found that a low-carbohydrate diet was more effective for weight loss than a low fat diet.

1. Nordmann AJ, Nordmann A, Briel M, et al. Effects of low-carbohydrate vs low fat diets on weight loss and cardiovascular risk factors: a meta-analysis of randomized controlled trials. *Arch Intern Med*. 2006;166:285–293.
2. Sacks FM, Bray GA, Carey VJ, et al. Comparison of weight-loss diets with different compositions of fat, protein, and carbohydrates. *N Engl J Med*. 2009;360:859–873.
3. Hall KD, Bernis T, Brychta R, et al. Calorie for calorie, dietary fat restriction results in more body fat loss than carbohydrate restriction in people with obesity. *Cell Metab*. 2015;10.1016/j.cmet2015.07.021
4. Bazzano L, Hu T, Reynolds, K. Effects of low-carbohydrate and low-fat diets: a randomized trial. *Ann Intern Med*. 2014;161:309–316.

Questions:
1. What are the advantages and disadvantages of following a carbohydrate restricted eating pattern?
2. After evaluating the evidence presented in these papers, how would you advise a DM patient regarding a weight loss diet?
3. What factors about your patient should you consider before recommending a specific dietary pattern?

---

glucose levels in comparison to either 50 g of glucose or 50 g of white bread. Foods are ranked in comparison to the ranking of glucose: low glycemic foods are designated as less than 55, intermediate GI foods have a designation of between 56 and 70, and those over 70 are considered to have a high GI.

Many variables affect the GI of a food. Fat, fiber, acidity level, the form in which it is consumed (solid, liquid), processing, and cooking can alter how quickly a food is digested. In general, those foods that contain greater amounts of fat and fiber have a lower GI. Although the GI can be a valuable tool for people with diabetes to refine their metabolic control, its use is not without certain caveats. Because fat plays such a seminal role in determining the GI of a food, some foods, such as candy bars, often have far lower GI rankings than more healthful foods such as skim milk, yet the latter is a better choice from a nutrition standpoint.

Glycemic Load

The GI of a food is the same no matter how much carbohydrate is consumed. The **glycemic load** (GL) attempts to reconcile the digestibility rate of foods with the amount of carbohydrate they contain. The GL is calculated by multiplying the GI ranking of the food by the number of grams of carbohydrate in a serving and then dividing by 100. A GL of 10 or less is low, 11 to 19 is medium, and greater than 20 is high. For example, the GI of a white bagel is 72; the GL of a 5-oz bagel is 51, and that of a 2.5-oz bagel is 25. There are approximately 75 g of carbohydrate in a 5-oz bagel versus 35 g of carbohydrate in a 2-oz bagel, and so:

$$72 \text{ (GI)} \times 75 \text{ (g of carbohydrate)} = 5400/100$$
$$= 54 \text{ GL (5-oz bagel)}$$
$$72 \text{ (GI)} \times 35 \text{ (g of carbohydrate)} = 2520/100$$
$$= 25 \text{ GL (2.5-oz bagel)}$$

It is important to remember that the GI and GL are based on individual foods, but that people eat mixed meals. The GI and GL of a mixed meal will be the average of all carbohydrate foods consumed. Foods that are primarily protein and fat do not have a GI. The GI is often an adjunct tool people with diabetes can use in addition to carbohydrate regulation. The response of glucose levels to the same quantity of different GI foods can be ascertained by checking blood glucose both before and 2 or 3 hours after eating. See **Table 9.6** for a sample of the GI and GL of a variety of foods.

It should be mentioned that there can be significant variability in the GI among the same foods due to differences in growing conditions, brand, and variety, as well as a wide range of responses to the same food in different individuals. Patients often need to take a trial and error approach to how specific foods will influence their glycemic control by checking their blood glucose after meals.

TABLE 9.6 GLYCEMIC INDEX AND GLYCEMIC LOAD OF SELECTED FOODS

Food	Serving Size in Grams	Glycemic Index	Glycemic Load
Bagel, white	70	72	25
Hamburger Bun	30	61	9
White Bread	30	71	10
Whole Wheat Bread	30	71	9
Oatmeal	55	250	13
Cornflakes	30	93	23
Raisin Bran	30	61	12
Corn on the Cob	150	60	20
Rice, white	150	89	43
Rice, brown	150	50	16
Pasta, white, boiled	180	46	22
Milk, whole	250 (ml)	41	5
Milk, skim	250 (ml)	32	4
Ice cream (regular fat)	50	57	6
Apple	120	39	6
Banana, ripe	120	62	16
Grapefruit	120	25	3
Orange	120	72	4
Potatoes, baked russet	150	111	33
Carrots	80	35	2

Data from "International tables of glycemic index and glycemic load values: 2008" by Fiona S. Atkinson, Kaye Foster-Powell, and Jennie C. Brand-Miller in the December 2008 issue of *Diabetes Care*, Vol. 31, number 12, pages 2281-2283.

Consistency in the timing and amount of carbohydrate eaten at meals has been shown to improve glycemic control in those people with type 1 and type 2 diabetes who use oral hypoglycemic medications or fixed or sliding scale insulin regimens.[33,34] Greater flexibility in carbohydrate intake and improved glycemic control have also been shown in people who match their insulin doses to the amount of carbohydrate they eat at meals.[35,36]

Fiber

Fiber is defined as the indigestible parts of plant products. Dietary fiber can be divided into two types: soluble and insoluble. From a practical standpoint, fiber has no caloric value, although metabolism of bacteria in the colon can contribute to energy requirements. Insoluble fiber provides bulk to the stool and reduces gut transit time, which can alleviate constipation. Soluble fiber can lower cholesterol

TABLE 9.7 SOURCES OF SOLUBLE AND INSOLUBLE FIBER

Soluble Fiber Sources	Insoluble Fiber Sources
Oat bran	Wheat bran
Citrus fruits	Carrots
Legumes	Cabbage
Apples	Corn

levels by two mechanisms. One is by binding to cholesterol and decreasing its absorption in the intestine. The second mechanism involves reducing enteroheptic recirculation of bile acids. Soluble fiber binds to cholesterol and bile acids in the intestine and promotes their excretion in the feces. The removal of bile acids leads to a decrease in the amount of bile acids in the recirculated bile acid pool. The liver must then produce additional bile acids to compensate for this loss. Since cholesterol is necessary to make bile acids, this deficit in the bile acid pool leads to a decrease in intracellular cholesterol stores which in turn increases catabolism of low density lipoprotein (LDL). Soluble fiber also slows gastric emptying, and dietary fiber can reduce glucose levels when consumed in quantities approaching 50 g.[37] Recommendations for fiber intake are between 25 and 35 g per day, with higher values for men and younger individuals, or 14 g of fiber per 1000 calories.[38] Actual fiber intakes for Americans are significantly below recommendations, in the range of 13 to 15 g per day.[39] See **Table 9.7** for examples of foods that are high in fiber.

Overall, it is important to encourage people with diabetes to choose carbohydrates from vegetables, fruits, whole grains, legumes, and low-fat dairy products over those that contain added sugars, fats, and sodium, such as sugar-sweetened beverages, bakery products, or frozen desserts

Sucrose and Other Nutritive Sweeteners

The time is long past where sucrose was a forbidden component in the diet of persons with diabetes. It has been well established that sucrose and other caloric sweeteners do not increase glycemic response any more than equivalent amounts of starch.[40,41] In fact, as foods containing sucrose may also have appreciable amounts of fat, the rise in glucose levels from these foods compared to equivalent amounts of carbohydrate from pure monosaccharide may be attenuated. However, caloric sweeteners such as sucrose, fructose, honey, corn syrup, and molasses contain four calories per gram, the same as most dietary carbohydrate. Many foods containing a significant amount of sucrose or other caloric sweeteners are high in calories and fat and lacking in micronutrients. Therefore, sucrose-containing foods should not replace calories supplied from foods from the major food groups in the diet. Substitution of fructose for glucose, which does have a lower glycemic index, does not appear to provide any dietary advantage. When consumed in excessive quantities, fructose can exacerbate hypertriglyceridemia or lead to further deterioration in glucose levels in those in poor metabolic control since fructose is converted to glucose when insulin is lacking.[42]

> **PRACTICE POINT**
>
> Sucrose can be incorporated as a part of the diet in persons with diabetes.

Protein

Protein has limited impact on glycemic response. In people with type 2 diabetes, protein causes an increase in insulin response without a corresponding rise in blood glucose levels.[43] It has been hypothesized that higher protein diets may be beneficial in the control of diabetes. Several studies have found a role of higher protein diets (28% to 40% of total energy) in the reduction of A1C and the improvement of lipid levels.[44,45] The influence of protein on insulin response and glucose excursions in persons with type 1 diabetes is less clear-cut.[46,47] Increasing protein intake may help with promoting satiety, which can aid in calorie reduction in people who need weight loss.[48,49]

The Academy of Nutrition and Dietetics Practice Guideline for type 1 and type 2 diabetes in adults recommends a usual protein intake of 15% to 20% of daily energy.[28] Note that the American Diabetes Association takes no position on the optimal amount of protein in the diet of people with diabetes other than to recommend that it be individualized to meet patient needs. On the other hand, the Joslin Diabetes Center believes that the evidence for higher protein intakes for people with type 2 diabetes who are overweight is convincing and recommends that protein make up between 20% and 30% of calories.[9]

Fat

The acceptable macronutrient range for fat set by the Institute of Medicine is between 20% and 35% of calories, although no tolerable upper intake level is given.[30] The Dietary Guidelines 2015 recommends limiting saturated fat to 10% of calories.[50]

Excess saturated fat has been linked to insulin resistance and metabolic syndrome.[51] Dietary fat consumed alone or as part of a mixed meal slows gastric emptying times and, when eaten in large enough quantities, increases insulin requirements.[52] Conversely, moderate amounts of healthful dietary fats may help prevent rapid spikes in blood glucose associated with large carbohydrate intakes. People using fast-acting insulin at mealtimes may need to adjust insulin doses upward and change insulin delivery times when dietary fat makes up a substantial portion of the meal.

People with diabetes are at two to four times the risk of cardiovascular disease compared to the general population. Cardiovascular disease (CVD) strikes at a younger age and puts those with diabetes at the same risk of CVD as those without diabetes who have preexisting cardiovascular damage.[53] Reduction in saturated and trans fats is associated with both an improvement in lipid profiles and better glycemic control. Several studies have also shown that a Mediterranean dietary pattern, which is lower in total carbohydrate and higher in monounsaturated fatty acids, may be beneficial in controlling cardiac risk factors, as well as glycemia even in the absence of weight reduction in persons with type 2 diabetes.[27,54] Omega-3 fatty acids help reduce triglyceride levels and cardiac arrhythmias, although there may be an accompanying rise in LDL cholesterol when supplements are used. The recommendation for people with diabetes, as well as the general public, is to eat foods high in long-chain omega-3 fatty acids such as fatty fish, nuts, and seeds.[55] Despite the improvement in lipid profiles, results of trials looking at the outcome of supplementing eicosapentaenoic and docosahexaenoic fatty acids have not shown a decrease in the rate of cardiovascular events.[55-57]

At 9 calories per gram, fat provides more than double the caloric density of protein and carbohydrate. Therefore, when weight loss is a goal, persons with diabetes may need to moderate total fat intake as part of a calorie-reduced meal plan.

Nonnutritive Sweeteners

Although caloric sweeteners are permitted as part of a food plan for persons with diabetes, the calorie and carbohydrate load associated with their use has encouraged the development of alternative, low-calorie sweeteners. Nonnutritive sweeteners, also known as artificial sweeteners, are often hundreds of times sweeter than their counterparts and require the use of only very small amounts to mirror the sweetness of sugar. They provide few, if any, calories or carbohydrate. All of the nonnutritive sweeteners on the market in the United States have undergone premarket safety testing or have been granted GRAS (generally regarded as safe) status by the Food and Drug Administration (FDA). Use of each of the sweeteners is permitted during pregnancy, although some healthcare providers discourage the consumption of saccharin because it crosses the placenta.

In the past few years, there have been a number of epidemiological studies linking of use of nonnutritive sweeteners, especially in diet sodas, to an increase in caloric intake and weight gain. Several theories have been postulated as to the mechanism of this phenomenon, including that consumption of liquids containing sweetness, but no calories, stimulates appetite receptors in the brain. At present there is inadequate evidence to support or refute these propositions.[58] Currently, the American Diabetes Association states that nonnutritive sweeteners can be used to reduce overall caloric intake associated with caloric sweeteners, presuming that intake does not compensate by consuming other caloric foods.[55] For all nonnutritive sweeteners, the FDA determines an acceptable daily limit (ADL) of intake.

See Table 9.8 for details. The ADL includes a 100-fold safety factor and generally exceeds the average intake of these sweeteners by people with diabetes.[59-61]

Alcohol

Moderate intake of alcoholic beverages has little effect on glycemic control, and there is a body of evidence that suggests that it may improve cardiovascular risk and overall glycemic control.[62,63] Alcohol is digested and absorbed in the body without the need for insulin. It interferes with gluconeogenesis and blunts the hormonal counter-regulatory response to **hypoglycemia** (undesirably low blood sugar, less than 70 mg/dL). The liver requires approximately an hour to process an ounce of alcohol. During this time, it effectively suspends its role in glucose replenishment; therefore, alcohol can induce hypoglycemia in people with diabetes who take insulin or oral insulin secretagogues. This may be undesirable because the body's response to alcohol in someone with diabetes can be quite complex. Many alcoholic beverages contain significant amounts of carbohydrate; a piña colada, for example, has approximately 30 grams of carbohydrate. Depending on the number and type of alcoholic beverages consumed, balancing the need for insulin to metabolize the carbohydrate against the glucose lowering effects of alcohol can be difficult. Counseling patients to limit and/or avoid alcoholic beverages with higher carbohydrate content is often advisable. Consuming alcohol with foods that contain carbohydrate can help prevent delayed hypoglycemia.

> **PRACTICE POINT**
>
> Alcohol can induce hypoglycemia in people with diabetes who take insulin or oral insulin secretagogues.

Although moderate alcohol consumption may bestow some metabolic benefits, intemperate intake is discouraged. Excess alcohol consumption (greater than three drinks a day) has been associated with both hyperglycemia and hypertension.[63] Alcohol is a source of nonnutritive calories, providing 7 calories per gram. Excess consumption of alcohol can displace the intake of nutrient-dense food in the diet and promote weight gain.

Persons with diabetes who choose to drink should be counseled to do so in moderation: no more than one alcoholic beverage per day for women and no more than two alcoholic beverages per day for men. One alcoholic beverage is defined as 1.5 oz of distilled spirits, 12 oz of beer, or 5 oz of wine. To reduce the risk of hypoglycemia, those persons taking insulin or oral secretagogues should be advised to eat carbohydrate-containing foods along with their alcoholic beverages.

Micronutrients

There is no evidence that suggests that people with diabetes who eat a balanced diet have micronutrient needs in excess of the general public. Although both chromium and magnesium play pivotal roles in glucose metabolism, and

TABLE 9.8 NONNUTRITIVE SWEETENERS

Generic Name	Brand Name	Sweetness Compared to Sucrose (Number of Times Sweeter)	ADI (mg/kg/day)	Number of 12-oz Soda Cans = to ADI for 150-lb (68-kg) Person	Number of Table-top Sweetener Packets = to ADI for 150-lb (68-kg) Person	Cooking and Baking Conversion for ½ cup Granular White Sugar	Heat Stable
Acesulfame-K	Sweet One, Sunett	200	15	25	20	6 packets	Yes
Aspartame	Equal, NutraSweet	200	40	14-17	68	½ cup	No
Neotame	Newtame	7000-13000	2	ND	200	0.125 cup	Yes
Saccharin	Sweet'N Low, Sweet Twin	300	5	42	9	½ cup	Yes
Sucralose	Splenda	600	15	15	30	¼ cup Splenda Sugar Blend	Yes
Stevia	Truvia, PureVia, Sweet Leaf	200-300	4	16	30	12 packets	Yes
Luo Han Guo	Nectresse, Monk Fruit in the Raw, PureLo	150	ND	ND	ND	12 packets	Yes

ADI = acceptable daily intake. ADI calculation is determined by dividing X mg/kg by 100, where X = daily dose that showed no effect.

ND = No Data Note: Beverages, sauces, puddings, and frozen desserts are better sweetened with nonnutritive sweeteners than cakes and cookies, which depend on sugar for moistness and tenderness as well as sweetness. Generally, no more than half the amount of sugar called for in the recipe should be replaced with artificial nonnutritive sweeteners.

Data from Nonnutritive Sweeteners: Current Use and Health Perspectives. A Scientific Statement from the American Heart Association and the American Diabetes Association Diabetes Care August 2012 vol. 35 no. 8 1798-1808; FDA Additional Information about High-Intensity Sweeteners Permitted for use in Food in the United States University of Illinois Extension Can You Cook and Bake with Artificial Sweeteners http://extension.illinois.edu/diabetes2/subsection.cfm?SubSectionID=34 Updated June 2014. http://www.fda.gov/Food/IngredientsPackagingLabeling/FoodAdditivesIngredients/ucm397725.htm.

supplementation for those individuals who are deficient in these nutrients is beneficial in restoring euglycemia, increasing intake in those with adequate reserves has not be proven efficacious.[64,65] Individuals who are infirm, elderly, pregnant, vegan, or following very-low-calorie diets may require supplementation of specific nutrients.

Recently, there has been great interest in the connection between vitamin D and insulin resistance. Vitamin D is associated with glucose-induced insulin secretion. Many persons with and without diabetes are vitamin D deficient, especially if they happen to live in climates far from the equator. The incidence of type 1 diabetes increases the farther people live from the equator.[66,67] Recommended Dietary Allowance for vitamin D for adults 19 to 70 years is 600 IU per day; for people older than 70 years, the requirement increases to 800 IU.[30] Because vitamin D is so poorly distributed in the food supply and sunscreen is ubiquitously used, recommending a vitamin D supplement to persons with diabetes, especially the elderly, may be appropriate.

Herbal and Dietary Supplements

A variety of dietary supplements, such as bitter melon, prickly pear cactus, and fenugreek, can have effects on glucose metabolism and insulin resistance. At present there are no large-scale, double-blind clinical trials for herbal or dietary supplements that have proven a consistent, reproducible effect on diabetes control.[68]

CASE STUDY REVISITED

One week later, Aubree returns to the outpatient clinic for medical nutrition therapy with a registered dietitian. As instructed at discharge, she brings with her a record of her blood glucose levels and diet recall for the past 24 hours. Her anthropometrics and insulin regimen are also shown below:

Anthropometric Data:
Height: 155 cm (61")
Weight: 44 kg (97 lbs)
BMI: 18 kg/m^2

Biochemical Data:
Blood glucose levels previous 24 hours
8 am: 290 (upon awakening/before breakfast)
11 am: 166 (before lunch)
2 pm: 170 (midday check, before snack)
4 pm: 188 (before dinner)
10 pm: 172 (before bed)

Clinical Data:
Medications:
Insulin Regimen for Home:
NPH 50 units (1.2 units/kg/day)
25 units at bedtime
25 units upon awakening
Lantus using the 1 unit per 15 g CHO

Dietary Data:
Dietary History: At home, Aubree has to get to school early so she does not have much time for breakfast. She has breakfast and lunch at school. Aubree is a good student. Mom describes her as detail oriented and conscientious about her health. Aubree expresses interest in self-management of her glycemia but she is stressed for time with this added to her busy schedule.
Typical Diet Recall:
8 am: Breakfast: bagel with cream cheese, juice
Typically no midmorning snack at school
12 pm: Lunch: school lunch (ham and cheese sandwich, pudding, potato chips, chocolate milk)
2 pm: Snack: brownie, milk
5 pm: Dinner: chicken (baked), rice or potato, cooked peas or corn
10 pm: Evening snack: kingsize candy bar and 12 oz Coke or Sprite to stay awake while doing homework
Physical activity: Plays on a soccer team (practice 3 times/week; games on Saturday)

Questions:
1. What is your assessment of Aubree's current glycemic control?
2. What additional questions might you ask to assess Aubree's understanding of the relationship between insulin and carbohydrate intake?
3. What is the appropriate meal plan for Aubree?
4. If Aubree requires 1800 kcals daily, use the carbohydrate counting method to calculate a meal plan and insulin regimen for Aubree.

Cinnamon

Cinnamon is the familiar spice used to give flavor to everything from French toast to Middle-Eastern poultry dishes. There are two types of cinnamon: Ceylon, which is native to Sri Lanka, and Cassia, which is the type commonly found in the United States. Cassia cinnamon contains coumarin, a compound that can be toxic to the liver if consumed in high doses. Cinnamon's use in diabetes control has been controversial for some time. It purportedly helps improve glycemic control by reducing insulin resistance. However, studies looking at the effects of cinnamon on glucose control, regardless of type used, have shown inconsistent results.[69,70]

A recent review,[71] which compared the results of 10 clinical trials, found that cinnamon was helpful in lowering both fasting glucose and cholesterol levels when taken in doses between 120 mg (0.02 teaspoons) to 6 g (1.2 teaspoons). The compound cinnamaldehyde, found in cinnamon, is thought to be responsible for its insulin-stimulating action. Cinnamon is generally considered safe in usual amounts consumed[71] and therefore could be suggested as a dietary measure with minimal cost and safety concerns to patients who want to use a dietary adjunct to their medications. Patients who want to give cinnamon a try in relatively high doses may want to opt for the Ceylon versions.

Medical Nutrition Therapy for Diabetes

Lifestyle intervention, including nutrition therapy, remains a foundational element in the management of diabetes. The most recent American Diabetes Association guidelines encourage self-management education and support for individuals with diabetes. The clinician should facilitate the development of knowledge and skills for on-going self-management in order to improve clinical outcomes and quality of life for their patients. Education should be patient centered and responsive to individualized needs and preferences. Goals for nutrition therapy in adult diabetes as defined by the American Diabetes Association are as follows[55]:

- To promote and support healthful eating patterns, emphasizing a variety of nutrient-dense foods in appropriate portion size
- Attain individualized glycemic, blood pressure, and lipid goals
- Achieve and maintain body weight goals
- Delay or prevent complications of diabetes
- To address individual nutrition needs based on personal and cultural preferences, health literacy and numeracy, access to healthful food choices, willingness and ability to make behavioral changes, and barriers to change
- To maintain the pleasure of eating by providing positive messages about food choices while limiting food choices only when indicated by scientific evidence
- To provide the individual with diabetes with practical tools for day-to-day meal planning rather than focusing on individual macronutrients, micronutrients, or single foods[55]

Medical nutrition therapy (MNT) is effective and recommended for all people with diabetes.[54] Studies have found that MNT can reduce A1C by 0.3% to 1% and 0.5% to 2% in type 1 and type 2 diabetes patients, respectively.[55] Patients benefit most when MNT is provided shortly after diagnosis.[28] Table 9.9 presents the Academy of Nutrition and Dietetics Evidence-based Practice Guideline for recommended nutrition visits.

The initial encounters with a patient generally will focus on nutritional assessment as well as establishing a good rapport, which will continue throughout several sessions. The nutritional assessment may also take several sessions in order to collect all of the essential data that provide the basis for nutrition interventions. Follow-up is important to evaluate the efficacy of intervention and establish new goals, with adjustment of nutrition therapy accordingly.

Nutrition Assessment

Nutritional assessment relies upon the usual data elements obtained through anthropometric measures, including waist circumference, weight and calculated BMI, biochemical analysis, clinical assessment, and diet history. Diet history and assessment of food intake should be comprehensive, with attention to meal patterns, meal preparation, food-shopping habits, and cultural values and beliefs of the patient. At this time, social and economic stressors should be assessed as well as knowledge and skill level, willingness for change, and barriers to dietary adherence. Diet recall and food records are used to evaluate overall energy intake and macronutrient distribution. Weight history and physical activity (frequency and intensity) is determined. Sleep patterns and quality of sleep should also be assessed, as these can impact glycemic control.[55] Clinical data, including biochemical indices related to glucose control and cardiac risk factors such as lipid profile and blood pressure, are obtained. Medications and their impact on glycemia is determined. Nutrition planning should coincide with glycemic goals, medical comorbidities, and patients' preferences and ability to adhere to recommendations.[72] Self-monitoring of

TABLE 9.9 RECOMMENDED NUTRITION VISITS FOR DIABETES DIAGNOSIS

Initial Encounters		Follow Encounters	
Number	Duration	Number	Duration
3 to 4	45 to 90 minutes	Once yearly	unspecified

Data from the Academy of Nutrition and Dietetics Evidence Based Practice Guidelines Franz, MJ, Powers, MA Leontes C. et al. *J Am Diet Assoc*. 2010;110:1852-1889.

blood glucose is important to overall glycemic control. As overweight and obesity is an overwhelming component of type 2 diabetes—half of all people with type 2 diabetes are obese[73]—a focus on modest weight loss, which includes an evaluation of calories consumed, is important.

Nutrition Intervention
Meal Planning

The best meal plan for a particular person is the one that they are willing to use. Determination of the appropriate method to employ is derived from a thorough nutrition assessment. As much as is feasible, the dietary regimen should be adjusted to fit the individual's preferences and lifestyle, not the other way around.[55]

> **PRACTICE POINT**
>
> Individuality in meal planning is necessary to assure willingness to comply.

A variety of meal planning methods, ranging from the very simplistic to those requiring the use of mathematical calculations, are available. Regardless of which method is employed, a basic focus on food/food groups as opposed to nutrients is usually a more effective teaching tool when instructing patients. For patients who take insulin and are on a fixed insulin dose, consistency in carbohydrate intake with respect to time and amount is helpful in maintaining blood glucose control. Patients on a flexible insulin dosing regimen may be prescribed carbohydrate counting to maximize glycemic control.[55] Patients taking oral agents that cause the pancreas to secrete insulin, such as sulfonylureas, also benefit from having fixed meal periods with standardized amounts of carbohydrate at each meal. As a starting point or for persons with low literacy or understanding, simple messages focusing on the content of the U.S. Dietary Guidelines 2015[50] may be appropriate. Guidelines directed at increasing consumption of fruits and vegetables, reducing excess sodium and added sugars, and aiming for consistency in carbohydrate intake and meal timing can be employed.

Plate Method

The "plate method," a visual rendering of the appropriate amounts of the major food groups to eat at each meal, has the benefits of incorporating all of the food groups, not simply those with carbohydrate. It is easy to understand, is reproducible in almost any dining situation, and enforces a basic method of portion control. Patients are instructed to divide their plate into three sections by bifurcating the plate and then bifurcating one of the halves again. The largest section, one-half of the plate, is filled with non-starchy vegetables and the other two sections are made up of protein and starchy foods, respectively. A glass of milk and a small piece of fruit accompany the plate. The American Diabetes Association, on their website, includes a step-by-step method to assemble a healthy plate: http://www.diabetes.org/food-and-fitness/food/planning-meals/create-your-plate/.[74]

Exchange Method

Meal plans based on exchange or substitution lists have been used over several decades. With this approach, foods that have similar calorie and macronutrient content are grouped together. Food groups include dairy, fat, fruits, vegetables, meats/proteins, and starches. Patients are prescribed a certain number of servings from each food group for each meal and snack. These food choice plans provide structure for the type and amount of food allowed at each meal, but give patients latitude in selecting the particular food(s) that will fill each group. This type of planning tool is often beneficial for those who need weight loss, because the total number of food groups assigned per day is based on a particular calorie level. **Table 9.10** provides a meal plan based on the exchange method for an 1,800-calorie diet.

Basic Carbohydrate Counting Method

Meal plans based on carbohydrate counting have become a popular and flexible method of meal planning. Basic carbohydrate counting involves adding up the total amount of carbohydrate, regardless of its source, to be eaten at a meal either in choices or in grams. One carbohydrate choice

---

CASE STUDY REVISITED

One month later, Aubree comes in for a nutrition visit. Your assessment of her knowledge indicates that she has improved her understanding of carbohydrate counting and her blood glucose levels are relatively well managed. Aubree has been highly motivated and would like to further control her glucose. With the help of the nurse practitioner, she recently started using the method of matching insulin to carbohydrate to dose her insulin.

Questions

1. Her insulin to carbohydrate ratio is 10 and her correction factor is 40. Aubree's current blood glucose reading is 280 mg/dL and her target is 120 mg/dL. She is planning to eat 90 g of carbohydrate at lunch. How many units of insulin should Aubree take?

TABLE 9.10 RECOMMENDED SERVINGS FOR AN 1,800-CALORIE PLAN

Meal	Food Group					
	Meat and Meat Substitutes (lean)	Starch	Fruit	Milk (skim)	Fats	Nonstarchy Vegetables
Breakfast	1	1	1	1	2	
Lunch	2	2			2	2
Dinner	6	3		1	2	2
Snack 1			1		2	
Snack 2		1		1		
Totals	8	7	2	3	7	4

Nutrient distribution: 1,805 calories; 191 g carbohydrate (42%); 115 g protein (25%); 66 g fat (33%)

Sample Menu

Breakfast
1 scrambled egg
1 slice whole grain toast
1 ¼ cups strawberries
1 teaspoon soft spread
1 cup low-fat milk

Lunch
1 small salad (1 cup mixed greens; 1 cup mixed cucumber, tomato, peppers)
2 tablespoons dressing
1 cup of lean meat–based chili with ¼ cup of low-fat cheddar cheese topping

Snack 1
1 small apple with 20 almonds

Dinner
6 oz of broiled halibut
1 cup of garlic roasted Brussels sprouts
1 medium sweet potato
2 teaspoons soft spread
1 8 oz cup of non-fat sugar-free yogurt

Snack 2
8 oz of low-fat milk
½ whole grain English muffin with 1 teaspoon low-sugar jam

---

provides 15 grams of carbohydrate. Patients are given a goal amount of carbohydrate to aim for at a meal; for example, a woman with type 2 diabetes may have 45 g to 60 g of carbohydrate to use at dinner. Basic carbohydrate counting allows for consistency in meal carbohydrate intake, but does not teach healthy eating guidelines or how to choose healthier carbohydrate selections. Combining the use of basic carbohydrate counting with the glycemic index can assist people with diabetes in selecting those carbohydrates that are digested slowly and will have less impact on blood glucose levels. More recently, the American Diabetes Association recommends protein and fat gram counting for better glycemic control in some individuals.[55]

> **PRACTICE POINT**
>
> Basic carbohydrate counting involves adding up the total amount of carbohydrate, regardless of its source, to be eaten at a meal either in choices or in grams.

Advanced Carbohydrate Counting or Matching Insulin to Carbohydrate Method

Those people who use multiple daily injections of insulin or wear an insulin pump may use an advanced method of carbohydrate counting known as matching insulin to carbohydrate. The amount of insulin given at a meal is a combination of the insulin units needed for both the carbohydrate content of the meal and the amount required to reduce the blood glucose into the target range. In this method, the **insulin to carbohydrate ratio** (ICR) defines the amount of carbohydrate processed by one unit of insulin. The correction factor (CF), also known as the sensitivity factor, defines the number of points one unit of insulin will lower the blood glucose.

A variety of equations exist for determining ICR and CFs. In general, they include variations of adding together all the insulin given on an average day, including both basal and bolus insulin (the total daily dose [TDD]), derived from continuous glucose monitoring to attempt to refine dosing guidelines.[76] In practice, 450 or 500 divided by the TDD is used to determine the ICR and 1,500 to 2,000 divided by the TDD for the CF. The larger the numerator, the greater the margin of safety. In addition, patients are given a target or goal blood glucose number. This can range from 100 mg/dL to 150 mg/dL depending on the patient's age, state of health, blood glucose control, and the frequency of and sensitivity to hypoglycemic reactions. Using this method (450 for the carbohydrate factor and 1,500 for the correction factor), assuming the TDD is 100, the insulin to carb ratio would be 4.5 (round up to 5) and the CF 15. For a meal containing 50 g of carbohydrate in which the pre-meal glucose value is 250 mg/dL and the goal glucose value is 100 mg/dL, the patient will take 20 units of insulin.

Insulin ratios can also be determined if patients have kept food and blood glucose records. The correction factor can be ascertained if the pre- and post prandial glucose values are available and if the number of units of insulin given is known. (To calculate the CF, subtract the postglucose number from the preglucose value and divide by the units of insulin injected.) For example, if 5 units of insulin were given to reduce the blood glucose by 100 points, the correction factor is 20. Initial calculations should be viewed as a jumping off point that will need further refinements through trial and error.

> **PRACTICE POINT**
>
> The total daily dose (TDD) is determined by adding together all the insulin given on an average day, including both basal and bolus insulin. The insulin carbohydrate ratio (ICR) is determined by dividing 450 or 500 by the TDD. The correction factor (CF) is calculated by dividing 1,500 to 2,000 by the TDD.

Matching insulin to carbohydrate allows flexibility in meal planning. Meals do not have to be eaten at fixed times, nor does the amount of carbohydrate need to remain constant. Although often used together at mealtimes, the CF can be used independently of the ICR ratio to bring the blood glucose levels down at times when they are elevated between meals. Patients may have one carbohydrate ratio for the day or their ratio may vary depending on the meal. Insulin sensitivity changes throughout the day and is also affected by the amount of fat consumed. Some people will have a smaller carbohydrate ratio at dinner simply because their dinner meal is often higher in fat than their breakfast or lunch meals. Often patients will also have an alternate correction factor that they use during the night when they are more sensitive to insulin.

> **Example:**
>
> **Determination of Insulin to Carbohydrate Ratio (ICR):**
> - Total daily dose of insulin (TDD): 100 units
> - Divide 450 by TDD: 450 ÷ 100 = 4.5 round up to 5
> - ICR is 1:5 (1 unit insulin:5 g carbohydrate)
>
> **Determination of Correction Factor (CF):**
> - Divide 1500 by TDD: 1500 ÷ 100 = 15
>
> Correction Factor (CF) = 15
>
> **Determination of total bolus insulin dose:**
>
> Current glucose = 250 mg/dL
>
> Goal glucose = 100 mg/dL
>
> Meal contains 50 g carbohydrate, how much total insulin is required?
>
> *How much insulin is needed to cover the meal?*
>
> With an insulin to carbohydrate ratio of 1:5, 1 unit of insulin is needed to process 5 g of carbohydrate. How much would be needed to cover 50 g of carbohydrate?
>
> $$\frac{1 \text{ unit insulin}}{5 \text{ g carbohydrate}} = \frac{X \text{ units insulin}}{50 \text{ g carbohydrate}}$$
>
> $$X = 10 \text{ units insulin}$$
>
> *How much insulin is needed to lower the glucose?*
>
> Current glucose – goal glucose = amount glucose needs to be lowered
>
> 250 mg/dL – 100 mg/dL = 150 mg/dL
>
> The glucose needs to be lowered by 150 mg/dL
>
> With a CF of 15, 1 unit of insulin will lower the glucose by 15.
>
> $$\frac{1 \text{ unit insulin}}{15} = \frac{X \text{ units insulin}}{150}$$
>
> $$X = 10 \text{ units insulin}$$
>
> Total bolus insulin needed: 10 units + 10 units = 20 units of insulin total

---

and dividing a constant or a multiple of body weight in pounds by the TDD to arrive at the ICR and CF. Davidson et al.[75] advocated the 1,700 rule for correcting insulin and using 2.8 times weight in pounds divided by the TDD to establish the ICR. Recently, researchers have used data

CASE STUDY REVISITED

Follow-up visit: Now that soccer season is in full swing, Aubree finds herself at times light-headed and anxious. Her blood glucose levels have been running on the low side, particularly on days of soccer practice. She asks whether she should be adjusting her insulin or carbohydrate intake in any way.

Questions

1. What physiologic explanations are there for Aubree's change in glycemic state? How does exercise alter Aubree's insulin requirements?
2. What signs and symptoms will you instruct Aubree to watch out for following exercise?
3. Describe your diet education plan for exercise management.

TABLE 9.11 USUAL AMOUNTS OF CARBOHYDRATE FOR PEOPLE WITH TYPE 2 DIABETES

	Men	Women
Active	60-75 grams	45-60 grams
Sedentary	45-60 grams	30-45 grams
For weight loss	45-60 grams	30-45 grams

Data from American Diabetes Association. Carbohydrate Counting. Retrieved from: http://www.diabetes.org/food-and-fitness/food/what-can-i-eat/understanding-carbohydrates/carbohydrate-counting.html.

PRACTICE POINT

Matching insulin to carbohydrate allows flexibility in meal planning.

In addition to glycemic control, nutrition interventions for people with diabetes should take into account risk reduction strategies for cardiovascular disease, high blood pressure and obesity where applicable. Eating patterns such as the Dietary Approaches to Stop Hypertension (DASH) diet have been found effective in improving glycemic control and ameliorating cardiovascular risk factors.[77] For those individuals requiring weight reduction, a meal plan designed to produce a calorie deficit of 250 to 500 calories less than the individual's current intake may be most appropriate.[78] Examples of usual amounts of carbohydrates recommended for men and women with type 2 diabetes are listed in **Table 9.11**.

Exercise

Exercise and physical activity are key components in the self-management guidelines for people with diabetes. Exercise improves cardiovascular health, sleep, and bone density; contributes to weight loss; and improves glucose control.

PRACTICE POINTS

Exercise and physical activity are key components in the self-management guidelines for people with diabetes.

Type 1 Diabetes

The normal response to moderate exercise in those without diabetes is a reduction in insulin output and an increase in glucagon secretion that results in glycogenolysis and gluconeogenesis.[79] In the presence of elevated circulating insulin, glycogenolysis is blunted and insulin-enhanced muscle glucose uptake is augmented, leaving the individual at risk for hypoglycemia. In addition, counter-regulatory mechanisms (catecholamines, growth hormone, and cortisol) present in healthy individuals that help prevent hypoglycemia during exercise may be curtailed by repeated episodes of low blood glucose in the person with type 1 diabetes.[80,81] Prolonged insulin sensitivity following moderate to vigorous exercise can induce hypoglycemia up to 36 hours after exercise in children with type 1 diabetes.[82]

CORE CONCEPT 6

During exercise, in the presence of elevated circulating insulin, glycogenolysis is blunted and insulin-enhanced muscle glucose uptake is augmented, leaving the individual at risk for hypoglycemia.

Although hypoglycemia is the most prevalent complication of exercise for people with type 1 diabetes, strenuous exercise, such as resistance training, can induce hyperglycemia and, in individuals whose diabetes is poorly controlled, diabetic ketoacidosis.[79] High-intensity exercise stimulates an increase in catecholamine levels, changing the balance between glucose generation and disposal toward greater glucose release. As endogenous insulin supplementation is not available, glucose levels increase temporarily, but generally decline in 1 to 2 hours.[84,83] In those persons with elevated blood glucose levels and ketone production, absolute insulin deficiency enhances additional ketone production and the risk of ketoacidosis.

Exercise provides many of the same benefits to people with type 1 diabetes as experienced by the general public and people with type 2 diabetes. However, the ability of exercise to improve A1C values is not well established.[85,66] This is likely due to the fact that although increased physical activity has been shown to improve insulin sensitivity and reduce the total quantity of insulin administered,[87,88] exercise can both induce hypoglycemia and hyperglycemia.

Type 2 Diabetes

Improvements in glycemic control stimulated by physical activity are generally due to reductions in insulin resistance in skeletal muscle. Studies have demonstrated that glucose uptake into skeletal muscle can increase by up to 50% in people with type 2 diabetes.[89] Insulin-dependent glucose uptake into muscle is accomplished through the translocation of glucose transporter protein type 4 (GLUT4), which is impaired in type 2 diabetes.[90,91] Exercise increases GLUT4 abundance and blood glucose transport, improving glycemic control.[92] Hypoglycemia in those persons not taking insulin or insulin secretagogues is usually rare, as the decline in endogenous plasma insulin levels exceeds transport of glucose into the muscle cells.[93] Reduction of glucose levels may continue up to 72 hours postexercise.[94]

> **CORE CONCEPT 7**
>
> Improvements in glycemic control stimulated by physical activity are generally due to reductions in insulin resistance in skeletal muscle.

The American Diabetes Association recommends that adults with diabetes perform at least 150 min/week of moderate-intensity aerobic physical activity spread over three days/week with no more than two consecutive days without exercise. In the absence of contraindications, adults with type 2 diabetes should be encouraged to perform resistance training at least twice per week.[21] In children and adolescents, and in those for whom weight loss is a priority, 60 minutes or more per day of physical activity may be required.[55,95]

In individuals with type 2 diabetes performing moderate exercise, glucose transport by muscle usually rises more than hepatic glucose production, causing blood glucose levels to decline.[96] There is a compensatory reduction in plasma insulin levels, making the risk of exercise-induced hypoglycemia in anyone not taking insulin or insulin secretagogues quite minimal, even with prolonged activity.[97] These improvements in insulin action can last between 24 and 72 hours. The benefits of moderate exercise persist whether the activity is accomplished all at once or is divided into multiple sessions throughout the day.[98] Prevention and management of hypoglycemia during exercise requires coordination between reduction in available insulin levels and increasing blood glucose levels with carbohydrate intake. In those individuals who are not taking insulin or insulin secretagogues, increases in carbohydrate consumption are not needed and, in the case of those with type 2 diabetes who are overweight or obese, not recommended. People who control their diabetes with an insulin pump or multiple daily injections of insulin can reduce bolus and or basal insulin to help prevent hypoglycemia. If exercise is completed postmeal, reduction of pre-meal bolus dose between 25% and 75% of usual is recommended.[79] Alternately or additionally, depending on the duration and intensity of exercise, pump basal rates can be reduced by 20% to 50% 1 to 2 hours before exercise, and basal rates can reduced or suspended during exercise.[79]

Carbohydrate Adjustment

The amount of carbohydrate necessary to prevent hypoglycemia is dependent on the intensity and duration of exercise. **Table 9.12** provides general guidelines for carbohydrate adjustment in exercise.

CASE STUDY REVISITED

At her routine nutrition counseling visit, Aubree is doing very well. Her blood glucose levels have ranged in the 140s. She is interested in knowing what the ideal glucose target range is for her. She would like to maintain tighter control. She also wants to know how often she should be monitoring her blood sugars.

Questions

1. What is the ideal glucose target range for Aubree?
2. What are the risks of tight glycemic control?
3. How often should Aubree be monitoring her glucose?

TABLE 9.12 EXERCISE AND CARBOHYDRATE ADJUSTMENT[99]

Duration and Intensity	Blood Glucose Levels	Carbohydrate Adjustment
30 minutes or less low intensity Leisurely walk, playing in the yard	<100 mg/dL	15 g
	100-200 mg/dL	0-15 g
	>200 mg/dL	No need for extra carbohydrate
30-60 minutes, moderate intensity Brisk walking, bike riding	<100 mg/dL	15-30 g
	100-200 mg/dL	Nothing to begin; then 15 for every 30 minutes of exercise
	200-300 mg/dL	No need for extra carbohydrate; increase fluids
	≥300 mg/dL	Test for ketones; if present, avoid exercise. Exercise with caution if no ketones present and keep well hydrated.
30-60 minutes, high intensity Soccer, field hockey, running	<100 mg/dL	30 g
	100-200 mg/dL	15 g
	200-300 mg/dL	No need for extra carbohydrate
>60 minutes, moderate intensity	<100 mg/dL	15 to 30 g in the first hour, then 15 g per hour of activity
	100 to 200 mg/dL	15 g per hour of activity
	200-300 mg/dL	No need for extra carbohydrate in the first hour, then 15 g per hour of activity

Data from Kosair Children's Hospital http://www.kosairchildrenhospital.com/carbohydrate-adjustment-for-activity. See chart with details. Accessed November 30, 2014.

Glycemic Targets and Self-Monitoring of Blood Glucose

Self-monitoring of blood glucose (SMBG) is an important tool for both patients and providers to determine appropriate meal and correction medication doses for those on insulin, to assess the efficacy of the treatment regimens, and to assist patients to respond to hyperglycemia and hypoglycemia. The frequency and timing of SMBG is related to the individual's medication regimen, their level of control, and the information being sought. Both the American Diabetes Association and the American Association of Clinical Endocrinologists endorse the practice of individuals with diabetes, who take insulin multiple times per day, checking their blood glucose on a regular basis. The American Diabetes Association is the more prescriptive, stating that SMBG in those using multiple dose injection insulin or an insulin pump should be performed prior to meals, at bedtime, prior to exercise, driving, occasionally postprandial, and whenever low blood glucose levels are suspected. In children with type 1 diabetes, more frequent self-monitoring is associated with lower A1C levels.[100]

The benefit of SMBG stems from maintaining better glycemic control. Sufficient evidence exists that lower A1C levels are associated with reduced microvascular complications and neuropathy and decreased cardiovascular events. However, the clinician should carefully consider the patient's risk for hypoglycemia and whether a lower glycemic target outweighs that risk. Patients who have a longer life expectancy and few comorbidities are ideal candidates, assuming that hypoglycemia is not a persistent obstacle. Table 9.13 lists the targets suggested by the American Diabetes Association for blood glucose monitoring.[100]

For those with type 2 diabetes who take oral agents or one dose of basal insulin per day, the results of self-monitoring of glucose control have been mixed. A photo demonstration of blood glucose monitoring by fingerstick

TABLE 9.13 GLYCEMIC TARGETS FOR INSULIN-DEPENDENT DIABETES

Glycemic Target Category	A1C	Mean Plasma Glucose mg/dL (Range)	Indicated Population
Stringent	<6.5%	122 (fasting) (112-127)	Long life expectancy, short-duration diabetes, type 2 diabetes treated with lifestyle or metformin, pregnant women*
Reasonable	<7%	126 (100-152)	Nonpregnant adults
Flexible	<7.5%	152 (143-162)	Children (all age groups); in setting goals, long-term benefits must be weighed against the risk of hypoglycemia
Less Stringent	<8%	183 (147-217)	History of hypoglycemia, limited life expectancy, extensive comorbidities or vascular complications, difficulty achieving goals due to lifestyle management

*During later pregnancy, in the second or third trimesters, A1C of <6% may be desirable if hypoglycemia is absent.

is shown in **Figure 9.4**. Several studies have demonstrated that self-monitoring of blood glucose is associated with improved problem-solving skills in hyperglycemia and hypoglycemia.[101,102] In order for SMBG to become a routine part of their treatment plan, patients must be educated on its purpose and use. Too often patients check their blood glucose without understanding the import of the numbers and SMBG becomes an exercise in busy work.

For many patients controlled on oral agents or taking one injection of basal insulin a day, checking once or twice per day is usually sufficient to extrapolate their control level. Bedtime and fasting numbers can be used to titrate the dose of basal insulin. SMBG can also help identify glucose patterns related to the quantity and types of food ingested. Paired tests, in which the patient checks blood glucose levels both prior to and 2 to 3 hours after a meal, are useful to help determine whether changes in food choices and or medication are indicated.

Acute and Chronic Complications of Diabetes

Acute Complications

The acute complications of diabetes are hyperglycemia and hypoglycemia. The causes of hyperglycemia and hypoglycemia are listed in **Table 9.14**, while the symptoms of both complications are shown in **Figure 9.5**. Hyperglycemia and hypoglycemia occur when there is a mismatch between the amount of insulin present in the blood and the available

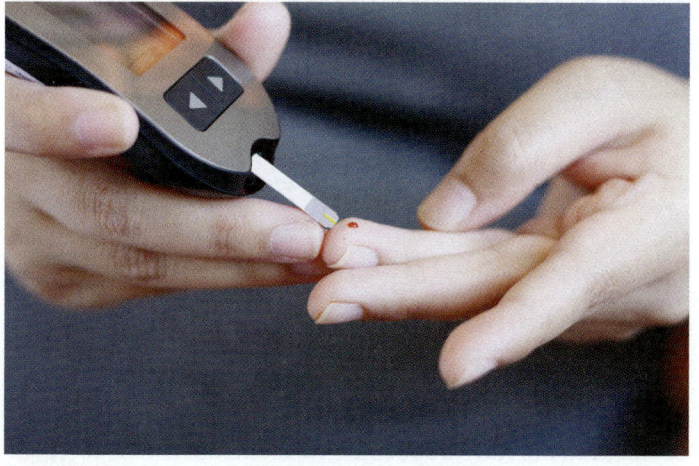

FIGURE 9.4 Demonstration of Blood Glucose Monitoring
©Kwangmoozaa/Shutterstock.

TABLE 9.14 CAUSES OF HYPERGLYCEMIA AND HYPOGLYCEMIA

Hypoglycemia Causes	Hyperglycemia Causes
Excessive diabetes medicine	Insufficient diabetes medicine
Inadequate carbohydrate	Excessive carbohydrate
Exercise	Exercise
Alcohol	Steroids
Illness resulting in suboptimal intake	Some psychiatric medications
	Critical illness and metabolic stress

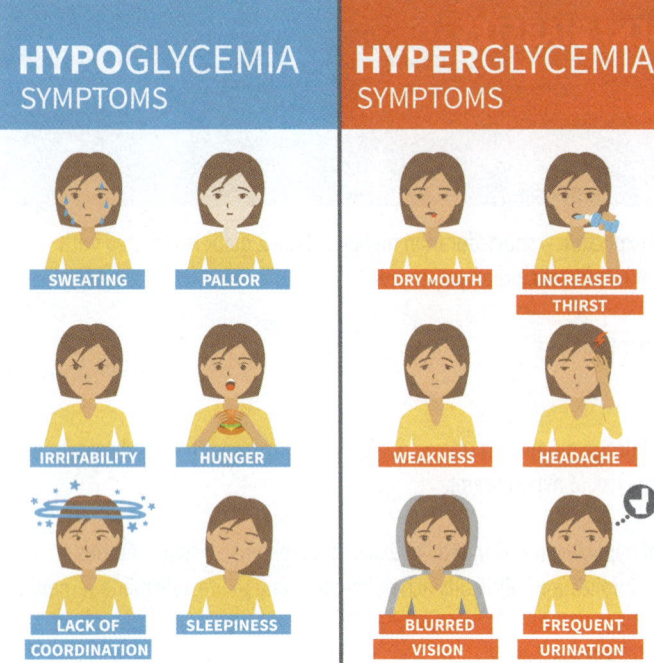

FIGURE 9.5 Symptoms of Hypo- and Hyperglycemia
© Irina Strelnikova/Shutterstock.

TABLE 9.15 DISTINGUISHING SYMPTOMOLOGY OF HYPOGLYCEMIA VERSUS HYPERGLYCEMIA

Symptoms of Hypoglycemia	Symptoms of Hyperglycemia
Andrenergic	Increased thirst
Sweating	Dry mouth or skin
Shakiness	Fatigue
Rapid heartbeat	Blurred vision
Anxiety	Increased infections
Hunger	
Weakness	
Tingling around the mouth	
Neurologic symptoms	
Headache	
Double vision	
Lack of coordination	
Confusion	
Seizures	
Inappropriate behavior	

TABLE 9.16 CLASSIFICATION OF HYPOGLYCEMIA LEVEL

Level	Classification	Threshold
1	Glucose alert level	≤ 70 mg/dL
2	Clinically significant hypoglycemia	< 54 mg/dL
3	Severe hypoglycemia	Not established

glucose concentration. Excessive glucose in relation to insulin results in hyperglycemia, while elevated levels of insulin in the absence of sufficient glucose predisposes to hypoglycemia. A comparison of hyperglycemia and hypoglycemia can be found in **Table 9.15**.

Hyperglycemia may be defined as a blood glucose level above 130 mg/dL after an 8-hour fast and a glucose level greater than 180 mg/dL 2 hours postprandially. Excessive carbohydrate intake, illness, certain medications such as corticosteroids, limited activity, strength training, and skipping insulin or oral hypoglycemics can all lead to hyperglycemia. Persistent hyperglycemia in the face of insulin deficiency can precipitate dehydration, ketone formation, and ketoacidosis in persons with type 1 diabetes and susceptible individuals with type 2 diabetes. People with type 2 diabetes can also develop hyperosmolar hyperglycemic nonketotic coma (HHNC). Persons with type 2 diabetes who develop HHNC usually are elderly with several comorbidities and have a diminished thirst sensation. Treatment for hyperglycemia is additional insulin and/or exercise.

The American Diabetes Association recognizes blood glucose levels below 70 mg/dL as consistent with hypoglycemia in those with diabetes.[100] Mild hypoglycemia can be disorienting to the person and often frightening to bystanders, while severe hypoglycemia can lead to serious consequences such as motor vehicle accidents and falls. The symptoms of hypoglycemia are divided into those that are derived from the autonomic nervous system, such as sweating and palpitations, and those that are due to the brain's glucose deprivation. Initial neuroglycopenic (shortage of glucose in the brain) symptoms may include difficulty concentrating and the inability to perform simple mathematical computations. As hypoglycemia worsens, deterioration in the ability to think clearly, slurred speech, confusion, irrational behaviors, lethargy, seizures and loss of consciousness can occur. **Table 9.16** provides the classification for level of hypoglycemia, from alert levels 1 (minor) to 3 (severe). Severe hypoglycemia does not have a specific threshold, but can be defined as hypoglycemia that results in severe cognitive impairment that requires medical intervention.

TABLE 9.17 TREATMENT OF HYPOGLYCEMIA
3 to 4 glucose tabs
1 tablespoon honey or sugar
4 oz of juice
6 oz regular soda
8 jelly beans
8 oz of skim milk

Symptoms of hypoglycemia can also occur even if the blood glucose level is above 70 mg/dL. This often happens if the glucose level falls rapidly from a higher value to a much lower value. When those whose blood glucose is in poor control have their glucose levels brought into the normal range rapidly, they may also feel the symptoms of hypoglycemia due to the release of epinephrine.

The treatment for low blood glucose is carbohydrate, which is described in more detail in **Table 9.17**. All carbohydrate will eventually raise glucose levels, but carbohydrate that contains excess fiber or fat should be avoided because it will slow digestion. Use of the "15/15" rule is recommended in clinical practice. Specifically, it is recommended for patients to eat 15 grams of carbohydrate and wait 15 minutes. For glucose levels of 50 mg/dL to 70 mg/dL, consuming 15 g of carbohydrate, such as 4 oz of juice, 6 oz of regular soda, or 3 to 4 glucose tabs will usually bring glucose levels back to target range. Blood glucose levels less than 50 mg/dL often require at least 30 g of carbohydrate to return blood glucose values back to target range. After waiting 15 minutes, blood glucose should be re-checked to make sure levels have risen above 80 mg/dL. Because protein increases insulin response without raising blood glucose, protein-containing foods should not be used to treat hypoglycemia. Additional treatment is required if glucose levels have not reached targets. Severe hypoglycemia that produces unconsciousness may require the use of a glucagon injection into fatty tissue, such as the buttocks. Injectable glucagon raises blood glucose by releasing glucose stored in the liver. It can also induce nausea and vomiting, requiring that the person be placed on his or her side to avoid aspiration.

Chronic Complications

Uncontrolled diabetes leads to a host of microvascular, macrovascular, and neurological complications. Both the Diabetes Control and Complication Trial and the United Kingdom Prospective Diabetes Study support the role of intensive control of glucose in reducing the risk of complications.[103,104] For every 1% drop in blood glucose levels, there is a corresponding reduction in risk of complications of approximately 40%.[16] Chronic complications of diabetes are outlined in **Figure 9.6**.

> **CORE CONCEPT 8**
>
> For every 1% drop in blood glucose levels, there is a corresponding reduction in risk of complications of approximately 40%.

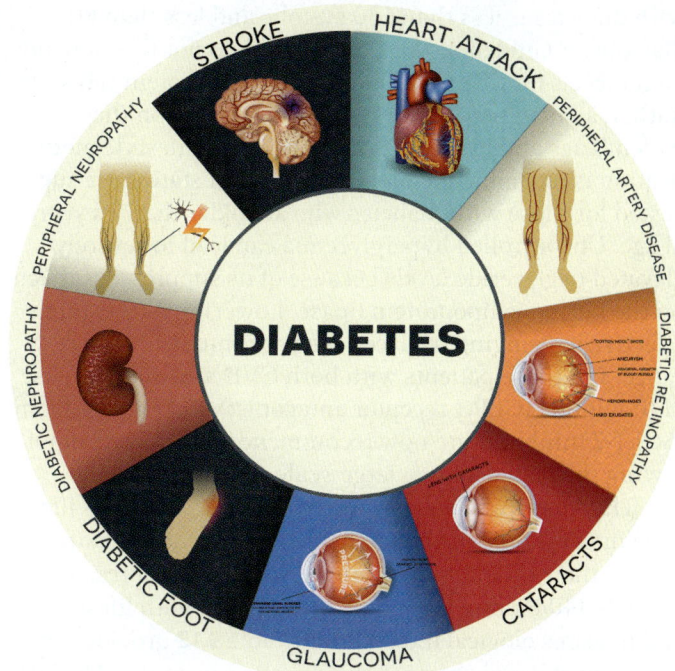

FIGURE 9.6 Chronic Complications of Diabetes
© Tefi/Shutterstock.

Psychological Complications

Diabetes distress refers to the intense stress related to the experience of living with diabetes. Patients with diabetes often have negative psychological effects from the constant worry of daily medication management, dietary specifications, and blood glucose monitoring, as well as the long-term concern of disease progression. Data on diabetes distress estimates a prevalence of 18% to 45% in those with diabetes. To make matters worse, those with diabetes distress are more likely to have higher A1C levels, nutritionally inadequate diets, lower exercise levels, and lower self-efficacy. The American Diabetes Association recommends provision of additional specific diabetes education to address any areas of concern for the patient, followed by referral to a mental health specialist who is ideally familiar with diabetes management.[55]

Macrovascular Complications

Macrovascular complications include heart disease, stroke, and peripheral vascular disease. Unlike the impressive reductions seen in the risk of microvascular damage with intensive glycemic control, intensive control of blood glucose does not completely reduce the risk of developing macrovascular complications in persons with diabetes. One of the defining features of CVD is endothelial dysfunction. Insulin resistance and hyperglycemia contribute to endothelial dysfunction, which diminishes the normal anti-atherogenic properties of the endothelial cells.[105] Endothelial dysfunction is often present in people with prediabetes and metabolic syndrome and is an independent risk factor for CVD. Persons with diabetes often have the independent CVD risk factors of hypertension and dyslipidemia in addition to diabetes. Target blood pressure for people with diabetes is less than 130 systolic and less than 80 diastolic.[106] Guidelines for lipid control do not recommend target levels for LDL and high-density lipoprotein (HDL).[107] Rather, a target percentage reduction is based on the patient's age and initial LDL starting level. Lifestyle modification is recommended for everyone, but statins are suggested for those with diabetes who are older than 40 years of age. Uncontrolled hyperglycemia can lead to severely elevated triglyceride levels because of its suppressive effects on the hormone lipoprotein lipase. Lowering A1C is often effective in bringing triglycerides back into the target range. For those patients with both CVD and diabetes, use of liraglutide (GLP-1 receptor antagonist) and empaglifozin (SGLT-2 inhibitor) are now recommended as treatment following the results of two large-scale clinical trials.[108]

The American Diabetes Association recommends lifestyle intervention for those persons with blood pressure greater than 120/80 mm Hg; those whose blood pressure exceeds 140/80 mm Hg should be managed with lifestyle and pharmacological intervention. **Table 9.18** provides an overview of blood pressure classification in adults. The 2017 American Diabetes Association Standard of Medical Care in Diabetes has expanded to provide four options of blood pressure–reducing medications to treat those with both hypertension and diabetes. These medications include ACE inhibitors, thiazide-like diuretics, angiotension receptor blockers, and dihydropyridine calcium channel blockers.[108] Studies have shown positive effects on lipid parameters and blood pressure of diets that limit saturated fat, trans fat, cholesterol, and sodium intake.[109,110] In addition, Mediterranean diets have shown promise in helping those with diabetes lower cardiac risk.[111] The DASH diet, which promotes a diet low in sodium (<1,500 mg/day) and saturated fat (6% of calories) but high in potassium (4,700 mg), has been proven effective in lowering blood pressure.[112]

> **PRACTICE POINTS**
>
> Dietary interventions include limiting saturated fat to <7% of calories, minimizing or eliminating artificial trans fats, increasing fiber intake, including 2 g of plant stanols and sterols, and including of omega-3 fatty acids in the form of fatty fish or plant sources.

Microvascular Complications

Nephropathy In the United States in 2008, diabetic **nephropathy** (damage to the kidneys due to diabetes) accounted for 44% of new cases of end-stage renal disease.[16] Approximately one-third of people with type 1 diabetes will develop nephropathy within 20 years of being diagnosed with diabetes. Although far fewer people with type 2 diabetes will develop end-stage nephropathy, the sheer number of people who have type 2 diabetes means that the burden of treating those who will need dialysis could become overwhelming.[1] The 2007 Kidney Disease Outcomes Quality Initiative (KDOQI) guidelines divided kidney disease into five stages.[113] The loss of glomerular filtration rate (GFR) and the recommended nutrition intervention per stage of kidney disease is given in **Tables 9.19** and **9.20**. In the initial stages, the concentrating ability of the kidneys is not affected and blood urea nitrogen (BUN) and creatinine are normal. Often, microalbuminuria is the first indication that the kidneys are functioning abnormally. **Microalbuminuria** is defined as greater than 30 mg but less than 300 mg daily of albumin in the urine. Overt proteinuria correlates closely with a more rapid rate of progression to end-stage renal disease.[114] Lifestyle interventions concentrate on controlling hyperglycemia and blood pressure. Dyslipidemia is often a concurrent finding in those with diabetes and

TABLE 9.18 BLOOD PRESSURE CLASSIFICATION IN ADULTS

	American College of Cardiology/American Heart Association 2017 Guideline for High Blood Pressure Levels in Adults		
Category	Systolic[†] (mm Hg)		Diastolic[†] (mm Hg)
Normal	Less than 120	And	Less than 80
Elevated	120–129	And	Less than 80
Hypertension Stage 1	130–139	Or	80–89 or higher
Hypertension Stage 2	≥ 140	Or	≥ 90

*For adults ages 18 and older who are not on medicine for high blood pressure and do not have a short-term serious illness. Source: http://www.acc.org/guidelines/hubs/high-blood-pressure
[†]If systolic and diastolic pressures fall into different categories, overall status is the higher category.
http://www.nhlbi.nih.gov/health/public/heart/hbp/dash/new_dash.pdf . Box 2.
Data from American College of Cardiology/American Heart Association 2017 Guideline for High Blood Pressure Levels in Adults.

TABLE 9.19 STAGES OF CHRONIC KIDNEY DISEASE[113,119,122]

Stage	GFR	Description	Symptoms	Action for Individuals with DM
1	90 or greater	Normal kidney function with structural or urine abnormalities	None usually	Observation Healthy lifestyle Testing of blood and urine parameters, control of blood pressure and blood glucose
2	60-89	Mild CKD	None usually	Observation Healthy lifestyle Testing of blood and urine parameters, control of blood pressure and blood glucose
3a	45-59	Moderate CKD	Possible fatigue, fluid retention, anemia, high blood pressure	Control of blood pressure and blood glucose. More frequent estimation of creatinine, Hb, and urinary protein
3b	30-44	Moderate CKD	Possible fatigue, fluid retention, anemia, high blood pressure	Control of blood pressure and blood glucose. Six-month estimation of creatinine, Hb, and urinary protein
4	15-29	Severe CKD	Development of bone disease, high blood pressure, anemia, cardiac disease, possible uremia, hyperkalemia, and hyperphosphatemia	Planning for end-stage disease. Control of blood pressure and blood parameters. Three-month estimation of creatinine, Hb, urinary protein, potassium, and phosphorus
5	<15	End-stage CKD	Uremia if not on dialysis	Dialysis

Data from http://www.renal.org/information-resources/the-uk-eckd-guide/ckd-stages#sthash.uZIAxEQg.iukIA4B8.dpbs and KDOQI Clinical Practice Guidelines and Clinical Practice Recommendations for Diabetes and Chronic Kidney Disease.

TABLE 9.20 NUTRITION RECOMMENDATIONS FOR DIABETES AND CHRONIC KIDNEY DISEASE[113]

Nutrient	Chronic Kidney Disease Stage	Recommendation
Protein	1-4	0.8 g/kg/day
Phosphorus	1-2	1.7 g/day
	3-4	0.8-1.0 g/kg/day
Potassium	1-2	>4 g/day
	3-4	2.4 g/day
Sodium	1-4	<2.3 g/day

Data from KDOQI Clinical Guidelines and Clinical Practice Recommendations for Diabetes and Chronic Kidney Disease http://www2.kidney.org/professionals/KDOQI/guideline_diabetes/guide5.htm.

renal disease and is a major risk factor for cardiovascular events. Control of lipid levels through dietary modification along with appropriate medications has become a more pressing concern as more evidence has accumulated linking the dyslipidemia of diabetic renal disease to increased morbidity and mortality. People with diabetes in the early stages of kidney disease can often continue to follow the same healthful dietary patterns suggested for controlling diabetes and other chronic diseases such as a Mediterranean or DASH diet, both low in saturated fats, added sodium, and sugars and plentiful in fruits and vegetables.[115]

In the past, aggressive protein restriction was thought to preserve kidney function and extend the time prior to the onset of dialysis. Secondary analyses of the data from the Modification in Diet in Renal Disease, the largest multicenter study to address the relationship between protein intake and kidney function, indicated that protein restriction does have a role in slowing diabetic and nondiabetic renal disease.[116] However, the results of newer studies evaluating whether protein restriction prevents decline in albumin excretion rate (AER) and in GFR have been mixed.[117,118] Although clinical trials have shown a reduction in AER, reducing protein has not been as effective in preventing the decline in GFR, and very low levels of dietary protein restriction can lead to malnutrition. Plant-based protein sources may be encouraged for early stage kidney disease as they contain less saturated fat and provide a better fiber source than animal proteins. Despite the fact that evidence supporting protein restriction remains limited, clinical guidelines developed by the major renal and diabetes organizations often still call for protein modifications for people with diabetes and renal disease. The 2012 Kidney Disease Improving Global Outcomes Practice Guideline for the Evaluation and Management of Chronic Kidney Disease suggests 0.8 g/kg/day of protein in adults with diabetes and GFR <30 mL/min/173/m² and avoidance of intake >1.3 g/kg in adults with chronic kidney disease (CKD) at risk of progression.[119] The Academy of Nutrition and Dietetics nutrition guidelines suggest an intake of 0.6 to 0.8 g/kg body weight with at least 50% coming from high biological value protein sources particularly in patients with diabetes.[120] The American Diabetes Association, in its 2014 guidelines, has moved to a more liberal approach suggesting patients maintain usual levels of dietary protein intake.[121]

As damage to the kidneys continues, their ability to remove waste products is diminished and dietary modifications of the minerals potassium and phosphorus in addition to sodium are required. The stages of kidney disease are discussed in **Table 9.19**. Persons with diabetes taking angiotensin converting enzyme inhibitors or angiotension receptor blockers may be predisposed to higher potassium levels and need a modification of these nutrients sooner than is customarily required. **Table 9.20** outlines the nutrition recommendations for individuals with diabetes and CKD. When patients reach Stage 5 (GFR <15 mL/min/1.73 m²), the kidneys can no longer eliminate waste products effectively without mechanical intervention. Hemodialysis or peritoneal dialysis (PD) is initiated. In addition to modifications in minerals and macronutrients, dialysis patients must restrict fluid and the patient using PD must take into account the glucose absorbed from the dialysis solution when calculating carbohydrate and energy needs. Blood glucose levels should be monitored closely when patients start or change dialysis solutions.

Retinopathy Diabetes is the leading cause of new cases of blindness in adults age 20 years to 70 years.[16] After 20 years of diabetes, most people will have some evidence of diabetic eye disease. There are four stages of **retinopathy**, but retinopathy can be broadly divided into two major categories: nonproliferative and proliferative retinopathy. In nonproliferative retinopathy, high blood glucose causes the lining of the blood vessels in the retina to thicken and leak. Leakage of blood and fluid into the center of the retina, called macular edema, can result in loss of central vision. In proliferative retinopathy, new, fragile cells grow on the surface of the retina, obscuring vision. If left untreated, proliferative retinopathy can cause blindness. Because of the pressure exerted on the retina by scar tissue, advanced proliferative retinopathy may also lead to retinal detachment. The manifestations of diabetic retinopathy are shown in **Figure 9.7**.

Retinopathy cannot be cured, but it can be treated with laser photocoagulation and vitrectomy surgery. Diabetic eye disease does not usually cause vision loss until it is well

DIABETIC RETINOPATHY

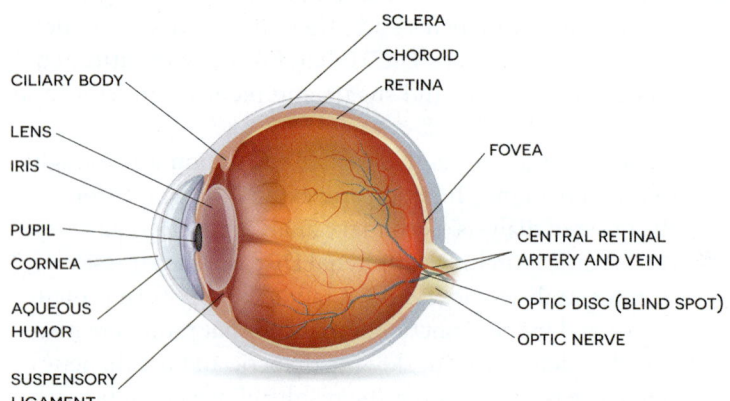
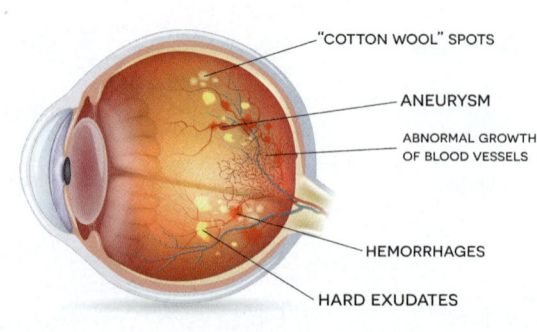

FIGURE 9.7 Manifestations of Diabetic Retinopathy
© Tefi/Shutterstock.

advanced. Quitting smoking and controlling blood glucose levels, cholesterol levels, and blood pressure are key to preventing and slowing the progression of retinopathy. People with diabetes are also at higher risk of eye conditions that affect people without diabetes, such as cataracts and age-related macular degeneration. The Age-Related Eye Disease Study (AREDS), conducted in 2001, found that daily high doses of vitamins C and E, beta-carotene, and the minerals zinc and copper can help slow the progression to advanced AMD. In 2006, a second, 5-year study, called AREDS2, determined that the AREDS formulation with the addition of lutein and zeaxanthin and the removal of beta-carotene, reduced the risk of AMD.[123,124]

Dental Disease Blood glucose control and optimal dental care are important in maintaining good oral health and euglycemia. High glucose levels in the oral mucosa are associated with increased levels of bacteria and the development of periodontal disease. People with high glucose levels often have dry mouth due to reduction in saliva output. Lack of saliva, which provides both a chemical and mechanical barrier to bacterial infection, can hasten the development of sores and tooth decay. Uncontrolled periodontal disease increases cytokine production, worsening insulin resistance and destabilizing glucose control.[125] Poor oral health, which can lead to discomfort and pain when chewing and swallowing, may impinge on the adequate consumption of nutrients, contributing both to malnutrition and glycemic deterioration.[126]

Neuropathy Diabetic neuropathy is caused by elevated glucose levels, which damage the nerves throughout the body. There are four types of diabetic neuropathy: peripheral neuropathy, autonomic neuropathy, radiculoplexus neuropathy (diabetic amyotrophy), and mononeuropathy. The most common type is peripheral neuropathy, which affects nerves in the extremities, the feet, legs, hands, and arms. **Figure 9.8** demonstrates a diabetic foot check, which is helpful to determine any abnormalities in patients with neuropathy who may not otherwise feel or notice the condition. Symptoms include tingling or burning, loss of ability to feel pain or sensation in the affected limb, muscle weakness, and foot deformities. Although incurable, there are a variety of medications available to treat peripheral neuropathies.

Many gastrointestinal problems, including constipation, diarrhea, bloating, and heartburn, arising from diabetes are the result of autonomic neuropathy. One of the most difficult to treat diabetic complications is **gastroparesis**. Delayed gastric emptying is present in 25% to 55% of individuals with type 1 diabetes mellitus and 30% of type 2 diabetes mellitus patients.[127]

In gastroparesis, the nerves enervating the GI tract are affected and there is delayed gastric emptying in the absence of a mechanical gastric outlet obstruction. **Figure 9.9** illustrates the damaged vagus nerve and its effect on delayed gastric emptying. Gastroparesis compromises the delivery of food to the small intestine in a consistent manner. People with gastroparesis may experience early satiety, nausea and vomiting, bloating, abdominal pain, and constipation. The focus of treatment is on the control of symptoms, although the severity of symptoms does not correlate well with the degree of nerve damage, and the prevention or alleviation of malnutrition.[128] Both soluble fiber and fat can slow the pace of digestion, and therefore diets for gastroparesis are low in both of these nutrients. Small, frequent feedings are preferred over fewer, larger meals to prevent bloating and early satiety. Liquids, which empty faster than solids from the stomach, are usually better tolerated and patients with more severe symptoms may find a completely liquid diet easier to digest. Because early satiety, nausea, and vomiting can lead to poor intake and malnutrition, patients with severe symptoms and unintentional weight loss of 5% to 10% of usual body weight in 3 to 6 months may need to be managed wholly on enteral, or in rare cases, parenteral, nutrition.[128,129] Monitoring of weight status is, therefore, essential in gastroparesis.

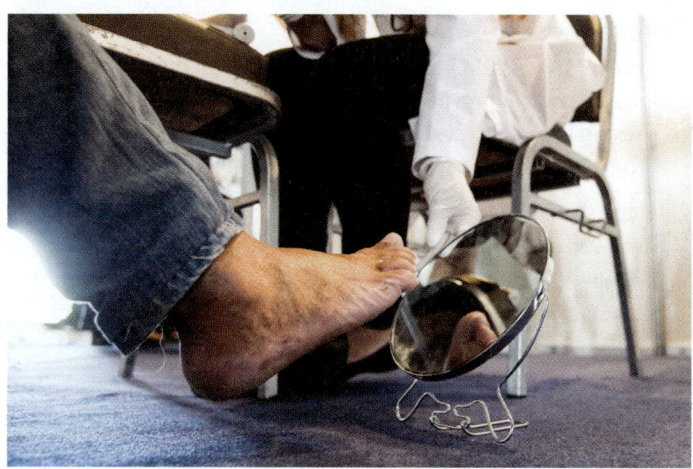

FIGURE 9.8 **Demonstration of Diabetic Foot Check**
© CP DC Press/Shutterstock.

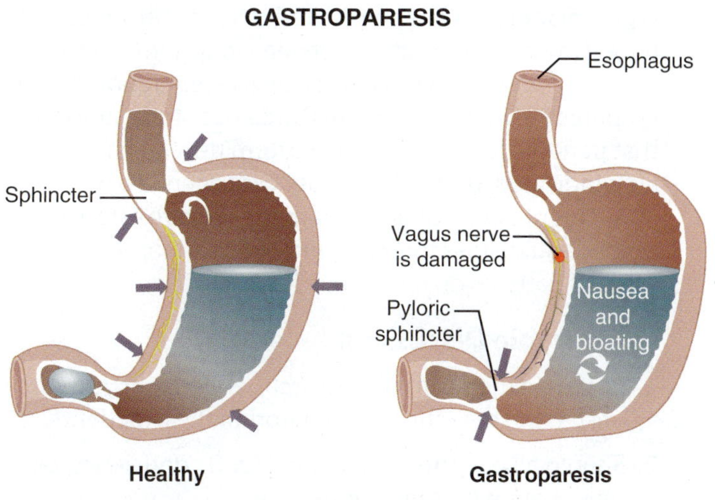

FIGURE 9.9 **Delayed Gastric Emptying**

In addition to adjustments in food intake, gastroparesis often requires modifications to the timing of medications. In patients taking insulin or insulin secretagogues, delayed gastric emptying can cause hypoglycemia. Changing the timing of insulin administration to 30 minutes after meals for those taking injections, or using an insulin pump to deliver an extended bolus, in which a portion of the insulin dose is given prior to the meal and the remainder is given over a set time period, has been shown to improve glycemic control.[129]

Medical Treatment of Diabetes

Although diet and exercise remain the cornerstone of diabetes management, all people diagnosed with type 1 diabetes will require insulin as a life-long treatment modality. Most of those with type 2 diabetes will also find the need for pharmacological intervention. Type 2 diabetes is a chronic disease whose natural history includes the slow, progressive loss of beta cell function.

> **CORE CONCEPT 9**
>
> Although diet and exercise remain the cornerstone of diabetes management, all people diagnosed with type 1 diabetes will require insulin as a life-long treatment modality.

> **PRACTICE POINTS**
>
> The role of drug therapy for type 2 diabetes to "achieve clinical and biochemical targets with as few adverse consequences as possible."

The American Association of Clinical Endocrinologists defines the role of drug therapy for type 2 diabetes to "achieve clinical and biochemical targets with as few adverse consequences as possible." Currently available hypoglycemic agents provide the same glucose-lowering capacity, decreasing A1C between 0.5% and 2%.[23] Decisions on the appropriate agent to use are based on the current level of glucose intolerance, the patient's weight and comorbidities, convenience, and patient preference.

The landscape for medications for patients with type 2 diabetes has changed significantly in the last 20 years. Whereas in the early 1990s there were only two choices of oral medication available in the United States, the sulfonylureas and the byguanides, there are now 11 categories of drugs, often with several choices among each category. As our understanding of diabetes as a disease affecting multiple organ systems has grown, so has the diverse avenues of pharmacological management multiplied.

New medications are being developed every day. As a practicing professional in the field of nutrition, familiarity with the different classes of drugs, understanding how they function, their side effects and contraindications, and how they interact with food intake is vital. **Table 9.21** reviews currently available oral and injectable noninsulin medications.

Insulin

Insulin is the one drug that is appropriate for use in all types of diabetes. Previously derived from pork or beef pancreas, all insulin currently in use in the United States is made in the laboratory from recombinant DNA. Insulins are categorized on the basis of their strength, onset of

Clinical Roundtable

Topic: Metformin and Vitamin B_{12} Deficiency

Background: Initiation of metformin monotherapy is recommended for all individuals newly diagnosed with type 2 diabetes. While considered safe, numerous studies have shown an association between long-term metformin use and vitamin B_{12} deficiency. A recent report by the Diabetes Prevention Program Outcomes Study suggests that periodic testing of B_{12} in metformin-treated individuals is indicated, particularly those with anemia or neuropathy. This presents clinicians with the need to establish practice guidelines for screening, monitoring, and treatment of patients on metformin for B_{12} deficiency.

Roundtable Discussion

1. Based on the results of research, what might you suggest as best practice for monitoring these patients?
2. Should all patients be screened for B_{12} deficiency, or only those with symptoms?
3. What other criteria might you put in place to be most efficient in monitoring for this drug nutrient interaction?

References

1. Aroda VR, Edelstein SL, Goldberg RB, et al. and the Diabetes Prevention Program Research Group. Long-term metformin use and vitamin B_{12} deficiency in the Diabetes Prevention Program Outcomes Study. *Endocr J.* 2013;60(12):1275-1280.
2. Sato Y, Ouchi K, Funase Y, Yamauchi K, Aizawa T. Relationship between metformin use, vitamin B_{12} deficiency, hyperhomocysteinemia and vascular complications in patients with type 2 diabetes. *Endocr J.* 2013;60(12):1275-1280.
3. Chapman LE, Darling AL, Brown JE. Association between metformin and vitamin B_{12} deficiency in patients with type 2 diabetes: A systematic review and meta-analysis. *Diabetes Metab.* 2016;42(5):316-327. doi: 10.1016/j.diabet.2016.03.008.

TABLE 9.21 ORAL AND INJECTABLE NON-INSULIN MEDICATIONS[130]

Class	Product	Primary Mechanism of Action	Advantages	Side Effects	Dose	Cost	A1C Reduction
Biguanides	Metformin	Reduction in hepatic glucose production	No hypoglycemia Reduction in CVD episodes Long history of safe use	Gastrointestinal distress (diarrhea, gas, cramping) B_{12} deficiency Lactic acidosis (rare) Cannot be used in significant CKD	500 to 2,500 mg	Low	1%-2%
Sulfonylurea (second generation)	Glyburide Glipizide Glimepiride	Increases insulin secretion	Long history of use Possible decrease in microvascular risk	Hypoglycemia, enhanced in elderly Weight gain Loses effectiveness over time Blunts myocardial ischemic preconditioning	Glyburide 1.25 to 20 mg Glipizide 5 to 15 mg Glimepiride 1 to 8 mg	Low	1%-1.5%
Meglitinides	Repaglinide Nateglinide	Increase insulin secretion	Dosing flexibility Decrease postprandial glucose excursions	Hypoglycemia Weight gain Blunts myocardial ischemic preconditioning	Repaglinide 0.5 to 4 mg Nateglinide 60 to 540 mg	Moderate	0.5%-1.0%
Thiazolidinediones	Pioglitazone	Increase peripheral glucose uptake by enhancing insulin action Decrease hepatic glucose output	No hypoglycemia Efficacy Acceptable in renal insufficiency Well tolerated Once-daily dosing	Weight gain (can be significant) Fluid gains Decrease triglycerides (TGs) Increase HDL-C Fracture risk is doubled	Pioglitazone 15 to 45 mg taken once daily without regard to meals Rosiglitaz 4 to 8 mg once daily without regard to meals	Low	1%-1.5%

(continues)

TABLE 9.21 ORAL AND INJECTABLE NON-INSULIN MEDICATIONS[130] (Continued)

Class	Product	Primary Mechanism of Action	Advantages	Side Effects	Dose	Cost	A1C Reduction
a-Glycosidase inhibitors	Acarbose Miglitol	Slows intestinal carbohydrate digestion/absorption	No hypoglycemia Decreased postprandial glucose excursions Decreased CVD events Weight neutral	Modest A1C reduction Major dose-related gastrointestinal intolerance (10%-35%) Compliance issues (must be taken with first bite of meal)	25-150 mg/day Acarbose must be taken with the first bite of a meal	Moderate	0.5%-1%
DPP-4 inhibitors	Sitagliptin Vildagliptin Saxagliptin Linagliptin Alogliptin	Increase insulin secretion (glucose dependent) Decrease glucagon secretion (glucose dependent)	No hypoglycemia Well tolerated No weight gain Fewer safety concerns than with the glitazones Once daily dosing	A1C reduction somewhat less than metformin, sulfonylureas, and glitazones Long-term efficacy and safety unknown Pancreatitis Expensive	Linagliptin 5 mg once daily Saxagliptin 5 mg once daily Sitagliptin 100 mg once daily	High	0.5%-1%
Bile acid sequestrants	Colesevelam	Decrease hepatic glucose production Increase incretin levels	No hypoglycemia Decrease LDL-C	Modest A1C reduction Constipation Increase TGs May decrease absorption of other medications	1,875 mg (three tablets) orally twice a day with meals or 3,750 mg (six tablets) orally once a day with a meal	High	0.5%
Dopamine-2 agonists	Bromocriptine	Modulates hypothalamic regulation of metabolism Increases insulin sensitivity	No hypoglycemia Decreased CVD events	Modest A1C reduction Dizziness Nausea Fatigue Rhinitis	0.8 to 4.8 mg once daily within 2 hours of waking	High	0.5%

(continues)

TABLE 9.21 ORAL AND INJECTABLE NON-INSULIN MEDICATIONS[130] (Continued)

Class	Product	Primary Mechanism of Action	Advantages	Side Effects	Dose	Cost	A1C Reduction
SGLT2 inhibitors	Canagliflozin Dapagliflozin Empagliflozin	Blocks glucose reabsorption by the kidney, increasing glucosuria	No hypoglycemia Weight reduction Decreased blood pressure	Genitourinary infections Polyuria Volume depletion Increased LDL-C	Canagliflozin 100-300 mg Dapagliflozin 5-10 mg Empagliflozin 10-25 mg	High	0.7%-1%
GLP-1 receptor agonists	Exenatide Exenatide extended release Liraglutide Albiglutide Lixisenatide Dulaglutide	Increase insulin secretion (glucose dependent) Slow gastric emptying Decrease glucagon secretion	No hypoglycemia Weight reduction Decreased postprandial glucose excursions	Long-term efficacy unknown Long-term safety unknown (possible link to thyroid cancer) In pancreatitis: caution if GFR <50 Must be injected Major dose-related gastrointestinal intolerance	Exenatide is injected twice daily 0-60 min before breakfast and supper, 5 mcg to 10 mg SC BID Liraglutide is injected once daily without regard to mealtimes, 0.6 mg SC 1.8 mg/day	High	0.8%-1.8%
Amylin mimetics	Pramlintide	Decrease glucagon secretion Increase satiety Slow gastric emptying	Decreased postprandial glucose excursions Weight reduction	Modest A1C reduction gastrointestinal side effects (nausea & vomiting) Injectable Frequent dosing schedule	15-120 mcg given with meals	High	0.5%-0.7%

SC = subcutaneous.
Data from Inzucchi S, Bergenstel, RM, Buse JB. Management of hyperglycemia in type 2 diabetes, 2015: a patient-center approach: update to a position statement of the American Diabetes Association and the European Association for the study of diabetes. Diabetes Care. 2015;38(1);140-149.

action, peak action, and duration of action. Most insulins in the United States are U100, which means that there are 100 units of insulin dissolved in 1 mL of liquid; however, U500, which is five times as strong, is available for those people who are severely insulin resistant. Table 9.22 reviews the characteristic of available insulins.

Most insulins can be divided into two major categories: those that are used as basal insulin and those used for bolus therapy. Basal insulins are long-acting insulins (16-24 hours) that provide insulin replacement throughout the day and help reduce excess glucose secretion from the liver. They are usually given as either one or two injections in the morning and either at dinner or bedtime. Bolus (short- or fast-acting) insulin is used to cover the blood glucose excursion following meals and to correct or reduce blood glucose elevations due to a mismatch between available

TABLE 9.22 INSULIN ACTION TIMES[131]

Category	Insulin	Start Time	Peak	Durations
Rapid	Lispro, Aspart, Glulisine	15 min	30 to 90 min	3 to 5 hours
Short-acting	Regular (R)	30 min	2 to 3 hours	5 to 8 hours
Intermediate-acting	NPH	2 to 4 hours	4 to 8 hours	12 to 16 hours
Long-acting	Detemir, Glargine	2 to 3 hours	–	24 hours
Pre-mixed NPH (intermediate-acting) and regular (short-acting)	70% NPH and 30% Regular	30 to 60 minutes	Varies	10 to 16 hours
	50% NPH and 50% Regular	30 to 60 minutes	Varies	10 to 16 hours
Pre-mixed insulin lispro protamine suspension (intermediate-acting) and insulin lispro (rapid-acting)	75% lispro protamine and 25% lispro	10 to 15 minutes	Varies	10 to 16 hours
	50% lispro protamine and 50% insulin lispro	10 to 15 minutes	Varies	10 to 16 hours
Pre-mixed insulin aspart protamine suspension (intermediate-acting) and insulin aspart (rapid-acting)	70% aspart protamine and 30% aspart	5 to 15 minutes	Varies	10 to 16 hours

Data from National Diabetes Clearinghouse Types of Insulin http://diabetes.niddk.nih.gov/dm/pubs/medicines_ez/insert_C.aspx.

insulin and glucose levels such as can occur with the dawn effect (rise in blood glucose in the early morning caused by release of counter-regulatory hormones).

Premixed insulins are combinations of analogs of long-acting insulin and fast-acting insulin. These preparations do not achieve the tight glucose control provided by basal and bolus insulin taken separately, but they are more convenient to use, because they generally do not require patients to take insulin injection in the middle of the day. The most common side effect of insulin is hypoglycemia, although in rare instances people can be allergic to either the insulin or the ingredients added to the insulin to maintain a balanced pH and retard bacterial growth.

CORE CONCEPT 10

The most common and serious side effect of insulin therapy is hypoglycemia.

There are a variety of insulin delivery devices on the market, including vial and syringe, pens, insulin pumps, and hybrid pen/pumps. Insulin pumps are the most complicated to use, but provide the most precise simulation of normal insulin delivery in the body.

People with type 1 diabetes are usually initiated on a basal bolus insulin regimen. Those with type 2 diabetes whose disease has progressed beyond the control of oral agents usually begin with one injection of basal insulin per day. As their beta cells continue to fail, they may require coverage of meals with prandial insulin. Prandial insulin can be dosed in a variety of ways, from fixed dose and sliding scale to the use of ratios. Patients using a fixed dose regimen will take the same amount of insulin at meals regardless of the blood glucose level or the amount of carbohydrate eaten. Those using a sliding scale will vary their amount of insulin based on their preprandial glucose level, while those using matching insulin to carbohydrate titrate their dose based on both their preprandial glucose level and the amount of carbohydrate they intend to consume.

Nutritional management is key to effective insulin use. The proper timing of insulin doses can affect how well the postprandial elevation in glucose is controlled. Regular insulin should be taken one-half hour before meals, whereas food must be taken within 15 minutes of taking fast-acting insulin. Consistency of carbohydrate intake is seminal to avoiding erratic blood glucose patterns in those using fixed dose or sliding scale insulin regimens. Both the glycemic index of the meal and its fat content will determine when it is best to inject insulin. For example, a breakfast of a highly processed cereal may require that fast-acting insulin be given up to 30 minutes before the meal to match the rapid rise in blood glucose caused by the easily digested carbohydrate. On the other hand, for a meal of fettuccine alfredo, splitting the total insulin between two injections given at the beginning of the meal and 2 hours later can help to adjust insulin delivery so that it coincides with the delay in glucose appearance in the bloodstream caused by the meal's high fat content.

Surgical Treatment Options

Metabolic Surgery

An interesting approach to treatment of type 2 diabetes is metabolic surgery. Gastrointestinal operations, such as the roux-en-Y gastric bypass surgery, have been shown to cause drastic effects on those with diabetes, including improved glycemic control and reduced CVD risk. Randomized controlled trials have shown diabetes remission in 30% to 63% of patients with follow-up of 1 to 5 years; however, 35% to 50% of patients have recurrence with an estimated remission period of 8.3 years following roux-en-Y gastric bypass.[132] The high cost and long-term concerns of gastrointestinal operations, such as dumping syndrome, lifelong need of vitamin and mineral supplements, and postprandial hypoglycemia, certainly are of concern if considering this treatment option. The 2017 recommendations for metabolic surgery in diabetes are listed in **Table 9.23**, provided that the patient is assessed for mental health and ability to follow nutrition and lifestyle recommendations postsurgery.

TABLE 9.23 INDICATIONS FOR METABOLIC SURGERY IN ADULTS WITH TYPE 2 DIABETES

BMI Cutoff	Indication
≥ 40 kg/m^2 (≥ 35 kg/m^2 if Asian American)	Regardless of level of glycemic control or medication use
35 to 39.9 kg/m^2 (32.5 to 37.4 kg/m^2 if Asian American)	If hyperglycemia is inadequately controlled despite optimal medical therapy and lifestyle changes
30.0 to 34.9 kg/m^2 (27.5 to 32.4 kg/m^2 if Asian American)	If hyperglycemia is inadequately controlled despite optimal medical therapy through oral and/or injectable medication (including insulin)

Data from American Diabetes Association. Obesity management for the treatment of type 2 diabetes. Sec. 7. In Standards of Medical Care in Diabetes 2017. Diabetes Care 2017;40(Suppl. 1):S57–S63.

Hospitalization and Illness for Patients with Diabetes

As a patient with diabetes ages, hospitalization is common. Factors to consider include new management of insulin based on changes in nutritional intake or clinical status, monitoring of blood glucose levels, and awareness of risk factors that can alter glycemia. Control of hyperglycemia and hypoglycemia is an important consideration for patients in the hospital setting. While both are associated with adverse outcomes (increased mortality in hospitalized patients), hypoglycemia is difficult to detect and

CASE STUDY REVISITED

Aubree suffered a soccer injury and is planned to come to the hospital for repair of a torn anterior cruciate ligament. Based on the complexity of her tear, she will need open surgery, thus requiring her to stay in the hospital. She is expected to have nothing by mouth after midnight prior to the surgery, which is scheduled early in the morning.

Questions

1. How must Aubree's diet and insulin regimen be altered?
2. What is your recommendation to the inpatient medical team regarding an appropriate glycemic target?
3. What laboratory indices should be drawn upon Aubree's admission?
4. What triggers for hypoglycemia should be monitored?

acutely dangerous.[133] Previously, tight control of glucose levels below a target of 110 mg/dL was recommended for patients in the hospital setting.[134-136] However, more recent studies have either failed to show benefit or have concluded that too-intensive treatment of elevated glucose levels leads to higher rates of mortality.[137] The American Society for Parenteral and Enteral Nutrition, in its clinical guidelines for nutrition support of adult patients with hyperglycemia; the American Association of Clinical Endocrinologists; and the American Diabetes Association Consensus Statement recommend a goal range of blood glucose between 140 mg/dL and 180 mg/dL.[138,139]

Noncritical Patients with Diabetes Admitted to the Hospital

For planned admissions, a baseline A1C should be measured (if none in the past 3 months). In addition, the patient's home regimen, ability to self-manage, and overall knowledge and behavior should be assessed ideally prior to admission. For patients requiring insulin who are noncritically ill, a basal insulin dose should be given along with bolus correction if necessary. Studies indicate that this basal bolus method is associated with fewer complications than a sliding scale. Typical insulin dosing may change from the patient's usual regimen if their nutritional intake declines or while they are ill.

A protocol for monitoring and prevention of hypoglycemia should be in place. Awareness of triggering events for hyperglycemia such as emesis, change in steroid medication, interruption of intake, or alteration in meal schedule is necessary. For patients with poor intake, a fast-acting insulin given immediately after the patient eats, or based on carbohydrate counting, can be effective. Once a patient's appetite improves, insulin injections should align with meals and in accordance of point of care testing of blood glucose.[140]

Management of Patients with Diabetes Requiring Nutrition Support

Enteral Nutrition

Enteral nutrition is the preferred method of feeding for all patients with a functioning gastrointestinal tract, including in the ICU setting.[141] Some common formulas and their nutrient content are listed in **Table 9.24**.

Both regular and diabetes-specific enteral feeding formulations have been used in patients who are not able to tolerate oral feedings. Diabetes-specific formulations are lower in total carbohydrate and higher in total fat (and sometimes protein). Micronutrient composition is similar to standard enteral feedings. The carbohydrate sources in these formulas (e.g., isomaltulose and sucromalt) often have a low glycemic index. Diabetes-specific formulations may also contain appreciable amounts of fiber and many provide fat in the form of monounsaturated and omega-3 fatty acids. Both the fiber and fat content of these formulas slow gastric emptying, thereby blunting excessive glucose rise. Several studies have found a benefit in glycemic control as well as a diminution in the amount of insulin required to maintain euglycemic when these feedings are used.[142-144] However, the latest iteration of the American Society for Enteral and Parenteral Nutrition Clinical Guidelines: Nutrition Support of Adult Patients with Hyperglycemia does not endorse diabetes-specific formulations over standard formulas for use in hospitalized patients with hyperglycemia. It is important to remember that specific diabetes formulas may not be appropriate for all patients with hyperglycemia. Comorbidities such as renal disease and gastroparesis may exclude the use

TABLE 9.24 NUTRIENT CONTENT OF FORMULAS DERIVED FROM MANUFACTURERS' WEBSITES

Formula	Density (calories/mL)	Protein (%)	Carbs (%)	Fat (%)	Fiber (g)	Carb Source	Meets RDA (mL)
Glucerna 1.0	1.0	16.7	34.3	49	14.4	Corn maltodextrin, fructose, short-chain fructoliogsaccharides	1,420
Glucerna 1.2	1.2	20	35	45	16	Corn maltodextrin, fructose	1,250
Glucerna 1.5	1.5	22	33	45	17	Corn maltodextrin, fructose, short-chain fructoliogsaccharides	1,000
Diabetisource AC	1.2	20	36	44	15.2	Pureed fruits and vegetables	1,250
Glytrol	1.0	18	40	42	15.2	Modified cornstarch	1,500

of these feedings due to electrolyte imbalances and the need to limit fat and fiber content.

Medication in enteral feeding Outside of critical care units, subcutaneous insulin administration is a more common method of insulin delivery. Scheduled subcutaneous insulin should consist of basal, meal, and correction components (with the latter two being administered before meals). Prolonged use of sliding scale insulin as the sole method of glucose control is discouraged.[23]

In stable patients, either in the hospital, nursing home, at home a basal bolus approach to insulin therapy, similar to that used for oral feeding, can be instituted. Basal insulin doses can be given with either long-acting insulin once per day or intermediate-acting insulin twice a day. Short-acting or rapid-acting insulin, in conjunction with food, can be provided to account for glucose excursions following nutrient intake.

In patients on continuous enteral infusion, half the total daily dose of insulin can be given as basal insulin with the rest provided as regular or short-acting given four to six times per day.

Parenteral Nutrition (PN)

Parenteral nutrition is administered in those patients who are malnourished or at risk for malnutrition whose gastrointestinal tract is compromised. Hyperglycemia is a frequent finding in patients both with and without diabetes.[145] The stress of illness, especially infection, promotes insulin resistance. In addition, dextrose supplied intravenously circumvents the normal incretin response, adding to the hyperglycemic milieu.[146] As many patients receiving PN are malnourished, reduction in muscle mass also contributes to insulin resistance.

PN solutions should provide adequate carbohydrate to spare protein for tissue synthesis while avoiding hyperglycemia. Carbohydrate is usually initially limited to 1.5 mg/kg to 2 mg/kg of body weight per minute to avoid hyperglycemia.[146] This translates into 100 to 150 g of carbohydrate given over 24 hours. Once glycemic control has been established and electrolytes stabilized, the dextrose in the PN can be advanced to a maximum of 4 mg/kg/min.[147] Patients in the ICU on PN can be maintained on 80% of calculated energy requirements to avoid insulin resistance.[141] For obese patients, calorie intake should be kept at 60% to 70% of estimated needs.[147] However, in patients fed hypocaloric solutions, an increase in the protein content to 2 g/kg body weight may be indicated to aid in protein sparing.[148] Although higher fat levels in PN displace carbohydrate calories and may decrease the risk of hyperglycemia, normalization in blood glucose levels may also be derived by decreasing the fat content of the PN. High circulating levels of fatty acids and muscle fat content increase insulin resistance and may induce immunosuppression.[149] For this reason, lipid emulsions above 1.3 g/kg/day are not recommended.

> **PRACTICE POINT**
>
> High circulating levels of fatty acids and muscle fat content increase insulin resistance and may induce immunosuppression. For this reason, lipid emulsions above 1.3 g/kg/day are not recommended.

Most patients with diabetes require insulin to control hyperglycemia while on PN. Until PN dose is established, IV infusion of insulin is preferred. This allows immediate titration of the insulin dose without having to wait until the next bag of PN is hung.[150] Once the dextrose in the PN is advanced to goal, insulin can be added to the bags of PN. When intravenous insulin is not possible, insulin can be added to the PN. One method of determining a starting insulin dose is to provide 0.05 to 0.1 units of regular insulin per gram of dextrose in the PN. Breakthrough hyperglycemia is controlled by subcutaneous insulin injection and one-half to two-thirds of the amount of subcutaneous insulin used that day is added to the next day's PN formulation. This procedure continues until blood glucose levels are stabilized.

Chapter Summary

Diabetes is a complex disease that can only be managed through the support from medical, psychological, and nutritional interventions. Patients with both type 1 and type 2 diabetes require support from the care team to increase self-efficacy and take charge in management of this disease. The acute complications of diabetes, hypoglycemia and hyperglycemia, must be managed daily in both the inpatient and outpatient setting. More threatening in the long term are the chronic complications of diabetes, which may be minimized or avoided through a daily pharmacological and lifestyle regimen. As the research continues to grow on the best practices for diabetes managment, clinicians must strive to ensure patients have the best comprehensive care and follow the most up-to-date recommendations to feel better and live longer.

Key Terms

polyuria, polydispia, polyphagia, acetone, acetoacetic acid, beta-hydroxybutyric acid, hyperglycemia, diabetic ketoacidosis, Kussmaul's respirations, euglycemia, gluconeogenesis, glycogenolysis, insulin resistance, gestational diabetes, glycemic index, glycemic load, hypoglycemia, insulin to carbohydrate ratio, diabetes distress, nephropathy, retinopathy, neuropathy, gastroparesis, miroalbuminuria

References

1. Centers for Disease Control and Prevention. *National Diabetes Statistics Report: Estimates of Diabetes and Its Burden in the United States, 2017*. Atlanta, GA: US Department of Health and Human Services; 2017. Updated July 217 2017. Accessed November 13, 2017.

2. Treatment and Care for American Indians/Alaska Natives: American Diabetes Association Web site. http://www.diabetes.org/living-with-diabetes/complications/native-americans.html. Updated April 1, 2014. Accessed September 20, 2014

3. Karvonen, M, Viik-Kajander M, Moltchanova, E, et al. Incidence of childhood type 1 diabetes worldwide. Diabetes Mondiale (DiaMond) Project Group. *Diabetes Care.* 2000;23(10):1516-1526.

4. Keenan HA, Sun JK, King GL, et al. Residual insulin production and pancreatic β-Cell turnover after 50 years of diabetes. *Diabetes.* 2010;59(11):2846-2853. doi: 10.2337/db10-0676

5. Gan MJ, Albanese-O'Neill A, Haller MJ. Type 1 diabetes: current concepts in epidemiology, pathophysiology, clinical care, and research. *Curr Probl Pediatr Adolesc Health Care.* 2012;42(10):269-291.

6. Triplitt CL. Understanding the kidneys' role in blood glucose regulation. *Am J Manag Care.* 2012;(suppl 1):S11-S16.

7. Kitabchi AE, Umpierrez GE, Murphy MB, et al. Hyperglycemia crises in diabetes. *Diabetes Care.* 2004;27(suppl 1):S94-102.

8. Wajchenberg BL. Beta-cell failure in diabetes and preservation by clinical treatment. *Endocr Rev.* 2007;(2):187-218.

9. Kasuga, M. Insulin resistance and pancreatic β cell failure. *J Clin Invest.* 2006;116(7):1756-1760. doi: 10.1172/JCI29189

10. Diabetes Risk Factors. National Diabetes Education Program website. http://ndep.nih.gov/am-i-at-risk/DiabetesRiskFactors.aspx. Updated November 2016. Accessed November 13, 2017.

11. Kelsey MM, Forster JE, Van Pelt RE, Reusch JE, Nadeau KJ. Adipose tissue insulin resistance in adolescents with and without type 2 diabetes. *Pediatr Obes.* 2014;5:373-380. doi: 10.1111/j.2047-6310.2013.00189.

12. Boden G. Effects of free fatty acids (FFAs) on glucose metabolism: significance for insulin resistance in type 2 diabetes. *Exp Clin Endocrinol Diabetes.* 2003;111(3):121-124.

13. Meier J, Nauck A. Is the diminished incretin effect in type 2 diabetes just an epiphenonimen of impair beta cell function? *Diabetes.* 2010;59(5):1117-1125.

14. Cavaghan M. The beta cell and first-phase insulin secretion: phases of insulin secretion. In Medscape Diabetes & Endocrinology: Incretin Hormones Expert column. https://www.medscape.org/viewarticle/483307_2. Accessed November 13, 2017.

15. American Diabetes Association. Diagnosis and classification of diabetes mellitus. *Diabetes Care.* 2009;32(Suppl 1):S62-S67.

16. Centers for Disease Control and Prevention. National Diabetes Fact Sheet: National estimates and general information on diabetes and prediabetes in the United States, 2011. Atlanta, GA: U.S. Department of Health and Human Services, Centers for Disease Control and Prevention; 2011.

17. Barbour LA, McCurdy CE, Hernandez TL, Kirwan JP, Catalano PM, Friedman JE. Cellular mechanisms for insulin resistance in normal pregnancy and gestational diabetes. *Diabetes Care.* 2007;30 (Suppl 2):S112-S119.

18. American Diabetes Association. Gestational diabetes mellitus. *Diabetes Care.* 2003;26(Suppl 1):S103-S105.

19. HAPO Study Cooperative Research Group, Metzger BE, Lowe LP, et al. Hypoglycemia and adverse pregnancy outcomes. *New Eng J Med.* 2008;358(19):1191-2002. doi: 10.1056/NEJMoa0707943.

20. International Association of Diabetes and Pregnancy Study Groups Consensus Panel, Metzger BE, Gabbe SG, Persson B, et al. International association of diabetes and pregnancy study groups recommendations on the diagnosis and classification of hyperglycemia in pregnancy. *Diabetes Care.* 2010;33:676-682. doi: 10.2337/dc09-1848.

21. American Diabetes Association. Classification and diagnosis of diabetes. Sec. 2. In: Standards of Medical Care in Diabetes 2017. *Diabetes Care.* 2017;40(suppl 1):S11-S24.

22. Committee opinion no. 504: Screening and diagnosis of gestational diabetes mellitus. *Obstet. Gyncol.* 2011;188(3):751-753. doi: 10.1097/AOG.0b013e3182310cc3.

23. Handelsman Y, Mechanick JI, Blonde L, et al. American Association of Clinical Endocrinologists Medical Guidelines for Clinical Practice for developing a diabetes mellitus comprehensive care plan. *Endocr Pract.* 2011;17(suppl 2):1-53. Table 4

24. Wheeler MI, Dunbar SA, Jacks LM, et al. Macronutrient, food groups and eating patterns in the management of diabetes: a systematic review of the literature 2010. *Diabetes Care.* 2012;35(2):434-445.

25. Kirk JK, Graves DE, Craven TE. Restricted carbohydrate diets in patients with type 2 diabetes a meta-analysis. *J Am Diet Assoc.* 2008;108(1):91-110.

26. Salas-Salvadó J, Bulló M, Babio N, et al. Reduction in the incidence of type 2 diabetes with a Mediterranean diet. *Diabetes Care.* 2011;34(1):14-19.

27. Estruch R, Ros E, Salas-Salvadó J, et al. Primary prevention of cardiovascular disease with a Mediterranean diet. *N Engl J Med.* 2013;368(14):1279-1290.

28. Franz MJ, Powers MA, Leontos C, et al. The evidence for medical nutrition therapy for type 1 and type 2 diabetes in adults. *J Am Diet Assoc.* 2010;110(12):1852-1889.doi:0.1016/j.jada.2010.09.014.

29. Clinical Nutrition Guideline for Overweight and Obese Adults with type 2 diabetes, prediabetes, or a high risk for developing type 2 diabetes. Joslin Diabetes Center Web site. Published August 7, 2011. Accessed November 13, 2017.

30. Institute of Medicine. *Dietary Reference Intakes: energy, carbohydrate, fiber, fat, fatty acids, cholesterol, protein and amino acids.* Washington DC: National Academies Press; 2002.

31. Jenkins DJ, Wolever TM, Taylor RH, et al. Glycemic index of foods: a physiological basis for carbohydrate exchange. *Am J Clin Nutr.* 1981;34(3):362-366.

32. Atkinson FS, Foster-Powell KS, Brand-Miller JC. International tables of glycemic index and glycemic load values. *Diabetes Care.* 2008;31(12):2281-2283.

33. Wolever TMS, Hamad S, Chiasson JL, et al. Day-to-day consistency in amount and source of carbohydrate intake associated with improved glucose control in type 1 diabetes. *J Am Coll Nutr.* 1999; 18:242-247.

34. Boden G, Sargrad K, Homko C, et al. Effect of a low-carbohydrate diet on appetite, blood glucose levels, and insulin resistance in obese patients with type 2 diabetes. *Ann Intern Med.* 2005;142:403-411.

35. DAFNE Study Group. Training in flexible, intensive insulin management to enable dietary freedom in people with type 1 diabetes: dose adjustment for normal eating (DAFNE) randomised controlled trial. *Br Med J.* 2002;325:746-751.

36. Lowe J, Linjawi S, Mensch M, James K, Attia J. Flexible eating and flexible insulin dosing in patients with diabetes. Results of an intensive self-management course. *Diabetes Res Clin Pract.* 2008; 80:439-443.

37. Chandalia M, Garg A, Lutjohann D, von Bergmann K, Grundy SM, Brinkley LJ. Beneficial effects of high dietary fiber intake in patients with type 2 diabetes mellitus. *N Engl J Med.* 2000;342(19):1392-1398.

38. Trumbo P, Schlicker S, Yates AA, Poos M. Dietary reference intakes for energy, carbohydrate, fiber, fat, fatty acids, cholesterol, protein and amino acids. *J Am Diet Assoc.* 2002;102(11):1621-1630.

39. Clemens R, Kranz S, Mobley AR, et al. Filling America's fiber intake gap: summary of a roundtable to probe realistic solutions with a focus on grain-based foods. *J Nutr.* 2012;142(7):1390S-401S. doi: 10.3945/jn.112.160176
40. Bantile JP, Swanson JE, Thomas W, Laine DC. Metabolic effects of dietary sucrose in type 2 diabetes subjects. *Diabetes Care.* 1993;16:1301-1305.
41. Peterson DB, Lambert J, Gerring S, et al. Sucrose in the diet of patients with diabetes-just another carbohydrate? *Diabetologia.* 1986;29:216-220.
42. Schaefer EJ, Gleason JA, Dansinger M. Dietary fructose and glucose differentially affect lipid and glucose homeostasis. *J Nutr.* 2009;139(6):1257S-1262S. doi: 10.3945/jn.108.098186.
43. Gannon MC, Nuttall JA, Damberg G, Gupta V, Nuttall FQ. Effect of protein ingestion on the glucose appearance rate in people with type 2 diabetes. *J Clin Endocrinol Metab.* 2001;86:1040-1047.
44. Gannon MC, Nuttall FQ, Saeed A, Jordan K, Hoover H. An increase in dietary protein improves the blood glucose response in persons with type 2 diabetes. *Am J Clin Nutr.* 2003;78:734-741.
45. Parker B, Noakes M, Luscombe N, Clifton P. Effect of a high-protein, high-monosaturated fat weight loss diet on glycemic control and lipid levels in type 2 diabetes. *Diabetes Care.* 2002;25:425-430.
46. Gray RO, Butler PC, Beers TR, Kryshak EJ, Rizza RA. Comparison of the ability of bread vs. bread plus meat to treat and prevent subsequent hypoglycemia in patients with insulin-dependent diabetes mellitus. *J Clin Endocrinol Metab.* 1996;81:1508-1511.
47. Peters AL, Davidson MB. Protein and fat effects on glucose responses and insulin requirements in subjects with insulin-dependent diabetes mellitus. *Am J Clin Nutr.* 1993;58:555-560.
48. Hamdy O, Horton ES. Protein content in diabetes nutrition plan. *Curr Diab Rep.* 2011;11(2):111-119.
49. Brinkworth GD, Noakes M, Parker B, Foster P, Clifton PM. Long-term effects of advice to consume a high protein, low-fat diet, rather than a conventional weight-loss diet, in obese adults with type 2 diabetes: 1-year follow-up of a randomized trial. *Diabetologia.* 2004;47:1677-1686.
50. U.S. Department of Health and Human Services and U.S. Department of Agriculture. *2015 – 2020 Dietary Guidelines for Americans.* 8th ed. Washington DC: U.S. Government Printing office; December 2015. http://health.gov/dietaryguidelines/2015/guidelines/ Accessed October 19, 2017
51. Riccardi G, Giacco R, Rivellese AA. Dietary fat, insulin sensitivity and the metabolic syndrome. *Clin Nutr.* 2004;23(4):447-456.
52. Wolpert HA, Atakov-Castillo A, Smith SA, Steil GM. Dietary fat acutely increases glucose concentrations and insulin requirements in patients with type 1 diabetes: implications for carbohydrate-based bolus dose calculations and intensive diabetes management. *Diabetes Care.* 2013;36:810-816. doi: 10.2337/dc12-0092.
53. Buse JB, Ginsberg HN, Bakris GL, et al. Primary prevention of cardiovascular disease in people in people with diabetes mellitus: scientific statement from the American Heart Association and the American Diabetes Association. *Diabetes Care.* 2007;30:162-172. doi: 10.2337/dc07-9917.
54. Estruch R, Martinez-Gonzalez M, Corelia D, et al. Effects of Mediterranean-style diet on cardiovascular risk factors; a randomized trial. *Ann Intern Med.* 2006;145(1):1-11.
55. American Diabetes Association. Lifestyle management. Sec. 4. In Standards of Medical Care in Diabetes 2017. *Diabetes Care.* 2017;40(suppl 1):S33-S43.
56. Holman RR, Paul S, Farmer A, et al. Atrovastatin in factorial with omega-3EE90 risk reduction in diabetes (AFORRD): a randomised controlled trial. *Diabetologia.* 2009;52:50-59. doi: 10.1007/s00125-008-1179-5.
57. ORIGIN Trial Investigators, Bosch J, Gerstein HC, et al. n-3 Fatty acids and cardiovascular outcomes in patients with dysglycemia. *N Engl J Med.* 2012;367:309-318. doi: 10.1056/NEJMoa1203859
58. Gardner C, Wylie-Rosett J, Gidding SS, et al. Nonnutritive sweeteners: current use and health perspectives: a scientific statement from the American Heart and American Diabetes Association. *Diabetes Care.* 2012;35(8):1798-1808.
59. Butchko HH, Stargell WW. Aspartame: scientific evaluation in the post-marketing period. *Regul Toxicol Pharmacol.* 2001;34(3):221-233.
60. Nonnutritive sweeteners: current use and health perspectives. a scientific statement from the American Heart Association and the American Diabetes Association. *Diabetes Care.* 2012;35(8)1798-1808.
61. Additional Information about High-Intensity Sweeteners Permitted for Use in Food in the United States. U.S. Food and Drug Administration Web site. http: www.fda.gov/food/ingredientspackaginglabeling/foodadditivesingredients/ucm397725.htm. Updated May 24, 2015. Accessed November 13, 2017.
62. Shai I, Wainstein J, Harman-Boehm I, et al. Glycemic effects of moderate alcohol intake among patients with type 2 diabetes: a multicenter, randomized, clinical intervention trial. *Diabetes Care.* 2007;30(12):3011-3016.
63. Howard AA, Amsten JH, Gourevitch MN. Effect of alcohol consumption on diabetes mellitus: a systematic review. *Ann Intern Med.* 2004;140:211-219.
64. Balk EM, Tatsioni A, Lichtenstein AH, Lau J, Pittas AG. Effect of chromium supplementation on glucose metabolism and lipids: a systematic review of randomized controlled trials. *Diabetes Care.* 2007;30(8):2154-2163.
65. Geil P, Shane-McWorter C. Dietary supplements in the management of diabetes: potential risks and benefits. *J Am Diet Assoc.* 2008;108(4 suppl 1):S59-65. doi: 10.1016/j.jada.2008.01.020.
66. Gillespie KD. Type 1 diabetes pathogenesis and prevention: a systematic review and meta-analysis 2006; *CMAJ.* 2006;175(2):165-170.
67. Zipitis CS, Kobegn A. Vitamin D supplementation in early childhood and risk of type 1 diabetes. *Arch Dis Child.* 2008;93(6):512-517. doi: 10.1136/adc.2007.128579.
68. Diabetes and Dietary Supplements: In Depth. National Center for Complementary and Alternative Medicine Web site. http://nccam.nih.gov/health/diabetes/supplements. Updated July 2015. Accessed November 13, 2017.
69. Khan A, Safdar M, Ali Khan MM, Khattak KN, Anderson RA. Cinnamon improves glucose and lipids of people with type 2 diabetes. *Diabetes Care.* 2003;(12)26:3215-3218.
70. Baker W, Kluger T, Gutierrez-Williams G, White CM, Kluger J, Coleman CI. Effect of cinnamon on glucose control and lipid parameters. *Diabetes Care.* 2008;31(1):41-43.
71. Allen RW, Schwartzman E, Baker WL, Coleman CI, Phung OJ. Cinnamon use in Type 2 diabetes: an updated systematic review and meta-analysis. *Ann Fam Med.* 2013;11(5):452-459. doi: 10.1370/afm.1517.
72. Academy of Nutrition and Dietetics Evidence Analysis Library. 2015 Diabetes Type 1 and Type 2 Evidence-Based Nutrition Practice Guideline. https://www.andeal.org/topic.cfm?menu=5305&cat=5595Accessed November 13,2017.
73. Nguyen NT, Nguyen XM, Lane J, Wang P. Relationship between obesity and diabetes in a US population: findings from the national health and nutrition examination survey 1999-2006. *Obes Surg.* 2011;(21):351-355. doi: 10.1007/s11695-010-0335-4.

74. American Diabetes Association. Create Your Plate. http://www.diabetes.org/food-and-fitness/food/planning-meals/create-your-plate. Updated September 14, 2016. Accessed November 13, 2017.
75. Davidson PC, Hebblewhite HR, Bode BW, et al. Statistically based CSII parameters: correction factor, (CR (1700 rule), carbohydrate-to-insulin ratio, CIR (2.8 rule), and basal-to-bolus ratio. *Diabetes Technol Ther*. 2003;3:237.
76. King, AB. How much do I give? Reevaluation of insulin dosing estimation formulas using continuous glucose monitoring. *Endocr Pract*. 2010;15(3)428-32 doi: 10.4158/EP09308.
77. Shirani F, Salehi-Abargouei A, Azadbakht L. Effects of Dietary Approaches to Stop Hypertension (DASH) diet on some risk for developing type 2 diabetes: a systematic review and meta-analysis on controlled clinical trials. *Nutrition*. 2013;29(7-8):939-947. doi: 10.1016/j.nut.2012.
78. Carbohydrate Counting. American Diabetes Association Web site. http://www.diabetes.org/food-and-fitness/food/what-can-i-eat/understanding-carbohydrates/carbohydrate-counting.html Updated August 30, 2017. Accessed October 20, 2017
79. Chu L, Hamilton J, Riddell MC. Clinical management of the physically active patient with type 1. *Phys Sports Med*. 2011;39(2):64-77. doi: 10.3810/psm.2011.05.1896
80. Ertel AC, Davis SN. Evidence for a vicious cycle of exercise and hypoglycemia in type diabetes mellitus. *Diabetes Metab Res Rev*. 2004;20(2):124-130.
81. Davis, SN, Galassetti P, Wasserman DH Tate D. Effects of antecedent hypoglycemia on subsequent counterregulatory responses to exercise. *Diabetes*. 2000;49(1):73-81.
82. MacDonald MJ. Postexercise late-onset hypoglycemia in insulin dependent diabetic patients *Diabetes Care*. 1987;10(5):584-588.
83. Riddell MC, Perkins BA. Type 1 diabetes and vigorous exercise: applications of exercise physiology to patient managament. *CJD*. 2006;30(1):63-71.
84. Iscoe KE, Riddell MC. Continuous moderate intensity exercise with or without intermittent high-intensity work: effects on acute and late glycemia in athletes with type 1 diabetes mellitus. *Diabetes Med*. 2011;28(7):824-32. doi: 10.1111/j.1464-5491.2011.03274.x.
85. Robertson K, Adolfosson P, Scheiner G, Hanas R, Riddell MC. Exercise in children and adolescents with diabetes. *Pediatr Diabetes*. 2009;10(suppl 12):154-168.
86. Michaliszyn SF, Shaibi GQ, Quinn, L. Fritschi C, Faulkner MS. Physical fitness, dietary intake, and metabolic control in adolescents with type 1 diabetes. *Pediatr Diabetes*. 2009;10(6)389-394. doi: 10.1111/j.1399-5448.2009.00500.x
87. Wallberg-Hendriksson H, Gunnarsson R, Henriksson J, et al. Increased peripheral insulin sensitivity and muscle mitochondrial enzymes but unchanged blood glucose control in type 1 diabetics after physical training. *Diabetes*. 1982;31(12):1044-1050.
88. Giannini C, Mohn A, Chiarelli F. Physical exercise and diabetes during childhood. *ACAT Biomed*. 2006;77(suppl 1):18-25.
89. DeFronzo RA, Gunnarsson R, Bjoorkman O, Olsson M, Wahren J. Effects of insulin on peripheral and spanchnic glucose metabolism in non-insulin dependent type 2 diabetes mellitus. *J Clin Invest*. 1985;76(1)149-155.
90. Thomas E, Sevilla L, Palacin M, Zorzano A. The insulin-sensitive GLUT4 storage compartment is a post-endocytic and heterogeneous population recruited by acute exercise. *Biochem Biophys Res Commun*. 2001;284(2):490-495.
91. Goodyear LJ, Kahn BB. Exercise, glucose transport, and insulin sensitivity. *Annu Rev Med*. 1998;49:235-261.
92. Wang Y, Simar D, Fiatarone Singh MA. Adaptations to exercise training within skeletal muscle in adults with type 2 diabetes or impaired glucose tolerance: a systematic review. *Diabetes Metab Res Rev*. 2009;25(1):13-40. doi: 10.1002/dmrr.928.
93. Asano RY, Sales MM, Browne RA, et al. Acute effects of physical exercise in type 2 diabetes: A review. *World J Diabetes*. 2014;15; 5(5):659-665. doi: 10.4239/wjd.v5.i5.659
94. King DS, Baldus PJ, Sharp RL, Kesl LD, Feltmeyer TL, Riddle MS. Time course for exercise-induced alterations in insulin action and glucose tolerance in middle-aged people. *J Appl Physiol*. 1995;78(1):17-22.
95. Exercise and type 2 diabetes: American College of Sports Medicine and the American Diabetes Association: joint position statement. *Med Sci Sports Exercise*. 2010;42(12):2282-2303.
96. Minuk HL, Vranic M, Marliss EB, Hanna AK, Albisser AM, Zinman B. Glucoregulatory and metabolic response to exercise in obese noninsulin-dependent diabetes. *Am J Physiol*. 1981;240(5):E458-E464.
97. Sigal RJ, Kenny GP, Wasserman GH, Castaneda-Sceppa C. Physical activity/exercise and type 2 diabetes. *Diabetes Care*. 2004;2(10): 2518-2539.
98. Baynard T, Franklin RM, Goulopoulou S, Carhart R Jr, Kanaley JA. Effect of a single vs multiple bouts of exercise on glucose control in women with type 2 diabetes. *Metabolism*. 2005;54(8):989-994.
99. Kosair Children's Hospital. http://www.kosairchildrenshospital.com/carbohydrate-adjustment-for-activity. Accessed November 30, 2014.
100. American Diabetes Association. Glycemic targets. Sec. 6. In Standards of Medical Care in Diabetes 2017. *Diabetes Care*. 2017;40(suppl 1):S48-S56.
101. Wang J, Zgibor J, Matthews JT, Charron-Prochownik D, Sereika SM, Siminerio L. Self-monitoring of blood glucose is associated with problem-solving skills in hyperglycemia and hypoglycemia. *Diabetes Educ*. 2012;38(2):207-218.
102. Farmer AJ, Perera R, Ward A, et al. Meta-analysis of individual patient data in randomized trials of self-monitoring of blood glucose in people with non-insulin treated type 2 diabetes. *BMJ*. 2012;344:e486. doi: 10.1136/bmj.e486
103. Workgroup on Hypoglycemia, American Diabetes Association. Defining and reporting hypoglycemia in diabetes: a report from the American Diabetes Association Workgroup on Hypoglycemia. *Diabetes Care*. 2005;28(5):1245-1249.
104. UK Prospective Diabetes Study (UKPDS) Group. Intensive blood-glucose control with sulphonylureas or insulin compared with conventional treatment and risk of complications in patients with type 2 diabetes (UKPDS 33). *Lancet*. 1998;352(9131):837-853.
105. Hadi AR, Carr CS, Al Suwaidl J. Endothelial dysfunction: cardiovascular risk factors, therapy, and outcome. *Vasc Health Risk Manag*. 2005;1(3):183-198.
106. Whelton PK, Carey RM, Aronow WS, et al. 2017 ACC/AHA/AAPA/ABC/ACPM/AGS/APhA/ASH/ASPC/NMA/PCNA Guideline for the prevention, detection, evaluation, and management of high blood pressure in adults, *J Am Coll Cardiol*. 2017. doi: 10.1016/j.jacc.2017.11.006.
107. Stone A, Robinson J, Lichtenstein A. 2013 ACC/AHA guideline on the treatment of blood cholesterol to reduce atherosclerotic cardiovascular risk in adults: a report of the American College of Cardiology/American Heart Association task force on practice guidelines. *Circulation*. 2014;129(25 suppl 2):S1-S45. doi: 10.1161/01.cir.0000437738.63853.7a

108. American Diabetes Association. Pharmacologic approaches to glycemic treatment. Sec 8. In Standards in Medical Care in Diabetes 2017. *Diabetes Care.* 2017;40(suppl 1):SS64-S74.

109. Vedovato M, Lepore G, Coracina A, et al. Effect of sodium intake on blood pressure and albuminuria in Type 2 diabetic patients: the role of insulin resistance. *Diabetologia.* 2004;47(2):300-303.

110. Van Horn L, Coin M, Kris-Etherton P, et al. The evidence for dietary prevention and treatment of cardiovascular disease. *J Am Diet Assoc.* 2008;108(2):287-331. doi: 10.1016/j.jada.2007.10.050.

111. Mantzoros CS, Williams CJ, Manson JE, Meigs JB, Hu FB. Adherence to the Mediterranean dietary pattern is positively associated with plasma adiponectin concentrations in diabetic women. *Am J Clin Nutr.* 2006;84(2):328-335.

112. What Is the DASH Eating Plan? National Heart, Lung and Blood Institute Web site. http://www.nhlbi.nih.gov/health/health-topics/topics/dash/lifestyle.html. Published September 16, 2015. Accessed November 13, 2017.

113. National Kidney Foundation. KDOQI Clinical Practice Guidelines and Clinical Practice Recommendations for Diabetes and Chronic Kidney. *Am J Kidney Dis.* 2007;49(2):Supp 2.

114. Turin TC, James M, Ravani P, et al. Proteinuria and rate of change in kidney function in a community-based population. *J Am Soc Nephrol.* 2013;24(10):1661-1667. doi: 10.1681/ASN.2012111118

115. National Kidney Foundation. KDOQI clinical practice guideline for diabetes and CKD: 2012; *Am J Kidney Dis.* 2012;60(5):850-886. doi: 10.1053/j.ajkd.2012.07.005.

116. Pedrini MT, Levey AS, Lau J, Chalmers TC, Wang PH. The effect of dietary protein restriction on the progression of diabetic and nondiabetic renal diseases: A meta-analysis. *Ann Intern Med.* 1996;124(7):627-632.

117. Dussol B, Iovanna C, Raccah D, et al. A randomized trial of low-protein diet in type 1 and in type 2 diabetes mellitus patients with incipient and overt nephropathy. *J Ren Nutr.* 2005;15(4):398-406.

118. Pijls LT, de Vries H, van Eijk JT, Donker AJ. Protein restriction, glomerular filtration rate and albuminuria in patients with type 2 diabetes mellitus: a randomized trial. *Eur J Clin Nutr.* 2002;56(12);1200-1207.

119. Kidney Disease Improving Global Outcomes (KDIGO) CKD Workgroup. KDIGO 2012 Clinical Practice Guideline for the Evaluation and Management of Chronic Kidney Disease. *Kidney Int.* 2013;3(1):1-163.

120. Beto JA, Ramirez WE, Bansal VK. Medical nutrition therapy in adults with chronic kidney disease: integrating evidence and consensus into practice for the generalist registered dietitian nutritionist. *J Acad Nutr Diet.* 2014;114(7):1077-1087.

121. Evertt A, Boucher J, Cypress M, et al. Nutrition therapy recommendations for the management of adults with diabetes. *Diabetes Care.* 2014;37(suppl 1):S120-S143.

122. The Renal Association. http://www.renal.org/information-resources/the-uk-eckd-guide/ckd-stages#sthash Accessed November 13, 2017.

123. Age-Related Eye Disease Study 2 Research Group. Lutein/Zeaxanthin and Omega-3 fatty acids for age-related macular degeneration. The age-related eye disease study 2 (AREDS2) controlled randomized clinical trial. *JAMA.* 2013;15;309(19):2005-2015. doi: 10.1001/jama.2013.4997.

124. Age-Related Eye Disease Study 2 (AREDS2) Research Group, Chew EY, SanGiovanni JP, et al. Lutein/zeaxanthin for the treatment of age-related cataract: AREDS2 randomized trial report no. 4. *JAMA Ophthalmol.* 2013;131(7):843-850. doi: 10.1001/jamaophthalmol.2013.4412.

125. Gulati M, Anand V, Jain N, et al. Essentials of Periodontal medicine in preventive medicine. *Int J Prev Med.* 2013;4(9)988-994.

126. Touger-Decker R, Mobley C, Academy of Nutrition and Dietetics. Oral health and nutrition Academy of Nutrition and Dietetics Position Statement. *J Acad Nutr Diet.* 2013;113(5):693-701. doi: 10.1016/j.jand.2013.03.001.

127. Shin A, Camilleri M. Diagnostic assessment of diabetic gastroparesis. *Diabetes.* 2013;62(8):2667-2673. doi: 10.2337/db12-1706.

128. Sadiya A. Nutritional therapy for the management of diabetic gastroparesis: clinical review. *Diabetes Metab Syndr Obes.* 2012;5:329-335. doi: 10.2147/DMSO.S31962.

129. Parrish CR. Nutrition intervention in the patient with gastroparesis. *Prac Gastroenterol.* 2003;3:53-66.

130. Inzucchi S, Bergenstel RM, Buse JB. Management of hyperglycemia in type 2 diabetes, 2015: a patient-center approach: update to a position statement of the American Diabetes Association and the European Association for the study of diabetes. *Diabetes Care.* 2015;38(1);140-149.

131. Insulin, Medicines, and Other Diabetes Treatments. National Diabetes Clearinghouse. http://diabetes.niddk.nih.gov/dm/pubs/medicines_ez/insert C.aspx. Updated November 2016. Accessed November 13, 2017.

132. American Diabetes Association. Obesity management for the treatment of type 2 diabetes. Sec. 7. In Standards of Medical Care in Diabetes 2017. *Diabetes Care.* 2017;40(suppl 1):S57-S63.

133. Nasraway SA Jr. Hypoglycemia during critical illness. *J Parenter Enteral Nutr.* 2006;30(3):254-258.

134. Van Den Berghe G, Wouters P, Weekers F, et al. Intensive insulin therapy in critically ill patients. *N Engl J Med.* 2001;345(19):1359-1367.

135. Krinsley JS. Effect of an intensive glucose management protocol on the mortality of critically ill adults. *Mayo Clin Proc.* 2004;79(8):992-1000.

136. Van Den Berghe G, Wilmer A, Hermans G, et al. Intensive insulin therapy in the medical ICU. *N Engl J Med.* 2006;354(5):449-461.

137. NICE-SUGAR Study Investigators, Finfer S, Chittock DR, et al. Intensive vs. conventional glucose control in critically ill patients. *N Engl J Med.* 2009;360(13):1283-1297. doi: 10.1056/NEJMoa0810625

138. McMahon MM, Nystrom E, Braunschweig C, et al. A.S.P.E.N Clinical Guidelines: Nutrition Support of adult patients with hyperglycemia. *J Parenter Enteral Nutr.* 2013;37(1):23-36. doi: 10.1177/0148607112452001

139. Moghissi ES, Korytkowski MT, DiNardo M, et al. American Association of Clinical Endocrinologists and American Diabetes Association Consensus Statement on Inpatient Glycemic Control. *Diabetes Care.* 2009;32(6):1119-1131. doi: 10.2337/dc09-9029

140. American Diabetes Association. Diabetes care in the hospital. Sec. 14. In Standards of Medical Care in Diabetes 2017. *Diabetes Care.* 2017;40(suppl 1):S120-S127.

141. McClave SA, Martindale RG, Vanek VW, et al. Guidelines for the provision and assessment of nutrition support therapy in the adult critically ill patients. *J Parenter Enteral Nutr.* 2009;33(3):277-316. doi: 10.1177/0148607109335234.

142. Pohl M, Mayr P, Mertl-Roetzer M, et al. Glycemic control in patients with type 2 diabetes mellitus with a disease-specific enteral formula: stage II of a randomized, controlled multicenter trial. *J Parenter Enteral Nutr.* 2009;33(1):37-49. doi: 10.1177/0148607108324582.

143. Vanschoonbeek K, Lansink M, van Laere KJM, Senden JM, Verdijk LB, van Loon LJ. Slowly digestible carbohydrate sources can be used to attenuate the postprandial glycemic response to the ingestion of diabetes specific enteral formulas. *Diabetes Educ.* 2009;35(4):631-640. doi: 10.1177/0145721709335466

144. Ellia M, Ceriello A, Laube H, Sinclair AJ, Engfer M, Stratton RJ. Enteral nutrition support and use of diabetes-specific enteral formulas for patients with diabetes. *Diabetes Care.* 2005;28(9)2267-2279.

145. Pasquel FJ, Spiegelman R, McCauley M, et al. Hyperglycemia during total parenteral nutrition: an important marker of poor outcome and mortality in hospitalized patients. *Diabetes Care.* 2010;33(4):739-741. doi: 10.2337/dc09-1748.

146. Via MA, Mechanick JI. Inpatient enteral and parenteral [corrected] nutrition for patients with diabetes. *Curr Diab Rep.* 2011;11(2):99-105. doi: 10.1007/s11892-010-0168-5.

147. ASPEN Board of Directors and the Clinical Guidelines Task Force. Guidelines for the use of parenteral and enteral nutrition in adult and pediatric patients. *J Parenter Enteral Nutr.* 2002;26(suppl):1SA-138SA.

148. Hoffer LJ, Bistrian BR. Appropriate protein provision in critical illness: a systematic and narrative review. *Am J Clin Nutr.* 2012;96(3): 591-600.

149. Liu Z, Liu J, Jahn LA, Fowler DE, Barrett EJ. Infusing lipid raises plasma free fatty acids and induces insulin resistance in muscle microvasculature. *J Clin Endocrinol Metab.* 2009;94(9):3543-3549.

150. Clement S, Braithwaite SS, Magee MF, et al. Management of diabetes and hyperglycemia in hospitals. *Diabetes Care.* 2004;27 (2):553-591.

Chapter 10

Nutrition in Cardiovascular Disease

Alexis Madej

Chapter Outline

Core Concepts
Introduction
Cardiac Physiology in Health and Disease
CVD Clinical Course
Nutritional Management in CVD
Hypertension Clinical Course

Nutritional Management in Hypertension
Obesity and CVD Clinical Course
Heart Failure Clinical Course
Nutritional Management in Heart Failure
Nutrition Assessment in Heart Failure
Nutrition Support in CVD

CORE CONCEPTS

1. Cardiovascular disease (CVD) encompasses several conditions affecting the heart and blood vessels, including atherosclerosis, coronary artery disease (CAD), myocardial infarction (MI), stroke, peripheral artery disease (PAD), hypertension (HTN), and heart failure (HF).

2. CVD occurs when the proper function of the heart and circulatory system is interrupted.

3. Many CVD risk factors are modifiable and can be prevented or improved with early intervention; these include dyslipidemia, diabetes mellitus (DM), elevated blood pressure, obesity/overweight, physical inactivity, diet, and smoking.

4. Dyslipidemia refers to alterations in the normal transport of lipids and lipoproteins that contribute to atherosclerosis and CVD risk. Modifiable risk factors for dyslipidemia include diet choices, weight gain, and physical inactivity.

5. Outcomes associated with HTN include stroke, HF, MI, kidney failure, and death. HTN increases the risk of HF by two-fold in men and three-fold in women.

6. Modifiable factors for HTN include obesity, stress, excessive alcohol intake, high salt intake, and smoking.

7. An elevated body mass index (BMI) increases risk of morbidity and mortality from cardiovascular events.

8. HF refers to the heart's inability to provide the body with adequate oxygenated blood. HF can be caused by damage to the heart tissue from CAD, MI, and HTN.

9. Cardiac cachexia is an uncontrollable loss of weight that includes muscle, fat, and eventually bone loss. It is associated with a 50% mortality rate at 18 months. The condition is not reversible with nutrition intervention, but adequate nutrition may diminish negative outcomes.

Learning Objectives

1. Explain the normal function of the cardiovascular system.
2. Describe the pathophysiology of cardiovascular disease (CVD) and related conditions.
3. Discuss the significance of CVD prevention and the most recent American Heart Association and American College of Cardiology (AHA/ACC) guidelines.
4. Develop evidence-based nutrition interventions for individuals with dyslipidemia, hypertension, and/or heart failure.
5. Identify nutrition-related implications of medications used in the treatment of CVD.
6. Recognize the significance of obesity and malnutrition in CVD progression and related outcomes.
7. Determine when it is appropriate to initiate nutrition support in the CVD population, and explain the best method for providing nutrition support and monitoring outcomes.

Introduction

Cardiovascular disease (CVD) encompasses several conditions affecting the heart and blood vessels, including atherosclerosis, coronary artery disease (CAD), myocardial infarction (MI), stroke, peripheral artery disease (PAD), hypertension (HTN), and heart failure (HF). Many of these conditions stem from each other. For example, **atherosclerosis**, the hardening and narrowing of arteries due to plaque build-up, can lead to blood vessel blockages. Depending on the location of the blocked artery, the result may be MI, CAD, stroke, or PAD.[1]

Heart disease accounts for 1 out of 4 deaths in the United States each year, and costs over $207 billion per year when considering cost of health care, medications, and lost productivity.[2] CVD is the leading cause of death across most ethnic and racial groups in the United States, with CAD, the most common type of heart disease, killing 365,000 people in 2014.[2,3] Globally, CVD causes 17.3 million deaths per year. Preventive treatment that includes dietary patterns with emphasis on types of fat, physical activity, and lifestyle interventions can prevent and help treat CVD through their effects on modifiable risk factors such as HTN, weight, and blood lipid parameters.[4,5]

> **CORE CONCEPT 1**
>
> Cardiovascular disease (CVD) encompasses several conditions affecting the heart and blood vessels, including atherosclerosis, coronary artery disease (CAD), myocardial infarction (MI), stroke, peripheral artery disease (PAD), hypertension (HTN), and heart failure (HF).

Cardiac Physiology in Health and Disease

The cardiovascular system is responsible for the transport of oxygen-rich blood and nutrients throughout the body, and for the removal of carbon dioxide and waste products. Its vital role is to maintain interstitial homeostasis.[6] The cardiovascular system is composed of the heart and blood vessels. The heart is made up of three layers: the epicardium (outer layer), **myocardium** (middle layer), and endocardium (inner layer). The heart is divided into four chambers. The top chambers are the right and left atria, and the bottom chambers are the right and left ventricles. The right atrium collects oxygen-poor blood delivered from two large veins, the superior vena cava and the inferior vena cava. Blood flows down from the right atrium to the right ventricle through the tricuspid valve. The blood is then pumped from the right ventricle through the pulmonary valve and pulmonary artery to the lungs to become oxygenated. Oxygen-rich blood is delivered from pulmonary veins to the left atrium and flows to the left ventricle through the mitral valve. From the left ventricle, blood is pumped through the aortic valve and the aorta to fuel the entire body through a network of arteries, arterioles, and capillaries. The cycle repeats itself as venules and veins return oxygen-depleted blood back to the superior and inferior vena cava and finally to the heart.[7] **Figure 10.1** illustrates the pathway of blood flow through the heart.

Each cardiac cycle has a period of **systole** and **diastole**. Systole refers to active pumping of blood out of the heart by the ventricles. Diastole is when the ventricles are relaxed and blood flows from the atria to refill the ventricles. There are several equations used to measure the proper function of the cardiovascular system. **Stroke volume** is the amount of blood pumped per heartbeat. It can be calculated as the blood volume in the ventricle at the end of diastole (end-diastolic volume) minus the blood volume in the ventricle at the end of systole (end-systolic volume). **Cardiac output** is a measure of blood pumped per minute that is calculated by multiplying the stroke volume by the heart rate. **Ejection fraction (EF)** is typically used to measure heart function or contractility in HF patients (Box 10.1). It represents the amount of blood being pumped out of the ventricle each time it contracts. EF is the percentage of blood in the ventricle at the end of diastole that is pumped out during systole; the equation is stroke volume (amount of blood pumped out) divided by end-diastolic volume (amount of blood left in the chamber). A normal EF is between 55% and 80%. **Mean arterial pressure (MAP)** is defined as the average pressure that pushes blood through the arteries during a cardiac cycle. MAP is a product of cardiac output and **total peripheral resistance** (resistance of blood flow in systemic circulation). MAP can also be approximated as diastolic pressure plus one-third of the difference between systolic and diastolic pressures.[6] These measurements make it possible to closely monitor the effects of diseases of the cardiovascular system.

CASE STUDY INTRODUCTION

Carl is a 55-year-old male referred for medical nutrition therapy (MNT) after being diagnosed with dyslipidemia. At his initial MNT visit he discloses that he works over 60 hours per week as an accountant and relies on fast food choices for meals during the day. His wife prepares family meals for dinner, and he does not want to complain or change her cooking habits. He admits that he does not exercise, but tries to play outside with his daughters on the weekends.

Anthropometric Data:
Weight: 95 kg (210 lbs)
Height: 178 cm (60")
BMI: 30 kg/m^2
Waist circumference: 107 cm (42")

Biochemical Data:
Total cholesterol (TC) 299 (Desirable: < 200 mg/dL)
Low-density lipoprotein cholesterol (LDL-C) 179 (Desirable: <100 mg/dL)
High-density lipoprotein cholesterol (HDL-C) 28 (Desirable: ≥40 mg/dL)
Triglycerides 155 (Desirable: <150 mg/dL)

Clinical Data:
Past Medical History: HTN, dyslipidemia (newly diagnosed)
Medications: metoprolol
Vital Signs: Blood pressure 160/73 mm Hg, Temperature 98.6°F, Heart rate 70 beats/min
Nutrition-focused Physical Exam: Appears well nourished, apple-shaped body type

Dietary Data:
24-hour Diet Recall
Breakfast (6 am): 2 cups of coffee (cream and sugar added)
Lunch (12 pm): Large steak and cheese sandwich, snack-sized chips, 12 ounces of soda
Snack (3 pm): 2 cookies, or a donut, or a fruit cup
Snack (6 pm): Peanut butter and jelly sandwich or bologna (2 slices) and cheese (1 slice) with a little mayonnaise on white bread
Dinner (8 pm): Large serving of spaghetti and meatballs (3 large homemade ricotta meatballs), homemade marinara sauce, 2 dinner rolls with butter, garden side salad (lettuce, cucumber, tomato) with ranch dressing, 8 ounces of water, sometimes wine (15 ounce glass)
Snack (10 pm): Ice cream with fruit (large bowl)

Questions

1. What risk factors does Carl have for CVD at this point?
2. How would you interpret Carl's biochemical data?
3. Assess Carl's diet recall. Make notes regarding his eating pattern and food/beverage choices. What recommendations can be made? What goals can be set?
4. Plan a nutrition intervention to help Carl improve his lipid panel.
5. Is it possible to encourage Carl to follow up? What is the benefit of follow-up MNT visits?

In order for the heart to effectively pump blood throughout the body, electrical activity (action potential) exists within a network of intercalated discs between **myocytes** (heart cells). Electrical activity is started at the sinoatrial (SA) node, which causes the left and right atrium to contract by means of depolarization. The electrical impulse travels to the atrioventricular (AV) node, atrioventricular bundle (bundle of His), right and left bundle branches, and finally to **Purkinje fibers** that spread throughout the right and left ventricles. An **electrocardiogram** can be used to measure the heart's electrical activity by placing electrodes on the body surface that can detect the activity in the extracellular fluid.[6] **Figure 10.2** illustrates the cardiac conduction system, and **Figure 10.3** shows the stages of an electrocardiogram measuring the heart's electrical activity.

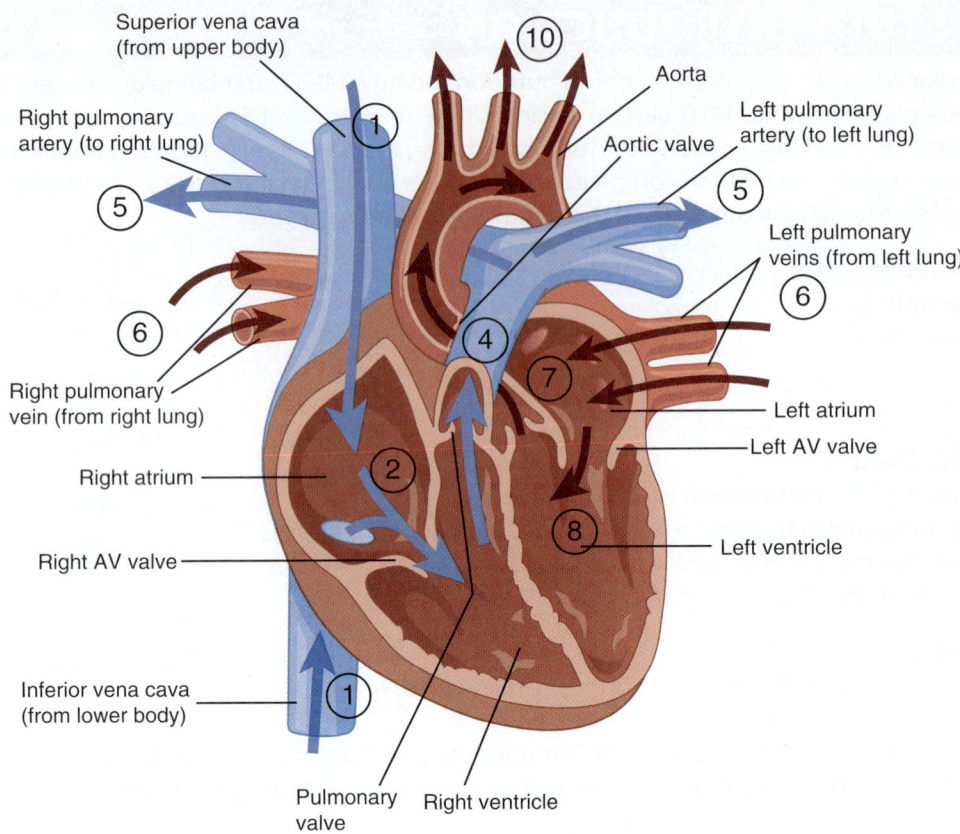

FIGURE 10.1 Pathway of Blood Flow Through the Heart.

CVD describes a collection of conditions in which the proper function of the heart and circulatory system is interrupted. One modifiable pathway that is a culprit for the disruption of cardiovascular function is atherosclerosis. Atherosclerosis describes an active inflammatory process leading to the buildup of plaque that narrows and thickens artery walls and restricts normal blood flow. The location of plaque and potential rupture determines the CVD outcome, which can include MI, CAD, stroke, and PAD.[2] The inflammation associated with atherosclerosis assaults the inner endothelial lining of the arteries. As the endothelium becomes weakened from continued exposure to stressors (high serum cholesterol levels, cigarette toxins, hemodynamic disturbance), it is more likely to host high levels of low-density lipoprotein cholesterol (LDL-C). High levels of LDL-C embedded in the endothelial cells undergo enzymatic alterations, become oxidized, and cause cell death within the endothelium. This triggers an inflammatory cascade, activating release of lymphocytes and monocytes. The monocytes become macrophages and engulf the oxidized LDL-C to form **foam cells** and the

Box 10.1
Equations Measuring Cardiac Function

Stroke volume (SV) = End Diastolic Volume (EDV) − End Systolic Volume (ESV)

Cardiac Output = SV × Heart Rate (HR) in beats per minute (bpm)

Ejection Fraction = SV/EDV

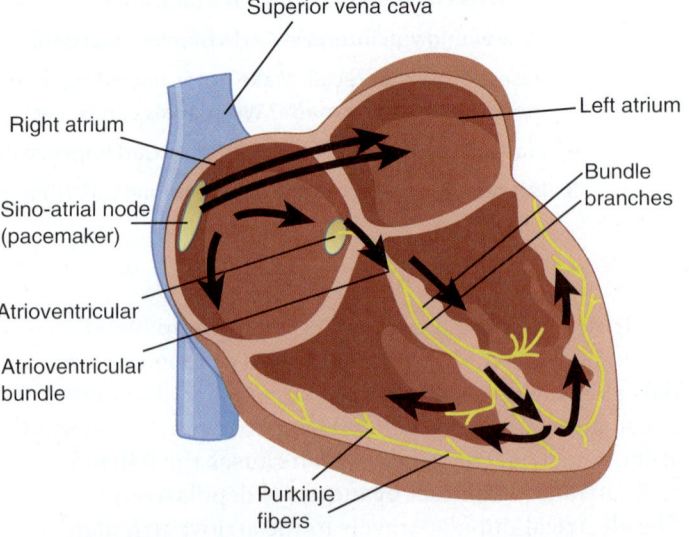

FIGURE 10.2 Cardiac Conduction System.

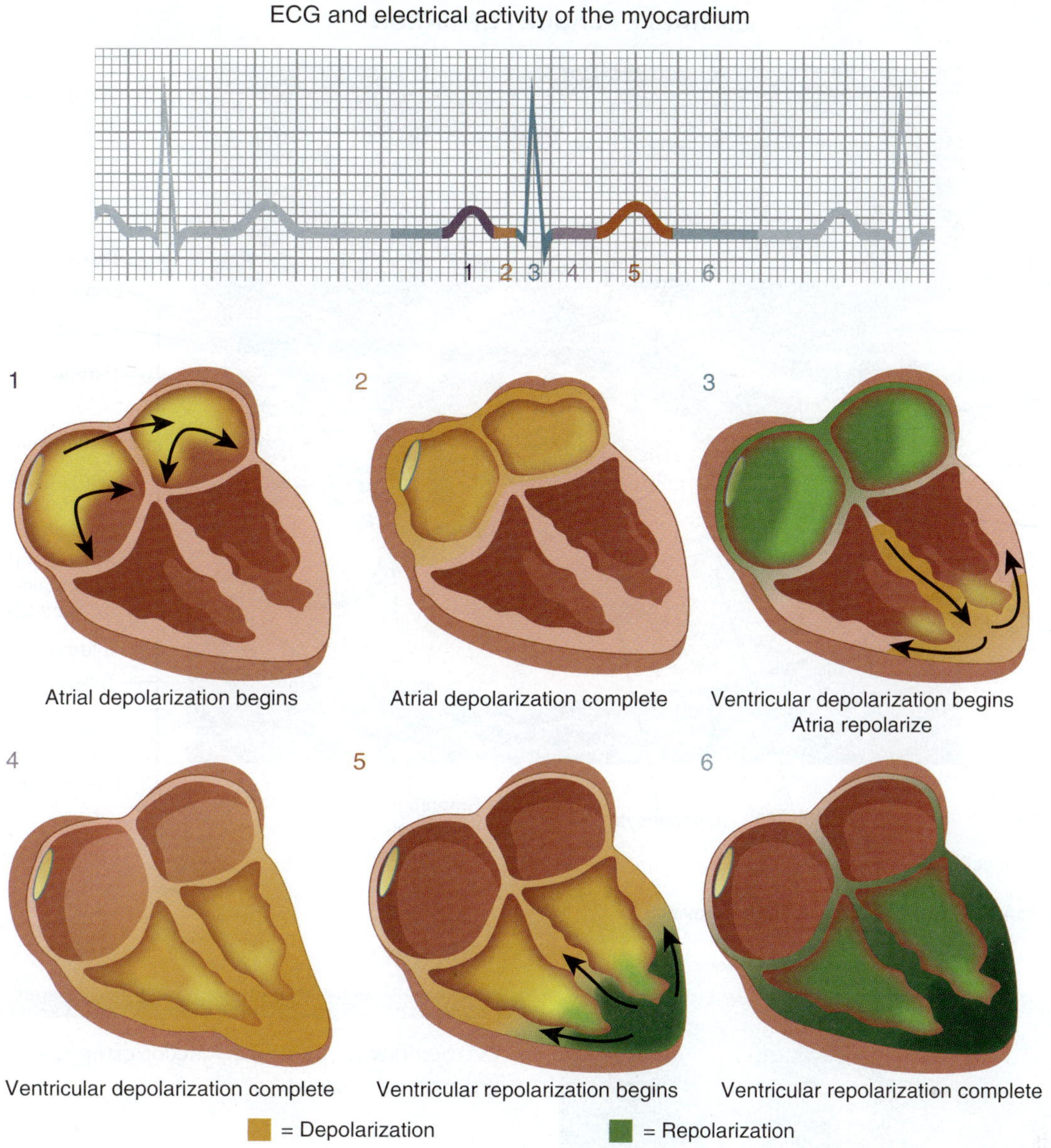

FIGURE 10.3 Electrocardiogram and Electrical Activity of the Myocardium.

lipid core of atherosclerotic plaque. A fibrous cap covers the core. If the fibrous cap is thin and the lipid core is thick, the plaque is said to be vulnerable. **Vulnerable plaque** is a thin-cap fibroatheroma and it is the most at risk of rupture.[8] **Figure 10.4** illustrates vulnerable plaque formation. Plaque can become calcified, narrowing the artery and causing stenosis.[6] If vulnerable plaque ruptures, the outcome is **thrombosis**, the formation of a blood clot that interferes with normal blood flow. A blood clot that breaks free and travels to another area of the body is referred to as an **embolism**.[8] The final location of the blockage determines the CVD event.

It is estimated that a heart attack occurs every 43 seconds in the United States. Each year, 735,000 Americans suffer from a heart attack. Prevention matters; while the rate of deaths caused by CVD remains significant, the number of these deaths in the United States has decreased by about 17% from the year 2000 to 2010. The stroke death rate has decreased by 23% during this same time period. These statistics show the effect of preventative measures, such as smoking cessation programs, in combination with the early management of diabetes mellitus (DM), dyslipidemia, and elevated blood pressure. Early management of these conditions involves nutrition and physical activity interventions.[4]

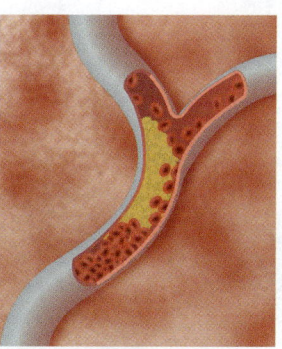

Cholesterol Accumulation and Plaque Formation.
Reproduced from CDC https://www.cdc.gov/cholesterol/facts.htm.

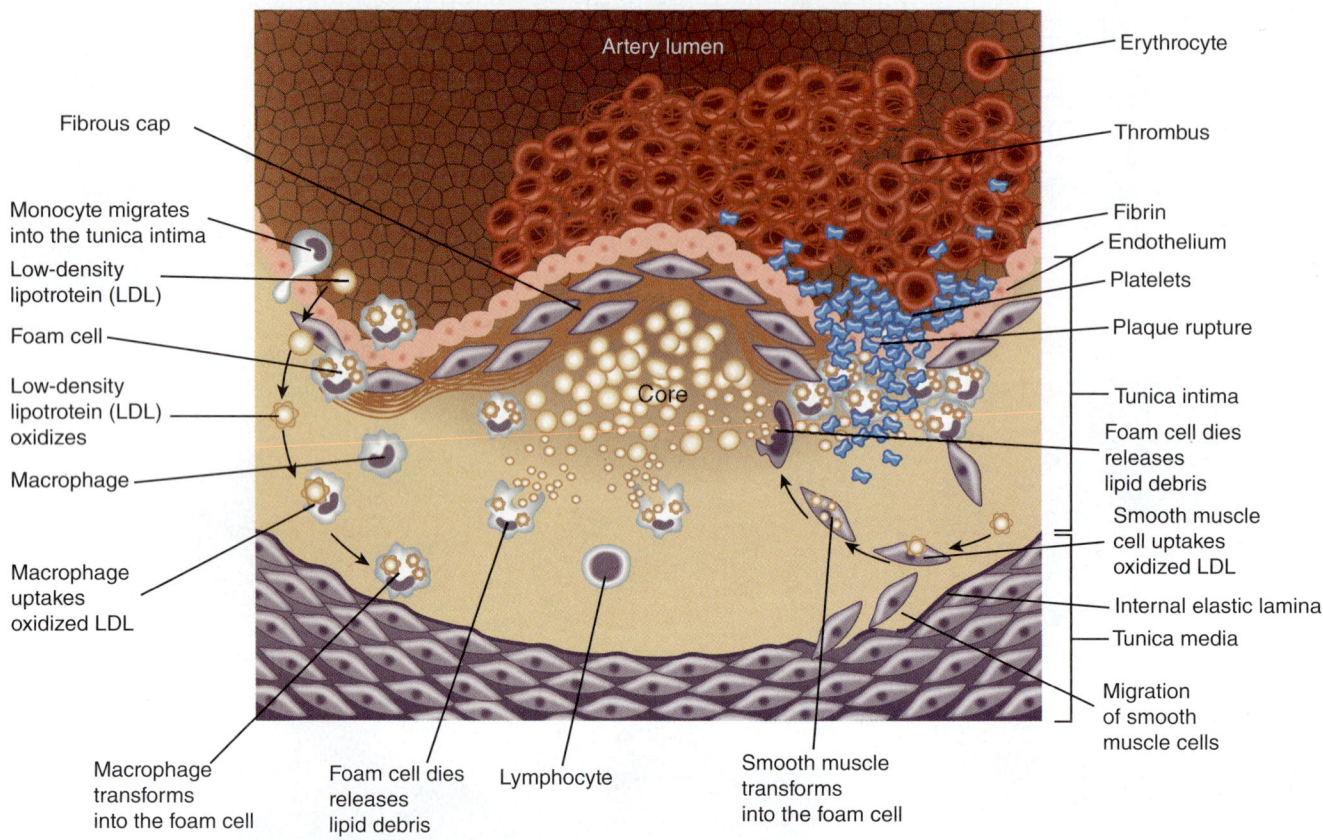

FIGURE 10.4 Factors Associated with Vulnerable Plaque Formation.

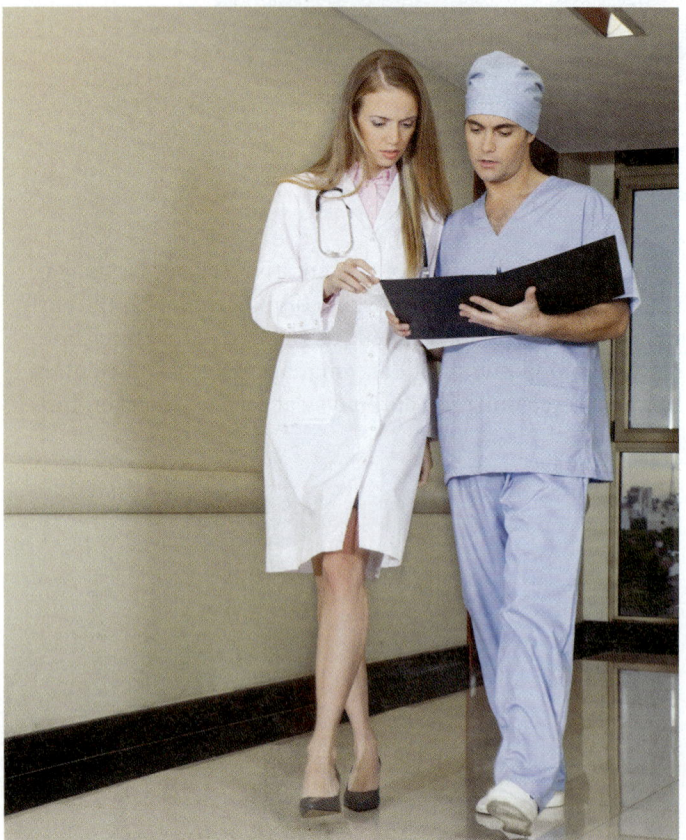

CORE CONCEPT 2

CVD occurs when the proper function of the heart and circulatory system is interrupted.

CVD Clinical Course

The most recent American Heart Association and American College of Cardiology (AHA/ACC) guidelines recommend using a 10-year and lifetime CVD risk calculator that is available for download and use at the AHA website. The calculator uses the following CVD risk factors: male gender, older age, race, dyslipidemia, DM, elevated blood pressure, and smoking status.[9] Additional CVD risk factors include obesity and overweight, physical inactivity, and diet. Many of these risk factors are modifiable and can be prevented or improved with early intervention; see **Table 10.1**. The Academy of Nutrition and Dietetics (AND) recommends that medical nutrition therapy (MNT) is provided by a registered dietitian (RD) for the following CVD risk factors: overweight/obesity, abnormal lipid profiles, DM, and/or HTN.[10] This chapter will provide a review of the nutrition management of dyslipidemia and high blood pressure for the prevention of CVD. This text has additional chapters dedicated to MNT for obesity and DM.

TABLE 10.1 MODIFIABLE VERSUS NONMODIFIABLE RISK FACTORS FOR CVD[4,9]

Modifiable Risk Factors	Nonmodifiable Risk Factors
Diabetes	Male gender
Diet	Older age
Dyslipidemia	Race
Elevated blood pressure	
Obesity and overweight	
Physical inactivity	
Smoking	

CORE CONCEPT 3

Many CVD risk factors are modifiable and can be prevented or improved with early intervention; these include dyslipidemia, DM, elevated blood pressure, obesity/overweight, physical inactivity, diet, and smoking.

Dyslipidemia

Lipid molecules include cholesterol, triglycerides, and phospholipids. Cholesterol is a necessary part of cell membranes, steroid hormones, and bile acids, and it is composed of four carbon rings and a carbon ring tail.[5] Triglycerides are essential for the transport of fat. They are structurally made up of a three-carbon glycerol backbone and three fatty acid chains. Both cholesterol and triglycerides travel as part of the core of **lipoproteins** (**Figure 10.5**).

Phospholipids are essential components of cell membranes, and they consist of a glycerol molecule and two fatty acid chains. Phospholipids and free cholesterol join with protein molecules (**apolipoproteins**) to make up the outer layer of lipoproteins.[11] Lipoproteins are responsible for the transport and delivery of fatty acids; there are several types classified by density.[5] Triglyceride-rich lipoproteins are the least dense; examples include chylomicrons, chylomicron remnants, and very-low-density lipoprotein (VLDL). VLDL is produced in the liver and transports fatty acids and LDL-C.[5,11] VLDL eventually breaks down into intermediate-density lipoprotein (IDL). IDL can be accepted by receptors in liver cells or broken down to LDL-C. Higher density lipoproteins include LDL-C, HDL-C, and lipoprotein(a). Normal lipoprotein transport moves triglycerides from the intestine to the liver and then on to storage sites such as fat tissue and utilization sites mainly muscle.[11]

Dyslipidemia refers to alterations in the normal transport of lipids and lipoproteins that contribute to atherosclerosis and CVD risk. Dyslipidemia is diagnosed when a blood test detects abnormal levels of circulating lipids. **Table 10.2** illustrates how lipid lab values are interpreted. Dyslipidemias

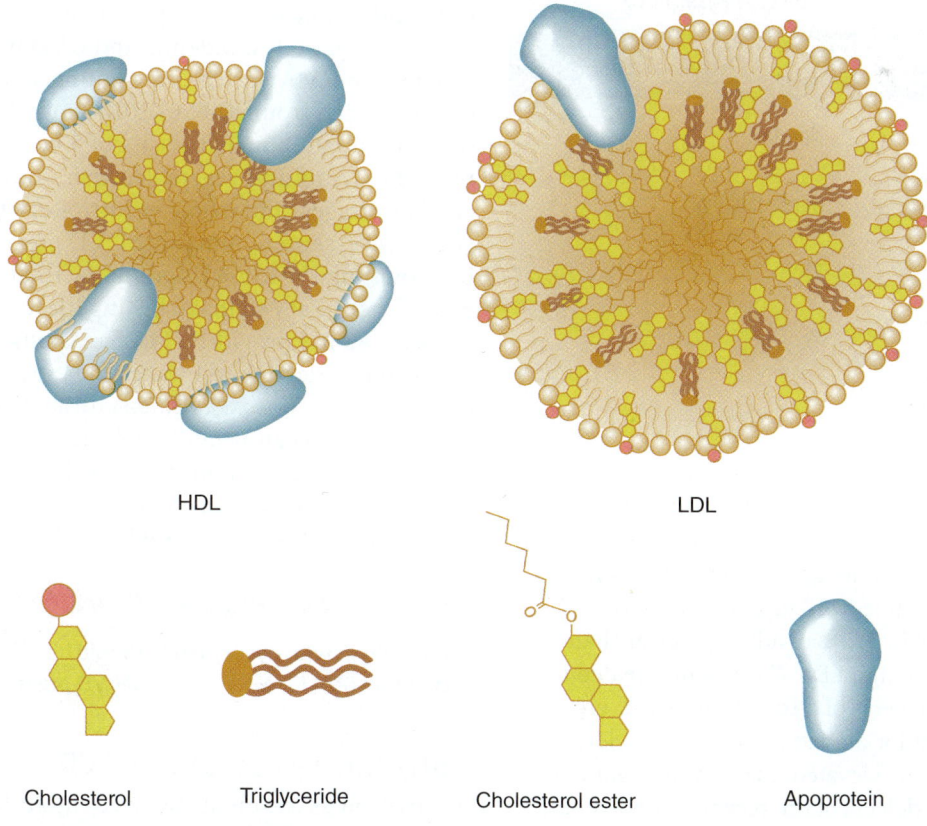

FIGURE 10.5 The Structure of Lipoproteins.

TABLE 10.2 INTERPRETING LIPID LABORATORY VALUES

Total Cholesterol Level	Category
<200 mg/dL	Desirable
200-239 mg/dL	Borderline high
≥240 mg/dL	High

LDL Cholesterol Level	Category
<100 mg/dL	Optimal
100-129 mg/dL	Near optimal/Above optimal
130-159 mg/dL	Borderline high
160-189 mg/dL	High
≥190 mg/dL	Very high

HDL Cholesterol Level	Category
<40 mg/dL	A major risk factor for CVD
40-59 mg/dL	Normal
≥60 mg/dL	Protective against CVD

Triglycerides	Category
<150 mg/dL	Normal
150-199 mg/dL	Borderline high
200-499 mg/dL	High
≥500 mg/dL	Very high

Courtesy of National Heart, Lung, and Blood Institute.

that involve elevated total cholesterol (TC) and LDL-C are associated with increased risk of CVD, and more specifically CAD.[11] Nearly 31 million adults in the United States have a total serum cholesterol value ≥240 mg/dL. Elevated LDL-C >130 mg/dL is prevalent in 31.7% of adults.[3] Fewer than 1 out of 3 individuals with high LDL-C are being treated for it.[12] As mentioned, high levels of circulating LDL-C create a favorable environment for oxidation and atherosclerosis. Serum LDL-C can become elevated due to weight gain, diet choices, inactivity, and defects of the receptors on liver and peripheral cells that usually bind LDL-C.[5] Elevated levels of HDL-C are protective against CAD. HDL-C facilitates reverse transport of cholesterol from the bloodstream to the liver for conversion to bile acids and elimination, and thus prevents LDL-C oxidation and atherosclerosis.[5,11]

Nonmodifiable risk factors for dyslipidemia include genetics and increasing age. One genetic disorder, **familial hypercholesterolemia (FH)**, is caused by defective LDL-C receptors leading to LDL-C levels greater than the 95th percentile for age and gender.[5,13] FH is diagnosed with a combination of LDL-C levels, family history of premature CAD, and **xanthomas** (subcutaneous yellow patches caused by deposits of excess lipids).[5] FH, if left untreated, can result in significant increased risk of CAD; 85% of men and 50% of women with untreated FH will have a coronary event before reaching 65 years of age.[13] Modifiable risk factors for dyslipidemia include diet choices, weight gain, and physical inactivity. MNT for dyslipidemia addresses these risk factors.

> **CORE CONCEPT 4**
>
> Dyslipidemia refers to alterations in the normal transport of lipids and lipoproteins that contribute to atherosclerosis and CVD risk. Modifiable risk factors for dyslipidemia include diet choices, weight gain, and physical inactivity.

Nutritional Management in CVD

Lifestyle changes, including weight loss, diet modification, and physical activity, play a pivotal role in the early management of dyslipidemia and CVD prevention. Unfortunately, many Americans are falling short of dietary goals; data collected from 2009 to 2010 show that less than 1% of the population met at least 4 of 5 healthy eating goals related to fruits and vegetables, fish, sodium, sugar-sweetened beverages, and whole grains.[4] Registered dietitians (RDs) are essential in making CVD prevention a reality by providing the knowledge and facilitating the behavior change necessary to make lasting lifestyle changes. Working with an RD providing MNT sessions over 6 to 12 weeks can lead to a decreased intake of energy (232 to 710 kcal/day), total fat (5% to 8%), and saturated fat (2% to 4%). These changes can result in a decrease of TC (7% to 21%), LDL-C (7% to 22%), and triglycerides (11% to 31%). A greater improvement in cholesterol levels is seen as more time is spent at MNT visits with an RD.[14]

> **PRACTICE POINT**
>
> Individuals with dyslipidemia should be referred to a registered dietitian (RD) for MNT as part of CVD prevention.

Nutrition Assessment in CVD

A nutrition assessment involves the collection of information related to the following categories: food/nutrition intake and related history; anthropometric measurements; biochemical data, medical tests, and procedures; nutrition-focused physical findings; and client history. In the patient with dyslipidemia, it is important to acquire a complete recall of food/beverage intake and to identify choices high in saturated and trans fat. During the recall, additional information is collected regarding medication and herbal supplement use, food allergies/intolerances, knowledge/beliefs/attitudes towards nutrition and diet change, eating behaviors, frequency of eating out, access to food, and physical activity. Anthropometric data includes height, weight, usual body weight (UBW), weight history, body mass index (BMI), waist circumference (WC), and waist-to-hip ratio (WHR). WC and WHR are essential to collect because BMI does not accurately predict CVD in adults older than 65 years of age. Elevated BMI, WC, and WHR increase the risk of CVD. In this population, biochemical data include TC, HDL-C, LDL-C, triglycerides, blood pressure, and fasting glucose. Additional labs may include lipoprotein(a), hemoglobin A1c, 25-OH vitamin D, thyroid function tests, and C-reactive protein. The physical exam should include observation of fat distribution; fluid retention; and presence of xanthomas, xanthelasma, corneal arcus, and palmar discolorations. Finally, client history involves a review of medical, family, and social history.[14] **Table 10.3** summarizes the information collected during the nutrition assessment for patients with dyslipidemia and/or HTN.

Medications in CVD

The nutrition assessment involves a review of a patient's medication regimen. Classes of medications used to treat dyslipidemias include statins, bile acid absorption inhibitors, cholesterol absorption inhibitors, fibrates, and nicotinic acid. Statins interfere with the enzyme HMG-CoA reductase and the production of cholesterol. Statins also decrease C-reactive protein and have anti-inflammatory effects. This class of medication is preferred for the treatment of dyslipidemia. Bile acid absorption inhibitors block the reabsorption of bile acids in the intestine, allowing them to bind to and remove circulating cholesterol. A side effect of this mechanism is the potential for decreased absorption of fat, fat-soluble vitamins, calcium, iron, zinc, magnesium, beta-carotene, and folate. Cholesterol absorption inhibitors decrease cholesterol absorption at the intestinal level. Fibrates are used in the case of hypertriglyceridemia. Nicotinic acid is a form of niacin (vitamin B3) that can be used to decrease cholesterol and triglycerides, but may also increase blood glucose levels.[11]

The 2013 AHA/ACC guidelines on the treatment of blood cholesterol to reduce atherosclerotic cardiovascular risk in adults recommend statin therapy for the following four groups: individuals with clinical atherosclerotic cardiovascular disease (ASCVD), LDL-C ≥190 mg/dL, ages 40 to 75 years with diabetes type 1 or 2, and ages 40 to 75 years with 7.5% estimated 10-year ASCVD risk. The statin therapies recommended are either high-intensity (daily dose lowers LDL-C by about 50%) or moderate-intensity (daily dose lowers LDL-C by about 30% to 50%). These guidelines focus on the maximum of statin therapy

TABLE 10.3 NUTRITION ASSESSMENT FOR DYSLIPIDEMIA AND/OR HYPERTENSION[14]

Nutrition Assessment Category	Data Collected
Food/nutrition intake and related history	• Usual recall of food/beverage intake • Food choices high in saturated fat, trans fat, sodium, and added sugar • Frequency of eating out/convenience foods • Medication and dietary supplement regimen • Knowledge/beliefs/attitudes towards nutrition; readiness to change • Food allergies/intolerances • Symptoms of nausea, vomiting, diarrhea, constipation • Eating behaviors • Access to food • Physical activity recall
Anthropometric measurements	• Height, weight • Weight history, UBW • BMI • WC • WHR
Biochemical data, medical tests, and procedures	• TC • HDL-C • LDL-C • TG • Blood pressure • Lipoprotein(a) • Fasting glucose, hemoglobin A1c • 25-OH vitamin D • Thyroid function tests • C-reactive protein (CRP) • Glomerular filtration rate (GFR)
Nutrition-focused physical findings	• Fat distribution pattern • Fluid retention • Xanthomas, xantelasma, corneal arcus, palmar discoloration
Client history	• Medical history • Family history • Social history

rather than providing specific LDL-C and HDL-C targets.[15] Correcting dyslipidemia with statins can result in a 21% decrease in the rate of CAD progressing to HF. **Table 10.4** illustrates the nutrition implications of medications used for the treatment of elevated blood cholesterol. The AHA/ACC guidelines do not include the use of plant stanols, sterol esters, stanols, stanol esters, or red yeast Chinese rice supplements for the treatment of dyslipidemia. If a patient reports the use of alternative therapies, the RD should ensure that the patient's physician and pharmacist are aware of these therapies and that the risks versus the potential benefits are addressed.

Energy Needs in CVD

The nutrition assessment includes a calculation of energy needs. The gold standard for estimating energy needs for individuals with dyslipidemia is indirect calorimetry. When this method is not possible, predictive equations can be used.[14]

> **PRACTICE POINT**
>
> The gold standard for estimating energy needs in CVD patients is indirect calorimetry. When this method is not possible, predictive equations can be used.

Nutrition Intervention in CVD

MNT for dyslipidemia focuses on the achievement of a healthy body weight and normal lipid values with a combination of increased physical activity and a meal plan that emphasizes fruits, vegetables, whole grains, lean protein, low-fat dairy, and heart-healthy fats. These goals confer with new CVD prevention clinical practice guidelines from the AHA/ACC and the National Heart, Lung, and Blood Institute (NHLBI). These guidelines were designed to update the previous Adult Treatment Panel III (ATP III) report from the National Cholesterol Education Program (NCEP).[4] The AHA/ACC recommendation for LDL-C lowering is a diet pattern that emphasizes vegetables, fruits, and whole

TABLE 10.4 CHOLESTEROL MEDICATIONS AND NUTRITION IMPLICATIONS[11,15,16]

Medication	Potential Side Effect	Nutrition Intervention
Statins (atorvastatin, simvastatin)	• Nausea, abdominal pain, constipation, diarrhea, indigestion, gas • Medication metabolism is effected by grapefruit juice	• Monitor gastrointestinal symptoms and make diet recommendations for symptom relief; consider small, frequent meals • Encourage avoidance of grapefruit juice
Bile acid absorption inhibitors (cholestyramine)	• Anorexia, weight change, tongue irritation, nausea, vomiting, abdominal pain, constipation, diarrhea, indigestion, gas • May decrease absorption of fat-soluble vitamins (A, D, E, K), calcium, iron, zinc, magnesium, beta-carotene, and folate	• Monitor weight and gastrointestinal symptoms and make diet recommendations for symptom relief; consider small, frequent meals • Monitor levels of fat-soluble vitamins, calcium, iron, zinc, magnesium, and folate and replete as needed • Educate on food sources of nutrients that may need to be consumed in larger quantities and separate from medication to prevent deficiencies
Cholesterol absorption inhibitors (ezetimibe)	• Diarrhea	• Monitor for diarrhea and make diet recommendations for symptom relief
Fibrates (gemfibrozil)	• Taste changes, nausea, vomiting, abdominal pain, constipation, diarrhea, indigestion, gas	• Monitor gastrointestinal symptoms and make diet recommendations for symptom relief; consider small, frequent meals
Niacin (nicotinic acid)	• Dry mouth, nausea, vomiting, diarrhea, indigestion, peptic ulcer, cramps, gas • May increase blood glucose	• Monitor gastrointestinal symptoms and make diet recommendations for symptom relief; consider small, frequent meals • Monitor blood glucose to maintain within normal limits; educate on blood glucose control

grains; includes low-fat dairy products, poultry, fish, legumes, nontropical vegetable oils, and nuts; and limits intake of sweets, sugar-sweetened beverages, and red meats.[3] In addition to recommended diet patterns, the Academy of Nutrition and Dietetics Evidence Analysis Library (EAL) provides recommendations with regards to macronutrient intake for individuals with dyslipidemia. The EAL recommends 25% to 35% calories from fat (<7% calories from saturated fat), 15% to 20% calories from protein, and 45% to 60% calories from carbohydrates, with an emphasis on high-fiber choices.[14] Diet recommendations require consideration of estimated energy needs, personal and cultural food preferences, and medical history. An RD is critical in individualizing these general guidelines and ensuring long-term diet compliance for best outcomes. Along with nutrition education, an RD can facilitate behavior change by using motivational interviewing, addressing barriers to change, and allowing the patient to establish personal diet goals that are meaningful and achievable.

Replacement of Saturated/Trans Fats with Other Fats or Carbohydrates

For patients with dyslipidemia, the EAL recommends <7% daily calories from saturated fat, and the AHA/ACC further reduce the goal to 5% to 6% of daily calories. The current national average consumption is 11% of calories from saturated fat. Both the EAL and AHA/ACC recommend reducing calories from trans fat as low as possible. Calories from saturated/trans fats should be replaced with polyunsaturated fatty acids (PUFA), followed by monounsaturated fatty acids (MUFA), and finally high-fiber carbohydrates for the largest benefit.[4,5,14]

These recommendations are justified by a review of evidence from clinical trials. Randomized controlled trials (RCTs) have illustrated that a modified diet can result in a decrease of LDL-C by 11 to 13 mg/dL or 11% when a diet consisting of 5% to 6% saturated fat, 26% to 27% total fat, 15% to 18% protein, and 55% to 59% carbohydrate is compared to a diet consisting of 14% to 15% saturated fat, 34% to 38% total fat, 13% to 15% protein, and 48% to 51% carbohydrate.[4,5] Additional RCTs have shown that a 1% decrease in calories from saturated fat correlates with a 1.2 to 1.8 mg/dL decrease in LDL-C. The largest decrease in LDL-C is seen when saturated fat is replaced with PUFA. Replacing saturated fat with PUFA also lowers triglycerides by about 0.4 mg/dL and HDL-C by about 0.2 mg/dL. When MUFA are used to replace saturated fat, triglycerides increase by about 0.2 mg/dL and HDL-C is lowered by about 1.2 mg/dL. If saturated fat is replaced with carbohydrates, triglycerides increase by 1.9 mg/dL and HDL-C is lowered by about 0.4 mg/dL. If 1% of calories from trans fat are replaced with MUFA or PUFA, LDL-C is lowered by 1.5 mg/dL and 2.0 mg/dL, respectively. Additionally, triglycerides are lowered by about 1.2 mg/dL and 1.3 mg/dL, and HDL-C is increased by 0.4 mg/dL and 0.5 mg/dL, respectively.[4] A meta-analysis of prospective cohort studies concluded that as little as a 2% increase in calories from trans fat correlates with a 23% increased risk of CHD.[17] Although previous guidelines have also encouraged a reduction in dietary cholesterol intake, the AHA/ACC review of current evidence concluded that there are insufficient findings to suggest that decreasing dietary cholesterol decreases LDL-C.[4]

An online consumer research study of 1,000 adults conducted by the AHA in 2006 found that less than half of participants could identify a food source of trans fat and less than 70% could identify at least three food sources of saturated fat.[18] An RD can assist in education related to fats and facilitate lasting behavior change. The message for dyslipidemia patients is to consume saturated and trans fats less often. Nutrition intervention involves the identification of food sources of the different types of fats. Saturated fats include high-fat meats, fried meats, full-fat dairy (whole milk, cream, cheese), butter, and lard. Trans fat sources include some fried foods and processed foods (depending on the fat used), stick margarine, traditional vegetable shortening, and any food containing the ingredient "partially hydrogenated oil." Trans fat is also found in small amounts in meat and dairy products due to the fermentation process in animals' rumens.[18] The nutrition facts label is mandated by the United States Food and Drug Administration (FDA) to list quantity of both saturated fat and trans fat. MNT includes education related to interpreting nutrition facts labels to choose foods with zero grams trans fat and less than 3 grams of saturated fat per serving.

In order for patients to make diet changes, tasteful and easy alternatives need to be provided. An RD can work with patients to develop a meal plan that emphasizes heart-healthy fats: poly- and monounsaturated fats. Examples include fish high in omega-3 fatty acids, olive and canola oil, nuts, seeds, and avocados. Instead of simply instructing patients to eliminate foods high in saturated/trans fat, ideas can be provided for substitutions—for example, replacing butter with olive oil, grilling salmon burgers instead of traditional burgers, and trying low-fat Greek yogurt instead of sour cream. Table 10.5 shows suggestions for choosing heart-healthy fats. Table 10.6 illustrates ways to decrease saturated fat intake.

Omega-3 Fatty Acids

Two or more servings per week of fatty fish is associated with 30% to 45% reduced risk of death from cardiac events in the general population. This benefit is attributed to the omega-3 fatty acids eicosapentaenoic acid (EPA) and docosahexaenoic acid (DHA). Suggested mechanisms of EPA and DHA include a modest decrease in atherosclerosis, blood pressure, left ventricular mass, and heart rate with an increase in stroke volume.[14,19-24] The EAL recommendation for omega-3 FAs for the prevention of heart disease is two 4-ounce servings of fatty fish per week. In patients with heart disease, the recommendation increases to two or more 4-ounce servings of fatty fish per week. The dose of 1 g/day EPA + DHA has been shown to decrease risk of death from cardiac events in patients with heart disease.[14,21,22,25] It is important to note that there is a risk of

TABLE 10.5 GUIDELINES FOR INCREASING UNSATURATED FAT INTAKE

Easy Ways to Choose More Unsaturated Fats Each Day

- Add a couple slices (3 tbsp) of avocado to a sandwich
- Order grilled or baked salmon when eating out
- Make tuna salad using chunk light tuna and light mayonnaise
- Snack on trail mix made with 2-3 tbsp of nuts (almonds, walnuts, peanuts), 2 tbsp dried fruit, and ½ cup whole grain cereal
- Spread an apple half with 1-2 tbsp of peanut butter, or have a handful of almonds with a piece of fruit for a quick snack
- Add 2 tbsp of crushed walnuts or almond slivers to yogurt or cereal
- Try 1 tbsp olive oil and vinegar as a topping on sandwiches and salads
- Sprinkle 2 tbsp of sunflower or pumpkin seeds onto salads or cooked veggies
- Add 1 tbsp of flaxseed to oatmeal or hot cereal
- Try 1-2 tbsp of almond butter on wheat crackers as a snack

TABLE 10.6 GUIDELINES FOR DECREASING SATURATED FAT INTAKE

Low Saturated Fat Choose MORE Often	High Saturated Fat Choose LESS Often
1% or skim milk	Whole milk, cream, half & half
Low-fat yogurt, low-fat Greek yogurt	Whole milk yogurt
Cheese made with 1% or skim milk	Whole milk cheese
Low-fat sour cream	Sour cream
Lean animal meats (loin, leg, round, extra lean hamburger, venison)	High-fat animal meats (ribs, T-bone steak, regular hamburger meat, bacon, sausage, pepperoni, salami, hot dogs)
Light meat poultry without skin	Dark meat poultry with skin
Grilled, baked, broiled, steamed, braised, boiled, roasted foods	Fried foods
Olive, canola oil	Palm, palm kernel oil
Heart-healthy spread	Stick butter

exposure to mercury, polychlorinated biphenyls (PCBs), and other contaminants from some types of seafood. The AHA states that as long as fish is consumed within the guidelines set by the Food and Drug Administration (FDA) and Environmental Protection Agency (EPA), the benefits of eating fish outweigh the risks for middle-aged and older men and postmenopausal women. High-risk populations (pregnant women, children) are advised to avoid fish high in mercury and choose up to 12 ounces per week of fish lower in mercury. There are online resources available from the AHA, FDA, and EPA to classify fish that are high in omega-3 fatty acids and low in mercury, such as salmon, sardines, and anchovies.

If unable to meet recommendations from dietary sources and no contraindications exist, supplementation of 850 mg/day EPA+DHA may be warranted (1 g fish oil supplement provides 200 to 800 mg EPA+DHA).[14,25] Fish oil supplementation is contraindicated in patients with angina and implantable cardioverter defibrillators (ICDs). Studies have shown increased cardiac mortality and sudden death rates in patients with angina taking 3 g/day fish oil supplementation. Studies have also shown an increased incidence of arrhythmia in patients with ICDs taking 1.8 g/day fish oil supplementation.[14,26,27] The potential adverse effects of fish oil supplementation are a reason to recommend food sources before supplements.

Fiber

The EAL fiber recommendations are 25 to 35 grams daily, including 7 to 13 grams of soluble fiber.[3,19] Meeting fiber goals, in addition to other guidelines discussed above, can further reduce TC by 2% to 3% and LDL-C by up to 7%.[14] A meta-analysis of 10 prospective cohort studies found an increase of 10 g/day of fiber to be associated with a 12% decrease in cardiac events and a 30% decrease in cardiac deaths.[19] A study including 68 men and women found that an intake of 30 g/day fiber with 13 g/day soluble fiber resulted in decreased TC and LDL/HDL ratio.[28] A study of 36 overweight men who increased fiber intake to 30 g/day illustrated a 17% decrease in small LDL-C, 6.2% decrease in LDL-C, and 5% decrease in LDL/HDL ratio.[28] When providing MNT for dyslipidemia, an RD will identify and encourage consumption of fiber-rich foods such as whole grains, fruits, vegetables, nuts, seeds, and beans.

Nuts

Nuts can be recommended as a source of unsaturated fat that may help to improve dyslipidemia when used to replace saturated/trans fats. The EAL states that there is fair evidence to suggest that the consumption of 5 ounces of nuts per week is associated with reduced risk of MI based on results from the Nurses' Health Study.[14]

Plant Stanols and Sterols

Plant stanols and sterols have been considered for individuals with dyslipidemia because they compete with cholesterol for absorption in the small intestine. Intake levels that may result in reduced triglycerides and LDL-C are 0.8 to 3 g/day.

The average intake from natural sources of nuts, vegetable oils, fruits, and vegetables is only 0.2 g/day. Fortified spreads contain 0.5 to 1.7 grams per tablespoon.[19,29]

Added Sugar

Added sugar contributes to weight gain, which is a risk factor for dyslipidemia. The AHA recommends reducing added sugar to no more than 100 calories per day for women and 150 calories per day for men.[30] MNT for dyslipidemia includes the identification and reduction of sugars and syrups that are added to foods during processing, preparation, or at the table.

Physical Activity

As a part of MNT for dyslipidemia, the EAL recommends at least 2 days/week of resistance exercise and moderate intensity physical activity for at least 30 minutes on most days of the week.[14] The AHA/ACC guidelines for CVD prevention recommend physical activity 3 to 4 times per week for an average of 40 minutes at moderate to vigorous intensity. This level of physical activity can reduce LDL-C by 3 to 6 mg/dL.[4] The AHA/ACC concludes that the entire population of the United States was physically active, incidence of CHD could be reduced by 6%.[4]

> **PRACTICE POINT**
>
> Physical activity on most days of the week is recommended as part of MNT for CVD prevention.

Antioxidant Supplements

The EAL states that vitamin E, vitamin C, and/or beta-carotene supplements should not be recommended because there is no evidence of CVD benefit and there is the potential for harm.[14]

Alcohol

In moderation, alcohol consumption may reduce the risk of CVD. The EAL guidelines define moderation as one drink per day for women and two drinks per day for men. Individuals who do not currently consume alcohol should not be encouraged to start.[14]

Smoking Cessation

Smoking cessation is an important element of CVD prevention. During MNT, an RD can refer a patient to the appropriate smoking cessation programs.

> **PRACTICE POINT**
>
> As part of MNT for dyslipidemia, recommendations for LDL-C lowering include a reduction of calories from saturated and trans fat, and a diet pattern that emphasizes vegetables, fruits, whole grains, low-fat dairy, lean protein, and unsaturated fats.

Nutrition Monitoring/Evaluation in CVD

The monitoring and evaluation portion of MNT for dyslipidemia involves a review of the nutrition assessment categories: food/nutrition intake and related history; anthropometric measurements; biochemical data, medical tests, and procedures; nutrition-focused physical findings; and client history. Refer to Table 10.3. This allows the RD to monitor patient progress towards established goals and outcomes.

Hypertension Clinical Course

Hypertension (HTN) is chronic high blood pressure. Primary (essential) HTN refers to high blood pressure that is not the result of another disease; it accounts for 95% of HTN cases.[31] One-third of all adults in the United States have HTN. The prevalence is highest among African American adults (44%).[3] HTN has been referred to as a silent killer because there are usually no symptoms associated with high blood pressure, but the outcomes can be severe, including stroke, HF, MI, kidney failure, and death. HTN causes vascular stress, which creates an environment for atherosclerosis and thrombosis.[31] Chronic elevated blood pressure results in myocyte hypertrophy, myocardial scarring, and loss of myocardial contractile tissue in the incidence of MI; these conditions promote the development of HF. HTN increases the risk of HF by two-fold in men and three-fold in women.[12]

HTN is a condition in which the force of blood pushing against artery walls is increased. **Systolic blood pressure** is the force caused when the heart is actively pumping blood. **Diastolic blood pressure** is the force when the heart is at rest. A blood pressure (BP) reading lists systolic above diastolic blood pressure. Normal BP is defined as less than 120/80 mm Hg. "Elevated BP" is the range of 120-129 mm Hg systolic and <80 mm Hg diastolic. Recently, the ACC/AHA have lowered the threshold for defining HTN. Currently, stage 1 HTN is BP of 130-139 mm Hg systolic or 80-89 mm Hg diastolic. Stage 2 HTN is BP of ≥ 140 mm Hg systolic or ≥ 90 mm Hg diastolic.[32] Conditions that may promote elevated BP include sympathetic nervous system hyperactivity, abnormal cardiovascular or renal development, renin-angiotensin system activity, defect in natriuresis (which usually brings BP back to normal after high salt intake), and increased intracellular sodium and calcium. Obesity may lead to HTN by causing increased intravascular volume, elevated cardiac output, and activation of the renin-angiotensin system.[31] Risk factors for HTN include African American ethnicity, obesity, stress, excessive alcohol intake, high salt intake, family history of HTN, DM, and smoking.[32,33]

> **CORE CONCEPT 5**
>
> Outcomes associated with HTN include stroke, HF, MI, kidney failure, and death. HTN increases the risk of HF by two-fold in men and three-fold in women.

CASE STUDY REVISITED

Six weeks after his initial visit, Carl returns to see the RD at the lipid clinic. His data are as follows:

Anthropometric Data:
Weight: 100 kg (220 lbs)
Height: 178 cm (70")
BMI: 30 kg/m^2
Waist circumference: 109 cm (43")

Biochemical Data:
Total cholesterol (TC) 280 (Desirable: < 200 mg/dL)
Low-density lipoprotein cholesterol (LDL-C) 167 (Desirable: <100 mg/dL)
High-density lipoprotein cholesterol (HDL-C) 25 (Desirable: ≥40 mg/dL)
Triglycerides 180 (Desirable: <150 mg/dL)

Clinical Data:
Medications: metoprolol, Lasix (recently added)
Vital Signs: Blood pressure 150/68 mm Hg, Temperature 98.6°F, Heart rate 89 beats/min
Nutrition-focused Physical Exam: Well-nourished, apple-shaped body type

Dietary Data:
24-hour Diet Recall
Breakfast (6 am): 2 cups of coffee (2% milk and sugar added), 2 cups sweetened whole grain cereal with 2% milk
Lunch (12 pm): Large turkey and cheese sub, snack-sized potato chips, 12 ounces of soda, oatmeal cookie
Snack (3 pm): Apple slices with 4 tbsp peanut butter, cheese and crackers
Dinner (8 pm): 6 to 9 oz grilled salmon, 3 cups pasta primavera (olive oil and about 1 cup vegetables), 2 slices of garlic bread, large salad (lettuce, tomato, cucumber, olives, chickpeas, feta cheese, low-fat ranch dressing), 8 ounces of water
Snack (10 pm): 1½ cups low-fat frozen yogurt (sometimes the entire pint), fruit
Physical activity: Remains sedentary

Questions

1. How does Carl's diet compare to his last visit?
2. Identify changes that he has made and how they relate to his anthropometric and laboratory data.
3. What are your nutrition priorities and recommendations for Carl?

CORE CONCEPT 6

Modifiable risk factors for HTN include obesity, stress, excessive alcohol intake, high salt intake, and smoking.

Nutritional Management in Hypertension

Studies have shown that counseling patients to reduce sodium intake by about 1,150 mg/day results in lowering BP by 3 to 4 mm Hg systolic and 1 to 2 mm Hg diastolic.[4] MNT for HTN involves educating patients on reduced sodium intake and the DASH (Dietary Approaches to Stop Hypertension) diet pattern, as well as motivational interviewing to facilitate behavior change. A patient's readiness to change and personal motivators drive MNT sessions.

PRACTICE POINT

Individuals with HTN should be referred to an RD for MNT as part of CVD prevention.

Nutrition Assessment in Hypertension

The nutrition assessment categories for the HTN population are the same as those described for dyslipidemia. Table 10.3 identifies data collected during the assessment of patients with dyslipidemia and/or HTN.

Medications in Hypertension

A detailed assessment of the patient's medication regimen is useful to address the many food/nutrient–medication interactions associated with antihypertensive medications.[34] The 2014 Evidence-Based Guideline for the Management of High Blood Pressure in Adults from the Eighth Joint National Committee recommends the use of a thiazide-type diuretic, calcium channel blocker (CCB), angiotensin-converting enzyme inhibitor (ACEI), or angiotensin receptor blocker (ARB) as initial antihypertensive treatment in the general non–African American population. In the general African American population, initial therapy should be with a thiazide-type diuretic or CCB.[35] **Table 10.7** provides an overview of antihypertensive medication classes and nutrition implications.

Energy Needs in Hypertension

Similar to dyslipidemia, the MNT for HTN involves assessing energy needs using indirect calorimetry or predictive equations (Mifflin–St Jeor, Harris–Benedict).

Nutrition Intervention in Hypertension

The dietary pattern recommended by the AHA/ACC for blood pressure lowering is a combination of the DASH diet and reduced sodium intake. Individually, both the DASH diet and reduced sodium intake have the potential to lower BP; the benefit is maximized with a combination of both.[4,34]

DASH Diet and Sodium Reduction

The DASH diet emphasizes whole grains, fruits, vegetables, low-fat dairy, nuts, fish, lean meats, and unsaturated fats. It is high in calcium, fiber, potassium, and magnesium, and low in total fat, saturated fat, cholesterol, and sodium.[39,40] **Table 10.8** illustrates the components of the DASH diet. The diet is supported by clinical trials; an RCT of 412 individuals found that when comparing a high-sodium control diet to a low-sodium DASH diet, the reduction in systolic BP was 7.1 mm Hg in those without HTN and 11.5 mm Hg in those with HTN.[40] Another RCT of 144 overweight or obese patients with high BP achieved the following reductions in BP: 16.1/9.9 mm Hg with the DASH diet and weight management; 11.2/7.5 mm Hg with the DASH diet alone; and 3.4/3.8 mm Hg with a control diet. The DASH diet plus weight management group also benefited from reduced left ventricular mass.[41]

A high sodium intake is associated with elevated BP and negative effects on the blood vessels, heart, and kidneys.[42] The evidence compiled by the AHA/ACC illustrates that in adults with a baseline BP of 120 to 150/80 to 95 mm Hg, reducing sodium intake to 2,400 mg/day or 1,500 mg/day (from 3,300 mg/day) decreases BP by 2/1 mm Hg and

TABLE 10.7 ANTIHYPERTENSIVE MEDICATION CLASSES AND NUTRITION IMPLICATIONS[16,21,36-38]

Medication	Potential Side Effect	Nutrition Intervention
Thiazide-type diuretics	• K+, Mg+ depletion • Elevated blood glucose (BG) • Elevated lipids	• Monitor and replete K+ and Mg+; educate on food sources of each • Maintain BG within normal limits; educate on BG control • Monitor lipids; provide MNT for dyslipidemia
Loop Diuretics	• K+, Mg++, Ca++ depletion • Elevated BG • Anorexia, nausea, vomiting	• Monitor and replete K+, Mg++, Ca++; educate on food sources of each • Maintain BG within normal limits; educate on BG control • Educate on small frequent meals as tolerated; monitor adequacy of oral intake
Calcium channel blockers (CCBs)	• Metabolism is effected by grapefruit juice	• Encourage limited grapefruit juice consumption
Angiotensin-converting enzyme inhibitors (ACEIs)	• Hyperkalemia • Nausea, vomiting, abdominal pain	• Educate on <2,000 mg/day K+; provide a list of foods containing K+; monitor serum K+ • Educate on small frequent meals as tolerated; monitor adequacy of oral intake
Angiotensin receptor blockers (ARBs)	• Hyperkalemia • Zinc deficiency	• Educate on <2,000 mg/day K+; provide list of foods containing K+; monitor serum K+ • Monitor and replete zinc; educate on food sources of zinc
Beta-blockers	• Hyperkalemia	• Educate on <2,000 mg/day K+; provide a list of foods containing K+; monitor serum K+

TABLE 10.8 THE DASH DIET

Food Group	Servings Per Day			Serving Sizes	Examples and Notes	Significance of Each Food Group to the DASH Eating Plan
	1,600 Calories	2,000 Calories	2,600 Calories			
Grains*	6	6-8	10-11	1 slice bread 1 oz dry cereal[†] ½ cup cooked rice, pasta, or cereal	Whole wheat bread and rolls, whole wheat pasta, English muffin, pita bread, bagel, cereals, grits, oatmeal, brown rice, unsalted pretzels and popcorn	Major sources of energy and fiber
Vegetables	3-4	4-5	5-6	1 cup raw leafy vegetable ½ cup cut-up raw or cooked vegetable ½ cup vegetable juice	Broccoli, carrots, collards, green beans, green peas, kale, lima beans, potatoes, spinach, squash, sweet potatoes, tomatoes	Rich sources of potassium, magnesium, and fiber
Fruits	4	4-5	5-6	1 medium fruit ¼ cup dried fruit ½ cup fresh, frozen, or canned fruit ½ cup fruit juice	Apples, apricots, bananas, dates, grapes, oranges, grapefruit, grapefruit juice, mangoes, melons, peaches, pineapples, raisins, strawberries, tangerines	Important sources of potassium, magnesium, and fiber
Fat-free or low-fat milk and milk products	2-3	2-3	3	1 cup milk or yogurt 1½ oz cheese	Fat-free (skim) or low-fat (1%) milk or buttermilk; fat-free, low-fat, or reduced-fat cheese; fat-free or low-fat regular or frozen yogurt	Major sources of calcium and protein
Lean meats, poultry, and fish	3-6	6 or less	6	1 oz cooked meats, poultry, or fish 1 egg	Select only lean meats; trim away visible fat; broil, roast, or poach; remove skin from poultry	Rich sources of protein and magnesium
Nuts, seeds, and legumes	3 per week	4-5 per week	1 daily	⅓ cup or 1½ oz nuts 2 tbsp peanut butter 2 tbsp or ½ oz seeds ½ cup cooked legumes (dry beans and peas)	Almonds, hazelnuts, mixed nuts, peanuts, walnuts, sunflower seeds, peanut butter, kidney beans, lentils, split peas	Rich sources of energy, magnesium, protein, and fiber
Fats and oils[§]	2	2-3	3	1 tsp soft margarine 1 tsp vegetable oil 1 tbsp mayonnaise 2 tbsp salad dressing	Soft margarine, vegetable oil (such as canola, corn, olive, or safflower), low-fat mayonnaise, light salad dressing	The DASH study had 27% of calories as fat, including fat in or added to foods
Sweets and added sugars	0	5 or less per week	<2 daily	1 tbsp sugar 1 tbsp jelly or jam ½ cup sorbet, gelatin 1 cup lemonade	Fruit-flavored gelatin, fruit punch, hard candy, jelly, maple syrup, sorbet and ices, sugar	Sweets should be low in fat

Reproduced from NIH Your Guide to Lowering Your Blood Pressure with DASH https://www.nhlbi.nih.gov/files/docs/public/heart/dash_brief.pdf (PAGE 3 Table).

*Whole grains are recommended for most grain servings as a good source of fiber and nutrients.

[†] Serving sizes vary between ½ cup and 1¼ cups, depending on cereal type. Check the product's Nutrition Facts label.

[§] Fat content changes serving amounts for fats and oils. For example, 1 tbsp of regular salad dressing equals one serving; 1 tbsp of a low-fat dressing equals one-half serving; 1 tbsp of a fat-free dressing equals zero servings.

Abbreviations: oz = ounce; tbsp = tablespoon; tsp = teaspoon

7/3 mm Hg, respectively.[4] This reduction in BP is seen in both genders as well as African American and non–African American adults. A recent meta-analysis of 167 trials concluded that in patients with HTN, a reduced-sodium diet decreased systolic BP by about 5, 6, and 10 mm Hg in white, African American, and Asian participants, respectively.[43] Another meta-analysis of 28 RCTs found that modestly reducing sodium intake resulted in reducing systolic BP by about 5 mm Hg in patients with HTN and by about 2 mm Hg in individuals without HTN.[44] An RCT of 20 individuals with untreated HTN showed that BP fell from 163/100 mm Hg to 147/91 mm Hg when sodium intake was decreased from 11,200 mg/day to 2,900 mg/day.[45] There is a clear relationship between the reduction of dietary sodium intake and improvements in BP, and therefore modification of a risk factor of CVD.

High sodium intake has also been found to be associated with left ventricular hypertrophy, which is a risk factor for CVD outcomes.[33] Three studies have illustrated that reducing sodium intake decreases left ventricular mass; the sodium reductions ranged from 2,000 to 5,000 mg/day and the study durations from 6 weeks to 4 years. Two of the studies combined reduced sodium intake with additional diet and lifestyle changes.[46-48]

In addition to illustrating that decreased sodium intake modifies risk factors for CVD, studies have also shown a direct relationship between sodium intake and CVD. A meta-analysis of 13 prospective cohort studies found that an increase in sodium intake of 5,000 mg/day was associated with a 23% increase in the risk of stroke and a 14% increase in the risk of CVD.[49] In a meta-analysis of seven RCTs, individual trials showed a trend towards reduced sodium intake and decreased CVD and stroke events; when data were pooled, the result was a statistically significant 20% reduction in CVD and stroke events.[50] This confers with data from a long-term follow-up of phase I and phase II of the Trials of Hypertension Prevention. An analysis of 3,126 participants from both trials found that a sodium reduction led to a significant 25% decrease in CVD and stroke events.[51] A challenge has come from recent observational studies that have suggested a relationship between sodium reduction and increased risk of CVD and stroke.[52,53] The AHA reviewed the evidence and published a statement that the findings were based on secondary analysis from studies not originally intended to suggest a relationship between sodium intake and CVD/stroke. Suggested reasons for careful consideration of the results include measurement error, residual confounding, and reverse causality.[42] The current AHA guidelines continue to recommend reduced sodium intake for the prevention of CVD.

The AHA recommendation is a sodium intake of <1,500 mg/day for the entire population.[42] The Dietary Guidelines for Americans 2015 recommends <2300 mg/day sodium intake for all adults; African Americans; and individuals with HTN, DM, and/or chronic kidney disease (CKD).[54] The EAL guideline is also to consume <2,300 mg/day of sodium initially, followed by a further reduction to <1,600 mg/day as needed.[33] Estimations of national sodium intake from 2003 to 2008 National Health and Nutrition Examination Survey (NHANES) data show that 90.7% of adults in the United States consume more than 2,300 mg/day of sodium.[55]

MNT provided by an RD is critical for the HTN population. The nutrition intervention provides the necessary education and support needed for successful diet change. The DASH diet is complex when observed by the untrained eye. An RD can make this diet pattern easy to follow by creating individualized meal plans that meet the cultural considerations, food preferences, and additional nutrient needs unique to each patient.

Advice to follow a sodium restriction can be overwhelming given the plethora of high-sodium food choices in grocery stores and restaurants. Much of the sodium consumption in the United States can be attributed to processed foods such as breads, grains, cereals, soups, sauces, and cured meats.[42] An RD can address barriers to change, such a busy lifestyle, by providing ideas and recipes to illustrate that cooking fresh, healthy foods can be a fast and easy alternative to relying on high-sodium convenience foods. Another common barrier is the misconception that a low-sodium diet is a bland diet; this can be overcome by showing ways to preserve the flavor and appeal of food with a variety of herbs and spices when cooking.

The education piece of MNT for HTN incorporates information regarding daily sodium goals, food sources of sodium, low- and high-sodium choices, and a meal plan that meets the DASH diet guidelines. Important goals are to replace salt with other spices (just 1 tsp of added salt contains 2,300 mg of sodium) and to read food labels to choose foods with less than 140 to 300 mg of sodium per serving. Education tools include handouts with diet guidelines and a comparison of low- and high-sodium foods. See **Table 10.9** for a list of food choices that can be suggested to replace high-sodium foods. Over the course of several MNT sessions an RD can provide the education and motivation for behavior change that is essential for the nutrition management of HTN.

Potassium Supplementation

The latest guidelines by the ACC and AHA for lifestyle management of HTN have recently incorporated potassium supplementation as a recommendation for non-pharmacologic intervention of HTN. Increased potassium intake should be preferably be in the form of diet modification and may be contraindicated for some patients with CKD. A high potassium:sodium ratio has been a cornerstone of the Dash diet.[32]

Alcohol Intake

Excessive alcohol intake is a risk factor for HTN. A reduction in alcohol intake may reduce systolic BP by 2 to 4 mm Hg. Individuals with HTN should be instructed to only consume alcohol in moderation (one drink per day for women and two drinks per day for men).[34]

TABLE 10.9 SUBSTITUTIONS FOR HIGH SODIUM FOOD CHOICES

Low Sodium Choose MORE Often	High Sodium Choose LESS Often
Fresh meat, poultry, fish	Breaded and processed meats, poultry, fish
Low-sodium deli meat, rinsed tuna	Deli meat, canned tuna
Swiss cheese, mozzarella cheese	Hard cheese, cottage cheese
Low-sodium bread & rolls	Salted bread & rolls
Rice, pasta	Commercial pasta or rice mixes
Fresh or frozen fruits & veggies	Canned goods, pickled veggies
Low-sodium soup	Soup and bouillon
Vinegar, low-sodium dressing	Salad dressing, soy sauce

Physical Activity

As part of MNT for HTN, the EAL recommendation for physical activity is 30 minutes on most days of the week.[34] The AHA/ACC guidelines recommend physical activity 3 to 4 times per week for an average of 40 minutes at moderate to vigorous intensity. This level of physical activity can reduce systolic BP by 2 to 5 mm Hg and diastolic BP by 1 to 4 mm Hg.[3]

Smoking Cessation

Smoking cessation is an important element of HTN treatment and CVD prevention. During MNT, an RD can refer a patient to the appropriate smoking cessation programs.

> **PRACTICE POINT**
>
> MNT for HTN involves educating patients on reduced sodium intake and the DASH (Dietary Approaches to Stop Hypertension) diet pattern; individually, both the DASH diet and reduced sodium intake have the potential to lower BP, the benefit is maximized with a combination of both.

Nutrition Monitoring/Evaluation in Hypertension

Similar to dyslipidemia, the monitoring and evaluation portion of MNT for HTN involves a review of the nutrition assessment categories described in Table 10.3. Specific goals and outcomes can be monitored and evaluated at each follow-up visit. Examples for the HTN patient include BMI, waist circumference, diet recall, sodium intake, and BP (EAL guidelines recommend a BP goal of <130/80 mm Hg).[34]

Obesity and CVD Clinical Course

Obesity is a risk factor for dyslipidemia, HTN, DM, CAD, stroke, and HF. An elevated BMI increases risk of morbidity and mortality from cardiovascular events.[56,57] Obesity can be defined as a BMI >30 kg/m². Abdominal obesity is a WC of >35 inches in women and >40 inches in men. WC is an important measure because it distinguishes between android (apple-shaped body) and gynoid (pear-shaped body) obesity. Android obesity is associated with an increased risk of CVD.

A review of the evidence by AHA/ACC shows that a weight loss of 3% to 5% can lead to clinically significant reduction in some CVD risk factors.[57] A 3-kg weight loss has been associated with a 15-mg/dL decrease in triglycerides; a 5-to 8-kg weight loss can lead to a 5-mg/dL decrease in LDL-C and a 2- to 3-mg/dL increase in HDL-C; and a 5% weight loss correlates with a 3 and 2 mm Hg reduction in systolic and diastolic blood pressures respectively.[57] Studies have shown that the most effective weight loss interventions are in person and of high intensity. These interventions include more than 14 sessions over 6 months with a trained interventionist and can be in an individual or group setting. Interventions usually include a 500 kcal/day deficit, increased physical activity, and behavior change strategies to increase adherence. The longer the intervention duration, the better the results. In this scenario, 35% to 60% of individuals maintain at least a 5% weight loss after 2 years.[57] In contrast, low- to moderate-intensity interventions provided by a primary care practitioner alone have not been shown to be effective.[57] This shows the importance of referral to an RD for weight loss MNT.

> **CORE CONCEPT 7**
>
> An elevated body mass index (BMI) increases risk of morbidity and mortality from cardiovascular events.

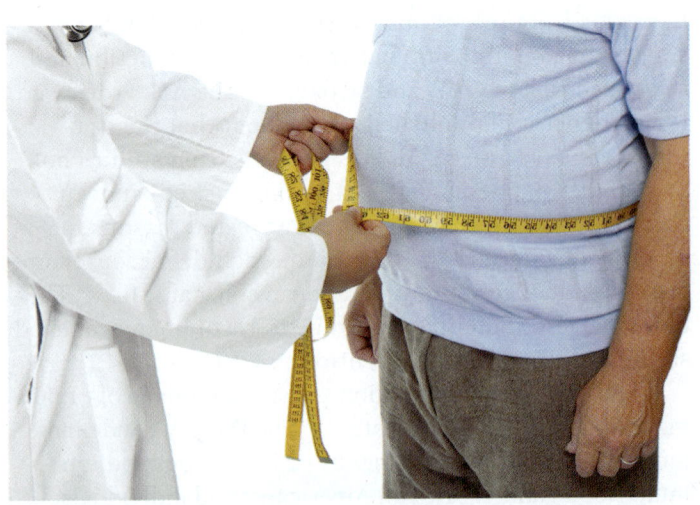

© kurhan/Shutterstock.

> ### CASE STUDY REVISITED
>
> One year later, Carl returns for another follow-up visit with his RD. He reports a lot of stress at work and an inability to maintain his nutritional goals as previously established. Over the past year he had bouts of chest pain and angina. A cardiac catheterization was performed, showing 90% occlusion in his left anterior descending coronary artery. An angioplasty was performed at the time of the exam. In addition to his other medications, his doctor added atorvastatin. Carl believes that dietary modification is no longer necessary because he is now on these medications.
>
> #### Questions
> 1. How would you explain to Carl the importance of lifestyle change in combination with pharmacotherapy for dyslipidemia and HTN?
> 2. Describe how MNT can be tailored to address both dyslipidemia and HTN.

> **PRACTICE POINT**
>
> A weight loss of 3% to 5% can lead to clinically significant reduction in some CVD risk factors.

CVD Outcomes

The CVD outcomes of HTN and atherosclerosis can result in the further outcomes of stroke, PAD, CAD, and HF. If atherosclerosis leads to an embolism in the cerebral arteries that supply the brain, the result can be an ischemic **stroke**. Stroke causes 1 in every 19 deaths in the United States.[12] Atherosclerosis can also narrow the arteries that deliver blood to the legs, arms, stomach, or kidneys in the case of **peripheral artery disease (PAD)**. The early stages of PAD in the extremities can cause cramping, pain, and discomfort. Untreated PAD can result in gangrene and limb amputation.[58]

Advanced Coronary Artery Disease Diagnosis and Surgical Treatment

Coronary artery disease (CAD) accounts for 1 in every 6 deaths in the United States.[2] CAD refers to atherosclerosis affecting the arteries that supply blood to the heart. CAD is also referred to as coronary heart disease (CHD) and **ischemic heart disease**. **Angina**, or chest pain, is a symptom of CAD, but individuals may be asymptomatic until a coronary event. When a blockage occurs in one or several of the coronary arteries that supply blood to the heart, the result can be a **myocardial infarction (MI)**, often referred to as a heart attack. An MI can be fatal. Nonfatal MI increases the risk of developing HF by decreasing functional heart myocytes, scaring heart tissue, causing left ventricular remodeling, and breaking down myocardium (heart muscle).[2] **Ischemic cardiomyopathy** is a type of HF in which the left ventricle is enlarged because of decreased blood supply to the heart muscle due to CAD and MI.

CAD can be diagnosed using CT scans, magnetic resonance imaging, cardiac catheterization, and angiography. Cardiac catheterization is a common yet invasive procedure where a catheter is inserted into a large blood vessel leading to the heart. Measures of blood pressure and flow can be used to assess heart function and parameters such as ejection fraction. Cardiac catheterizations commonly include an angiogram, where a contrast dye that can be seen on x-ray is injected through the catheter. The flow of contrast dye can be followed to determine stenosis or narrowing of specific arteries. When significant stenosis is found, **percutaneous coronary intervention (PCI)** or **coronary angioplasty** is performed by expanding a balloon-tipped catheter at the site and placing a stent.[6] **Figure 10.6** illustrates cardiac catheterization and angioplasty.

If PCI is not possible, a surgical option is **coronary artery bypass graft (CABG)**, in which the stenosis is bypassed with the placement of an artificial or saphenous vein graft.[6] Patients should receive a nutrition assessment prior to cardiac surgery. Obesity (BMI >30 kg/m^2) is associated with an increased rate of postoperative deep sternal wound and saphenous vein harvest site infections.[59,60] Malnutrition is a risk factor for morbidity and mortality in cardiac surgery patients. A study of 5,168 patients found that

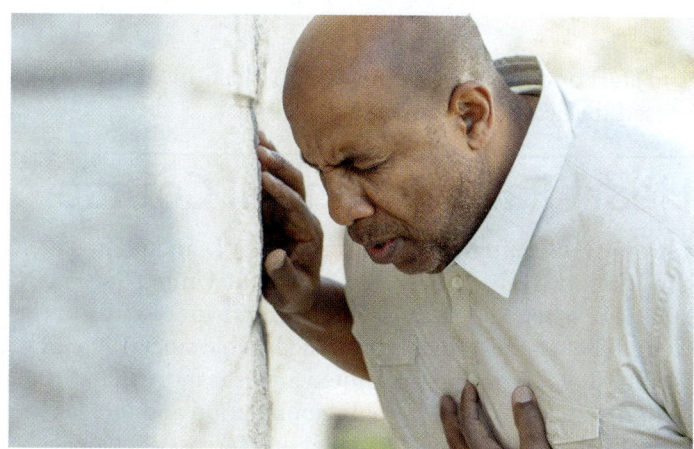
© pixelheadphoto digitalskillet/Shutterstock.

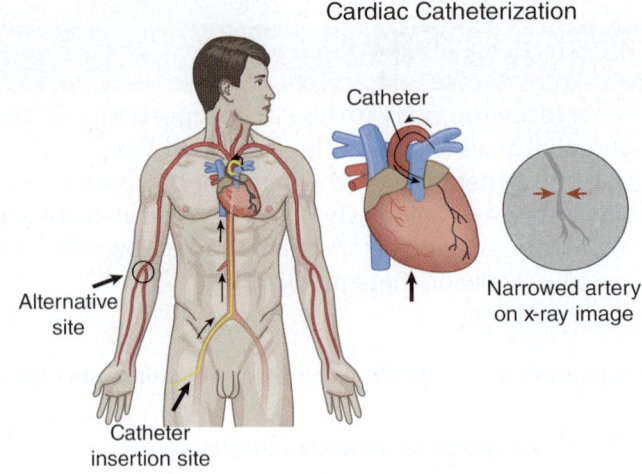

FIGURE 10.6A Cardiac Catheterization with Angiogram.

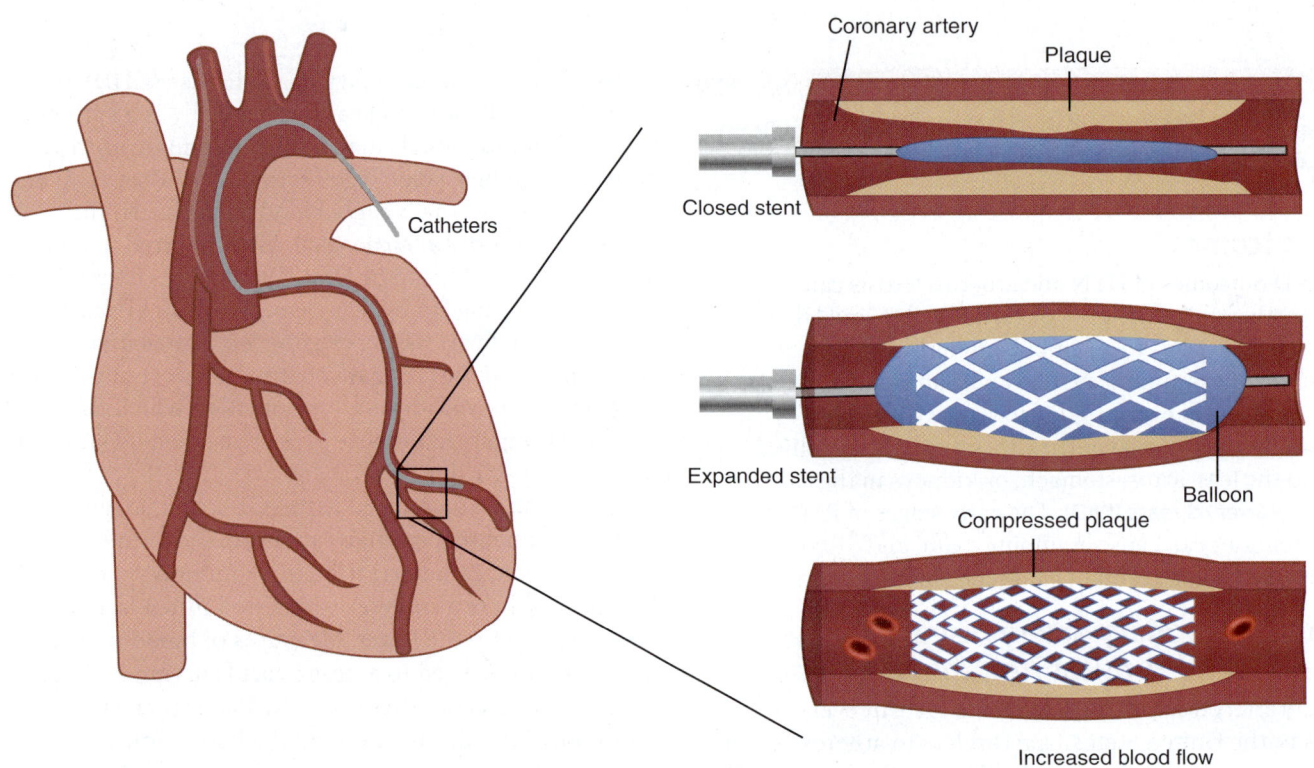

FIGURE 10.6B Stent Angioplasty.

BMI <20 kg/m² was associated with increased mortality after cardiopulmonary bypass.⁶⁰ Nutrition support may be warranted for malnourished cardiac patients before and/or after surgery. Nutrition support is discussed later in this chapter.

During CABG surgery, **cardiopulmonary bypass** is used to perform the work of the heart and lungs temporarily. Associated risks include ischemic damage to the bowel and bacterial translocation.⁵⁹ For this reason, it is important to monitor postoperative gastrointestinal (GI) function before advancing a patient's diet. After CABG, a cardiac patient is instructed to consume a high-protein, low-sodium diet for wound healing. The long-term MNT for a CABG patient is to start or continue to follow a heart-healthy diet as discussed in the dyslipidemia MNT section.

Heart Failure Clinical Course

Chronic HF is often the final stage of CVD and related conditions. The lifetime risk of HF in the United States is 20%.² HF is listed as a cause of death in 1 in 9 deaths in the United States; this rate has remained stable since 1995. The total cost of HF care in the United States is more than $30 billion annually.³¹ With an aging population and increasing rate of CVD, the stage is set for an increased incidence of HF; the number of individuals 65 years of age or older is

CASE STUDY REVISITED

Acute Hospital Admission Note
Several years later, Carl is now 60 years old and experiences an episode of increasing chest pain and dyspnea accompanied by nausea, vomiting, and feeling "unwell." He presents to the Emergency Deparment where an ECG is done indicating ST-elevation myocardial infarction. This is confirmed by elevated troponin levels. Upon hospital admission, a cardiac catheterization reveals 100% occlusion in his left and right coronary arteries. His EF = 35%.
Carl's wife passed away and his daughter is now away at college. He lives alone although his siblings live nearby.

Anthropometric Data:
Weight: 110 kg (242 lbs)
Height: 178 cm (70")
BMI: 34.7 kg/m^2

Biochemical Data:
Sodium 134 (135-145 mEq/L)
Potassium 3.5 (3.6-5.0 mEq/L)
Chloride 99 (98-110 mEq/L)
Carbon dioxide 23 (20-30 mEq/L)
Blood urea nitrogen 20 (6-24 mg/dL)
Creatinine 0.8 (0.4-1.3 mg/dL)
Glucose 130 (70-139 mg/dL)

Calcium 8.9 (8.5-10.5 mEq/L)
Phosphorus 4.5 (2.7-4.5 mg/dL)
Magnesium 1.7 (1.3-2.1 mEq/L)
Albumin 4.0 (3.5-5.0 g/dL)
Prealbumin 26 (17-36 g/dL)

Clinical Data:
Past Medical History: HTN, dyslipidemia, CAD, s/p angioplasty, obesity, depression
Medications: Metoprolol, atorvastatin, Lasix, gemfibrozil, Coumadin
Vital Signs: Blood pressure 159/80 mm Hg, Temperature 99.9°F, Heart rate 90 beats/min
Nutrition-focused Physical Exam: Patient demonstrates shortness of breath

Dietary Data:
24-hour Diet Recall
Since his wife passed away, Carl has relied primarily on convenience foods. Appetite remains good.
Breakfast (9 am): 1 cup coffee with 2% milk and sugar, 2 cups unsweetened whole grain cereal with 1 cup 2% milk, banana
Lunch (12 pm): Canned tomato soup and cheese sandwich, or cheese and crackers, or tuna sandwich with mayo
Snack (3 pm): Chocolate pudding or granola bar
Dinner (6 pm): Frozen pizza; or macaroni and cheese with canned peas; or spaghetti with canned tomato sauce, frozen broccoli, and frozen garlic bread

Diet prescription: 2 gm sodium, heart-healthy diet

Questions
1. Assess the sodium content of Carl's diet.
2. Outline the components of the nutrition education that would be provided to Carl after his CABG surgery.

---

predicted to increase from 35 to 70.3 million from the year 2000 to 2030.[2] HF can be caused by damage to the heart tissue from CAD, MI, and HTN. About 60% to 65% of HF is attributed to CAD, and 90% of HF patients have a history of HTN.[36,61]

HF refers to the heart's inability to provide the body with adequate oxygenated blood. Right-sided HF is when the heart cannot pump adequate blood to the lungs in order to be oxygenated. Left-sided HF is when the heart is unable to pump adequate oxygenated blood to the entire body. HF can also be distinguished as systolic and diastolic. Systolic HF refers to ventricular hypertrophy that leads to decreased pumping during systole. The result is HF with a reduced ejection fraction, defined as less than

40%. HF can also exist with a preserved EF; this is usually in the case of diastolic HF. Diastolic HF is classified as a thickening of the ventricle cavity as opposed to an enlargement of the whole ventricle. The reduced cavity size results in decreased filling capacity during diastole. While there are many ways to differentiate HF, it is also possible for many types of HF to occur at the same time.[6,62,63]

In the case of HF, cardiac output and arterial pressure are decreased. The inability to increase cardiac output leads to the symptoms of fatigue and decreased exercise tolerance. Fluid accumulation occurs in an effort to compensate for decreased arterial pressure and results in edema and **dyspnea** (shortness of breath).[6] **Acute decompensated heart failure (ADHF)** is a rapid onset of HF symptoms that requires immediate treatment.

Major HF risk factors include older age, HTN, MI, DM, valvular heart disease, and obesity. Additional risk factors are dyslipidemia, smoking, sleep-disordered breathing, chronic kidney disease, dietary factors, and sedentary lifestyle. Many of the modifiable risk factors associated with HF are the same for CVD. For this reason, the AHA/ACC recommends using similar preventative measures for both CVD and HF. The focus is on starting prevention at the earliest stage of HF.[4]

Heart failure has been classified by both the New York Heart Association (NYHA) and the AHA/ACC. The NYHA classes are based on functional capacity, while the AHA/ACC stages range from high risk for the development of HF to end-stage HF; **Table 10.10** shows these classification systems.[64]

Early treatment of HF involves pharmacotherapy along with placement of an ICD and/or cardiac resynchronization therapy (CRT) when appropriate. The gold standard treatment of end-stage HF is heart transplantation.[62] An option for patients awaiting heart transplantation and those who suffer acute cardiogenic shock is the implantation of a ventricular assist device (VAD). A VAD can also be used as destination therapy in HF patients who are not eligible for heart transplantation. The most common type of VAD is a **left ventricular assist device** (LVAD); this is a surgically implanted mechanical pump that supports the heart function by pumping blood from the left ventricle to the

TABLE 10.10 HEART FAILURE CLASSIFICATION[64]

New York Heart Association (NYHA) Functional Classification

Class	Patient Symptoms
Class I (Normal)	No limitation of physical activity. Ordinary physical activity does not cause symptoms of HF.
Class II (Mild)	Slight limitation of physical activity. Ordinary physical activity results in symptoms of HF.
Class III (Moderate)	Marked limitation of physical activity. Comfortable at rest, but less than ordinary activity causes symptoms of HF.
Class IV (Severe)	Unable to carry out any physical activity without symptoms of HF, or symptoms of HF at rest.

ACC/AHA Classification

Stage	Description
A (High risk for developing HF)	At high risk for HF but without structural heart disease or symptoms of HF.
B (Asymptomatic HF)	Structural heart disease but without signs or symptoms of HF.
C (Symptomatic HF)	Structural heart disease with prior or current symptoms of HF.
D (Refractory end-stage HF)	Refractory HF requiring specialized interventions.

CASE STUDY REVISITED

Four years later, Carl's CVD has progressed to end-stage HF. He presents to the hospital with SOB, fatigue, decreased exercise tolerance, and a recent weight loss. Diagnosis is ADHF. He reports that he no longer has an interest in food since his wife passed away and he has been instructed by his RD to follow a low-sodium diet. He recalls that he used to be a "big guy," but now the weight is melting off.

Anthropometric Data:
Weight: 65 kg (142 lbs)
Height: 178 cm (70 in)
Estimated dry weight: 63 kg (139 lbs)
Weight history
70 kg (6 months ago); 75 kg (12 months ago); 95 kg (15 years ago)

Biochemical Data:
Sodium 134 (135-145 mEq/L)
Potassium 3.2 (3.6-5.0 mEq/L)
Chloride 99 (98-110 mEq/L)
Carbon dioxide 23 (20-30 mEq/L)
Blood urea nitrogen 17 (6-24 mg/dL)
Creatinine 0.7 (0.4-1.3 mg/dL)
Glucose 110 (70-139 mg/dL)

Calcium 9.0 (8.5-10.5 mEq/L)
Phosphorus 4.0 (2.7-4.5 mg/dL)
Magnesium 1.5 (1.3-2.1 mEq/L)
Albumin 3.5 (3.5-5.0 g/dL)
Prealbumin 8 (17-36 g/dL)

Clinical Data:
Past medical history: HTN, dyslipidemia, CAD, s/p angioplasty, MI, CABG, obesity, depression, end-stage HF
Medications: metoprolol, atorastatin, Lasix, gemfibrozil, Coumadin, multivitamin/mineral supplement
Nutrition-focused physical exam: Bilateral temporal muscle wasting, lower extremity edema

Dietary Data:
24-hour Dietary Recall
Breakfast (9 am) 1 cup of coffee (cream and sugar added), toast with butter
Lunch (12 pm) usually skips lunch
Snack (3 pm) crackers and peanut butter, 8 ounces of milk
Dinner (6 pm) frozen dinner (meat or chicken with rice and vegetable), usually eats about 50%

Questions

1. What additional nutrition assessment data can be collected as part of subjective global assessment (SGA)? Why is SGA useful in Carl's current situation?
2. How would you describe Carl's nutritional status and nutritional risk factors?
3. How would you estimate Carl's current protein and energy needs?
4. Develop a nutrition intervention to present to Carl and his medical team. What data will be useful to monitor and evaluate?

---

aorta to circulate oxygen-rich blood throughout the body. **Figure 10.7** shows an LVAD.

Other types of VADs include right ventricular assist devices (RVADs) and bi-ventricular assist devices (BIVADs). Advances in VAD technology have made the devices smaller, more reliable, and longer lasting. VADs can be used for both temporary treatment and destination therapy at various stages of HF. In the case of heart transplantation, the VAD is removed and replaced with a donor organ.[63,65]

> **CORE CONCEPT 8**
>
> Heart failure (HF) refers to the heart's inability to provide the body with adequate oxygenated blood. HF can be caused by damage to the heart tissue from CAD, MI, and HTN.

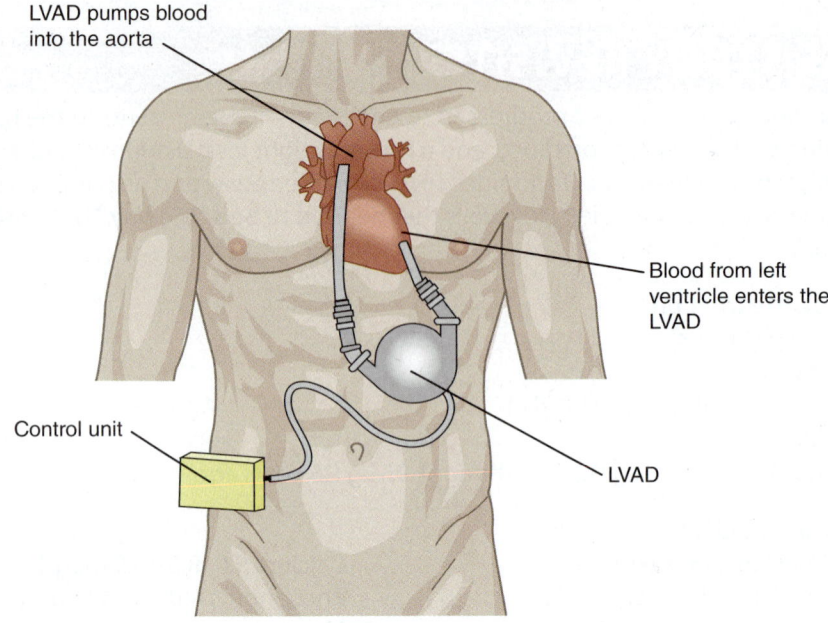

FIGURE 10.7 Left Ventricular Assist Device (LVAD).

Nutritional Management in Heart Failure

The EAL recommends that all HF patients be referred to an RD for MNT. An initial visit (at least 45 minutes) and one to three follow-ups (at least 30 minutes each) can result in improvements in dietary pattern, quality of life, edema, and fatigue.[66]

> **PRACTICE POINT**
>
> MNT for HF can result in improvements in dietary pattern, quality of life, edema, and fatigue.

Nutrition Assessment in Heart Failure

The nutrition assessment of the HF patient includes the following: food/nutrition intake and related history; anthropometric measurements; biochemical data, medical tests, and procedures; nutrition-focused physical findings; and client history. Table 10.3 describes data collected for each category for patients at risk of HF. In addition to these data, the assessment of the HF patient will include the following biochemical data: chem-10 lab panel (sodium, potassium, chloride, bicarbonate, blood urea nitrogen, creatinine, blood glucose, calcium, magnesium, phosphorus), hemoglobin, hematocrit, albumin, and prealbumin. Albumin and prealbumin should be measured and monitored because they correlate with disease outcome in several studies. However, albumin and prealbumin are influenced by several factors not related to nutrition status, and should not be used as independent nutrition markers. Additional anthropometric measurements in this patient population include EDW and ideal body weight (IBW).

A useful assessment tool for the HF population is **subjective global assessment (SGA)**. SGA evaluates weight change, dietary intake, GI symptoms, functional impairment, muscle wasting, and fat loss.[37,67] **Table 10.11** illustrates the components of SGA. The Mini Nutrition Assessment (MNA) from Nestle Health Science is another assessment tool, which screens for change in food intake, weight loss over 3 months, mobility, recent psychological stress, recent acute disease, and neuropsychological problems. See **Figure 10.8**.[68,69] SGA and the MNA help to classify HF patients as well-nourished, at risk of malnutrition, and malnourished.

> **PRACTICE POINT**
>
> A useful assessment tool for the HF population is subjective global assessment (SGA). SGA evaluates weight change, dietary intake, GI symptoms, functional impairment, muscle wasting, and fat loss.

Medications in Heart Failure

HF patients are often prescribed multiple medications with nutrition-related implications. Table 10.7 in the HTN section lists classes of medications that may be taken by HF patients; additional classes of medications are shown in **Table 10.12**. Possible drug–nutrient interactions are assessed to prevent and address potential adverse reactions.

Indirect calorimetry is the ideal way to assess energy needs in HF patients. When this method is not available, appropriate energy needs calculations such as Mifflin–St Jeor or Harris–Benedict can be used. A stress factor

TABLE 10.11 SUBJECTIVE GLOBAL ASSESSMENT[37,67]

Components of Subjective Global Assessment

Weight change	• Weight change over 2 weeks, 6 months, and 1 year • Intentional versus unintentional weight change • Actual weight and clothing size changes
Dietary intake	• Changes over time • Restrictions
Gastrointestinal symptoms	• Nausea, vomiting, diarrhea • Anorexia, dysphagia
Functional impairment	• Hand grip strength
Muscle wasting & subcutaneous fat loss	• Muscle stores: bicep, tricep, quadricep, deltoid, temple • Fat stores: tricep, chest, eyes, perioral, interosseous, palmar
Edema	• Hands, sacral, lower extremities

should be added to account for increased resting energy expenditure in HF patients. The EAL suggests calculating daily protein needs as 1.2 g/kg/day in well-nourished HF patients and 1.37 g/kg/day in nutritionally depleted HF patients.[66] Actual protein delivery will need to be modified in the case of the HF patient with acute renal insufficiency, depending on treatment method.

Assessing for Obesity

Obesity increases the risk of heart failure by two-fold.[56] The prevalence of overweight and obesity in the HF population is 65%. Factors that contribute to weight gain in HF patients include decreased exercise tolerance, excessive calorie intake, volume overload, and medications.[29,70] Obesity can be identified in the HF population with the anthropometric measurements of BMI (based on EDW), WC, and WHR. The outcomes associated with overweight and obesity include infection and poor wound healing, as well as increased incidence of comorbidities such as dylipidemia, HTN, and insulin resistance.[29,70] While elevated BMI has associated risks, it has also been found to be linked to a decreased mortality rate in the HF population. The protective effect of elevated BMI in HF patients has been termed the "**obesity paradox**."[71] A meta-analysis of 9 observational studies concluded that overweight (BMI 25-29.9 kg/m^2) and obesity (BMI ≥30 kg/m^2) were associated with a decreased risk of all-cause mortality and cardiovascular mortality when compared to normal BMI.[71] The Digitalis Investigation Group Trial followed 7,767 HF patients over 37 months, and found that a BMI of >30 kg/m^2 was associated with a mortality rate of 28%, as compared to 45% in those with a BMI of 18.5 to 25 kg/m^2 and 38% in those with a BMI <18.5 kg/m^2.[21,70]

The reason for the protective effect of obesity in HF is not well understood. One suggested reason is that HF may be found earlier in patients with an elevated BMI as compared to those with a lower BMI; low BMI may be indicative of disease progression. Another possible explanation is that a greater metabolic reserve allows obese individuals to handle metabolic stress better than those with a lower BMI. Increased adipose tissue in obese patients may play a role in neutralizing the effects of **tumor necrosis factor-alpha**, which typically contributes to muscle wasting in HF patients. The difficulty with using BMI to classify HF patients in these studies is that it is not possible to identify whether protective factors are related to increased lean body mass or increased fat tissue.[71] The role of the RD is to weigh the risks and benefits of each patient's BMI when performing nutrition assessments.

> **PRACTICE POINT**
>
> While elevated BMI has associated risks, it has also been found to be linked to a decreased mortality rate in the HF population. The protective effect of elevated BMI in HF patients has been termed the "obesity paradox."

Assessing for Cardiac Cachexia

Hippocrates (ca. 460-377 BC) described cardiac cachexia as follows: "The flesh is consumed and becomes water . . . the shoulders, clavicles, chest and thighs melt away. This illness is fatal."[72] **Cardiac cachexia** is an uncontrollable loss of weight that includes muscle, fat, and eventually bone loss. This condition effects an estimated 4% to 13% of HF patients and is associated with a 50% mortality rate at 18 months.[21,70,73,74] An observational prospective analysis of 208 patients previously hospitalized due to HF found that malnutrition (identified using the MNA) was an independent risk factor for mortality. The findings were mortality rates of 56%, 23.5%, and 11.3% after 12 months in the malnourished, at risk of malnutrition, and adequate nutrition status groups, respectively. After 32 months, the mortality rates increased to 80.8%, 42.4%, and 26.6% in each group, respectively. Associations were found between malnutrition and cognitive impairment, low prealbumin levels, and low BMI.[75] Similar results were found in a retrospective analysis of 154 HF patients; the mortality rates were 26.5% in the malnourished group, 42% in the at risk of malnutrition group, and 6.7% in the well-nourished group.[68]

Contributing factors to cardiac cachexia include metabolic malfunction, decreased calorie intake (due to anorexia, early satiety, volume overload, nausea, depression, medications, taste changes, and increased cytokine levels), loss of lean body mass (from decreased intake, tissue hypoxia, aging, decreased exercise, inflammation,

Mini Nutritional Assessment
MNA®

Nestlé NutritionInstitute

Last name:		First name:	
Sex:	Age:	Weight, kg:	Height, cm:	Date:

Complete the screen by filling in the boxes with the appropriate numbers. Total the numbers for the final screening score.

Screening

A Has food intake declined over the past 3 months due to loss of appetite, digestive problems, chewing or swallowing difficulties?
0 = severe decrease in food intake
1 = moderate decrease in food intake
2 = no decrease in food intake

B Weight loss during the last 3 months
0 = weight loss greater than 3 kg (6.6 lbs)
1 = does not know
2 = weight loss between 1 and 3 kg (2.2 and 6.6 lbs)
3 = no weight loss

C Mobility
0 = bed or chair bound
1 = able to get out of bed / chair but does not go out
2 = goes out

D Has suffered psychological stress or acute disease in the past 3 months?
0 = yes   2 = no

E Neuropsychological problems
0 = severe dementia or depression
1 = mild dementia
2 = no psychological problems

F1 Body Mass Index (BMI) (weight in kg) / (height in m)^2
0 = BMI less than 19
1 = BMI 19 to less than 21
2 = BMI 21 to less than 23
3 = BMI 23 or greater

IF BMI IS NOT AVAILABLE, REPLACE QUESTION F1 WITH QUESTION F2.
DO NOT ANSWER QUESTION F2 IF QUESTION F1 IS ALREADY COMPLETED.

F2 Calf circumference (CC) in cm
0 = CC less than 31
3 = CC 31 or greater

Screening score
(max. 14 points)

12-14 points: ☐ Normal nutritional status
8-11 points: ☐ At risk of malnutrition
0-7 points: ☐ Malnourished

®Société des Produits Nestlé S.A., Vevey, Switzerland, Trademark Owners.
1. Vellas B, Villars H, Abellan G, et al. Overview of the MNA® - Its History and Challenges. J Nutr Health Aging 2006;10:456-465.
2. Rubenstein LZ, Harker JO, Salva A, Guigoz Y, Vellas B. Screening for Undernutrition in Geriatric Practice: Developing the Short-Form Mini Nutritional Assessment (MNA®-SF). J Geront 2001;56A: M366-377.
3. Guigoz Y. The Mini-Nutritional Assessment (MNA®) Review of the Literature - What does it tell us? J Nutr Health Aging 2006; 10:466-487. Page 2
4. Kaiser MJ, Bauer JM, Ramsch C, et al. Validation of the Mini Nutritional Assessment Short-Form (MNA®-SF): A practical tool for identification of nutritional status. J Nutr Health Aging 2009; 13:782-788 (Short Form only)"

FIGURE 10.8 Mini Nutrition Assessment.
© Nestlé, 1994, Revision 2009. N67200 12/99 10M., For further information visit, www.mna-elderly.com.

TABLE 10.12 DRUG–NUTRIENT INTERACTIONS[16, 21]

Medication Class	Potential Side Effect	Nutrition Intervention
Anticoagulants (warfarin) Prevent blood clots	• Interact with vitamin K • Interact with additional herbs & supplements	• Educate on consistent intake of foods high in vitamin K; provide a list of foods containing vitamin K • Encourage patients to talk with their physician before taking vitamin E, fish oil, or herbal supplements
Inotropes (digoxin) Stimulate the heart to contract	• Hypo- or hyperkalemia • Decreased Ca+, Mg+ • Interactions with herbal supplements • Anorexia, weight loss, nausea, vomiting, diarrhea • Arrhythmias when combined with Ca+/Vitamin D supplementation	• Monitor K+; replete or restrict as indicated; educate on food sources • Monitor Ca++ and Mg++; replete as indicated; educate on food sources • Avoid St. John's wort; caution with aloe, foxglove, hawthorn • Educate on small frequent meals as tolerated; monitor adequacy of oral intake • Use caution with Ca++/vitamin D supplementation; educate on food sources as an alternative

and medications), malabsorption (due to intestinal edema and decreased GI perfusion), and increased losses (from diarrhea and diuresis).[21,70,73,76] Cardiac cachexia does not have a standard definition. A nutrition assessment should look for the criteria of more than 5% to 7.5% unintentional weight loss over 6 to 12 months and BMI <20 kg/m² (in patients younger than 65 years) or BMI <22 kg/m² (in patients older than 65 years). In addition, patients with cardiac cachexia will have at least three of the following: albumin <3.5 g/L, decreased total protein levels, anemia, elevated triglycerides, elevated glucose, elevated lactic acid, decreased muscle strength, fatigue, anorexia, decreased lean body mass, and ongoing inflammation (elevated norepinephrine, epinephrine, cortisol, and tumor necrosis factor-alpha).[74,76,77]

Cardiac cachexia is thought to involve the function of the immune, metabolic, and neurohormonal systems within the body. An inflammatory response caused from hypoxia, decreased heart function, and increased GI permeability from bowel edema results in an elevation of tumor necrosis factor-alpha. Tumor necrosis factor-alpha stimulates catabolic processes that result in muscle breakdown, anorexia, and decreased exercise tolerance. The muscle breakdown exacerbates further inflammatory response.[74] Patients with cardiac cachexia have been found to have increased levels of the stress hormones norepinephrine, epinephrine, and cortisol.[78] This explanation of the mechanism of cardiac cachexia progression helps to explain why the condition is not reversible with nutrition intervention. Adequate nutrition will not reverse cardiac cachexia, but it does have the potential to diminish the negative outcomes of the condition.[74]

Cardiac cachexia should be addressed as early as possible to mitigate the outcomes of increased rate of infection, poor wound healing, decubitus ulcers, bacterial overgrowth, malabsorption, loss of lean body mass, and overall morbidity and mortality.[21,70]

> **CORE CONCEPT 9**
>
> Cardiac cachexia is an uncontrollable loss of weight that includes muscle, fat, and eventually bone loss. It is associated with a 50% mortality rate at 18 months. The condition is not reversible with nutrition intervention, but adequate nutrition may diminish negative outcomes.

Nutrition Intervention in Heart Failure
The overall goal of MNT in the HF patient is to achieve optimal nutrition status to manage current HF, slow disease progression, and prepare for best surgical outcomes if/when LVAD and/or heart transplantation are indicated. An RD will ensure adequate daily calorie and protein intake and compliance with diet recommendations. In the case that a HF patient is unable to meet nutrition needs with oral intake, nutrition support may be warranted.

Sodium and Fluid Restrictions
The AEAL recommends 1.4 to 1.9 L/day of fluid and <2,000 mg/day of sodium for the HF population. The EAL highlights that this sodium restriction has been shown to improve NYHA functional class, sleep disturbance, physical activity tolerance, edema, B-type natriuretic peptide, and blood pressure in four clinical studies.[66] The Dietary Guidelines for Americans 2015 recommends <2300 mg/day sodium intake for all adults; African Americans; and individuals with HTN, DM, and/or CKD.[54] According to patient report in the NHANES sample of 574 adults over age 50 years with HF, sodium restriction adherence rates ranged from 20% to 71%. The average daily sodium intake was 2,729 mg/day. Only 18.7% achieved a sodium intake of <1,500 mg/day, and 15.4% had a sodium intake of >4,000 mg/day. Male gender and lower income were associated with higher sodium intake.[79]

A diet high in sodium and fluid can contribute to edema and ADHF.[33] A prospective cohort study of 123 ambulatory patients with systolic HF showed that patients consuming a high-sodium diet (≥2,800 mg/day) had a 2.5-fold increased risk of ADHF and an increased risk of hospitalization and mortality when compared to patients consuming lower amounts of sodium.[15] Another study of 97 HF patients concluded that a three-fold increase in 90-day hospital readmission rate was associated with low knowledge of dietary sodium.[80] MNT provided by an RD has the potential to increase patient knowledge and compliance. A 6-month nutrition intervention with 65 HF patients led to decreased calorie and fluid intake, decreased edema, and increased quality of life. Another 9-month nutrition intervention with 79 HF patients resulted in significant decreases in sodium and fluid intake and increased quality of life.[81,82]

The role of the RD is to educate patients and encourage compliance with a well-balanced, sodium/fluid restricted diet. The education piece includes identifying low- versus high-sodium foods, suggesting replacements for the salt shaker (herbs, spices, citrus), encouraging patients to cook fresh foods instead of processed foods, reviewing nutrition labels to identify sodium content, and developing an individualized meal plan. With regard to fluid, the RD can explain the reason for the restriction, illustrate fluid goals in terms that make sense to patients (2 L equals 8 cups), and identify foods that count as fluids (all foods that are liquid at room temperature such as soup, ice cream, popsicles, and ice chips). In addition to providing nutrition information, the importance of decreasing sodium and fluid intake can be explained with motivators that matter to each patient (increased quality of life, less sick days, more time with family). An RD can provide positive reasons for change, highlight ways to preserve the taste of food, discuss strategies for overcoming cravings and thirst, give tips on enjoying social events, show cultural sensitivity, and gain support from family and friends. The overall goal is to assist patients in adhering to sodium and fluid restrictions to achieve increased quality of life, decreased HF symptoms, and decreased hospitalizations.

Heart-healthy Eating

The reason for emphasizing heart-healthy eating in the HF population is to decrease the risk of cardiac events and prevent/manage the comorbidities of HTN, CAD, and DM. The dyslipidemia section of this chapter has a detailed review of heart-healthy eating. An RD can help combine recommendations for multiple conditions. An example is Table 10.13, which illustrates a sample heart-healthy meal plan with less than 1,500 mg/day of sodium and less than 2 L/day of fluid.

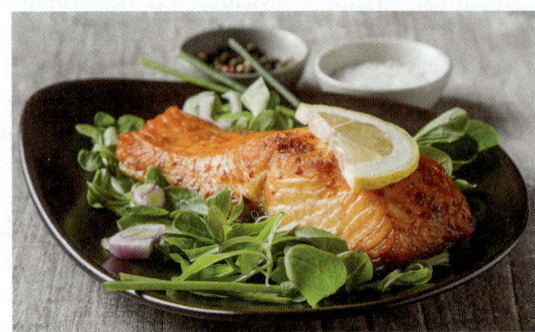
© Gaus Alex/Shutterstock.

TABLE 10.13 MEAL PLAN: HEART HEALTHY, <1500 MG/DAY SODIUM, <2 L/DAY FLUID

Breakfast
1 cup oatmeal, 1 tsp cinnamon
1-2 tbsp almond slivers
1 banana or 1 cup blueberries
1 cup low fat milk

Snack
6 oz Greek yogurt (0% fat)
½ cup strawberries
1 cup water

Lunch
2 slices whole grain bread
3 oz roast turkey, lettuce, tomatoes
2 tsp low-fat mayo
½ - 1 cup veggie sticks
1 orange, 1 cup seltzer water

Snack
1 mozzarella string cheese
6 whole grain crackers
1 cup lemon water

Dinner
4 oz grilled salmon with lemon zest
1-2 cups spinach salad
(2 tsp vinegar, 1 tbsp olive oil, 2 tbsp cranberries, 2 tbsp walnuts)
1 cup brown rice

Snack
Baked apple slices with cinnamon
1-2 tbsp natural peanut butter
1 cup water

Blood Glucose Management

Patients with HF benefit from BG management to decrease complications. An increase of hemoglobin A1c of 1% correlates with an 8% to 16% increase in the risk of hospitalization for HF and death.[21]

Nutrient Deficiencies

MNT for HF includes addressing possible nutrient deficiencies. Reasons for nutrient deficiencies in the HF population include overall decreased dietary intake and losses from diuretics.[83] Table 10.14 explains possible nutrient deficiencies and treatment. One goal of MNT is to ensure adequate micronutrient stores to reduce adverse events.

Dietary Supplements

An estimated one in every three HF patients takes complimentary alternative medicines. It is the role of the medical team, including the RD, to assist patients in evaluating nutrition supplement claims.[66,87] Precautions should be taken to avoid possible supplement–medication interactions. Evaluating dietary supplement regimens can help to prevent adverse reactions in HF patients.

Coenzyme Q

The theory is that coenzyme Q may improve systolic heart function, but there is limited evidence to support this claim. Coenzyme Q should not be taken with

TABLE 10.14 POSSIBLE NUTRIENT DEFICIENCIES IN THE HF POPULATION

Zinc Deficiency[16,21]

Risk factors for deficiency	ACE inhibitors, ARBs, thiazide diuretics, diarrhea, alcoholism
Symptoms	Dysguesia, poor wound healing, dry skin, poor appetite, weakness, facial rash (butterfly shape)
Treatment	220 mg/day zinc sulfate
Food sources	Wheat germ, liver, turkey, beef, pork, beans, cashews, soy nuts, sunflower seeds

Thiamine Deficiency[16,21,77,79,84]

Risk factors for deficiency	Alcoholism, loop diuretic use, malnutrition, older age, HF, vomiting/diarrhea, malabsorption, gastric bypass, frequent hospitalization
Symptoms	Cardiovascular, GI, and nervous system impairment *Wet Beriberi:* sodium retention, peripheral vasodilation, biventricular HF
Treatment	100 to 200 mg/day thiamine for 4 weeks; 100 mg/day IV or IM for 5 days if symptomatic deficiency
Food sources	Enriched grains, organ meats, wheat germ, pork, peas, peanuts, sunflower seeds, rice bran, soybeans, soy milk, tofu, brewer's yeast, beans

Vitamin D Deficiency[21,85,86]

Risk factors for deficiency	Poor oral intake, malabsorption, decreased sun exposure, steroid administration
Symptoms	Osteopenia, secondary hyperparathyroidism, cardiomyopathy, alteration of renin-angiotensin axis, may affect vascular endothelium (inflammation, thrombosis, cell proliferation), altered Ca+ channel fluxes
Treatment	50,000 IU ergocalciferol once weekly for 6 to 8 weeks
Food sources	Fatty fish, egg yolk, liver, fortified dairy products

gemfibrozil, tricyclic antidepressants, or warfarin due to interactions. Adverse reactions associated with coenzyme Q are transient nausea, maculopapular rash, epigastric pain, dizziness, photophobia, and irritability. Current research does not support the use of coenzyme Q in HF patients.[66,87]

Hawthorne

In a meta-analysis of eight RCTs, hawthorne was found to improve maximal workload, pressure-heart rate products, and symptoms of fatigue and dyspnea with doses ranging from 160 to 1,800 mg/day. The risks associated with hawthorne in the HF population include interactions with beta-blockers, calcium channel blockers, digoxin, and nitrates. Adverse reactions include dizziness and vertigo. At this time there is limited evidence to support the use of hawthorne in HF patients.[66,87]

B-Complex Vitamins

While B-complex vitamins have been shown to decrease homocysteine levels, studies have failed to show any significant reduction in cardiovascular morbidity or mortality. In addition, there has been evidence to support the risk of restenosis in patients with a history of MI or recent stent who were taking either 0.8 to 1.2 mg/day folic acid or 0.06 to 0.4 mg/day B12 supplementation in combination with other vitamins. At this time, routine supplementation of B vitamins is not recommended for HF patients. Exceptions include the case of micronutrient deficiencies, alcoholic cardiomyopathy, and macrocytic anemia.[21,66]

Antioxidants

A review of RCTs does not support the use of vitamin E, vitamin C, or beta-carotene supplements in HF patients.

Clinical Roundtable

Topic: Nutritional Management of Poor Intake with End Stage Heart Failure

Background: End-stage heart failure symptoms often lead to decreased appetite and inadequate food/beverage intake. Given the risk of malnutrition in this population, interventions aimed at adequate energy and protein intake are common. Increasing nutritional intake in patients with multiple dietary restrictions prescribed for heart failure can be a challenge for the RD.

Roundtable Discussion

What would you recommend to address this issue? Would you prescribe nutrition supplement drinks when a patient is on a fluid restriction? Would you suggest using appetite stimulants? Which medication would you recommend? How will you illustrate the benefits versus the potential risks? How would you monitor for measurable outcomes based on your recommendations?

Food sources of antioxidants should be encouraged rather than supplementation.[21]

Vitamin E

The risks of vitamin E supplementation in HF patients outweigh the benefits. Observational studies suggest decreased risk of CHD associated with vitamin E, but RCTs fail to support the theory. An increased incidence of HF was found to be associated with 400 IU/day vitamin E supplementation in the HOPE trial. This trial included 9,541 adults with a 7-year follow-up. High doses of vitamin E supplementation (>400 IU/day) may be associated with mortality. For these reasons, vitamin E supplementation is not recommended for the HF population.[21,88]

Nutrition Intervention in the Case of Cardiac Cachexia

MNT for cardiac cachexia will not reverse the condition, but it can aid in the prevention of further loss of muscle, fat, and bone mass.[21,70] The RD will ensure that the cardiac cachexia patient meets estimated energy, protein, and nutrient needs. A calorie count is helpful to monitor oral intake. Decreased intake and early satiety can be addressed with small/frequent meals; nutrition supplement drinks/snacks; and an appetite-stimulating medication, such as megestrol acetate (Megace). Studies have shown that a dose of 160 mg/day of megestrol acetate may improve appetite within 1 week, but potential weight gain requires a higher dose (480-800 mg/day) for a longer duration. Side effects include edema, elevated BG, adrenal suppression, elevated liver enzymes, and increased risk of deep vein thrombosis.[74] If a patient is unable to meet at least 60% of calorie and protein needs with oral intake, nutrition support is warranted.

Nutrition Monitoring/Evaluation in Heart Failure

The monitoring and evaluation portion of MNT for HF involves a review of all data collected during the nutrition assessment. Patient progress towards desired goals and outcomes will be documented. Monitoring and evaluation of the HF patient may include the following: weight change, hand grip strength, muscle and fat stores, edema, adequacy of protein/energy intake, compliance with sodium/fluid restrictions, activity tolerance, medication/dietary supplement regimen, symptoms related to food intake, chem-10 lab panel, albumin, prealbumin, and nutrition quality of life.

> **PRACTICE POINT**
>
> The overall goal of MNT in the HF patient is to achieve optimal nutrition status to manage current HF, slow disease progression, and prepare for best surgical outcomes if/when left ventricular assist device and/or heart transplantation are indicated.

Nutrition Support in CVD

Nutrition support is initiated at times when the CVD patient is otherwise unable to meet calorie, protein, fluid, and nutrient needs with oral intake. Nutrition support may be warranted in the case of malnutrition and cardiac cachexia, or intubation due to ADHF and/or **cardiogenic shock**. Cardiogenic shock is a severe, life-threatening condition of systemic hypoperfusion. This can be an outcome of MI or end-stage HF, in addition to multiple other causes.[89] Damage to the heart muscle leads to decreased cardiac output and MAP. Shock results in pulmonary congestion, systemic inflammation, and acidosis. Treatment usually includes mechanical ventilation, fluid resuscitation, **vasopressors**, and **intra-aortic balloon pump (IABP)** support. Vasopressors increase BP and MAP by constricting blood vessels. Examples include norepinephrine, dopamine, and dobutamine. An IABP provides short-term mechanical support to increase cardiac output. A balloon is placed in the aorta via the femoral artery without the need for invasive surgery. In the case of MI, treatment may continue with PCI or CABG. In the case of HF, treatment may continue with the placement of a VAD.[89] Special consideration should be made when providing nutrition support to this patient population. Cardiogenic shock decreases blood supply to the gut, therefore increasing gut permeability and bacterial

CASE STUDY REVISITED

Carl's condition has worsened during his hospital admission. He is now requiring mechanical ventilation as a result of pulmonary edema. The team is planning for LVAD surgery while he awaits a heart transplant.

Questions

1. Update the nutrition care plan for Carl given his current status. What data need to be collected to reassess Carl's nutrient needs? Explain scenarios in which nutrition support is indicated and contraindicated. If indicated, what nutrition support recommendations should be provided to the medical/surgical team?
2. Carl's CVD progression has been followed from his initial dyslipidemia diagnosis to the complications of end-stage HF. What can be learned from his case in its entirety?

translocation. In addition, the following factors increase risk of bowel ischemia: vasopressors; IABP; mechanical ventilation; decreased cardiac output; renal insufficiency; and history of MI, PAD, or stroke.[59]

Enteral nutrition (EN) is the recommended route of feeding for cardiac patients, as long as normal GI function exists. This guideline is supported by the Critical Care Guidelines from the American Society of Parenteral and Enteral Nutrition (A.S.P.E.N.) and the Society of Critical Care Medicine (SCCM), along with the Academy of Nutrition and Dietetics' EAL. EN decreases the rate of infection and complications when compared to parenteral nutrition (PN).[90,91] When provided appropriately, EN in a preoperative cardiac patient population can improve left ventricular end-diastolic volume and immune defense. In the postoperative patient population, EN can decrease infection rate, preserve renal function, prevent mucosal atrophy, preserve GI microbiota balance, improve gut perfusion, and decrease length of hospital stay.[92,93] A trial that provided EN to nine cardiac patients on the first postoperative day found the following results: increased cardiac index and splanchnic blood flow, decreased MAP by 10%, stable heart rate, and tolerance of EN. These patients received 130% of measured energy expenditure while medically managed with dobutamine and norepinephrine to maintain MAP of 70 mm Hg.[94] An additional study illustrated that EN was tolerated in postoperative cardiothoracic patients medically managed with dopamine and norepinephrine when EN was started within 2 to 3 days of surgery, and advanced slowly over 4 to 6 days.[95]

When estimating calorie and protein needs in the intubated cardiac patient, the recommendation is to use the Penn State equation, or the modified Penn State equation in patients older than 60 years with a BMI >30 kg/m². In the nonintubated cardiac patient, indirect calorimetry is the gold standard for estimating calorie needs. Protein needs for cardiac patients requiring nutrition support can be estimated as 1.5 to 2 g/kg/day UBW, or IBW in patients with a BMI >30 kg/m².[59] A.S.P.E.N./SCCM and the EAL recommend starting EN within 24 to 48 hours of intensive care unit (ICU) admission following fluid resuscitation.[90,91] In the cardiac patient, EN should only be initiated when a patient is hemodynamically stable, vasopressor dose is decreased, MAP is 60 to 70 mm Hg, and intra-abdominal pressure is >20 mm Hg. A feeding tube can be placed in the stomach or small bowel; small-bowel feedings are recommended in the cases of high aspiration risk, supine position, heavy sedation, and high gastric residuals.[59,90,91] A fluid-restricted formula is usually required in this population due to the presence of edema. Additional protein modulars may be used to meet elevated protein requirements to achieve positive nitrogen balance. The A.S.P.E.N./SCCM recommendation is to initiate EN at 10 to 20 mL/hour and advance to reach goal rate within 48 to 72 hours as tolerated.[59,90] EN patients are monitored for the following: MAP, vasopressor doses, ventilatory requirements, abdominal pain/distention, nasogastric tube output, gastric residuals (>500mL or >250mL on two consecutive occasions), absence of stool/flatus/bowel sounds, ileus, diarrhea, dilated and thickened bowel loops, and metabolic acidosis. Some of these symptoms can be resolved with troubleshooting. In the case of high gastric residuals, EN route should be into the small bowel

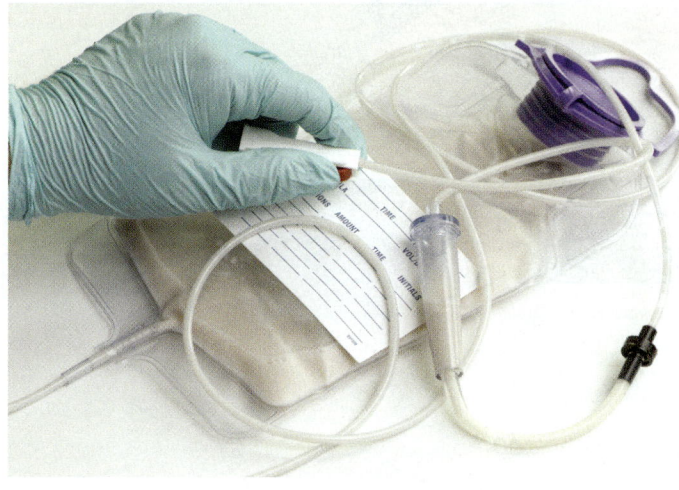

⚠ Clinical Controversy

Saturated Fat and Risk of CVD

A Presidential Advisory was recently issued by the American Heart Association on dietary fat and risk of CVD. In their report they describe the evidence supporting that a reduction in saturated fat intake can decrease risk of CVD. This is despite the fact that a recent meta-analysis claimed a lack of evidence for guidelines recommending lowering consumption of saturated fat. The AHA Advisory claims that studies used in this analysis did not sufficiently look at macronutrient type that replaced saturated fat. Their review of pooled studies analysis such as those conducted by Farvid et al[9], which looked at the linoleic acid and the benefit of replacing saturated fat with polyunsaturated fat, confirmed that current dietary recommendations are valid and evidence based.

As an RD in an established lipid clinic, what is your position or rationale when advising patients amidst these conflicting results? Based on your review of the papers referenced, determine the rationale for your dietary interventions and how you might explain this to your patients.

References

1. Chowdhury R, Warnakula S, Kunutsor S, et al. Association of dietary, circulating, and supplement fatty acids with coronary risk a systematic review and meta-analysis. *Ann Intern Med*. 2014;160:398-406.
2. Farvid MS, Ding M, Pan A, Sun Q, et al. Dietary linoleic acid and risk of coronary heart disease: A systematic review and meta-analysis of prospective cohort studies. *Circulation*. 2014;130:1568-1578.

---

and prokinetic agents such as metoclopramide and erythromycin can be provided.[90,91] Diarrhea can be addressed with a hypo-osmolar, fiber-free formula; other causes of diarrhea should always be explored (sorbitol-containing medications, antibiotics, *Clostridium difficile*, and large volumes of fluid to the small intestine).[90] In the case of sudden worsening of hemodynamic status or GI function, EN should be held.[59] EN protocols can establish standards for initiating and advancing EN, monitoring for tolerance, troubleshooting common side effects, and holding EN. Having an EN protocol in place reduces ICU and hospital length of stay and number of days of ventilation.[96]

PN is indicated in the case of mesenteric ischemia, GI dysfunction, or intolerance of adequate energy from EN.[97] Due to the risk of infection, A.S.P.E.N./SSCM guidelines state that PN should not be started until 7 days postoperatively in well-nourished patients. An earlier start can be considered in malnourished patients. Once initiated, the risk of infection can be decreased with intensive insulin therapy for blood glucose management and protocols for preventing central line bacteremia. In the cardiac population, care should be taken to minimize PN volume and ensure that triglycerides remain <400 mg/dL.[59,96] Finally, A.S.P.E.N./SCCM recommend the use of glutamine supplementation in critically ill cardiothoracic patients because of the potential for reduced hospital and ICU stay, infectious complications, and mortality.[90]

Once a cardiac patient is no longer requiring mechanical ventilation and GI function is confirmed, an oral diet can be advanced as tolerated. Intake is monitored with calorie counts, and nutrition support can be discontinued when the patient is able to meet at least 60% of energy and protein needs with oral intake.

PRACTICE POINT

Nutrition support is initiated at times when the CVD patient is otherwise unable to meet calorie, protein, fluid, and nutrient needs with oral intake. Nutrition support may be warranted in the case of malnutrition and cardiac cachexia, or intubation due to acute decompensated heart failure and/or cardiogenic shock.

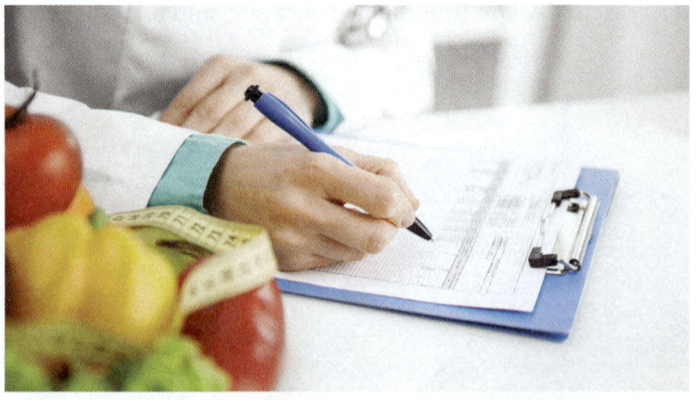
© Stasique/Shutterstock.

Chapter Summary

Cardiovascular disease (CVD) describes conditions that are caused by an interruption of the normal function of the heart and circulatory system. Types of CVD include atherosclerosis, coronary artery disease (CAD), myocardial infarction (MI), stroke, peripheral artery disease (PAD), hypertension (HTN), and heart failure (HF). CVD is currently the number one cause of death worldwide. Prevention and early management are critical to improving outcomes. Medical nutrition therapy (MNT) is an integral part of the prevention and management of CVD and related conditions.

Key Terms

atherosclerosis, myocardium, systole, diastole, stroke volume, cardiac output, ejection fraction, mean arterial pressure, total peripheral resistance, myocytes, Purkinje fibers, electrocardiogram, foam cells, vulnerable plaque, thrombosis, embolism, lipoproteins, apolipoproteins, dyslipidemia, familial hypercholesterolemia, xanthomas, hypertension, systolic blood pressure, diastolic blood pressure, stroke, peripheral artery disease, coronary artery disease, ischemic heart disease, angina, myocardial infarction, ischemic cardiomyopathy, percutaneous coronary intervention, coronary angioplasty, coronary artery bypass graft, cardiopulmonary bypass, dyspnea, acute decompensated heart failure, left ventricular assist device, subjective global assessment, obesity paradox, cardiac cachexia, tumor necrosis factor-alpha, cardiogenic shock, vasopressor, intra-aortic balloon pump

References

1. Kusumoto FM. Cardiovascular disorders: Heart disease. In: Hammer GD, McPhee SJ, eds. *Pathophysiology of Disease: An Introduction to Clinical Medicine*. 7th ed. New York, NY: McGraw-Hill; 2013.
2. Mozzafarian D, Benjamin EJ, Go AS, et al. on behalf of the American Heart Association Statistics Committee and Stroke Statistics Subcommittee. Heart disease and stroke statistics—2016 update: a report from the American Heart Association. *Circulation*. 2016;133:e38-e360.
3. Mozaffarian D, Benjamin EJ, Go AS, et al. Heart disease and stroke statistics—2015 update: a report from the American Heart Association. *Circulation*. 2015;131:e29-322.
4. Eckel RH, Jakicic JM, Ard JD, et al. 2013 AHA/ACC Guideline on Lifestyle Management to Reduce Cardiovascular Risk. A Report of the American College of Cardiology/American Heart Association Task Force on Practice Guidelines. *Circulation*. 2014;129:S76-S99.
5. Dietary fats and cardiovascular disease. A presidential advisory of the American Heart Association. *Circulation*. 2017;135. https://doi.org/10.1161/CIR.0000000000000510
6. Mohrman DE, Heller L. The peripheral vascular system. In: Mohrman DE, Heller L, eds. *Cardiovascular Physiology*. 8th ed. New York, NY: McGraw-Hill; 2014. http://accessmedicine.mhmedical.com.ezproxy.library.tufts.edu/content.aspx?bookid=843&Sectionid=48779654 Accessed October 4, 2017.
7. Gray, H. *Anatomy of the human body*. Philadelphia, PA: Lea & Febiger, 1918; Bartleby.com, 2000. www.bartleby.com/107/. Accessed October 4, 2017.
8. Stephanadis C, Antoniou CK, Tsiachris D, Pietri T. Coronary atherosclerotic vulnerable plaque: Current perspectives. *Journal of the American Heart Association*. 2017;6:e005543
9. American Heart Association. *2013 Prevention Guidelines Tools: CV Risk Calculator*. http://professional.heart.org/professional/GuidelinesStatements/PreventionGuidelines/UCM_457698_Prevention-Guidelines.jsp. Accessed October 4, 2017. .
10. Academy of Nutrition and Dietetics. Evidence Analysis Library. http://www.andeal.org/a_z_index.cfm. Accessed October 4, 2017.
11. Mann, DL. Braunwald's heart disease: A *textbook of cardiovascular medicine*. 10th ed. Philadelphia, PA: Elsevier Saunders, 2015.
12. Centers for Disease Control and Prevention. National Health Report: Leading Causes of Morbidity and Mortality and Associated Behavioral Risk and Protective Factors—United States, 2005–2013. *MMWR*. 2014;63(04);3-27.
13. Civeira F, Pocovi M, Alegria E, et al. Guidelines for the diagnosis and management of heterozygous familial hypercholesterolemia. *Atherosclerosis*. 2004;173(1):55-68.
14. Academy of Nutrition and Dietetics. Evidence Analysis Library. *Disorders of Lipid Metabolism: Major Recommendations (2011)*. http://www.andeal.org/topic.cfm?menu=5300&cat=4530. Accessed October 4, 2017.
15. Stone NJ, Merz CNB, Blum FCB, et al. 2013 ACC/AHA Guideline on the Treatment of Blood Cholesterol to Reduce Atherosclerotic Cardiovascular Risk in Adults. *J Am Coll Cardiol*. 2013. http://unmfm.pbworks.com/w/file/fetch/77279762/2013%20ACC_AHA%20Cholesterol%20Guidelines.pdf. Accessed October 4, 2017.
16. Pronsky ZM, Elbe D, Ayoob K. Food Medication Interactions. 18th ed. Birchrunville, PA: Food-Medication Interactions; 2015.
17. Mozaffarian D, Katan MB, Ascherio A, Stampfer MJ, Willett WC. Trans fatty acids and cardiovascular disease. *N Engl J Med*. 2006;354:1601–1613.
18. Eckel RH, Borra S, Lichtenstein AH, Yin-Piazza SY. Understanding the complexity of trans fatty acid reduction in the american diet, American Heart Association Trans Fat Conference 2006: Report of the Trans Fat Conference Planning Group. *Circulation*. 2007;115(16):2231-2246.
19. Van Horn L, McCoin M, Kris-Etherton PM, et al. The evidence for dietary prevention and treatment of cardiovascular disease. *J Am Diet Assoc*. 2008;108:287-331.
20. Davy BM, Davy KP, Ho RC, Beske SD, Davrath LR, Melby CL. High-fiber oat cereal compared with wheat cereal consumption favorably alters LDL-cholesterol subclass and particle numbers in middle-aged and older men. *Am J Clin Nutr*. 2002;76:351-358.
21. Dunn SP, Bleske B, Dorsch M, Macaulay T, Van Tassell B, Vardeny O. Nutrition and heart failure: impact of drug therapies and management strategies. *Nutr Clin Pract*. 2009;24:60-75.
22. Mozaffarian D, Gottdiener JS, Siscovick DS. Intake of tuna or other broiled or baked fish versus fried fish and cardiac structure, function, and hemodynamics. *Am J Cardiol*. 2006;97(2):216.
23. Bucher HC, Hengstler P, Schindler C, Meier G. n-3 polyunsaturated fatty acids in coronary heart disease: A meta-analysis of randomized controlled trials. *Am J Med*. 2002;112(4):298-304.
24. Mozaffarian D. Fish and n-3 fatty acids for the prevention of fatal coronary heart disease and sudden cardiac death. *Am J Clin Nutr*. 2008;87(6):1991S-6S.
25. Wang C, Harris WS, Chung M, et al. n-3 Fatty acids from fish or fish-oil supplements, but not alpha-linolenic acid, benefit cardiovascular disease outcomes in primary- and secondary-prevention studies: a systematic review. *Am J Clin Nutr*. 2006;84(1):5-17.

26. Burr ML, Ashfield-Watt PA, Dunstan FD, et al. Lack of benefit of dietary advice to men with angina: results of a controlled trial. *Eur J Clin Nutr.* 2003;57(2):193-200.
27. Raitt MH, Connor WE, Morris C, et al. Fish oil supplementation and risk of ventricular tachycardia and ventricular fibrillation in patients with implantable defibrillators: A randomized controlled trial. *JAMA.* 2005;293(23):2884-2891.
28. Jenkins DJ, Kendall CW, Vuksan V, et al. Soluble fiber intake at a dose approved by the US Food and Drug Administration for a claim of health benefits: Serum lipid risk factors for cardiovascular disease assessed in a randomized controlled crossover trial. *Am J Clin Nutr.* 2002;75:834-839.
29. Retelny VS, Neuendorf A, Roth J. Nutrition protocols for the prevention of cardiovascular disease. *Nutr Clin Pract.* 2008;23:468-476.
30. Johnson RK, Appel LJ, Brands M, et al. Dietary sugars intake and cardiovascular health a scientific statement from the American Heart Association. *Circulation.* 2009;120(11):1011-1020.
31. Sutters M. Systemic hypertension. In: Papadakis MA, McPhee SJ, Rabow MW, eds. *Current Medical Diagnosis & Treatment 2018.* New York, NY: McGraw-Hill; 2017. http://accessmedicine.mhmedical.com.ezproxy.library.tufts.edu/content.aspx?bookid=2192&sectionid=168192419. Accessed October 4, 2017.
32. Whelton PK, Carey RM, Aronow WS, Casey DE, Collins KJ, Dennison Himmelfarb C, et al, 2017 ACC/AHA/AAPA/ABC/ACPM/AGS/APhA/ASH/ASPC/NMA/PCNA Guideline for the Prevention, Detection, Evaluation, and Management of High Blood Pressure in Adults. Hypertension. 2017;HYP.0000000000000065, originally published November 13, 2017. https://doi.org/10.1161/HYP.0000000000000065. Accessed November 29, 2017.
33. He FJ, Burnier M, MacGregor GA. Nutrition in cardiovascular disease: salt in hypertension and heart failure. *Eur Heart J.* 2011;32(24):3073-3080.
34. Academy of Nutrition and Dietetics. Evidence Analysis Library. *Hypertension Major Recommendations.* http://www.andeal.org/topic.cfm?menu=5285&cat=3261. Accessed October 4, 2017.
35. James PA, Oparil S, Carter BL, et al. 2014 evidence-based guideline for the management of high blood pressure in adults: report from the panel members appointed to the Eighth Joint National Committee (JNC 8). *JAMA.* 2014;311(5):507-520.
36. Atkins G, Rahman M, Wright JT, Jr. Diagnosis and treatment of hypertension. In: Fuster V, Walsh RA, Harrington RA, eds. *Hurst's The Heart.* 13th ed. New York, NY: McGraw-Hill; 2011. http://accessmedicine.mhmedical.com.ezproxy.library.tufts.edu/content.aspx?bookid=376&Sectionid=40279802 AccessedOctober 4, 2017..
37. Charney P, Malone A. *ADA pocket guide to nutrition assessment.* Chicago, IL: American Dietetic Association; 2004.
38. Pujol TJ, Barnes JT, Sucher K. Diseases of the cardiovascular system. In: Nelms M, Sucher KP, Lacey K, Long Roth S, eds. *Nutrition therapy and pathophysiology.* 3rd ed. Boston, MA: Cengage Learning; 2016:292-341.
39. U.S. Department of Health and Human Services and National Institutes of Health, National Heart, Lung, and Blood Institute. *Your guide to lowering blood pressure.* http://www.nhlbi.nih.gov/files/docs/public/heart/hbp_low.pdf Accessed October4, 2017.
40. Sacks FM, Svetkey LP, Vollmer WM, et al. Effects on blood pressure of reduced dietary sodium and the Dietary Approaches to Stop Hypertension (DASH) diet. DASH-Sodium Collaborative Research Group. *N Engl J Med.* 2001;344:3-10.
41. Blumenthal JA, Babyak MA, Hinderliter A, et al. Effects of the DASH diet alone and in combination with exercise and weight loss on blood pressure and cardiovascular biomarkers in men and women with high blood pressure: the ENCORE study. *Arch Intern Med.* 2010;170(2):126-135.
42. Whelton PK, Appel LJ, Sacco RL, et al. Sodium, blood pressure, and cardiovascular disease further evidence supporting the American Heart Association sodium reduction recommendations. *Circulation.* 2012;126(24):2880-2889.
43. Graudal NA, Hubeck-Graudal T, Jurgens G. Effects of low-sodium diet vs. high-sodium diet on blood pressure, renin, aldosterone, catecholamines, cholesterol, and triglyceride (Cochrane Review). *Am J Hypertens.* 2012;25:1-15.
44. He FJ, MacGregor GA. Effect of modest salt reduction on blood pressure: a meta-analysis of randomized trials: implications for public health. *J Hum Hypertens.* 2002;16:761-770.
45. MacGregor GA, Markandu ND, Sagnella GA, Singer DR, Cappuccio FP. Double-blind study of three sodium intakes and long-term effects of sodium restriction in essential hypertension. *Lancet.* 1989;334:1244-1247.
46. Ferrara LA, de Simone G, Pasanisi F, Mancini M. Left ventricular mass reduction during salt depletion in arterial hypertension. *Hypertension.* 1984;6:755-759.
47. Liebson PR, Grandits GA, Dianzumba S, et al. Comparison of five antihypertensive monotherapies and placebo for change in left ventricular mass in patients receiving nutritional-hygienic therapy in the Treatment of Mild Hypertension Study (TOMHS). *Circulation.* 1995;91:698-706.
48. Jula AM, Karanko HM. Effects on left ventricular hypertrophy of long-term non-pharmacological treatment with sodium restriction in mild-to-moderate essential hypertension. *Circulation.* 1994;89:1023-1031.
49. Strazzullo P, D'Elia L, Kandala NB, Cappuccio FP. Salt intake, stroke, and cardio-vascular disease: Meta-analysis of prospective studies. *BMJ.* 2009;339:b4567.
50. Taylor RS, Ashton KE, Moxham T, Hooper L, Ebrahim S. Reduced dietary salt for the prevention of cardiovascular disease: a meta-analysis of randomized controlled trials (Cochrane Review). *Am J Hypertens.* 2011;24:843–853.
51. Cook NR, Cutler JA, Obarzanek E, et al. Long-term effects of dietary sodium reduction on cardiovascular disease outcomes: observational follow-up of the Trials of Hypertension Prevention (TOHP). *BMJ.* 2007;334:885-892.
52. Ekinci EI, Clarke S, Thomas MC, et al. Dietary salt intake and mortality in patients with type 2 diabetes. *Diabetes Care.* 2011;34:703–709.
53. Stolarz-Skrzypek K, Kuznetsova T, Thijs L, et al. European Project on Genes in Hypertension (EPOGH) Investigators. Fatal and nonfatal outcomes, incidence of hypertension, and blood pressure changes in relation to urinary sodium excretion. *JAMA.* 2011;305:1777-1785.
54. U.S. Department of Health and Human Services and U.S. Department of Agriculture. *2015 – 2020 Dietary Guidelines for Americans.* 8th Edition. Washington DC: U.S. Government Printing office, December 2015. http://health.gov/dietaryguidelines/2015/guidelines/
55. Cogswell ME, Zhang Z, Carriquirey, AL, et al. Sodium and potassium intakes among US adults: NHANES 2003-2008. *Am J Clin Nutr.* 2012;96:647–657.
56. Kenchaiah S, Evans JC, Levy D, et al. Obesity and the risk of heart failure. *N Eng J Med.* 2002;347:305-313.
57. Jensen MD, Ryan DH, Hu FB, et al. 2013 AHA/ACC/TOS Guideline for the Management of Overweight and Obesity in Adults. *J Am Coll Cardiol.* 2013. https://doi.org/10.1161/01.cir.0000437739.71477.ee
58. American Heart Association. *Answers by heart. Cardiovascular conditions. What is peripheral vascular disease?* http://www.heart.org/idc/groups/heart-public/@wcm/@hcm/documents/downloadable/ucm_300323.pdf Accessed October 4, 2017.

59. Cresci G, Hummell AC, Raheem SA, et al. Nutrition intervention in the critically ill cardiothoracic patient. *Nutr Clin Pract*. 2012;27(3):323-334.
60. Engelman D, Adams DH, Burne JG, et al. Impact of body mass index and albumin on morbidity and mortality after cardiac surgery. *J Thorac Cardiovasc Surg*. 1999;118:866-873.
61. Chobanian AV, Bakris GL, Black HR, et al. Seventh report of the Joint National Committee on Prevention, Detection, Evaluation, and Treatment of High Blood Pressure. *Hypertension*. 2003;42:1206-1252.
62. Yancy CW, Jessup M, Bozkurt B, et al. 2013 ACCF/AHA Guideline for the Management of Heart Failure: A Report of the American College of Cardiology Foundation/American Heart Association Task Force on Practice Guidelines. *J Am Coll Cardiol*. 2013;62(16):e147-e239.
63. Fuster V, Walsh RA, Harrington RA, eds. *Hurst's The Heart*. 13th ed. New York, NY: McGraw-Hill; 2011.
64. Yancy CW, Jessup M, Bozkurt B, et al. 2013 ACCF/AHA Guideline for the Management of Heart Failure: A Report of the American College of Cardiology Foundation/American Heart Association Task Force on Practice Guidelines. *J Am Coll Cardiol*. 2013;62(16):e147-e239.
65. National Heart, Lung, and Blood Institute. *How Is Heart Failure Treated?* http://www.nhlbi.nih.gov/health/health-topics/topics/hf/treatment.html. Updated June 22, 2015. Accessed October 4, 2017.
66. Academy of Nutrition and Dietetics. Evidence Analysis Library. *Heart Failure Major Recommendations*. http://www.andeal.org/topic.cfm?menu=5289. Accessed August 15, 2014.
67. Detsky AS, McLaughlin JR, Baker JP, et al. What is subjective global assessment of nutritional status? *JPEN J Parenter Enteral Nutr*. 1987;11:8–13.
68. Aggarwal A, Kumar A, Gregory MP, et al. Nutrition assessment in advanced heart failure patients evaluated for ventricular assist devices or cardiac transplantation. *Nutr Clin Pract*. 2013;28(1):112-119.
69. Nestle Nutrition Institute. *Mini Nutrition Assessment*. http://www.mna-elderly.com. Accessed October 4, 2017.
70. Lennie TA. Nutrition self-care in heart failure, state of the science. *J Cardiovasc Nurs*. 2008;23(3):197-204.
71. Oreopoulos A, Padwal R, Kalantar-Zadeh K, Fonarow GC, Norris CM, McAlister FA. Body mass index and mortality in heart failure: a meta-analysis. *Am Heart J*. 2008;156(1):13-22.
72. Katz AM, Katz, PB. Disease of the heart in the works of Hippocrates. *Brit Heart J*. 1962;24(3):257-264.
73. Gottschlich, MM. *The A.S.P.E.N. Nutrition support core curriculum: A case-based approach—The adult patient*. Silver Spring, MD: American Society of Parenteral and Enteral Nutrition; 2007.
74. Carlson H, Dahlin CM. Managing the Effects of Cardiac Cachexia. *J Hosp Palliat Nurs*. 2014;16(1):15-20.
75. Bonilla-Palomas JL, Gámez-López AL, Anguita-Sánchez MP, et al. Impact of malnutrition on long-term mortality in hospitalized patients with heart failure. *Revista Española de Cardiología (English Edition)*. 2011;64(9):752-758.
76. Anker SD, Coats A J. Cardiac cachexia syndrome with impaired survival and immune and neuroendocrine activation. *CHEST*. 1999;115(3):836-847.
77. Sandek A, Doehner W, Anker SD, von Haehling S. Nutrition in heart failure: an update. *Curr Opin Clin Nutr Metab Care*. 2009;12:384-391.
78. Anker SD, Chua TP, Ponikowski P, et al. Hormonal changes and catabolic/anabolic imbalance in chronic heart failure and their importance for cardiac cachexia. *Circulation*. 1997;96(2):526-534.
79. Lemon SC, Olendzki B, Magner R, et al. The dietary quality of persons with heart failure in NHANES 1999-2006. *J Gen Intern Med*. 2009;25(2):135-140.
80. Kollipara UK, Jaffer O, Amin A, et al. Relation of lack of knowledge about dietary sodium to hospital readmission in patients with heart failure. *Am J Cardiol*. 2008;102:1212-1215.
81. Ramirez EC, Martinez LC, Tejeda AO, Gonzalez VR, David RN, Lafuente EA. Effects of a nutritional intervention on body composition, clinical status, and quality of life in patients with heart failure. *Nutrition*. 2004;20:890-895.
82. Kuehneman T, Saulsbury D, Splett P, Chapman DB. Demonstrating the impact of nutrition intervention in a heart failure program. *J Am Diet Assoc*. 2002;102(12):1790-1794.
83. Azizi-Namini P, Ahmed M, Yan AT, Keith M. The role of B vitamins in the management of heart failure. *Nutr Clin Pract*. 2012;27(3):363-374.
84. Wooley JA. Characteristics of thiamin and its relevance to the management of heart failure. *Nutr Clin Pract*. 2008;(23):487-493.
85. U.S. Department of Health and Human Services and National Institutes of Health, Office of Dietary Supplements. *Dietary Supplement Fact Sheet: Vitamin D*. http://ods.od.nih.gov/factsheets/VitaminD-QuickFacts/. Updated April 15, 2016. Accessed October 4, 2017.
86. Fiscella K, Franks P. Vitamin D, Race, and Cardiovascular Mortality: Findings From a National US Sample. *Ann Fam Med*. 2010;8:11-18.
87. Escott-Stump S. *Nutrition diagnosis-related care*. Philadelphia, PA: Lippincott Williams & Wilkins; 2008.
88. Jialal I, Devaraj S. Vitamin E supplementation and cardiovascular events in high-risk patients. *N Engl J Med*. 2000;342:154-60.
89. Hochman JS, Ingbar DH. Cardiogenic shock and pulmonary edema. In: Kasper DL, Fauci AS, Hauser SL, Longo DL, Jameson J, Loscalzo J. eds. *Harrison's Principles of Internal Medicine*. 18th ed. New York, NY; McGraw-Hill; 2014:2232-2237
90. McClave S, Martindale RG, Vanek VW, et al. Guidelines for the provision and assessment of nutrition support therapy in the adult critically ill patient: Society of Critical Care Medicine (SCCM) and American Society for Parenteral and Enteral Nutrition (A.S.P.E.N). *JPEN Parenter Enteral Nutr*. 2009;33:277-316.
91. Academy of Nutrition and Dietetics. Evidence Analysis Library. *Critical Illness: Major Recommendations (2012)*. http://www.andeal.org/topic.cfm?menu=5302&cat=4801. Accessed October 4, 2017.
92. Visser M, Davids M, Verberne HJ, et al. Rationale and design of a proof-of-concept trial investigating the effect of uninterrupted perioperative parenteral nutrition on amino acid profile, cardiomyocytes structure, and cardiac perfusion and metabolism of patients undergoing coronary artery bypass grafting. *J Cardiothorac Surg*. 2011;6:36-43.
93. Tepaske R, Velthius H, Oudemans-van Straaten HM, et al. Effect of preoperative oral immune enhancing nutritional supplement on patients at high risk of infection after cardiac surgery: a randomized placebo controlled trial. *Lancet*. 2001;358:696-701.
94. Revelly J, Tappy L, Berger MM, Gersbach P, Cayeux C, Chioléro R. Early metabolic and splanchic responses to enteral nutrition in postoperative cardiac surgery patients with circulatory compromise. *Intens Care Med*. 2001;27(3):540-547.
95. Berger M, Revelly JP, Cayeux MC, Chiolero R. Enteral nutrition in critically ill patients with severe hemodynamic failure after cardiopulmonary bypass. *Clin Nutr*. 2005;24(1):124-132.
96. Widlicka A. Enteral nutrition in the cardiothoracic intensive care unit: challenges and considerations. *Nutr Clin Pract*. 2008;23:510-520.
97. Mechanick J, Scurlock C. Glycemic control and nutritional strategies in the cardiothoracic surgical intensive care unit—2010: state of the art. *Semin Thorac Surg*. 2010;22(3):230-235.

Chapter 11

Nutrition in Oral Health

Haley Hooks
Carole Palmer

Chapter Outline
Core Concepts
Introduction
Background
Nutrition and Oral Health Interrelationships
Nutrition and Development of the Oral Cavity
Effects of Diet and Dietary Habits on Common Oral Diseases
Oral Health During the Life Cycle

CORE CONCEPTS

1. While nutrition and diet affect the health of the oral cavity, the status of the oral cavity may also affect one's ability to consume an adequate diet and achieve nutritional balance.
2. Dental caries is a chronic, multifactorial disease that results from an interplay of factors including a susceptible tooth, dental plaque, diet, and saliva.
3. The cariogenicity of a food depends on its composition, carbohydrate content, frequency and duration of exposure to teeth, and form and consistency.
4. Demineralization, or tooth decay, begins when cariogenic bacteria metabolize fermentable carbohydrates and produce organic acids that lower the salivary pH to below 5.5.
5. Fluoride prevents and controls dental caries through inhibiting demineralization, enhancing remineralization, and inhibiting caries-promoting bacteria.
6. Periodontal disease is a chronic, inflammatory disease that is systemic in nature and results from an interaction of microbial, genetic, and lifestyle factors.
7. Edentulism and the use of dentures can have a significant effect on masticatory function and ultimately dietary habits and nutritional adequacy.
8. Oral infections are strongly associated with immunosuppression and may result in poor nutritional status.
9. Early childhood caries, the most common oral health condition of American children, is associated with microbial, environmental, and dietary factors including frequent, long-term use of baby bottles containing fermentable carbohydrates.
10. The nutritional status of older adults is often negatively affected by compromised dentition due to periodontal disease, xerostomia, edentualism, and wearing dentures.

Learning Objectives

1. Outline how general nutrition status can affect and be affected by the health of oral tissues and structures.
2. Assess the nutritional status and nutritional risk of patients using the oral cavity and structures.
3. Describe the pathophysiology of the different oral diseases.
4. Explain the role of nutrition in the development and prevention of oral diseases.
5. Develop a nutrition therapy plan for the prevention and treatment of oral diseases.
6. Identify the oral diseases most common during pregnancy, infancy, childhood, adulthood, and older adulthood.

Introduction

The interrelationship between nutrition and dietary patterns is relevant to common oral conditions, including dental caries, periodontal disease, edentulism, and oral infections. An understanding of pathophysiology and nutritional implications of oral health during pregnancy, infancy, childhood, adolescence, adulthood, and older adulthood is important to appreciate its impact on health. Knowledge of various oral diseases and chronic health conditions is helpful to establish goals for nutritional counseling and an important consideration of social, environmental, and lifestyle factors.

Background

The relationship between diet and oral health and disease has been recognized for centuries. Over 2,000 years ago, Aristotle noted that figs caused teeth to rot. In 1746, Pierre Fauchard, the "father of dentistry," recognized that sugars caused tooth decay.[1] It is now well understood that nutrition, dietary patterns, and food choices play a notable role in oral health and disease. Diet and nutrition affect and are affected by the health of the oral cavity. Good nutrition is the foundation for general oral health. Because the oral cavity is the pathway to the rest of the body, problems in the mouth can significantly impact diet and nutritional status. The Surgeon General of the United States' critical report, *Oral Health in America*, stresses the crucial, but often overlooked, fact that one cannot be healthy without a healthy mouth.[2]

The relationship between oral health and nutrition requires the attention of all health professionals, including those working in nutrition. Nutrition professionals are in the ideal position to recognize the potential oral health concerns that accompany systemic disease and dietary patterns. Nutrition-focused physical examinations including the oral cavity may reveal problems that require the attention of dental professionals. Conversely, when nutrition counseling and dietary intervention are warranted, dental professionals may refer individuals with oral health conditions impacting eating ability or nutritional status to nutrition professionals for nutrition therapy.[3]

Nutrition and Oral Health Interrelationships

Nutrition and oral health have a synergistic relationship. Adequate nutrition is essential for the development of all tissues and structures in the body, including those in the oral cavity. Nutritional insults that occur during the critical periods of growth and development may have lifelong consequences.[4] Systemic diseases with oral manifestations, as well as oral infections, impact functional ability to eat and may result in poor diet and undermine nutritional status. In turn, poor nutritional status can increase susceptibility to oral diseases, such as periodontal disease.

Nutrition and Development of the Oral Cavity

The primary teeth begin developing around 6 weeks' gestation, while mineralization of the protein matrix begins around 3 to 4 months' gestation. Although the timing of tooth development varies from child to child, primary teeth typically begin erupting around 6 months of age, with the majority of primary teeth erupting by 2 to 3 years of age. Most permanent teeth typically erupt completely by age 16 years. The **enamel**, the hard mineralized surface of teeth, and **dentin**, the bony tissue forming the bulk of tooth beneath the enamel, are composed of **hydroxyapatite**, a crystalline structure that is a naturally occurring form of calcium and phosphorus. When fluoride is available prenatally, **fluoroapatite** is formed, which is a more-resistant crystalline structure than hydroxyapatite. Once the tooth erupts into the oral cavity, mineralization of outer layers of tooth enamel continues topically throughout life from minerals in saliva and diet. The consistent availability of fluoride from fluoridated water, fluoride oral rinses, and other sources has proven to be more important to enamel resistance over time than that provided pre-eruptively.[5]

Optimal nutrition is particularly important during the early phases of growth and development of the oral cavity. Nutritional status has a notable effect on teeth pre-eruptively.[5] Vitamin D is essential to the process by which calcium and phosphorus are incorporated into hydroxyapatite crystals. Deficiencies in vitamins D and A and protein-energy malnutrition are associated with hypomineralization and **enamel hypoplasia**, which is enamel deficiency that increases tooth vulnerability to damage. Protein-energy malnutrition and vitamin A deficiency are also associated with salivary gland atrophy. Both salivary gland atrophy and enamel hypoplasia result in increased susceptibility to dental caries.[5] Malnutrition can result in delayed and abnormal development of teeth and surrounding structures and result in increased caries risk for developing dentition.[4] Once teeth erupt into the mouth, systemic effects of nutritional aberrations have

CASE STUDY INTRODUCTION

Elsie is an 85-year-old woman who was diagnosed with osteoporosis 15 years ago. In addition to her osteoporosis, she has arthritis and tooth loss secondary to periodontal disease. She also has a history of type 2 diabetes mellitus, hyperlipidemia, and hypertension, which are controlled with medications. Elsie has a complete upper denture and partial lower dentures that were made at her last dental appointment 5 years ago. Elsie is widowed and lives alone. She has two children who visit once every few weeks and help out with grocery shopping and meal preparation. The following clinical information was collected when she visited her primary care provider.

Anthropometric Data:
Height: 163 cm (64")
Weight: 47.7 kg (105 lbs)
BMI: 18.1 kg/m^2
Weight History
Elsie reports a stable weight over the past 3 years.

Biochemical Data:
Hemoglobin A1C 6.8% (4.3-5.8%)
Albumin 3.5 (3.5-5.0 g/dL)
Prealbumin 16 (17-36 g/dL)
Calcium 9 (8.5-10.5 mEq/L)
25-hydroxy vitamin D 20 ng/dL (20-100 ng/dL)
Low-density lipoprotein (LDL-C) 125 (Desirable <100 mg/dL)
High-density lipoprotein (HDL-C) 45 mg/dL (Desirable ≥40 mg/dL)

Clinical Data:
Past Medical History: Type 2 diabetes mellitus, hyperlipidemia, hypertension, osteoarthritis
Medications: Simvastatin, metoprolol, metformin, glipizide, Fosamax, aspirin, calcium carbonate 600 mg with breakfast and lunch, vitamin D$_3$ 800 IU daily
Vital Signs: Blood pressure: 135/90 mm Hg, Temperature 98.4°F, heart rate 77 beats/min
Nutrition-focused Physical Exam: Appears frail with diminished fat stores and temporal muscle wasting. Skin feels cold to touch. Elsie has a complete upper denture and partial lower denture. Normal tongue noted. Gums appear red and swollen.

Dietary Data:
Dietary History: Elsie has been instructed to follow a carbohydrate-controlled, low–saturated fat, low-sodium diet. Compliance is questionable due to reliance on convenience foods for most meals.

Questions
1. How would you describe Elsie's nutritional status?
2. What are Elsie's nutritional risk factors?
3. What additional information might you need?

---

little effect on teeth other than topically. The oral bone and soft tissue undergo remodeling throughout life, making poor nutrition a risk factor for oral infections and impaired tissue growth, regeneration, and healing.

Effect of Oral Health on Diet and Nutrition

The oral cavity is often referred to as the "gatekeeper for nutrition" because poor oral health can have a significant impact on food choices, nutritional status, and overall health (**Figure 11.1**).[5] Mouth pain from dental caries, poorly fitting dentures, gum disease, or oral infection can result in decreased appetite and can lead to food avoidances due to a lack of desire and/or ability to eat. In children, pain and discomfort from dental caries can result in reduced intake and poor food choices, which may lead to failure to thrive.[1]

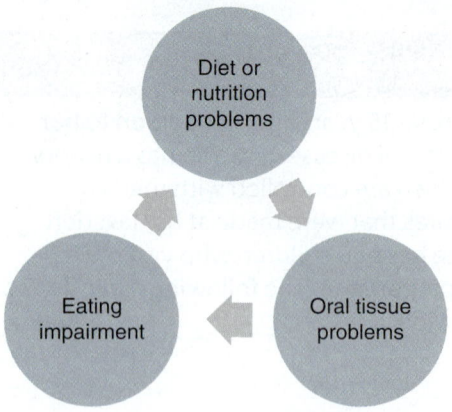

FIGURE 11.1 Interrelationship Between Nutrition and Oral Health

In the face of decreased mastication, instead of eating fresh fruits, vegetables, and whole grains, food choices tend toward foods that are easier to chew, but are often low in nutritional quality, such as cakes and processed foods. These food choices are often high in calories, fat, carbohydrates, or sodium, which are associated with an increased risk for chronic diseases and some cancers.[1]

CORE CONCEPT 1

While nutrition and diet affect the health of the oral cavity, the status of the oral cavity may also affect one's ability to consume an adequate diet and achieve nutritional balance.

Effect of Systemic Nutrition Deficiency or Excess on the Oral Cavity

The oral cavity is often referred to as a "mirror of overall health" because the earliest clinical manifestations of nutritional or other health disorders are often first visible in the oral cavity (**Table 11.1**). The oral mucosal cells have a more rapid turnover (3 to 7 days) than other tissues in the body.[6] Because of this rapid tissue turnover, immediate tissue needs for nutrients are often greater in the oral cavity and signs of deficiencies and toxicities often appear first in the oral cavity before becoming clinically evident elsewhere in the body.[1,6]

Deficiencies in water-soluble vitamins, protein, and iron are more readily visible in the oral cavity, compared to other nutrients.[3] For instance, one of the first clinical signs

TABLE 11.1 IDENTIFICATION OF NUTRIENT DEFICIENCIES IN THE FACE AND ORAL CAVITY

Body Part	Symptom	Nutrient Implication
Face	Dark skin over cheeks and under eyes	Inadequate niacin, riboflavin, and/or vitamin B_6
	Temporal wasting	Inadequate calories and/or protein
	Pallor	Inadequate iron
	Dry, flaky, scaly skin (seborrheic dermatitis)	Riboflavin, niacin, vitamin B_6, and/or essential fatty acid deficiency
Lips	Cheilosis	Inadequate niacin and/or riboflavin
	Angular fissures	Inadequate niacin, vitamin B_6, riboflavin, and/or iron
Tongue	Glossitis	Folate, niacin, riboflavin, iron, vitamin B_6, and/or vitamin B_{12}, and/or may be associated with protein-calorie malnutrition
	Pale, atrophic, smooth/slick	Inadequate iron, vitamin B_{12}, niacin, and/or folate
	Magenta or purple color	Advanced riboflavin deficiency
	Macroglossia	Inadequate niacin
	Glossodynia (burning mouth syndrome)	Folate, iron, vitamins B_6 and B_{12}, and/or zinc deficiency
Gums	Spongy, bleeding, abnormal redness	Vitamin C deficiency

Modified from Touger-Decker, R., & Mobley, C. (2013). Position of the Academy of Nutrition and Dietetics: oral health and nutrition. *J Acad Nutr Diet*, 113(5), 693-701. doi:10.1016/j.jand.2013.03.001.

of vitamin C deficiency is gingival bleeding and redness. Vitamin B-complex deficiencies are associated with cracks in the corner of the mouth.[1] Nutrient toxicities, while rare, also have oral implications. Excess vitamin A intake may impair oral-tissue healing and cause **xerostomia**, or reduced or absent saliva flow, and impair tooth formation. Although rarely seen in humans, vitamin D toxicity can cause pre-eruptive enamel hypoplasia and defective calcification of the tooth pulp in children.[1]

Systemic nutrition also plays an important role in dental diseases, including periodontal disease and oral infections. Periodontal disease results from a bacterial infection of the gum tissue surrounding the teeth. Gums become red, swollen, puffy, and readily bleed and the alveolar bone may recede, which increases the risk for tooth loss. While nutritional deficiency does not cause periodontal disease, nutrition can play a pivotal role in its prevention, initiation, progression, severity, and response to treatment. Malnutrition may reduce host resistance and increase the susceptibility to periodontal infection. Deficiencies in calcium, vitamin D, and phosphorus are all associated with alveolar bone loss and may increase the risk of tooth loss. On the other hand, optimal nutrition status enhances immune function, increases tissue resistance to periodontal pathogens, and promotes periodontal healing.[1]

Effects of Diet and Dietary Habits on Common Oral Diseases

Dental Caries

Dental caries (**Figure 11.2**), also known as cavities, is one of the most common infectious diseases. Despite the widespread decline in caries prevalence and severity in developed nations, disparities remain and many children and adults still develop caries. In the United States, caries is the most common chronic disease of childhood; it is five times more common than asthma.[7] Dental caries is also increasing in frequency among the elderly, as more people are retaining more teeth throughout their lifespan. The burden of dental caries lasts a lifetime; once a tooth is affected, it requires restoration and maintenance throughout life.[7]

Pathophysiology

Dental caries is a slowly progressing, multifactorial chronic disease that results from the interaction between the host (susceptible tooth), agent (dental plaque), and environmental factors (diet and saliva).[1] Wherever dental **plaque**, or colonized bacteria on tooth surfaces, adheres to tooth enamel surfaces, enamel demineralization and its sequelae, dental caries, can occur.

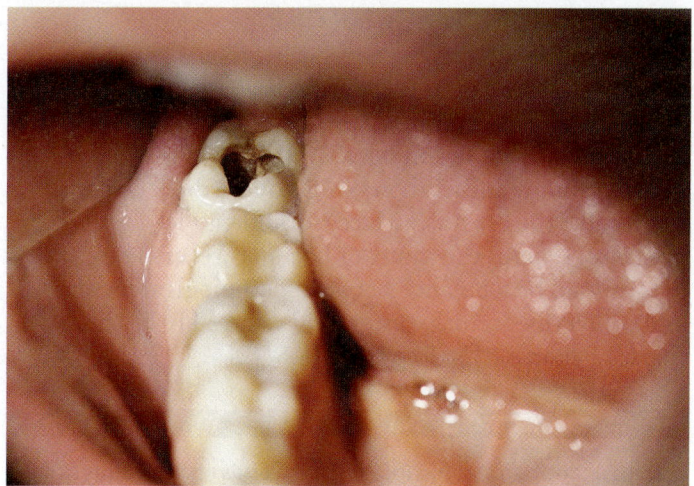

FIGURE 11.2 Dental Caries
©Kyrylo Glivin/Shutterstock.

The decay process begins when cariogenic bacteria in dental plaque metabolize fermentable carbohydrates, primarily mono- and disaccharides, and produce organic acids on tooth enamel surfaces. When the pH at the enamel surface is lowered to below 5.5, these organic acids begin the **demineralization** of tooth enamel surfaces, which is the chemical process by which minerals are removed from the teeth. When the demineralization has progressed to the point that the enamel has been totally penetrated, exposing a much more susceptible layer of dentin, the bacteria themselves can penetrate into the protein of the dental layer, destroying it through proteolysis as the acid continues to destroy the enamel rods that are in the dentin. If untreated, this bacterial infection can penetrate into the bloodstream via the pulp of the tooth, destroy the dentin, and allow infection to progress throughout the body. Thus, the caries process is a two-step process. The first step is demineralization of the enamel outer layer of the tooth. If this demineralization is halted before it reaches the dentin beneath it, remineralization by fluoride and other remineralizing minerals can help reverse the process. The second step, when the bacteria invade the dentin layer of the tooth, is not reversible. If the disease progresses into the dentin, it must be restored by dental treatment.[7,8] Demineralization without the second step can occur when acids are present in contact with tooth enamel over time for any reason, such as excessive sipping of acidic beverages, frequent consumption of acidic foods, acid regurgitation from gastrointestinal reflux disorders or eating disorders, or loss of salivary protection via use of anti-sialogogic medications, or medications that inhibit saliva flow.

Remineralization is the body's natural repair process for noncavitated carious lesions, which is a demineralized lesion without evidence of cavitation. Calcium and phosphorus, primarily from saliva, diffuse back into demineralized lesions in teeth and help rebuild the enamel crystals. When topical fluoride, calcium, and phosphate are available, the rebuilt crystals are more resistant to acid demineralization than from the calcium and phosphate remineralization alone. The crystal surface is much less soluble than the initial carbonated hydroxyapatite mineral, making it more difficult for acid to dissolve the crystal surface.[8] Whether a lesion will progress, remain the same, or becomes reversed is determined by a balance between pathological factors and protective factors, commonly referred to as the "caries balance."[7,8]

> **CORE CONCEPT 2**
>
> Dental caries is a chronic, multifactorial disease that results from an interplay of factors including a susceptible tooth, dental plaque, diet, and saliva.

Etiologic Factors

Four factors must be simultaneously present for caries to occur: (1) a susceptible host or tooth surface; (2) cariogenic bacteria including *Streptococcus* or *Lactobacillus* in the dental plaque or oral cavity; (3) a substrate for the bacteria (fermentable carbohydrates); and (4) time in the mouth for bacteria to metabolize the fermentable carbohydrates, produce acids, and cause a drop in salivary pH to below 5.5, also called the "critical pH." Once the pH is acidic, oral bacteria can initiate the demineralization process that leads to dental caries (**Figure 11.3**).

Susceptible Tooth The development of dental caries requires a tooth susceptible to attack. Vulnerability depends on the composition of the tooth and enamel, the location of the tooth, quantity and quality of saliva, and the presence and extent of pits and fissures in the tooth crown. While acidic saliva increases susceptibility to decay, alkaline saliva may have a protective effect.

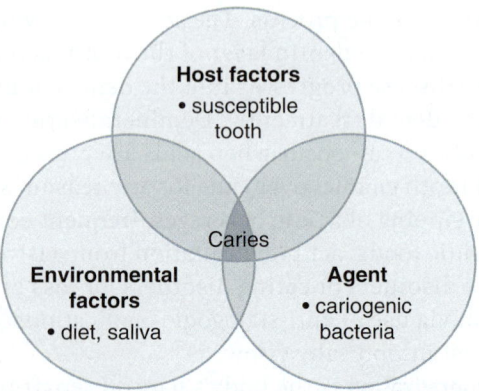

FIGURE 11.3 An Etiological Model of Dental Caries: Caries Occurs Through the Interaction of Host Factors (Tooth, Saliva Flow, and Composition), Dietary Factors, and Bacterial Factors

Microorganisms Certain microorganisms, namely, *Streptococcus mutans* and, to a lesser extent, *Streptococcus sanguis* and *Lactobacillus*, are essential to the dental decay process. These bacteria metabolize fermentable carbohydrates and produce weak acids as a byproduct, which causes local pH to fall below 5.5. The acidic pH then causes the tooth to demineralize, which may eventually lead to caries development as described above.[7]

Substrate–Dietary Factors Cariogenic bacteria can metabolize any fermentable carbohydrate, including all monosaccharides and disaccharides. **Cariogenicity** refers to the caries-promoting properties of a diet or food. The cariogenicity of a diet varies depending on the composition of the food consumed, the amount of carbohydrates consumed, the frequency and duration of the carbohydrate's exposure on teeth, and the form and consistency of the food consumed.[5]

Food Composition: Cariogenic Foods Cariogenic foods are those that contain fermentable carbohydrates, which, when in contact with microorganisms in the mouth, can cause a drop in salivary pH to 5.5 or less and stimulate the caries process (See **Table 11.2**). While starchy foods, including rice, pasta, potatoes, and bread, are generally of low cariogenicity, their caries-promoting potential increases if they are finely ground, heat-treated, or high in sucrose.[5] Examples of grains and starches that are cariogenic by nature of their fermentable carbohydrate composition include pretzels, crackers, chips, cereals, and breads.

Fruit drinks, sodas, sweetened teas, and other sugar-sweetened beverages are also cariogenic. While lactose has low cariogenicity, dairy products sweetened with fructose, sucrose, or other added sugars are cariogenic. The causal relationship between dental caries and sucrose consumption is also well established.[5] All dietary forms of sugar, including honey, molasses, agave nectar, brown sugar, and corn syrup, are cariogenic and can be used by oral bacteria to produce acid. Cariogenic bacteria can metabolize all simple carbohydrates, including glucose, fructose, galactose, maltose, lactose, and sucrose.[5] Starches may also be cariogenic if retained in the mouth long enough to be hydrolyzed into simple sugars by salivary amylase.[1] Uncooked starch and cooked stable starchy foods, such as rice, potatoes, whole grains, and unrefined plant foods, are generally considered to be of lower cariogenicity when consumed at mealtimes or snacks.[5] While fruits are often acidogenic, when consumed as part of a mixed diet, fruit is not considered a major factor in development of dental caries.[5] Fruits with higher water content, such as watermelon, have lower cariogenicity than others such as bananas and dried fruits. Noncarbohydrate components of food can also modulate the cariogenic potential of foods. Dietary fiber can stimulate saliva production. Water also helps to decrease the amount of time

TABLE 11.2 DIETARY PATTERNS THAT AFFECT CARIES RISK

Increase Caries Risk	Decrease Caries Risk
Frequent or prolonged between-meal snacking	Limiting between-meal snaking to 2 to 3 times per day
Frequent or prolonged between-meal sipping on sweetened beverages	Drinking, rather than sipping, sweetened and acidic beverages. Limit sugared or sugar-free carbonated beverages to meal times only
Frequent between-meal use of cariogenic foods like desserts	Having sweets with meals rather than between meals
Chewing sugar-sweetened gum	Chewing sugar-free gum (particularly those with sugar alcohols like xylitol)
Using slowly dissolving hard candies like breath mints and cough drops	Consuming fruits, vegetables, dairy products, and nuts as between-meal snacks
Eating sticky foods like dried fruits or fruit roll-ups	Using water frequently to clean mouth of food debris

Modified from Palmer, C. A., Burnett, D. J., & Dean, B. (2010). Its More Than Just Candy. *Nutrition Today*, 45(4), 154-164. doi:10.1097/nt.0b013e3181ec963b.

foods remain in the mouth, thereby counterbalancing the cariogenic potential of foods.[1]

Food Amount Epidemiologic evidence demonstrates that there is a strong association between the amount of sugar consumed and the risk for dental caries on a population level.[5] Many of these studies were conducted at times when sugar availability was increased or decreased. Populations with higher sugar intakes have a higher rate of dental caries as compared to similar populations with lower sugar intakes.[5] Conversely, when population consumption of sugars is less than 10 kg/person/year, the level of dental caries is low, such as during wartime rationing.[9] However, this type of research applies to overall populations, not individuals. Because dental caries is a direct contact disease of the oral cavity, population-based information is of limited value for individuals.

> **PRACTICE POINT**
>
> The most critical dietary factor for the development of dental caries is the amount of time that any fermentable carbohydrate is in contact with dental plaque, rather than the total amount of sugar consumed.[1]

Frequency and Duration of Exposure The primary evidence for the association between frequency of sugar consumption and risk for dental caries comes from the Vipeholm study, which was conducted after World War II between 1945 and 1953.[10] The study found that sugars, even when consumed in large amounts, had little effect on caries development if consumed up to a maximum of four times per day and at meal times only. Increased consumption of sugar between meals was also associated with a significant increase in dental caries.[10]

Another study conducted in 5-year-old Icelandic children found that when sugars were consumed more than four times per day, the presence of caries increased markedly.[11] A higher frequency of fermentable carbohydrate consumption, especially if it involves nibbling or sipping of foods and beverages, is caries promoting. Eating fermentable carbohydrates at bedtime is also discouraged because saliva production diminishes during sleep.

Foods that tend to be retained in the mouth for longer periods of time, such as hard candy or dried fruit, increase the exposure time of teeth to bacterial acids. Conversely, foods that are quickly eliminated from the mouth are potentially less damaging than those that are retained for longer. For example, a sugary drink consumed rapidly is less cariogenic than if it is sipped over a long period of time. Overall, caries risk increases as the number or length of eating or drinking occasions increases.[1]

Form and Consistency The cariogenicity of a food is also related to its physical form and consistency. Food form determines the retention time, or adhesion, of a food in the mouth. Solid foods such as cookies, chips, crackers, and pretzels can stick between teeth in interproximal spaces and have high adherence capacity. Liquids generally have lower adherence because they are rapidly cleared from the mouth. Consistency also affects adherence. Chewy foods such as gumdrops and marshmallows, although high in sugar, stimulate saliva production and have lower adherence than solid, sticky foods such as chips, bagels, or bananas.

Clinical Roundtable

Topic: Sugar Intake in Caries Development

Background: The classic Vipeholm study provides the primary evidence for the effects of high sugar consumption on dental caries. The study was conducted shortly after the Second World War in an adult mental institution in Sweden between 1945 and 1953. Working with 633 individuals, it investigated the effects of consuming sugary foods of varying stickiness (oral retention times) and at different times throughout the day on the development of dental caries.

The study measured caries increment in subjects that consumed:

1) Refined sugars with a slight tendency to be retained in the mouth, at meal times only
2) Refined sugars with a strong tendency to be retained in the mouth, at meal times only
3) Refined sugars with a strong tendency to be retained in the mouth, between meals

The study found that sugars, even when consumed in large amounts, had little effect on caries development if consumed up to a maximum of four times per day and at meal times only. Increased consumption of sugar between meals was associated with a significant increase in dental caries.

Roundtable Discussion

1. Discuss the relationship between frequency of sugar consumed versus quantity of sugar consumed.
2. How does timing of sugar consumption impact dental caries risk?
3. How might this study raise questions about research ethics?

Reference

1. Gustafsson BE, Quensel C, Lanke LS, et al. The effect of different levels of carbohydrate intake on caries activity in 436 individuals observed for five years. *Acta Odontologica Scandinavica.* 1953;11(3-4):232-364. doi:10.3109/00016355308993925

CORE CONCEPT 3

The cariogenicity of a food depends on its composition, carbohydrate content, form, consistency, and frequency and duration of exposure to teeth.

Cariostatic Foods Cariostatic foods do not contribute to decay, are not metabolized by microorganisms, and do not cause a drop in salivary pH to 5.5 or less within 30 minutes. Protein foods such as eggs, seafood, meats, poultry, and nuts, along with fats and oils such as margarine, butter, and seeds, are cariostatic. Foods that stimulate salivary flow, including whole grain foods, peanuts, hard cheeses, and chewing gum, also protect against decay.[5,12] Common nonnutritive sweeteners, including acesulfame potassium, aspartame, and sucralose, are not metabolized by oral bacteria, so they are not cariogenic.[13]

CORE CONCEPT 4

Demineralization, or tooth decay, begins when cariogenic bacteria metabolize fermentable carbohydrates and produce organic acids that lower the salivary pH to below 5.5.

Anticariogenic foods are cariostatic foods that prevent plaque from recognizing cariogenic foods. Cow's milk and aged cheese are anticariogenic due to their calcium, phosphorus, and casein content.[5] Xylitol, a five-carbon sugar alcohol, is also anticariogenic because bacteria cannot metabolize five-carbon sugars in the same manner as six-carbon sugars like glucose, sucrose, and fructose. Because xylitol is not recognized by salivary amylase, it does not cause a decrease in salivary pH. Furthermore, *S. mutans* cannot metabolize xylitol and is inhibited by it. Chewing gum also stimulates saliva, which increases the buffering capacity of saliva and the clearance of fermentable carbohydrates from the tooth surface.[13]

Food Combinations There is evidence that combining foods has potential anticaries efficacy. Remineralization potential is enhanced when cariogenic foods are eaten with dairy products. For instance, bananas, which are cariogenic due to their fermentable carbohydrates and adherence capability, are less cariogenic when eaten with cereal and milk than when eaten alone.[5] Due to the anticariogenic properties of cheese, combining cheese with sugary snacks or snacks with high adherence is also beneficial. Consuming cheese following a sugary snack virtually eliminates the usual fall in pH that occurs with sugar consumption.[5] Crackers eaten with cheese are also less cariogenic than when eaten alone. Cariogenic beverages and sweets are also less cariogenic when consumed with a meal than when consumed alone. The additional foods stimulate saliva and provide a buffering effect, thereby decreasing the cariogenic potential of the substrate.[1] The sequence of eating foods during a meal also affects the magnitude of the change in the pH. Eating acidogenic foods between cariostatic or anticariogenic foods and eating chewy foods that simulate saliva flow with foods that have minimal effect on saliva flow can reduce demineralization. Table 11.2 provides an overview of dietary patterns that affect caries risk.

Caries Treatment and Prevention

Dental caries is usually clinically managed through restorative treatment. Restorations are temporary in nature, and caries can form at the margins of existing restorations, if the etiologic factors are not eliminated or controlled. Although the development of carious lesions is generally a slow process, caries development is more rapid in some circumstances (e.g., in young children, where newly erupted teeth are less highly mineralized than in older people, or in any condition resulting in lack or diminution of protective saliva). Tooth structure may be successfully preserved through removal of dental plaque, application of fluoride, or placement of sealants.[7]

Dental caries is a disease that must be prevented throughout the lifetime. Successful caries prevention requires management of all of the host, agent, and environmental factors.

Managing the Host/Agent/Environment

Diet A healthy diet is important prenatally during dental formation and will help ensure optimal tooth and other oral tissue development before birth. Teeth that are not optimally mineralized before birth are more susceptible to acid destruction once erupted into the mouth. After birth and throughout life, a nutritious diet will also help foster oral tissue growth, development, regeneration, and healing of oral bone and soft tissue. Managing the dietary patterns and factors that initiate and promote the caries process is crucial to preventing and/or minimizing the caries process. This includes focusing on a balanced diet and modifying the sources and quantity of fermentable carbohydrates. Positive habits should be encouraged, including snacking on anticariogenic or cariostatic foods, chewing sugarless gum after consuming cariogenic items, and having sweets with meals rather than as snacks.

Plaque Control Daily removal of dental plaque through toothbrushing and flossing breaks up the virulent bacterial colonies or plaque that initiate caries as well as infect gums. Simply telling patients they can eat whatever they want, as long as they brush their teeth afterwards, is inappropriate, particularly because acid is formed within seconds when plaque bacteria are provided a carbohydrate food source.

Fluoride

Fluoride is a natural element that is important to the integrity of bone and teeth. Fluoride is the most extensively studied community health measure in recent history, and the use of fluoride for the prevention of dental caries is regarded as the most effective dental public health practice in existence.[14] Fluoride is beneficial to all age groups throughout the life cycle (**Table 11.3**). Despite the unquestioned scientific evidence of the overwhelming benefits of fluoride, an antifluoridation movement is still active, especially where community water fluoridation is on the local ballot for public vote. Antifluoridationists argue water fluoridation is associated with adverse health consequences, namely, acquired immune deficiency syndrome (AIDS) and cancer, and is an infringement on freedom of choice. Although the antifluoride charges are unfounded, they can have a powerful influence on the public.

Mechanisms of Fluoride Action Fluoride functions to prevent and control dental caries in several ways. It inhibits tooth demineralization, enhances tooth remineralization, and inhibits caries-promoting plaque bacteria.[15,16] Fluoride is concentrated in saliva and plaque; it inhibits the demineralization of sound enamel and enhances the remineralization of demineralized enamel. As cariogenic bacteria metabolize carbohydrates and produce acid, fluoride is released from the dental plaque in response to a lower pH.[15] The demineralized enamel selectively takes up the released fluoride, along with fluoride, calcium, and phosphorus in saliva. This process improves the structure of the enamel and inhibits future dissolution of tooth mineral by acid.[15,16] The process of demineralization and remineralization continues throughout the lifetime of the tooth (**Figure 11.4**). Fluoride also affects oral plaque bacteria. As fluoride concentrates in dental plaque, it interferes with acid production by inhibiting essential enzyme activity, thus reducing the potential for enamel destruction.[16]

TABLE 11.3 DIETARY REFERENCE INTAKE FOR FLUORIDE

Age	Reference weight*		Adequate intake[†]	Tolerable upper intake[§]
	kg	lbs	mg/day	mg/day
0-6 months	7	16	0.01	0.7
6-12 months	9	20	0.5	0.9
1-3 years	13	29	0.7	1.3
4-8 years	22	48	1.1	2.2
≥9 years	40-76	88-166	2.0-3.8	10.0

*Values based on data collected during 1988 to 1994 as part of the third National Health and Nutrition Examination Survey
[†]Intake that maximally reduced occurrence of dental caries without causing unwanted side effects, including moderate fluorosis.
[§]Highest level of nutrient intake that is likely to pose no risks for adverse health effects in almost all persons.
Data from Dietary Reference Intakes for Calcium, Phosphorus, Magnesium, Vitamin D, and Fluoride. (1997). 288-313. doi:10.17226/5776.

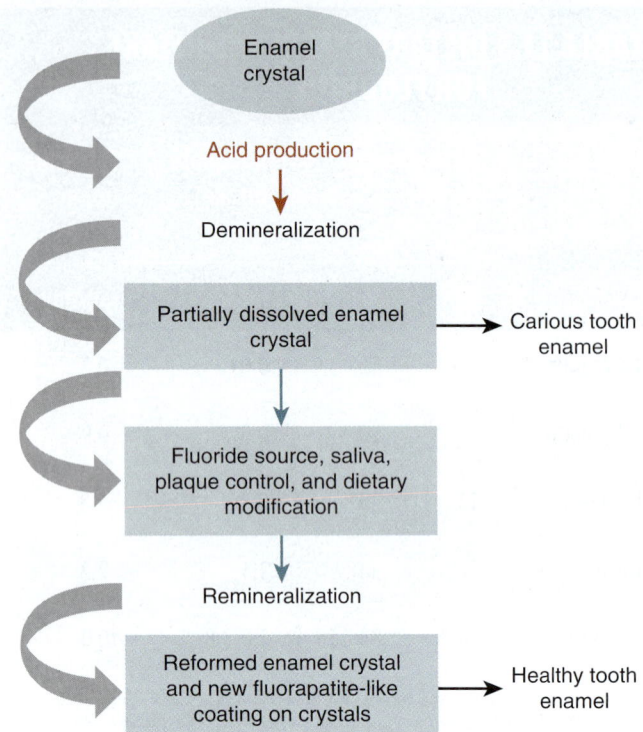

FIGURE 11.4 The Demineralization and Remineralization Process Lead to Remineralized Enamel Crystals with Surfaces Rich in Fluoride and Lower in Solubility

Modified from Selwitz, R. H., Ismail, A. I., & Pitts, N. B. (2007). Dental caries. *The Lancet*, 369(9555), 51-59. doi:10.1016/s0140-6736(07)60031-2 and Featherstone, J. D. (1999). Prevention and reversal of dental caries: role of low level fluoride. *Community Dentistry and Oral Epidemiology*, 27(1), 31-40. doi:10.1111/j.1600-0528.1999.tb01989.x

CORE CONCEPT 5

Fluoride prevents and controls dental caries through inhibiting demineralization, enhancing remineralization, and inhibiting caries-promoting bacteria.

Systemic Versus Topical Fluoride Fluoride exposure can be both systemic and topical. Systemic fluoride exposure occurs through the supplementation or dietary intake of fluoride. When fluoride is consumed, it is absorbed into the bloodstream and subsequently deposited into developing bones and teeth or excreted in urine.[14] During tooth development, or the pre-eruptive phase, fluoride from the diet and saliva is incorporated into the mineral structure of teeth and helps increase resistance to acid demineralization. After tooth eruption, or the posteruptive phase, ingested fluoride is secreted in saliva and contributes topically to tooth protection. The systemic benefits of fluoride on developing teeth occur from birth until all teeth have erupted.[14]

In the earliest days of fluoride research, it was believed that fluoride exposure was most important during the prenatal period and during childhood. It was widely believed that fluoride affects enamel and inhibits dental caries only when systemically incorporated into developing dental enamel. Recent research indicates that fluoride's predominant effect is topical and posteruptive.[15] It is now understood that fluoride works mainly after teeth have erupted, especially when small amounts are maintained consistently in the dental plaque and saliva. Adults also benefit from fluoride, rather than exclusively children, as was historically assumed. The maximum benefit for caries prevention occurs when both systemic and topical sources of fluoride are used.[14]

Sources of Fluoride Sources of fluoride include fluoridated drinking water; foods and beverages made with fluoridated water; oral health products, such as fluoride-containing toothpaste, fluoride rinses, topically applied gels and foams; and dietary fluoride supplements. Fluoridated drinking water and fluoride toothpaste are the most common sources of fluoride in the United States and are largely responsible for caries prevention in this country.[15] While fluoride has significantly reduced caries in children, it has not entirely eliminated them; the association between sugar intake and caries still persists.[17]

Topical fluoride sources, including toothpastes, rinses, gels, foams, varnishes, and pastes, are highly effective and easily administered.[14] Over-the-counter fluoride products carrying the American Dental Association seal of approval on the product label have undergone extensive clinical testing to ensure their safety and effectiveness.[18]

Children should not swallow products meant for topical use due to the risk of fluorosis. **Fluorosis** occurs when excessive fluoride is ingested during pre-eruptive tooth mineralization, resulting in defective tooth mineralization. Fluorosis can only occur while teeth are developing in the jaw and mineralizing. The American Dental Association does not recommend children younger than age 6 years use fluoride mouth rinses to avoid the overingestion of fluoride.[19] Children aged 2 to 6 years should brush with a pea-sized amount of fluoride toothpaste only and be supervised while brushing and taught to spit out rather than swallow toothpastes, rinses, or gels.[20] Parents of children younger than 2 years should consult with the child's dentist or physician before using fluoride toothpaste.

Dental professionals often utilize more concentrated fluoride solutions in the form of gels, foam, varnishes, and pastes.[14,15] The use of fluoride varnishes in school-based oral health programs and private practice is increasing, as research shows it is an effective and easily applied method for providing topical fluoride therapy.[21] Studies comparing various combinations of fluoride modalities show that their effectiveness in preventing dental caries is additive.[15]

Total fluoride intake is difficult to determine because of the wide availability of fluoride sources, the variation in levels of fluoride in foods and beverages, the effects of home water treatments and filtration systems, and the variability of fluoride intake. The effect of the water supply avlone is further complicated by the diffusion of fluoride into nonfluoridated areas through bottled beverages, processed foods, and other sources.[14]

Water Fluoridated drinking water contains a fluoride concentration effective for preventing and controlling dental caries. This concentration either occurs naturally or is reached through water fluoridation, which is the controlled addition of fluoride to a community water supply.[15] Fluoridation of public water supplies is the most effective dental public health measure in existence. It has the benefit of reaching all segments of the population, regardless of socioeconomic status or age. In most communities, every $1 invested in fluoridation saves $38 or more in treatment costs. Federal fluoridation guidelines, maintained by the Public Health Service since 1962, state that community drinking water should be maintained at 0.7 to 1.2 ppm fluoride.[15]

Recent studies show community water fluoridation reduces childhood dental caries by 18% to 40%.[15] Water fluoridation also reduces socioeconomic disparities in dental caries, as it is particularly beneficial for individuals living in communities with fewer resources, who have a high burden of dental caries and less access to oral health care.[14,16]

Recently, there has been a trend toward consumption of less tap water and more bottled water. The U.S. Food and Drug Administration does not require water bottle companies to list the fluoride content of bottled water, but it does require fluoride additives to be listed. Most bottled water in the United States contains less than 0.3 ppm fluoride. A person substituting bottled water for fluoridated tap water will not receive the caries prevention benefits of community water fluoridation. The fluoride content of individual well water also varies considerably and should be tested. Home water purification and filtration systems may also affect the fluoride content of water.[14]

Foods and Beverages Overall, water and water-based beverages provide approximately 80% of a person's fluoride intake.[14] Examples include carbonated beverages, beer, ready-to-drink juices, and drinks prepared with fluoridated water. Most foods contain minimal amounts of fluoride, except for brewed tea, which has approximately 1.4 ppm.[22] In general, it is difficult to estimate amounts of fluoride consumed due to the wide variations of fluoride content in foods and beverages.[16]

Dietary Supplements Fluoride supplements should be recommended **only** for children at high risk of developing dental caries and whose primary source of drinking water is deficient in fluoride. The following factors should be used to determine whether or not a fluoride supplement is indicated[14]:

1. Determination of the fluoride level of the primary drinking water
2. Potential sources of dietary fluoride
3. Children's caries risk

When indicated, the recommendation for fluoride supplementation applies to children up to 16 years of age.

Due to risk of fluorosis, fluoride supplements are **not** recommended for formula-fed or breastfed infants who live in fluoridated communities and receive drinking water between feedings. If the infant does not receive drinking water between feedings or drinks bottled water when on a diet of exclusive breast milk, he or she should be supplemented according to the fluoride supplement guidelines (refer to **Table 11.4**). The

Clinical Roundtable

Topic: The Antifluoridation Movement

Background: While the American Dental Association and the Academy of Nutrition and Dietetics have endorsed community water fluoridation as a public health measure, there is a growing anti–water fluoridation movement. Because decisions to fluoridate public water are often made at the local level through public referenda, opponents of water fluoridation often use this public decision process to influence water fluoridation legislation. The messages and appeals of anti–water fluoridationists can have a strong influence on the public. Although opponents have gained publicity in their attempt to create an illusion of scientific controversy over water fluoridation, their claims are largely unproven. Today, the challenges to increasing and maintaining community water fluoridation include the following:

- Lack of awareness of the importance of water fluoridation and lack of recognition of the current oral problems of society by those who vote on fluoride legislation
- Misconception that fluoridation is no longer needed or effective
- Difficulty navigating the political processes needed for the adoption of water fluoridation
- Unsubstantiated claims or fear tactics made by fluoridation opponents that influence public opinion against fluoridation
- An unsupportive political environment from a fiscal standpoint. Because many of the public water systems that are not fluoridated serve small populations, this increases the per-capita cost of fluoridation

Roundtable Discussion

1. Discuss ways to educate the patient and community about the importance of fluoride using rationale that will impact their health.
2. How might you promote the importance of fluoridation to an individual who believes that the public water supply should not be fluoridated?

Reference

1. Palmer CA, Gilbert JA. Position of the Academy of Nutrition and Dietetics: the impact of fluoride on health. *J Acad Nutr Diet*. 2012;112(9):1443-1453. doi:10.1016/j.jand.2012.07.012

TABLE 11.4 DIETARY FLUORIDE SUPPLEMENT SCHEDULE

Age	Fluoride Ion Level in Drinking Water (ppm)*		
	<0.3 ppm	0.3-0.6 ppm	>0.6 ppm
Birth to 6 months	None	None	None
6 months to 3 years	0.25 mg/day[†]	None	None
3 to 6 years	0.50 mg/day	0.25 mg/day	None
6 to 16 years	1.0 mg/day	0.5 mg/day	None

*1ppm = 1 mg/L
[†]2.2 mg of sodium fluoride contains 1 mg of fluoride ion
Modified from American Academy of Pediatric Dentistry. (2014). Guideline on Fluoride Therapy. 38(6), 181-184.

child's physician or dentist must prescribe the fluoride supplements as they are not available over the counter.[23]

Fluorosis Fluorosis is excessive fluoride ingestion before tooth eruption, resulting in hypomineralization of tooth enamel and mottled enamel (**Figure 11.5**). Clinically, fluorosis can range from mild to severe and present as hardly noticeable white spots to severe, apparent dark spots on teeth.

Recently, there has been an increase in prevalence of mild fluorosis in the United States and other developed nations. This is attributed to a variety of factors, including misuse of dietary fluoride supplements, swallowing of fluoride toothpastes and rinses, use of powdered infant formula reconstituted with fluoridated water, and the "halo" effect of increased fluoride from foods and beverages processed with fluoridated water.[14] Mild fluorosis results in teeth that have increased resistance to acid, but have white areas of enamel, which may be unsightly. According to the Centers for Disease Control and Prevention, 23% of children in the United States have some form of fluorosis, and 2.45% of children have moderate to severe forms.[24] Although this level of fluorosis is not considered a public health problem, measures should be taken to minimize this condition. Adherence to

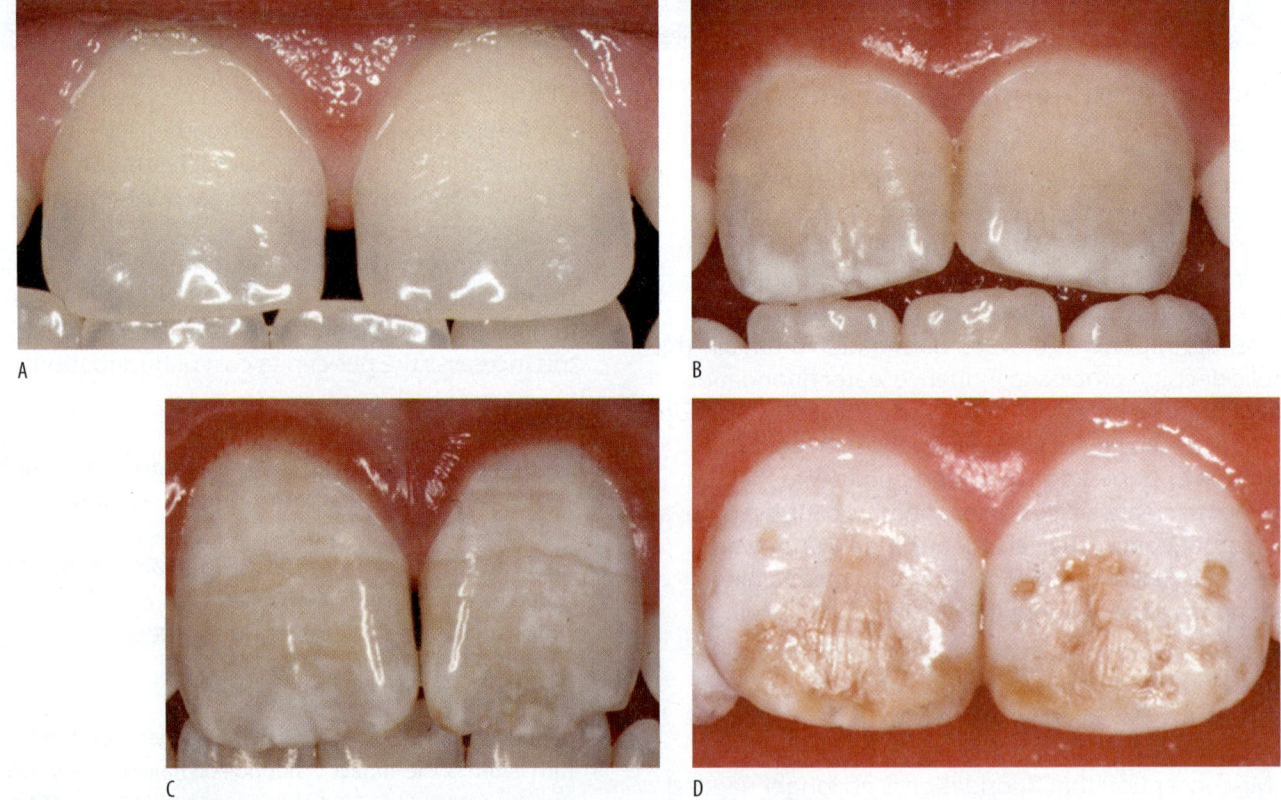

FIGURE 11.5 Dental Fluorosis. A. Normal B. Mild Fluorosis C. Moderate Fluorosis D. Severe Fluorosis

Reproduced from CDC http://www.cdc.gov/fluoridation/faqs/dental_fluorosis.

Chapter 11 Nutrition in Oral Health 341

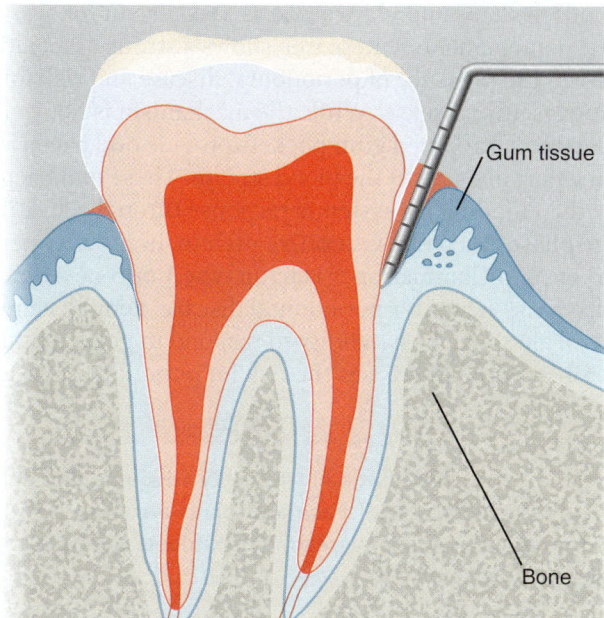

FIGURE 11.6 Use of Probe to Measure Periodontal Pocket Depth

Reproduced from National Institute of Dental and Craniofacial Research, National Institutes of Health. Use of Probe to Measure Periodontal Pocket Depth. (n.d.). Retrieved from https://www.nidcr.nih.gov/imagegallery/oralhealth/PeriodontalPocketDepth.htm.

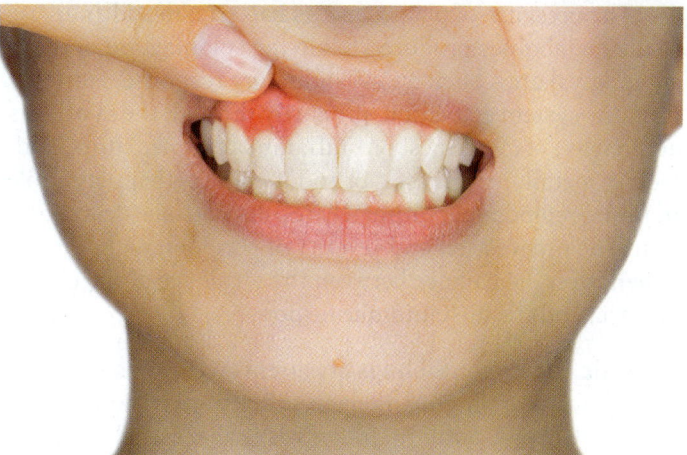

FIGURE 11.7 Gingivitis
©Stefano Garau/Shutterstock.

the American Dental Association recommendations regarding fluoride use for children aged 6 years and younger will reduce the prevalence and severity of enamel fluorosis.[15]

Periodontal Disease

Periodontal disease, or gum disease, is a chronic infection of the hard and soft tissue supporting the teeth.[25] It is generally characterized by gingival recession and bleeding, formation of deep pockets between the **gingiva** (gums) and tooth, and loss of alveolar bone that supports the teeth.[3] The severity of periodontal disease is categorized as mild, moderate, or severe based on measurements of periodontal pocket depth (**Figure 11.6**), attachment loss, and gingival inflammation around the teeth.[25]

Periodontal diseases are a collection of inflammatory processes that range from gingivitis to periodontitis. Gingivitis is a common, mild, and reversible form of periodontal disease characterized by infected, red, swollen, and bleeding gums (**Figure 11.7**). In the absence of proper oral hygiene, gingivitis may develop into periodontal disease, which is a chronic inflammatory disease of the supporting tissues of the teeth. In addition to red, swollen, and bleeding gums, teeth may show exposed tooth surfaces, and alveolar bone loss may occur due to the inflammatory process. Chronic periodontitis progresses slowly and is usually diagnosed during adulthood. If the disease manifests quickly during adolescence and post-adolescence, it is referred to as aggressive periodontitis.[26]

Pathophysiology

Microbial Factors Certain oral bacteria, most notably *Porphyromonas gingivalis, Aggregatibacter actinomycetemcomitans, Tannerella forsythia, Treponema deticola, Prevotella intermedia,* and *Fusobacterium nuceatum,* must be present for the development of periodontal disease. These bacteria colonize the subginigival pocket, or the area around the teeth below the gum line, and form dental plaque. Microbial factors differ considerably among people with periodontal disease. Different patients exhibit various mixes of oral pathogens.[26]

CASE STUDY REVISITED

Upon further interview, Elsie states that she first showed signs of periodontal disease at a dental visit 25 years ago, when she was 60 years old. At the time she smoked one pack of cigarettes per day until she quit smoking at the age of 65 years. She also reports life-long lactose intolerance and subsequently avoids dairy products. Elsie was diagnosed with osteoarthritis 20 years ago. She reports that she brushes her teeth daily, but rarely flosses due to her arthritic hands. Because of lack of dental insurance coverage, Elsie did not visit the dentist again until she was 75 years old.

Questions

1. What oral health, socioeconomic, and dietary factors likely contributed to the development and progression of Elsie's periodontal disease?
2. What lifestyle recommendations do you have for Elsie?

The presence of plaque and its bacteria, in addition to the metabolites produced following colonization of the subgingival area, elicit an inflammatory response. Host immune system activation, primarily through the synthesis and release of cytokines, pro-inflammatory mediators, and matrix metalloproteinases, or endopeptides, that play a role in tissue remodeling, ultimately results in tissue destruction. The progression and severity of periodontal disease depends on the balance between the virulence of the plaque bacteria and the host immune response.

Genetic Factors Siblings of patients with aggressive periodontitis are highly likely to suffer from periodontal disease. Chronic adult periodontitis is also estimated to have 50% heritability.[26]

> **PRACTICE POINT**
>
> Genetics are recognized as a key determinant of periodontal disease progression.

Lifestyle Factors Smokers are at increased risk for periodontal disease; suffer from a more severe, progressive form of the disease; and have more severe periodontal breakdown than nonsmokers. While it is unclear why smokers are more susceptible to periodontal disease, it may be related to compromised resistance and immunological functions.[26] While diet plays a part in the prevention of periodontal disease, there is little evidence that it has a significant role in the development and progression of the disease.

> **PRACTICE POINT**
>
> Smoking is the most significant lifestyle factor in periodontitis.

> **CORE CONCEPT 6**
>
> Periodontal disease is a chronic, inflammatory disease that is systemic in nature and results from an interaction of microbial, genetic, and lifestyle factors.

Relationships with Systemic Conditions Periodontal disease is systemic in nature, meaning that it is modulated by body systems and plays a role as a risk factor for systemic derangements.[27] Research shows a strong association between the presence of periodontal disease and risk for cardiovascular disease. While the mechanism is not well understood, inflamed gum pockets provide oral bacteria with a port of entry to the blood stream. These oral bacteria may then modulate a systemic response through elevating acute phase reactants, C-reactive protein, or other systemic markers of inflammation.[26] Having type 1 or type 2 diabetes is also a risk factor for periodontal disease. Poor glycemic control alters the host's ability to respond to periodontal microbes, which increases the risk for periodontal disease.[27]

> **PRACTICE POINT**
>
> Although it is clear that a nutritionally adequate diet helps prevent periodontal disease and plays a role in positive outcomes for periodontal treatment, nutrients alone are not a cure for the disease.[28]

Prevention and Management

A nutritionally sound diet can prevent dental disease, and certain nutrients may exert a protective effect. Vitamin C and other antioxidants, including beta-carotene and vitamin E, for instance, buffer the production of free radicals seen in periodontal disease. Aside from severe vitamin C deficiency in scurvy-related periodontitis (**Figure 11.8**), there is little evidence in support of an association between antioxidants and periodontal disease.[12] There is a relationship between osteoporosis and periodontal disease, as both are associated with bone loss. Dairy foods are a rich source of calcium and vitamin D, which are essential for bone health. There appears to be an inverse association between increased dairy intake and periodontal disease.[28] Periodontal disease also seems to progress more rapidly in undernourished populations, likely due to the importance of nutrition in maintaining the host's immune response.[12] Nutrition recommendations for maintaining periodontal health are the same as those for caries prevention.

Severe periodontal disease may be treated surgically. Before surgery, it is important for patients at nutritional risk,

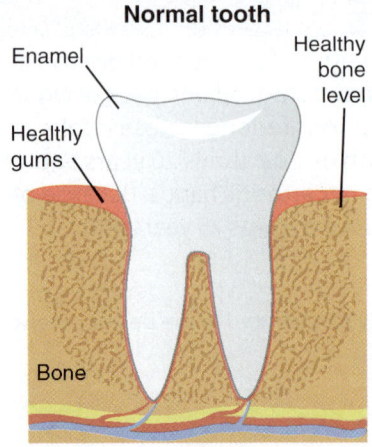
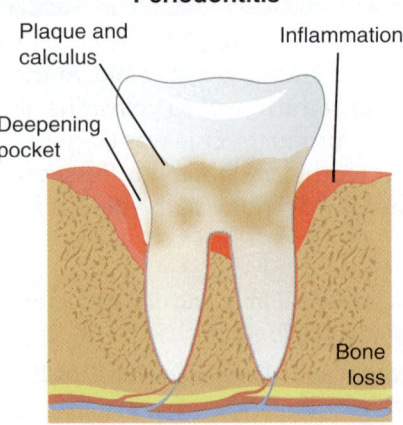

FIGURE 11.8 Periodontitis

⚠ Clinical Controversy

Does oral health care reduce the risk of ventilator-associated pneumonia (VAP)?

Pneumonia, particularly ventilator-associated pneumonia (VAP), is one of the most common hospital-acquired infections and is one of the leading causes of morbidity and mortality in critically ill patients. Oral health is correlated with VAP and oral health care appears to play a role in VAP prevention. Liao et al. studied 199 mechanically ventilated patients who received either routine nursing care (which included mouth care with a sponge and tap water) or an evidence-based oral health care program (which included oral assessment that dictated the frequency of oral care, 5 minutes of mouth care, treatment with chlorhexidine, and keeping the head of the bed elevated higher than 30°) for 4 consecutive days. The incidence of VAP in the intervention group was significantly lower than in the control group. Haghighi et al. studied 100 participants who received either standard oral care or more frequent oral care. Both cares included brushing with toothpaste, using antiseptics, and moistening lips. No significant difference was found in the incidence rate of VAP between the control and intervention group, although markers of oral health and mucosal plaque index were improved in the intervention group.

Questions

1. What are the potential advantages and disadvantages of instituting an evidence-based oral healthcare routine for critically ill patients?
2. Describe the risks and benefits of instituting such a program.

References

1. Centers for Disease Control and Prevention. Health care associated infections: Ventilator-associated pneumonia. https://www.cdc.gov/hai/vap/vap.html. Accessed December 10, 2017.
2. Liao, YM, Tsai JR, Chou FH. The effectiveness of an oral health care program for preventing ventilator-associated pneumonia. *Nurs Crit Care*. 2015;20(2):89-97
3. Haghighi A, Shafipour V, Bagheri-Nesami M, Gholipour Baradari A, Yazdani Charati J. The impact of oral care on oral health status and prevention of ventilator-associated pneumonia in critically ill patients. *Aust Crit Care*. 2017;30(2):69-73

---

including those with poor nutrition status and diabetes, to receive proper nutrition support to ensure optimal surgical outcomes. Postoperative nutrition requirements increase due to blood loss, increased catabolism, tissue regeneration, and host defense activities. If the ability to consume one's regular diet is compromised, a diet of modified consistency may be used. Oral nutrition supplements may be used if nutrient intake is inadequate.

Edentulism and Dentures

Pathophysiology

Edentulism, or tooth loss, can result from trauma, dental caries, or periodontal disease.[29] Edentulism and removable prostheses (dentures; **Figure 11.9**) can have a significant effect on the process of chewing, also known as **masticatory function**, ultimately impacting dietary habits and nutritional adequacy. Masticatory function decreases with compromised dentition, which leads to a tendency to favor softer, more processed foods. This may then result in a diet low in vitamins, minerals, protein, and fiber.[30] Tooth loss and subsequent dietary changes may increase the risk for a variety of chronic disease.[30]

> **CORE CONCEPT 7**
>
> Edentulism and/or the use of dentures can have a significant effect on masticatory function and ultimately dietary habits and nutritional adequacy.

Treatment and Prevention

While dentures have long been the standard treatment for edentulism, they are not a perfect substitute for natural dentition. Removable dentures may be partial (replacing a few teeth) or full (replacing either the maxillary and or mandibular arch of teeth). Compared to individuals with natural teeth, those with dentures experience poor nutrient composition and eating-related quality of life.

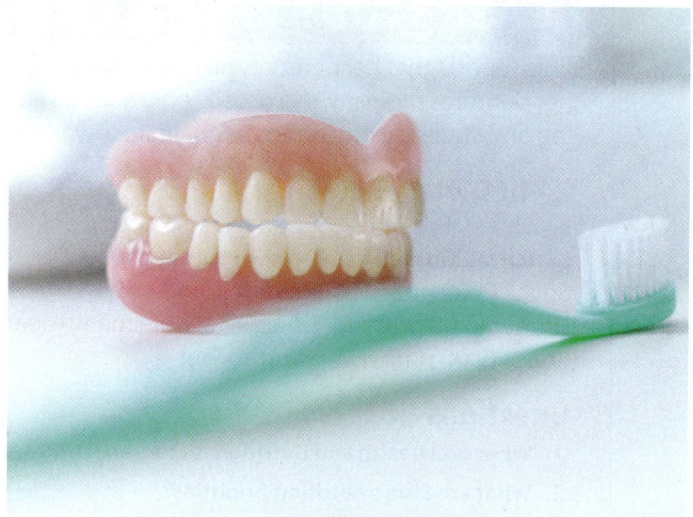

FIGURE 11.9 Dentures
© Adam Gault/Getty Images.

Chewing capacity with regular dentures is only approximately 20% to 25% of natural teeth.[3] Individuals with full dentures tend to bite and chew larger sized pieces of food and avoid foods difficult to chew, including fresh fruits and vegetables, steak, and hard-crusted breads. Dentures may also make it difficult to sense where food is in the mouth and whether it is fully chewed, thereby increasing choking risk.[6] The fit of dentures may be altered by changes in body weight or alveolar bone. Poor-fitting dentures may also adversely affect dietary intake and nutritional adequacy. The potential for these nutritional concerns to result in malnutrition is high, particularly in the elderly population.[3] Edentulism may also be treated with dental implants. Dental implants are metal posts surgically implanted into the jaw and covered with a crown to simulate a natural tooth. Unlike dentures, they are typically not associated with eating difficulties.[3]

> **PRACTICE POINT**
>
> Edentulous individuals often regard harder, coarser foods such as whole grains, fruits, vegetables, and meats, as difficult or nearly impossible to chew.

It is prudent for edentulous patients and denture-wearing patients to receive a dietary assessment and nutritional counseling. Simple measures, including using a knife and a fork as teeth to cut food into smaller pieces and moistening tough-to-chew food, should be emphasized.[3] While the provision of implants improves chewing efficiency, dietary improvement is not an inevitable outcome.[30] Patients with dentures or dental implants should receive dietary counseling that reinforces the importance of a balanced diet. These guidelines can help enhance eating pleasure and diet quality, ultimately improving nutritional status.

Oral Infections

Pathophysiology

Oral fungal infections are strongly associated with immunosuppression.[31] Predisposing factors for oral candidiasis, the most common oral fungal infection in humans, include extremes of age; HIV/AIDS or leukemia; and the use of oral antibiotics, immunosuppressive therapy, and corticosteroids.[32] To prevent denture-related candida infection, it is essential to remove dentures nightly and frequently clean them with an antimicrobial rinse.[31]

Candida is a normal inhabitant of the mouth and generally causes no problems in healthy individuals. *Candida* overgrowth can lead to oral discomfort, an altered taste sensation, and dysphasia, resulting in poor nutrition.[32] If left untreated, candidal infection can cause malnutrition by impairing intake. Malnutrition and oral candidiasis may be interrelated because malnutrition can suppress the immune system and facilitate fungal growth.[33] The ulcers that accompany other oral viral infections such as herpes simplex and cytomegalovirus can also cause pain and lead to reduced oral intake.

> **CORE CONCEPT 8**
>
> Oral infections are strongly associated with immunosuppression and may result in poor nutritional status.

Treatment and Prevention

The oral manifestations of fungal and viral infection can exacerbate poor nutritional intake. Nutritional intervention, in addition to dental care, is essential to preventing patients from becoming severely malnourished.[9] Once the type and extent of oral manifestations are identified, a tailored nutrition care plan should be developed.

CASE STUDY REVISITED

Elsie reports that her dentures no longer fit properly. She states that while she tries to remember to clean her dentures regularly, she usually only does so about once a month. Elsie complains of difficulty chewing and states that she tends to gravitate towards soft, "mushy" foods. Her food recall is as follows:

24-hr Dietary Recall

Breakfast (9:30 am):	1 banana and 1 cup cooked grits
Lunch (12:00 pm):	1 can of tomato soup
Snack (3:00 pm):	1 cup Jello
Dinner (6:00 pm):	1 microwavable meal: meat patty with mashed potatoes and gravy
Snack (9:00 pm):	1 cup sorbet

Questions

1. What oral health and nutrition factors are contributing to Elsie's underweight status?
2. What are Elsie's nutrition priorities?
3. What dietary recommendations do you have for Elsie?

> **PRACTICE POINT**
>
> Patients with oral infections may find that spices, tart or sour foods, and very hot and cold foods cause pain. Patients may find symptom relief with minimizing intake of these foods. Temperate, moist, and mild foods may be better tolerated. The consumption of small, frequent meals, followed by brushing to reduce caries risk, should be encouraged.

Oral high-calorie, high-protein supplements may be helpful in meeting nutrient needs and optimize healing. While probiotics have been shown to reduce *Candida* load, their long-term ability to modulate microflora is unknown.[31] It also appears that a diet high in carbohydrates may be a risk factor for oral candidiasis, and substitution with xylitol may be of value in controlling infection. However, more research is needed before this intervention is recommended.[32]

Oral Health During the Life Cycle

Pregnancy

Oral Health Concerns

Good nutrition and oral health is essential, yet often overlooked, during pregnancy. Pregnancy is a time when preventive oral care should be increased. However, the majority of women in the United States do not consult a dentist during pregnancy, and only about half of pregnant women attend to dental problems when they occur. Barriers to dental care during pregnancy include inadequate dental insurance, persistent myths about the effects of pregnancy on oral health, and concerns for fetal safety during dental treatment.[34]

Various hormonal and dietary factors contribute to an increased risk of oral health problems during pregnancy, most notably gingivitis, periodontal disease, and dental caries. Hormonal alternations during pregnancy may lead to an increased susceptibility to gingivitis and periodontal disease.[35] Periodontal disease is the most common oral disease in pregnancy, affecting nearly 60% to 75% of pregnant women. While the exact mechanism is unclear, studies have found periodontal disease in pregnant women to be a clinically significant risk factor for a preterm, low-birthweight neonate.[34]

During pregnancy, the oral cavity is exposed more often to gastric acid, increasing the risk for tooth erosion and caries. Frequent vomiting and a lax esophageal sphincter leading to acid reflux increase the acidity of the oral cavity.[34] Common eating habits and cravings during pregnancy, such as frequent snacking of candy and decay-promoting foods, also increase caries risk (Table 11.5). Dental caries may then subsequently interfere with the intake of a nutrient-rich diet.[35]

Nutritional Management

Women are recommended to see a dentist before pregnancy. Limiting the intake of cariogenic foods and beverages, especially snacks between meals, will further help to reduce the risk of dental caries. Fluoride recommendations do not change during pregnancy. While fluoride crosses the placenta, no evidence shows that it prevents cavities in children. Ideally, women are recommended to see a dentist and complete any needed dental treatment before pregnancy. Pregnant women without previous dental care should be recommended to see their dentist within the first trimester. Generally, only emergency dental treatment and maintenance care are given during pregnancy. Dietitians are in the prime position to screen pregnant women and refer those needing dental care to a dentist.[35]

Infancy and Early Childhood

Oral Health Concerns

Oral health problems in infancy and early childhood may predict future dental problems and interfere with growth and cognitive development.[36] Early childhood caries, formerly often referred to as baby-bottle tooth decay, is the most common oral health condition of American children.[1] The most recent data show that 42% of children in the United States between the ages of 2 and 11 years have dental caries in their primary teeth, and 17.5% of children aged 5 to 18 years have untreated dental caries. This is just

TABLE 11.5 DIETARY SUGGESTIONS FOR ORAL PROBLEMS DURING PREGNANCY

General Guidelines	Potential Issues	Diet and Nutrition Guidelines
Visit dentist prior to becoming pregnant and visit dentist at least once during pregnancy	• Pregnancy gingivitis increases risk for low-birth-weight infants • Vomiting and gastroesophageal reflux may lead to tooth erosion • Frequent snacking may lead to caries	• Follow the dietary guidelines MyPlate for Americans • Take prenatal vitamin/mineral supplement per obstetrician's recommendation • Limit quantity and frequency of cariogenic foods and those high in fermentable carbohydrate

Modified from Palmer CA, Burnett DJ, Dean B. It's more than just candy: Important relationships between nutrition and oral health. *Nutrition Today*. 2010; 45(4):154-164.

slightly under the obesity rates for children aged 6 to 12 years.[37] The prevalence of dental caries in the primary teeth of children aged 2 to 4 years increased from 18% in 1988 through 1994 to 24% in 1999 through 2004. During this same time period, caries prevalence in the primary teeth of 6 to 8 year olds also increased. A significant disparity of caries prevalence exists, with more caries being reported in non-Hispanic black and Mexican-American children than non-Hispanic white children.[38] Healthy People 2020 outlines specific measures aimed to promote the oral health of young children (**Table 11.6**).[39] Greater attention to the oral health of this age group is essential if these objectives are to be met.

Early Childhood Caries (ECC)

Early childhood caries (EEC) is defined as the presence of at least one decayed tooth, a missing tooth, or a tooth surface that has been filled in any primary tooth in a child 6 years or younger (**Figure 11.10**).[40] In children younger than 3 years of age, presence of dental caries is termed severe ECC. Dietary factors play an important role in ECC. Prolonged use of a sweetened pacifier and breast-feeding at will also increase the risk for ECC. Environmental factors related to ECC include caregivers' social status, poverty, ethnicity, years of education, and dental insurance coverage.[41]

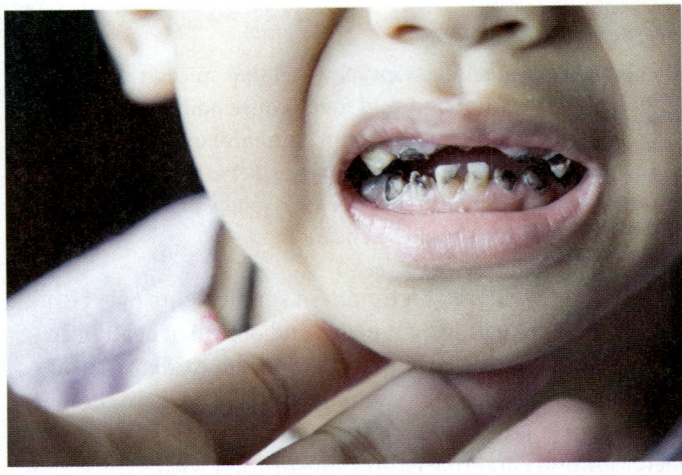

FIGURE 11.10 Early Childhood Caries
©Noppadon stocker/Shutterstock.

> **PRACTICE POINT**
>
> ECC risk is increased with frequent, long-term use of baby bottles or sippy cups containing fermentable sugars, including cow's milk, formula, fruit juice, soda, or other sweetened beverages.

ECC may begin developing before teeth have fully erupted. While the lower incisors (lower front teeth) are protected by the tongue, the upper incisors are particularly vulnerable. In severe cases, the decayed crowns may break off and the permanent developing teeth may be damaged. Children with ECC may be negatively affected by premature tooth loss, oral pain, feeding problems, speech disorders, failure to thrive, and low self-esteem.[35]

> **CORE CONCEPT 9**
>
> Early childhood caries, the most common oral health condition of American children, is associated with microbial, environmental, and dietary factors including frequent, long-term use of baby bottles containing fermentable carbohydrates.

Nutritional Management

Early childhood caries is preventable and reversible in its earliest stages.

TABLE 11.6 HEALTHY PEOPLE 2020 ORAL HEALTH OBJECTIVES IN INFANCY AND EARLY CHILDHOOD

OH-1 Reduce the proportion of children and adolescents who have dental caries experience in their primary or permanent teeth	
OH-1.1	Reduce the proportion of children aged 3 to 5 years with dental caries experience in their primary teeth
OH-1.2	Reduce the proportion of children aged 6 to 9 years with dental caries experience in their primary and permanent teeth
OH-1.3	Reduce the proportion of adolescents aged 13 to 15 years with dental caries experience in their permanent teeth
OH-2 Reduce the proportion of children and adolescents with untreated dental decay	
OH 2.1	Reduce the proportion of children aged 3 to 5 years with untreated dental decay in their primary teeth
OH 2.2	Reduce the proportion of children aged 6 to 9 years with untreated dental decay in their primary and permanent teeth
OH 2.3	Reduce the proportion of adolescents aged 13 to 15 years with untreated dental decay in their permanent teeth

Modified from US Department of Health and Human Services. Oral health. http://www.healthypeople.gov/2020/topicsobjectives2020/objectiveslist.aspx?topicId=32. Accessed April 7, 2014.

> **PRACTICE POINT**
>
> Management of ECC includes diet modification and oral hygiene education and counseling for parents, guardians, and caregivers.[42] Messages should focus on health behaviors including brushing a child's teeth at least daily, limiting frequent use of bottles and sippy cups with sugar-sweetened beverages, and ensuring children have adequate exposure to fluoride.[35]

Dietary guidelines include removal of nighttime bottles and modifying the frequency and content of daytime bottles. Infants should never be put to bed with a bottle. Bottle content should be limited to water, milk, or formula. Gums and teeth should be cleaned with a gauze or washcloth after feedings. Children should be weaned from a bottle by 1 year of age and transitioned to regular cups, not sippy cups or juice boxes. Cariogenic foods should be limited to mealtimes and followed by tooth brushing or mouth rinsing.[35] Dietary recommendations must be realistic and focus on a healthy, balanced diet (Table 11.7). The goal should be to help caregivers develop the life-long habits needed to promote oral health for themselves and for those whom they influence.

Adolescence

Oral Health Concerns

Adolescents have distinctive oral health and nutritional needs due to unique social and psychological circumstances. Dental caries, eating disorders, and periodontal disease are important oral health concerns.[43] While the prevalence of dental caries in adolescents has declined significantly over the past decade, it remains unnecessarily high at 59%.[37,38] This high prevalence is influenced by various dietary patterns common during adolescence. Frequent intake of cariogenic foods including sugar-sweetened beverages, sweets, and convenience foods, in addition to between-meal snacking, increase the risk for dental caries. Teenagers may also be unaware that acidic sugar-free beverages can also cause tooth demineralization.[1]

Eating disorders, especially bulimia, also present significant risks to oral health. Many of the first clinical signs of an eating disorder appear in the oral cavity.[3] Frequent purging of acidic gastrointestinal contents leads to tooth erosion of the lingual and occlusal surfaces on maxillary teeth.[1] Patients may complain that tooth enamel appears to be flaking off, and that the teeth and gingiva are sensitive or painful. Patients may also present with swollen glands, xerostomia, or even mucosal trauma (from objects used to induce vomiting). Xerostomia results in a loss of the protective effect of saliva.[1]

Adolescents have a higher prevalence of gingivitis than prepubertal children or adults. Available evidence shows that tissue damage from periodontal disease may start in late adolescence. The increased prevalence is likely caused by the rise in hormones during adolescence.[43]

Nutritional Management

Treatment of the adolescent patient can be multifaceted and complex. In order to provide the best nutrition education and counseling, care providers must understand the unique social and psychological concerns of this age group (Table 11.8). Messages should be positive and personalized.[43]

> **PRACTICE POINT**
>
> Guidelines include minimizing between-meal snacking; limiting consumption of juice, soda, and acid-containing beverages; and minimizing slowly dissolving, sweet foods. Adolescents should be encouraged to choose noncariogenic foods as snacks and eat cariogenic foods with meals.[1]

A diet based on the U.S. Department of Agriculture's MyPlate will support dietary adequacy and overall oral health. If an eating disorder is present, a interprofessional approach is critical and should include medical, psychiatric, dental, and nutritional professionals.

TABLE 11.7 DIETARY SUGGESTIONS FOR ORAL PROBLEMS DURING INFANCY AND EARLY CHILDHOOD

General Guidelines	Potential Issues	Diet and Nutrition Guidelines
Have first dental visit at age 12 months and subsequent visits biannually	• Early childhood caries in primary teeth • Prolonged bottle feeding with fermentable carbohydrates	• Use bottles containing only water for pacifiers, naps, and bedtime and only if necessary • Learn to identify cariogenic foods and those with fermentable carbohydrates • Avoid continuous use of sippy cups, unless containing only water • Minimize excessive between-meal snacks • Clean teeth after taking sugar-sweetened medication • Rise mouth with water after eating

Modified from Palmer CA, Burnett DJ, Dean B. It's more than just candy: Important relationships between nutrition and oral health. *Nutrition Today*. 2010; 45(4):154-164.

TABLE 11.8 DIETARY SUGGESTIONS FOR ORAL HEALTH PROBLEMS DURING ADOLESCENCE

	General Guidelines	Potential Issues	Diet and Nutrition Guidelines
Older Children	Visit dentist biannually	• Caries in primary and permanent teeth • Frequent cariogenic snacks	• Minimize between-meal snacks • Eat cariogenic foods with meals and choose noncariogenic foods as snacks
Teenagers	Visit dentist biannually	• Gingivitis and periodontal disease • Dental caries • Caries or enamel erosion from bulimia nervosa purging • Nutrient deficiencies related to disordered eating • Frequent cariogenic snacks • Soda displacing milk, limiting calcium and vitamin D consumption	• Minimize consumption of juice, regular and sugar-free carbonated drinks, and acid-containing beverages • Choose whole fruits, vegetables, sandwiches, nuts, and low-fat dairy products as between-meal snacks • Minimize slowly dissolving, sweetened foods • Ensure adequate calcium and vitamin D intake

Modified from Palmer CA, Burnett DJ, Dean B. It's more than just candy: Important relationships between nutrition and oral health. *Nutrition Today*. 2010; 45(4):154-164.

Adulthood

Oral Health Concerns

The most prevalent oral health concern during adulthood is periodontal disease, which usually is manifest in midlife. In 2010, approximately 47% of adults aged 30 years and older in the United States had periodontal disease.[25] Periodontal disease is directly associated with lower levels of education and higher levels of poverty; marked racial and ethnic disparities exist, with non-Hispanic blacks and Mexican American having a similar prevalence of periodontitis but a higher prevalence than non-Hispanic whites.[25]

Periodontal disease may result in recession of the gingival tissues around the teeth. The newly exposed tooth surface is less mineralized than enamel and more susceptible to acid demineralization. This recession and acid demineralization increases the risk for **root caries**, or decay on the root surface of the tooth.[1] According to the third National Health and Nutrition Survey conducted from 1999 to 2004, the prevalence of root caries among adults between 20 to 34 years of age was 10.4%, rising to 30.8% among adults ages 50 to 64 years.[44] The risk for root caries also increases with medication use, as many of the medications used by adults and the elderly can cause xerostomia. When saliva production is decreased, the cariogenicity of the diet increases because food is cleared more slowly from the mouth and the enamel is less readily remineralized.[1]

CASE STUDY REVISITED

Elsie complains of dry mouth and states that in addition to problems chewing food, she also has issues swallowing food and sensing taste. She takes various medications for her diabetes, hyperlipidemia, hypertension, and osteoporosis. Her medication regimen is as follows:

Hydrochlorothiazide	50 mg once per day
Simvastatin	20 mg once a day
Metoprolol	200 mg once a day
Metformin	500 mg with breakfast and dinner
Glipizide	5 mg with breakfast and dinner
Fosamax	10 mg once a day, first thing in the morning
Calcium carbonate	600 mg with breakfast and lunch
Vitamin D_3	800 IU once a day

Questions

1. Which medications are likely causing Elsie to experience xerostomia?
2. What dietary and oral health recommendations would you give Elsie to help ameliorate her dry mouth?

Nutrition Management

As previously emphasized, periodontal disease appears to be only slightly associated with diet. A dietary pattern that supports periodontal health is similar to the dietary pattern for caries prevention (Table 11.9). Nutrition counseling and education should emphasize the importance of a balanced diet that follows the Dietary Guidelines for Americans.[1] The high prevalence of root caries in middle-aged adults reinforces the importance of strategies to prevent root caries. At the patient level, dental professionals must emphasize optimal oral health behaviors, including brushing and flossing teeth and attending regular dental visits. Nutrition professionals should encourage patients to reduce their intake of cariogenic foods.

Geriatrics

> **CORE CONCEPT 10**
>
> The nutritional status of older adults is often negatively affected by compromised dentition due to periodontal disease, xerostomia, edentulism, and wearing dentures.

Oral Health Concerns

Individuals aged 65 years and older are the fastest growing group in the United States today.[45] In 2008, this age group represented 13% of the United States population, and it is projected to increase to approximately 20% by 2030.[45] Approximately one-third of the elderly population has untreated dental caries, and about 40% has periodontal disease. About 25% of those 65 years and older have no natural teeth; those living in poverty are twice as likely to be edentulous when compared to those with higher incomes. Access is an important issue, as minority, low-income, and institutionalized/homebound older adults are the most likely to have oral disease, but the least likely to receive services.[45]

Older adults have unique oral health needs. Older adults experience higher rates of chronic diseases and they consume more medication associated with increased risk for xerostomia and root caries.[1,46] The most common cause of xerostomia in older adults is the use of prescription and nonprescription medications, and 80% of the most commonly prescribed medications cause xerostomia (Table 11.10).[46] Medication-induced xerostomia is common in the geriatric patients because this population is more vulnerable to medication side effects.

TABLE 11.10 XEROSTOMIA IN OLDER ADULTS

Drug classes likely to cause complaints of dry mouth:
- Anticholinergic drugs
- Antidepressants
- Sedatives and tranquilizers
- Antihistamines
- Antihypertensives (alpha and beta blockers, diuretics, calcium channel blockers, angiotensin-converting enzyme inhibitors)
- Cytotoxic agents
- Anti-Parkinsonism drugs
- Antiseizure drugs

Modified from Sreebny, L. M., & Schwartz, S. S. (1997). A reference guide to drugs and dry mouth - 2nd edition. *Gerodontology*, 14(1), 33-47. doi:10.1111/j.1741-2358.1997.00033.x.

> **PRACTICE POINT**
>
> The older population may become handicapped by their dentition. Adequate dietary intake is a challenge for aging patients who report having poor oral health, periodontal disease, xerostomia, edentulism, and wearing dentures.[30]

As masticatory efficiency declines, elderly generally avoid eating foods that are difficult to chew, including raw, fibrous vegetables; some fruits; and nuts. These nutrient-dense foods are often replaced by easily chewed, calorically dense foods that are high in saturated fat. This shift in dietary patterns may result in a diet low in key nutrients. Poor oral

TABLE 11.9 DIETARY SUGGESTIONS FOR ORAL HEALTH PROBLEMS DURING ADULTHOOD

General Guidelines	Potential Issues	Diet and Nutrition Guidelines
Visit dentist biannually	• Periodontal disease • Root carries • Cariogenic and acidic food and beverage consumption	• Ensure adequate calcium and vitamin D intake • Use water for treating dry mouth instead of hard candy

Modified from Palmer CA, Burnett DJ, Dean B. It's more than just candy: Important relationships between nutrition and oral health. *Nutrition Today*. 2010; 45(4):154-164.

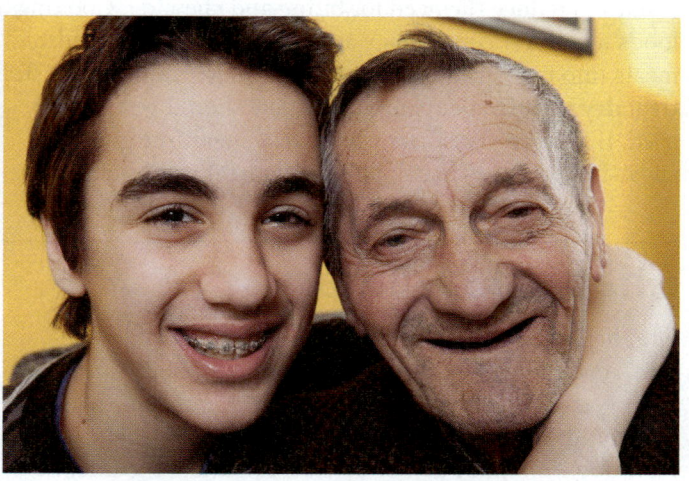

FIGURE 11.11 Good Oral Health is Important Across the Life Cycle
©videnko/Shutterstock.

TABLE 11.11 DIETARY SUGGESTIONS FOR ORAL HEALTH PROBLEMS IN GERIATRICS

General Guidelines	Potential Issues	Diet and Nutrition Guidelines
Visit dentist biannually	• Periodontal disease • Root caries • Edentulism • Xerostomia	• Ensure adequate calcium and vitamin D intake • Use water for treating dry mouth instead of hard candy • Ensure appropriately fitting dentures • Adapt nutritious foods in the face of chewing difficulties (e.g., choose applesauce instead of whole apple) • Drink adequate fluids and/or chew sugar-free gum for dry mouth • Choose appropriate multivitamin/mineral supplement

Modified from Palmer CA, Burnett DJ, Dean B. It's more than just candy: Important relationships between nutrition and oral health. *Nutrition Today*. 2010; 45(4):154-164.

health status is also associated with an increased risk for malnutrition.[47]

Nutritional Management

Dietary and nutritional management for elders with compromised oral health must be individualized and concurrently address chronic health conditions, disabilities, and oral health concerns (Table 11.11). It is essential for nutrition professionals to integrate oral health in the nutrition care process for older adults.[3] Dietary management strategies include ensuring proper-fitting dentures and adapting nutritious foods to the appropriate consistency for chewing. Patients should be guided to peel and chop fruits and vegetables to reduce the need for biting and chewing. Cooking foods to a softer consistency and cutting vegetables and meats into bite-sized pieces may also make eating easier. To treat dry mouth, adequate fluid intake should be encouraged. If fluid restriction is warranted, sugar-free gum or sugar-free lozenges may help stimulate saliva production.

Chapter Summary

Oral health can affect and be affected by diet and nutrition. As a gateway to the rest of the human body, the oral cavity can have a significant effect on overall health and wellbeing. Similarly, compromised nutritional status resulting from poor diet or disease can affect the integrity of the oral cavity. Emerging research is revealing important relationships among nutrition, oral disease, and chronic conditions such as diabetes and cardiovascular disease. While most oral health diseases are not life threatening, the emphasis should be placed on prevention rather than treatment. Nutrition professionals should promote good oral health through good nutrition. Nutritionists have the responsibility to identify oral health concerns in patients and modify the nutrition therapy plan accordingly. As the understanding of the association between nutrition and oral disease continues to grow, nutrition professionals are uniquely qualified to integrate oral health screening, education, and referrals into their everyday practice.

Key Terms

enamel, dentin, hydroxyapatite, fluorapatite, enamel hypolpasia, xerostomia dental caries, plaque, demineralization, remineralization, cariogenicity, cariogenic, cariostatic, anticariogenic, fluoride, fluorosis, periodontal disease, gingiva, edentulism, masticatory function, early childhood carries (ECC), root caries

References

1. Palmer CA, Burnett DJ, Dean B. It's more than just candy: Important Relationships between nutrition and oral health. *Nutr Today*. 2010;45(4):154-164. doi:10.1097/NT.0b013e3181e98969
2. U.S. Department of Health and Human Services. *Oral health in America: A report of the surgeon general*. Rockville, MD: U.S. Department of Health and Human Services, National Institute of Dental and Craniofacial Research, National Institutes of Health; 2000.
3. Touger-Decker R, Mobley C. Position of the Academy of Nutrition and Dietetics: oral health and nutrition. *J Acad Nutr Diet*. 2013;113(5):693-701. doi:10.1016/j.jand.2013.03.001
4. So M, Ellenikiotis YA, Husby HM, Paz CL, Seymour B, Sokal-Gutierrez, K. Early childhood dental caries, mouth pain, and malnutrition in the Ecuadorian Amazon Region. *Int J Environ Res Public Health*. 2017;14(5):550. doi:10.3390/ijerph14050550
5. Moynihan P, Petersen PE. Diet, nutrition and the prevention of dental diseases. *Public Health Nutr*. 2004;7(1a):201-226.
6. Palmer CA, Boyde LD. *Diet and nutrition in oral health*. 3rd ed. Upper Saddle River, NJ: Pearson Education; 2017.
7. Selwitz RH, Ismail AI, Pitts NB. Dental caries. *Lancet*. 2007;369(9555):51-59. doi:10.1016/s0140-6736(07)60031-2
8. Struzycka I. The oral microbiome in dental caries. *Pol J Microbiol*. 2014;63(2):127-135.
9. WHO Guidelines Approved by the Guidelines Review Committee. *Guideline: Sugars Intake for Adults and Children*. Geneva, Switzerland: World Health Organization; 2015.
10. Gustafsson BE, Quensel CE, Lanke LS, et al. The Vipeholm dental caries study; the effect of different levels of carbohydrate intake on caries activity in 436 individuals observed for five years. *Acta Odontol Scand*. 1954;11(3-4):232-264.
11. Holbrook WP, Arnadottir IB, Takazoe I, Birkhed D, Frostell G. Longitudinal study of caries, cariogenic bacteria and diet in children just before and after starting school. *Eur J Oral Sci*. 1995;103(1):42-45.

12. Moynihan PJ. The role of diet and nutrition in the etiology and prevention of oral diseases. *Bull World Health Organ.* 2005;83(9):694-699. doi:/S0042-96862005000900015
13. Thabuis C, Cheng CY, Wang X, et al. Effects of maltitol and xylitol chewing-gums on parameters involved in dental caries development. *Eur J Paediatr Dent.* 2013;14(4):303-308.
14. Palmer CA, Gilbert JA. Position of the Academy of Nutrition and Dietetics: the impact of fluoride on health. *J Acad Nutr Diet.* 2012;112(9):1443-1453. doi:10.1016/j.jand.2012.07.012
15. Recommendations for using fluoride to prevent and control dental caries in the United States. Centers for Disease Control and Prevention. *MMWR Recomm Rep.* 2001;50(Rr-14):1-42.
16. Guideline on fluoride therapy. *Pediatr Dent.* 2013;35(5):E165-168.
17. Scardina GA, Messina P. Good oral health and diet. *J Biomed Biotechnol.* 2012;720692. doi:10.1155/2012/720692
18. American Dental Association. ADA seal of acceptance program and products. http://www.ada.org/sealprogramproducts.aspx. Accessed September 4, 2017.
19. American Dental Association. Mouthrinses. http://www.ada.org/en/public-programs/advocating-for-the-public/fluoride-and-fluoridation/fluoridation-faq. Accessed September 4, 2017.
20. American Dental Association. Fluoridation FAQs. http://www.ada.org/en/~/media/ADA/Publications/ADA%20News/Files/fluoridation_facts. Accessed September 4, 2017.
21. Marinho VC, Worthington HV, Walsh T, Clarkson JE. Fluoride varnishes for preventing dental caries in children and adolescents. *Cochrane Database Syst Rev.* 2013;7:Cd002279. doi:10.1002/14651858.CD002279.pub2
22. Lussi A, Hellwig E, Klimek J. Fluorides—mode of action and recommendations for use. *Schweiz Monatsschr Zahnmed.* 2012;122(11):1030-1042.
23. Rozier RG, Adair S, Graham F, et al. Evidence-based clinical recommendations on the prescription of dietary fluoride supplements for caries prevention: a report of the American Dental Association Council on Scientific Affairs. *J Am Dent Assoc.* 2010;141(12):1480-1489.
24. Beltran-Aguilar ED, Barker L, Dye BA. Prevalence and severity of dental fluorosis in the United States, 1999-2004. *NCHS Data Brief.* 2010;(53):1-8.
25. Thornton-Evans G, Eke P, Wei L, et al. Periodontitis among adults aged ≥30 years—United States, 2009-2010. *MMWR Suppl.* 2013;62(3):129-135.
26. Laine ML, Crielaard W. Functional foods/ingredients and periodontal diseases. *Eur J Nutr.* 2012;51 Suppl 2:S27-30. doi:10.1007/s00394-012-0325-5
27. Oppermann RV, Weidlich P, Musskopf ML. Periodontal disease and systemic complications. *Braz Oral Res.* 2012;26(Suppl 1):39-47.
28. Najeeb S, Zafar MS, Khurshid Z, Zohaib S, Almas K. The role of nutrition in periodontal health: an update. *Nutrients.* 2016;8(9). doi:10.3390/nu8090530
29. Nascimento GG, Leite FR, Conceicao DA, Ferrua CP, Singh A, Demarco FF. Is there a relationship between obesity and tooth loss and edentulism? A systematic review and meta-analysis. *Obes Rev.* 2016;17(7):587-598. doi:10.1111/obr.12418
30. Gil-Montoya JA, de Mello AL, Barrios R, Gonzalez-Moles MA, Bravo M. Oral health in the elderly patient and its impact on general well-being: a nonsystematic review. *Clin Interv Aging.* 2015;10:461-467. doi:10.2147/cia.s54630
31. Williams DW, Kuriyama T, Silva S, Malic S, Lewis MA. Candida biofilms and oral candidosis: treatment and prevention. *Periodontol 2000.* 2011;55(1):250-265. doi:10.1111/j.1600-0757.2009.00338.x
32. Singh A, Verma R, Murari A, Agrawal A. Oral candidiasis: an overview. *J Oral Maxillofac Pathol.* 2014;18(Suppl 1):S81-85. doi:10.4103/0973-029x.141325
33. Poisson P, Laffond T, Campos S, Dupuis V, Bourdel-Marchasson I. Relationships between oral health, dysphagia and undernutrition in hospitalised elderly patients. *Gerodontology.* 2016; 33(2):161-168. doi:10.1111/ger.12123
34. Steinberg BJ, Hilton IV, Iida H, Samelson R. Oral health and dental care during pregnancy. *Dent Clin North Am.* 2013;57(2):195-210. doi:10.1016/j.cden.2013.01.002
35. Fitzsimons D, Dwyer JT, Palmer C, Boyd LD. Nutrition and oral health guidelines for pregnant women, infants, and children. *J Am Diet Assoc.* 1998; 98(2):182-186,189;quiz 187-188. doi:10.1016/s0002-8223(98)00044-3
36. Alkarimi HA, Watt RG, Pikhart H, Sheiham A, Tsakos G. Dental caries and growth in school-age children. *Pediatrics.* 2014;133(3):e616-623. doi:10.1542/peds.2013-0846
37. National Institutes of Health, National Institute of Dental and Craniofacial Research. Dental Caries (Tooth Decay) in Adolescents (Aged 12-19), and in Children (Aged 2-11). www.nidcr.nih.gov/DataStatistics/FindDataByTopic/DentalCaries/DentalCariesAdolescents12to19.htm. Accessed September 4, 2017.
38. Dye BA, Mitnik GL, Iafolla TJ, Vargas CM. Trends in dental caries in children and adolescents according to poverty status in the United States from 1999 through 2004 and from 2011 through 2014. *J Am Dent Assoc.* 2017; doi:10.1016/j.adaj.2017.04.013
39. US Department of Health and Human Services. Oral health. http://www.healthypeople.gov/2020/topicsobjectives2020/objectiveslist.aspx?topicId=32. Accessed September 4, 2017.
40. Policy on Early Childhood Caries (ECC): Classifications, consequences, and preventive strategies. *Pediatr Dent.* 2016;38(6):52-54.
41. Sun HB, Zhang W, Zhou XB. Risk factors associated with early childhood caries. *Chin J Dent Res.* 2017;20(2):97-104. doi:10.3290/j.cjdr.a38274
42. Tinanoff N, Palmer CA. Dietary determinants of dental caries and dietary recommendations for preschool children. *J Public Health Dent.* 2000;60(3):197-206; discussion 207-209.
43. Guideline on Adolescent Oral health care. *Pediatr Dent.* 2016;38(6):155-162.
44. Dye BA, Tan S, Smith V, Lewis BG, et al. Trends in oral health status: United States, 1988–1994 and 1999–2004. National Center for Health Statistics. *Vital Health Stat.* 2007;11(248).
45. Centers for Disease Control and Prevention, National Center for Health Statistics. New series of reports to monitor health of older Americans. http://www.cdc.gov/nchs/pressroom/01facts/olderame.htm. Accessed September 4 2017.
46. Sreebny LM, Schwartz SS. A reference guide to drugs and dry mouth, 2nd ed. *Gerodontology.* 1997;14(1):33-47.
47. Walls AW, Steele JG, Sheiham A, Marcenes W, Moynihan PJ. Oral health and nutrition in older people. *J Public Health Dent.* 2000;60(4):304-307.

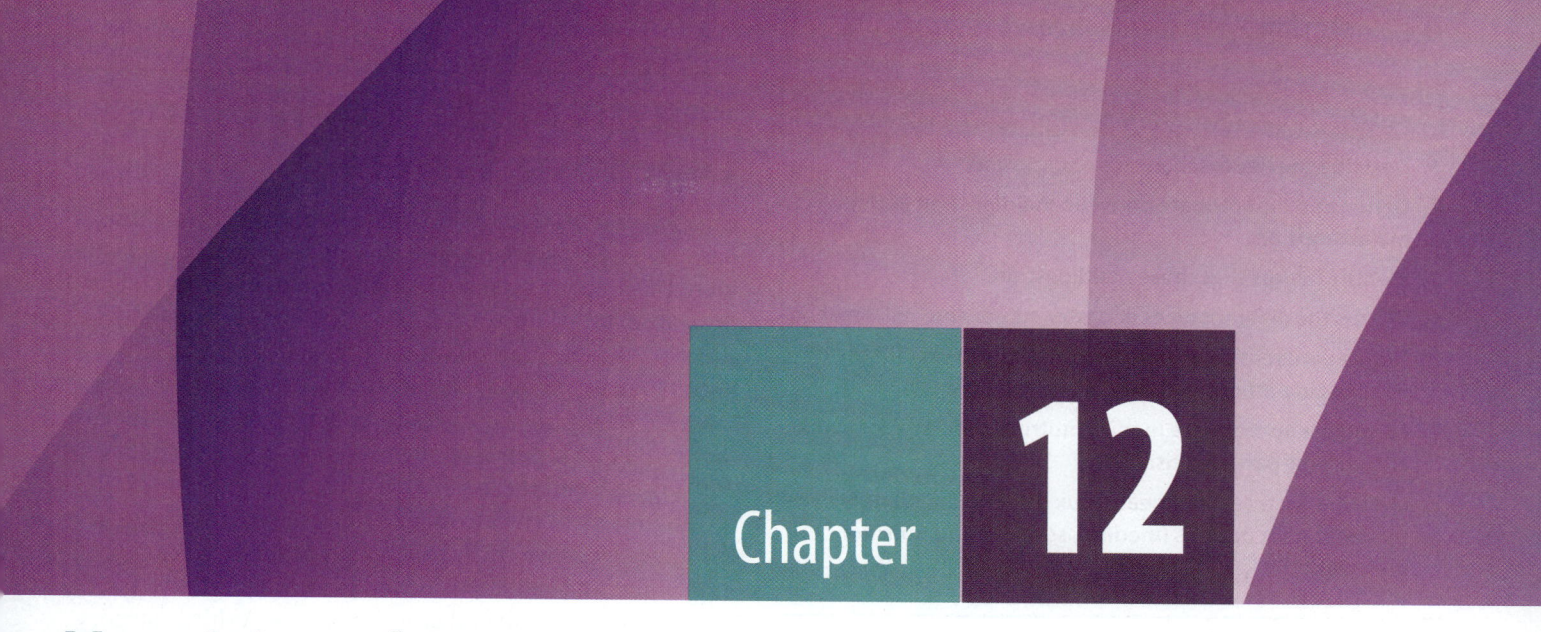

Chapter 12

Nutritional Management of Gastrointestinal Maldigestion

V. Paige Murphy
Rachel Wilkinson

Chapter Outline

Core Concepts
Introduction
Functional Anatomy of the Digestive System
Overview Of Digestion And Absorption
Key Mechanisms of Digestion
Medical Nutrition Therapy for Disorders of Digestion

CORE CONCEPTS

1. Any disease state that impairs normal digestion or absorption requires medical nutrition therapy at all stages of treatment to improve quality of life and prevent any secondary nutritional deficiencies.

2. The digestive system relies on the cooperation of a complex network of gastrointestinal and accessory organs in order to accomplish its functions in digestion and absorption.

3. Although digestion must first occur to allow for proper absorption, the two processes are entirely distinct in purpose and function.

4. While maldigestion and malabsorption are distinguishable in a pathophysiological sense, the two disorders often occur together clinically.

5. Gastric surgery indicates a number of concerning nutritional implications that may occur during the postoperative period. Nutrition interventions should be tailored to each individual depending on the symptoms and clinical manifestations that arise.

6. Acute pancreatitis and chronic pancreatitis differ substantially in their respective nutritional requirements. For both disease states, it is crucial to provide sufficient energy to meet increased needs, adapt care plans in regard to individual symptoms, and intervene with nutrition support when necessary.

7. Any changes to the integrity of the GI anatomy will alter function and impact how the body digests and ultimately absorbs nutrients.

8. GERD is a common condition with various possible medical, surgical, and nutritional treatments. It is important for dietitians to be well versed in the most up-to-date treatment options for these patients, individualizing interventions to target the cause of reflux.

Learning Objectives

1. Describe the key mechanisms of digestion.
2. Define and differentiate between maldigestion and malabsorption.
3. Identify factors that cause maldigestion.
4. Discuss the different types of gastric surgery for maldigestion.
5. Define pancreatitis (acute and chronic) and explain the differences in pathophysiology.
6. Formulate appropriate medical nutrition therapy for acute and chronic pancreatitis.
7. Describe gastroesophageal reflux disease and identify various treatment options (medical, surgical, and nutrition/lifestyle).

Introduction

There is no bodily system more readily involved in maintaining nutritional status than the gastrointestinal (GI) tract and its accessory organs. Together, these structures form a digestive system with one true purpose—to extract nutrients from food that is consumed (digestion) and relay them to the body in a usable form (absorption).[1] Normal digestion and absorption occur at numerous points along the tract, encompassing all of the structures from mouth to anus, and require integration of the nervous, endocrine, and circulatory systems.[2] Given this complexity, there are countless areas where the system can fail. Thus, a wide range of diagnoses may account for an individual's poor nutritional status through impairment of digestion, absorption, or both.

Pathology of the digestive system hovers near the top of the list of most commonly treated healthcare complaints in the United States, accounting for nearly 50 million ambulatory visits and more than 20 million hospitalizations annually.[3] For all disease states affecting digestion and absorption, nutrition therapy is a crucial component of both prevention and treatment.[4] Given the complexity of GI disorders and treatment, this chapter will cover the nutritional management of maldigestion, while Chapter 13 will detail nutritional management of malabsorption.

> **CORE CONCEPT 1**
>
> Any disease state that impairs normal digestion or absorption requires medical nutrition therapy at all stages of treatment to improve quality of life and prevent any secondary nutritional deficiencies.

Note: The digestive system is an immensely complex system and, there are many disorders that arise when the system fails. This chapter addresses those that most directly influence nutritional status by impairing normal digestion. There are several other conditions involving the digestive system that most often occur secondary to disease states. As these may not have as direct of an impact on the body's utilization of foods, they are covered elsewhere in the text.

Functional Anatomy of the Digestive System

The body's digestive system is a powerhouse. At the most basic level, this system maintains an individual's nourishment through four interreliant processes: ingestion, digestion, absorption, and excretion.[2] Efficiency in completing these processes relies on interaction and cooperation within a network of GI and accessory organs (**Figure 12.1**).[5]

Essentially, the GI tract (also referred to as the alimentary canal or the gut) is a long muscular tube with openings at the mouth and the anus. This continuation of the external environment can be divided into two main categories: the upper digestive tract, which includes the oral cavity, esophagus, and the stomach, and the lower digestive tract, comprising the small and large intestines. A third category supports digestion and absorption by providing the secretions necessary for these processes to occur. This group, which consists of the salivary glands, the liver, the gallbladder, and the pancreas, is collectively referred to as the accessory organs; each connects to the GI system at a specific point along the tract via ducts that allow for transfer of the secretions.[1,2,5] For example, pancreatic juices empty into the proximal portion of the small intestine (the **duodenum**) through the sphincter of Oddi. This relationship is critical, as digestive enzymes contained in the solution are required

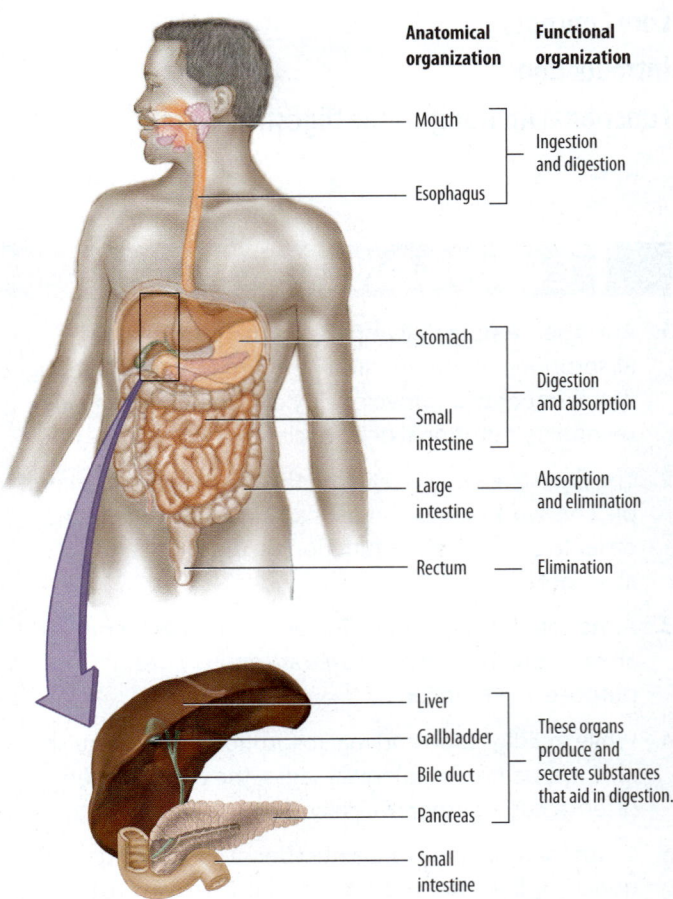

FIGURE 12.1 Anatomic and Functional Organization of the GI Tract

CASE STUDY INTRODUCTION

Janice is a 36-year-old female who is admitted for an evaluation as a candidate for a Roux-en-Y gastric bypass surgery. Given her body mass index (BMI), comorbidities, and previous attempts to lose weight, in addition to an interprofessional assessment, she is considered suitable for this surgery. Janice works as an administrative assistant in a medical office. Her information is below.

Anthropometric Data:
Weight: 112 kg (246 lbs)
Height: 165 cm (69")
BMI: 36.7 kg/m2

Biochemical Data:
Sodium 137 (135-145 mEq/L)
Potassium 4.1 (3.6-5.0 mEq/L)
Chloride 100 (98-110 mEq/L)
Carbon dioxide 22 (20-30 mEq/L)
Blood urea nitrogen 16 (6-24 mg/dL)

Creatinine 1.0 (0.4-1.3 mg/dL)
Glucose 145 (70-139 mg/dL)
Calcium 9.2 (8.5-10.5 mEq/L)
Phosphorus 4.1 (2.7 to 4.5 mg/dL)
Magnesium 1.7 (1.3 to 2.1 mEq/L)

Clinical Data:
Past Medical History: Obesity, hypertension, prediabetes, gastroesophageal reflux disease (GERD), hyperlipidemia
Medications: Prevacid, Diuril, atorvastatin
Vital Signs: Blood pressure: 160/79 mm Hg; Temperature: 97.8°F
Nutrition-focused Physical Exam: Patient appears alert and obese with adiposity consistent with gynoid body type, Pitting edema noted on bilateral lower extremities. Oral exam reveals good dentition and normal tongue and mucosa. Abdominal exam is unremarkable. Skin is warm and intact with no wounds noted. Fingernails are normal with good capillary refill.

Dietary Data:
Dietary History: Janice reports a good appetite, enjoys most foods
24-hr Diet Recall:
Breakfast (7:30 am): 5oz bagel with cream cheese; Coffee with cream and 2 sugars
Lunch (1pm): 12 inch burrito with chicken, cheese, rice, pinto beans, guacamole and sour cream diet soda
Snack (4pm): 1 cup potato chips and sour cream dip; 10 grapes
Dinner (7pm): Frozen entree (includes macaroni and cheese, or lasagna), small salad of lettuce and tomatoes with olive oil, one glass of red wine.

Questions
1. What are the postoperative nutrition implications of this surgical procedure?
2. What symptoms might Janice experience?
3. What micronutrient deficiencies might Janice be at risk for?
4. Provide a postoperative nutrition care plan for Janice.

---

by half of all ingested carbohydrates and protein and almost all ingested lipids.[2]

The pancreas is vital to the digestive system. This complex organ has both exocrine and endocrine functions, illustrated in (**Figure 12.2**). The endocrine cells, made up of the islets of Langerhans, release hormones into the blood stream.[6] These hormones include insulin and glucagon. The exocrine pancreas makes up most of the organ. These cells, called acinar cells, produce enzymes that assist with digestion, including protease, pancreatic lipase, and amylase.[6]

A number of anatomical characteristics separate the digestive system from other organ structures and allow for completion of its unique functions. First, four distinct layers comprise the gut wall throughout the entirety of the tract: (1) mucosa, (2) submucosa, (3) muscularis externa, and (4) serosa. Each layer has a specific responsibility when moving ingested food particles through the digestion and absorption processes, including the secretion of enzymes and control of muscle movement and blood flow. Second, the enlarged surface area of the small intestine, created by the

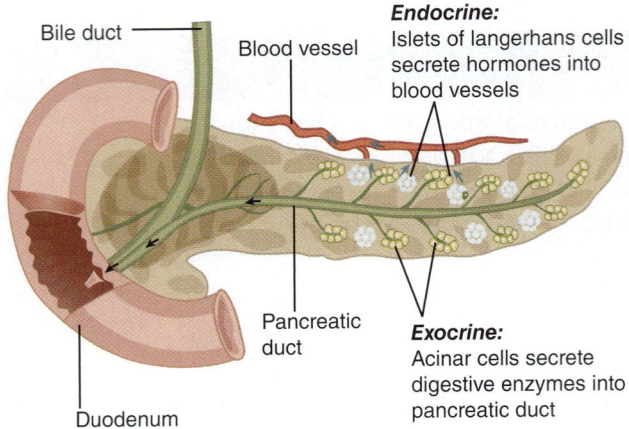

FIGURE 12.2 **The Pancreas Performs Both Endocrine and Exocrine Functions**

folds of Kerckring, the villi, and the microvilli's **brush border** (an array of microvilli on the membrane of epithelial cells), maximizes the capacity for absorption. Third, the contraction of both smooth (involuntary) and striated (voluntary) muscles allows for passage of food particles (via **peristalsis** the involuntary contraction and constriction of smooth muscle in wavelike patterns to propel a food bolus down the esophagus and upper GI tract), as well as for the opening and closing of sphincters, down the tract. Neural involvement in GI function, which regulates both muscle movement and secretions, is made possible by the enteric nervous system and its strategic positioning within the walls of the GI tract.[2,7] Each characteristic is fundamentally necessary for completing the normal processes of digestion and absorption.

> **CORE CONCEPT 2**
>
> The digestive system relies on the cooperation of a complex network of gastrointestinal and accessory organs in order to accomplish its functions in digestion and absorption.

Overview of Digestion and Absorption

The pathways through which the body obtains usable nutrients are unavoidably intertwined; absorption cannot occur without digestion as a precursor., Although the two processes are coordinated in action, they are distinctly separate. **Digestion** can be defined as the mechanical or enzymatic breakdown of food to its constituents. The term **absorption** describes the movement of these digested particles from the external environment and into the cells of the GI tract to be utilized by the body.[2] Understanding the mechanisms of normal nutrient digestion and absorption will yield greater understanding of the nutritional implications that arise when these processes are impaired.

> **CORE CONCEPT 3**
>
> Although digestion must first occur to allow for proper absorption, the two processes are entirely distinct in purpose and function.

Pathophysiological Distinction: Maldigestion versus Malabsorption

Impaired digestive processes decrease the body's ability to maintain its nutritional status. Just as digestion and absorption are two separate processes, maldigestion and malabsorption are physiologically distinct. The term **maldigestion** is used in cases when the breakdown of macronutrients is impaired[8]—theoretically, it is the failure of the enzymatic processes of digestion. Thus, maldigestion often denotes the inability of the digestive system to access or utilize digestive enzymes (as would occur in gastric surgery or pancreatitis).[9] **Malabsorption**, however, occurs as a result of defective mucosal uptake or transport of inadequately digested nutrients.[8,9] There are a range of diagnoses linked to the presence of malabsorption, and addressing each would extend beyond the scope of this chapter. The majority of associated disorders involve pathophysiology of the small intestine,[10] where the greatest amount of absorption occurs,[2] but are also seen in diseases of the pancreas, liver, biliary tract, and stomach.[10] Understand that both maldigestion and malabsorption occur from damage to the normal anatomy of one or more of the many components of the digestive system.

Differentiating between maldigestion and malabsorption is important in a pathophysiologic sense. Understanding the mechanisms behind the disease progression—and thus whether the symptoms are occurring from issues with digestion or absorption—is helpful in determining the best course of treatment. **Table 12.1** provides a list of signs and symptoms of both maldigestion and malabsorption. However, the distinction is not always useful clinically: maldigestion and malabsorption present with similar clinical markers. **Table 12.2** lists biochemical abnormalities common to both cases.[10] Because digestive and absorptive processes are so intimately connected, the term **malassimilation** may be used to describe cases where both maldigestion and malabsorption occur.[9] Note that although maldigestion and malabsorption are two separate conditions, they often occur in tandem in a clinical context.

> **CORE CONCEPT 4**
>
> While maldigestion and malabsorption are distinguishable in a pathophysiologic sense, the two disorders often occur together clinically.

Key Mechanisms of Digestion

The breakdown of food into absorbable nutrients begins in the oral cavity and progresses through the remaining GI tract structures in sequence:

1. The swallowing mechanism passes digesta into the esophagus as a **bolus** (a ball of food).
2. The bolus moves through the stomach, where it mixes with gastric juices to become **chyme**.

TABLE 12.1 COMMON SIGNS AND SYMPTOMS OF MALDIGESTION AND MALABSORPTION

Signs and Symptoms

- Diarrhea
- Steatorrhea
- Weight loss
- Flatulence
- Bloating, distention
- Abdominal pain
- Glossitis
- Cheilosis
- Stomatitis
- Ascites
- Blood in stool
- Weakness
- Fatigue
- Cachexia
- Edema
- Bone pain
- Muscle weakness
- Signs of bleeding
- Easy bruising

TABLE 12.2 BIOCHEMICAL ABNORMALITIES OF MALDIGESTION AND MALABSORPTION

Biochemical Abnormalities

Anemia:
1. Microcytic anemia
   - Iron deficiency
2. Macrocytic anemia
   - Vitamin B_{12} deficiency
   - Folate deficiency

- Hypoalbuminemia
- Hypocalcemia
- Hypokalemia
- Hypomagnesemia
- Hypophosphatemia
- Hypotriglyceridemia
- Elevated alkaline phosphate
- Elevated serum bilirubin
- Elevated serum folate levels
- Fat-soluble vitamin deficiency

3. Chyme passes into the small intestine, where the majority of digestive processes occur.
4. Any remaining undigested matter moves into the large intestine (colon).

Digestive processes take place in both the lumen of the GI tract and on the brush border. At each location, digestive enzymes act on the carbohydrates, protein, and lipids contained in food, reducing the digesta into forms the body is capable of utilizing. The various necessary enzymes are secreted by the mouth, stomach, pancreas, and small intestine.

Ultimately, carbohydrates are reduced to the monosaccharides glucose, fructose, and galactose; lipids to glycerol, free fatty acids, and monoglycerides; and proteins, which are first broken down into polypeptides, and then to individual amino acids.[1,2,7]

Medical Nutrition Therapy for Disorders of Digestion

Gastric Surgery

A typical gastric surgery involves a resection of the stomach as indicated for treatment of trauma or disease to the upper GI tract and the reconstructive procedure that follows. The three most common initial surgical procedures include vagotomy, pyloroplasty, and gastric resection.[11] A **selective vagotomy** eliminates innervation from the vagus nerve to parietal cells of the proximal stomach, decreasing the secretion of gastric acid and reducing cellular response to gastrin.[11-13] In a **total (truncal) vagotomy**, parietal cell innervation is severed and the portion of the vagus nerve that controls gastric emptying is eliminated. To correct for complications related to decreased gastric emptying, total vagotomy procedures are completed with a **pyloroplasty** which enlarges the pyloric sphincter.[11,13] The decision to use the final option, gastric resection, depends on the extent of the damaged stomach that would require removal.[13]

Pyloroplasty and gastric resection procedures are always followed by subsequent reconstruction, generally through a gastroduodenostomy (Billroth I), a gastrojejunostomy (Billroth II), or a Roux-en-Y. **Figure 12.3** depicts Billroth I and Bilroth II, while **Figure 12.4** details a Roux-en-Y procedure. A Billroth I procedure involves partial **gastrectomy** or pyloroplasty with a reconstruction consisting of an **anastomosis** of the proximal end of the duodenum to the distal end of the stomach.[11,13] Billroth II procedures create a similar anastomosis, but instead connect the proximal end of the jejunum to the distal end of the stomach following a partial gastrectomy. A "blind loop" of the duodenum is created in order to facilitate continued flow of bile salts and pancreatic enzymes.[14] The Roux-en-Y (gastric bypass), although most recently popularized for its use in treatment of obesity, began as a treatment for gastric disease.[13] This procedure yields similar results to the Billroth II, but creates a small pouch following the gastric resection with anastomosis of the jejunum to the upper portion of the stomach.[11]

In most cases, gastric surgeries occur as the result of refractory peptic ulcer disease[16] that does not respond to medical management, such as proton pump inhibitor medication. A second common diagnosis that may indicate a surgical procedure is malignancy; gastrectomy procedures serve as the primary treatment for localized gastric cancers.[15] Additionally, elective bariatric surgeries used in the treatment of extreme obesity continue to increase in popularity.

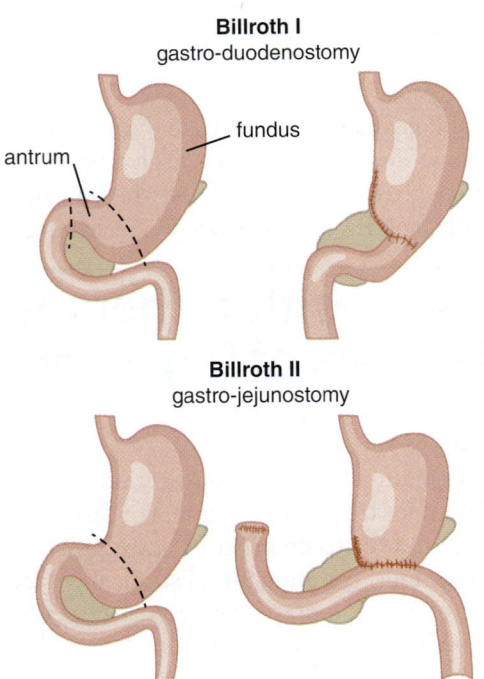

FIGURE 12.3 Pyloroplasty and Gastric Resection Procedures are Always Followed by Subsequent Reconstruction, Generally Through a Gastroduodenostomy (Billroth I), a Gastrojeju- Nostomy (Billroth II)

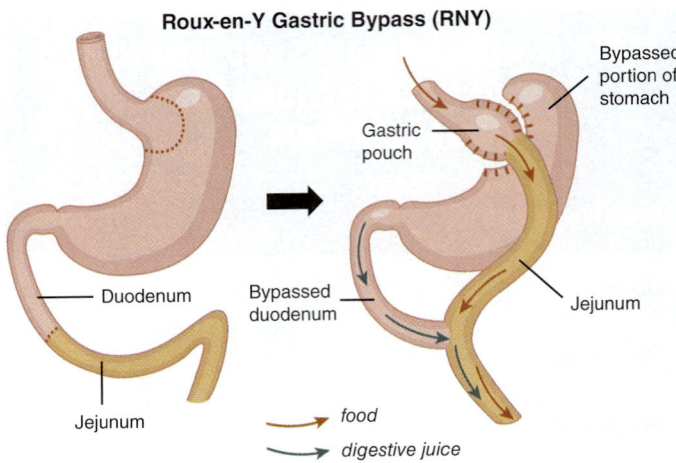

FIGURE 12.4 The Roux-En-Y Creates a Small Gastric Pouch by Removing the Top Part of the Stomach from It's Remaining Portion. The Jejunum is Anastomosed to This Newly Created Gastric Pouch

Though these procedures are not outwardly addressed in this chapter, they include many of the same surgical techniques used to treat GI disorders. Thus, a bariatric surgery patient is at risk for similar nutritional complications and should follow a comparable medical nutrition therapy plan as an individual who underwent a nonelective gastric surgery.[11]

Medical Nutrition Therapy

Nutritional Implications: Postoperative Nutrition-Related Complications When portions of the stomach are resected or rerouted during a gastric surgery, normal digestive mechanisms may be altered or lost altogether. Changes to the stomach that affect holding capacity, gastric emptying, and enzyme secretion are responsible for the most common nutrition-related postoperative complications. Those with significant nutritional implications include gastric stasis, fat maldigestion, select nutrient deficiencies, and dumping syndrome (to be described below).[14] Symptoms may be prevented, reduced, or eliminated through appropriate nutrition interventions.

Gastric Stasis The occurrence of **gastric stasis** is a concern for all patients during the postoperative period, but is most common in surgical procedures that include a total vagotomy. Gastric stasis, or **gastroparesis**, is the delayed gastric emptying that occurs when vagus innervation, and thus control, are eliminated. Patients typically present with nausea and vomiting, anorexia, bloating, and/or early satiety—all of which severely limit oral intake. In addition, those who present with gastric stasis are at an increased risk for developing small intestine bacterial overgrowth, which will be discussed later in the chapter.[14]

The management of gastric stasis typically involves the use of prokinetic and antiemetic medications combined with careful nutrition interventions.[14] Dietary modifications are made based on the individual and their symptoms. Consuming small, frequent meals throughout the day will help to decrease bloating, early satiety, and the severity of nausea and vomiting. Many patients may experience exacerbated symptoms when consuming solid foods but have no difficulty with liquid intake. For this subgroup, it is necessary to increase calories from liquids or pureed foods. In many cases, an oral nutritional supplement may be recommended. If symptoms persist, patients will likely benefit from the adoption of a low-fat, low-fiber diet since foods of this nature tend to have faster gastric emptying rates than their high-fat, high-fiber counterparts. However, liquid fats do not pose a problem and should not be excluded; most are well tolerated and serve as a source of extra calories. In addition, patients should avoid the intake of alcohol and carbonated beverages, which are known to slow gastric emptying. Light exercise postprandially may help to speed up gastric emptying rates and facilitate proper digestion.[14,15]

> **PRACTICE POINT**
>
> Patients who present with gastric stasis should consume small, frequent meals and will likely require increased calories in liquid forms. Although solid fats are not often well tolerated, fats will provide necessary energy in liquid form.

Fat Maldigestion In a functioning digestive system, chief cells of the stomach secrete gastric lipase to initiate lipid digestion. Following gastric resection and/or reconstruction, there is a marked decrease in gastric secretions and thus the necessary digestive enzymes. When lipids cannot be digested properly and are not subsequently absorbed, patients present with the symptoms of fat malabsorption. This manifests primarily as greasy, foul-smelling diarrhea known as **steatorrhea** which indicates undigested fat excretion in the stool. Patients may also report cramping and abdominal pain.[14]

For many patients, it will be necessary to initiate a low-fat diet. This recommendation is often paired with the inclusion of a **medium-chain triglyceride** (MCT) oil supplement.[16] MCTs are indicated for patients with fat maldigestion and malabsorption because they do not follow the conventional channels for lipid digestion; instead, MCTs are absorbed directly into portal circulation and immediately transported to the liver for oxidation.[17] Regardless, the amount of caloric intake from dietary lipids should be no higher than 30% for all individuals experiencing steatorrhea. The use of exogenous lipase may be initiated to aid in digestive processes. For cases of prolonged fat maldigestion, it is of the utmost importance to monitor the status of the fat-soluble vitamins A, D, E, and K and replete deficiencies as necessary.[14,16]

> **PRACTICE POINT**
>
> Although fat intake should provide no more than 30% of caloric intake for patients with fat malabsorption, it remains an important source of energy. MCT oil supplements may be indicated for patients with severe or chronic fat malabsorption.

Nutrient Deficiencies For many patients, the changes to digestive processes that occur following gastric surgery lead to the maldigestion and malabsorption, and thus deficiency, of a number of micronutrients. Most often, patients present clinically with iron, folate, and/or vitamin B_{12} deficiency, but other common nutrient deficiencies include calcium, copper, thiamin, zinc, and vitamin D.[18] Note that micronutrient deficiencies develop slowly and may not manifest until years after the gastric procedure. Continued monitoring of the nutrients of concern is necessary.[19]

It is common for postoperative patients to develop iron-deficiency anemia, pernicious anemia, or macrocytic anemia[11]; anemias arise due to inadequate intake or malabsorption of iron, vitamin B_{12}, and/or folate. Although clinicians monitor for any and all symptoms of deficiency-related anemias, members of the medical team are highly attuned to those associated with vitamin B_{12} and iron because the mechanisms for occurrence are so well understood.[14]

Vitamin B_{12} becomes an issue when secretion of **intrinsic factor**, which typically occurs via the parietal cells of the stomach, is diminished following gastric surgery. Intrinsic factor is necessary for absorption of the vitamin.[2,14] Iron deficiency, the most common postoperative deficiency, may be attributed to one or two factors. First, gastric surgeries (specifically, gastrectomies) can lead to rapid transit of food particles through the duodenum, decreasing absorption time. Second, gastric acid that is secreted by the stomach is a key player in the conversion of ferric ions to ferrous ions—the form of iron most easily absorbed.[14] Some patients report a new intolerance and thus avoidance of red meat following surgery, one of the primary sources of heme iron.[20] Regardless of the cause, all deficiencies are treated through supplementation, whether orally or via injection.[11,14,19]

Dumping Syndrome Dumping syndrome (DS) is not only the most common complication of gastric surgery—it is the most intrusive. DS describes a range of symptoms that occur when stomach contents are released too quickly and in too large of a volume into the small intestine. This creates a hyperosmolar overload, which the body overcompensates for by drawing excess fluid into the intestine. DS is subdivided into two forms: early and late; classification depends on the length of time following ingestion of a meal that symptoms arise. It is likely the result of a combination of factors, including changes in gastric emptying, changes to innervation of the stomach, and changes in the function of the pyloric sphincter.[11,14]

Early DS, which accounts for more than 75% of cases, manifests 10 to 30 minutes postprandially as a combination of GI and vasomotor symptoms. The typical GI symptoms—abdominal pain, bloating, nausea, vomiting, and explosive diarrhea—occur as a direct result of the hyperosmolar content and influx of fluid into the intestine. Vasomotor symptoms include headache, flushing, fatigue, dizziness, perspiration, palpitations, and hypotension, and are likely the consequence of hormone fluctuations. The expression of these symptoms will vary based on the individual.[14,21]

The remaining 25% of cases are classified as late DS (patients rarely experience symptoms common to both categories). Late dumping manifests anywhere from 1 to 3 hours after a meal with systemic, vascular symptoms. It is thought to be the result of reactive hypoglycemia: the rapid delivery of carbohydrates to the small intestine is followed by rapid absorption of glucose into circulation, which the body counters with an exaggerated release of insulin. Associated symptoms include perspiration, weakness, confusion, and shakiness.[11,14,21]

The majority of patients with DS respond to a course of treatment that includes nutrition therapy. Pharmacologic agents like acarbose and octreotide can be used to correct hypoglycemia, delay gastric emptying, decrease postprandial vasodilation, and increase the absorption of water in the intestine. Regardless, dietary modifications are unavoidable. Patients will work to identify foods that trigger episodes of dumping. Generally, foods that exacerbate symptoms and should be avoided are those containing lactose or the simple sugars sucrose, fructose, or sugar alcohols (xylitol, mannitol, and sorbitol). Carbohydrate intake should instead consist primarily of complex carbohydrate choices. Including protein and fat at each meal in increased amounts will counterbalance the caloric deficit created by the decreased carbohydrate intake. It is crucial that patients continue to meet daily energy needs to avoid unintentional weight loss.[14,21]

Distributing daily intake into small, frequent meals, along with slow and thorough chewing, will help to prevent large amounts of undigested foods from reaching the small intestine too quickly. Fluid intake should be limited, if not completely restricted, during mealtimes. Patients should wait at least 30 minutes after finishing a meal to drink liquids.[14,21] It may be helpful for patients to lie in the supine position postprandially to delay gastric emptying and minimize vasomotor symptoms. For those who experience severe hypoglycemic episodes, supplementation of dietary fibers has been proven effective to delay glucose absorption and prolong transit time.[21]

> **CORE CONCEPT 5**
>
> Gastric surgery indicates a number of concerning nutritional implications that may occur during the postoperative period. Nutrition interventions should be tailored to each individual depending on the symptoms and clinical manifestations that arise.

Nutrition Assessment All patients recovering from gastric surgery are at nutritional risk. Throughout the postoperative period, individuals are monitored for the physical manifestations and biochemical indicators of the nutritional complications, including unexplained weight loss, inadequate intake, food intolerances, or other parameters consistent with malnutrition.[11] Weight loss following a gastric procedure is well documented, and unintended weight loss is of nutritional concern for non-elective procedures. Postprandial fullness is the main culprit, but weight loss may also result from inadequate intake due to DS symptoms or malabsorption.[14]

A complete nutrition assessment should address the patient's dietary history, anthropometric values and other physical indicators of nutritional status, biochemical indices, and clinical parameters. Evaluation of dietary habits that typically exacerbate symptoms, including consumption of simple carbohydrates, caffeine, dairy foods, and/or fluids with meals is critical. Symptoms that would interfere with normal eating patterns, such as nausea, vomiting, constipation, and diarrhea, may be addressed through nutrition interventions. Biochemical assessments should consider values associated with anemia, fluid and electrolyte status, and the micronutrients of concern. Finally, continue to evaluate for any manifestations of malnutrition, as well as albumin and prealbumin levels.[11]

Nutrition Intervention As gastric procedures modify the anatomy of the digestive tract, all patients, regardless of the presence of the associated complications, will require dietary modifications. An individual's postoperative status, including prior medical history, will have a significant impact on their current nutritional requirements.[11] Thus, nutrition interventions should be individualized and will require adjustments based on the development of new or alleviation of existing symptoms.[14] A nutrition intervention should first ensure that the patient continues to maintain daily energy needs. Adequate caloric and protein intakes are necessary to promote optimal postoperative healing. This is accomplished through small, frequent meals that exclude foods known to exacerbate symptoms. See **Table 12.3** for a list of common foods to be limited or avoided altogether. If progression to solid food is delayed, it may be necessary to recommend appropriate nutrition support.[11,22] Studies have shown that, if warranted, postoperative early enteral nutrition is safe and well tolerated.[23]

It is always easier to prevent the occurrence of a nutritional complication than to correct it. For example, vitamin B_{12} supplementation is initiated for all patients following a gastric surgery, before the manifestations of pernicious anemia arise.[24] Nutrition education should also be provided that minimizes the symptoms of micronutrient deficiency, early and late DS, and maldigestion or malabsorption.[11]

Pancreatitis

Pancreatitis, in both its acute and chronic forms, is an inflammatory disorder of the pancreas. Both disease states require different approaches to nutritional management.[25] Although acute pancreatitis has less of an impact on digestive functions than chronic pancreatitis, pancreatic exocrine functions are more impacted by disease progression in chronic pancreatitis. All patients with acute pancreatitis require nutrition intervention, while many may require nutritional support. Chronic pancreatitis, on the other hand, has a direct impact on the digestive and absorptive abilities of the GI system, negatively affecting the patient's nutritional status. Any abnormality involving the exocrine functions of the pancreas will have considerable nutritional implications.

TABLE 12.3 FOODS TO LIMIT OR AVOID FOLLOWING GASTRIC SURGERY

Food Group	Foods to Limit or Avoid
Dairy Products	• Chocolate milk or other dairy products made with added sugar – It may be necessary to choose lactose-free products or soy milk.
Protein Foods	• Fried meat, poultry, or fish • Deli meats • Sausage, hot dogs, bacon • Tough or chewy meats • Dried beans and peas • Nuts and chunky nut butters
Vegetables	• All raw vegetables (excluding lettuce) • Any cooked vegetables served with skins or seeds • Beets • Gas-producing vegetables, including broccoli, Brussels sprouts, cabbage, and cauliflower • Collards, mustard, and turnip greens • Corn • Potato skins
Fruits	• All raw fruits except banana and melons • Dried fruits, including prunes and raisins • Any fruit juice • Canned fruit in sugar or syrup
Beverages	• Any caffeinated or carbonated beverage • Alcoholic beverages • Beverages made with sugar, corn syrup, or honey • Fruit juices and other fruit drinks – Do not drink milk or other beverages with meals or snacks. After consuming solid foods, wait a minimum of 30 minutes before having a beverage.
Other	• Sugar • Honey, syrup • Sorbitol, xylitol

Modified from Academy of Nutrition and Dietetics. Gastric surgery nutrition therapy. Nutrition Care Manual, Client Education Material. 2015.

TABLE 12.4 COMMON ETIOLOGIES FOR ACUTE PANCREATITIS*

Etiology	Susceptibility Factor
Lifestyle Factors	• Chronic alcoholism (>2 drinks per day) • Obesity (BMI >30) • Heavy smoking history • Illegal drug use
Duct Obstruction	• Gallstones of biliary sludge • Postendoscopic cholangiopancreatography (ERCP) • Tumors • Anatomical abnormalities • Parasites
Metabolic Abnormalities	• Hyperlipidemia • Hypercalcemia • Acidosis
Medications (*partial list*)	• Acetaminophen • Azathioprine • Erythromycin • Estrogen • Hydrochlorothiazide • Nonsteroidal anti-inflammatory drugs • Tetracycline
Genetic Factors	• Cystic fibrosis gene (*CFTR*) • Trypsinogen gene (*PRSS1*) • Pancreatic secretory trypsin inhibitor gene (*SPINK1*)
Infectious	• Viral infection • Bacterial infection
Trauma	• Blunt or penetrating • Surgical

*A number of cases (20%) are idiopathic[29].
Data from Papachristou G, Singh V, Whitcomb DC. Acute pancreatitis. In: Textbook of clinical gastroenterology and hepatology. Wiley-Blackwell; 2012:518-524. Accessed 1/23/2016 11:41:00 AM. 10.1002/9781118321386.ch69.

Acute Pancreatitis

Acute pancreatitis (AP) is an extremely common disorder of the digestive system, most often the result of a biliary tract obstruction or chronic alcoholism. See **Table 12.4** for a more comprehensive list of common etiologies.[25,26]

Regardless of the initial cause, all cases of AP manifest as inflammation of the pancreas, as seen in (**Figure 12.5**). This figure depicts a gallstone blockage, which is a common, but not the only, cause of acute pancreatitis. Although the exact mechanism of pancreatic injury in AP is not fully understood, the most common theory involves irregular activation of pancreatic digestive enzymes. Premature stimulation of trypsin within the pancreas results in autodigestion of the pancreatic cells, triggering a immune response.

ACUTE PANCREATITIS

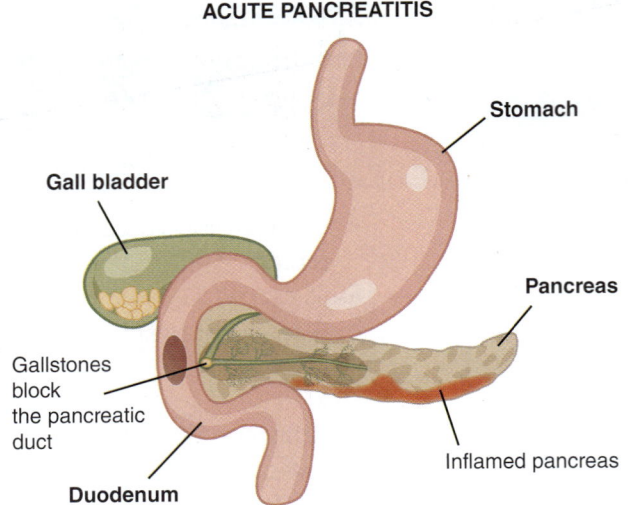

FIGURE 12.5 Acute Pancreatitis is Represented here as the Result of Gallstones Blocking the Pancreatic Duct

The enzymes released by the destroyed cells eventually move into circulation, to be later detected by elevated serum amylase and lipase levels. Patients typically present clinically with abdominal pain that may radiate to the back, nausea, vomiting, and steatorrhea.[25, 27-29]

A clinical diagnosis is made upon admission based on the presence of at least two of the following three criteria:

1. Sudden onset of abdominal pain characteristic of AP
2. Serum amylase and/or lipase levels three (or more) times the upper limit of normal values
3. Findings characteristic of AP on abdominal imaging studies (contrast-enhanced computed tomography, magnetic resonance imaging, or transabdominal ultrasound)

Additionally, although the vast majority of AP cases resolve without causing significant harm, it is not uncommon for immune system involvement to extend beyond the pancreas and trigger a systemic inflammatory response. The 15% of patients who develop multi-organ involvement and/or pancreatic necrosis within the first 72 hours of diagnosis have prolonged hospital stays, as well as significant increases in morbidity and mortality.[25,29]

Classification Once AP is determined as the definitive diagnosis, a scoring system is then used to classify the severity of the disease state. Of the many classification tools available, most consider both the level of systemic inflammation and the level of extra-pancreatic organ dysfunction. Although there are a number of useful systems—including Ranson's Criteria, APACHE II, and BISAP—the newly revised Atlanta classification is the most applicable system in the clinical setting. Under this method, clinical severity is stratified into three categories: mild, moderate, and severe. The revised Atlanta clarification is described in more detail in **Table 12.5**.[29,30]

If the patient improves rapidly without organ failure or systemic complications, the disease falls into the mild AP category. If local or systemic complications arise, but cannot be classified as persistent (lasting more than 48 hours), the disease is defined as moderate AP. Finally, if persistent

TABLE 12.5 REVISED ATLANTA CLASSIFICATION SYSTEM WITH CLINICAL IMPLICATIONS

	Revised Atlanta Classification (2012)	Implications
Mild	• No organ failure • No systemic inflammation or local complications	• Typically does not require abdominal imaging • Frequently discharged within 3 to 7 days of onset of illness
Moderate	• Transient organ failure (defined as organ failure lasting <48 hours) • Local systemic complications without persistent organ failure (>48 hours)	• Organ failure includes respiratory, cardiovascular, and renal failure • Local complications include interstitial pancreatitis and necrotizing pancreatitis • May require a longer hospital stay • Typically associated with a higher mortality rate
Severe	• Persistent organ failure (>48 hours)	• Persistent organ failure may affect single or multiple organs • Patients with persistent organ failure usually present with one or more local complications • Associated with increased risk of death (mortality reported to be as great as 50%)

Data from Banks PA, Bollen TL, Dervenis C, et al. Classification of acute pancreatitis—2012: revision of the atlanta classification and definitions by international consensus. Gut. 2013;62(1):102-111.

organ failure affecting single or multiple organ(s) occurs, the disease is regarded as severe AP and is associated with high morbidity and mortality rates.[25,30] Classification guides provide guidance for determining the best course of treatment. When the Atlanta system is used, the mild, moderate, and severe classifications help determine the necessary extent of dietary intervention. Most notably, these levels provide the most reliable indication of patients who will require nutrition support.[25,29]

Treatment The primary treatment for AP involves early, aggressive fluid resuscitation and pain treatment immediately upon admission. The treatment plan will also provide management of respiratory and renal function; treatment of infection; and, when warranted, nutrition support.[25,28,30] For an AP patient, it is absolutely critical to prevent stimulation of the pancreas and thus reduce the release of its digestive secretions. Pancreatic rest is accomplished through the implementation of **NPO** (*nil per os*, or nothing by mouth) status; without food entering the digestive tract, there is no trigger prompting pancreatic stimulation.[28]

Pancreatitis represents a highly catabolic state in body.[29] For the majority of patients, this is not terribly concerning, as mild AP will have little impact on metabolism or nutritional status.[26] In addition, oral intake is typically restored within 3 to 5 days of hospitalization, when the symptoms of nausea, vomiting, and abdominal pain resolve.[25,29] Past studies have suggested feedings should begin first with clear liquids and progress to foods as tolerated.[27,29] However, the 2016 ASPEN guidelines recommend patients with mild disease advance to a normal diet rather than a clear liquid diet initially, as this has been shown to decrease hospital length of stay.[31]

Patients classified with severe AP have elevated nutrition needs as a result of increased energy expenditure and high protein catabolism rates.[26] Nutrition support is recommended early in the course of the disease. When initiated within the first 48 hours, enteral nutrition (EN) has been shown to improve overall outcomes in these patients.[28,29]

Nutrition Support Nutrition support is indicated for all patients with severe necrotizing pancreatitis and in more moderate cases if oral nutrition is not possible due to pain or other symptoms after more than 5 days.[26] EN is preferred over parenteral nutrition (PN) because it is associated with reduced infectious and systemic complications and hospital length-of-stay, and is less expensive.[29,32] In addition, strong evidence suggests that the risks of multi-organ failure and mortality are significantly less for patients given EN when compared to those receiving PN.[32]

Both the American Society for Parenteral and Enteral Nutrition (A.S.P.E.N.) and the European Society for Parental and Enteral Nutrition (E.S.P.E.N.) emphasize that there are no specific contraindications for EN use in the clinical setting. Position statements from both societies confirm that tube feeding can be executed successfully even when severe AP is accompanied by complications such as pseudocysts, ascites, and/or **fistulas**, which are abnormal passages or connections between two body parts.[26,32] Most patients tolerate standard polymeric intact protein enteral formulas although a peptide based, MCT oil containing formula may be indicated if significant maldigestion is present.[28,31]

The recommendation for route of EN is slightly controversial. Some clinicians feel that nasojejunal (NJ) tube placement is superior to nasogastric (NG) tube placement because it provides greater pancreatic rest (see **Figure 12.6**).[29] However, substantial evidence indicates that NG feeding—which is simpler, less expensive, and easier to implement—is equally as effective as NJ feeding for patients with severe AP.[27,32-35] Regardless of the route implemented, the timing of EN support is also considered important. When started within the first 48 hours of admission, EN may reduce the risk of multi-organ involvement and infection.[25,32] However this is not a consistent finding, and requires further study.

In some cases, EN may need to be supplemented with or replaced by PN. Although associated with greater complications, PN is associated with a lower risk of death than if no supplementary nutrition is provided. This route is indicated only for patients unable to tolerate the EN route or when complications to the digestive tract render EN administration impossible.[25,26,36]

Oral feeding can be attempted once symptoms normalize, if it does not result in pain or further complications. This typically begins with initiation of liquids, then a low-fat solid diet, progressing to a more normalized intake as tolerated. EN or PN feedings may be gradually weaned as oral intake improves over time.[26,28]

> **PRACTICE POINT**
>
> Enteral nutrition, whether via a nasogastric or nasojejunal route, is the preferred method of nutrition support for patients with severe acute pancreatitis and should be started within 48 hours of admission. Energy requirements are approximately 25 to 35 kcal/kg/day with protein requirements between 1.2 g and 1.5 g protein/kg/day.

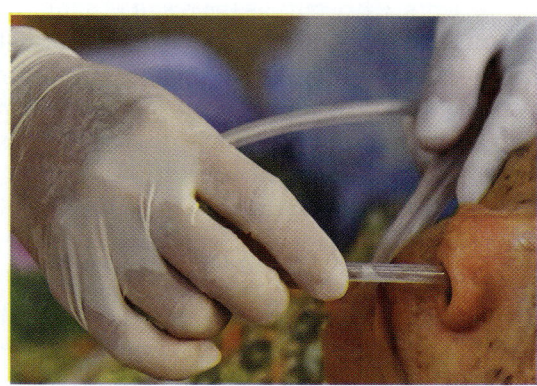

FIGURE 12.6 Placement of Nasogastric Tube for Feeding During Acute Pancreatitis
© Anukool Manoton/Shutterstock.

> ## ⚠ Clinical Controversy
>
> ### Early versus Delayed Enteral Feeding in Acute Pancreatitis
>
> A recent meta-analysis by Yao et al. confirms that enteral nutrition (EN) is associated with lower mortality (RR = 0.36, 95%; CI = 0.20-0.65, P = 0.001) and rate of multiple organ failure (RR = 0.39, 95% CI 0.21-0.73, P = 0.003). EN during acute pancreatitis is the optimal mode of feeding these critically ill patients and may even alter the course of this inflammatory condition if provided early. Recently, Jin et al. demonstrated that EN when given within 72 hours of onset was associated with reduced secondary infections and improved serum albumin. However, this is in contrast to a systematic review by Vaughn et al. One study reported in that review, by Bakker et al., found no benefit to early EN as compared to resumption of an oral diet after 72 hours. Similarly, Stimac et al. demonstrated no benefit to early nasojejunal EN when compared to no intervention with EN. Because nutrition support is so important in acute pancreatitis, determining the optimal timing of initiation is important.
>
> Read the supporting review articles and the difference in original works described above. Compare study design and findings. What would your recommendation be regarding the timing of EN in acute pancreatitis?
>
> ### References
>
> 1. Yao H, He C, Deng L and Liao G. Enteral versus parenteral nutrition in critically ill patients with severe pancreatitis: a meta-analysis. *Eur J Clin Nutr.* 2017; doi:10.1038/ejcn.2017.139.
> 2. Jin M, Zhang H, Lu B, Li Y, Wu D, Qian J, Yang H. The optimal timing of enteral nutrition and its effect on the prognosis of acute pancreatitis: apropensity score matched cohort study. Pancreatology. 2017;17(5):651-657.
> 3. Vaughn, VM; Shuster, D Mary Rogers, AM, Mann, J Conte, ML, Saint, S, Chopra, V. Early versus delayed feeding in patients with acute pancreatitis A Systematic Review. *Ann Intern Med.* 2017;166:883-892. doi:10.7326/M16-2533.
> 4. Stimac D, Poropat G, Hauser G, Licul V, Franjic N, Valkovic Zujic P, et al. Early nasojejunal tube feeding versus nil-by-mouth in acute pancreatitis: a randomized clinical trial. *Pancreatology.* 2016;16:523-8.
> 5. Bakker OJ, van Brunschot S, van Santvoort HC, Besselink MG, Bollen TL, Boermeester MA, et al. Dutch Pancreatitis Study Group. Early versus on-demand nasoenteric tube feeding in acute pancreatitis. *N Engl J Med.* 2014;371:1983-93.

Chronic Pancreatitis

The hallmark of chronic pancreatitis (CP) is progressive, long-standing inflammation of the pancreas leading to fibrosis and gradual loss of both exocrine and endocrine functions. CP presents as one of two recognized forms—small-duct or large-duct—and can take several years to develop. However, the disease is complex and pathogenesis is controversial. The most common cause, responsible for upwards of 80% of cases, is excessive alcohol consumption. However, there are a number of other contributing factors. For many patients, CP occurs as the result of a mixture of environmental factors (alcohol abuse, tobacco use, suboptimal nutrition, and/or occupational chemical exposure) and genetic predisposition. In addition, CP may accompany a hereditary conditions or autoimmune disease. Approximately 20% of cases are classified as idiopathic.[28,37-39]

For all patients with CP, the continuous inflammation causes irreversible damage. Fibrous tissue replaces the normal parenchyma of the pancreas and results in the loss of islets and acinar cells. The resulting loss of function manifests as diabetes mellitus (type 3c) and/or as decline in pancreatic exocrine function in varying degrees, respectively. These changes to pancreatic structure wreak havoc on the normal digestion and absorption of nutrients. In addition, almost all patients with CP report significant upper abdominal pain that may radiate to the back. See **Table 12.6** for the most common clinical presentations of CP.[28,37-40]

Medical and Nutrition Therapy of Clinical Features All treatment of CP begins with conservative, noninvasive measures for pain control and nutrition management to correct the consequences of exocrine insufficiency. This will include counseling against any exacerbating factors. Patients should receive thorough education on abstinence from alcohol, smoking cessation, and limiting excessive dietary fat. More extreme measures, including endoscopic treatment or surgical intervention, are only considered when conventional therapy fails to control pain or other complications.[28,38] The therapy required by each of the primary complications will be discussed in detail in the following sections.

Abdominal Pain Almost all patients with CP experience debilitating abdominal pain. It serves as the primary reason many seek initial medical care, but it is also the most difficult to correct. This type of pain typically worsens postprandially, especially following the consumption of a high-fat meal. Both recurrent and continuous abdominal pain are associated with decreased appetite, weight loss, and eventual malnutrition.[37,38,41]

TABLE 12.6 CLINICAL FEATURES OF CHRONIC PANCREATITIS[37,38]

Abdominal Pain	• In upper abdomen, may radiate to the back • Exacerbated by eating and/or drinking (especially alcohol) • **Type A Pain:** recurrent episodic pain • **Type B Pain:** continuous pain
Pancreatic Exocrine Insufficiency (PEI)	• Maldigestion • Steatorrhea • Weight loss
Diabetes Mellitus (DM)	• Type 3c diabetes mellitus • Endocrine hormone deficiencies – Insufficient glucagon and insulin
Rare Complications	• Pseudocysts • Splenic vein thrombosis • Nausea and vomiting • Jaundice • Pale, clay-colored stools

Data from 37. Afghani E, Sinha A, Singh VK. An overview of the diagnosis and management of nutrition in chronic pancreatitis. Nutr Clin Pract. 2014;29(3):295-311; and Berberat PO, Ceyhan GO, Dambrauskas Z, Büchler MW, Friess H. Chronic pancreatitis. In: Textbook of clinical gastroenterology and hepatology. Wiley-Blackwell; 2012:525-532.

Although abdominal pain may be corrected interventionally or surgically, the first line of treatment is always non-narcotic analgesics and/or nonsteroidal anti-inflammatory agents for pain relief. For those with severe pain that does not subside after initial intervention, narcotic analgesics are prescribed; most will require this route for pain management. Because medical therapy is largely ineffective, many patients ultimately require endoscopic or surgical treatment. Surgical procedures indicated by intractable abdominal pain involve drainage and/or resection and will be discussed later in the chapter.[37,38] Interestingly, there is strong evidence that exogenous enzymes supplementation for pancreatic insufficiency can be used to treat pain in CP patients. The mechanism by which enzyme therapy alleviates pain is thought to occur through a reduction in pancreatic secretions and thus ductal pressure.[37,41]

Pancreatic Exocrine Insufficiency The primary nutritional concern for patients with CP is maldigestion due to deficiency of pancreatic enzymes. Pancreatic exocrine insufficiency (PEI) formally defined as a reduction in pancreatic enzyme activity below the threshold necessary for normal digestion, is directly related to destruction of acinar cell mass and the associated decrease in levels of the enzymes lipase, amylase, and trypsin.[37,42]

The most common and reliable indication of exocrine insufficiency is bulky, foul-smelling stools indicative of excess excretion of fat. As pancreatic lipase is responsible for 90% of all lipid digestion, PEI is primarily associated with maldigestion of fat leading to steatorrhea. Decreased secretion of amylase impacts carbohydrate metabolism and may lead to starch excretion in the feces (**amylorrhea**), abdominal distention, and/or flatulence. In addition, the loss of pancreatic trypsin leads to maldigestion of protein, which can manifest as edema, ascites, and/or **azotorrhea** (excess nitrogen in the urine or feces). However, because the body has additional mechanisms for carbohydrate and protein breakdown that do not require pancreatic enzymes, fat maldigestion remains the primary concern. Any maldigestion and subsequent malabsorption can cause unintentional weight loss, micronutrient deficiencies, and malnutrition. Early diagnosis of PEI is crucial in order to prevent or reduce these complications.[28,37,38]

The vast majority of patients can be managed by dietary interventions to reduce steatorrhea and supplement calories. This generally includes maintenance of adequate intake, with the highest level of fat that will not result in steatorrhea or abdominal pain. Most importantly, all patients with PEI will benefit from supplementation with exogenous **pancreatic enzyme replacement therapy** (PERT). Nutrition therapy will focus on alleviating PEI-related symptoms, limiting both weight loss and micronutrient deficiencies, and, above all, preventing malnutrition.[37,38,42,43]

Pancreatic Enzyme Replacement Therapy The best way to improve the nutritional status of a patient with PEI is by initiating PERT immediately upon diagnosis. Supplementation with exogenous pancreatic enzymes is associated with alleviation of symptoms (steatorrhea and abdominal pain) and improvement in body weight; in addition, because the enzymes are safe, well tolerated, and easy to administer, PERT has become the gold standard of treatment for the maldigestion associated with CP.[28,38,41,43]

Pancreatic enzymes with each oral feeding ensure adequate digestion and absorption, allowing patients with PEI to consume a regularly normal diet without consequence. **Pancreatic enzyme preparations** (PEP), called pancrelipase or pancreatin, contain a mixture of the digestive enzymes amylase, lipase, and protease. The enteric-coated tablets are taken orally and designed to withstand the acidic environment of the stomach to prevent denaturation of the enzymes before reaching the duodenum.[28,41,43,44] Refer to **Table 12.7** for a more detailed list of PEP.

Administration dose should be individualized per patient and per meal, according to body weight, severity of exocrine insufficiency, and fat composition of food. Initial dosage usually includes 20,000 units of lipase, but most patients require between 25,000 and 75,000 units per meal; generally approximately 2,000 units of lipase are needed per gram of fat.[37,41] While correct dosing allows for optimal digestion in the gut lumen, timing of administration is

TABLE 12.7 PANCREATIC ENZYME PREPARATIONS (PEP) APPROVED FOR USE[37,41,45]

- Creon
  - Enteric
  - Delayed-release capsule
- Zenpep
  - Enteric
  - Delayed-release capsule
- Pancreaze
  - Enteric
  - Delayed-release capsule
- Ultresa
  - Enteric
  - Delayed-release capsule
- Pertzye
  - Enteric
  - Delayed-release capsule
- Viokace
  - Nonenteric*
  - Tablet

*Primarily used for pain treatment.
Data from Afghani E, Sinha A, Singh VK. An overview of the diagnosis and management of nutrition in chronic pancreatitis. Nutr Clin Pract. 2014;29(3):295-311; Muniraj T, Aslanian HR, Farrell J, Jamidar PA. Chronic pancreatitis, a comprehensive review. part II: Diagnosis, complications, and management. Dis Mon. 2015;61(1):5-37; and U.S. Food and Drug Administration. Updated questions and answers for healthcare professionals and the public: Use an approved pancreatic enzyme product (PEP). FDA Drug Safety and Availability Web site. http://www.fda.gov/Drugs/DrugSafety/PostmarketDrugSafetyInformationforPatientsandProviders/ucm204745.htm#q3. Published May 17, 2012. Updated 2012. Accessed January 31, 2016.

equally as important. Enzymes must be taken to facilitate interaction with both nutrients and the intestinal lumen at the same time. There is evidence that the optimal timing of PEP dosing in relation to food consumption with pancreatitis is during and after a meal, and not prior (which is the standard with PERT therapy in cystic fibrosis).[37,44]

When administered in the correct dose and with correct timing, PERT will aid in the digestion of fats, protein, and carbohydrates; increase absorption of micronutrients; alleviate steatorrhea; and help to maintain normal nutritional status for patients with PEI.[37]

> **PRACTICE POINT**
>
> Every patient with PEI should be treated with pancreatic enzyme replacement therapy (PERT). A dose ranging from 20,000 to 75,000 USP units of lipase per meal and about half of that amount (~20,000 USP units) per snack should be initiated. The most important parameter for monitoring success is body weight.

Nutrient Deficiency and Malnutrition Patients with CP, especially those also diagnosed with PEI, are at increased risk for nutrient deficiency and malnutrition as a result of maldigestion, malabsorption, and poor oral intake. Because the etiology for most cases of CP is chronic alcoholism, many patients enter the disease state with an already-impaired nutritional status.[46] The development and severity of malnutrition is two-fold. First, maldigestion and malabsorption force the body to deplete its energy and nutrient stores. Second, there is increased metabolic activity as a result of the disease process; patients with CP have resting energy expenditure 30% to 50% above normal.[37,40]

Thorough nutritional screening will identify all patients at risk for nutrient deficiencies and malnutrition. The major cause—maldigestion of macronutrients—is corrected in large part by the initiation of PERT. However, nutrition interventions must ensure sufficient intake to meet the increased caloric needs of the patient. Typically, a diet providing at least 35 kcal/kg of body weight/day through small, frequent meals will meet the energy demands of CP. Most patients will not require a fat restriction due to supplementation with exogenous pancreatic enzymes; however, if fat intake is not fully tolerated, MCTs can be added to the diet without exacerbation because they do not require lipase for digestion.[28,37,40]

Nutrition therapy for patients with CP must always include monitoring for and repletion of any micronutrient deficiencies. Nutrients of concern are primarily the fat-soluble vitamins A, D, E, and K; deficiency of these vitamins correlates directly with severity of steatorrhea, but may also be the result of suboptimal intake. Increased losses and malabsorption may also contribute to deficiencies of vitamin B_{12}, calcium, zinc, magnesium, copper, folate, and/or thiamin.[28,37,40,46]

More than 80% of patients with CP can be treated adequately with normal oral food intake and pancreatic enzymes. Approximately 10% to 15% may require additional calories and protein through an oral nutritional supplement. Tube feeding is indicated in only 5% of patients with CP, and fewer than 1% will need nutrition support through PN.[26,37]

> **PRACTICE POINT**
>
> It is critical to provide adequate protein (1.2-1.5 g protein/kg/day) and energy intake (35 kcal/kg/day) to meet the increased demands of CP and prevent the development of malnutrition.

> **CORE CONCEPT 6**
>
> Acute pancreatitis and chronic pancreatitis differ substantially in their respective nutritional requirements. For both disease states, however, it is crucial to provide sufficient energy to meet increased needs, adapt care plans in regard to individual symptoms, and intervene with nutrition support when necessary.

Pancreatic Surgery

Pancreatic procedures that alter the GI anatomy are massively complex and associated with a number of surgical complications and debilitating nutritional implications postoperatively. Surgery of this nature is indicated in one of two cases: to treat pancreatic malignancies or when pain management in CP cannot be controlled through noninvasive treatment.[47] See Table 12.8 for the common CP complications that require surgical intervention.

There are two primary categories of procedures used for patients with pancreatitis: those that involve decompression (or drainage) and those that involve resection. A growing area of surgical intervention combines the two mechanisms. See Table 12.9 for the most frequently used techniques. Regardless of the method, the goal for surgical intervention is first, to eliminate pain and second, to preserve as much of the pancreatic anatomy as possible.[38,47]

As with any procedure, patients require postoperative nutrition care to prevent or decrease potential for surgical complications. In addition, because of the altered digestive anatomy and changes to normal pancreatic function, patients are subject to delayed gastric emptying, fat malabsorption, and hyperglycemia. For many patients, early satiety and poor appetite lead to decreased oral intake, further compromising nutrition status. Significant unintended weight loss is common following surgical intervention. Finally, as a result of the preexisting disease state that necessitated the intervention, many patients have poor nutritional status long before surgical intervention. Each implication culminates to considerable risk for malnutrition.[47]

Nutrition Implications Disruption to the anatomy of the digestive system has a substantial impact on normal digestive and absorptive processes.[47] Many of the associated complications will look similar to those seen in patients in the postoperative period for gastric surgery. Here, it will be helpful to consider the instrumental role of pancreatic exocrine and endocrine functions for utilization of nutrients, as well as the implications of involving the small intestine in reconstructive procedures, when studying the nutritional implications of pancreatic surgery. For example, note that a large number of patients with CP also suffer from PEI preoperatively. The disruption to pancreatic structure that occurs during

TABLE 12.8 INDICATIONS FOR SURGICAL INTERVENTION IN CHRONIC PANCREATITIS[37,38,47]

Chronic Abdominal Pain	• Pain does not resolve with conservative medical treatment • Prolonged medication use results in narcotic dependency
Obstruction	• Common bile duct and/or pancreatic duct obstruction • Duodenal obstruction • Portal and/or splenic vein obstruction
Malignancies	• Mass lesion in pancreatic head • Suspected pancreatic cancer
Pancreatic Complications	• Ductal rupture • Persistent or symptomatic pseudocyst • Pancreatic fistula unresponsive to other therapy • Pancreatic ascites unresponsive to medical therapy

"Data from Afghani E, Sinha A, Singh VK. An overview of the diagnosis and management of nutrition in chronic pancreatitis. Nutr Clin Pract. 2014;29(3):295-311; Berberat PO, Ceyhan GO, Dambrauskas Z, Büchler MW, Friess H. Chronic pancreatitis. In: Textbook of clinical gastroenterology and hepatology. Wiley-Blackwell; 2012:525-532. Accessed 1/23/2016 11:41:00 AM. 10.1002/9781118321386.ch70; and Berry AJ. Pancreatic surgery: Indications, complications, and implications for nutrition intervention. Nutr Clin Pract. 2013;28(3):330-357."

TABLE 12.9 COMMON METHODS FOR PANCREATIC PROCEDURES[38,47]

Drainage Procedures	• Pancreaticojejunostomy – Puestow procedure – Partington-Rochelle procedure • Reduce intra-pancreatic pressure by draining the main pancreatic duct • Prevent the loss of pancreatic function by preserving pancreatic tissue
Procedures Involving Resection	• Pancreaticoduodenectomy – Classic Whipple procedure (see Figure 12.7) – Pylorus-preserving procedure – Left pancreatic resection • Indications: contracted duct, inflamed pancreatic mass, suspicious of pancreatic carcinoma
Procedures Combining Resection *and* Drainage	• Pancreatic head resection – Duodenum-preserving: Beger operation – Local: Frey operation – Central: Büchler-Farkas operation • Extremely effective for pain management (90% long-term success rate for relief) • Allows for good preservation of pancreatic function

Data from Berberat PO, Ceyhan GO, Dambrauskas Z, Büchler MW, Friess H. Chronic pancreatitis. In: Textbook of clinical gastroenterology and hepatology. Wiley-Blackwell; 2012:525-532. Accessed 1/23/2016 11:41:00 AM. 10.1002/9781118321386.ch70; and Berry AJ. Pancreatic surgery: Indications, complications, and implications for nutrition intervention. Nutr Clin Pract. 2013;28(3):330-357.

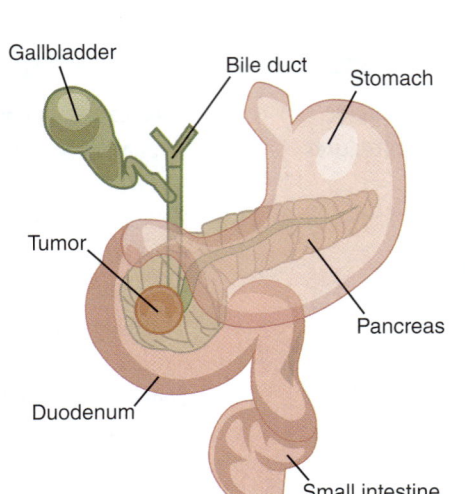
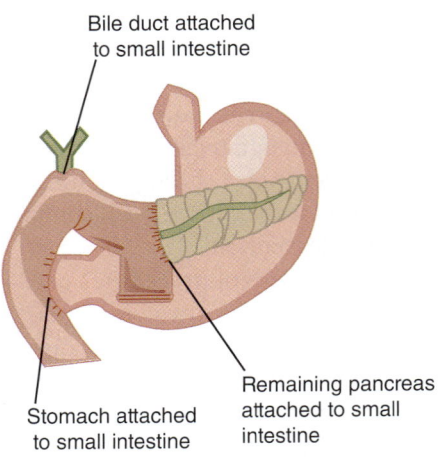

FIGURE 12.7 Pancreaticoduodenectomy Using the Classic Whipple Procedure

surgery does little to remedy the insufficiency—instead, existing conditions will often worsen and a number of new cases will arise.[47] Upwards of 80% of individuals will experience some degree of PEI following pancreatic resection and all will require PERT to achieve normal fat digestion and absorption.[48,49] If unrecognized and untreated, patients are at risk for unintentional weight loss and nutrient deficiencies. In addition, compromising the structural integrity of the pancreas will affect endocrine functions; 20% to 50% of patients develop diabetes from decreased insulin production following surgery and will require thorough education on the management of blood glucose.[50]

The leading cause of postoperative complications for pancreatic surgery patients is delayed gastric emptying (DGE). The exact pathophysiology of DGE is largely unknown, and there are a number of hypothesized causes. Regardless, DGE can have a severe impact on a patient's nutritional status, and can delay initiation of oral feedings and prolong the hospital stay.[47] Symptoms of concern include nausea, vomiting, bloating, early satiety, and abdominal pain.[50] The medical nutrition therapy for these patients is nearly identical to those who experience DGE following gastric resection: maintain intake to meet energy needs through small, frequent meals high in protein and low in solid fats and fiber.[51]

Nutrition Interventions General operative nutrition guidelines recommend small, frequent meals that include protein and limit fat to less than 30% of total caloric intake. In addition, eating slowly and chewing foods thoroughly will help to facilitate proper digestive progresses in the gut. Avoid simple sugars, as well as sugar alcohols, in both foods and drinks. Fluid intake should be limited at mealtime; the majority should occur 30 to 40 minutes postprandially. Finally, early identification and management of malnutrition improves quality of life for postoperative patients; often, interventions include nutrition support in the form of EN and/or PN.[50]

> **CORE CONCEPT 7**
>
> Any changes to the integrity of the GI anatomy will alter function and impact how the body digests and ultimately absorbs nutrients.

Gastroesophageal Reflux Disease

Gastroesophageal reflux disease (GERD) is a common digestive disorder, with estimated prevalence between 10% and 20% in the Western world.[52] Normally, the lower esophageal sphincter opens when food passes from the esophagus to the stomach, and then immediately closes to prevent any food or stomach acid from moving back into the esophagus. **Figure 12.8** shows a relaxed or weakened lower esophageal sphincter, which is now open and allowing reflux to occur.

Typically, symptoms of GERD include heartburn and regurgitation of stomach acid. Other symptoms may include abdominal pain, bad breath, epigastric pressure, cough, sore throat, dental erosions, wheezing, or difficulty swallowing.[52,53] Diagnosis may be made based on history and symptoms, although further testing may be necessary to rule out further complications. Over time, untreated GERD can lead to erosive esophagitis, pulmonary disease, esophageal adenocarcinoma, Barrett's esophagus, and peptic stricture.[52] Treatment can include medication, surgery, and/or nutrition and lifestyle modifications.

Medical and Surgical Treatment Medical treatment of GERD typically involves the use of acid-suppressing medications, such as proton-pump inhibitors (PPIs). This medication is taken 30 to 60 minutes prior to eating a meal to reduce the production of acid in the stomach.[52] If the

CASE STUDY REVISITED

Janice presents for a regularly scheduled follow-up appointment with her surgeon in clinic 3 months later. Although she is very happy with the results of her surgery, she admits to having a problem of nausea and continued acid reflux. After asking about the foods that Janice has been preparing at home, the surgeon asks you, the dietitian, to consult with the patient.

Anthropometric Data:
Current weight: 100 kg (220 lbs)
Preoperative weight: 112 kg (246 lbs)
Height: 165 cm (69")
BMI: 36.7 kg/m^2

Clinical Data:
Medications: Prevacid, Diuril, atorvastatin, vitamin B$_{12}$ (sublingual), vitamin D$_3$, calcium citrate plus vitamin D, multivitamin with minerals
Vital Signs: Blood pressure: 120/76 mm Hg, Temperature: 97.9°F
Nutrition-focused Physical Exam: Patient appears fatigued, but otherwise healthy. Frequently experiencing a dry cough.

Dietary Data:
Dietary History: Janice trying her best to follow a "healthy diet" that was discussed in her preoperative nutrition classes. She admits that when she is rushed at dinnertime, she often chooses a frozen meal with a small glass of chocolate milk before going to bed.
24-hour Diet Recall:
Breakfast (8 am): Carnation instant breakfast with low-fat milk, English muffin with jelly, coffee
Lunch (12 pm): Tuna or turkey sandwich with lettuce, tomato, whole wheat bread, mayonnaise; iced tea.
Dinner (6 pm): Frozen meal or spaghetti with marinara sauce (2 cups), cooked broccoli (1 cup), orange juice (6 oz)

Questions

1. What do you think is the cause of her symptoms?
2. What foods do you tell her may be causing her symptoms, particularly at dinnertime?
3. What other strategies might she incorporate to reduce her acid reflux symptoms?

---

patient's symptoms do not improve with medical therapy, surgical options may be considered.

Surgical intervention can be beneficial for patients who do not have symptom improvement with medication, do not wish to take medication daily, have additional complications such as hiatal hernia or morbid obesity, or show symptoms of continued erosion despite treatment. A **Nissen Fundoplication** is a procedure where the top portion of the stomach is wrapped around the lower esophagus to improve the integrity of the lower esophageal sphincter and reduce reflux.[54] **Figure 12.9** illustrates how the sphincter is now reinforced and tightened. For morbidly obese patients, gastric bypass may be recommended as a treatment for GERD, as Nissen Fundoplication has been shown to be less beneficial in these patients.[52] The Roux-en-Y gastric bypass has been shown to be most favorable in reduction of GERD symptoms as well as other obesity-related comorbidities.

Nutrition Assessment and Intervention When a patient complains of reflux, it is helpful to get a detailed dietary recall in order to assess any potential trigger foods in the diet. Foods that may cause increased reflux include fatty foods, chocolate, alcohol, mint, spicy foods, caffeine, and acidic foods.[53] Consuming smaller, more frequent meals as opposed to larger meals may reduce reflux as well.[53,55]

Accurate anthropometric measurements are also helpful in assessing whether the reflux may be related to obesity, as increasing BMI has been shown to be associated with increasing GERD symptoms. In fact, weight loss of up to 10% has been shown to be effective in reducing chronic medication use and improving the effects of the patient's current PPI.[56,57]

Other than weight loss and avoidance of trigger foods, there are a few other strategies that can help patients improve symptoms. Quitting smoking and wearing

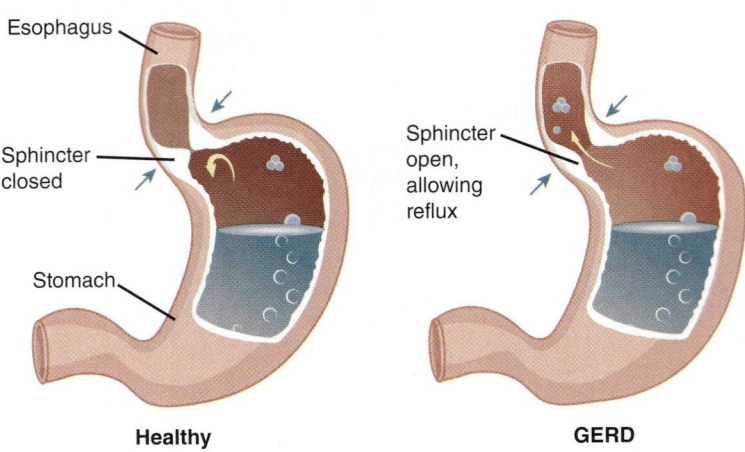

FIGURE 12.8 Gastroesophageal Reflux Disease is Characterised by an Open Esophageal Sphincter, Allowing Reflux into the Esophagus

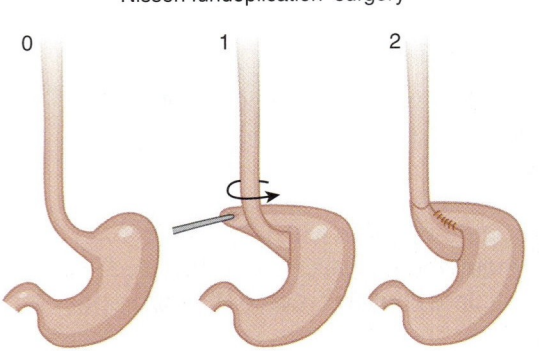

FIGURE 12.9 The Nissen Fundoplication Surgery Wraps the Stomach Around the Lower Esophagus to Improve the Integrity of the Lower Esophageal Sphincter to Reduce Reflux

loose-fitting clothing may be beneficial. Notably, waiting at least 3 hours after eating to lie down and elevating the head of the bed have been shown to decrease reflux.[53] Patients may need instruction on meal timing and meal planning to improve satiety and avoid late night meals and snacks.

CORE CONCEPT 8

GERD is a common condition with various possible medical, surgical, and nutritional treatments. It is important for dietitians to be well versed in the most up-todate treatment options for these patients, individualizing interventions to target the cause of reflux.

Clinical Roundtable

Topic: Nutrition and lifestyle interventions for gastroesophageal reflux disease (GERD)

Background: Frequent GERD symptoms are becoming more common and afflict up to 20% of North Americans. GERD is one of the most common gastro-intestinal disorders, negatively impacting productivity and healthcare costs. Dietary modifications commonly proposed include avoidance of certain foods such as fat, chocolate, alcohol, mint, citrus, tomato, coffee, tea, and large meals. Lifestyle changes include weight reduction and succession of smoking. Pharmacological interventions with acid-reducing medications (antacids) are common, contributing to the financial burden of the disease. In addition, the long-term consequences of GERD on quality of life and health, including the risk of esophageal adenocarcinoma, support the need for better management of this disorder. Unfortunately, individuals with moderate to severe symptoms of GERD commonly follow some (avoiding citrus and tomato products, and certain types of alcohol), but not all dietary modifications. This suggests that progress can be made in lifestyle management techniques. At the same time, lack of adherence to recommended dietary changes is concerning. Furthermore, the combination of weight reduction and smoking cessation may be challenging for many patients. What would be your approach to nonpharmacological management of GERD?

References

1. Kubo1 A, Block G, Quesenberry CP, Buffler P, and Corley DA. Dietary guideline adherence for gastroesophageal reflux disease. *BMC Gastroenterol.* 2014;14:144.

Chapter Summary

Proper digestion is crucial to obtaining adequate levels of nutrients from the foods we eat. Problems with digestion can occur at any point in the GI tract, leading to a wide variety of conditions. Dietitians have the opportunity to take the lead in treatment of theses patients, providing the support they need to maintain their weight and overall nutritional status while dealing with complex diseases. Chapter 13 will continue the discussion of the GI tract, focusing on disorders of absorption.

Key Terms

duodenum, brush border, peristalsis, digestion, absorption, maldigestion, malabsorption, malassimilation, bolus, chyme, selective vagotomy, total vagotomy, pyloroplasty, gastrectomy, anastomosis, gastric stasis, gastroparesis, steatorrhea, medium-chain triglyceride, intrinsic factor, dumping syndrome, NPO, fistula, pancreatic exocrine insufficiency, pancreatic enzyme preparations, amylorrhea, azotorrhea, pancreatic enzyme replacement therapy, gastroesophageal reflux disease (GERD), Nissen Fundoplication

References

1. Joneja JMV. *Digestion, diet, and disease: Irritable bowel syndrome and gastrointestinal function.* New Brunswick, NJ: Rutgers University Press; 2004.
2. Gropper SS, Smith JL. The digestive system: Mechanism for nourishing the body. In: *Advanced nutrition and human metabolism.* 6th ed. Belmont, CA: Wadsworth Cengage Learning; 2013:33-62.
3. Digestive diseases statistics for the United States. U.S. Department of Health and Human Services, National Institute of Diabetes and Digestive and Kidney Diseases. http://www.niddk.nih.gov/health-information/health-statistics/Pages/digestive-diseases-statistics-for-the-united-states.aspx. Updated 2014. Accessed January 22, 2016.
4. Montgomery SC, Williams CM, Maxwell IV PJ. Nutritional support of patient with inflammatory bowel disease. *Surg Clin North Am.* 2015;95(6):1271-1279.
5. Barrett KE. Functional anatomy of the GI tract and organs draining into it. In: *Gastrointestinal Physiology.* 2nd ed. New York, NY: McGraw Hill; 2014.
6. The Pancreas. John Hopkin's University. http://www.pathology.jhu.edu/pancreas/basicoverview1.php?area=ba. Updated 2016. Accessed July 12, 2017.
7. Towers E, Tischler M. *Gastrointestinal Physiology: A Clinical Approach.* Switzerland: Springer International Publishing; 2014.
8. Rogers AI, Madanick RD. Maldigestion and malabsorption. In: *Textbook of Clinical Gastroenterology and Jepatology.* Hoboken, New Jersey; Wiley-Blackwell; 2012:279-287. 10.1002/9781118321386.ch39.
9. WGO practice guideline: Malabsorption. 2015. World Gastroenterology Organization (WGO). http://www.worldgastroenterology.org/guidelines/global-guidelines. Accessed November 26, 2017.
10. Högenauer C, Hammer HF. Maldigestion and malabsorption. In: Feldman M, Friedman LS, Brandt LJ, eds. *Sleisenger and Fordtran's Gastrointestinal and Liver Disease.* 10th ed. Philadelphia, PA: Elsevier, Saunders; 2016:1788-1823.
11. Academy of Nutrition and Dietetics. *Nutrition Care Manual.* Gastric surgery. https://www.nutritioncaremanual.org/topic.cfm?ncm_category_id=1&lv1=5522&lv2=19309&lv3=268431&ncm_toc_id=268431&ncm_heading=Nutrition%20Care. Accessed November 26, 2017.
12. Jamieson GG, Devitt P, Coventry BJ. Gastric surgery. In: Coventry BJ, ed. *Upper abdominal surgery: Complications, risks and consequences.* London, UK: Springer; 2014:43-80.
13. Nelms MN. Diseases of the upper gastrointestinal tract. In: Nelms M, Sucher KP, Lacey K, Roth SL, eds. *Nutrition Therapy & Pathophysiology.* 2nd ed. Belmont, CA: Brooks/Cole CENGAGE Learning; 2011:340-375.
14. Rogers C. Postgastrectomy nutrition. *Nutr Clin Pract.* 2011;26(2):126-136.
15. Jones J. Gasroparesis. *Today's Dietitian.* 2014;16(7):16.
16. Marcason W. What are the dietary guidelines following bariatric sugery? *J Am Diet Assoc.* 2004;104(3):487-488.
17. St-Onge M, Jones PJH. Physiological effects of medium-chain triglycerides: Potential agents in the prevention of obesity. *J Nutr.* 2002;132(3):329-332.
18. O'Donnell K. Small but mighty: Selected micronutrient issues in gastric bypass patients. *Pract Gastroenterol.* 2008;XXXII(5):37-48.
19. Shikora SA, Kim JJ, Tarnoff ME. Nutrition and gastrointestinal complications of bariatric sugery. *Nutr Clin Pract.* 2007;22:29-40.
20. Handzlik-Orlik G, Holecki M, Orlik B, Wylezol M, Dulawa J. Nutrition management of the post-bariatric surgery patient. *Nutr Clin Pract.* 2015;30(3):383-392.
21. Ukleja A. Dumping syndrome: Pathophysiology and treatment. *Nutr Clin Pract.* 2005;20(517):525.
22. Academy of Nutrition and Dietetics. *Nutrition Care Manual.* Client Education Material. Gastric surgery nutrition therapy. 2015. https://www.nutritioncaremanual.org/client_ed.cfm?ncm_client_ed_id=167. Accessed November 26, 2017.
23. Braga M, Gianotti L, Gentilini O, Liotta S, Di Carlo V. Feeding the gut after digestive surgery: Results of a nine-year experience. *Clin Nutr.* 2002;21(1):69-65.
24. Collene AL, Hertzler S. Metabolic outcomes of gastric bypass. *Nutr Clin Pract.* 2003;18:136-140.
25. Lankisch PG, Apte M, Banks PA. Acute pancreatitis. *Lancet.* 2015;386(9988):85-96.
26. Meier R, Ockenga J, Pertkiewicz J, et al. ESPEN guidelines on enteral nutrition: Pancreas. *Clin Nutr.* 2006;25(2):275-284.
27. Petrov M, S., McIlroy K, Grayson L, Phillips ARJ, Windsor JA. Early nasogastric tube feeding versus nil per os in mild to moderate acute pancreatitis: A randomized controlled trial. *Clin Nutr.* 2013;32(5):697-703.
28. Academy of Nutrition and Dietetics. *Nutrition Care Manual.* Pancreatitits. https://www.nutritioncaremanual.org/topic.cfm?ncm_category_id=1&lv1=5522&lv2=19869&lv3=268935&ncm_toc_id=268935&ncm_heading=Nutrition%20Care. Accessed November 25, 2017.
29. Papachristou G, Singh V, Whitcomb DC. Acute pancreatitis. In: *Textbook of clinical gastroenterology and hepatology.* Hoboken, New Jersey: Wiley-Blackwell; 2012:518-524.
30. Banks PA, Bollen TL, Dervenis C, et al. Classification of acute pancreatitis—2012: revision of the atlanta classification and definitions by international consensus. *Gut.* 2013;62(1):102-111.
31. McClave S, Taylor B, Martindale R, et al. Guidelines for the Provision and Assessment of Nutrition Support Therapy in the Adult Critically Ill Patient: Society of Critical Care Medicine (SCCM) and American Society for Parenteral and Enteral Nutrition (A.S.P.E.N.). *J Parenter. Enteral. Nutr.* 2016;40(2):185-186.

32. Olah A, Romics Jr. L. Enteral nutrition in acute pancreatitis: A review of the current evidence. *World J Gastroenterol*. 2014;20(43):16123-16131.

33. Kumar A, Singh N, Prakash S, Saraya A, Joshi Y. K. Early enteral nutrition in severe acute pancreatitis: A prospective randomized controlled trial comparing nasojejunal and nasogastric routes. *J Clin Gastroenterol*. 2006;40(5):431-434.

34. Eatock FC, Chong P, Menezes N, et al. A randomized study of early nasogastric versus nasojejunal feeding in severe acute pancreatitis. *Am J Gastroenterol*. 2005;100(2):432-439.

35. Singh N, Sharma B, Sharma M, et al. Evaluation of early enteral feeding through nasogastric and nasojejunal tube in severe acute pancreatitis: A noninferiority randomized controlled trial. *Pancreas*. 2012;41(1):153-159.

36. Gianottia L, Meierb R, Loboc DN, et al. ESPEN guidelines on parenteral nutrition: Pancreas. *Clin Nutr*. 2009;28(4):428-435.

37. Afghani E, Sinha A, Singh VK. An overview of the diagnosis and management of nutrition in chronic pancreatitis. *Nutr Clin Pract*. 2014;29(3):295-311.

38. Berberat PO, Ceyhan GO, Dambrauskas Z, Büchler MW, Friess H. Chronic pancreatitis. In: *Textbook of Clinical Gastroenterology and Hepatology*. Hoboken, New Jersey: Wiley-Blackwell; 2012:525-532. Accessed 1/23/2016 11:41:00 AM. 10.1002/9781118321386.ch70.

39. Braganza JM, Lee SH, McCloy RF, McMahon MJ. Chronic pancreatitis. *Lancet*. 2011;377(9772):1184-1197.

40. Rasmussen HH, Irgun O, Olesen SS, Drewes AM, Holst M. Nutrition in chronic pancreatitis. *World J Gastroenterol*. 2013;19(42):7267-7275.

41. Muniraj T, Aslanian HR, Farrell J, Jamidar PA. Chronic pancreatitis, a comprehensive review. part II: Diagnosis, complications, and management. *Dis Mon*. 2015;61(1):5-37.

42. Muniraj T, Aslanian HR, Farrell J, Jamidar PA. Chronic pancreatitis, a comprehensive review and update. part I: Epidemiology, etiology, risk factors, genetics, pathophysiology, and clinical features. *Dis Mon*. 2014;60(12):530-550.

43. Sikkens ECM, Cahen DL, Kuipers EJ, Bruno MJ. Pancreatic enzyme replacement therapy in chronic pancreatitis. *Best Pract Res Clin Gastroenterol*. 2010;24(3):337-347.

44. Berry AJ. Pancreatic enzyme replacement during pancreatic insufficiency. *Nutr Clin Pract*. 2014;29(3):312-321.

45. U.S. Food and Drug Administration. Updated questions and answers for healthcare professionals and the public: Use an approved pancreatic enzyme product (PEP). FDA Drug Safety and Availability. http://www.fda.gov/Drugs/DrugSafety/PostmarketDrugSafetyInformationforPatientsandProviders/ucm204745.htm#q3. Published May 17, 2012. Accessed January 31, 2016.

46. Duggan SN, Smyth ND, O'Sullivan M, Feehan S, Ridgway PF, Conlon KC. The prevalence of malnutrition and fat-soluble vitamin deficiencies in chronic pancreatitis. *Nutr Clin Pract*. 2014;29(3):348-354.

47. Berry AJ. Pancreatic surgery: Indications, complications, and implications for nutrition intervention. *Nutr Clin Pract*. 2013;28(3):330-357.

48. Domínguez-Muñoz JE. Pancreatic enzyme replacement therapy: Exocrine pancreatic insufficiency after gastrointestinal surgery. *HPB*. 2009;11(Suppl. 3):3-6.

49. Friess H, Michalski CW. Diagnosing exocrine pancreatic insufficiency after surgery: When and which patients to treat. *HPB*. 2009;11(Suppl. 3):7-10.

50. Marcason W. What is the whipple procedure and what is the appropriate nutrition therapy for it? *J Acad Nutr Diet*. 2015;115(1):168.

51. Parrish CR. Nutritional considerations in the patient with gastroparesis. *Gastroenterol Clin North Am*. 2015;44(1):83-95.

52. Badillo R, Francis D. Diagnosis and treatment of gastroesophageal reflux disease. *World J Gastrointest Pharmacol Ther*. 2014;5(3):105-112.

53. Johnson A. *What You Need to Know About GERD*. Academy of Nutrition and Dietetics. http://www.eatright.org. Published June 25, 2015. Accessed July 12, 2017.

54. GERD Surgery. Mayo Clinic. http://www.mayoclinic.org/diseases-conditions/gerd/multimedia/gerd-surgery/img-20006950. Updated 2017. Accessed July 12, 2017.

55. Jarosz M, Taraszewska A. Risk factors for gastroesophageal reflux disease: the role of diet. *Prz Gastroenterol*. 2014;9(5):297-301.

56. de Bortoli N, Guidi G, Martinucci I et al. Voluntary and controlled weight loss can reduce symptoms and proton pump inhibitor use and dosage in patients with gastroesophageal reflux disease: a comparative study. *Dis Esophagus*. 2014;29(2):197-204.

57. Ness-Jensen E, Hveem K, El-Serag H et al. Lifestyle intervention in gastroesophageal reflux disease. *Clin Gastroenterol Hepatol*. 2016;14(2):175-182.

Chapter 13

Nutrition Management of Gastrointestinal Malabsorption

V. Paige Murphy
Rachel Wilkinson

Chapter Outline

Core Concepts
Introduction

Key Mechanisms of Absorption
Medical Nutrition Therapy for Disorders of Absorption

CORE CONCEPTS

1. Celiac disease, once diagnosed, can be managed with careful adherence to the gluten-free diet. This requires extensive patient education and monitoring. Until patients reach an asymptomatic state and the damage is allowed to heal, there are a number of deficiencies and/or intolerances that may occur.

2. There is no set diet recommendation that can be made for patients diagnosed with irritable bowel syndrome (IBS). An individualized plan—ensuring adequate intake while allowing for any patient intolerances—must be put in place.

3. Patients with non-celiac gluten sensitivity (NCGS) may also benefit from a gluten-free diet. Although there is no current best practice guideline for medical nutrition therapy for NCGS, dietitians can help patients create an individualized diet that minimizes the symptoms.

4. Inflammatory bowel disease is associated with a wide range of nutritional implications that center on malnutrition. Adequate intake, whether in the form of nutritional support or oral intake, is required.

5. Careful assessment of the patient's nutritional status and GI symptoms will direct nutritional intervention in leaky gut syndrome, such as limiting alcohol and practicing stress management. Clinicians should be wary of "easy fix" fad diets that patients may be following.

6. Deficiencies in iron, vitamin C, vitamin A, alpha-tocopherol, vitamin B_{12}, folic acid, nickel, and selenium are possible in patients with *H. pylori*. Patients with this infection should be monitored closely for both nutrient deficiency and unintentional weight loss.

7. Small intestinal bacterial overgrowth is often associated with and occurs concurrently with a number of other disorders related to maldigestion and malabsorption. Nutrition therapy plays a critical role in the treatment of this patient population.

8. In surgical resections of the GI tract, the amount of bowel removed and remaining and the location from which the resection is made are key determinants as to whether digestive and absorptive processes can be maintained postoperatively and if prolonged nutrition intervention is necessary.

Learning Objectives

1. Describe the key mechanism of absorption.
2. Identify factors that cause malabsorption.
3. Define the abnormalities leading to celiac disease and their manifestations.
4. Describe medical nutrition therapy for individuals with celiac disease.
5. Explain potential medical nutrition therapy approaches for patients with irritable bowel syndrome.
6. Distinguish key differences between ulcerative colitis and Crohn's disease.
7. Discuss nutritional implications during and following medical treatment for inflammatory bowel disease.
8. Discuss the dietitian's role in treatment of patients with Helicobacter pylori infection.
9. Identify risk of malnutrition and specific deficiencies associated with short bowel syndrome.
10. Recognize the phases of intestinal adaptation to short bowel syndrome and discuss associated medical nutrition therapy.

Introduction

The gastrointestinal (GI) tract functions to both digest and absorb nutrients. This chapter will focus on absorption, which moves digested particles of food from outside the cells into the cells of the GI tract for further utilization. Malabsorption can occur as a result of two things: (1) inadequately digested nutrients are transported or (2) mucosal uptake of nutrients is flawed. Medical nutrition therapy is a key part of treatment for patients with malabsorptive conditions, and registered dietitians have a recognized and important role in implementing these strategies.

Key Mechanisms of Absorption

Absorption Sites

Once food particles have been broken down into their simplest constituents via digestion, these nutrients cross the barrier between the lumen of the GI tract and the internal environment of the body. This is the process of absorption.[1]

Although select components of the digesta are absorbed within the stomach (water, alcohol, and select minerals), the vast majority of absorption occurs in the small intestine. See **Figures 13.1** and **13.2** for a visual representation of absorption sites. Absorptive processes for most micro- and macronutrients begin in the duodenum and continue throughout the middle and distal portions of the small intestine—the **jejunum** and the **ileum**, respectively.[2] Finger-like projections (the villi) of the gut wall

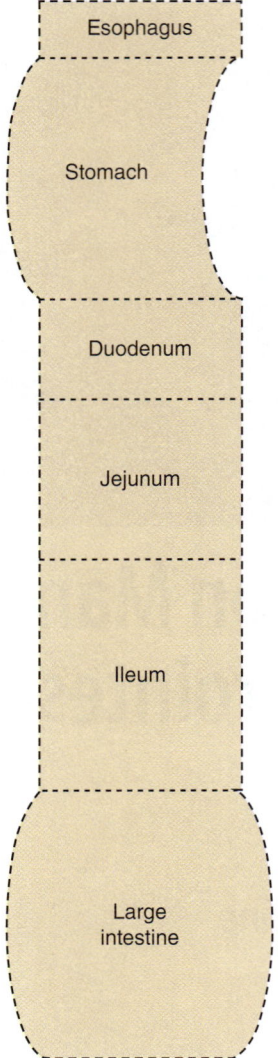

FIGURE 13.1 Absorptive Sites Within the Gi Tract

contain intestinal absorptive cells called **enterocytes**. The mechanism by which nutrients are absorbed into enterocytes depends on a number of factors: (1) the solubility of the nutrient, (2) the concentration or electrical gradient, and (3) the size of the molecule to be absorbed.[2] The majority of food components pass into circulation after binding to transport proteins, crossing the epithelium through the process of diffusion.[1] Other absorption methods include facilitated diffusion and active transport; occasionally, nutrients enter through pinocytosis, endocytosis, or a paracellular route.[2]

The remaining digesta empties from the ileum into the cecum of the large intestine. From there, the matter continues through the ascending, transverse, descending, and sigmoid sections, where colonic epithelial cells work to absorb primarily water, sodium, and chloride. When this process is complete, any unabsorbed materials have been dehydrated to form feces and pass through the distal end of the tract, the anus. Normal defecated material will contain *only* sloughed GI cells; inorganic matter; water; and insignificant amounts of unabsorbed nutrients, constituents of digestive juices, fiber, and bacteria.[1,2]

CASE STUDY INTRODUCTION

Daniel is a 24-year-old male who was referred to the gastroenterology outpatient clinic by his primary care physician. The patient presents with complaints of excessive diarrhea for the past 3 weeks. Daniel contacted his physician when the episode did not respond to over-the-counter anti-diarrheal medications. The following clinical information was taken during his initial appointment.

Anthropometric Data:
Current Weight: 62.8 kg (138 lbs)
Height: 175 cm (69")
BMI: 20.5 kg/m^2
Weight history
UBW: 75 kg (165 lbs)

Biochemical Data:
Sodium 156 (135-145 mEq/L)
Serum osmolality 327 (275-295 mOsm/kg)

Clinical Data:
Past Medical History: none
Medications: Imodium anti-diarrheal caplets OTC
Vital Signs: Blood pressure: 127/83 mm Hg   Temperature: 101.5°F
Nutrition-focused Findings:
Patient appears pale and fatigued. Abdominal exam reveals distention and patient reports pain when mild abdominal pressure applied. Skin is dry, intact and warm to touch; no wounds noted. Oral exam reveals dry mucosa and tongue. No lesions seen. Good dentition noted.

Dietary Data:
Diet History: Typically follows a diet with no restrictions. Patient reports that he has been limiting his intake to "mild, easy to digest" foods to avoid exacerbating the stomach pain and diarrhea.
24-hr Diet Recall:
Breakfast (6:30 am): 1 slice of toast with jelly, coffee with cream.
Lunch(12:30pm): 1 bowl of elbow macaroni (about 1 and 1/2 cups cooked); butter (1 tbs), parmesan cheese (1 tbs).
Dinner (6:30pm): Baked chicken, 1 cup of white rice, 1/2 cup carrots, water.

Questions
1. What are your concerns regarding Daniel's nutritional status?
2. What might explain his sodium and osmolality as measured?
3. What additional information would you request?
4. Based on his symptoms, do you believe that he presents with a disorder associated with maldigestion, malabsorption, or both?

Medical Nutrition Therapy for Disorders of Absorption

Celiac Disease (CD)

Perhaps the most well-understood autoimmune disorder, **celiac disease** (CD) is characterized by inflammatory injury to the intestinal mucosa following gluten ingestion. An inappropriate immune response is triggered by specific sequences of amino acids found in the **prolamin** fractions of wheat, barley, and rye. Of note, CD pathogenesis can only occur in individuals with an incredibly specific genetic profile that includes human leukocyte antigen (HLA)-DQ2 or DQ8 alleles.[3,4]

Damage to the mucosal surface appears in a "patchy," sporadic pattern, most evident in the proximal portion of the small intestine. Structural changes to the normal villous structure flatten the epithelial wall, decreasing the surface area and thus capacity for absorption, as seen in (**Figure 13.3**). As a result, undiagnosed or untreated CD is

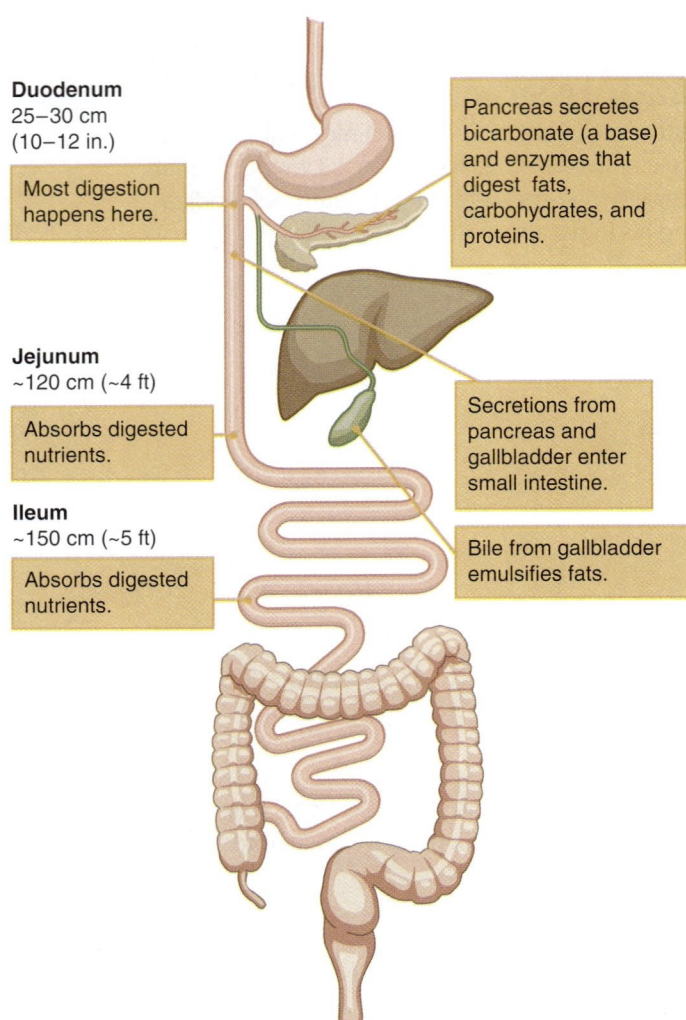

FIGURE 13.2 **The Small Intestine** The Duodenum is Mainly Responsible for Digesting Food; The Jejunum and Ileum Primarily Deal with Absorption of Food. The Duodenum Secretes Mucus, Enzymes, and Hormones Along with Other Digestive Juices from Assisting Organs to Aid Digestion. All Along the Intestinal Walls, Nutrients are Absorbed into Blood and Lymph. Undigested Materials are Passed on to the Large Intestine.

associated with significant malabsorption of both macro- and micronutrients.[3,4]

Diagnostic procedures begin with an initial assessment of serologic values. The highly sensitive and specific immunoglobulin A-transglutaminase assay is the most readily used approach when CD is suspected. Other important measures include tissue transglutaminase, endomysial antibody, and/or deamidated antigliadin peptide. All individuals with positive values will have the diagnosis confirmed by a duodenal biopsy. During the procedure, several specimens are taken to account for the intermittent nature of the disease. CD diagnoses are supported by clinical improvement after a gluten-free diet is implemented.[3,4]

Clinical Manifestations

The clinical manifestations of CD exist on a wide spectrum of both GI and extraintestinal manifestations. See **Figure 13.4** for a list of manifestations by location in the body. Symptoms present in children and adults at similar rates, the severity of which varies greatly among individuals and on the degree of affected intestine, as described in **Table 13.1**. Although there is a classic profile for CD, marked by chronic diarrhea, weight loss, and fatigue, the vast majority of patients present with atypical symptoms and some report no GI symptoms whatsoever.[3,4]

As a result of the broad range of presentations, one of the biggest clinical barriers for patients with CD is misdiagnosis. For more than 50% of new patients, CD is initially undiagnosed or misdiagnosed. Most often, patients will report multiple, mild symptoms common to a number of other GI disorders. Without appropriate serologic testing and/or biopsy procedures, a false conclusion is easy to make. The most common misdiagnosis for patients with CD is irritable bowel syndrome.[3,4]

Nutrition Interventions

The only effective treatment for patients with CD is a lifelong commitment to avoidance of dietary gluten. A strict gluten-free diet (GFD) allows the intestinal mucosa to heal and prevents any future symptoms or complications from occurring. Because as little as 50 mg of gluten per day can cause continued enteropathy, patients with CD require extensive education on foods containing the offensive prolamins of wheat, barley, and rye (gliadin, hordein, and secalin, respectively). See **Table 13.2** for a list of safe and unsafe food sources for individuals following a GFD. In addition, counseling should include information on label reading and cross-contamination. First, gluten is present in many of the ingredients widely used in processed foods. There are a number of nonfood items, including supplements, medications, and make-up such as mascara and lip stick, that can be sources of gluten. Second, the potential for cross-contamination in processing, storage, and transport both in industry and at home is significant. Complete elimination of gluten from the diet is difficult and requires diligence to maintain.[3-5]

Due to the varying degrees of damage that can occur to the small intestine, patients with new diagnoses of CD may present with varying degrees of malabsorption. Many patients present with micronutrient deficiencies—most often as iron, calcium, vitamin D, vitamin B_{12}, and/or folate—which are responsible for the anemias and/or bone disorders many patients experience. Nutrient deficiencies of this kind occur because the proximal portion of the intestine, where CD causes the most significant damage, is the primary location for absorption. In addition to the GFD, all patients with clinical evidence of malabsorption should be supplemented to replete any deficiencies. Many eating patterns within the GFD are also associated with deficiency, depending on the level of patient reliance on processed, low-nutrient-density

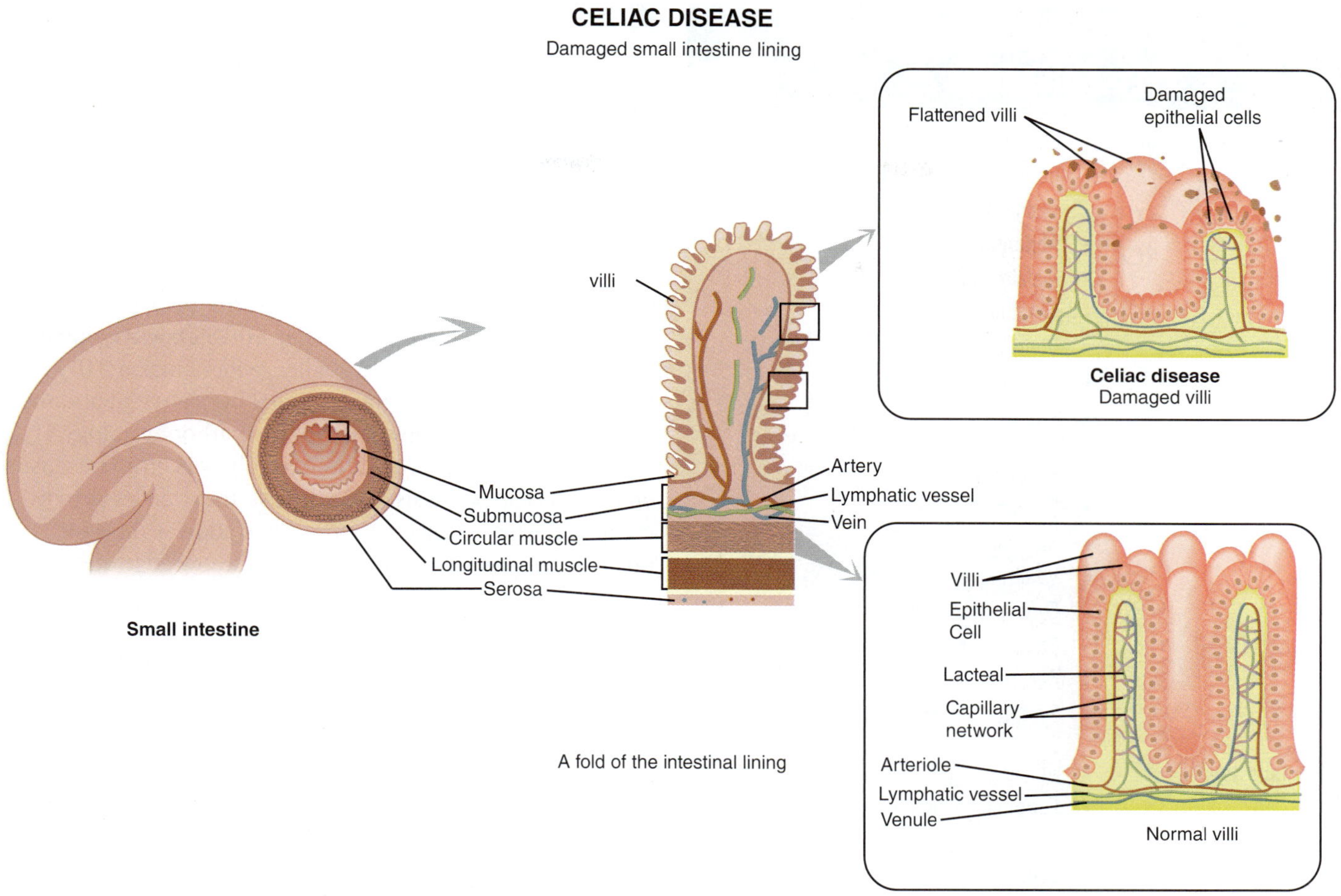

FIGURE 13.3 Structural Changes to the Normal Villous Structure Flatten the Epithelial Wall, Decreasing the Surface Area and Thus Capacity for Absorption

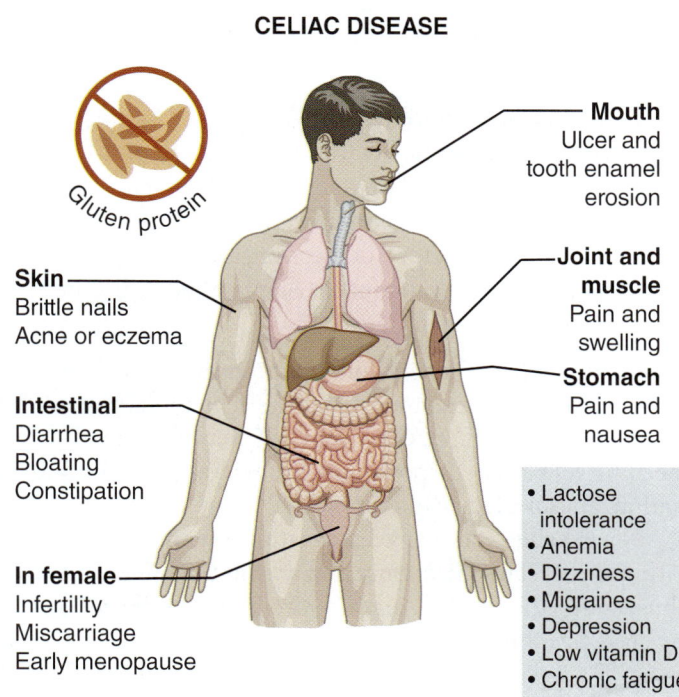

FIGURE 13.4 Manifestations of Celiac Disease by Location in the Body

foods. As most prepacked gluten-free foods are made with refined flours, these products are not enriched with the B vitamins and iron, nor do they provide sufficient amounts of fiber. Patients should be educated on meal planning tips that are both in accordance with the GFD and allow for adequate nutrient intake.[3,4,7,8]

A number of patients with CD also develop with secondary lactose intolerance. For many, the reduced levels of the enzyme lactase are temporary and will regenerate as the GFD allows the intestine to heal. For these individuals, it is beneficial to follow a lactose-free diet until their symptoms have resolved. Given 3 to 6 months of treatment (and thus mucosal repair), dairy products can be reintroduced if tolerated. Vitamin D and calcium levels should be carefully monitored.[3,4,7]

PRACTICE POINT

The gluten-free diet is the only treatment for patients with celiac disease. With careful adherence, most individuals will begin to notice symptomatic improvement within only 48 hours and full clinical remission after 3 to 6 months.

TABLE 13.1 CLINICAL MANIFESTATIONS OF CELIAC DISEASE[3,4]

Classical Presentation	• Chronic diarrhea • Iron-deficiency anemia • Weight loss • Abdominal pain • Malaise and fatigue • Irritability • Depression • Abdominal distention • Anorexia
Gastrointestinal	• Flatulence • Dyspepsia • Bloating • Vomiting • Constipation • Steatorrhea • Recurrent or severe aphthous stomatitis • Symptomatic lactose intolerance
Extraintestinal	• Ataxia • Peripheral neuropathy • Muscle weakness • Sensory loss • Macrocytic anemia (folate deficiency) • Elevated prothrombin time (vitamin K deficiency) • Hypocalcemia • Vitamin D deficiency • Osteopenic bone disease • Arthralgia • Dental enamel defects • Male and female infertility, miscarriage • Malignancies
Superficial	• Short stature • Clubbing • Edema • Dermatitis herpetiformis
Pediatric-Specific	• Impaired growth • Weight faltering (previously failure to thrive) • Delayed puberty • Hypotonia • Behavioral problems, such as poor academic performance

Data from Leffler DA, Cárdenas A, Kelly CP. Celiac disease. In: Textbook of clinical gastroenterology and hepatology. Wiley-Blackwell; 2012:288-298. Accessed 1/23/2016 11:41:00 AM. 10.1002/9781118321386.ch40; and Academy of Nutrition and Dietetics. Celiac disease. Nutrition Care Manual.

> **CORE CONCEPT 1**
>
> Celiac disease, once diagnosed, can be managed with careful adherence to the gluten-free diet. This requires extensive patient education and monitoring. Until patients reach an asymptomatic state and the damage is allowed to heal, there are a number of deficiencies and/or intolerances that may occur.

Irritable Bowel Syndrome (IBS)

As the most frequently diagnosed digestive disorder, yet one of the most complex and controversial, **irritable bowel syndrome** (IBS) presents an interesting challenge for clinicians. IBS is a functional GI disorder characterized by recurrent abdominal pain and altered bowel habit, the pathophysiology of which is only partially understood. There is little consensus on the true pathogenesis of the disease and even less agreement on the best treatment approach to address the wide range of symptoms. It is necessary to acknowledge that the science surrounding IBS continues to evolve.[9,10]

In addition, although there are dietary components to both the manifestations and treatment of the disease, IBS does not fit neatly into a discussion on digestion and absorption. However, nutrition therapy is at the center of current research. Given both the increasingly high prevalence and debate surrounding the syndrome, this chapter would be incomplete without a discussion of IBS.

Fundamentals of IBS

Common etiology indicates that IBS has peak incidence in the 20-year and 30-year age groups; occurs predominantly in females; and is preceded by anxiety, depression, and/or a severe adverse life event in more than half of patients. However, there is no single, agreed-upon cause. Instead, the symptoms of IBS are thought to result from both central brain and peripheral gut abnormalities. Current evidence supports four main contributing factors:

1. Abnormal GI motility
2. **Visceral hypersensitivity** (the experience of pain within the internal organs)
3. Altered brain-gut communication
4. Psychosocial factors: depression, anxiety, and/or **somatization** (complaint of recurrent medical symptoms of unknown cause)

The relationship among irregular gut motility, sensation, and the brain is dependent on the enteric nervous system and its regulation of the GI system. IBS may also be influenced by genetic predisposition, chronic low-grade inflammation, and/or dietary intolerances.[9,11,12]

Bowel habits vary between constipation and diarrhea within the IBS classification, often within the same patient. Thus, an IBS diagnosis is further specific as one the following classifications:

1. IBS-C: Constipation Predominant
2. IBS-D: Diarrhea Predominant

TABLE 13.2 SAFE AND UNSAFE FOODS AND INGREDIENTS FOR THE GLUTEN-FREE DIET[4-6]

Contain Gluten (Unsafe)	Processed Foods that May contain Gluten (Unsafe)	Gluten-Free Foods (Safe)

- Wheat
  - All varieties, including einkorn, emmer, spelt, and kamut
  - Wheat starch, wheat bran, wheat germ, cracked wheat, hydrolyzed wheat protein
- Barley
- Rye
- Triticale (cross-breed of wheat and rye)
- Brewer's yeast
- Dextrin
- Malt
- Modified food starch
- Starch
- Most flour varieties
  - Bromated flour, durum flour, enriched flour, farina, graham flour, phosphated flour, self-rising flour, semolina, white/wheat flour
	- Bouillon cubes
	- Brown rice syrup
	- Candy
	- Chewing gum
	- Communion wafers
	- French fries
	- Gravy varieties
	- Imitation fish
	- Matzo, matzo meal
	- Potato chips
	- Prepared sauces
	- Processed meats
	- Rice mixes
	- Seasoned tortilla chips
	- Soups
	- Soy sauce
	- Vegetables in sauce
		- Amaranth
		- Arrowroot
		- Buckwheat
		- Cassava (manioc)
		- Corn
		- Finger millet (ragi)
		- Flax
		- Legumes
		- Lentils
		- Mesquite
		- Millet
		- Montina
		- Nuts
		- Oats*
		- Potatoes
		- Quinoa
		- Rice
		- Sago
		- Seeds
		- Sorghum
		- Soy
		- Tapioca
		- Teff (or tef)
		- Wild rice
		- Yucca

*Oats are often contaminated by wheat or barley because of growing and processing practices. It is generally recommended that newly diagnosed patients abstain from consuming oats, while all CD patients should purchase oats designated as gluten-free.

Data from Academy of Nutrition and Dietetics. Celiac disease. Nutrition Care Manual; See JA, Kaukinen K, Makharia GK, Gibson PR, Murray JA. Practical insights into gluten free diets. Nat Rev Gastroenterol Hepatol. 2015;12(10):580-591; and National Institute of Diabetes and Digestive and Kidney Disorders. Celiac disease. U.S. Department of Health and Human Services, Health Information Web site. http://www.niddk.nih.gov/health-information/health-topics/digestive-diseases/celiac-disease/Pages/facts.aspx#examples. Published June 2015. Updated 2015. Accessed February 1, 2016.

3. IBS-M: Mixed, Constipation and Diarrhea
4. IBS-U: Unspecific

Individuals may alternate between the classifications over time. However, given the varying classifications and an abundance of additional GI and non-GI symptoms, the presentation of IBS is often confusing and contradictory. Clinicians use the Rome III Diagnostic Criteria, as described in **Table 13.3**, to eliminate differential diagnoses and confirm the presence of IBS. Diagnosis via the Rome III Criteria relies heavily upon the clinical manifestations of IBS.[9,13]

Clinical Presentation

As indicated by the varying classifications of IBS, there is extreme irregularity in terms of bowel habits, frequency, and consistency for this population. Patients will present with constipation, diarrhea, or both, most often accompanied by lower abdominal pain and uncomfortable

TABLE 13.3 ROME III DIAGNOSTIC CRITERIA* FOR IRRITABLE BOWEL SYNDROME[13]

Recurrent abdominal pain or discomfort** at least 3 days per month in the last 3 months associated with *two or more* of the following:
1. Improvement with defecation
2. Onset associated with a change in frequency of stool
3. Onset associated with a change in form (appearance) of stool

*Criteria fulfilled for the last 3 months with symptom onset at least 6 months prior to diagnosis
**Discomfort denotes an uncomfortable sensation not described as pain
Reprinted with permission from the Rome Foundation; all Rights Reserved.
Rome III diagnostic criteria for functional gastrointestinal disorders. Rome III Disorders and Criteria Web site. http://www.romecriteria.org/assets/pdf/19_RomeIII_apA_885-898.pdf. Updated 2006. Accessed February 2, 2016.

distention. Other common GI-related symptoms include incomplete fecal evacuation, straining or difficulty with bowel movements, mucus in the stool, excessive flatulence, urgency, and/or incontinence.[9,12,14]

Episodic abdominal pain is one of the most common physical manifestations seen in IBS and is often the reason individuals seek initial medical consultation. For many, the pain is described as severe and debilitating, but cannot be pinpointed to a specific location. Instead, patients describe bilateral pain in the general abdominal area that often radiates to the back and/or perianal region. Exacerbation of pain is often associated with eating, accompanied by increased urgency of bowel movements following a meal. Pain of this nature may be relieved by defecation, but this is not consistent throughout the IBS population.[12] Many researchers feel that this exhausting pain can be attributed to the initial presentation of visceral hypersensitivity. Theoretically, patients would experience an enhanced sensitivity to colonic distention in the gut, resulting in a reduced threshold for pain.[15]

There is a wide range of non-GI, psychological symptoms seen in patients with IBS. Extraintestinal manifestations are not often associated with other GI disorders, so their presence may help to influence the initial IBS diagnosis. As previously mentioned, anxiety, depression, and somatization are common concurrent conditions. Other non-GI symptoms include medically unexplained headaches; fatigue; lethargy; palpitations; sleep disturbances; and neck, chest, and/or back pain.[9,12]

> **PRACTICE POINT**
>
> Be mindful that because of the strong influence of psychological factors on IBS presentation, there is an unfortunate stigma surrounding the disorder. Many patients are made to feel that the symptoms they experience are simply the result of hypochondriasis. However, both the GI and non-GI symptoms experienced by patients with IBS are very real and can be debilitating.

Treatment

Unfortunately, because of the varying manifestations of IBS, current interventions are not uniformly successful. There are a number of treatments that can be used to minimize symptoms. The most common approach is a combination of pharmacologic, psychosocial, and nutritional therapies. Medication use may include antidiarrheal agents, antispasmodics, antidepressants, and/or selective serotonin reuptake inhibitors, among others, all of which work to control abdominal pain, bloating, or consistency of the stool. The efficacy of pharmacologic intervention is inconsistent and many IBS patients rely on complementary therapies. For example, some individuals will find relief with cognitive behavior therapy or gut-directed hypnotherapy.[9,10,14] Most patients (approximately 70%), however, believe that intolerance to specific foods and/or the overall act of eating is responsible for their symptoms. Diet modifications are extremely prevalent in the IBS population, and nutrition interventions continue to be of interest.[16]

Medical Nutrition Therapy

It is understandable why there is no one specific dietary intervention used in cases of IBS. The varying components of effective nutrition therapy are based on the patient's presenting symptoms, identification of food intolerances and/or potential allergies, and adjustment for energy and nutrient needs. The symptoms of IBS often lead to changes in oral intake, which can subsequently result in nutrient deficiencies, dehydration, and unintentional weight loss.[9] Many different dietary approaches have been utilized in both clinical and academic settings, but few controlled trials exist to support their use. Current recommendations are based on observed effects rather than on scientific evidence.[11]

Based on the subjective association between intake and exacerbation of GI symptoms, patients identify many food items as important triggers. For example, IBS is historically associated with lactose intolerance. Patients may also present with aversions to gluten, caffeine, alcohol, and/or high-fat foods. As a result, nutrition therapy must involve the identification of foods not tolerated. The diet may then be adjusted to allow for a trial elimination of these foods. It is important to closely monitor the patient's presenting symptoms; ongoing elimination diets that are shown to have little impact on symptoms are unnecessary and may ultimately impact nutrition status. There is warranted concern regarding nutritionally inadequate diets in this population.[9,11,12]

Other, more general, nutrition recommendations include normalizing eating patterns and consuming 5 to 6 small meals each day to ensure adequacy of all nutrients. Increasing fiber through whole grains, fresh fruits and vegetables, seeds, and nuts may be beneficial for some patients, but will worsen symptoms in others. If an increase in dietary fiber is favorable, increase fluids accordingly. A low-fat diet is often better tolerated in this population. Patients will also benefit from omitting foods that increase gas and flatulence (for example, beans, cabbage, and onions). Finally, depending on the adequacy of oral intake, it may be necessary to implement a general multivitamin or other micronutrient supplementation in accordance with any identified deficiencies.[9,11,17,18]

Two interventions that have attracted considerable attention recently include implementation of the low FODMAP diet and introduction of probiotics to the diets of IBS patients.[9,12,18] Although no definitive recommendations can be made based on the current evidence, research in both areas continues to progress.

> **CORE CONCEPT 2**
>
> There is no set diet recommendation that can be made for patients diagnosed with irritable bowl syndrome (IBS). An individualized plan—ensuring adequate intake while allowing for any patient intolerances—must be put in place.

Low FODMAP Diet The acronym FODMAP represents Fermentable Oligo-, Di-, and Monosaccharides and Polyols—carbohydrates grouped together based on the length of their chains.[18] Researchers at Monash University in Melbourne,

Australia, theorized that ingestion of any one of the FODMAP constituents would worsen the symptoms of digestive disorders, including IBS, and the **low FODMAP diet** was born (see **Figure 13.5**). Short-chain carbohydrates (FODMAPs) are poorly absorbed by the small intestine and thus pass into the colon, where they can trigger GI symptoms through two separate mechanisms. First, the highly osmotic nature of FODMAPs draws excess fluid into the lumen of the intestine. Second, colonic bacteria rapidly ferment any unabsorbed FODMAPs, inducing gas production. Both occurrences cause luminal distention, contributing to the excess bloating, flatulence, cramping, and diarrhea seen in IBS.[11,18-20]

Oligosaccharides are carbohydrates of 3-10 linked monosaccharide units found in foods as fructans and galactans. They pose an issue for patients with IBS because the human body does not produce the enzymes necessary for their digestion. The specific **disaccharide** (two monosaccharides-linked) of concern is lactose, which is only considered a FODMAP if there is insufficient levels of lactase. Free fructose is a simple sugar (**monosaccharide**); as one of the simplest constituents of carbohydrates, fructose requires no digestion. However, fructose becomes a FODMAP when the amount ingested exceeds that of glucose. In a functioning gut, absorption of fructose would follow an alternative mechanism and there would be little to no issue. However, in individuals with IBS, this route is often impaired, resulting in fructose malabsorption. Finally, **polyols** are sugar alcohols. Finally, the absorption of polyols (or sugar alcohols) across the intestinal barrier is slow; moreover, the gut is capable of absorbing only approximately one-third of what is consumed.[21] See **Table 13.4** for the foods highest in each of the FODMAP constituents.

Research in this area is relatively new and still ongoing. The rationale supported by many studies, however, is that avoidance of foods high in FODMAPs will reduce fermentation and distention in the gut and thus a number of the associated symptoms. Evidence from a number of trials supports the reduction of symptoms in patients with IBS who closely adhere to the low FODMAP diet. The research does not present the low FODMAP diet as a cure, but instead supports its use as the first line of treatment for improving quality of life. However, researchers and clinicians do express some concern with the safety of long-term FODMAP restriction, primarily in regard to the nutritional inadequacies associated with any form of elimination diet. Clinicians recommend a gradual stepwise reintroduction of small amounts of individual FODMAP foods to assess tolerance. The goal is to determine appropriate tolerance amounts so that some FODMAP foods can be consumed in the diet long term. Regardless, the current evidence for the low FODMAP diet presents markedly more strengths than weaknesses with the majority of studies supporting its role in symptom relief for patients with IBS.[9,11,12,18,21,22]

Probiotics **Probiotics** are live microorganisms often sold as dietary supplements or as components of foods (for example, yogurt) that are intended to have health benefits through interaction with the body's normal flora. Research on general probiotic use is still evolving, but there is preliminary evidence that specific strains may be useful in alleviating the symptoms associated with IBS.[23,24]

The relationship between a functioning human gut and the complex community of bacteria it houses is mutually beneficial. A number of studies suggest that imbalances or abnormalities in this normal flora may influence the severity of the GI-related symptoms common to IBS.[24,25] Theoretically, this indicates the potential for probiotic supplementation as a corrective treatment. There are a number of proposed ways through which probiotics may positively influence IBS pathophysiology:

- Stimulation of goblet cells to produce mucus that enhances gut barrier function, normalizes bowel movements, and reduces visceral hypersensitivity
- Improvement of gut motility and/or acceleration of transit time
- Protection against pathogenic bacteria
- Modulation of the gut inflammatory response and colonic fermentation
- Stabilization of intestinal permeability and the colonic microbiota

There is still much to be understood in terms of how probiotics affect gut function; thus, because the exact pathophysiological mechanism(s) that probiotics impact has yet to be determined, their use is typically recommended for all subtypes in the IBS population (IBS-C, IBS-D, IBS-M, and IBS-U). Despite the many unknowns, an increasingly large body of research has shown improvement

Dairy	
Cow milk	
Soft cheeses	
Butter	
Yogurt	
Cream	
Non-dairy milk	
Lactose-free products	
Hard cheeses	

Vegetables	
Asparagus	Corn
Avocado	Broccoli
Red onion	Brussel sprouts
Cabbage	Mushrooms
Tomato	Peas
Potato	Bell pepper
Cucumber	Carrots
Squash	Olives

Grains	
Bulgur wheat	Pasta
Rye	Wheat
Bread	
Milk	Quinoa
Polenta	Rice
Oats	

Fruits	
Pears	Grapes
Apples	Cantaloupe
Cherries	Plums
Watermelon	Peaches
Strawberries	Pineapple
Bananas	Blueberries
Limes	Oranges
Lemons	

Drinks	
Fruit juices	Lagers
Beer	Ciders
Fizzy drinks	
Tea	Water
Coffee	Wine

Proteins	
Chickpeas	Kidney beans
Lentils	Baked beans
Soybeans	
Chicken	Eggs
Fish	Peanuts

Treats	
High fructose corn syrup	Dark chocolate
Artificial sweeteners	Maple syrup
Honey	Golden syrup
Chocolate	Sugar

FIGURE 13.5 Low FODMAP Diet Chart

Reproduced from YorkTest Laboratories.

TABLE 13.4 FODMAP COMPONENTS WITH HIGH FODMAP FOODS TO AVOID[18,19,21]

Oligosaccharides	Disaccharides	Monosaccharides	Polyols
Fructans, Galactans	**Lactose**	**Fructose**	**Sorbitol, Mannitol, Maltitol, Xylitol, Erythritol, Polydextorse, Isomalt**

• Apples
• Artichokes
• Asparagus
• Barley
• Beets
• Brussels sprouts
• Broccoli
• Cabbage
• Chickpeas
• Fennel
• Garlic
• Leeks
• Legumes
• Lentils
• Okra
• Onions
• Peaches
• Peas
• Persimmon
• Pistachios
• Rye
• Shallots
• Watermelon
• Wheat
	• Dairy foods
	  – Cheese (soft and fresh)
	  – Custard
	  – Ice cream
	  – Milk (cow, goat, and sheep; regular and low-fat)
	  – Yogurt
		• Apples
		• Artichokes
		• Asparagus
		• Canned fruits in natural juice
		• Cherries
		• Honey
		• High fructose corn syrup
		• Mangoes
		• Peaches
		• Pears
		• Sugar snap peas
		• Watermelon
		• *Large total fructose dose*: concentrated fruit sources, large servings of fruit, dried fruit, fruit juice
			• Apples
			• Apricots
			• Artificial sweeteners
			• Avocado
			• Cauliflower
			• Cherries
			• Mushrooms
			• Nectarines
			• Peaches
			• Pears
			• Plums
			• Prunes
			• Snow peas
			• Watermelon

Data from Marcason W. What is the FODMAP diet? J Acad Nutr Diet. 2012;112(10):1696; Low FODMAP diet for irritable bowel syndrome. Monash University - Medicine, Nursing, and Health Sciences Web site. http://www.med.monash.edu/cecs/gastro/fodmap/. Published January 18. Updated 2016. Accessed February 5, 2016; and Mansueto P, Seidita A, D'Alcamo A, Carroccio A. Role of FODMAPs in patients with irritable bowel syndrome. Nutr Clin Pract. 2015;30(5):665-682.

in abdominal distention, pain and/or discomfort, flatulence, and altered bowel movements.[14,25-28]

The general consensus in clinical and academic settings is that, because probiotics are both safe and have been shown effective in the treatment for IBS, recommending their use to patients is reasonable.[9] That being said, which species or strains that are the most beneficial for this population remains unclear.[26,27] Although the most widely used species of probiotics are *Lactobacillus* and *Bifidobacterium*, there are a number of individual strains that have been shown to impact different components of IBS. See **Table 13.5** for a more comprehensive list of probiotic strains.[29]

In addition to the disagreement regarding the best probiotic strain, there is no set dosage for use in IBS. In light of current evidence, probiotics may be used to supplement other forms of primary treatment; they are not meant to serve as the only method for symptom relief. When making a patient recommendation, refer to the most current clinical evidence and reevaluate after a minimum of 4 weeks of consistent use.[9,18,26,31]

> **PRACTICE POINT**
>
> Research surrounding diet interventions for IBS continues to evolve. Implementing the low FODMAP diet and/or the use of probiotics should occur on a trial basis, with careful monitoring of how each may affect the patient's symptoms. Always consult the most current evidence before making any recommendations.

Non-Celiac Gluten Sensitivity

The GFD is not only popular among those with celiac disease, but also with patients who have **non-celiac gluten sensitivity (NCGS)**. This condition is both controversial and not well defined in the literature.[32,33] Evidence has not been able to pinpoint how gluten might cause gastrointestinal symptoms without inflammation of the gut. Because NCGS does not appear to cause intestinal damage, malabsorption is less likely. There is some speculation that NCGS is closely related to IBS, as both the GFD and low FODMAP diet have provided symptom relief in recent trials.[32]

TABLE 13.5 PROBIOTIC STRAINS FOR USE IN INFLAMMATORY BOWEL SYNDROME[14,24,25,29,30]

- *Bifidobacterium* species
  - *B. animalis*
  - *B. bifidum*
  - *B. breve*
  - *B. infantis*
  - *B. longum*
- *Lactobacillus* species
  - *L. acidophilus*
  - *L. bulgaricus*
  - *L. casei*
  - *L. paracasei,*
  - *L. plantarum*
  - *L. rhamnosus*
  - *L. salivarius*
- *Saccharomyces* species
  - *S. boulardii*
- *Streptococcus* species
  - *S. thermophiles*

It is important for the care team to first eliminate celiac disease as the cause of symptoms, as that will determine whether strict avoidance of gluten is necessary.[33] Once this disease is ruled out, the dietitian can assist in helping the patient reduce symptoms with dietary intervention.

Medical Nutrition Therapy

Nutrition assessment in these patients should include a detailed dietary recall to help pinpoint nutrients of concern. The dietary recall can also help assess whether the patient is adequately following the GFD. A food and symptom log can help to find any patterns between food intake and GI symptoms.

The goal of nutrition intervention for patients with NCGS is symptom relief. Some patients may benefit from strict elimination of gluten, while others may be able to tolerate some level of this protein.[33] The low FODMAP diet can also be trialed in this population with the help of an experienced dietitian.[32] Frequent reassessment of nutritional status and gastrointestinal symptoms will help direct interventions. This heavily debated condition presents a unique opportunity for dietitians to become involved in research to find the best diet for these patients.

> **CORE CONCEPT 3**
>
> Patients with non-celiac gluten sensitivity (NCGS) may also benefit from a gluten-free diet. Although there is no current best practice guideline for medical nutrition therapy for NCGS, dietitians can help patients create an individualized diet that minimizes their symptoms.

Inflammatory Bowel Disease (IBD)

Among the many complex disorders covered within this chapter, **inflammatory bowel disease** (IBD) is perhaps one of the most intricate and involved. Much of the etiology behind this group of disorders remains unclear, making it difficult for researchers and practitioners to target specific treatments or therapies. In terms of nutrition, the existing evidence base (which is often unclear, conflicting, or weak) is a source of significant confusion. It is abundantly clear that diet plays a pivotal role in the disease process for these patients, both as a potential component of the pathogenesis and in the subsequent treatment.[34] This patient population often presents with strong, predetermined beliefs about the impact of diet on the IBD clinical course and in exacerbating or alleviating symptoms.[35] When considered in the context of the documented toll that the natural progression of IBD takes on nutritional status, these reasons indicate the importance of the dietitian in prevention and management.

IBD encompasses a group of chronic, relapsing-remitting immune disorders that originate in the GI tract. The two major forms of IBD—**ulcerative colitis** (UC) and **Crohn's disease**—represent intrinsically distinct conditions that share a number of overlapping features. The pathomechanisms behind IBD are largely undefined, although a single cause-and-effect relationship is improbable. As with many inflammatory disorders, IBD is thought to arise from an inappropriate interaction among genetic factors, environmental influences, and other endogenous modifiers. Within this context, diet has been proposed as a potential modulator in the disease process. While a full discussion on the pathophysiology of IBD is outside of the scope of this chapter, the key takeaway from current data is the theory that gut microbiota activate the intestinal immune system in a genetically susceptible host, triggering cycles of inflammation and healing.[34,36-40]

Distinguishing Features of Ulcerative Colitis and Crohn's Disease

Although similar in many aspects of clinical presentation, UC and Crohn's disease are fundamentally different disorders. The most prominent distinction is the location of the inflammatory process; UC is characterized by inflammation that is limited to the mucosal layer of the colon, while Crohn's disease triggers transmural inflammation that can affect any organ of the GI tract from mouth to anus. See **Table 13.6** for the most commonly involved sites. **Figure 13.6** demonstrates these key differences between Crohn's disease and UC. As a result, each disorder has a notably different impact on its respective patient population, meaning discernable disease courses and chief complaints (these differences, of course, impact all other components of the disease process, including nutritional implications and treatment options). For example, the cardinal symptom of UC, identified in over 90% of patients at presentation, is chronic, bloody diarrhea. However, because of the variability in disease location that occurs with

Clinical Roundtable

Topic: Diet as an Etiological Factor in IBD[36-38]

Background: The increase in worldwide incidence of IBD, especially in recently industrialized nations, has led to an interesting discussion on the role of diet as an environmental factor in the largely unidentified etiology of the disease. Why? The sharp rise in the incidence trend has paralleled the social and economic advances that are accompanied by a shift towards a more Western lifestyle; this includes, of course, dietary changes.[3-5] Within a nutrition-related text, this is worth discussing.

The surge in new cases in accordance with increased consumption of more refined and processed foods (the so-called "Western diet") suggests a strong role of diet in the pathogenesis of IBD. There are several proposed mechanisms that may explain why dietary factors have such a significant impact:

- Direct effect of dietary antigens on inflammatory processes
- Diet-induced alterations of gene expression that affect the transcription factors involved in regulation of intestinal inflammation
- Changes to the composition or homeostasis of gut microbiome
- Shifts in GI permeability secondary to diet composition[35-38,41-44]

Researchers now agree that dietary factors play an underestimated role in the pathogenesis and course of IBD. The question arises about which foods may be involved? Components of the Western diet, which is high in fat and protein but low in fruits and vegetables, have taken much of the blame.[35,43,44] A number of studies have further identified the dietary components that can be considered risk factors for IBD development:

- **Cow's milk:** Data suggest a likely relationship between hypersensitivity to cow's milk at an early age and subsequently development of IBD, particularly UC.
- **Refined carbohydrates:** As one of the first dietary factors to be implicated, high intakes of sugar and refined carbohydrates are associated with increased risk of both UC and Crohn's; in addition, a high intake of overall carbohydrates has been linked to increased risk for onset of Crohn's.
- **Dietary fat:** Both the type and the amount of fat are linked to increased risk of UC and Crohn's—this includes high dietary intakes of total fat and high ratios of omega-6 to omega-3 fatty acids, particularly a high intake of linoleic acid, which is metabolized to arachadonic acid and has pro-inflammatory properties.
- **Animal proteins:** Increased consumption of high-fat meats has been suspected as a risk factor for both Crohn's and UC.
- **Fast food:** Studies have identified an increase relative risk of IBD when individuals consume fast food at least twice per week.
- **Preservatives:** A number of additives used for the preservation of foods, like dietary sulfur, have been linked with increased numbers of UC cases[34-36,38,40-43,45]

Roundtable Discussion

The identification of food components that impact IBD development have significant implications for necessary shifts in dietary patterns, and are important considerations for those already diagnosed (whether in remission or periods of relapse). How might this be incorporated into your education and care plan for a patient with IBD? How will you evaluate the efficacy of avoiding these dietary components?

Crohn's, the presenting symptoms are less consistent than those seen in UC. In general, nonspecific symptoms like fatigue, prolonged diarrhea (not typically accompanied by blood), abdominal pain, weight loss, and fever are the hallmarks of Crohn's disease. Carefully examine **Table 13.7** for a comprehensive comparison of UC and Crohn's disease.[37,46,47]

Both UC and Crohn's occur as intermittent exacerbations of symptoms followed by periods of remission; the length of time spent in either of the phases is extremely individual and cannot be predicted.

The severity of symptoms will range from mild to severe; this can change on a person-to-person basis or over time within the same disease course. Although objective measures for disease activity exist (indices like Truelove and Witt's for use in UC and the Crohn's Disease Activity Index), most clinicians do not utilize any formal activity index in daily practice and instead focus on GI and extraintestinal manifestations. Disease severity has important implications for predicting clinical outcomes. Patients with UC typically experience long periods of completely asymptomatic remission; two-thirds of patients will have at least one relapse in the 10 years following diagnosis, with a very small percentage experiencing continued symptoms with no complete remission. According to guidelines published by the American College of Gastroenterology, the disease course is similar for those with Crohn's: two-thirds of patients will have a combination of years in relapse and years in remission, with 20% of all patients experiencing annual relapses, 13% following a relapse-free course, and less than 5% with a continuous course of the disease.[37,46,47]

Medical Management of IBD With no specific, curative treatments identitifed, the management of IBD instead involves pharmacologic and nutritional measures. The

TABLE 13.6 COMMON LOCATIONS OF GI INVOLVEMENT FOR CROHN'S DISEASE PATIENTS[46]

Location of Affected Tract	Percentage of Presenting Patients
Small bowel (typically distal ileum, or ileitis)	80%; 30% have ileitis exclusively
Ileum and colon (ileocolotis)	50%
Colon	20%
Perianal disease	30%
Mouth	5%–15%
Gastroduodenal	5%–15%
Esophagus	>5%
Proximal small bowel	>5%

Data from Peppercorn MA, Kane SV. Clinical manifestations, diagnosis and prognosis of crohn disease in adults. UpToDate Web site. Published December 17. Updated 2015. Accessed June 16, 2016.

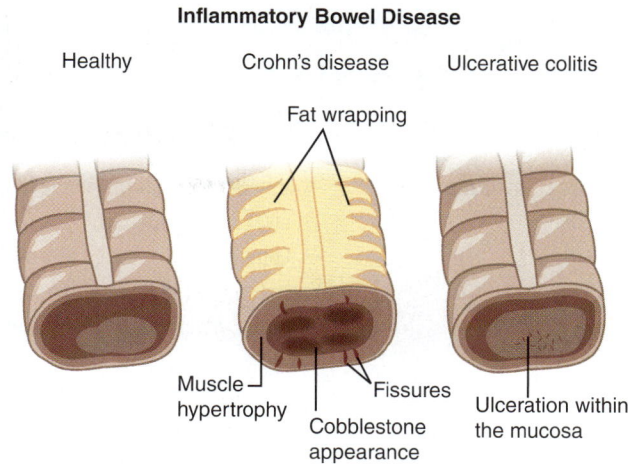

FIGURE 13.6 Key Differences Between Crohn's disease and Ulcerative Colitis

overarching goal of treatment is to induce and maintain remission, with secondary, but significant objectives that include correction of nutritional status, prevention of complications, and facilitation of mucosal healing. While the accomplishment of each goal contributes to improved quality of life, a more concrete outcome is the avoidance of surgical intervention. This, however, is often inevitable.[34,37]

Induction of Remission   The bulk of IBD's medical management emphasizes anti-inflammatory and/or immunosuppressive pharmacotherapy. Due to the relapsing nature of the disease, patients with IBD will require treatment that is highly individualized to fit the needs of the initial presentation or current flare. Pharmacologic therapy to induce remission includes a carefully monitored combination of systemic aminosalicylates, corticosteroids, immunosuppressive agents, antibiotic treatment, and other biological therapies like anti-tumor necrosis factor (anti-TNF) drugs. These agents may also be effective

CASE STUDY REVISITED

At the gastroenterology clinic, the medical team begins a diagnostic workup to identify the source of Daniel's excessive diarrhea and unintentional weight loss. The team probes for his medical history, which reveals no previous gastrointestinal disorder or surgery. In addition, Daniel confirms that although his stool is watery and frequent, there are no signs of excess fat in the feces that would indicate steatorrhea. There is no presence of blood in the stool. Daniel also reveals that his diarrhea is accompanied by considerable abdominal pain that is not always relieved by defecation. In addition, his bowel movements are preceded by extreme urgency.

When questioned on his personal history, Daniel does not report any alarming psychosocial abnormalities. He reports experiencing fatigue and moderate stress at his job, but no symptoms of anxiety or depression. Daniel claims no history of substance abuse, but does have a 4-year history of tobacco use and consumes alcohol on occasion.

Questions

1. Think back to the case presentation. Do you agree with your original description of Daniel's illness?
2. There are many sources of malabsorption that are indicated by excessive diarrhea and weight loss. What distinguishing features of Daniel's symptoms are important? Are there any specific questions you would ask, biochemical lab values you would consider, or other procedures you would require to confirm a diagnosis?

TABLE 13.7 CLINICAL DISTINCTION BETWEEN ULCERATIVE COLITIS AND CROHN'S DISEASE[37,39,46,47]

	Ulcerative Colitis	Crohn's Disease
Disease Distribution	<ul><li>Inflammatory process limited to the mucosal layer of the colon</li><li>Commonly involves the rectum, may extend proximally (but only within the large intestine)</li><li>Inflammation is continuous and circumferential</li></ul>	<ul><li>Inflammatory process occurs transmurally from mouth to anus</li><li>Patchy, asymmetrical involvement</li><li>Unlike UC, often extends into perianal disease (anal fissures and/or anorectal abscess) but with rectal sparing</li></ul>
Clinical Presentation	*Onset of symptoms is gradual and intermittent:*<ul><li>Diarrhea, typically bloody</li><li>Frequent bowel movements, small in volume secondary to rectal inflammation</li><li>Colicky abdominal pain</li><li>Urgency associated with defecation</li><li>**Tenesmus** (cramping, rectal pain)</li><li>Incontinence</li><li>Patients with primarily distal disease may present with constipation accompanied by blood and/or mucus discharge</li></ul>	*Symptoms may exist for years before diagnosis:*<ul><li>Cramp-like abdominal pain</li><li>Prolonged diarrhea without bleeding, may fluctuate over time</li><li>Transmural inflammation is linked with **sinus tracts** that can lead to:<ul><li>Fistula formation (common, unlike in UC); symptoms depend on the site of the fistula</li><li>*Phlegmon* formation</li><li>*Abscess* formation</li></ul></li><li>*Perianal disease*:<ul><li>Perianal pain, drainage from large skin tags, anal fissures, perirectal abscesses, and anorectal fistulas</li></ul></li><li>Other potential GI involvement:<ul><li>Oral: aphthous ulcers, pain</li><li>Esophageal: odynophagia, dysphagia</li><li>Gastroduodenal: upper abdominal pain</li><li>Gallstones may form secondary to reduced bile acid</li></ul></li></ul>
Systemic Symptoms	<ul><li>Fever</li><li>Chronic fatigue</li><li>Unintended weight loss</li><li>Dyspnea or palpitations<ul><li>Secondary to anemia</li></ul></li></ul>	<ul><li>Chronic fatigue</li><li>Unintended eight loss</li><li>Fever (occurs less frequently)</li></ul>
Physical Examination	<ul><li>Evidence of blood in rectum</li><li>Mild to moderate UC:<ul><li>Otherwise normal</li></ul></li><li>Moderate to severe UC:<ul><li>Abdominal tenderness to palpitation</li><li>Hypotension</li><li>Tachycardia</li><li>Pallor</li></ul></li><li>For those with prolonged diarrhea:<ul><li>Evidence of muscle wasting</li><li>Loss of subcutaneous fat</li><li>Peripheral edema resulting from weight loss and malnutrition</li></ul></li></ul>	<ul><li>May be normal or show nonspecific signs (pallor, weight loss)</li><li>*More specific signs:*<ul><li>Perianal lesions</li><li>Perianal skin tags</li><li>Sinus tracts</li><li>Abdominal tenderness</li></ul></li></ul>

TABLE 13.7 CLINICAL DISTINCTION BETWEEN ULCERATIVE COLITIS AND CROHN'S DISEASE[37,39,46,47] (continued)

	Ulcerative Colitis	Crohn's Disease

Diagnosis	• Presence of diarrhea for ≥4 weeks
	• Evidence of active inflammation on endoscopy and chronic changes on biopsy
	• Exclusion of other causes of colitis by
	  – History (i.e., recent travel, nonsteroidal anti-inflammatory drug [NSAID]/medication exposure)
	  – Laboratory studies (i.e., stool studies for toxins to rule out infection, serologic testing for sexually transmitted diseases)
	  – Endoscopy and biopsy (see below)
		• Established with endoscopic findings or imaging studies in a patient with a compatible clinical history
		• Colonoscopy is the most appropriate initial test for those with predominant diarrhea, while imaging studies are used for patients with abdominal pain
		• Exclude differential diagnoses

Endoscopic Findings	• Punctate (i.e., studded) ulceration appears, may become confluent and leaves islands of inflammatory tissue
	• Erythematous appearance (i.e., redness): loss of vascular markings due to engorgement of the mucosa
	• Mucosa also appears granular, hyperaemic, and friable (bleeds easily)
	• **Pseudopolyps** ("inflammatory polyps") and mucosal bridging may develop
	• Over time, shortening of the colon and a reduction in diameter occur as a result of thickening/contracture of mucosal layer
	• Additional findings may include:
	  – Petechiae (small red and/or purple spots)
	  – Exudate (fluid secretions)
	  – Edema
	  – Erosions
		• Ileocolonic involvement:
		  – Focal ulcerations adjacent to areas of normal appearing mucosa
		  – Polypoid mucosal changes give "cobblestone" appearance
		• Skip areas of involvement
		  – Segments of normal-appearing bowel interrupted by large areas of disease
		  – Different from the continuous involvement seen in UC
		• Transmural nature of inflammation results in fibrotic strictures and fistulas
		• Pseudopolyps (as seen in UC) are often present

Histologic Features (via Biopsy)	• Crypt cell abnormalities
	  – Crypt branching
	  – Shortening and disarray
	  – Crypt atrophy
	  – Crypt abscesses: collections of neutrophils that migrate across crypt epithelium into the lumen
	• Epithelial cell abnormalities
	  – Goblet cell mucin depletion
	  – Paneth cell metaplasia
	• Inflammatory features
	  – Increased lamina propria cellularity
	  – Basal plasmacytosis
	  – Basal lymphoid aggregates
	  – Lamina propria eosinophils
		• Focal ulcerations
		• Abnormal mucosal architecture
		• Increased cellularity of the lamina propria with infiltration of neutrophils
		• **Granulomas** (seldom found in UC)
		  – "Histological hallmark"
		  – A collection of monocytes and/or macrophages and other inflammatory cells with or without giant cells
		  – Reported in as many as 70% of patients with Crohn's disease

(continues)

TABLE 13.7 CLINICAL DISTINCTION BETWEEN ULCERATIVE COLITIS AND CROHN'S DISEASE[37,39,46,47] (continued)

	Ulcerative Colitis	Crohn's Disease

Extraintestinal Manifestations	• **Musculoskeletal**
	  – Peripheral arthritis
	  – Spondyloarthropathy, which may progress to ankylosing spondylitis
	  – Osteoporosis, osteopenia, and osteonecrosis
	• **Ocular**
	  – Uveitis, iritis, or episcleritis
	• **Dermatological**
	  – Erythema nodosum and/or pyoderma gangrenosum
	• **Hepatobiliary**
	  – Sclerosing cholangitis
	  – Fatty liver
	  – Autoimmune liver disease
	• **Hematopoietic**
	  – Venous and arterial thromboembolism
	  – Anemia	

Acute and Chronic Complications	• Severe bleeding and/or massive hemorrhage
	• Fulminant colitis
	  – ≥10 stools per day
	  – Continuous bleeding
	  – Abdominal pain
	  – Distention
	  – Acute, severe toxic symptoms: fever and anorexia
	  – High risk of developing toxic megacolon
	• **Toxic megacolon**: colonic diameter >6 cm or cecal diameter >9 cm and the presence of systemic toxicity
	• Perforation
	  – Typically the result of toxic megacolon
	  – May occur during the first episode of UC due to the lack of scarring from prior episodes of colitis
	• Strictures: narrowing of the colon, may cause symptoms of obstruction
	• Dysplasia and colorectal cancer: increased risk related to severity and duration of disease
		• **Fibrostenosis** (narrowing), which may result in small bowel obstruction
		• Short bowel syndrome (SBS), if multiple surgeries are necessary secondary to reoccurrence
		• Dysplasia and colorectal cancer: increased risk related to severity and duration of disease
		• Fistulae formation between the lumen of the gut and mesentery and/or another organ or the abdominal wall or skin
		• Abscess formation
		• Bleeding
		  – While diarrhea is characteristically nonbloody, rapid bleeding is an uncommon but life-threatening complication
		• Malnutrition
		• Bone disease
		  – Osteopenic bone disease and osteoporosis

for maintenance of remission—see Table 13.8. However, many of the aforementioned medications are potentially toxic and often cause incredibly damaging side effects. For example, corticosteroids, which present a wide range of negative repercussions when used long term, are prescribed at high dosages when necessary to induce remission in moderate-to-severe disease courses. Once remission has been reached and maintained, the goal then becomes to taper steroids and avoid future use.[34,37,39]

Of extreme importance, enteral nutrition (EN) has been identified as a strategy to both induce and maintain remission in patients with Crohn's disease, although not for those with UC. Some studies have demonstrated remission rates equal to or beyond that of corticosteroid use.[36] This will be discussed in further detail in a subsequent section.

Maintenance of Remission Once remission is achieved, the long-term goals are to maintain an asymptomatic state

TABLE 13.8 PHARMACOLOGIC AGENTS FOR INDUCTION OR MAINTENANCE OF REMISSION IN INFLAMMATORY BOWEL DISEASE[37,39]

	Ulcerative Colitis	Crohn's Disease
Aminosalicylates	**For Mild to Moderate:** cornerstone treatment of active disease and for maintenance of remission	**For Mild to Moderate:** effective in induction of remission and maintenance of remission
Corticosteroids	**For Moderate to Severe:** prescribed at high dosage to bring condition under control, then tapered	**For Severe Active Disease:** effective in induction of remission
Immuno-suppressants	**Cyclosporine, for Severe:** used because of its rapid action, but must be closely supervised; not to be used as a routine oral therapy or long term	**Azathioprine, for Maintenance of Remission:** maintenance therapy shown effective in clinical trials compared to placebo **Methotrexate, for Maintenance of Remission:** used as second-line for patients unresponsive to azathioprine (may also be used for improving symptoms in active disease)
Antibiotics (metronidazole, ciprofloxacin)		**For Mild to Moderate:** used for antibacterial action despite no identification of a causative microorganism
Anti-TNF-α (infliximab)	**For Severe:** safer (but more expensive) alternative to cyclosporine; effective rescue therapy for induction of remission	**For Severe Active Disease:** effective in induction of remission, useful for retreatment after relapse

Data from Shanahan F. Ulcerative colitis. In: Textbook of clinical gastroenterology and hepatology. Wiley-Blackwell; 2012:355-371. Accessed 1/23/2016 11:41:00 AM. 10.1002/9781118321386.ch49; and Vermeire S, Van Assche G, Rutgeerts P. Crohn's disease. In: Textbook of clinical gastroenterology and hepatology. Wiley-Blackwell; 2012:372-393. 10.1002/9781118321386.ch50.

for as long as possible and, similarly, to minimize the frequency and/or severity of relapses. Most patients with IBD can be successfully maintained—meaning a return to a normal function and high quality-of-life—with aminosalicylates and an occasional course of corticosteroid treatment. There is a potential role for nutritional support in the maintenance of remission to be discussed later.[36,37]

Surgical Intervention Alhough surgical intervention (in the form of bowel resection and/or reconstruction) is often considered the last resort for patients with IBD, it should not be delayed if there is clear clinical decline despite aggressive pharmacologic therapy or failure of pharmacologic therapy altogether. In addition, acute complications (like toxic megacolon in UC) or evidence of dysplasia indicating colorectal cancer are well-defined indications for surgery. Modest approximations suggest that one-fifth of all IBD patients will require intestinal resection on the basis of intractable symptoms, bowel obstruction, or perforation.[37,39,46,47] Surgical intervention involving bowel resection causes significant changes to the integrity of the GI tract, which introduces new challenges to an already-complicated nutritional status. Refer to the section of this chapter entitled Bowel Surgery and Short Bowel Syndrome (SBS) for more information on this topic.

Medical Nutrition Therapy An IBD diagnosis is accompanied by various nutritional challenges. At the most basic level, the common sequelae of the inflammatory process (uncontrolled pain, nausea, fever, and/or diarrhea) are associated with a number of consequences that negatively affect nutritional status: loss of appetite, decreased dietary intake, malabsorption, and/or altered nutrient metabolism.[48,49] Because the inflammatory process of Crohn's disease can occur at any point along the GI tract, with specific involvement of the small intestine (where the majority of absorption occurs), nutritional implications are generally more drastic for this patient population when compared to those with UC.[45]

Nutrition Implications

The disruption of GI tract function and the associated symptoms of pain, nausea, and diarrhea contribute to significant reductions in dietary intake and impaired nutrient utilization. Important challenges related to these changes include malabsorption, unintended weight loss, malnutrition, micronutrient deficiencies, and impaired bone health.[48]

Malabsorption The specific type of malabsorption—bile acid or bile salt malabsorption—that results from the inflammatory processes of IBD is seen primarily in patients with

Crohn's disease that have involvement of the small intestine. In a healthy GI tract, the vast majority of bile acids will be absorbed by receptors in the distal ileum after they are used for the digestion and absorption of dietary lipids. Bile salt malabsorption will occur when more than 50 cm of terminal ileum is diseased. Unabsorbed bile salts travel into the colon and draw increased fluid into the lumen, resulting in secretory diarrhea. More importantly, however, if more than 100 cm of the terminal ileum is affected, the amount of bile salts lost from malabsorption will deplete all stores and outweigh the body's ability to compensate, triggering a dangerous cascade of fat maldigestion/malabsorption, steatorrhea, weight loss, and ultimately malnutrition.[34,36,46]

Weight Loss and Reduced Muscle Mass Although unintended weight loss and reductions in muscle mass are becoming increasingly less common due to advances in nutrition therapy, these implications remain important indicators of nutritional status for this patient population. General weight loss, observed in up to 70% of patients with IBD, is largely related to malabsorption, decreased oral intake, or a combination of the two. It is most pronounced in those with acute exacerbations of or widespread Crohn's disease.[36,45,46] In addition, some degree of lean body mass (LBM) depletion is estimated to occur in more than half of individuals with IBD, with significant muscle wasting observed in one-fifth of patients with prolonged symptomatic periods. Reductions in muscle mass are directly related to disease activity, as the inflammatory process amplifies protein catabolism; reductions may also be due, in part, to corticosteroid treatment and/or decreased physical activity. Regardless, loss of LBM beyond 10% is associated with increased morbidity for this patient population.[34,36,49]

Malnutrition Although malnutrition is most readily identified in those with Crohn's disease affecting the small intestine, its effects are widespread and can impact any individual within the IBD patient population, even during periods of remission. Malnutrition, recognized as protein-energy malnutrition (PEM), is one of the most influential factors on poor clinical outcomes associated with the disease process. As it depends largely on disease activity, PEM is reported in 20% to 85% of patients. Malnutrition (accompanied by weight loss) is the third most common clinical feature identified in Crohn's disease, preceded only by diarrhea and abdominal pain. The typical factors that contribute to malnutrition, related to both the pathology and treatment of IBD, are summarized in Table 13.9.[4,34,36,45,49]

Micronutrient Deficiencies In the context of reduced intake, chronic diarrhea, malabsorption, and GI blood loss, a variety of micronutrient deficiencies are common to IBD. Evidence suggests that even patients who appear well nourished according to anthropometric measures, even during periods of remission, can mask baseline vitamin and mineral deficiencies. Of the many deficiencies observed in this population, listed in Table 13.10, those most commonly identified nutrient deficiencies:

TABLE 13.9 CONTRIBUTING FACTORS TO MALNUTRITION IN INFLAMMATORY BOWEL DISEASE[4,34,36,45,49,50]

Etiologies of Malnutrition

Inadequate intake secondary to anorexia, nausea, and vomiting

Nutrient maldigestion and/or malabsorption secondary to location and extent of disease

Increased GI or nutrient losses secondary to diarrhea and/or fistula protein losses

Enhanced nutritional requirements secondary to catabolic effects of inflammation

Drug–nutrient interactions

Bowel resection and/or reconstruction

TABLE 13.10 MICRONUTRIENT DEFICIENCIES COMMON TO INFLAMMATORY BOWEL DISEASE[4,34,36,51]

Water-Soluble Vitamins

Vitamin B$_{12}$
Folic acid
Niacin
Vitamin B$_6$
Vitamin C

Fat-Soluble Vitamins

Vitamin D
Vitamin A
Vitamin E
Vitamin K

Minerals

Calcium
Iron
Copper
Magnesium
Phosphate
Potassium
Selenium
Zinc

1. **Disease activity**: Iron-deficiency anemia, which occurs secondary to chronic GI blood loss, is present in up to 80% of UC patients
2. **Disease location**: Patients with Crohn's disease centralized in the terminal ileum will be more likely to experience vitamin B_{12} deficiency due to the loss of absorption site and/or fat-soluble vitamin deficiency (fat malabsorption attributed to bile acid deficiency)

Beyond the pathophysiology of IBD, some pharmacological treatments can contribute to further complications by either causing or exacerbating deficiencies. The most common and well-documented micronutrient deficiencies in IBD are iron, folic acid, and vitamin B_{12}.[4,36,45,48,50,51]

Bone Disease

Due to the high prevalence of malnutrition and micronutrient deficiencies, osteoporosis and/or osteomalacia are common problems for the IBD patient population; nearly 50% of all IBD patients are affected by some degree of bone disease. First, the most plausible explanation for reductions in bone mineral density is malabsorption of calcium and vitamin D. Second, long-term use of glucocorticoid therapy is associated with significant bone loss; in fact, it is the most common cause of secondary osteoporosis. Third, self-imposed restrictions of dairy products are widespread; inadequate calcium intake is reported in more than one-third of patients, accompanied by inadequate vitamin D intakes and low serum vitamin D concentrations. This represents a critical area for nutrition intervention.[4,34,48,51]

Nutrition Interventions

Originally, the main focus of dietary interventions was to maximize or correct nutritional status, to maintain adequate macro- and micronutrient intake levels, and to assist in identifying and avoiding foods that may exacerbate symptoms. Preserving nutritional status is critical in the prevention of long-term health consequences and in minimizing the potential for relapse. While these primary goals remain critical to the treatment of all patients with IBD, nutrition therapy now extends beyond its role as a supportive measure. For patients with Crohn's disease, evidence suggests that nutrition support can act in adjunct or replace pharmacologic agents as a primary therapy for induction and maintenance of remission.[38,38,43,49]

Nutrition Support

In the context of IBD management, nutrition support can be divided into three basic categories with fundamentally different objectives: enteral nutrition for correcting malnutrition, enteral nutrition as a tool to modify the underlying disease process (to induce or maintain remission), and recourse parenteral nutrition when enteral support is contraindicated.[45]

Enteral Nutrition—Role in Correcting Malnutrition

EN support is indicated to improve or correct the nutritional status of all patients who present with signs of malnutrition. This recommendation is supported by both well-documented clinical outcomes and the ESPEN guidelines for enteral nutrition (which list indications for EN as the prevention and treatment of undernutrition and/or inadequate nutritional intake for UC and Crohn's disease). EN may be given in addition to oral intake or as exclusive enteral nutrition (EEN) based on the current status of the patient.[36,38,49,52-54]

> **PRACTICE POINT**
>
> EN is justified and necessary on the basis of malnutrition for those who have lost >5% of normal body weight, those with a BMI of <18.5 kg/m², and those with continuing weight loss despite pharmacologic intervention.[45]

Enteral Nutrition—Role in Inducing or Maintaining Remission

EEN has illustrated efficacy in inducing remission in patients with active Crohn's disease and is now considered a mainstay of treatment. Although the evidence is not yet strong enough to support the complete replacement of corticosteroid therapy, several studies have indicated that EN achieves remission rates comparable to or surpassed that of corticosteroid use. The expected clinical remission rate is well over 50%.[4,34,36,38,45,49,52]

> **PRACTICE POINT**
>
> EN given as the sole source of nutrition (EEN) can induce clinical remission in Crohn's disease.[38,55,56]

In addition, EN may also be used as an additive strategy to maintain clinical remission and prevent relapses for this same patient population. Current evidence shows lower recurrence rates in patients supplemented with EN when compared to those who return to a normal diet during asymptomatic periods. Assessment of mucosal cytokine profiles indicates that EN is able to maintain remission through the alleviation of mucosal inflammation, although the exact mechanism remains undefined.[34,36,38,45,49,56]

> **PRACTICE POINT**
>
> EN given as at least 50% of calories during asymptomatic periods has been proven effective in maintaining clinical remission of Crohn's disease. The quantity of enteral formula is directly related to remission rates, with higher amounts of formula associated with higher remission rates.[38,55,56]

> **PRACTICE POINT**
>
> There is no difference in therapeutic efficacy among elemental, semi-elemental, and polymeric formulas for the induction or maintenance of remission in Crohn's disease. Consider, however, that polymeric feeds are generally less hyperosmolar and are easier to flavor if consumed orally.[34,38,45,55,57]

One of the biggest differences between remission maintained by pharmacologic treatment and remission maintained via EN is mucosal healing. While corticosteroids fail to stimulate mucosal healing (one of the treatment goals of IBD), there is evidence that EN support decreases disease activity and downregulates mucosal pro-inflammatory cytokines to actively reduce intestinal inflammation. Normalization of numerous inflammatory markers (c-reactive protein, interleukin 6, insulin-like growth factor 1) begins almost immediately. In addition to inducing or maintaining remission, this effectively promotes mucosal healing. These results are not seen in patients treated with corticosteroids alone. The bottom line: EN allows a GI tract otherwise plagued by inflammation to heal.[4,34,36,45,57]

> **PRACTICE POINT**
>
> Remember, the use of nutrition support as a means of inducing or maintaining remission applies only to those with Crohn's disease. There is no evidence that EN is an effective therapy for active UC, so it is not recommended for use in this context. Nutrition support is only indicated for patients with UC for the purpose of correcting malnutrition.[35,36,38,45,54,55]

Parenteral Nutrition The use of parenteral support is—as it is for many chronically ill patients—controversial for the IBD population. PN should only be used for UC or Crohn's disease patients when EN is contraindicated or attempts at enteral feeding have failed. Special circumstances that call for the use of PN include cases of severe malnutrition, high-output fistulas, obstruction, or toxic megacolon, or during the preoperative period. Traditionally, PN was used to induce bowel rest in patients with debilitating and/or long-standing flare-ups, but this practice is no longer recommended. Research and clinical outcomes have illustrated that the use of PN during a period of bowel rest is not effective for either UC or Crohn's disease. Instead, PN should serve as a short-term solution until nutritional status is corrected and/or until conversion to EN becomes appropriate.[4,34,55]

> **PRACTICE POINT**
>
> Indications for PN include those with intractable vomiting, severe stenotic disease, and short bowel syndrome or a perforated GI tract.[45]

There are several shortcomings to PN use in the clinical setting. First, PN is associated with significant risks for the patient (including line sepsis) and much higher medical costs. Second, PN does not have the same therapeutic effects on the intestinal lumen that are seen when EN is employed as a remission induction or maintenance treatment; PN is not indicated as a therapy for UC and Crohn's disease. Although PN may be necessary as a means to correct nutritional deficiency, it is important to consider about the risks of using PN for an extended period of time. Careful monitoring is required.[4,38,49,55]

> **PRACTICE POINT**
>
> If indicated, PN should be introduced cautiously and progressively with close monitoring, as in all other high-risk contexts; many patients who require PN for malnutrition may have had prolonged malnutrition and may be at high risk for refeeding syndrome.[45]

Micronutrient Supplementation Given the high prevalence of micronutrient deficiencies noted in both UC and Crohn's disease patients, a daily multivitamin supplement should be instituted immediately following diagnosis. Keep in mind that these deficiencies are observed at all degrees of disease severity, even in patients who show no sign of malnutrition according to anthropometric measures.[49-51] Supplementation beyond the daily multivitamin may also be necessary depending on the course of the disease. Additional supplements often used in this population include iron, calcium, vitamin D, vitamin B_{12}, and folate. Any supplement recommendation should be accompanied by careful consideration of the type, brand, and dosage. Many ingredients in vitamin and mineral supplements can cause additional GI symptoms in those with IBD (lactose, sugar alcohol, artificial coloring, etc.). The biggest challenge in this arena is iron supplementation, which is necessary based on the incredibly high incidence of deficiency. Approximately 25% of patients will react poorly to an oral iron supplement, which manifests as worsening symptoms or disease activity.[48,49]

> **PRACTICE POINT**
>
> For mild IBD activity with mild-to-moderate anemia (Hgb 10-12 g/dL for women or Hgb 10-13 g/dL in men), iron supplementation can be attempted by the oral route. IV supplementation should be used in adults with moderate-to-severe anemia or for those who do not tolerate oral iron.[51]

> **PRACTICE POINT**
>
> All IBD patients must be monitored for appropriate calcium and vitamin D intake due to the high potential for osteoporosis and/or osteomalacia. Recommended intake levels for calcium should fall between 1,000 and 1,500 mg.[51] Several studies have shown positive outcomes with vitamin D supplementation of at least 1,000 IU.[58]

Individualized Diets Counseling this population on oral intake, both during times of remission and active flare-ups of the disease, can be problematic. There is no single recommendation that can be made for a specific diet. Instead, patients will require special tailoring to develop a plan that ensures sufficient intake (in terms of both energy and nutrients) and identifies any trigger foods. In addition, this plan must take the disease course, the type of pharmacology used, and past surgical history into consideration.[43,54]

It is common for patients to self-restrict and/or avoid certain foods or food groups in an attempt to alleviate ongoing symptoms or prevent triggering active disease. Trigger foods will be identified as exacerbations of symptoms or the disease course. This can be done safely using a supervised elimination diet; this process involves removing foods from the diet and assessing for the presence of symptoms during that time. Studies indicate that elimination diets help to eliminate the possibility of adverse food reactions and significantly lower relapse rates.[4,35,37,48,49,54]

> **PRACTICE POINT**
>
> Elimination diets are safest and most effective when the patient is concurrently receiving supplemental or total EN, as this ensures that diet quality will be maintained as foods are removed.[49]

> **CORE CONCEPT 4**
>
> Inflammatory bowel disease is associated with a wide range of nutritional implications that center on malnutrition. Adequate intake, whether in the form of nutritional support or oral intake, is required.

While trigger foods are largely individual, the most commonly recognized are dairy products and fiber-containing foods. Other problematic foods include processed meat, soft drinks, citrus fruits, and alcoholic beverages. Any food identified as a trigger should be avoided, particularly during a flare. Nevertheless, this is difficult to generalize—what prompts a symptom in one patient may be well tolerated in another. As a result of the tendency to avoid certain foods, these patients are at a high risk for insufficient dietary intake. An important component of nutrition therapy will be to help patients identify these foods and compose a plan that limits these foods without sacrificing diet quality. Overall, a well-balanced diet with as minimal restrictions as possible is encouraged.[4,35,37,43,48,49,54,57,59]

Defined Diets An area of expanding IBD research centers around **defined diets**, which are dietary regimens based on an underlying theory or ideology of how food interacts with the body. Although the evidence is still highly controversial and lacks rigorous scientific backing, the use of such diets has grown in the patient population due to the lay literature and online searching. It is important to be aware of the several defined diets that have been publicized as successful antidotes to intestinal inflammation, which are described in more detail in **Table 13.11**. At a practical level, these diets are difficult to follow, may cause unnecessary financial burden, and are associated with a high deficiency risk due to their restrictive nature.[42,56]

The Bottom Line This population is often receptive to nutrition counseling and may actively seek professional guidance. Patients with both UC and Crohn's disease will have a strong interest in any dietary modifications that can be made as part of the management plan. However, data indicate that while up to 90% of IBD patients consider dietary guidance an important factor, only 20% feel they receive adequate information. It is of the utmost importance that careful time and consideration is spent with each patient, developing a plan that all parties involved feel meets the needs of the individual.[4,38,54]

Leaky Gut

Increased intestinal permeability, or **leaky gut** syndrome, is a highly debated condition in nutrition and gastroenterology. A quick Internet search of "leaky gut" will lead to a plethora of fad diets promising relief, but research on this syndrome has only just begun.

While we know that the cells lining the small intestine allow for transport of molecules into the bloodstream, we do not know exactly how inflammation is related to larger molecules and microorganisms progressing through this barrier.[62] Some research has shown that this increased permeability may be related to IBD, as the dysfunctional structure and integrity of the gut can lead to increased inflammation and therefore worse IBD outcomes.[63] The protein zonulin functions to open spaces between intestinal cells and allow substances to pass, while keeping out harmful bacteria and toxins. Interestingly, this protein is unregulated in both celiac disease and type 1 diabetes.[62] Whether this is a cause or an effect of leaky gut remains to be discovered.

Other contributing factors to leaky gut syndrome include NSAID use, excessive alcohol intake, radiation and chemotherapy, bacterial infections, and increased stress.

Medical Diagnosis

A lactulose-mannitol challenge may be used as a test to determine presence of leaky gut. A patient would come into clinic and consume a solution that includes both sugars, then supply urine over the course of 6 hours. The aim of the test is to assess the ratio of lactulose to mannitol recovered in the urine, with a normal result being less than 0.03%. A higher rate may indicate increased permeability of these sugars from the small intestine into the bloodstream, leading to a potential diagnosis of leaky gut. The issue with this test is that many factors can influence the test, such as patient size, duration of urine collection, and geographical location.[62]

The 51-chromium-labeled ethylenedaminetetraacetic acid (51-Cr-EDTA) permeability test has a similar aim as the lactulose-mannitol challenge. In this test, a patient ingests

CASE STUDY REVISITED

Daniel is diagnosed with Crohn's disease as the explicit source of malabsorption.

Questions

1. What typical features differentiate Crohn's disease from ulcerative colitis?
2. How will this change the nutrition therapy you choose to initiate?

TABLE 13.11 DEFINED DIETS: ADDITIONAL DIETARY MODIFICATIONS CONSIDERED FOR USE IN INFLAMMATORY BOWEL DISEASE

There are a number of modifications to oral intake, including both restrictions and supplementations, that have been proposed as therapeutic options for patients with IBD. The changes listed in this table, although insufficiently backed by conflicting or weak evidence, but are increasing in popularity in either patient use or in the literature.

Dietary Regimen	Underlying Theory

The Low FODMAP Diet[42,45,54-56]	• As previously discussed in the context of IBS, dietary FODMAPs are short-chain carbohydrates that are poorly absorbed in the small intestine, causing GI symptoms that are also common to IBD
	• An association between incompletely or malabsorbed FODMAPs and IBD has thus been postulated
	   – Early trials indicate a reduction of symptoms in more than 50% of patients with Crohn's disease and 33% of patients with UC
	   – This may be particularly useful in patients with "IBS-type" functional symptoms like bloating or osmotic diarrhea

The Specific Carbohydrate Diet (SCD)[34,49,54,56,60]	• Originally proposed to treat celiac disease, the SCD proposes strict elimination of all complex carbohydrates (disaccharides and polysaccharides) on the basis that bacterial fermentation of maldigested carbohydrates contributes to intestinal inflammation and/or bacterial and yeast overgrowth – Monosaccharides are the only permitted carbohydrates • Despite case reports that suggest that the SCD may be an effective tool in IBD, there are no published results that support its use (and long-term adherence is challenging).
The Paleolithic Diet[42,54,56]	• Based on the theory that the digestive tract is poorly evolved to handle the modern diet (i.e., the introduction of new foods beyond what was consumed in Paleolithic-era hunter-gatherer societies) – Diet is high in protein and polyunsaturated fatty acids and low in saturated fat; also devoid of grains, refined sugar, and dairy. • Although popular in the patient population (self-imposed), there are currently no published studies evaluation its efficacy in IBD.
High-Fiber Diet[36,49,54]	• Fiber has a beneficial effect on gut bacteria. – In addition, dietary fiber that metabolizes into short-chain fatty acids can stimulate water and sodium absorption in the colon and promote mucosal healing • Several studies have identified a fiber-rich, unrefined-carbohydrate diet as a key factor in reducing rates of hospital admission and surgeries for patients with Crohn's. • Other trials suggest that fiber supplementation (with Plantago ovate seeds) is as effective as pharmacologic treatment for maintaining remission. • Other studies have failed to demonstrate clinically-significant reductions in symptoms with a high-fiber diet.

Supplementation with Omega-3 (n-3) Fatty Acids[36,49,55,61]	• Fatty acids are mediators in the inflammatory cascade.
	   – Omega-3 fatty acids are believed to have immunomodulary properties, thus their proposed role in resolving IBD symptoms associated with inflammation.
	   – Despite the theoretical evidence that n-3 fatty acids (particularly fish oil) might be beneficial in both Crohn's and UC, this has not been reproduced and current evidence is weak.
	• Currently, although there is little sufficient evidence in favor of n-3 fatty acids as a maintenance therapy for IBD patients, their role in attenuating the general inflammatory process is well established.

Prebiotic and Probiotic Use[38,49,55]	• The proposed relationship between IBD and alterations in the gut microbiota has a considerable amount of evidential support, indicating potential for prebiotic and/or probiotic use in this patient population.
	• Prebiotics: Current evidence is insufficient in human IBD trials, but promising nonetheless and will likely continue to gain popularity
	• Probiotics: Potential effect for use only in UC patients, with no efficacy shown for Crohn's disease patients; effects are strain specific
	   – For use reducing the activity of mild-to-moderate UC: **VSL #3** (*B. breve, B. longum, B. infantis, L. acidophilus, L. casei, L. delbrueckii, L. plantarum,* and *Streptococcus salivarius subsp. thermophilus*)
	   – Additional strains for consideration: *S. boulardii, L. GG, B. bifidum, B. breve,* and *L acidophilus*.

radio-labeled EDTA and urine is again collected over time to assess whether the chemical is recovered in the urine. Similar issues arise with the accuracy of this test, suggesting its use may or may not be clinically relevant.[62]

Larazotide acetate is a medication currently being considered for treatment in patients who have celiac disease and symptoms suggestive of leaky gut despite strict adherence to the gluten-free diet. This medication serves as a tight-junction regulator.[62] Clinical trials are currently underway, making this an exciting area of preliminary research.

Nutrition Intervention

Because leaky gut syndrome is not well defined or studied in the literature development of nutrition intervention recommendations are in the initial stages. Some practical suggestions may include the following:

1. Provide instruction and support for patients with celiac disease to ensure they follow the GFD strictly
2. Utilize MyPlate to promote an overall healthy diet
3. Promote stress management techniques
4. Review alcohol intake
5. Recommend patient discuss NSAID usage with their physician if this is a regularly taken medication[62]

As more is discovered in research about leaky gut syndrome etiology and treatment, dietitians will have the ability to provide more up-to-date recommendations to help these patients reduce symptoms.

> **CORE CONCEPT 5**
>
> Careful assessment of the patient's nutritional status and GI symptoms will direct nutritional intervention in leaky gut syndrome, such as limiting alcohol and practicing stress management. Clinicians should be wary of "easy fix" fad diets that patients may be following.

Helicobacter pylori

Helicobacter pylori (*H. pylori*) is a bacterial infection that colonizes the stomach by moving through the mucosal lining, attaching to gastric epithelial cells, and releasing cytotoxins to allow for generation of more bacteria.[64,65] This infection can lead to a host of medical conditions, from general gastritis to peptic or duodenal ulcer, mucosal-associated lymphoid tissue lymphoma, and gastric cancer. In fact, *H. pylori* infection is implicated in 75% of gastric cancer cases worldwide.[64] (**Figure 13.7**) shows the bacteria penetrating the mucosal lining and leading to an ulcer. Transmission of these bacteria is due to inter-human contact and is strongly associated with low socioeconomic status.

Medical Treatment

Medical therapy for elimination of *H. pylori* infection is a 7-day combination therapy of four drugs: a proton-pump inhibitor (PPI) and three antibiotics (clarithromycin, amoxicillin, and metronidazole. The use of multiple types of antibiotic medications reflects the discovery of antibiotic resistance with certain strains of *H. pylori*. The eradication of *H. pylori* is

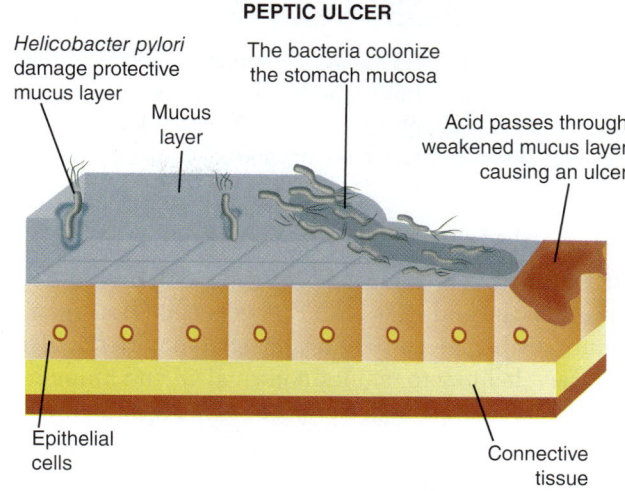

FIGURE 13.7 Bacterial Penetration of the Mucosal Lining Leads to Peptic Ulcer

important for prevention of secondary diseases as well as the standard therapy for treating peptic ulcer disease.[66]

Besides the use of PPI and antibiotics, probiotics have received some support for an additional benefit in the treatment of *H. pylori* and peptic ulcer disease.[67] The mechanism behind this theory is that probiotics are able to attach to the gastric epithelial cells and provide immune system support. In patients with diarrhea, probiotic use was able to decrease this symptom. Although this is a promising addition to the current accepted treatment regimen, future studies must assess the most beneficial probiotic strain, frequency, dose, and length of treatment.

Nutrition Assessment

Assessment of nutrient status is important to determine whether a patient will require any supplementation. *H. pylori* has been known to cause deficiencies in iron, vitamin C, vitamin A, alpha-tocopherol, vitamin B_{12}, folic acid, zinc, nickel, and selenium.[64,65] The infection has been speculated to affect insulin resistance, obesity, and lipid profiles.[65] Perhaps most importantly, *H. pylori* has been linked to malnutrition, particularly in children of developing nations. It is imperative that the dietitian assess whether a patient has any signs of nutrient deficiency or unintentional weight loss.

Nutrition Intervention

Eradication of *H. pylori* through the use of PPI and antibiotic combination therapy usually corrects micronutrient deficiencies because the bacteria are no longer sequestering these nutrients for their own proliferation. It is still important to monitor these micronutrient levels and provide supplementation as necessary. Limited research has suggested that avoidance of high levels of zinc, nickel, and iron may assist in quicker elimination of the bacteria as *H. pylori* requires these minerals to grow[64]; however, this must be weighed against the detrimental effects of becoming deficient in these nutrients.

In the case of unintentional weight loss, nutritional advice should be provided to help the patient safely regain weight and improve overall nutritional status through a general healthy diet.

> **CORE CONCEPT 6**
>
> Deficiencies in iron, vitamin C, vitamin A, alpha-tocopherol, vitamin B_{12}, folic acid, nickel, and selenium are possibly in patients with *H. pylori*. Patients with this infection should be monitored closely for both nutrient deficiency and unintentional weight loss.

Small Intestinal Bacterial Overgrowth (SIBO)

The human gut is home to more than 10 times more bacteria than the body has cells.[68] This normal flora is part of a mutually beneficial relationship shared with the digestive tract, helping to maintain normal GI and immune functions. The vast majority of bacteria are contained in the colon, with smaller amounts found in the small intestine, where abnormal amounts would interfere with the digestion and absorption of food. If a disproportionate number of bacteria (typically of the colonic nature) invade the small intestine, the overgrowth competes with the body for ingested nutrients and can impair the individual's nutritional status. This condition is referred to as **small intestinal bacterial overgrowth** (SIBO).[68-71]

SIBO occurs secondary to a number of clinical conditions, such as those listed in Table 13.12, and is typical in cases of diminished gastric acid secretion or disordered GI motility. Most bacteria that enter the digestive tract via ingestion are eliminated within the acidic environment of the stomach. Any that survive long enough to pass into the small intestine are subsequently cleared; normal motility is thus a major defense system against bacterial colonization of the small intestine, due in part to the action of the **migrating motor complex** (MMC). The MMC, or "intestinal housekeeper," produces a cleansing wave every 90 to 120 minutes during times of fasting. This wave sweeps the contents of the small intestine towards the colon, effectively removing any unwanted bacteria from the area. As such, one of the most common underlying causes of SIBO is impairment of the MMC—reduced frequency or complete loss of MMC movements occurs in an estimated 70% of patients with SIBO.[68-72]

SIBO is formally defined when >100,000 colony-forming units of bacteria per milliliter of intestinal juice are found in the proximal small intestine.[70,72] Although the bacterial strains are typically nonpathogenic in nature, such dramatic changes in the normal flora have a massive impact on nutritional status. The clinical manifestations that occur are primarily the result of malabsorption, caused by both bacterial competition for ingested nutrients and damage to the small intestinal epithelium. SIBO is also responsible for a number of nonspecific GI symptoms that often times contribute to an initial misdiagnosis.[68-71]

Diagnosis

Typically, bacterial abnormalities are identified using direct culture—the gold standard for diagnosis. As the intestinal bacterial flora is often out of reach of instrumentation, this method is not appropriate when assessing for SIBO. The SIBO diagnosis is made using a lactulose breath test. During the test, patients are given a predetermined amount of lactulose and all gases exhaled are measured over the course of several hours. Theoretically, any small intestinal bacteria will feed off of the lactulose; this bacterial fermentation produces methane and/or hydrogen gas, depending on the type of bacteria present. The gases are subsequently expelled by the lungs. Because the human body is unable to produce methane or hydrogen gas, their presence in the breath is indicative of SIBO; the test is positive if the patient produces a minimum of 20 ppm hydrogen and/or methane within the first 2 hours following administration.[68-71]

Consequences of Overgrowth on Absorption

Some degree of nutrient malabsorption is virtually guaranteed with the SIBO diagnosis. While there are a number of reasons why it occurs, malabsorption is primarily attributed to competition for nutrients and/or damage to absorptive surfaces.[70]

TABLE 13.12 CLINICAL CONDITIONS ASSOCIATED WITH SMALL INTESTINAL BOWEL OVERGROWTH[68-72]

Disturbances in Small Intestinal Transit and/or Motility	• Autonomic visceral neuropathy • Blind loops of the small intestine • Changes with aging • Chronic intestinal pseudo-obstruction • Disordered migrating motor complex • Intestinal stricture • Surgical alteration of normal small intestinal anatomy
Disturbances in Gastric Acid Secretion	• Achlorhydria • Acid suppression via medication • Chronic atrophic gastritis • Gastric resection
Associated Diagnoses	• Acute and chronic pancreatitis • Celiac disease • Chronic radiation enteropathy • Diabetes mellitus • Diverticulosis/diverticulitis • End-stage renal disease • End-stage liver disease • Fibromyalgia • Gastroesophageal reflux disease • Hypothyroidism • Immunodeficiency syndrome(s) • Inflammatory bowel disease (primarily Crohn's disease) • Irritable bowel syndrome • Recurrent antibiotic use • Short bowel syndrome

One of the most common complications of SIBO is fat malabsorption. As part of the normal absorptive process, digested lipids (monoglycerides and fatty acids) combine with phospholipids and bile acid to form **micelles**. Micelles transport the otherwise poorly absorbed substrates to the surface of the enterocyte, where they are taken up by the body. In the presence of SIBO, intraluminal bacteria cause the deconjugation of bile acid; if the concentration of conjugated bile acids drops below the threshold necessary for micellar formation, as is often the case, absorption of fats is impaired. It is thus extremely common for patients to present with chronic steatorrhea. Improper micellar formation and/or fat malabsorption will often lead to deficiencies of the fat-soluble vitamins.[70,72]

Bacterial activity in the gut lumen has been shown to indirectly damage the absorptive mucosa; when this occurs, carbohydrate and protein absorption may also be affected. Mucosal injury and decreased brush border enzyme activity interfere primarily with carbohydrate uptake; in this case, bacterial flora ferment the carbohydrate substrates before they are made available to the host. Though severe protein malnutrition is extremely rare in SIBO patients, gut bacteria similarly compete with the host for protein substrates. Overall absorptive dysfunction and mucosal injury, along with decreased levels of the enterokinases necessary for pancreatic protease activation, contribute to decreased amino acid and peptide uptake.[70,72]

Finally, SIBO's effect can extend beyond macronutrient malabsorption, inhibiting uptake of several micronutrients. As mentioned, fat malabsorption is linked with deficiencies of the fat-soluble vitamins (primarily vitamins A, D, and E; because vitamin K is actually synthesized by the bacterial microflora, deficiency is rarely seen). In addition, bacteria within the intestinal lumen readily utilize vitamin B_{12} before it can be absorbed. Deficiencies of thiamine and nicotinamide, although less common, have also been reported for similar reasons. In contrast, folate levels are often elevated in this population; the gut bacteria synthesize the vitamin, which is subsequently absorbed by the body.[70,72]

Clinical Presentation

Symptoms will vary depending on both the type of bacteria colonizing the small intestine and the nature of any underlying intestinal abnormality that preceded SIBO. There are a number of clinical features common to most SIBO cases: excess intestinal gas, abdominal distention and bloating, diarrhea, and pain or discomfort. Refer to **Table 13.13** for a more comprehensive patient profile.[68-73]

The classical manifestations of SIBO are largely the result of bacterial interaction with ingested food; within this context, symptoms may be exacerbated postprandially or may occur secondary to malabsorption. For example, bacteria that prefer to metabolize carbohydrates will produce excess gas and cause significant intestinal distention, while those that metabolize bile salts and therefore inhibit fat absorption will contribute to chronic steatorrhea. When these symptoms reduce or alter normal food intake, as is often the case, the disease state is further complicated. The vast majority of patients identify postprandial bloating and/or nausea as the culprits behind decreased oral intake. Correcting nutritional status remains a priority.[70-72]

TABLE 13.13 CLINICAL CHARACTERISTICS OF SMALL INTESTINAL BOWEL OVERGROWTH[68,73]

Gastrointestinal Symptoms	• Abdominal discomfort, pain, and/or cramping • Belching Constipation • Diarrhea and/or steatorrhea • Distention (especially postprandial bloating) Early satiety • Flatulence • Lactose intolerance • Nausea • Weight loss
Extraintestinal Symptoms	• Anemia • Depression • Eczema • Fatigue • Headaches or loss of concentration • Impaired night vision • Joint pain • Neuropathy • Osteomalacia

Biochemical Abnormalities	• Micronutrient deficiencies
	  – Vitamin A
	  – Vitamin B_{12}
	  – Vitamin D
	  – Vitamin E
	  – Iron
	• Hypoproteinemia, hypoalbuminemia

Medical Treatment

There are three primary components to the treatment of SIBO:

1. Correct (or treat) the underlying cause.
2. Eliminate bacterial overgrowth via antibiotic therapy.
3. Address any nutritional implications, including deficiencies.

Regardless of the pathogenesis behind the diminished acid production and/or motility impairment that ultimately resulted in SIBO, any excess bacteria colonizing the small intestine must be eradicated. Therefore, antibiotic therapy forms the cornerstone of treatment. In some cases where antibiotic use is contraindicated (allergies and/or limited response), patients are fed with an **elemental formula**. Elemental formulas provide nutrients in predigested forms and are thought to be absorbed within the first few feet of the small intestine. Research shows that, because the nutrients are absorbed before reaching the bacteria, which are subsequently starved, elemental diets provide a safe and effective alternative to treating the overgrowth. The vast majority of patients are prescribed Rifaximin because of its efficacy within the digestive tract: 99.6% will remain in the gut without being absorbed. SIBO has a high recurrence rate (nearly 50%) within 9 months following antibiotic treatment if the underlying cause is not also addressed.[68,70,73,74]

Nutrition Therapy

Nutrition interventions are critical to successful management of SIBO. While there are a number of overarching goals to be met through nutrition therapy—symptom management, correction of nutritional deficiencies, and recurrence prevention—all interventions should be individualized to meet the patient's specific needs.[68,72]

Although symptoms associated with malabsorption may begin to improve shortly after treatment begins, it is important for patients to initially avoid foods that contribute to intestinal fermentation. The damage caused by SIBO results in decreased secretion of the brush border enzymes lactase, sucrase, and maltase; because the epithelium takes time to repair and regenerate, the reduction in these enzymes may continue after the overgrowth has been treated. Undigested and unabsorbed lactose, sucrose, and maltose become substrates for bacterial fermentation; thus, restricting intake of sugars and starches can help prevent prolonged bloating and abnormal bowel movements while the intestine heals. Preliminary research has shown that a low FODMAP diet, as previously discussed in the context of IBS therapy, is useful in reducing the symptoms associated with fermentation. For all patients, the dietitian can help to identify problematic foods using a careful and supervised elimination diet. This allows for a symptom management plan that is customized per individual tolerances.[68,71,75]

There are a number of other dietary modifications that can be made to reduce specific symptoms. For example, for patients with persistent steatorrhea, a decrease in or restriction of fat intake may be beneficial in the beginning of treatment.[72] Others who present with enduring and/or uncomfortable flatus may find relief from eliminating nonabsorbable sugar alcohols (sorbitol, aspartame, and saccharine) from the diet. Aerophagia—the involuntary swallowing of air—occurs in all individuals via normal activities such as chewing gum or drinking beverages through a straw. This, however, may be irritating to the SIBO patient population and can be avoided to help reduce abdominal distention.[75]

> **PRACTICE POINT**
>
> Encourage patients to maintain a log that will track intake and symptoms. This provides for identification of foods or food groups that continue to exacerbate the symptoms of malabsorption, which can be avoided in the beginning of treatment through a careful elimination diet and reintroduced once symptoms resolve.

It may be difficult to correct nutrient deficiencies when digestive symptoms persist, as this indicates that a certain degree of the brush border of the intestinal tract remains damaged. In patients with documented steatorrhea, the use of MCTs can help to facilitate absorption of fatty acids. As symptoms subside, however, all nutrient deficiencies should be identified and corrected. Again, SIBO typically interferes with the fat-soluble vitamins A, D, and E; vitamin B_{12}; and iron, but other deficiencies are not uncommon.[68,72,75]

> **PRACTICE POINT**
>
> When recommending supplementation of micronutrients, be sure to select brands without fillers or other ingredients such a as gluten and/or sugars that may continue intestinal fermentation and/or irritation.[68]

Finally, nutrition therapy can play a role in promoting the actions of the MMC. This will be critical in preventing recurrence of bacterial overgrowth. Because the MMC is deactivated when eating, the most important consideration will be meal spacing. Individuals prone to SIBO should be encouraged to distribute meals evenly throughout the day, typically every 3 to 5 hours, and to avoid or limit between-meal snacking; both modifications will allow sufficient time for the cleansing wave to remove waste from the small intestine.[68,71]

The goal of nutritional intervention for this population is the same as that for all disease states: the optimization of nutritional status. In severe cases of SIBO, individuals may present with weight loss and/or malnutrition. For these patients, nutritional supplements should be provided and careful monitoring of weight and markers of nutrition status is necessary. Although uncommon, PN may be indicated to provide nutrition to the severely malnourished patient; however, this is associated with a number of secondary complications and should only be used when all other options for nutrient repletion have been exhausted.[70,72] The bottom line remains: the dietitian plays an integral role in helping patients with SIBO to alleviate symptoms, optimize digestion, and improve nutritional status.[68]

> **PRACTICE POINT**
>
> When evaluating clients with undiagnosed GI complains, SIBO should always be on the dietitian's radar. The most important concerns when working with this population include maintaining adequate nutritional intake through a customized dietary approach, correcting nutrient deficiencies, and maximizing digestion.[71]

> **CORE CONCEPT 7**
>
> SIBO is often associated with and occurs concurrently with a number of other disorders related to maldigestion and malabsorption. Nutrition therapy plays a critical role in the treatment of this patient population.

⚠ Clinical Controversy

Do probiotics have a place at the table for SIBO treatment?

Although antibiotic use currently serves as the first line of treatment for eliminating inappropriate bacterial overgrowth of the small intestine, it is not a guaranteed solution. The most common concerns with antibiotic treatment in the context of SIBO involve poor patient tolerance and diminished efficacy with long-term use. More importantly, there is a large potential for rebound colonization after treatment is stopped. Interest in the use of probiotics as a potential treatment for SIBO and as a means for preventing recurrence has grown. However, the evidence is largely preliminary and is, in many cases, controversial.[76,77]

The biggest barrier to probiotic use in this population is the limited availability of high-quality trials specific to SIBO patients. As clinicians in an evidenced-based practice, this is certainly cause for apprehension for many dietitians. There is sufficient evidence demonstrating the benefit of probiotic use to the disordered GI tract at large. There are several identified mechanisms for how these benefits occur:

1. Competition with pathogens for adherence to the intestinal epithelium and mucosa
2. Production of bacteriocins (produced by bacteria to kill or inhibit bacterial strains closely related to produced bacteria)
3. Inhibition of bacterial translocation
4. Enhancement of mucosal barrier function
5. Downregulation of inflammatory processes
6. Modulation of gut motor and sensory responses and signaling between luminal bacteria, the intestinal epithelium, and the immune system[77,78]

The results from preliminary and pilot trials are encouraging. Most studies have focused on bacterial strains from the genus *Lactobacillus*, which have been proven effective for other GI-related conditions.[78,79] For example, one small study using *L. casei* and *L. acidophilus* illustrated a statistically significant reduction in chronic diarrhea related to bacterial overgrowth.[77]

Similar results were seen in a study investigating the effect of probiotics on SIBO secondary to chronic liver disease. Researchers found that probiotic therapy, which was a combination of five bacterial species (*Bifidobacterium bifidum, B. longum, L. acidophilus, L. rhamnosus,* and *Streptococcus thermophilus*) showed a statistically significant reduction in GI symptom relief when compared to the placebo group. In addition, for 24% of individuals in the therapy group, the bacterial growth was eradicated altogether.[80]

In another pilot study assessing *L. casei*, 64% of patients receiving the treatment no longer tested positive for the lactulose breath test given at the end of the 6-week intervention period. However, there were no significant improvements in abdominal symptoms seen in this trial.[76]

Additional trials, although small, have directly compared probiotic use to antibiotic use. In one study, patients were randomized to receive either a combination probiotic or the antibiotic Metronidazole as treatment for SIBO. The probiotic contained *L. casei, L. plantarum, S. faecalis,* and *B. brevis*. Based on the statistically significant reduction of symptoms seen in the intervention group, the study conclusions favored probiotic use over antibiotic use.[76]

The most promising results have come from a study that using a **synbiotic**—a product containing both prebiotic and probiotic strains. This study enrolled individuals with chronic stomach pain and/or changes in bowel movements secondary to SIBO with no other anatomical or functional diagnoses. Thirty cases confirmed with a breath test were randomized in a double-blind manner into either the synbiotic group or the control group. The synbiotic, Lactol, is a combination of *L. sporogenes* (probiotic) and fructo-oligosaccharides (prebiotic). At the end of the 6-month treatment period, all subjects in the synbiotic group reported complete disappearance of stomach pain. This group also reported considerably less bloating and diarrhea when compared to the control group. In addition, almost all (93.3%) of participants in the treatment group tested negative in the breath test given at the end of the study.[78]

Although promising, these studies are difficult to compare due to the vast differences in study populations, probiotic species used, and clinical outcomes. These limitations, when combined with the small sample sizes of each study, hamper the generalization of the results.[77]

The beneficial effects of prebiotics need to be confirmed with double-blind, randomized, placebo-controlled trials of notably larger sample sizes. Before the recommendation for probiotic use in this patient population can be solidified, these trials must demonstrate the following:

1. The most favorable bacterial strain and/or combination of strains
2. Appropriate dosage and dose effects
3. The therapeutic role of probiotics as initial therapy or in maintenance/suppression
4. Clinical relevance[76-78]

⚠ Clinical Controversy (continued)

Because antibiotic therapy cannot correct the underlying microflora imbalances in SIBO, recurrences of overgrowth and the accompanying symptoms following this treatment method are common. Probiotics appear to be viable alternatives or adjuncts to conventional treatment of SIBO by helping to rebalance the gut flora and improving overall function of the GI tract.[79-81] Current evidence shows support for the reduction of symptoms and overall reduction of inappropriate bacterial overgrowth, but the use of probiotics within this population necessitates further research.[81]

Read the two articles below. Critique their study design and findings. How do they compare? What is the clinical relevance of their findings? What are your recommendations based on the findings of these papers?

References

1. Khalghi AR, Khalighi, MR, Behdani, R., et al. Evaluating the efficacy of probiotic on treatment in patients with small intestinal bacterial overgrowth (SIBO) - A pilot study. *Indian J Med Res*. 2014;140(5):604-608.

2. Kwak DS, Jun DW, Seo JG, et al. Short-term probiotic therapy alleviates small intestinal bacterial overgrowth, but does not improve intestinal permeability in chronic liver disease. *Eur J Gastroenterol Hepatol*. 2014;26(12):1353-1359.

Bowel Surgery and Short Bowel Syndrome (SBS)

As with any disease state, surgical interventions for disorders of the small and large intestines are used only when more conventional methods of care fail. If extensive damage to the bowel occurs as the result of chronic disease or obstruction, function in that area is understandably lost and that section requires removal.[82] For example, it is common for a patient with Crohn's disease to require surgery related to uncontrolled inflammation or for complications secondary to the disease progression.[39] In any case, surgical management typically involves resection to remove the damaged bowel and a reconstruction to allow digestive processes to occur with as much normalcy as possible. The extent of resection and procedure of choice depends on the preemptive diagnosis and degree of damage. The nutritional implications and necessary interventions also depend on the area and amount of the bowel that is removed.[82] Different sections of the small and large intestines have different responsibilities in terms of digestion and absorption. Any changes to the integrity of the GI tract will have significant consequences on nutritional status postoperatively.

Bowel Resection

There are a number of diagnoses involving the GI tract that, when all other treatment approaches have been exhausted, warrant surgical intervention. These conditions often involve intestinal inflammation, obstruction, or acute injury. The magnitude of the refractory disease and

CASE STUDY REVISITED

Despite the efforts of the medical team, Daniel's Crohn's disease remains poorly controlled. He has a number of relapses that deplete his nutritional status quickly.

Two years after his diagnosis, Daniel has his first bowel resection surgery. Afterwards, he has approximately 120 cm of his small intestine remaining with an ileostomy, meaning his colon is not continuous with his GI tract.

During the first month after discharge from the hospital following the bowel resection and ileostomy procedure, Daniel has multiple admissions for dehydration and continued unintended weight loss. The dietitian completes a recall, which reveals that he is eating adequately. This means that his intake is not the source of his significant weight loss.

Questions

1. What additional diagnosis might Daniel present with?
2. List the potential nutritional implications of decreased bowel length and loss of colon continuity.
3. What might you recommend for Daniel to maintain his quality of life for the long term?

the extent of damage determine the amount of bowel to be resected. As portions of the small and/or large intestine are removed, the segments that remain may be reattached to one another, forming an **anastomosis**. When necessary, an artificial opening referred to as a **stoma** is created to form a new path for fecal excretion; this type of procedure, called an **ostomy**, will be discussed in more detail later in the chapter. (**Figure 13.8**) depicts a stoma formed from part of the colon brought through the abdominal wall. The goal is to leave as much functional bowel as possible and to facilitate relatively normal digestive processes.[82,83]

Although all patients are at high risk for malabsorption and subsequent malnutrition following bowel resection, the needs of each individual will vary greatly. The postoperative nutritional implications and thus the care plan to be implemented depend primarily on the location and amount of remaining bowel. The most obvious consideration is the difference in function at each segment of the GI tract, with careful attention to which area may have been lost. It is also critical to recognize that some portions of the intestine are more capable of adapting and compensating for loss of absorptive capacity than others. Accordingly, the three factors that most affect nutritional status in this patient population are as follows:

1. How much functional bowel remains?
2. What sections of the small and/or large bowel remain?
3. Is the ileocecal valve present?[82]

Absorption Affected by Resection Site The tasks of the small and large intestines differ. Each portion is designed specifically to facilitate the absorption of nutrients, fluid, and electrolytes. Considering the area of resection can help the clinician predict the nutritional challenges a patient will face postoperatively before any complications actually occur.[84]

Duodenal Resection The most proximal portion of the small intestine, the duodenum (approximately 25-30 cm in length), is a digestive dynamo. Not only is it the preferred site of absorption for many micronutrients, but it is also the location at which the pancreatic enzymes and bile salts enter the GI tract. Loss of the duodenum would be catastrophic to normal digestion and absorption. Fortunately, it is rarely resected or involved in bowel reconstructive procedures.[85]

Jejunal Resection More than 90% of nutrient absorption occurs within the first 100 to 150 cm of the small

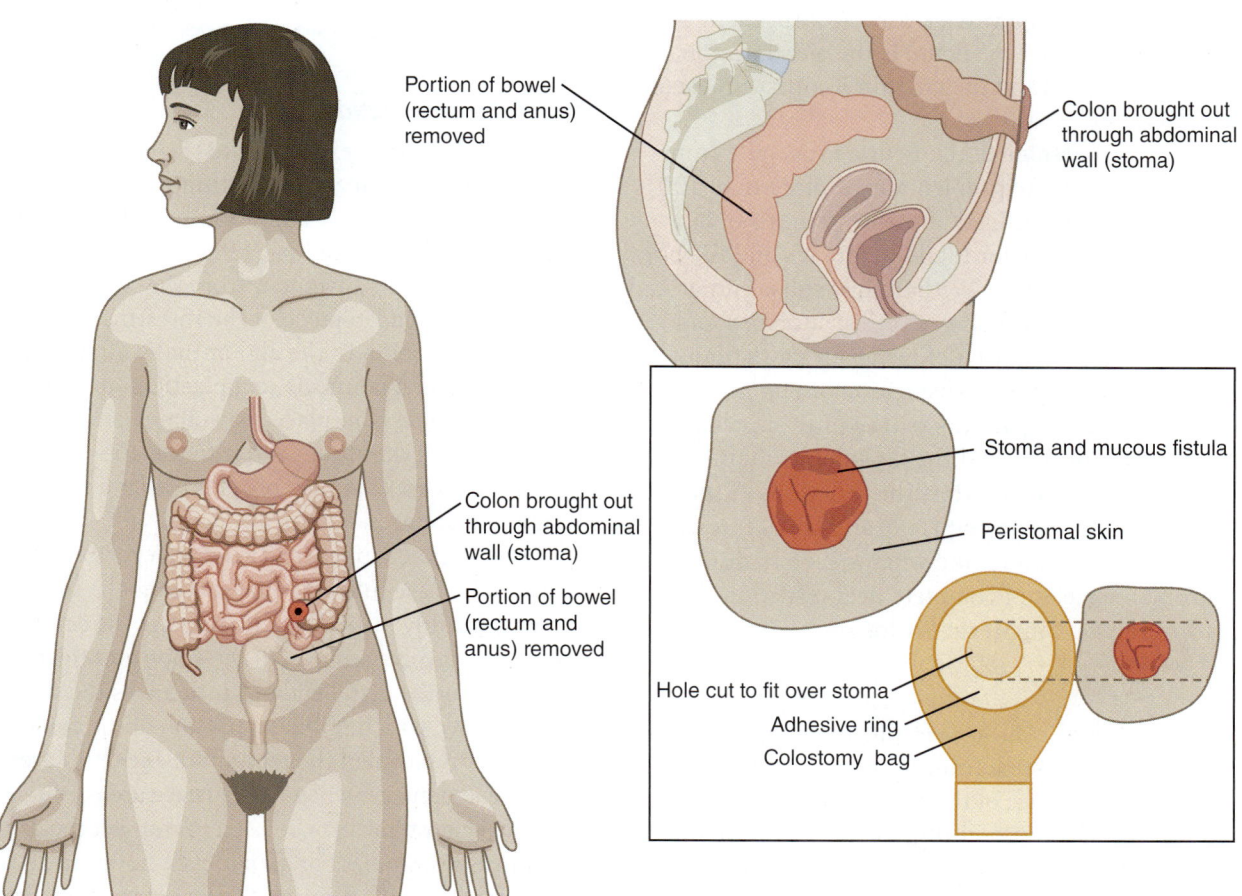

FIGURE 13.8 A Stoma is Created by Bringing the Colon Through the Abdominal Wall for Normal Fecal Excretion

intestine. This area encompasses the duodenum and the proximal portion of the jejunum, meaning that the jejunum (approximately 200-300 cm in length in its entirety) has a similarly critical role in facilitating absorptive processes. In addition, jejunal enterohormones (cholecystekinin, secretin, gastric inhibitory peptide, and vasoactive inhibitory peptide) are key to normal digestion and absorption. When segments of the jejunum are removed, the resulting reduction in surface area and decreased transit time indicates significant potential for impaired nutrient absorption.[85]

The ileum is capable of adapting both structurally and functionally to perform the lost functions of the jejunum. Jejunal resections are thus typically well tolerated when enough of the ileum remains to compensate. Documented patient outcomes are notably better for jejunal resections when compared to ileal resections.[85,86]

Ileal Resection The ileum (approximately 300-400 cm in length) has an absorptive capacity nearly double that of the jejunum with a much slower intrinsic motility. Here, an intestinal feedback mechanism known as the **ileal brake** is triggered when undigested nutrients enter into the ileum. Ileal brake activation delays gastric emptying and slows transit time in the proximal portions of the small intestine, allowing extended contact time between nutrients and the mucosa. This mechanism, which facilitates greater nutrient absorption, is one of the key factors allowing the ileum to compensate for any decreased absorption in the jejunum.[85-87] In addition, the ileum is the only location for absorption of bile salts and the vitamin B_{12}-intrinsic factor complex.[84-85]

Significant resections of the ileum, especially from the terminal portion, are problematic. If more than 100 cm of terminal ileum are lost, hepatic synthesis of bile salts cannot compensate for intestinal losses and the bile salt pool is not maintained. Without bile salts, undigested fat is excreted in feces, causing severe steatorrhea and potential fat-soluble vitamin deficiency. If more than 60 cm of terminal ileum is lost, absorption of vitamin B_{12} is readily impaired. Most patients will require supplementation of both vitamin B_{12} and the fat-soluble vitamins. Loss of the distal ileum and thus the functions of the ileal brake lead to rapid gastric emptying and small intestine transit time, closely mimicking what is seen in dumping syndrome. In cases of complete ileal resection, most patients will rely on long-term PN for sustenance and survival.[82,84,85,88,89]

The Ileocecal Valve The **ileocecal (IC) valve** separates the ileum of the small intestine from the cecum of the large intestine. The importance of the IC valve is twofold. First, it plays a pivotal role in preventing the reflux of colonic contents into the ileum. Second, the IC valve maintains slow control over the passage of digesta from the ileum into the colon, increasing nutrient/mucosa contact time in the small intestine.[85] When this crucial area is removed as part of the surgical resection, there is considerable loss of absorptive function. More importantly, however, loss of the IC valve places the patient at considerable risk for developing SIBO within whatever small intestine remains. The presence or absence of the IC valve is an essential consideration when determining nutritional implications postoperatively.[84,88]

Colonic Involvement Although little nutrient absorption occurs past the small intestine, the large intestine (approximately 160 cm in length) is the central site for fluid and electrolyte reabsorption. Whereas a normal colon recovers between 1 and 1.5 L of electrolyte-rich fluid daily, this capacity can increase by three- to five-fold if necessary for compensation. Regardless, preservation of the colon is imperative for the maintenance of hydration status. Of equal importance, the colon can help to compensate for decreased jejunal carbohydrate absorption if necessary; maintaining half (or more) of the colon is equivalent to maintaining 50 cm of functional small intestine. Outcomes are significantly better in patients able to retain colonic function.[85,86]

> **CORE CONCEPT 8**
>
> In surgical resections of the GI tract, the amount of bowel removed and remaining and the location from which the resection is made are key determinants as to whether digestive and absorptive processes can be maintained postoperatively and if prolonged nutrition intervention is necessary.

Bowel Reconstruction

If intestinal damage extends into the bowel, warranting removal of the colon and/or rectum, it will be necessary to surgically create a new pathway for fecal excretion. This type of procedure, referred to as an ostomy, removes colonic involvement from the digestive pathway altogether. Instead, a piece of the intestine is brought through an incision in the abdominal wall; this segment, called the stoma, connects to a plastic pouch **appliance**. Once the ostomy is in place, bowel movements naturally empty through the stoma and into the appliance. On an individual basis, ostomies provide either a temporary or a permanent solution.[90]

Ostomy procedures are further categorized based on the portion of the intestine that serves as the stoma. The two most readily utilized techniques are the **ileostomy**, which may involve removal of the colon and the rectum and connects the distal end of the ileum as the stoma, and the **colostomy**, which utilizes a portion of the colon as the stoma after removal of the rectum. In extreme cases of widespread damage, when ileal surface area or function is lost, a **jejunostomy** may be used to connect the distal jejunum as the stoma. For all patients, however, the extent of nutritional implications will relate more to the initial amount and type of bowel resection than to the presence of an ostomy itself. As previously addressed, a bowel resection will alter intestinal motility, absorptive capacity, and production of waste. While placement of the stoma will not exacerbate the nutritional consequences of the resection, its location does play a role in determining the type of fecal matter produced.[83,90,91]

Jejunostomy Patients who have received an end jejunostomy require the most intensive nutritional interventions because they lack both the ileum and the colon in continuity. The remaining jejunum is incapable of compensating for the loss of ileal and colonic function. Therefore, these patients are subject to significant malabsorption of macro- and micronutrients, as well as high-volume fluid and electrolyte losses.[84,92]

Ileostomy An ileostomy placement indicates resection of the terminal ileum and colon, and therefore loss of the important IC valve. Absence of the IC valve results in increased motility throughout the proximal small intestine, shortening the length of contact time between nutrients and absorptive mucosa. If transit time is sufficiently altered, absorption of both macro- and micronutrients will be impaired. The nutrient of most concern is vitamin B_{12}, which requires receptors located in the distal end of the ileum to be absorbed. Finally, and perhaps most importantly, patients with ileostomies struggle to maintain proper hydration status without a continuous colon to reabsorb water and electrolytes.[83]

Without the opportunity to pass through the colon, where fluid is reabsorbed and stool is shaped, ileostomy output manifests as watery, less-formed waste. In the initial weeks following surgery, output averages at 1,200 mL/day, but may settle to 600 mL/day as the body adjusts.[83]

Colostomy A colostomy is further specified as one of three types based on the portion of the colon that is used as the stoma. In an ascending colostomy—the least common of the three—the stoma is created using the ascending colon and exits via the right abdominal wall. This indicates that all but the first segment of the colon has been resected. Output from an ascending colostomy will be much more watery when compared to the remaining two procedures. The second variation, a descending colostomy, utilizes either the descending or the sigmoid colon to create the stoma, which will then exit through the left lower abdomen. **Figure 13.9** provides a visual image of a descending colostomy. Output is generally semi-formed or fully formed because it has passed through ascending and transverse sections of the colon. This is the most common of the colostomy procedures. Finally, a transverse colostomy can be created using one or two stomas from any portion of the transverse colon. If there are two openings, the procedure is referred to as a double-barrel colostomy, with one to pass semi-formed stool and the other to pass mucus.[91]

Nutritional Implications of Bowel Resection and Bypass: Common Guidelines

Any postoperative patient is at high risk for nutritional implications. This patient population is especially vulnerable considering the following:

1. The significant changes to the GI anatomy that will undoubtedly affect the processes of digestion and absorption
2. The strong potential for malnutrition from the preceding disease state that likely existed prior to surgery

The location at which the resection was made is extremely important. This, along with the amount of functional bowel remaining, will determine how well the patient is able to adapt and obtain nutrition following bowel surgery. Many patients, particularly those who have undergone multiple surgeries or who have received extensive bowel resection, will develop short bowel syndrome. This common condition will be discussed in its entirely in the following section and will guide much of the nutrition intervention patients will require. There is, however, a set of general guidelines that apply to all members of this patient population in the immediate postoperative period.[82]

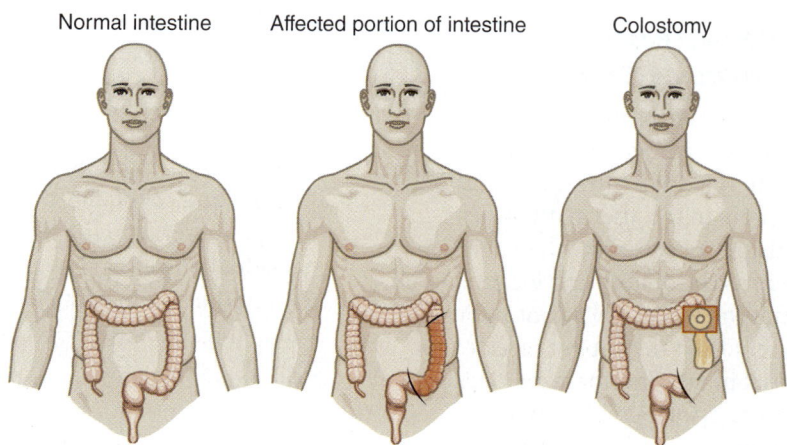

FIGURE 13.9 A Colostomy is Placed Depending on the Disease Affected Portion of the Colon. There are 3 Major Types of Colostomy, Ascending, Decending, and Transverse; Shown Here is a Decending Colostomy

Research and clinical experience support the initiation of oral intake as soon as can be tolerated postsurgery. This relies heavily on the individual patient and procedure. The traditional method involves progression from a clear liquid diet to a more normalized meal plan, but many patients with extensive resection will require nutrition support in the form of PN as the healing process begins. Clear liquids can be initiated when signs of bowel function return (flatus and/or a bowel movement), providing fluid and electrolytes and some stimulation to the GI tract with minimal digestion. Eventually, the patient will be advanced to a low-fiber diet that provides adequate energy, protein, fluid, and electrolytes. Smaller, more frequent meals are often better tolerated. As oral intake increases, adequate fluid intake is encouraged.[82,83,91]

Nutrition therapy will focus primarily on ensuring adequate absorption to optimize nutritional status postoperatively and promote healing. In addition, there are a number of diet modifications that can help in the alleviation of symptoms; for example, patients are encouraged to avoid gas- and/or odor-producing foods and foods that may exacerbate diarrhea. Other nutrition-related goals include decreasing the risk of obstruction and maintaining hydration status through proper fluid and electrolyte balance. As always, diet recommendations will be highly individualized. Patients should be considered at risk for developing malnutrition until able to consume a normalized diet without symptoms (which may include cramping, nausea, vomiting, excessive flatulence, or diarrhea).[83,91]

Nutrition support in the form of EN or PN is necessitated when patients are unable to meet energy needs orally or when postoperative complications, such as obstructions, fistulas, or anastomotic leaks, arise. It should not be surprising that cases of malnutrition are common. Be cognizant of indications that the patient requires supplemental or complete support, including evidence of malabsorption, fluid and electrolyte imbalance, weight loss, decreased muscle mass, and/or micronutrient deficiencies. PN use is not unusual in this population.[82]

Nutritional Implications of Bowel Resection and Bypass: Short Bowel Syndrome (SBS)

Short bowel syndrome (SBS) broadly encompasses any malabsorption related to decreased absorptive surface area and/or loss of functional capacity in the small intestine. For the vast majority of cases, SBS occurs in the aftermath of surgical resection or bypass; the degree of severity will depend on the length of resection, as well as the quality and location of remaining bowel. The presence or absence of a continuous colon (in other words, whether or not the patient received an ostomy) will also be influential in SBS development. Because of chronic fluid, nutrient, and electrolyte malabsorption, patients will rely on bowel adaptation and a combination of pharmacologic and nutritional therapies for survival.[84,89]

It is important to note that because of the extreme heterogeneity in this patient population, it is difficult to develop uniform scientific trials. Large, prospective, randomized studies do not exist. Therefore, all of the recommendations for SBS patients are based on best practice from small clinical trials and the guidance of experienced clinicians.[84]

Pathophysiology In a normal adult, the length of the small intestine varies between 300 and 800 cm, approximately half of which can be removed without significant issue. However, when extensive bowel resection is necessary, patients may be left with 100 cm or less of functioning small intestine. While there is no fixed bowel length necessary for SBS diagnosis, resections of this nature—with loss of two-thirds or more of the small intestine—loosely define the disorder. Within the context of bowel length, there are two clinical distinctions of SBS. The first contains patients with approximately 100 to 120 cm of remaining bowel without continuity of the colon (those with a small-bowel ostomy). The second encompasses those with continuity of the colon with 50 cm or less of remaining small bowel; for this group, the presence of the IC valve and functioning colon significantly improve absorptive capacity. These categorizations can be further divided based on which specific segments of the small intestine remain. Resection of the duodenum and terminal ileum will be more detrimental to patients than resection of the jejunum. Regardless, in the presence of any degree of SBS, severe malabsorption is inevitable. Both groups rely heavily on the ability of the remaining bowel to compensate for the lost absorptive surface and function; this process is known as intestinal adaptation.[84,85,88,89,93]

Intestinal Adaptation There are three phases of postoperative rehabilitation for bowel resection: the acute phase, the adaptation phase, and the maintenance phase. The acute phase begins immediately following surgery and generally lasts up to 4 weeks. As the patient stabilizes, they will enter into the most crucial period of recovery: the adaptation phase. This phase, which lasts 1 to 2 years,[94] is marked by both structural and functional changes in the remaining bowel to allow for compensation of lost surface area. The list of potential adaptations includes the following:

1. Villous hypertrophy: Significant increases in villi height and crypt depth
2. Slight increase in the length and diameter of the residual bowel
3. Alterations in motility, enzyme activity, and hormonal responses

While the exact mechanism of these changes remains unknown, the sum effect of the adaptation period is a sizeable increase in the remaining bowel's absorptive capacity. The dietitian plays a critical role: The adaptations occur only if nutrients are presented to the intestinal lumen. This importance cannot be overstated; a gradual increase in nutrient exposure through oral intake is the most powerful stimulus to intestinal adaptation. The time that the patient spends in the adaptation phase must be maximized to its full potential. Once an individual enters into the maintenance phase, it is unlikely that any other structural or functional changes will occur to the GI tract.[85,88,89]

> **PRACTICE POINT**
>
> Transition patients to a complex oral diet as early as possible in the postoperative recovery period to stimulate the necessary adaptive changes within the remaining intestinal tract.[88]

Management of SBS SBS manifestations are most aptly controlled through pharmacologic treatment and medical nutrition therapy. The overarching goal is the prevention of malnutrition and chronic dehydration through adequate absorption of nutrients and fluids. A number of medications, listed in **Table 13.14**, will help to slow intestinal transit, while others will minimize the gastric acid hypersecretion that is common to this patient population; management of both will improve absorption rates. This section will focus on the dietary modifications that, when made based on personal tolerance and procedure type, will ensure that the energy and fluid needs of the patient are met while minimizing any nutrition-related symptoms that arise.[84,88,89]

Nutrition support may be required either temporarily in the postoperative period or on a more long-term basis depending on the specific needs of the patient. A SBS diagnosis does not necessarily indicate **intestinal failure**, which is clinically defined when an individual is unable to maintain nutritional autonomy and thus requires long-term PN.[93]

Medical Nutrition Therapy For patients in the postoperative adaptation phase, the most prudent nutritional goal is stimulation through maximized use of remaining gut with provision of adequate energy, fluid, and electrolytes. It is common for patients to be fed via PN and supplemented with additional IV fluids in the period immediately following surgery. At this point, PN serves as the primary source of nutrition and hydration until the bowel begins to adapt. Ultimately, the intention is to wean all patients from nutrition support. Nutritional autonomy can be accomplished in many cases, especially for those with a colon in continuity and/or a minimum of 100 cm of functional small bowel remaining. Even if maximal adaptation of the bowel is achieved, the vast majority of patients will experience malabsorption of at least 30% of nutrients ingested.[84,85,94,95]

> **PRACTICE POINT**
>
> Encourage patients to consume nutrient-dense foods that are higher in calories than necessary to meet energy needs. Aim for 45 to 60 kcal/kg/day. Patients may need to ingest 200% to 400% over needs to offset the malabsorption experienced in this condition.[84,85,96]

> **PRACTICE POINT**
>
> Weaning from PN can be initiated when the patient tolerates oral nutrition without excessive stool or ostomy output. Continue to monitor output as the weaning process progresses, in addition to weight status to include either weight maintenance or appropriate weight gain. If necessary, oral intake can be supplemented with enteral feedings.[85,88,95]

The secondary nutritional goal for patients with SBS is management of symptoms related to both the postoperative recovery period and to malabsorption. This patient population is extremely heterogeneous; dietary modifications vary depending on differences in GI anatomy and functional capacity of the remaining mucosa. Depending on these factors, patients may present with nausea, vomiting, obstruction, diarrhea, and/or dehydration., Each symptom has its own dietary modification. For example, chronic diarrhea

TABLE 13.14 PHARMACOLOGICAL TREATMENT OPTIONS FOR SHORT BOWEL SYNDROME[88,89]

Drug Category	Action
Antimotility/Antidiarrheal Agents *Common examples:* loperamide, diphenoxylate, atropine, codeine, deodorized tincture of opium (DTO), clonidine	Used to slow peristalsis and improve absorption of fluid, electrolytes, and nutrients
Antisecretory Agents Histamine H_2 antagonists (H_2 blockers) *Common examples:* famotidine, ranitidine, cimetidine Proton pump inhibitors (PPIs) *Common examples:* omeprazole, lansoprazole, protonix Somatostatin analogues *Common examples:* octreotide	Used to decrease gastric acid secretion, diarrheal losses, and risk for peptic ulcer disease
Parenteral Infusion Therapy *May vary from saline infusions to full PN support*	Needed to maintain fluid and electrolyte balance postoperatively as bowel function normalizes

Data from Matarese LE, O'Keefe SJ, Kandil HM, Bond G, Costa G, Abu-Elmagd K. Short bowel syndrome: Clinical guidelines for nutrition management. Nutr Clin Pract. 2005;20:493-502; and Wall EA. An overview of short bowel syndrome management: Adherence, adaptation, and practical recommendations. J Acad Nutr Diet. 2013;113(9):1200-1208.

is exacerbated by a diet high in concentrated simple sugars, which should be avoided because of their increased hyperosmotic load.[82,88,91]

Diet Composition In terms of specific macronutrients, diet composition will vary depending on the location and length of remaining bowel. Currently, there are two specific sets of recommendations that were developed based on whether or not the patient has the colon in continuity. A summarization of the two sets is provided in **Table 13.15**.[129] There are also recommendations to be made for each individual macronutrient. The most important factor when developing an individual diet prescription is including complex and varied macronutrients that will stimulate the digestive tract.[85]

Both carbohydrate type and amount are incredibly important for this patient population. Complex carbohydrates, which are generally well tolerated, should comprise approximately 50% of the dietary intake, with an increased goal (closer to 60%) for patients with a colon in continuity. Fiber, in both the soluble and insoluble forms, is a crucial dietary inclusion. Soluble fiber plays a role in slowing gastric emptying and intestinal transit time, contributing to greater nutrient–mucosa exposure and thus increased absorption rates. Moreover, it is essential in promoting intestinal adaptation as the bowel adjusts postoperatively.[89]

Although insoluble fiber also slows intestinal transit time, it is generally more useful in bulking the stool for patients with watery fecal or ostomy output. The rationale for emphasizing carbohydrates—especially fiber—for those with an intact colon is a concept called **salvage absorption**: the normal flora will ferment any unabsorbed carbohydrates that enter the colon to short-chain fatty acids, which are subsequently absorbed and utilized. This can serve as a significant source of energy for patients with SBS; salvage absorption can add up to 500 calories daily. One final consideration in the context of carbohydrates is lactose intake, which is often avoided in this population because of concern regarding lactose intolerance. However, most patients will actually tolerate lactose in the diet, making restriction unnecessary.[88,89,93]

Most patients with SBS have little difficulty tolerating protein intake, meaning that normal consumption can be encouraged. The general guideline for patients with and without a colon in continuity is protein as 20% of daily energy intake. There is no evidence in the literature to support the benefit of one protein source over another, but high-biologic value sources will provide more absorbable and better utilized protein and overall calories when compared to plant sources.[88]

The level of optimal fat intake in the postoperative diet is heavily debated. Fat provides substantial energy and essential fatty acids. Patients with ostomies, or no colon in continuity, benefit from moderately high amounts of fat (30%-40% of daily calories) in the diet; consumption at this level helps to increase the potential that energy is absorbed. Levels should be lower for those with an intact colon (approximately 20%-30% of caloric intake) to maximize absorption and minimize output.[88,89] The controversy is that for many patients, especially those with an intact colon, fat malabsorption and steatorrhea can be severe. One of the long-term complications of chronic fat malabsorption is **oxalate nephrolithiasis**, or kidney stones. Normally, oxalate from food will bind to calcium, leaving very little that can be absorbed by the colon. However, if unabsorbed fatty acids enter the colon, they will bind to calcium in the lumen instead, meaning that oxalate ions are free to be absorbed. Eventually, free oxalate ions circulate through the kidney for excretion; increased levels tend to cause stones, reported in nearly 60% of those with an intact colon. For this reason, these patients are recommended to consume lower levels of fat (to decrease the risk of fat malabsorption) than their counterparts without a colon in continuity (who are not at increased risk for this complication) and to avoid foods high in oxalate, such as those listed in **Table 13.16**. As always, make recommendations based on individual needs and tolerance.[85,88,89]

Fluid and Electrolyte Needs Fluid and electrolyte management can be one of the most difficult components of nutrition care for this patient population because of the massive increase in losses. The trend seen throughout this

TABLE 13.15 DIET COMPOSITION FOR SHORT BOWEL SYNDROME, WITH AND WITHOUT COLON CONTINUITY[88,89,95]

	Small Bowel Ostomies (no colon in continuity)	Intact Colon (colon in continuity)
Meal Frequency and Distribution	4 to 6 small meals per day	3 meals + 2 snacks per day
Carbohydrates	40% to 50% total caloric intake	50% to 60% total caloric intake
Protein	20% to 30% total caloric intake	20% to 30% total caloric intake
Fat	30% to 40% total caloric intake	20% to 30% total caloric intake
Oxalate Restriction	Not generally required	Restriction necessary

Data from Matarese LE, O'Keefe SJ, Kandil HM, Bond G, Costa G, Abu-Elmagd K. Short bowel syndrome: Clinical guidelines for nutrition management. Nutr Clin Pract. 2005;20:493-502; Wall EA. An overview of short bowel syndrome management: Adherence, adaptation, and practical recommendations. J Acad Nutr Diet. 2013;113(9):1200-1208; and Fessler TA. A dietary challenge: Maximizing bowel adaptation in short bowel syndrome. Today's Dietitian. 2007;9(1):40.

TABLE 13.16 HIGH-OXALATE FOODS AND BEVERAGES TO LIMIT[85,96]

Beverages	Black tea, chocolate-containing beverages (chocolate milk, hot chocolate, cocoa, Ovaltine), cola, draft (dark) beers, instant coffee, juice made from high-oxalate fruits, soy beverages
Fruits	Apricots, blackberries, blueberries, cherries, concord grapes, currants, elderberries, figs, gooseberries, kiwi, lemons, limes, oranges, pear, plums, rhubarb, strawberries, tangerines
Nuts and Seeds	Almonds, cashews, peanuts, pecans, all variations of nut butters, sesame seeds, soy nuts, tahini
Starches	Amaranth, buckwheat, cereal (bran or other high fiber), fruit cake, grits, pretzels, taro, wheat bran, wheat germ, whole wheat bread, whole wheat flour
Vegetables	Artichoke, asparagus, beans (baked, green, dried, kidney, wax), beets, beet greens, carrots, celery, chicory, chives, collards, dandelion greens, eggplant, endive, escarole, kale, leeks, okra, olives, peppers (chili and green), potatoes, red cabbage, rutabaga, spinach, summer squash, sweet potato, Swiss chard, tomatoes, zucchini
Miscellaneous	Black pepper (>1 tsp), chocolate, marmalade, parsley, soy products

Data from Parrish CR. The clinician's guide to short bowel syndrome. Pract Gastroenterol. 2005;XXIX(9):67-106; and UPMC Nutrition Services. Low oxalate diet. University of Pittsburgh Medical Center Web site. http://www.upmc.com/patients-visitors/education/nutrition/Pages/low-oxalate-diet.aspx. Updated 2016. Accessed March 31, 2016.

section continues here: needs differ on an individual basis depending on the remaining GI anatomy.[95] Many patients with extensive resection will have a **net secretory response** to both dietary and fluid intake; these patients will excrete more water and sodium than can be ingested, resulting in increased dehydration and electrolyte depletion.[85,93] Those with small-bowel ostomies or with limited remaining colon length are at especially high risk and will have much higher fluid requirements than those with a colon in continuity.[84,88,93]

IV fluid support will be necessary in the period immediately following surgery. The volume of urine produced should guide the total amount of IV and oral fluid delivered. An additional consideration for determining requirements is the composition of stool output or ostomy effluent; account for any increased losses by increasing the fluid provided. Initial fluid and electrolyte needs will be greater until the bowel is given appropriate time to adapt. The goal for ostomy output following surgery is approximately 1 to 1.5 L/day; this may decrease to approximately 600 mL/day for patients with an ileostomy and to 200 to 600 mL/day for those with a colostomy.[83,84,91,95]

> **PRACTICE POINT**
>
> A guideline for determining IV fluid support for postoperative SBS patients is that those with >1.5 L stool output and <800 mL urine output in 24 hours will have difficulty maintaining hydration and electrolyte balance without IV infusion therapy. Set a goal for the patient to produce at least 1,200 mL of urine daily.[84,89]

As a general rule, oral fluid intake should always exceed losses (whether via stool or stoma output) to prevent dehydration. Patients at an increased risk for dehydration may require **oral rehydration solutions** (ORS)—dilute glucose–water mixtures containing electrolytes. Commercially available ORS drinks contain a specific ratio of water, glucose, and sodium to utilize the glucose–sodium active transport mechanism at the intestinal brush border. Because of this pathway, ORS can be absorbed even in the presence of significant diarrhea; ORS solutions are thus a very effective way to maintain hydration status.[84,85,88,95]

> **PRACTICE POINT**
>
> ORS that contains 70 to 90 mEq of Na and 20 g of glucose per liter has been shown to result in positive sodium and fluid balance. To maximize the benefit of ORS, patients should replace both hypertonic (juices, soft drinks) and hypotonic (plain water) beverages with ORS as much as possible.[95]

> **PRACTICE POINT**
>
> ORS beverages, although incredibly useful, are typically not considered palatable by patients. Begin with a goal of 1 L per day and increase the volume to meet needs (usually 2-3 L/day) if the patient demonstrates ability and/or willingness to sip throughout the day.[85]

Additional Micronutrient Considerations All postoperative SBS patients will require a daily multivitamin with minerals, preferably in a chewable or liquid form to facilitate maximum nutrient absorption. Any additional supplemental needs will vary on an individual basis. Deficiencies secondary to malabsorption are certainly not unusual.[88,89]

There are two specific nutrients (or groups of nutrients) that require careful attention. First, vitamin B_{12} becomes a concern for this population when >60 cm of terminal ileum has been removed; as previously discussed, this is the location of vitamin B_{12}-intrinsic factor complex absorption. Patients with ileal resections require routine monitoring of serum vitamin B_{12} and methylmalonic acid (a marker of B_{12} status), often needing injections to prevent or correct deficits.[88,89,93] Second, the divalent cations—calcium, magnesium, and zinc—are deficiency risks in the setting of decreased absorption and increased excretion.[88,89]

> **PRACTICE POINT**
>
> Use caution when supplementing magnesium, as certain forms are poorly absorbed and act as a cathartic. The safest forms of magnesium include the slow-releasing magnesium lactate or magnesium gluconate, which do not increase output or cause other GI symptoms as much as other forms of magnesium (especially magnesium oxide).[88,89]

> **PRACTICE POINT**
>
> Calcium supplementation at 1,000 to 1,500 mg/day can help to reduce the risk of oxalate nephrolithiasis by binding to dietary oxalate.[93]

Finally, be aware that osteoporosis, anemia, and fat-soluble vitamin deficiencies are also common for SBS patients on a long-term basis. Persistent monitoring of the associated nutrients can help to prevent these secondary conditions.[85]

Oral Diet Modifications For SBS patients able to consume an oral diet, there are some small, but effective, modifications that will help to minimize symptoms:

1. Take small bites when eating and chew thoroughly before swallowing to help facilitate full digestion by the altered GI tract.
2. Consume small, frequent meals, distributed evenly throughout the day.
3. Drink liquids separately from meals; sip slowly throughout the day.
4. Avoid simple or concentrated sugars, which may exacerbate osmotic diarrhea, in both food and beverages
5. Avoid practices and/or products that increase bloating through swallowed air, such as chewing gum, drinking through a straw, carbonated beverages, smoking, chewing tobacco, or eating meals too quickly.
6. Avoid foods that can cause increased gas formation and/or odor: alcohol, asparagus, beans, broccoli, Brussels sprouts, cabbage, cauliflower, eggs, fish, etc.
7. Increase consumption of foods that decrease odor, like buttermilk, cranberry juice, kefir, parsley, yogurt, etc.
8. Increase consumption of foods that help to thicken stool, including applesauce, bananas/banana flakes, cheese, pasta, pectin, potatoes, rice, etc.
9. Consuming the largest meal of the day mid-afternoon, versus in the evening, can help to decrease output overnight (for those who find this is an issue).
10. Liberalize added salt, especially for patients with small bowel ostomies.

Adding these simple adjustments into the normal pattern of eating can help increase patient comfort with oral feedings and will be advantageous to optimizing digestion and absorption.[83-85,91]

Role of Home Nutrition Support After the initial postoperative period—when PN support is necessary for all SBS patients as the lone source of energy, fluid, and electrolytes—approximately 50% of patients may gradually decrease dependence on PN/IV support with progression to the oral diet already discussed. Unfortunately, many cannot be fully weaned and will thus require long-term PN/IV support. This group is made up of those unable to absorb more than one-third of oral intake (when attempted) and/or those whose extensive resections left little functional bowel length remaining. Normally, long-term PN is necessary for the survival of ostomy patients with <100 to 140 cm of small bowel remaining or those with <40 to 60 cm of healthy small bowel but with colon continuity. Regardless, if full PN/IV support is required throughout the duration of the adaptation period, the likelihood of permanent intestinal failure (and thus long-term nutrition support) is 95%. The initiation of home PN/IV support as cycled infusions will maintain quality of life—and create a sort of normalcy—for these individuals.[84,86,88,89,94]

> **PRACTICE POINT**
>
> Support provided on a long-term basis at home will vary greatly from the short-term PN provided in the postoperative hospital setting in terms of delivery. Mimic the anticipated home PN regimen prior to discharge from the hospital to assess tolerance and make any necessary corrections.[85]

The Bottom Line SBS is a complex and highly individualized condition. Successful management requires coordination of medical, nutritional, and pharmaceutical therapies with the ultimate goal of providing the energy, nutrients, and fluid required for survival. Frequent follow-ups are required for close monitoring of the nutritional status of the patient. The dietary prescription will likely change as the adaptation period progresses and beyond, when necessary to treat nutrient deficiencies and/or potential complications common to this population.[89]

Chapter Summary

A functioning GI tract is necessary to maintain nutritional status and overall health. Any procedure or disease that damages the integrity of one or more of the many components of this system will have immense implications for the patient. The dietitian plays a critical role in providing highly individualized nutrition interventions that address both adequate intake and the etiology of the specific disease. Although sometimes challenging, the GI malabsorption disorders will require careful and thoughtful care. As the evidence continues to grow and new interventions are presented in the literature and the lay-press, it is important to remain cognizant and informed within this progressive field.

Key Terms

jejunum, ileum, enterocytes, celiac disease, prolamin, irritable bowel syndrome, somatization, visceral hypersensitivity, low FODMAP diet, oligosaccharide, disaccharide, monosaccharide, polyols, probiotics, non-celiac gluten sensitivity (NCGS), inflammatory bowel disease, Crohn's disease, ulcerative colitis, tenesmus, psuedopolyps, granulomas, toxic megacolon, fibrostenosis, defined diets, VSL#3, leaky gut, *Helicobacter pylori*, small intestinal bacterial overgrowth, migrating motor complex, micelles, elemental formula, synbiotic, anastomosis, stoma, ostomy, ileocecal (IC) valve, ileal brake, appliance, colostomy, ileostomy, jejunostomy, short bowel syndrome, intestinal failure, salvage absorption, oxalate nephrolithiasis, net secretory response, oral rehydration solutions

References

1. Joneja JMV. *Digestion, diet, and disease: Irritable bowel syndrome and gastrointestinal function.* New Brunswick, NJ: Rutgers University Press; 2004.
2. Gropper SS, Smith JL. The digestive system: Mechanism for nourishing the body. In: *Advanced nutrition and human metabolism.* 6th ed. Belmont, CA: Wadsworth Cengage Learning; 2013:33-62.
3. Leffler DA, Cárdenas A, Kelly CP. Celiac disease. In: *Textbook of clinical gastroenterology and hepatology.* Hoboken, New Jersey: Wiley-Blackwell; 2012:288-298.
4. Academy of Nutrition and Dietetics. *Nutrition Care Manual.* Celiac disease. https://www.nutritioncaremanual.org/topic.cfm?ncm_category_id=1&lv1=5522&lv2=22684&lv3=268009&ncm_toc_id=268009&ncm_heading=Nutrition%20Care. Accessed November 30, 2017.
5. See JA, Kaukinen K, Makharia GK, Gibson PR, Murray JA. Practical insights into gluten free diets. *Nat Rev Gastroenterol Hepatol.* 2015;12(10):580-591.
6. National Institute of Diabetes and Digestive and Kidney Disorders. Celiac disease. U.S. Department of Health and Human Services, Health Information. http://www.niddk.nih.gov/health-information/health-topics/digestive-diseases/celiac-disease/Pages/facts.aspx#examples. Published June 2015. Updated 2015. Accessed February 1, 2016.
7. Wierdsma NJ, van Bokhorst-de van der Scheuren, MAE., Berkenpas M, Mulder CJJ, van Bodegraven AA. Vitamin and mineral deficiencies are highly prevalent in newly diagnosed celiac disease patients. *Nutrients.* 2013;5:3975-3992.
8. García-Manzanares Á, Lucendo AJ. Nutritional and dietary aspects of celiac disease. *Nutr Clin Pract.* 2011;26(2):163-173.
9. Academy of Nutrition and Dietetics. Nutrition Care Manual Irritable bowel syndrome (IBS). https://www.nutritioncaremanual.org/topic.cfm?ncm_category_id=1&lv1=5522&lv2=19589&lv3=268517&ncm_toc_id=268517&ncm_heading=Nutrition%20Care. Accessed November 30, 2017.
10. Wald A, Rakel D. Behavioral and complementary approaches for treatment of irritable bowel syndrome. *Nutr Clin Pract.* 2008;23(3):284-292.
11. Böhn L, Störsrud S, Liljebo T, Collin L, Lindfors P, Törnblom H, Simren M. Diet low in FODMAPs reduces symptoms of irritable bowel syndrome as well as traditional dietary advice: A randomized control trial. *Gastroenterology.* 2015;149(6):1399-1407.
12. Spiller R. Irritable bowel syndrome. In: *Textbook of clinical gastroenterology and hepatology.* Hoboken, New Jersey: Wiley-Blackwell; 2012:472-481.
13. Rome Foundation. Rome III diagnostic criteria for functional gastrointestinal disorders. http://www.romecriteria.org/assets/pdf/19_RomeIII_apA_885-898.pdf. Updated 2006. Accessed February 2, 2016.
14. Didari T, Mozaffari S, Nikfar S, Abdollahi M. Effectiveness of probiotics in irritable bowel syndrome: Updated systematic review with meta-analysis. *World J Gastroenterol.* 2015;21(10):3071-3084.
15. Zhou Q, Verne GN. New insights into visceral hypersensitivity - clinical implications in IBS. *Nat Rev Gastroenterol Hepatol.* 2011;8(6):349-355.
16. Lacy BE. The science, evidence, and practice of dietary interventions in irritable bowel syndrome. *Clin Gastroenterol Hepatol.* 2015;13(11):1899-1906.
17. Academy of Nutrition and Dietetics. *Nutrition Care Manual.* Irritable bowel syndrome (IBS nutrition therapy. https://www.nutritioncaremanual.org/client_ed.cfm?ncm_client_ed_id=166. Accessed November 30, 2017.
18. Marcason W. What is the FODMAP diet? *J Acad Nutr Diet.* 2012;112(10):1696.
19. Low FODMAP diet for irritable bowel syndrome. Monash University - Medicine, Nursing, and Health Sciences. http://www.med.monash.edu/cecs/gastro/fodmap/. Published January 18 2016. Accessed February 5, 2016.
20. Gibson PR, Varney J, Malakar S, Muir JG. Food components and irritable bowel syndrome. *Gastroenterology.* 2015;148(6):1158-1174.
21. Mansueto P, Seidita A, D'Alcamo A, Carroccio A. Role of FODMAPs in patients with irritable bowel syndrome. *Nutr Clin Pract.* 2015;30(5):665-682.
22. Halmos EP, Power VA, Shepherd SJ, Gibson PR, Muir JG. A diet low in FODMAPs reduces symptoms of irritable bowel syndrome. *Gastroenterology.* 2014;146(1):67-75.
23. Probiotics: In depth. National Institutes of Health (NIH): National Center for Complementary and Integrative Health (NCCIH). https://nccih.nih.gov/health/probiotics/introduction.htm. Published January 11 2016. Accessed February 5, 2016.
24. Clauson ER, Crawford P. What you must know before you recommend a probiotic. *J Fam Pract.* 2015;64(3):151-155.
25. Spiller R. Review article: Probiotics and prebiotics in irritable bowel syndrome. *Aliment Pharmacol Ther.* 2008;28(4):385-396.
26. Santos AR, Whorwell PJ. Irritable bowel syndrome: The problem and the problem of treating it - is there a role for probiotics? *Proc Nutr Soc.* 2014;73(4):470-476.
27. Ford AC, Quigley EMM, Lacy BE, et al. Efficacy of prebiotics, probiotics, and synbiotics in irritable bowel syndrome and chronic idiopathic constipation: Systematic review and meta-analysis. *Am J Gastroenterol.* 2014;109(10):1546-1562.
28. Tiequn B, Guanqun C, Shuo Z. Therapeutic effects of lactobacillus in treating irritable bowel syndrome: A meta-analysis. *Intern Med.* 2015;54(3):243-249.
29. Mullin GE. Probiotics and digestive disease. *Nutr Clin Pract.* 2012;27(2):300-302.
30. Quigley EMM. Prebiotics and probiotics: Their role in the management of gastrointestinal disorders in adults. *Nutr Clin Pract.* 2012;27(2):195-200.

31. Moran C, Shanahan F. Editorial: Probiotics and IBS - where are we now? *Aliment Pharmacol Ther.* 2014;40(3):318.

32. Leung J, Crowe SE. Food allergy and food intolerance. In: Buckman A. et. *Nutrition care of the patient with gastrointestinal disease.* Boca Raton, FL: Taylor &Francis Group. 2015:63-88.33. Gibson PR, Skodje GI, Lundin KE. Non-coeliac gluten sensitivity. *J Gastroenterol Heptol.* 2017;32(1) 86-89.

34. Wędrychowicz A, Zajac A, Tomasik P. Advances in nutritional therapy in inflammatory bowel diseases: Review. *World J Gastroenterol.* 2016;22(3):1045-1066.

35. Hou JK, Lee D, Lewis J. Diet and inflammatory bowel disease: Review of patient-targeted recommendations. *Clin Gastroenterol Hepatol.* 2014;12(10):1592-1600.

36. Yamamoto T, Nakahigashi M, Saniabadi AR. Review article: Diet and inflammatory bowel disease - epidemiology and treatment. *Aliment Pharmacol Ther.* 2009;30(2):99-112.

37. Shanahan F. Ulcerative colitis. In: *Textbook of clinical gastroenterology and hepatology.* Hoboken, New Jersey: Wiley-Blackwell; 2012:355-371.

38. Durchschein F, Petrisch W, Hammer HF. Diet therapy for inflammatory bowel diseases: The established and the new. *World J Gastroenterol.* 2016;22(7):2179-2194.

39. Vermeire S, Van Assche G, Rutgeerts P. Crohn's disease. In: *Textbook of clinical gastroenterology and hepatology.* Hoboken, New Jersey: Wiley-Blackwell; 2012:372-393. 10.1002/9781118321386.ch50.

40. Spooren, C. E. G. M., Pierik MJ, Zeegers MP, Feskens EJM, Muscle AAM, Jonkers DMAE. Review article: The association of diet with onset and relpase in patients with inflammatory bowel disease. *Aliment Pharmacol Ther.* 2013;38(10):1172-1187.

41. Andersen V, Olsen A, Carbonnel F, Tjønneland A, Vogel U. Diet and risk of inflammatory bowel disease. *Dig Liver Dis.* 2012;44(3):185-194.

42. Hou JK, Abraham B, El-Serang H. Dietary intake and risk of developing inflammatory bowel disease: A systematic review of the literature. *Am J Gastroenterol.* 2011;106(4):563-573.

43. Owczarek D, Rodacki T, Domagala-Rodacka R, Cibor D, Mach T. Diet and nutritional factors in inflammatory bowel disease. *World J Gastroenterol.* 2016;22(3):895-905.

44. Issa M, Saeian K. Diet in inflammatory bowel disease. *Nutr Clin Pract.* 2011;26(2):151-154.

45. Forbes A, Goldesgeyme E, Paulon E. Nutrition in inflammatory bowel disease. *JPEN J Parenter Enteral Nutr.* 2011;35(5):571-580.

46. Peppercorn MA, Kane SV. Clinical manifestations, diagnosis and prognosis of crohn disease in adults. UpToDate. Updated April 25, 2017. https://www.uptodate.com/contents/clinical-manifestations-diagnosis-and-prognosis-of-crohn-disease-in-adults?source=search_result&search=Crohns%20disease&selectedTitle=2~150 Accessed November 30, 2017.

47. Peppercorn MA, Kane SV. Clinical manifestations, diagnosis, and prognosis of ulcerative colitis in adults. UpToDate Web site. https://www.uptodate.com/contents/clinical-manifestations-diagnosis-and-prognosis-of-ulcerative-colitis-in-adults?source=search_result&search=ulcerative%20colitis&selectedTitle=1~150. Updated August 21, 2017. Accessed November 30, 2017.

48. Vidarsdottir JB, Johannsdottir SE, Thorsdottir I, Björnsson E, Ramel A. A cross-sectional study on nutrient intake and status in inflammatory bowel disease patients. *Nutr J.* 2015;15(1):61-67.

49. DeLegge MH. Nutrition and dietary interventions in adults with inflammatory bowel disease. UpToDate Web site. https://www.uptodate.com/contents/nutrition-and-dietary-interventions-in-adults-with-inflammatory-bowel-disease?source=search_result&search=nutrition%20in%20IBD&selectedTitle=1~150.Updated. December 17 2015. Accessed November 30, 2017.

50. Vagianos K, Bector S, McConnell J, Bernstein C. Nutrition assessment of patients with inflammatory bowel disease. *JPEN J Parenter Enteral Nutr.* 2007;31(4):311-319.

51. Teitelbaum JE. Nutrient defiencies in inflammatory bowel disease. UpToDate Web site. https://www.uptodate.com/contents/nutrient-deficiencies-in-inflammatory-bowel-disease?source=search_result&search=nutrition%20deficiencies%20in%20IBD&selectedTitle=1~150 .Updated February 22, 2017. Accessed November 30, 2017.

52. Dray X, Marteau P. The use of enteral nutrition in the management of Crohn's disease in adults. *JPEN J Parenter Enteral Nutr.* 2005;29 (4 Suppl):S166-S169.

53. Lochs H, Dejong C, Hammarqvist F, et al. ESPEN guidelines on enteral nutrition: Gastroenterology. *Clin Nutr.* 2006;25(2):260-274.

54. Shah ND, Parian AM, Mullin GE, Limketkal B, N. Oral diets and nutrition support for inflammatory bowel disease: What is the evidence? *Nutr Clin Pract.* 2015;30(4):462-473.

55. Richman E, Rhodes JM. Review article: Evidence-based dietary advice for patients with inflammatory bowel disease. *Aliment Pharmacol Ther.* 2013;38(10):1156-1171.

56. Ruemmele FM. Role of diet in inflammatory bowel disease. *Ann Nutr Metab.* 2016;68(Suppl 1):33-41.

57. Brown AC, Ramphertab SD, Mullin GE. Existing dietary guidelines for Crohn's disease and ulcerative colitis. *Expert Rev Gastroenterol Hepatol.* 2011;5(3):411-425.

58. Reich KM, Fedorak RN, Madsen K, Kroeker K. Vitamin D improves inflammatory bowel disease outcomes: Basic science and clinical review. *World J Gastroenterol.* 2014;20(17):4934-4947.

59. Prince A, Whelan K, Moosa A, Lomer MCE, Reidlinger DP. Nutritional problems in inflammatory bowel disease: The patient perspective. *J Crohns Colitis.* 2011;5(5):443-450.

60. Kakodkar S, Farooqui AJ, Mikolaitis SL, Mutlu EA. The specific carbohydrate diet for inflammatory bowel disease: A case series. *J Acad Nutr Diet.* 2015;115(8):1226-1232.

61. Barbalho SM, Goulart RdA, Quesada K, Bechara MD, de Cássio Alves de Carvalho, A. Inflammatory bowel disease: Can omega-3 fatty acids really help? *Ann Gastroenterol.* 2016;29(1):37-43.

62. Stewart EA. Leaky gut syndrome – Learn about the causes, associated conditions, and treatments under research. *Today's Dietitian*; January 2016.

63. Michielan A, D'Inca R. Intestinal permeability in inflammatory bowel disease: Pathogenesis, clinical evaluation, and therapy of leaky gut. *Mediators Inflam.* 2015;1-10.

64. Haley PK, Gaddy JA. Nutrition and *Helicobacter pylori*: Host diet and nutritional immunity influence bacterial virulence and disease outcome. *Gastroenterol Res Pract.* 2016;1-10.

65. Franceschi F, Tortora A, Di Renzo T, et al. Role of Helicobacter pylori infection on nutrition and metabolism. *World J Gastroenterol.* 2014;20(36):12809-12817.

66. Hsu PI, Wu DC, Chen WC, et al. Randomized controlled trial comparing 7-day triple, 10-day sequential, and 7-day concomitant therapies for *Helicobacter pylori* infection. *Antimicrob Agents Chemother.* 2014;58(10):5936-5942.

67. Boltin D. Probiotics in *Helicobacter pylori*-induced peptic ulcer disease. *Best Pract Res Clin Gastoenterol.* 2016;30(1):99-109.

68. Jacob A. Treatment and management of SIBO - taking a dietary approach can control intestinal fermentation and inflammation. *Today's Dietitian.* 2012;14(12):16.

69. Rogers C. Postgastrectomy nutrition. *Nutr Clin Pract.* 2011;26(2):126-136.

70. Zaidel O, Lin HC. Uninvited guests: The impact of small intestinal bacterial overgrowth on nutritional status. *Pract Gastroenterol*. 2003;7:27-34.
71. Scarlata K. Small intestinal bacterial overgrowth - what to do when unwelcome microbes invade. *Today's Dietitian*. 2011;13(4):46.
72. DiBlaise JK. Nutritional consequences of small intestinal bacterial overgrowth. *Pract Gastroenterol*. 2008;69:15-28.
73. Shanab AA, Quera RM, Quigley EMM. Small intestinal bacterial overgrowth. In: *Textbook of clinical gastroenterology and hepatology*. Hoboken, New Jersey: Wiley-Blackwell; 2012:305-310.
74. Rezaie A, Pimental M, Rao SS. How to test and treat small intestinal bacterial overgrowth: An evidenced-based approach. *Curr Gastroenterol Rep*. 2016;18(2):8-19.
75. Bohm M, Siwiec RM, Wo JM. Diagnosis and management of small intestinal bacterial overgrowth. *Nutr Clin Pract*. 2013;28(3):289-299.
76. Grace E, Shaw C, Whelan K, Andreyev H.J.N. Small intestinal bacterial overgrowth: Prevalence, clinical features, current and developing diagnostic tests, and treatment. *Aliment Pharmacol Ther*. 2013;38(7):674-688.
77. Chen WC, Quigley EMM. Probiotics, prebiotics & synbiotics in small intestinal bacterial overgrowth: Opening up a new therapeutic horizon! *Indian J Med Res*. 2014;November:582-584.
78. Khalghi AR, Khalighi MR, Behdani R, et al. Evaluating the efficacy of probiotic on treatment in patients with small intestinal bacterial overgrowth (SIBO) - A pilot study. *Indian J Med Res*. 2014;140(5):604-608.
79. Gabrielli M, Sparano L, Roccarina D, Vitale G, Lauritano EC, Gasbarrini A. Treatment options for small intestinal bacterial overgrowth. *Dig Liver Dis*. ;3(2):50-53.
80. Kwak DS, Jun DW, Seo JG, et al. Short-term probiotic therapy alleviates small intestinal bacterial overgrowth, but does not improve intestinal permeability in chronic liver disease. *Eur J Gastroenterol Hepatol*. 2014;26(12):1353-1359.
81. Wolfson D. Probiotics and prebiotics in the treatment of small intestinal bacterial overgrowth. *Complementary Prescriptions Newsletter*. 2015;September.
82. Academy of Nutrition and Dietetics. *Nutrition Care Manual*. Bowel resection. https://www.nutritioncaremanual.org/topic.cfm?ncm_category_id=1&lv1=5522&lv2=144839&lv3=267423&ncm_toc_id=267423&ncm_heading=Nutrition%20Care. Accessed November 30, 2017.
83. Academy of Nutrition and Dietetics. *Nutrition Care Manual*. Ileostomy. https://www.nutritioncaremanual.org/topic.cfm?ncm_category_id=1&lv1=5522&lv2=19729&lv3=268561&ncm_toc_id=268561&ncm_heading=Nutrition%20Care. Accessed November 30, 2017.
84. Corrigan ML. Short bowel syndrome in adult PN patients. *Today's Dietitian*. 2015;17(12):30.
85. Parrish CR. The clinician's guide to short bowel syndrome. *Pract Gastroenterol*. 2005;XXIX(9):67-106.
86. Jeppesen PB. Spectrum of short bowel syndrome in adults: Intestinal insufficiency to intestinal failure. *JPEN J Parenter Enteral Nutr*. 2014;38(suppl 1):8S-13S.
87. van Avesaat M, Troost FJ, Ripken D, Hendriks HF, Masclee AAM. Ieal brake activation: Macronutrient-specfic effects on eating behavior? *Int J Obes (Lond)*. 2015;39(2):235-243.
88. Matarese LE, O'Keefe SJ, Kandil HM, Bond G, Costa G, Abu-Elmagd K. Short bowel syndrome: Clinical guidelines for nutrition management. *Nutr Clin Pract*. 2005;20:493-502.
89. Wall EA. An overview of short bowel syndrome management: Adherence, adaptation, and practical recommendations. *J Acad Nutr Diet*. 2013;113(9):1200-1208.
90. You YN. Ostomy expanded version. American Society of Colon and Rectal Surgeons. https://www.fascrs.org/patients/disease-condition/ostomy-expanded-version. Accessed April 1, 2016.
91. Academy of Nutrition and Dietetics. *Nutrition Care Manual*. Colostomy. https://www.nutritioncaremanual.org/topic.cfm?ncm_category_id=1&lv1=5522&lv2=19799&lv3=268598&ncm_toc_id=268598&ncm_heading=Nutrition%20Care. Accessed November 30, 2017.
92. Tappenden KA. Pathophysiology of short bowel syndrome: Considerations of resected and residual anatomy. *JPEN J Parenter Enteral Nutr*. 2014;38(suppl 1):14S-22S.
93. Jackson CS, Buchman AL. Short bowel syndrome. In: *Textbook of clinical gastroenterology and hepatology*. Hoboken, New Jersey: Wiley-Blackwell; 2012:299-304.
94. Keller J, Panter H, Layer P. Management of the short bowel syndrome after extensive small bowel resection. *Best Pract Res Clin Gastroenterol*. 2004;18(5):977-992.
95. Fessler TA. A dietary challenge: Maximizing bowel adaptation in short bowel syndrome. *Today's Dietitian*. 2007;9(1):40.
96. UPMC Nutrition Services. Low oxalate diet. University of Pittsburgh Medical Center. http://www.upmc.com/patients-visitors/education/nutrition/Pages/low-oxalate-diet.aspx. Updated 2016. Accessed March 31, 2016.

Chapter 14

Nutrition in Kidney Disease

Kathryn Wilson
Poonhar Poon

Chapter Outline

Core Concepts
Introduction
Renal Physiology in Health and Disease
Functions of the Kidney
Diseases of the Kidney
Nutrition Support in Kidney Disease
Nephrotic Syndrome

CORE CONCEPTS

1. The prevalence of chronic kidney disease is increasing due to the rising rates of risk factors such as diabetes and hypertension, as well as an aging population.

2. Prevention is a key component in the management of CKD and involves treatment of underlying conditions, such as diabetes.

3. Malnutrition risk increases as the glomerular filtration rate decreases, and may complicate the management of CKD due to protein, fluid, and/or micronutrient restrictions.

4. Medical nutrition therapy is a necessary component of CKD management and can improve outcomes by preventing malnutrition and slowing disease progression.

5. Protein is a necessary macronutrient in the diet of patients with kidney disease, and despite controversy regarding the possibility that protein restriction improves outcomes, these patients must be able to eat a balanced, palatable diet that provides adequate energy and protein to prevent loss of lean body mass.

6. Patients receiving renal replacement therapy can tolerate higher protein, fluid, and electrolyte levels than patients with CKD alone, so recommendations should be individualized to each patient.

Learning Objectives

1. Identify the magnitude and etiology of kidney disease.
2. Describe the progression of chronic kidney disease (CKD) and outline the importance of nutrition in its prevention and treatment.
3. Evaluate the relationship between malnutrition and each type of kidney disease.
4. Describe the different forms of renal replacement therapy and identify nutritional implications of each.

Introduction

An estimated 30 million people, or 15% of the United States' adult population, have chronic kidney disease (CKD).[1] The Centers for Disease Control and Prevention report that among those with severely reduced kidney function, almost 50% are unaware that they have the disease, and among those with mildly reduced kidney function, an overwhelming majority are unaware that they have the disease. CKD is more prevalent in women than in men and more common in non-Hispanic blacks than in non-Hispanic whites.[1] An estimated 8 million or more persons have a glomerular filtration rate (GFR) <60 mL/min/1.73 m^2, or stage 3 to 5 CKD, and risk increases with age.[2] CKD is a dangerous and life-altering diagnosis, and an increase in the prevalence of its risk factors, including diabetes mellitus and hypertension, signifies that the prevalence of CKD will likely continue to rise. Kidney disease increases risk of heart disease, stroke, immunosuppression, and depression, and lowers quality of life.[1] According to the United States Renal Data System 2016 report, the number of stage 5 CKD patients receiving treatment continues to increase, and did so by 3.5% in that year.[3] This coincides with falling mortality rates for dialysis and kidney transplant patients, decreasing by 32% and 44%, respectively, since 1996.[3]

> **CORE CONCEPT 1**
>
> The prevalence of chronic kidney disease is increasing due to the rising rates of risk factors such as diabetes and hypertension, as well as an aging population.

Renal Physiology in Health and Disease

The kidneys are two fist-sized organs located at the back of the abdomen in the retroperitoneal space. Known primarily for their role in eliminating waste and regulating fluid balance, the kidneys also maintain the chemical composition and stability of the blood, regulate blood pressure, and provide endocrine function to support bone and red blood cell formation. Each kidney consists of approximately one million **nephrons**, commonly referred to as the functional units of the kidney. These nephrons are responsible for filtering, secreting, and reabsorbing components of the blood in order to preserve necessary proteins and blood constituents while eliminating waste. Nephrons consist of two main components, the renal corpuscle and the renal tubule, each serving a unique function. The renal corpuscle is made up of the **glomerulus**, a mass of capillaries that are specifically responsible for filtering the plasma, and **Bowman's capsule**, a double layer of cells encapsulating the glomerulus, which collects the filtrate and opens up into the tubules. Filtration of the blood is a passive process that relies on blood pressure created by adequate cardiac output, which is the amount of blood pumped by the heart per minute, and the diameter of the renal artery, both of which determine the amount of blood flowing into the nephrons.[4] Initially, blood flows into the renal corpuscle of the nephron through the afferent arteriole and enters the glomerular space. The glomerulus allows fluid and waste to pass into the Bowman's capsule while preventing red blood cells and large macromolecules such as protein to get through (these return to the blood stream through the efferent arteriole). The resulting **ultrafiltrate**, (filtrate made once waste is filtered from the blood) proceeds to the second step of the filtration process by entering the renal tubules to be further modified. The **tubules**—which include the proximal convoluted tubule, the loop of Henle, and finally, the distal convoluted tubule—and the collecting duct reabsorb the ultrafiltrate. Each section of the tubule has a different permeability, secreting and absorbing different components of the ultrafiltrate (Table 14-1). For example, the proximal convoluted tubule is responsible for reabsorbing nutrients, while the descending loop of Henle reabsorbs water. Urine is produced and funneled into the collecting duct and renal pelvis, which narrows into a single ureter per kidney. The **ureters** bring urine to the bladder, which can then be released from the body.[4] Through this process the nephrons filter 1,600 L of blood per day, producing approximately 180 L of ultrafiltrate, resulting in approximately 1-2 liters of urine output daily depending on fluid intake.[4] The structure of the kidney and urinary system is illustrated in **Figure 14.1** and the structure of the nephron is illustrated in **Figure 14.2**.

While etiology of renal insult can be multifactorial in nature, kidney disease is characterized by an acute or progressive loss of functioning nephrons, which unfolds in a pattern of systemic hypertension, proteinuria and a gradual decline in **glomerular filtration rate (GFR)**, the amount of plasma filtered through the glomeruli within a given period.[5] Initially the kidneys can compensate for the loss of nephrons and maintain overall GFR. Because the same amount of blood must flow through the kidney despite now having fewer nephrons capable of filtering the blood, the kidneys activate the renin-angiotensin system to increase afferent arteriole vasodilation and concurrently constrict the efferent arteriole vessel.[6,7]

CASE STUDY INTRODUCTION

Dean is a 33-year-old African American male who presents to the hospital with reports of experiencing progressively worsening shortness of breath and weakness over the past 3 months. He attributes his fatigue to having a newborn child at home and studying for the bar exam. Three days prior to admission, Dean developed a cough, shortness of breath (orthopnea) that worsens at night (paroxysmal nocturnal dyspnea), and dyspnea with minimal exertion. He reports foamy, dark colored urine and increased frequency of nocturnal urination. Dean lives with his wife and infant daughter and recently graduated from law school. Dean states that his grandmother died of kidney disease at age 65 years.

Anthropometric Data:
Height: 175 cm (69")
Weight: 85 kg (189 lbs)
BMI: 28 kg/m^2
Weight history
Usual body weight 83 kg (183 lbs) 3 months ago

Biochemical Data:
Sodium 137 (135-145 mEq/L)
Potassium 5.5 (3.6-5.0 mEq/L)
Chloride 108 (98-110 mEq/L)
Carbon dioxide 21 (20-30 mEq/L)
Blood urea nitrogen 82 (6-24 mg/dL)
Creatinine 2.1 (0.4-1.3 mg/dL)
Glucose 98 (70-98 mg/dL)

Calcium 6.9 (8.5-10.5 mEq/L)
Phosphorus 5.8 (2.7-4.5 mg/dL)
Magnesium 2.5 (1.3-2.1 mg/dL)
Albumin 2.5 (3.5-5.0 g/dL)
Hemoglobin 7.7 (13.5-17.5 g/dL)
Hematocrit 22% (42%-52%)

Clinical Data:
Past Medical History: No significant past medical history
Medications: No medications
Vital Signs: Blood pressure: 178/96 mm Hg, Temperature 98.6°F, Heart rate 120 beats/min
Nutrition-focused Physical Exam: Dean appears well nourished and physically fit, with slight edema in his bilateral lower extremities. Skin appears dry; no wounds noted. Oral exam unremarkable with intact dentition, normal tongue.

Dietary Data:
24-hour Diet Recall:
Breakfast (5:30 am): 16 oz coffee with cream, bran muffin, banana, 6 oz orange juice
Lunch (12 pm): Cobb salad with 1 cup kale, 1 cup iceberg lettuce, 1 egg, 2 tablespoons bacon bits, ½ avocado, ¼ cup ranch dressing, 12 oz diet cola
Snack (4 pm): 20 oz blended sweetened coffee drink, blueberry scone
At home appetizer with wife (7 pm): cheese with crackers, two glasses wine
Dinner (8:30 pm): 8 oz baked chicken, 2 cups rosemary roasted potatoes, 1 cup zucchini sautéed in butter
Evening Snack (11 pm): 8 oz skim milk and 2 oatmeal cookies
Diet Prescription: No added salt diet (3-4 g Na) diet

Questions
1. What are Dean's CKD risk factors?
2. What are Dean's nutritional risk factors?
3. What physiologic complications of CKD does Dean exhibit?
4. How would you interpret Dean's labs?
5. What additional information would you like to obtain?

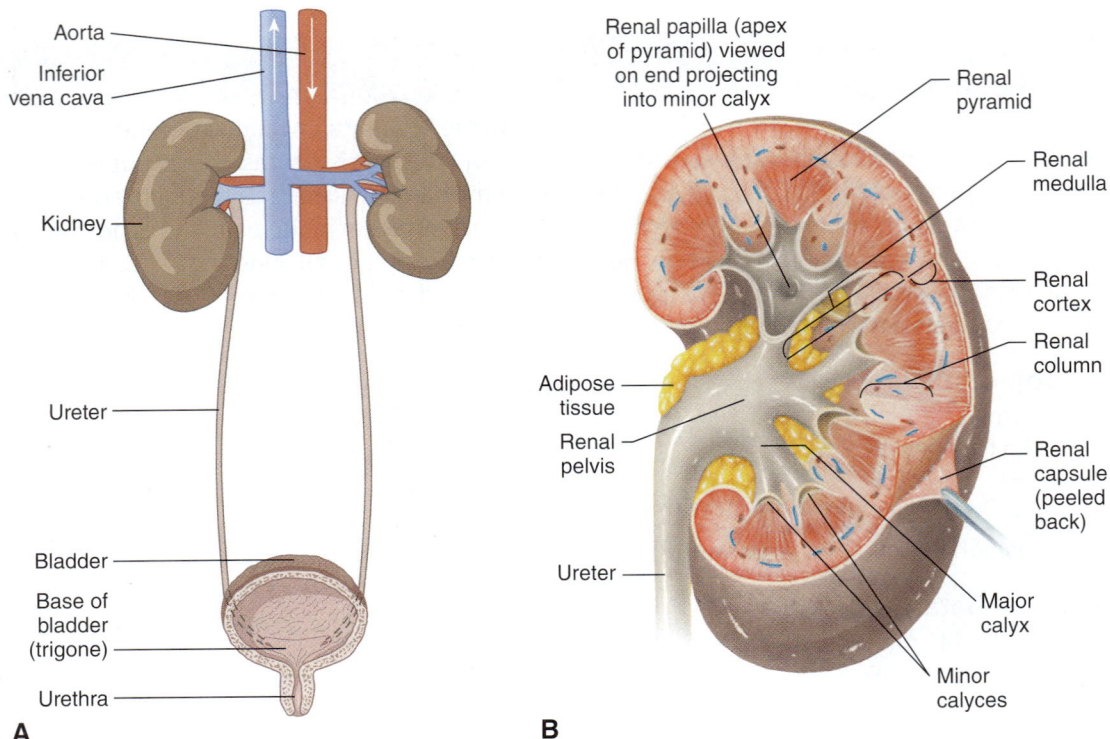

FIGURE 14.1 Anatomy of the Urinary System and Kidney

As a result, each remaining functional nephron takes on more pressure from the systemic circulation, a process known as **adaptive hyperfiltration**.[6,7] A sustained increase in blood volume and subsequent pressure leads to scaring (glomerulosclerosis) due to thickening of the walls and narrowing of the lumen of glomerular arterioles (arteriolosclerosis). In CKD, this syndrome of glomerular hypertrophy, glomerular hypertension with resulting macrophage infiltratation and accumulation of extracellular matrix components, eventually leads to loss of nephron

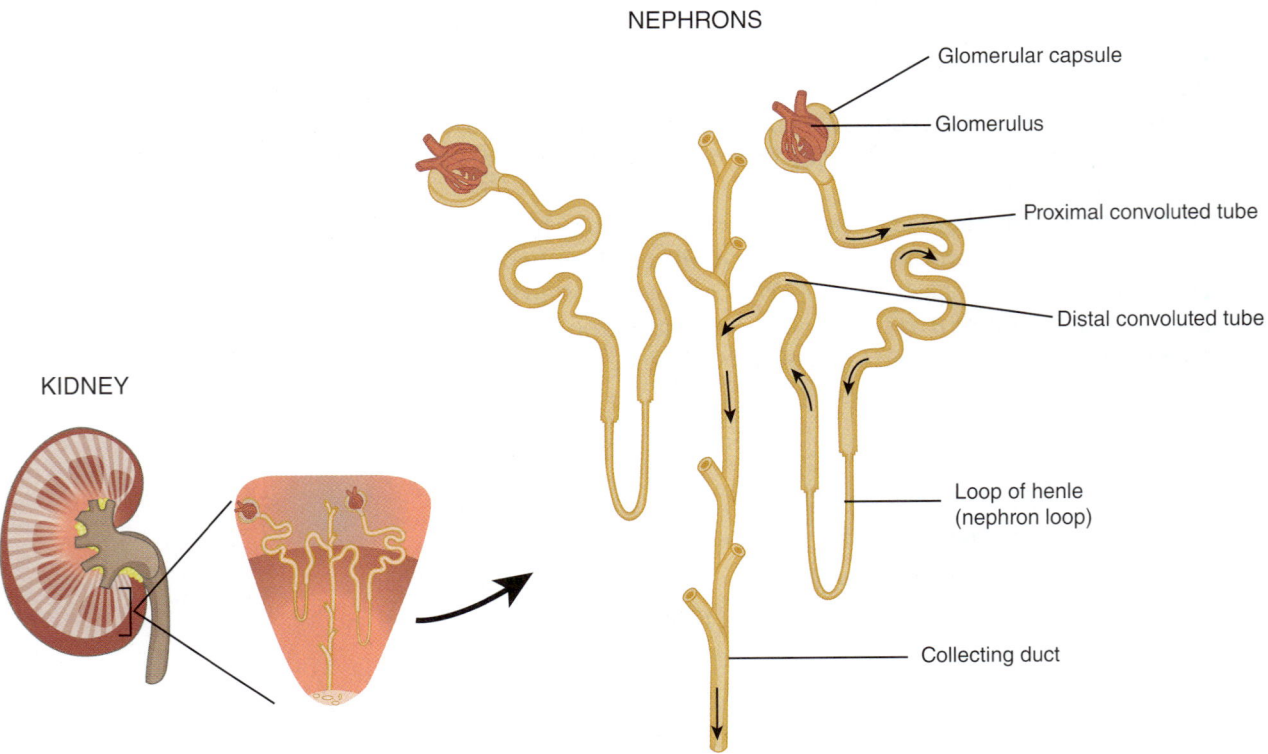

FIGURE 14.2 Physiology of a Nephron

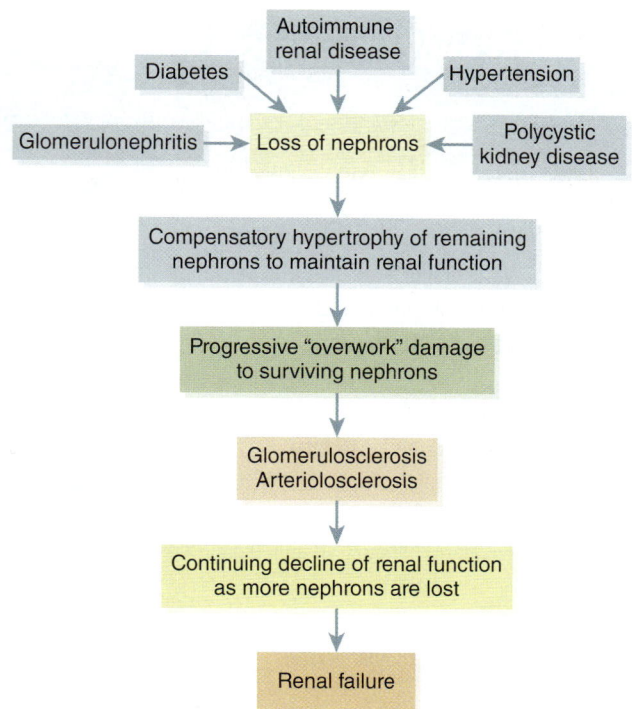

FIGURE 14.3 Progression of Chronic Kidney Disease

function, causing end-stage renal disease.[8] Disease progression is associated with uncontrolled diabetes, poorly controlled blood pressure, and high levels of protein in the urine, which contributes to continually decreasing GFR. A graphic representation of this process can be found in **Figure 14.3**.

Functions of the Kidney

As mentioned, the functions of the kidney include metabolic regulation, waste excretion, and hormone production. One of the key roles of the kidney is to maintain fluid and electrolyte balance by controlling the secretion and reabsorption of blood components regulating extracellular fluid (ECF) volume and osmolarity. The kidneys can concentrate urine up to 1,200 milliosmoles (mOsm) and can dilute urine to as little as 50 mOsm, depending on the volume of excess fluid present and the amount of solute that must be released. The kidney can excrete up to 12 L or as little as 500 mL of urine daily. This function of the kidney is critical for blood pressure regulation.

The kidneys can regulate blood pressure in two ways. If blood pressure is elevated or decreased, the kidneys can adjust the amount of urine formed in order to eliminate or conserve body fluid, a mechanism hormonally regulated through arginine vasopressin, also known as **antidiuretic hormone (ADH)**. The release of ADH is influenced by the osmolarity or solute concentration of ECF. Decreased ECF osmolarity inhibits ADH secretion, so the kidneys excrete more urine. Conversely, increased ECF osmolarity stimulates ADH secretion, so the kidneys reabsorb more fluid and excrete less urine, which can help to maintain appropriate blood pressure. The kidneys are also the main site of action of the renin-angiotensin-aldosterone system (RAAS). When there is a decrease in blood pressure, perfusion can be compromised, leading to reduced blood flow to body tissues, as well as the kidneys. **Figure 14.4** outlines the steps in the RAAS activation.

In addition to blood pressure regulation, the kidneys also play a role in blood pH regulation. Acids and bases are metabolically produced and a narrow parameter of pH must be maintained for appropriate organ system function. Primarily through the renal tubules, the kidneys maintain pH balance by excreting or reabsorbing acid or bicarbonate or producing new bicarbonate. For example, the kidney reabsorbs bicarbonate in the tubules and releases hydrogen ions in the urine when pH decreases below normal levels.

Another function of the kidney is to filter and eliminate waste products and toxins from the blood. Normal metabolism produces byproducts that must be removed from the body. At least 500 mL of urine output is necessary to rid the body of the average 600 mOsm of solute that is generated daily through normal metabolism.[9] The solute load includes **nitrogenous waste**, such as urea, creatinine, and ammonia, which are end products of protein metabolism.

Finally, the kidney produces and/or releases hormones, including those that control the production of red blood cells, activate vitamin D, and regulate

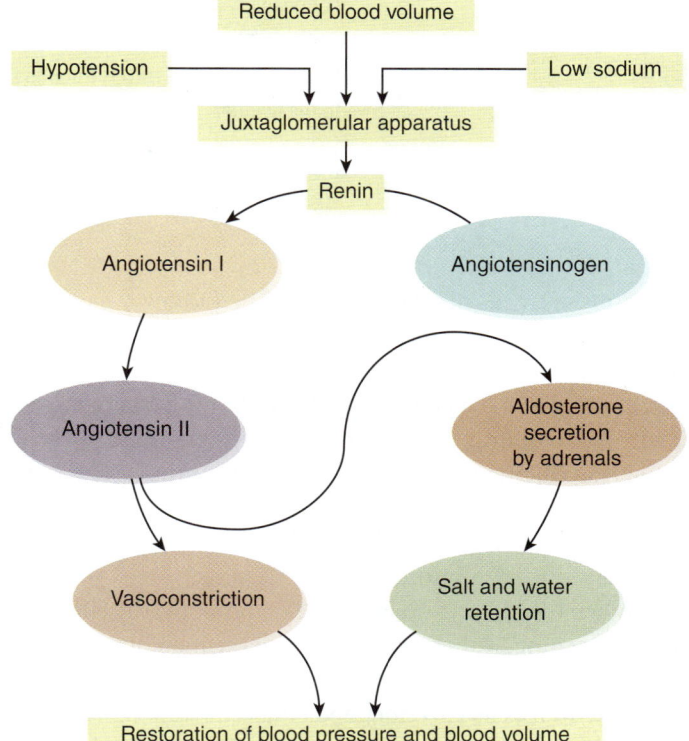

FIGURE 14.4 The role of the Kidney in the Regulation of Blood Pressure and Blood Volume

TABLE 14.1 FLOW OF FLUID THROUGH THE NEPHRON IN NORMAL AND COMPROMISED KIDNEY FUNCTION

Nephron Component	Normal Function	Compromised Function
Glomerulus	• Produces filtrate from blood	• Filtration is slow and incomplete • Waste products are unable to be eliminated • Proteins are lost through the pores of the glomerulus and are excreted in the urine
Proximal Convoluted Tubule	• Reabsorbs two-thirds of filtrate • Reabsorption site of glucose and amino acids • Reabsorbs a major fraction of sodium, bicarbonate, calcium, phosphorus, and potassium through active transport	• Impaired reabsorption of filtrate • Glucosuria, aminoaciduria • Renal tubular acidosis, bicarbonaturia, metabolic acidosis • Sodium and potassium wasting • Hypophosphatemia, vitamin D deficiency
Loop of Henle	Descending limb • Creates a concentration gradient. Reabsorbs water but is impermeable to sodium, with the purpose of concentrating urine Ascending limb • Reabsorbs electrolytes but is impermeable to water	• Dilute urine • Distal renal tubular acidosis
Distal Convoluted Tubule	• Concentrates urine when the body needs to conserve water, because it is permeable to water only in the presence of antidiuretic hormone (ADH)	• ADH is persistently present due to decreased blood flow through the kidneys • Kidneys conserve water to raise blood volume, leading to fluid retention
Collecting Duct	• Permeability regulated by ADH and aldosterone • Urine is formed and travels through the ureter to the bladder	• Insufficient removal of waste products from the blood enter the urine • Azotemia results

Data from Skorecki K, Chertow GM, Marsden PA, Taal MW, Yu ASL. *Brenner and Rector's The Kidney*. 10th ed. Philadelphia, PA: Elsevier; 2015.

blood pressure, as described above. The kidney secretes **erythropoietin** (EPO), the hormone that promotes red blood cell production in bone marrow upon detection of low oxygen levels. The kidney also activates 25-hydroxyvitamin D to 1,25-dihydroxyvitamin D_3, also known as calcitriol, the active form of vitamin D. The kidney further participates in bone homeostasis by regulating blood levels of calcium and phosphorus through parathyroid hormone regulation.

When the kidneys do not function properly, the effects are far reaching. Kidney failure leads to the inability of the kidney to perform its normal homeostatic control mechanisms, as well as its excretory and endocrine functions. This can lead to a buildup of waste products, fluid overload, electrolyte abnormalities, acid–base disturbances, anemia, and bone and mineral disorders, among other conditions.

Diseases of the Kidney

Kidney disease is the ninth leading cause of death in the United States.[10] Kidney disease may be hereditary or nonhereditary, and may be the result of direct insult or injury, drug toxicity, infection, as well as other disease states such as diabetes and hypertension. Most of the time, diseases of the kidneys effect the nephron. As the number of functioning nephrons declines, **oliguria**, or low urine volume, typically defined as less than 500 mL per day will occur. Oliguria gives rise to nitrogenous waste accumulation in the blood, a condition known as **azotemia**. Azotemia can cause physical symptoms such as shortness of breath and difficulty sleeping, as well as psychological symptoms such as confusion, depression, and anxiety.[11] Prolonged azotemia can progress to kidney failure.

> ## CASE STUDY REVISITED
>
> Dean is diagnosed with CKD. His age is 33 years, his creatinine is now 3.4 mg/dL, and his serum cystatin C is 2.0 mg/L (0.8-1.2 mg/L).
>
> Based on the MDRD equation, Dean's eGFR is 25 mL/min/1.73 m².
> Based on the CKD-EPI Creatinine equation, Dean's eGFR is 26 mL/min/1.73 m².
> Based on the CKD-EPI Cystatin C equation, Dean's eGFR is 35 mL/min/1.73 m².
>
> ### Questions
> 1. Compare the results. How do you account for the differences in eGFR?
> 2. What stage is Dean's CKD?

The two broad classifications of kidney disease are: **acute kidney injury (AKI)**, which refers to a rapid decline in kidney function, characterized by a sudden drop in GFR, and **chronic kidney disease (CKD)**, a decline in kidney function over time. The Kidney Disease Outcomes Quality Initiative (KDOQI) of the National Kidney Foundation (NKF) established guidelines for managing CKD in 2002. In 2003, a group of nephrology experts, **Kidney Disease: Improving Global Outcomes (KDIGO)**, was founded to provide a source of consolidated, evidence-based clinical practice guidelines to be used in all aspects of kidney disease treatment. By 2013, KDIGO had held 12 global conferences on kidney disease, and their guidelines, including medical nutrition therapy recommendations, are used frequently in clinical practice.[12,13]

Calculation of GFR

GFR is the best measure of kidney function and is used to stage the degree of kidney failure. GFR is estimated, also known as **estimated glomerular filtration rate (eGFR)**, based on various parameters and can be calculated by several equations: the Modification of Diet in Renal Disease study (MDRD) equation, the Chronic Kidney Disease Epidemiology (CKD-EPI) equation using creatinine, and the CKD-EPI equation using serum cystatin C. In adults, the MDRD study equation and the CKD-EPI creatinine equation are the most widely used to diagnose kidney disease.

MDRD Study Equation

The MDRD study equation estimates GFR based on age, ethnicity, sex, and serum creatinine level.[14] Creatinine is produced naturally by the body because it is a byproduct of creatine phosphate breakdown in the muscle. It is also used to estimate lean body mass, as creatine phosphate metabolism would increase proportionately to muscle mass, resulting in higher levels of creatinine in the blood and urine. Creatinine is not used by the body and is therefore cleared from the blood by the kidneys. This makes it a useful marker of kidney function, as a diseased kidney would not clear creatinine as effectively as a healthy kidney and resulting in higher serum creatinine (S_{cr}), or the measurement of creatinine in the serum. The MDRD study equation to calculate eGFR is as follows[14]:

$$eGFR = 175 \times (\text{creatinine mg/dL})^{-1.154} \times (\text{age in years})^{-0.203} \times (0.742 \text{ if female}) \times (1.210 \text{ if African American})$$

CKD-EPI Creatinine Equation

The CKD-EPI creatinine equation is appropriate for use if a GFR of 60 mL/min/1.73 m² or above is expected. This equation would not be appropriate for use in those who already have severely decreased kidney function.[14] The CKD-EPI Creatinine equation to calculate eGFR is as follows[15]:

$$eGFR = 141 \times \min(S_{cr}/\kappa, 1)^{\alpha} \times \max(S_{cr}/\kappa, 1)^{-1.209} \times 0.993^{\text{age}} \times (1.018 \text{ if female}) \times (1.159 \text{ if African American})$$

where S_{cr} is serum creatinine in mg/dL, age is reported in years, κ is 0.7 for females and 0.9 for males, α is -0.329 for females and -0.411 for males, min indicates the minimum of S_{cr}/κ or 1, and max indicates the maximum of S_{cr}/κ or 1.

CKD-EPI Cystatin C Equation

An estimated 3.6% of adults in the United States would technically be classified as having kidney disease if the only criterion for diagnosis was a GFR of 45 to 59 mL/min/1.73 m², determined through serum creatinine levels.[16] Cystatin C is a protein similar to creatinine, but unlike creatinine, this protein is not affected by body mass or diet. Cystatin C is an important marker of kidney function and can improve the accuracy of kidney disease diagnosis when evaluated in conjunction with creatinine and urine albumin.[15] The cystatin C equation is recommended as a confirmatory step in diagnosing kidney disease in patients who have a creatinine-based estimated GFR of 60 to 74 mL/min/1.73 m² and no presence of albuminuria.[16] Using this equation in addition to one of the creatinine-based GFR estimating equations may help clinicians to more accurately diagnose the disease. The CKD-EPI Cystatin C equation to calculate eGFR is as follows[16]:

$$eGFR = 133 \times \min(S_{cys}/0.8, 1)^{-0.499} \times \max(S_{cys}/0.8, 1)^{-1.328} \times 0.996^{Age} \times (0.932 \text{ if female})$$

where S_{cys} (standardized serum cystatin C) is reported in mg/L, min indicates the minimum of $S_{cys}/0.8$ or 1, max indicates the maximum of $S_{cys}/0.8$ or 1, and age is reported years.

Acute Kidney Injury

Acute kidney injury (AKI), historically referred to as acute renal failure or acute renal insufficiency, is a rapid decline in kidney function characterized by a sudden decrease in GFR.[17] AKI usually occurs in previously healthy kidneys, and patients with AKI may recover kidney function without long-term consequences. Although research is lacking in long-term follow-up of AKI patients, some small studies have reported between 60% and 70% of AKI patients recover completely.[18,19] AKI can last for days or weeks, sometimes longer, and if it persists, can progress to CKD.[20] Patients may need **renal replacement therapy (RRT)**, a treatment that replaces the normal blood-filtering function of the kidneys used to remove waste and fluid, while kidney function is impaired.

Etiology

There are many potential causes of AKI. **Prerenal AKI** causes involve inadequate renal perfusion and are the leading causes of AKI.[20] **Intrinsic AKI** causes are diseases within the renal parenchyma, and **postrenal AKI** causes involve urinary tract obstruction.[20] Major causes of AKI are sepsis, trauma, volume depletion, hypotension, intravenous contrast dye used for radiological procedures, medications, and preexisting chronic kidney disease.[21] Table 14.2 lists the prerenal, intrinsic, and postrenal causes of AKI and Table 14.3 identifies medications that have been associated with the onset of AKI.

Diagnosis

KDIGO defines AKI as an abrupt increase in serum creatinine of 0.3 mg/dL over the patient's baseline within 48 hours, a 50% increase of creatinine or more within 1 week, or urinary output of less than 0.5 mL/kg/hour for more than 6 hours.[12] To better define AKI, the RIFLE classification (Risk, Injury, Failure, Loss of kidney function, and End-stage kidney disease) were developed based on S_{cr}, GFR, and urine output determinants, and considers three severity classes of AKI (Risk, Injury, and Failure) according to the variations in S_{cr} and/or urine output, and two outcome classes (loss of kidney function and end-stage kidney disease).[22] Table 14.4 outlines characteristics of the three stages of AKI.

Medical Treatment

AKI may resolve or may have long-term consequences. Typically, drug-induced AKI is resolved once medication intake has ceased and the substance is removed from the body, although RRT may be required. Pharmacologic therapy, such as diuretics and vasopressors, may also be used for the treatment of AKI, but is dependent upon the cause.[20]

Medical Nutrition Therapy

Common side effects of decreased renal function in AKI patients include uremia, metabolic acidosis, and fluid and electrolyte imbalances, which may be managed in part

TABLE 14.2 CAUSES OF AKI

Prerenal	Intrinsic	Postrenal
Atherosclerosis	Contrast dye	Bladder cancer
Circulatory issues	Medications	Nephrolithiasis
Hypotension	Rhabdomyolysis	Prostate cancer
Severe dehydration	Sepsis	Urinary tract obstruction

Data from A.S.P.E.N. clinical guidelines: nutrition support in adult acute and chronic renal failure. *JPEN J Parenter Enteral Nutr.* 2010;34(4):366-377.

TABLE 14.3 MEDICATIONS ASSOCIATED WITH AKI

Acetaminophen	Antiretrovirals	Immunosuppressive agents
Acyclovir	Chemotherapeutic agents	Lithium
Aminoglycosides	Ciprofloxacin	Nonsteroidal anti-inflammatory drugs (NSAIDs)
Angiotensin converting enzyme (ACE) inhibitors	Contrast dyes	Proton-pump inhibitors
Angiotensin II receptor blockers (ARBs)	Foscarnet	Sulfa-based antibiotics
Antifungal agents	HMG-CoA reductase inhibitors (statins)	Vancomycin

Data from Pazhayattil GS, Shirali AC. Drug-induced impairment of renal function. *Int J Nephrol Renovasc Dis.* 2014;7:457-468.

TABLE 14.4 THREE STAGES OF AKI

Stage	Serum Creatinine	Percent Decrease in GFR	Urine Output (mL/kg/hour)
Stage 1: At risk for AKI	Increased 1.5 to 2x baseline	25%	<0.5 within 6 hours
Stage 2: Injury	Increased 2 to 3x baseline	>50%	<0.5 over 12 hours or longer
Stage 3: Kidney failure	Increased >3x baseline OR Increased by at least 4 mg/dL with an acute rise >0.5 mg/dL	75%	<0.3 for at least 24 hours OR Anuria for at least 12 hours

Data from Acute renal failure—definition, outcome measures, animal models, fluid therapy and information technology needs: the Second International Consensus Conference of the Acute Dialysis Quality Initiative (ADQI) Group. *Crit Care*. 2004;8:R204. https://doi.org/10.1016/S1470-2045(07)70246-3.

with nutritional intervention. Increased catabolism and increased protein needs are common if AKI is caused by or associated with infection or injury.[21] Administering medical nutrition therapy (MNT) to AKI patients is challenging due to the need to balance a patient's increased energy and protein needs with newly compromised protein metabolism that may lead to an unsafe accumulation of metabolic end products such as urea. Providing too much protein may result in metabolic acidosis due to retention of nitrogenous waste. Due to a lack of randomized, controlled trials demonstrating the efficacy of MNT in AKI, current recommendations are based on expert consensus from groups such as KDIGO and American Society of Parenteral and Enteral Nutrition (A.S.P.E.N.).[12,21]

> **PRACTICE POINT**
>
> In AKI, it is important to balance increased energy and protein needs with compromised protein metabolism.

Nutrition Assessment and Intervention

Nutrition assessment in AKI may be similar to that conducted for patients under metabolic stress, as AKI is often the result of trauma or stress. In AKI occurring without metabolic stress from sepsis or trauma, nutritional assessment involves evaluating anthropometrics, determining the presence of fluid retention, interpreting biochemical data, conducting a diet history, and completing a nutrition-focused physical assessment.

Energy The KDIGO guidelines recommend that patients receive 20 to 30 kcal/kg/day for all stages of AKI.[12] A.S.P.E.N. recommends using indirect calorimetry if possible, especially for patients who are critically ill.[21] Energy needs in AKI patients may be increased as much as 30%, so adequate calories from fat and carbohydrate are encouraged to prevent catabolism of dietary protein for energy.[23] Despite increased energy requirements, it is important to avoid overfeeding patients with AKI. A 2005 randomized trial comparing AKI patients receiving 30 kcal/kg/day to those receiving 40 kcal/kg/day found that 40 kcal/kg/day did not result in a more positive nitrogen balance than 30 kcal/kg/day. The higher calorie feeding was associated with a higher incidence of hypertriglyceridemia, hyperglycemia, and a greater fluid load.[24] These medical conditions should be avoided because dyslipidemia and insulin resistance are associated with both critical illness and kidney disease. Few specific guidelines are available for carbohydrate and fat intake, but recommended energy intake is 3 to 5 g/kg/day of carbohydrate and 0.8 to 1.0 g/kg/day of fat.[12]

> **PRACTICE POINT**
>
> Indirect calorimetry is the gold standard for determining energy requirements in AKI patients to avoid overfeeding.

Protein The KDIGO guidelines for protein recommend 0.8 to 1.0 g/kg/day of protein for AKI patients not on RRT, 1.0 to 1.5 g/kg/day for AKI patients on RRT, and up to 1.5 to 1.7 g/kg/day for hypercatabolic patients and those on **continuous renal replacement therapy (CRRT)**. CRRT is a type of dialysis utilizing hemofiltration, hemodialysis, or both, typically used in hospitalized patients with AKI. CRRT may result in increased protein losses and may necessitate some patients requiring up to 2.5 g/kg/day of protein.[25] Sixty percent of protein consumed should be of **high biological value (HBV)**, or foods containing all essential amino acids and readily available protein, to replace increased protein losses from CRRT.[12]

> **PRACTICE POINT**
>
> Acidosis and insulin resistance seen in critical illness and AKI stimulate protein catabolism and can lead to a negative nitrogen balance.

Fluid and Sodium When AKI and kidney disease results in decreased urine volume, fluid intake should be limited as much as possible while maintaining adequate protein and energy intakes.[26] Patients with anuria, or absence of urine formation, or who excrete less than 75 mL of urine daily are usually restricted to 1,000 mL to 1,200 mL of fluid per day. Sodium intake should be determined based on the patient's urine sodium output. Oliguria may decrease the amount of sodium lost in the urine, calling for a lower sodium intake.[26] Clinicians should be mindful of nondietary sources of sodium when implementing and enforcing sodium restriction in patients with AKI patients, as sodium can be found in many intravenous medications.

Potassium When tissue damage or trauma occurs, lysing of cells causes intracellular potassium to be released into the blood, putting patients at risk for hyperkalemia. Clinicians must closely monitor dietary potassium intake and serum potassium levels regularly throughout the disease course. Dietary allowances should be individualized based on serum potassium levels. These levels can change quickly due to the many processes that alter potassium levels, such as glucose, insulin, and bicarbonate administration, which all facilitate the drive of potassium intracellularly.[12] A summary of the nutritional guidelines for AKI can be found in Table 14.5.

Chronic Kidney Disease

Chronic kidney disease (CKD) is defined as a decline in renal function over time. CKD can be caused by various conditions, including AKI. It is defined using two criteria established by KDOQI[25]:

1. Kidney damage for more than 3 months as defined by structural or functional abnormalities of the kidney, with or without decreased GFR, manifest by either pathological abnormalities or markers of kidney damage, including abnormalities in the composition of the blood or urine, or abnormalities in imaging tests
2. GFR <60 mL/min/1.73 m² for ≥3 months, with or without kidney damage

Kidney damage leads to urinary protein losses through the glomerular filtration apparatus, which presents as an increased urinary albumin level.[26] In 2012, KDOQI and KDIGO advised that GFR and urine albumin levels be evaluated together to diagnose and assess CKD.[27]

CKD Classification

The classification of CKD is based on the level of kidney function demonstrated through the patient's GFR. Stages 1 and 2 CKD are marked by early signs of dysfunction such as proteinuria, hematuria, and anatomic abnormalities. Stages 3a, 3b, and 4 are the advanced stages of CKD, and progress to stages 5 and 5D, formerly known as **end-stage renal disease (ESRD)**. In these stages, the patient needs renal replacement therapy or a kidney transplant to survive. Stage 5D CKD is used to describe a patient with kidney failure on dialysis. **Table 14.6** outlines the criteria for CKD classification.

Etiology

CKD has various causes that may include a multitude of conditions. Chronic diseases that are increasingly prevalent in Western society, such as obesity, dyslipidemia, diabetes, and hypertension, are the most common factors that contribute to kidney damage.

TABLE 14.5 SUMMARY OF NUTRITIONAL GUIDELINES FOR AKI

	Stage 1	Stage 2	Stage 3	Notes
Energy (kcal/kg/day)	20-30	20-30	20-30	
Protein (g/kg/day)	0.8-1.0	0.8-1.5	1.5-1.7	RRT: 1.0-1.5 Hypercatabolic/CRRT: 2-2.5
Fluid (L/day)	Unrestricted	Unrestricted	1-1.2	Fluid restricted as much as possible during anuria
Sodium	Individualized based on urine output	Individualized based on urine output	Individualized based on urine output	Sodium will likely need to be limited during stage 3 due to decreased losses
Potassium	Individualized based on serum potassium levels Monitor potassium levels in the blood and restrict potassium if elevated			

Data from Kidney Disease: Improving Global Outcomes (KDIGO) Acute Kidney Injury Work Group. KDIGO Clinical Practice Guideline for Acute Kidney Injury. *Kidney Int* Suppl. 2012; 2: 1–138. Pannu N, Gibney RN. Renal replacement therapy in the intensive care unit. *Ther Clin Risk Manag.* 2005;1(2):141-150; and ASPEN Board of Directors and Clinical Guidelines Task Force. Guidelines for the use of parenteral and enteral nutrition in adult and pediatric patients. *JPEN J Parenter Enteral Nutr.* 2002;26(1 Suppl):1SA-138S.

CASE STUDY REVISITED

Dean's CKD continues to worsen. Six months later, his eGFR is 20 mL/min/1.73 m². He is admitted to the hospital and nutrition is consulted. Dean reports he has worsening edema in his legs and arms and continues to experience dyspnea at night and with minimal exertion. Due to his significant fatigue, he has put his studies on hold.

Anthropometric Data:
Weight: 88 kg (194 lbs)

Biochemical Data:
Sodium 127 (135-145 mEq/L)
Potassium 6.3 (3.6-5.0 mEq/L)
Chloride 117 (98-110 mEq/L)
Carbon dioxide 16 (20-30 mEq/L)
Blood urea nitrogen 95 (6-24 mg/dL)

Creatinine 4.2 (0.4-1.3 mg/dL)
Glucose 90 (70-98 mg/dL)
Calcium 6.4 (8.5-10.5 mEq/L)
Phosphorus 6.7 (2.7-4.5 mg/dL)

Dietary Data:
Diet Prescription: 2 g sodium and 2 g potassium diet

Questions

1. What stage is Dean's CKD now?
2. What are the nutrition priorities for Dean?
3. How are his labs a reflection of his physical presentation and anthropometric and clinical data?
4. How would you interpret Dean's weight trend in comparison to his original visit 6 months ago?
5. What additional information would you like to obtain?

Diabetes is the most common cause of CKD, followed by hypertension.[5] These two conditions account for 60% to 80% of all cases of CKD.[28,29] Hyperglycemia puts stress on the kidneys and can alter blood flow through the kidney. Over time, this can cause glomerular filters to lose their integrity and allow protein to be excreted in the urine. The loss of protein in the urine is called **microalbuminuria**. As with hyperglycemia, hypertension can stress the kidneys

TABLE 14.6 STAGES OF CHRONIC KIDNEY DISEASE

Stage	eGFR (mL/min/1.73m²)	Description	Estimated Kidney Function
1	90+	Normal kidney function; urine or other abnormalities point to kidney disease	90%-100%
2	60-89	Mildly reduced kidney function; urine or other abnormalities point to kidney disease	60%-89%
3a	45-59	Moderately reduced kidney function	45%-59%
3b	30-44	Moderately reduced kidney function	30%-44%
4	15-29	Severely reduced kidney function	15%-29%
5 or 5D	<15	Very severe, end-stage kidney failure Kidney failure on dialysis	<15%

Data from: National Kidney Foundation. Kidney Disease Outcomes Quality Initiative NKF-K/DOQI clinical practice guidelines for chronic kidney disease: evaluation, classification, and stratification. *Am J Kidney Dis*. 2002;39:S1-S266.

and damage the filtration, leading to microalbuminuria and, if untreated, CKD. Because insulin resistance and hypertension are potential complications of obesity, obesity is an independent risk factor for kidney disease.

Polycystic kidney disease (PKD) is an inherited disorder that causes cysts on the kidneys. The cysts can grow and multiply over time, causing the kidneys to enlarge and lose function. PKD is the fourth leading cause of CKD, representing about 5% of all kidney failure.[31] PKD can be autosomal dominant, which is the most common; autosomal recessive; or acquired (not genetic). Approximately 50% to 60% of individuals with PKD will develop CKD later in life.[31]

Other CKD risk factors include recurrent urinary tract infection, HIV infection, and immunological diseases such as lupus.[32] Many of the diseases that cause AKI can also lead to CKD. Risk of CKD has been reported to be twice as high in people with a history of nephrolithiasis.[33] Hyperoxalosis, which leads to hyperoxaluria, is a genetic condition that can also cause CKD.[34]

Medical Treatment

The main goals of treatment of CKD include delaying disease progression, treating complications, and providing RRT. Due to the large impact that other diseases have on the development and progression of CKD, treatment should also address comorbid conditions such as cardiovascular disease, diabetes, hypertension, and hyperlipidemia.

> **CORE CONCEPT 2**
>
> Prevention is a key component in the management of CKD and involves treatment of underlying conditions, such as diabetes.

Nutritional Concerns of CKD

Proper nutrition is important during CKD and it is deeply connected to the disease progression. The disease can impact nutritional status and, simultaneously, nutrition can impact disease progression. When GFR falls below 60 mL/min/1.73 m² (stages 3-5 CKD), nutritional status begins to deteriorate.[8] As the disease progresses, patients are at increased risk of malnutrition. The registered dietitian (RD) is an essential member of the interprofessional team for CKD patients because the risk of complications, morbidity, and mortality increases when CKD progresses to later stages and patients become at risk for malnutrition.[35]

> **CORE CONCEPT 3**
>
> Malnutrition risk increases as GFR decreases, and may complicate the management of CKD due to protein, fluid, and/or micronutrient restrictions.

Goals of Nutrition Intervention

The goals of nutrition intervention in CKD include preservation of kidney function by managing causes of CKD, such as diabetes and hypertension, and maintenance of adequate nutritional status. The key interventions for preserving kidney function in CKD progression are controlling blood pressure; preventing further damage from excessive protein intake; and managing diabetes, if present.[32] Maintaining adequate nutritional status includes achieving a stable weight with adequate body fat and muscle mass, normal visceral protein status, and sufficient dietary intake, as well as managing side effects of medications. Nutritional interventions should also be targeted toward associated conditions such as bone mineral disease, anemia, electrolyte and acid–base imbalances, and vitamin deficiencies. Each component is important for patient survival and quality of life in CKD.

Medical nutrition therapy provided by an RD is a necessary part of CKD treatment because there are numerous diet- and lifestyle-related causes of CKD, so MNT can be used to manage these underlying conditions. Because CKD is not often recognized until a patient presents with clinical symptoms, the RD can utilize MNT to manage CKD symptoms and complications. MNT may also be provided to prevent malnutrition caused by proteinuria, loss of appetite, medication side effects, and dialysis treatments.

> **CORE CONCEPT 4**
>
> Medical nutrition therapy is a necessary component of CKD management and can improve outcomes by preventing malnutrition and slowing disease progression.

Nutritional Assessment and Intervention

Nutritional assessment should include evaluation of anthropometric, biochemical, clinical, dietary, and environmental data, and physical/functional assessment. The KDOQI guidelines recommend that nutrition assessments be conducted every 6 to 12 months for stage 3 CKD patients, and every 1 to 3 months during stage 4 and 5 CKD.[28]

> **PRACTICE POINT**
>
> The ideal body mass index range for CKD is approximately 22 to 25.5 kg/m².[36]

Anthropometrics such as, height, weight, and weight history are important to assess fluid balance and determine the presence of malnutrition. The subjective global assessment can be used to help estimate fat and muscle status, as well as to identify malnutrition.[37] Evaluation of **standard body weight (SBW)** is another method used to detect malnutrition in CKD patients. Percentage of SBW is the patient's actual body weight expressed as a percentage of a defined normal body weight for Americans of a similar frame size, sex, height, and age[12,28]:

$$\%SBW = (actual\ weight\ /\ SBW) \times 100$$

The information used to determine "normal" weight comes from NHANES, the National Health and Nutrition

TABLE 14.7 INTERPRETATION OF PERCENTAGE OF STANDARD BODY WEIGHT[28]

% SBW	<70%	<90%	90%-110%	115%-130%	130%-150%	>150%
Nutritional Status	Severely malnourished	Mild to moderately malnourished	Well nourished; recommended target for maintenance dialysis patients	Mildly obese	Moderately obese	Severely obese

Data from National Kidney Foundation: NKF-K/DOQI Clinical practice guidelines for nutrition in chronic renal failure. *Am J Kidney Dis.* 2000;35:S1-S140.

Evaluation Survey (http://www2.kidney.org/professionals/kdoqi/guidelines_nutrition/nut_appx07a.html).[28]

Table 14.7 outlines the classifications of SBW interpretation. Standard body weight may also be used to estimate the **adjusted edema-free body weight (aBWef)** in patients undergoing dialysis with edema who are either obese or underweight.[28] This adjusted weight is important to use when determining energy and calorie intake goals for patients with edema, as failure to do so may result in over- or underestimation of needs, which could further complicate the disease process. The formula for calculating aBW_{ef} is as follows[28]:

$$aBW_{ef} = BW_{ef} + ([SBW - BW_{ef}] \times 0.25)$$

Biochemical tests commonly measured in CKD include sodium, potassium, chloride, carbon dioxide, blood urea nitrogen (BUN), creatinine, cystatin C, albumin, prealbumin, c-reactive protein (CRP), transferrin, corrected calcium, phosphorus, parathyroid hormone (PTH), vitamin D, hemoglobin, iron, ferritin, and percentage saturation of transferrin. Blood gas results, particularly pCO_2, can also be helpful. Because prealbumin is renally cleared and may be falsely elevated in renal failure, interpretation of prealbumin level must consider degree of renal function if it is to be used as a nutrition marker. Phosphorus, calcium, potassium, and sodium are also excreted in the urine, so their serum levels may be elevated due to decreased clearance by the diseased kidneys. Because AKI and CKD are associated with inflammation, which has a negative effect on nutritional status, both inflammation and nutrition status should be evaluated.[21]

Biochemical indices including eGFR, urine albumin-to-creatinine ratio (UACR), and urine protein may also be assessed. eGFR is a main determinant of CKD diagnosis and severity, but monitoring eGFR over time can help clinicians identify whether their interventions are working, with a stable eGFR indicating that treatment is effective.[32] Monitoring eGFR is important because as GFR declines, so does the patient's nutritional status.[38] UACR is used to determine whether a patient has albuminuria, a common biomarker of CKD progression. Normal levels are between 0 and 30 mg/g, with levels over 30 mg/g indicating albuminuria and CKD. Similar to eGFR, UACR monitored over time allows the clinician to know whether or not the nutritional intervention is helping slow the progression of disease.[32]

> **PRACTICE POINT**
>
> Consideration of fluid status is necessary when analyzing laboratory values of individuals with CKD.

A thorough diet history should be gathered from the patient using a 24-hour food recall or a 2-day food record. Patients on hemodialysis should ideally report one day of food records on a dialysis day and another on a nondialysis day to account for any changes in appetite, energy levels, or functional status impacting shopping and cooking ability attributable to treatment. Hand grip strength can also be measured to estimate any changes in functional status.[39] A CKD patient with good nutritional status will have a stable dry body weight, adequate fat and muscle stores, and sufficient appetite with adequate intake.[32,40] Several dietary components must be closely monitored in order to promote optimal nutrition status.

Energy The Academy of Nutrition and Dietetics' Evidence Analysis Library reports that an energy prescription of 23 to 35 kcal/kg/day is adequate for nondiabetic CKD patients on a protein-restricted diet.[41] KDOQI recommends 35 kcal/kg/day for patients in stages 4 to 5 CKD older than 60 years, and 30 to 35 kcal/kg/day for those younger than 60 years.[28] Calorie limits should be individualized for the patient based on energy expenditure and nutritional status.[28] For example, a CKD patient with rapid weight loss and high CRP levels, indicating inflammation, may need a greater amount of calories per kilogram than a more weight-stable patient.

Protein Protein restriction has been a controversial topic in renal nutrition because, although protein is a source of metabolic acid from nitrogenous waste, it is also necessary to maintain adequate nutritional status with sufficient lean body mass. Because it has been established that patients with more lean body mass have improved outcomes, adequate protein intake is imperative for CKD patients. Complications from excess nitrogenous waste and high phosphorus levels indicate that protein intake must be balanced to some degree during CKD. The goal of protein administration is to prevent lean body mass wasting while minimizing the impact of protein metabolism on GFR. According to the KDIGO guidelines, there is insufficient evidence to support routine protein restriction in all CKD patients; therefore, protein allowances should be individualized on a patient-by-patient basis.[29]

CASE STUDY REVISITED

During his hospitalization, Dean reports anorexia, nausea, and an "unpleasant taste in his mouth." He provides a recent diet intake.

Anthropometric Data:
Weight: 88 kg (194 lbs)

Biochemical Data:
Sodium 129 (135-145 mEq/L)
Potassium 5.9 (3.6-5.0 mEq/L)
Chloride 115 (98-110 mEq/L)
Carbon dioxide 19 (20-30 mEq/L)
Blood urea nitrogen 89 (6-24 mg/dL)

Creatinine 4.2 (0.4-1.3 mg/dL)
Glucose 99 (70-98 mg/dL)
Calcium 7.2 (8.5-10.5 mEq/L)
Phosphorus 8.8 (2.7-4.5 mg/dL)

Dietary Data:
24-hour Dietary Recall
Breakfast (8 am): 1 banana, 8 oz orange juice
Lunch (12 pm): ½ tuna sandwich on whole wheat bread, 12 oz diet cola
Snack (3 pm): Small coffee with cream and sugar, 3 oatmeal cookies
Dinner (7 pm): 1½ cups pasta with tomato sauce and 1 meatball; 1 cup garden salad with romaine lettuce, carrots, and tomatoes with Italian dressing; 16 oz water
Diet Prescription: 2 g sodium and 2 g potassium diet

Questions

1. Analyze the Dean's diet. How does it differ from his initial diet recall 6 months ago? What are your concerns?
2. The renal team is requesting your advice on his diet prescription. What would you recommend?
3. What specific diet changes do you suggest?

CORE CONCEPT 5

Protein is a necessary macronutrient in CKD patients' diets, and despite controversy regarding the possibility that protein restriction improves outcomes, patients must be able to eat a balanced, palatable diet that provides adequate energy and protein to prevent loss of lean body mass.

Fluid and Sodium Fluid and sodium balance become a concern in CKD because the renin-angiotensin-aldosterone system becomes compromised in any kidney disease.[6] Another concern is that GFR has been shown to decline more rapidly in those with higher blood pressure, making fluid and sodium balance even more important in slowing the progression of CKD.[7] Blood pressure goals, which are the same in hypertensive adults with and without CKD, are based on age and the presence or absence of both proteinuria and diabetes.[42] Medications typically used to treat hypertension in individuals with CKD are angiotensin converting enzyme inhibitors (ACEIs), angiotensin receptor blockers (ARBs), and diuretics or calcium channel blockers. Thiazide diuretics, typically prescribed in the non-CKD population with hypertension, are not as effective in patients with CKD, so use is limited.[43]

Fluid intake is not routinely restricted in all CKD patients, but sodium intake should not exceed 2.4 g/day.[44] Patients with CKD may already follow low-sodium diets because they are frequently used in the prevention and treatment of other conditions commonly associated with CKD, such as hypertension. All CKD patients should focus on limiting or eliminating high-sodium foods such as processed meats, cheeses, and packaged snack foods. Alternative methods to increase the palatability of low-sodium meals are needed to ensure adequate intake and compliance, especially in the hospital setting. Some techniques include using more spices during cooking and enhancing the visual appeal of meals by choosing foods with a variety of bright colors.

The most widely used, evidence-based low-sodium diet is the Dietary Approaches to Stop Hypertension (DASH) diet.[45] This diet, often used for hypertension management, emphasizes the importance of limiting saturated and hydrogenated fats while encouraging fruits, vegetables, dairy, whole grains, and omega-3 fatty acids. The DASH diet is high in magnesium and potassium and recommends more plant-based protein sources, which may not be appropriate for some CKD patients, particularly those following a low potassium, magnesium, and/or phosphorus diet. In addition, patients who take ACEIs or ARBs should closely monitor their potassium intake due to the possible potassium sparing nature of these medications, which can lead to hyperkalemia. After consideration of these dietary factors, the DASH diet may be a healthy potential option for stage 1 to 4 CKD patients.

Potassium Hyperkalemia can occur in advanced CKD because of reduced excretion by the kidneys, metabolic acidosis, and medications that inhibit potassium excretion such as ACEI and ARB, and may be compounded by increased consumption of potassium-containing foods. There are also additional potassium-sparing medications, such as diuretics, as well as potassium citrates that may be prescribed for some patients with kidney stones.[46] The serum potassium level should be monitored closely for patients who take these medications. Dietary interventions for hyperkalemia include limiting potassium-rich foods and avoiding salt substitutes containing potassium chloride. This is particularly important to remember for patients who are on a sodium-restricted diet, because they may be offered these salt substitutes to increase the palatability of their meals. Common high-potassium food sources can be found in **Figure 14.5**.

Calcium, Phosphorus, and Vitamin D Calcium, phosphorus, and vitamin D are important components of the diet of patients with CKD due to increased risk of mineral and bone disorder, also referred to as **renal osteodystrophy**, a condition that occurs when the kidneys are unable to maintain normal levels of blood calcium and phosphorus.[47] In health, bones utilize calcium, phosphorus, vitamin D, fibroblast growth factor 23, and parathyroid hormone to balance serum levels with bone viability. Parathyroid hormone (PTH) is a hormone released by the parathyroid glands to regulate calcium, phosphorus, and vitamin D in the blood. In the setting of increased phosphorus leading to low serum calcium, PTH is released into the blood and works to bring the levels back to normal by increasing calcium reabsorption in the body through releasing calcium from the bone through calcitonin production and decreasing calcium lost in the urine. PTH also facilitates the conversion of vitamin D from 25-hydroxyvitamin D to the active form, calcitriol or 1,25-dihydroxyvitamin D_3. Calcitriol will then enhance the absorption of calcium and phosphorus in the intestine. In normal physiology, these mechanisms will lead to an increase in serum calcium levels and, through negative feedback, PTH levels will decrease. **Figure 14.6** illustrates the process of calcium and phosphorus homeostasis by PTH regulation. **Fibroblast growth factor 23 (FGF23)** is a hormone produced by bone that acts in the kidney to regulate phosphorus and vitamin D metabolism by promoting phosphaturia and decreasing production of calcitriol, leading to decreased phosphorus levels.[46] FGF23 can decrease serum PTH; PTH and calcitriol can increase FGF23 production to regulate phosphorus levels.[48]

In CKD, calcium and phosphorus become imbalanced and vitamin D cannot be activated to calcitriol, which impedes the absorption of calcium in the intestine. The progression of mineral and bone disorder begins with decreased urinary phosphorus excretion by the diseased kidneys, which contributes to hyperphosphatemia. FGF23, which promotes phosphaturia, progressively increases beginning in early CKD to attempt to maintain normal phosphorus levels.[48] Low calcitriol levels hinder the body's ability to increase blood calcium concentrations, leading to prolonged elevation of serum PTH causing secondary hyperparathyroidism. FGF23 continues to increase as renal function declines, contributing to disordered phosphate homeostasis. This results in high bone turnover and bone disease.[49] Levels of phosphorus, calcium, vitamin D, and PTH should be monitored and controlled through medical and nutritional intervention to protect bone health in CKD.

Calcium As discussed, in CKD, calcium is decreased in blood due to low calcitriol. Calcium levels are often corrected to adjust for hypoalbuminemia in CKD because for every 1 g/dL fall in serum albumin, total calcium concentration falls by 0.8 mg/dL.[49] This may cause calcium levels to appear lower than they physiologically are. The target range for corrected serum calcium according to the KDOQI guidelines is 8.4 to 9.5 mg/dL.[49] It is recommended that CKD patients limit total elemental calcium intake (supplemental and dietary calcium) to 2,000 mg/day with a maximum 1,500 mg from phosphate binders.[49]

Phosphorus Serum phosphorus levels should be maintained between 2.7 and 4.6 mg/dL for stages 3 to 5 CKD

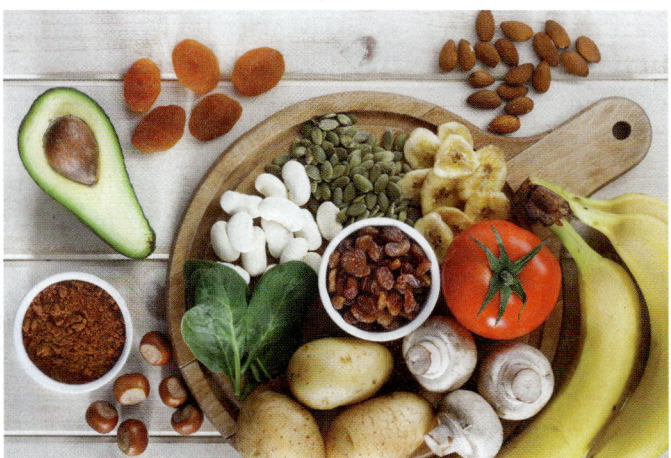

FIGURE 14.5 Dietary Sources of Potassium Include Bananas, Tomatoes, Potatoes, Dried Fruit, Spinach, Avocado, Pumpkin Seeds, Nuts, Cocoa Beans, and Mushrooms
© Evan Lorne/Shutterstock.

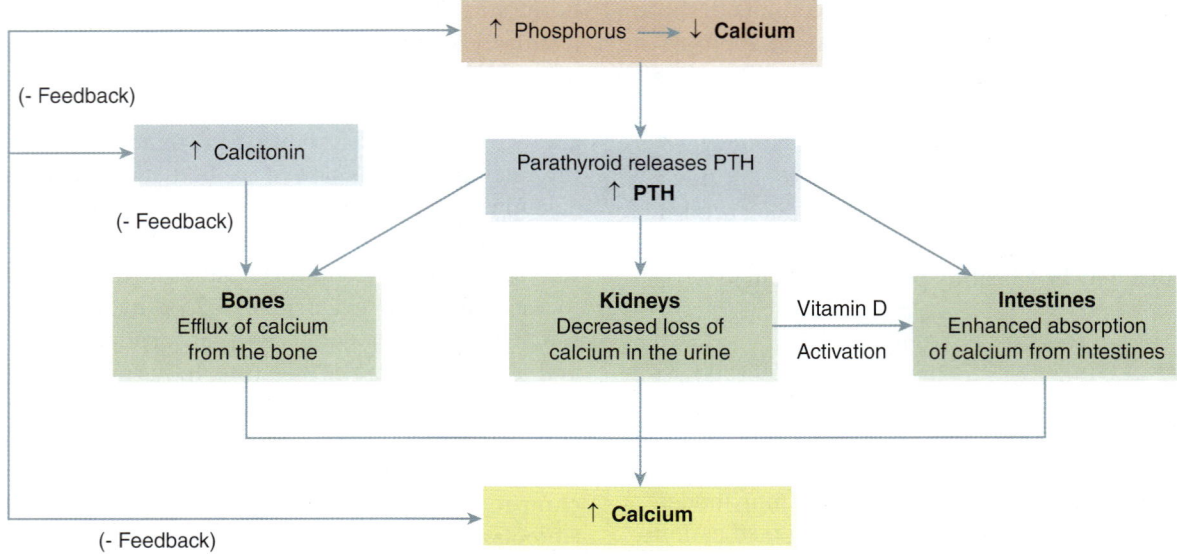

FIGURE 14.6 Mechanisms Involved in Calcium and Phosphorus Homeostasis in Normal Physiology
Data from Kraft MD. Phosphorus and calcium: A review for the adult nutrition support clinician. *Nutr Clin Pract*. 2015;30(1):21-33.

in order to prevent mineral and bone disorders.[49] Evidence shows that this is particularly important in dialysis patients, because mortality from cardiovascular disease and cardiovascular-related hospitalization is increased when phosphorus levels are greater than 5.5 mg/dL for patients with CKD stage 5 or 5D.[49]

Target phosphorus levels can be reached by limiting dietary protein intake and by using medications, known as **phosphate binders**, to reduce the small-intestinal absorption of phosphorus from foods. Phosphorus is abundant in most of the foods we eat, and is found in particularly high levels in animal proteins, plants, seeds, nuts, and legumes. **Table 14.8** lists foods with high, moderate, and low phosphorus content. Phosphate additives are frequently found in meat and dairy products as well as packaged foods, and are better absorbed than phosphorus from other foods.[47] Phosphorus from plant foods is less bioavailable than other sources because it comes in the form of phytate.[47] Because humans lack the phytase enzyme, the phosphorus in these foods is usually less than 50% absorbed.[46] Due to the limited information available about phosphorus content of food additives, patients limiting their phosphorus intake should choose fresh, nonpackaged foods rather than those that are packaged or processed. Patients experiencing fatigue or lacking the ability to cook or shop for themselves due to the symptoms of their illness are especially at risk of consuming additional phosphorus in the form of processed food additives. KDOQI guidelines recommend a limit on dietary phosphorus of 800 to 1,000 mg daily for patients with CKD to ensure a palatable diet and prevent malnutrition associated with decreased intake.[49]

Phosphate binders are used in conjunction with dietary phosphorus control to limit serum phosphorus levels. The KDOQI guidelines outline indications for initiating phosphate binder treatment.[49] Phosphate binder therapy is a logical treatment under the following conditions:

1. Serum phosphorus levels remain elevated after dietary phosphorus restriction is followed
2. Dietary phosphorus restriction interferes with the patient's intake of other critical nutrients
3. Serum PTH levels are elevated after dietary phosphorus restriction, even in the absence of elevated serum phosphorus levels

Phosphate binders are consumed at the time of eating to bind to phosphorus from foods and prevent its absorption. Use of phosphate binder should be individualized to the patient to ensure patient compliance and safety. The following is a list of the several different types of phosphate binders available on the market:

1. *Aluminum-based binders*. Aluminum-based binders, such as aluminum hydroxide, are effective but only indicated for use when the patient is unresponsive to other binders.[49] They are not recommended for long-term use due to the risk of aluminum toxicity and other gastrointestinal side effects, such as nausea, that may impact nutritional status.
2. *Calcium-based binders*. Calcium-based binders are the most commonly used phosphate binders on the market and are available in three forms: calcium carbonate, calcium acetate, and calcium citrate.

TABLE 14.8 LOW-, MEDIUM-, AND HIGH-PHOSPHORUS FOODS

Low (0-50 mg or <5% Daily Value)	Medium (51-150 mg or 5%-15% Daily Value)	High (>150 mg or >15% Daily Value)
Apple	Almond milk	Avocado
Beef, ground, extra lean	Bagel	Beans, baked
Bread, white	Bananas	Beef
Cabbage	Beans, black and pinto	Beer
Carrots, baby	Broccoli	Chickpeas
Cauliflower	Chicken	Chocolate
Cream cheese, 2 tablespoons	Cottage cheese, ½ cup	Dried fruit
Cucumber	Egg	Lamb
Egg white	English muffin	Lentils
Eggplant	Mayonnaise	Organ meats
Fruit cocktail	Oatmeal	Pork chop
Grapes	Parmesan cheese, 2 tablespoons grated	Processed meats
Grapefruit	Peaches	Salmon
Green beans	Peas	Split peas
Pasta, white	Shrimp	Soy milk
Pineapple	Spinach	Tea
Plums	Tortilla, flour and corn, 6-inch	Turkey, breast and thigh, skinless
Popcorn, unsalted	Tuna, canned	Whole grains
Strawberries		Yogurt
Sour cream		

Data from Academy of Nutrition and Dietetics. Nutrition Care Manual and Davita.com.

Calcium citrate is not recommended because evidence shows it increases aluminum absorption.[50] Calcium-based binders, which are available by prescription as well as over the counter, can be used in patients with normal calcium levels and are a less-expensive option, although risks include hypercalcemia and tissue calcification. Recent research has been aimed at finding an alternative phosphate binder formulation due to questions about calcium-based binder side effects. A 2013 meta-analysis found that patients taking non-calcium-based binders had a 22% reduction in all-cause mortality compared to patients on calcium-based phosphate binders, although the etiology is unclear.[50]

3. *Calcium-free and metal-free binders.* Sevelamer carbonate and sevelamer hydrochloride are prescription-only calcium-free and metal-free effective alternatives to other binders, and are especially appropriate for patients with hypercalcemia. Disadvantages include gastrointestinal side effects, especially nausea, and cost.[49] Patients on sevelamer have lower hospitalization rates and a lower risk of hypercalcemia compared to those on a calcium-based binder.[48]

4. *Lanthanum-based binders.* Lanthanum carbonate, which is available by prescription only, is a lanthanum-based binder appropriate for patients with hypercalcemia because it is also calcium free. Because lanthanum is a rare trace metal, there is a concern that lanthanum-based binders carry some risk of toxicity with long-term use.[51]

5. *Magnesium-based binders.* Magnesium carbonate is another binder with the potential to minimize calcium load; however, there are no long-term studies on its safety and efficacy. Patients on magnesium binders should have their serum magnesium levels monitored closely.

6. *Iron-based binders.* New U.S. Food and Drug Administration–approved iron-based phosphate binders, such as sucroferric oxyhydroxide and ferric citrate, have been developed and appear to be effective for use in stage 5D CKD patients. These binders have the potential to increase iron stores, a benefit for CKD patients with anemia, but long-term side effects are unknown at this time.[49,51]

> **PRACTICE POINT**
>
> Elevated serum phosphorus is an independent risk factor for heart disease and mortality.

Vitamin D Due to the kidneys' role in vitamin D activation, patients with kidney disease are at an increased risk for vitamin D deficiency. An estimated 70% to 80% of CKD patients are vitamin D deficient, typically defined as a serum level of less than 20 to 30 ng/dL.[52] Patients will not usually develop vitamin D deficiency until they reach stage 3 or 4 CKD.[49] KDOQI recommends that supplementation with active vitamin D (calcitriol, alfacalcidol, or doxercalciferol) be initiated when serum 25(OH)-vitamin D levels are less than 30 ng/dL and PTH levels are elevated.[49] In the early stages of CKD, PTH elevation may not be due to renal disease. Repletion of vitamin D in forms other than the active form can increase serum vitamin D levels in CKD patients because vitamin D can still be activated by other bodily tissues in addition to the kidney. Repletion of vitamin D should occur prior to initiating active vitamin D because the active form can elevate calcium and phosphorus levels in the blood.

Parathyroid Hormone (PTH) PTH levels may be elevated during CKD due to increased phosphorus and decreased calcitriol levels. Elevated PTH in secondary hyperparathyroidism can indicate abnormally high bone turnover rates. A healthy PTH level range is between 10 and 65 ng/mL; however, in CKD, the normal range is higher due to progressive skeletal resistance to the hormone. Additionally, hyperplasia of parathyroid cells seen in CKD causes the parathyroid gland to secrete more PTH than normal. Higher levels of PTH are expected and required to maintain normal bone turnover during uremia.[53,54]

Lipid Disorders

Alterations in lipoprotein metabolism occur more frequently in patients with CKD, which contributes to an increased risk for cardiovascular disease (CVD) for this patient population. About 50% of all CKD deaths are caused by CVD, making it imperative that the interprofessional team focus on preventing and treating those risk factors that may arise throughout the course of CKD.[55,56] Hypertriglyceridemia occurs in up to 70% of all CKD patients, and the pharmacological treatments available are meant to prevent pancreatitis, not treat the underlying lipid disorder.[57] Although the exact mechanisms are still being investigated, it is hypothesized that high cholesterol levels, particularly those of low density lipoprotein (LDL) and very low density lipoprotein, are caused by the increased inflammation, oxidative stress, and insulin resistance that accompany CKD.[58] Conversely, high LDL and triglyceride levels are independent risk factors for CKD.[58] Dietary and lifestyle techniques for prevention and management of dyslipidemia are necessary for CKD patients; however, no randomized controlled trials of diets low in saturated fat in these patients have been done. This is likely due to difficulty achieving a balanced, energy-dense low-saturated-fat diet with preexisting restrictions such as modified protein, low sodium, and low potassium. All CKD patients, especially those with dyslipidemia, should be encouraged to consume more unsaturated fatty acids. **Table 14.9** outlines the KDOQI dietary fatty acid composition guidelines for diabetes and CKD.[59]

TABLE 14.9 KDOQI RECOMMENDED DIETARY FATTY ACID COMPOSITION FOR INDIVIDUALS WITH DIABETES AND CKD

30% total energy from fat			
10% n-3 fatty acids	10% n-9 fatty acids	5% n-6 fatty acids	5% saturated fat

Data from KDOQI clinical practice guidelines and clinical recommendations for diabetes and chronic kidney disease. *Am J Kidney Dis.* 2007;49(suppl):S62-S73.

Registered dietitians should be aware that mortality risk factors in the CKD population are the opposite of that of the healthy population, as low serum total cholesterol levels are associated with an increased risk for mortality.[60,61] Because this is likely due to malnutrition, RDs must analyze a patient's nutritional status in conjunction with their cholesterol levels. A CKD patient with historically high cholesterol may present with recently lowered cholesterol, which may appear to be an improvement; however, it may be a reflection instead of underlying malnutrition and a consequently increased mortality risk.

Anemia

Anemia is a complication of CKD and is caused by insufficient EPO production by the damaged kidneys. It is universally present during stage 5 CKD and is a potential risk during all other stages.[62] The main biochemical assessment for anemia in CKD patients is hemoglobin, which has a recommended target level of 10 to 12 g/dL in CKD.[63,64] In the 1980s **erythropoietin stimulating agents (ESAs)**, such as recombinant human EPO, were developed; this alleviates CKD-related anemia but may introduce other problems, such as exacerbating hypertension.[62] In addition to EPO deficiency, decreased red blood cell survival is another contributor to anemia development in CKD. Iron-deficiency anemia during CKD is treated with intravenous or oral iron when transferrin is less than 20% saturated and serum ferritin is less than 500 ng/mL.[64] Although serum ferritin can be a component of anemia assessment, caution should be used when interpreting serum ferritin in CKD patients because it is a positive acute-phase protein and levels are increased by inflammation.[65] CKD patients should have acceptable iron status prior to starting ESAs for optimal response to therapy. Refer to **Table 14.10** for a summary of the nutrition guidelines for stages 3 to 5 CKD.

> **PRACTICE POINT**
>
> Oral iron supplements dosed at 200 mg two to three times daily may be prescribed to correct iron-deficiency anemia and support erythropoiesis.

TABLE 14.10 SUMMARY OF NUTRITION GUIDELINES FOR CKD PATIENTS STAGES 3 TO 5

	Stage 3-4	Stage 5	Comments
Protein (g/kg/day)	0.8	Individualize based upon patient	Avoid high protein intake (>1.3 g/kg); 50% of protein should be HBV protein
Energy (kcal/kg/day)	23-35	>60 years: 35 <60 years: 30-35	Individualize based on patient's nutrition status
Sodium (g/day)	<2.4	<2.4	Individualize based on patient's fluid status and blood pressure
Potassium (g/day)	<2.4 or individualize based on serum levels	<2.4	Limit high potassium foods in the diet and watch for salt substitutes. Individualize based on serum potassium levels.
Phosphorus (mg/day)	800-1,000 or 10-12 mg/g protein intake when serum phosphorus >4.6 mg/dL or PTH is elevated	800-1,000	Maintain serum phosphorus between 2.7 and 4.6 mg/dL for stage 3 and 4 CKD. Use phosphate binders as needed and limit high-phosphorus foods in the diet.
Calcium (mg/day)	<2,000	<2,000	Maximum 1,500 mg/day from phosphate binders. Maintain serum calcium between 8.4 and 9.5 mg/dL
Vitamin D	Supplement with oral calcitriol when serum vitamin D <30 ng/dL and PTH is elevated	Supplement with oral calcitriol when serum vitamin D <30 ng/dL and PTH is elevated	

Data from: National Kidney Foundation: NKF-K/DOQI Clinical practice guidelines for nutrition in chronic renal failure. Am J Kidney Dis. 2000;35:S1-S140.

End-Stage Renal Disease

Once patients progress to stage 5 CKD with a GFR of less than 15 mL/min/1.73 m², they are in end-stage renal disease (ESRD). Patients are now in kidney failure and cannot survive without a form of renal replacement therapy (RRT), such as dialysis or a kidney transplant. Stage 5 is referred to as stage 5D once a patient begins dialysis treatment. Stage 5D CKD costs the United States billions of dollars each year, with Medicare spending $34.3 billion in 2011 on this stage alone.[66] Nutrition restrictions become stricter as CKD progresses to stage 5 until the patient begins RRT.

Although these treatments are available, patients have the right to refuse RRT as a step toward ending their life in the setting of this debilitating, irreversible disease. If patients do not feel that their quality of life justifies undergoing this time-consuming and expensive treatment, they may decide to forego or withdraw the therapy and initiate the dying process. Many patients with stage 5 and 5D CKD also suffer from other diseases that may further diminish their quality of life. One large study found that stage 5D CKD patients who stopped dialysis and entered hospice survived for an average of 7.4 days without treatment.[67] This decision involves the RD because MNT may no longer be appropriate for the patient; they may wish to receive comfort measures including a liberal, unrestricted diet in their end-of-life care.

Renal Replacement Therapy

Renal replacement therapy, usually some form of dialysis, is used in kidney disease treatment to remove waste products and excess water and minerals from the blood in place of normal kidney function.[66] Pannu and Gibney define the five classic indications for dialysis as follows[25]:

1. Pulmonary edema that does not respond to diuretics
2. Hyperkalemia
3. Metabolic acidosis
4. Uremic complications such as pericarditis, encephalopathy, and bleeding
5. Toxicity of products that can be removed using dialysis, such as lithium, toxic alcohols, and salicylates

CASE STUDY REVISITED

Two years later, Dean is in Stage 5 CKD and has decided to initiate in-center hemodialysis.

Anthropometric Data:
Weight: 85 kg (187 lbs)

Biochemical Data:
Sodium 131 (135-145 mEq/L)
Potassium 5.6 (3.6-5.0 mEq/L)
Chloride 113 (98-110 mEq/L)
Carbon dioxide 17 (20-30 mEq/L)
Blood urea nitrogen 98 (6-24 mg/dL)
Creatinine 5.6 (0.4-1.3 mg/dL)
Glucose 79 (70-98 mg/dL)
Calcium 9.5 (8.5-10.5 mEq/L)
Phosphorus 4.9 (2.7-4.5 mg/dL)

Clinical Data:
Medications: Includes calcium acetate 3 with meals and 1 with snacks
Nutrition-focused Physical Exam: Dean appears tired with some notable edema in his upper and lower extremities.
Urine output: 1 L daily

Dietary Data:
24-hour Diet Recall:
Breakfast (8 am): 1 cup corn flakes with 4 oz low fat milk, 8 oz coffee with nondairy creamer
Lunch (12 pm): 1½ cups pasta with olive oil, green beans, 1 oz baked chicken, 12 oz ginger ale
Dinner (7 pm): 2 oz baked fish, 2 cups white rice, 6 spears fresh asparagus, 12 oz water
Diet prescription: 2 g sodium, 2 g potassium, low-phosphorus diet

Questions

1. How would you assess Dean's weight loss?
2. How would you assess Dean's labs?
3. What specific diet changes do you suggest for Dean as he initiates hemodialysis?

The mnemonic AEIOU can be used to remember these indications for RRT, referring to Acidemia (metabolic acidosis), Electrolyte abnormalities (hyperkalemia), Intoxications (toxicity of products requiring dialysis for clearance) Overload (volume overload such as pulmonary edema), and Uremia (uremic complications).[67] Some practitioners may also use persistent protein energy malnutrition as an indication that RRT should be initiated in patients with a GFR of <50 mL/min/1.73 m². This is recommended if there is no apparent cause for the malnutrition other than poor intake, as appetite may improve with adequate RRT.[28,32]

There are two main types of dialysis: hemodialysis and peritoneal dialysis.

Hemodialysis

In **hemodialysis (HD)**, blood is removed from the body and processed through a machine containing a dialysis membrane that acts as an artificial kidney (**Figure 14.7**).[69] HD is the more common form of dialysis, accounting for 90% of all dialysis modalities used by stage 5D CKD patients.

Hemodialysis can be done in a medical facility, requiring patients to visit the center several times weekly and undergo 3 to 5 hours of dialysis each visit. In-center

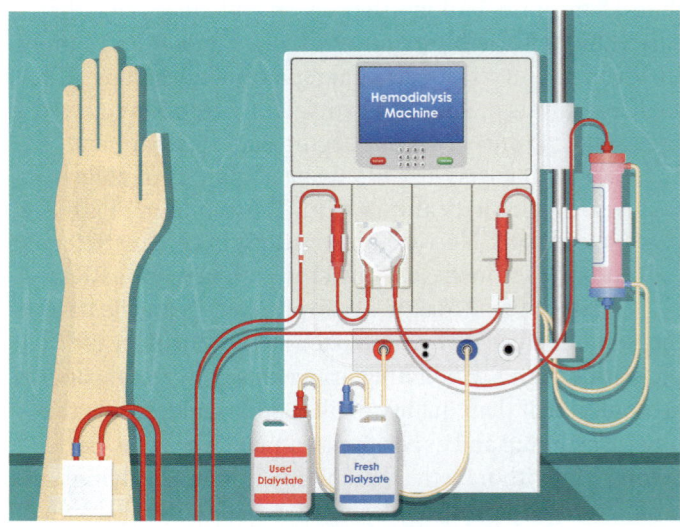

FIGURE 14.7 Hemodialysis
© rumruay/Shutterstock.

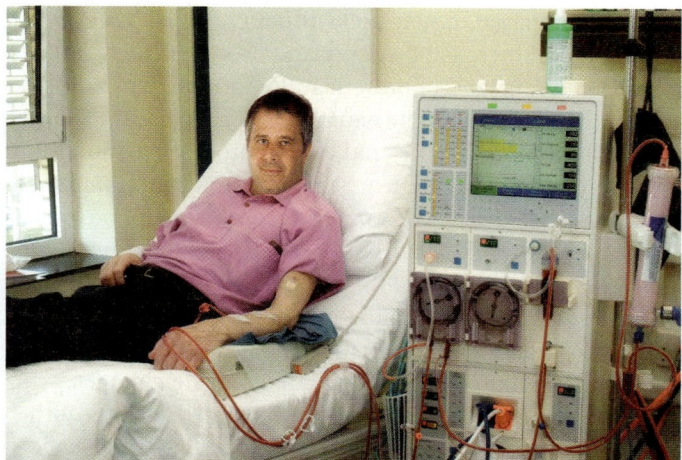

FIGURE 14.8 Patient Receiving In-center Hemodialysis
© gopixa/Shutterstock.

nocturnal HD (NHD) may provide a safe, convenient treatment for very sick and fatigued patients requiring close supervision.[70] This involves dialyzing over 6 to 10 hours overnight while the patient rests.

HD can also be performed in home (home hemodialysis [HHD]); however, it requires trained assistance, but gives more responsibility to the patient in exchange for increased freedom from visiting a hemodialysis center several times weekly (**Figure 14.8**). HHD is practiced by fewer than 2% of all stage 5D CKD patients on RRT.[70] The use of HHD is increasing in the United States, however, likely due to convenience and comfort factors that are not available from in-center HD treatments. As the disease progresses, it may become more difficult for patients to make it to the clinic several times weekly due to fatigue. HHD can be done as short daily HD, requiring the patient to dialyze 2 to 3 hours daily, or as NHD.

Kinetic Modeling

Kinetic modeling is used in hemodialysis to evaluate the effectiveness of dialysis in removing urea from the blood during treatment.[70] It is necessary to know how much urea is cleared during hemodialysis to ensure that the patient's blood levels of nitrogenous waste remain in the normal range. Kinetic modeling involves complex mathematical processes using computer systems, but the basic equation used is Kt/V, where K stands for dialyzer clearance or removal in milliliters per minute, t stands for the amount of time used for the dialysis treatment, and V stands for the patient's total body water volume. Kt would then be the total amount of urea cleared from the blood during the entire dialysis treatment.[71] The goal Kt/V per the KDIGO work group is 1.2 or greater.[71] Another method of determining dialysis efficacy is the calculation of the **urea reduction ratio (URR)**. This calculation indicates the reduction in the amount of urea as a result of the treatment, although it is not as accurate as Kt/V.[71] It is obtained by subtracting the end urea level from the starting urea level and then expressing it as a percentage of the starting urea level. A goal of at least 65% clearance is recommended.[71] Kt/V and URR are more useful when used to determine the weekly average after all dialysis treatments because the results can vary greatly depending on the patient and the day of treatment. An abnormally low Kt/V should not be a cause for concern if the patient's weekly average Kt/V meets the goal of 1.2.[71]

Peritoneal Dialysis

Peritoneal dialysis (PD) involves the use of the patient's own peritoneal membrane as the dialysis membrane. The peritoneal membrane lines the abdominal wall and is useful in dialysis because of its semipermeable nature. Dialysate is inserted into the abdominal cavity through a catheter in the abdomen, allowed to dwell for a period of time, and then drained and exchanged for fresh fluid (**Figure 14.9**). The dialysate absorbs waste and nutrients from the blood and uses the peritoneum as a filter, leaving blood free of the high amounts of wastes that build up during kidney failure. **Continuous ambulatory peritoneal dialysis (CAPD)** is a form of PD that requires three to five of these exchanges daily, while **continuous cycling peritoneal dialysis (CCPD)** uses a machine to carry out the exchanges overnight while the patient sleeps. Many patients choose to use CCPD because it gives them the most freedom during the day.

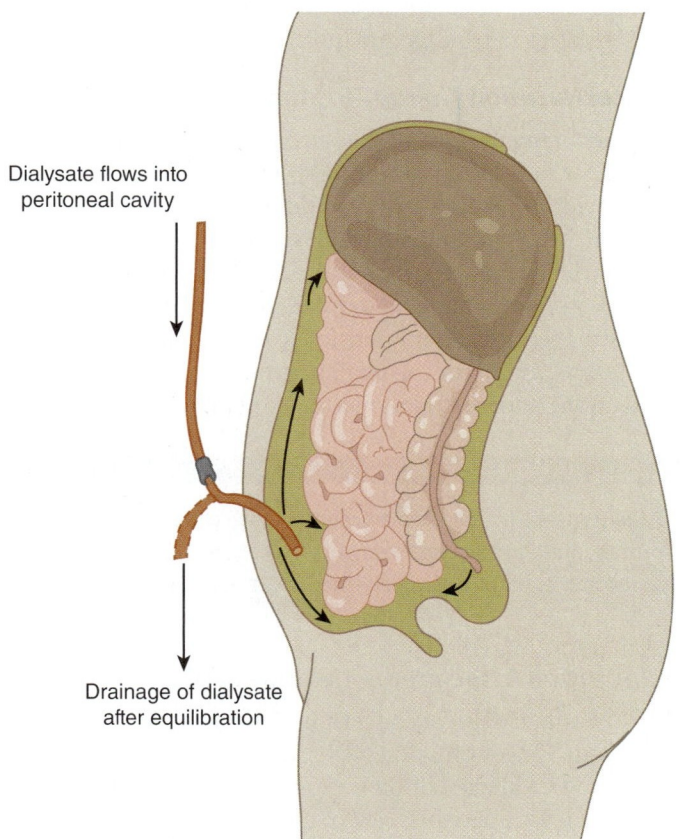

FIGURE 14.9 Peritoneal Dialysis

There are several disadvantages to PD in comparison to HD, which may explain why of home dialysis patients, the proportion of those on PD has decreased since the 1980s while those on HHD have increased.[69] These disadvantages include abdominal discomfort due to the volume of fluid infused into the abdomen and increased risk of peritonitis. Patients on manual exchanges must infuse one bag of dialysate into their abdomen per exchange, which can be 1.5, 2, 2.5, or 3 L at one time, depending on their needs.[72] This infusion may cause a sensation of fullness, which can impact the patient's mental health as well as their nutritional status, because the feeling of satiety several times per day is likely to interfere with hunger signals and can lead to decreased dietary intake.

Peritonitis, a potentially fatal peritoneal infection, can occur in chronic PD patients. This is usually due to bacterial contamination of the dialysate or an infection at the PD catheter site, where dialysate exits the body, and is treated with antibiotics.[73] Peritonitis poses a nutritional risk because infection increases energy and protein needs, so patients with peritonitis should be reevaluated at the time of diagnosis. Patients with malnutrition on PD are at a higher risk of developing peritonitis.[74]

Continuous Renal Replacement Therapy

Continuous renal replacement therapy (CRRT) is a slower form of RRT that may dialyze more blood daily than intermittent dialysis. Although some studies have found advantages of using CRRT, such as improved hemodynamic stability due to lower filtration rates and improved efficiency of solute removal, no evidence suggests that CRRT reduces morbidity and mortality.[25]

Medical Nutrition Therapy in Stage 5D CKD

There are many nutrition-related concerns for patients on dialysis, including significant treatment-related fatigue, nausea, vomiting, constipation, and increased risk of malnutrition. MNT goals during dialysis are to keep the patient well nourished and provide sufficient protein and energy to avoid protein catabolism for fuel, manage comorbidities such as diabetes and hypertension, prevent buildup of metabolic toxins, maintain fluid balance, prevent complications, and help the patient maintain a good quality of life.

> **CORE CONCEPT 6**
>
> Patients receiving renal replacement therapy can tolerate higher protein, fluid, and electrolyte levels than patients with CKD alone, so recommendations should be individualized to each patient.

Malnutrition Associated with Stage 5D CKD

Malnutrition is of great concern in dialysis patients, affecting 25% to 50% of those on HD[75,76] and 18% to 56% of those on PD.[77] Malnutrition in 5D CKD, as in other disease states, increases patients' risk of mortality.[78] Protein and energy requirements are usually increased for dialysis patients compared to non-dialysis patients with CKD.[27,79] In addition to increasing energy and protein needs, dialysis can facilitate the loss of protein and micronutrients such as calcium, magnesium, potassium, sodium, selenium, copper, and thiamin.[21] Additional contributors to malnutrition in dialysis patients include gastrointestinal symptoms such as nausea, delayed gastric emptying, and constipation, as well as psychosocial factors such as depression, loneliness, and economic adjustment to illness exacerbated by the extent to which the treatment interferes with the patient's life. Other causes of malnutrition include inadequate dialysis, insufficient dietary intake related to taste changes, unpalatable diets, early satiety, multiple medications with side effects, and/or metabolic acidosis. Patients with stage 5D CKD are also at high risk for inflammation, infection, and sepsis due to comorbidities related to underlying illness or hospitalizations. Refer to **Table 14.11** for factors related to malnutrition in stages 5 and 5D CKD.

Nutrition Assessment

Goals of MNT during RRT are achievement and maintenance of an appropriate body weight, adequate fluid and blood pressure management, sufficient protein and energy intake, and acceptable laboratory values. Nutrition assessment for stage 5D CKD patients includes anthropometric, biochemical, dietary, and physical assessments. The nutrition assessment for stage 5D CKD should include body weight, adjusted edema-free body weight, the patient's weight history throughout treatment, evaluation of lean body mass and appropriate intake using the Subjective Global Assessment, and laboratory values. Important laboratory measurements in stage 5D CKD are the same as those for other stages and should include serum electrolytes, especially sodium and potassium; water-soluble vitamins; bone mineral density assessment labs including calcium, phosphorus, PTH, and vitamin D; and anemia assessment labs including hemoglobin, hematocrit, iron, ferritin, and percentage saturation of transferrin.

Energy Energy needs vary greatly depending on the type of dialysis. Stage 5D CKD patients are recommended to consume 35 kcal/kg/day.[28] More care must be taken when determining energy needs for PD patients, because the glucose-containing dialysate may provide 300 calories or more daily depending on the PD regimen.[80] It is recommended that PD patients receive 35 kcal/kg/day from all nutrient sources, including dietary, dialysate, and other intake.[28]

Protein Protein is removed via the dialysate during every treatment, with the amount lost dependent on the duration of each treatment and the dextrose concentration of the dialysate. Approximately 0.2 g of amino acids are lost per liter of filtrate in both PD and CRRT, contributing to an overall 15 to 25 g of protein lost per treatment.[12] Several studies suggest that protein intake during CRRT should target between 2 and 2.5 g/kg/day.[80,81]

TABLE 14.11 FACTORS THAT CONTRIBUTE TO MALNUTRITION IN STAGE 5 AND 5D CKD

Hemodialysis-Related	Peritoneal Dialysis–Related	Non-Dialysis-Related
Decreased appetite	Decreased appetite	Decreased appetite (associated with uremia)
Increased protein clearance	Increased protein clearance	Protein restriction
Increased infection risk	Peritonitis/infection risk	Edema
Fatigue	Fatigue	Fatigue
Inconvenient dialysis schedule	Frequent dialysate exchanges	Sodium restriction
Increased nutrient needs	Increased nutrient needs	Chronic disease–associated increased nutrient needs
Nausea	Abdominal discomfort associated with dialysate in abdomen	Fluid restriction
Delayed gastric emptying	Delayed gastric emptying	Potassium restriction
Constipation	Constipation	Microalbuminuria

Data from Aparicio M, Cano N, Chauveau P, et al. Nutritional status of haemodialysis patients: a French national cooperative study. French Study Group for Nutrition in Dialysis. *Nephrol Dial Transplant.* 1999;14(7):1679-1686; National Kidney Foundation. Kidney Disease Outcomes Quality Initiative NKF-K/DOQI clinical practice guidelines for chronic kidney disease: evaluation, classification, and stratification. Aparicio M, Cano N, Chauveau P, et al. Nutritional status of haemodialysis patients: a French national cooperative study. French Study Group for Nutrition in Dialysis. *Nephrol Dial Transplant.* 1999;14(7):1679-1686; Combe C, Chauveau P, Laville M, et al. Influence of nutritional factors and hemodialysis adequacy on the survival of 1,610 French patients. *Am J Kidney Dis.* 2001;37(1):S81-S88; Dombros NV. Pathogenesis and management of malnutrition in chronic peritoneal dialysis patients. *Nephrol Dial Transplant.* 2001;16(suppl):111-113; Correia MI, Waitzberg DL. The impact of malnutrition on morbidity, mortality, length of hospital stay and costs evaluated through a multivariate model analysis. *Clin Nutr.* 2003;22(3):235-239.

Clinical Roundtable

Topic: Balancing Protein Restriction with Malnutrition in CKD

Background: Protein is an essential part of the human diet and is needed to maintain lean body mass. It is even more important to prevent malnutrition during chronic illness because malnutrition can contribute to poor outcomes. Consuming a diet high in animal proteins can increase the release of glucagon, insulin-like growth factor, and kinins, and can increase reabsorption of sodium in the proximal tubule, all of which have been shown to increase GFR.[84] An increase in GFR in kidney disease is not preferable, because this can put higher stress on the damaged kidneys and exacerbate the damage to cause an ultimate decline in kidney function. Some studies have shown that limiting dietary protein slows the progression of CKD and delays the need for renal replacement therapy,[84-87] and others have found that protein restriction may increase mortality risk.[88] Others have come up inconclusive, or have found that plant-based protein intake does not have as severe an effect on kidney function as animal protein sources.[89,90] In the absence of conclusive evidence as to whether or not protein restriction in CKD improves survival or increases malnutrition-related mortality, clinicians must analyze the available research and use their clinical judgment when following professional guidelines from sources such as KDIGO and KDOQI.

Roundtable Discussion: Consider the risks and benefits associated with dietary protein restriction during CKD.

1. Do you think protein should be restricted in all patients with CKD?
2. If not, are there any situations in which dietary protein restriction would benefit a patient?
3. How would you educate your patient on a protein restriction of 0.8 g/kg/day, and what are some techniques you could suggest to increase the palatability and caloric density of a protein-restricted meal plan?

KDOQI recommends a protein intake of 1.2 g/kg/day for HD patients, and 1.2 to 1.3 g/kg/day during PD.[28,83] Protein intake should be at least 50% HBV, ideally 60%. It is important to remember that although patients receiving CRRT and PD have about the same amino acid losses, protein needs are higher for patients on CRRT because net protein losses are greater with continuous filtration than periodic exchanges.

> **PRACTICE POINT**
>
> PD patients can generally consume a more liberalized diet in comparison to HD patients due to the increased frequency of dialysis.

Fluid and Sodium Fluid allowances for stage 5D CKD patients should be individualized to the patient considering their urine output. The general rule is to calculate fluid requirements at the patient's volume of urine output plus 1 L.[91] This is based on the assumption that insensible losses can be up to 1 L per day. Anuric patients excreting less than 75 mL of urine per day are typically fluid restricted to 1 to 1.2 L per day.[21] Hypertensive stage 5D CKD patients following a protein-restricted diet should have a sodium intake of less than 2 g per day, because blood pressure would ideally be controlled in order for protein restriction to be effective.[5]

Potassium Patients on dialysis should be monitored for hyperkalemia. Clinicians must be aware that a serum potassium of greater than 6 mEq/L is considered severe hyperkalemia and requires immediate medical attention, which may include emergent dialysis, to prevent the occurrence of cardiac events.[92] Hemodialysis recipients are more likely than peritoneal dialysis patients to experience hyperkalemia and are thus more likely to require a potassium-restricted diet.[80] HD patients are typically recommended to consume 2,000 mg daily or less, while PD patients may be advised to consume 3,000 to 4,000 mg daily or less.[80]

> **PRACTICE POINT**
>
> HD patients on a potassium-restricted diet may not be able to consume as many fruits, vegetables, and whole grains as are recommended to meet the dietary fiber goal of 20 to 30 g per day. Dietary counseling should focus on high-fiber, low-potassium foods as well as fiber supplementation if needed.

Phosphorus Dietary phosphorus restriction depends on serum phosphorus and PTH levels. In stage 5 and 5D CKD, an 800 to 1,200 mg daily phosphorus restriction should be initiated if serum phosphorus levels rise above 5.5 mg/dL or PTH levels are higher than 300 pg/mL.[21] Phosphate binders may also be used during stage 5D CKD to control serum phosphorus levels and protect bone health.

Micronutrients Stages 5 and 5D CKD patients should be monitored for hypercalcemia, defined as a corrected calcium greater than 10.2 mg/dL. If hypercalcemia is identified, dietary calcium, including calcium from any phosphate binders, should not exceed 2,000 mg per day.[49]

CKD patients are at greater risk for water-soluble vitamin deficiency due to poor intake and increased clearance of these vitamins by RRT.[6,91] Vitamin C supplementation at 125 mg daily is recommended for anyone receiving RRT; however, caution should be taken not to over-supplement, because doses greater than 200 mg daily have been shown to cause deposition of oxalate in the circulatory system and kidneys.[93-95] The B vitamins, specifically folate, pyridoxine, and thiamin, should also be supplemented for patients receiving RRT.[21] Several water-soluble multivitamin preparations with B vitamins and vitamin C are commercially available for dialysis patients. **Table 14.12** summarizes nutritional guidelines for patients with Stage 5D CKD.

Monitoring Nutritional Adequacy During Dialysis

Many changes, such as weight fluctuations and altered labs, may occur when dialysis is initiated after a period of impaired kidney filtration and azotemia. These changes, in addition to several potential side effects of dialysis, may put patients at risk for malnutrition. It is important that the RD monitor the patient's nutritional status and symptoms throughout treatment and adjust the treatment and the diet accordingly to prevent malnutrition.

Changes in the patient's weight throughout each treatment and over the course of treatments must be monitored closely. It is important to distinguish between the patient's actual weight and their true edema-free weight. Edema-free weight, also known as dry weight, is the patient's weight at which all or most excess body fluid has been removed and the weight at which the patient is without hypertension or hypotension. It is common to use a postdialysis weight as a dry weight.

Biochemical data can also be used in monitoring nutritional status during dialysis. Blood urea nitrogen is commonly used to assess the adequacy of dialysis treatment. A high BUN may indicate high dietary protein intake, decreased dialysis clearance, dehydration, or increased catabolism, while a low BUN may alert the clinician to poor dietary intake, low protein consumption, anabolism, or overhydration.[96] Electrolytes, specifically potassium, sodium, and chloride, are highly affected by kidney function. When dialysis begins to clear potassium, the risk of hyperkalemia should decrease. A high potassium level during dialysis may indicate that the dialysis is inadequate, making it an important tool in assessing dialysis treatment. Other lab parameters that may be helpful for the clinician to assess the

TABLE 14.12 SUMMARY OF NUTRITIONAL GUIDELINES DURING DIALYSIS

	Hemodialysis	Peritoneal Dialysis	Continuous Renal Replacement Therapy
Protein (g/kg/day)	≥1.2 and ≥50% HBV protein	1.2-1.3 and ≥50% HBV protein	1.8-2.5
Energy (kcal/kg/day)	>60 years old: 35 <60 years old: 30-35	35 (including calories from dialysate)	35
Sodium (g)	1-3 (individualize to patient's blood pressure and fluid status)	2-4 (individualize to patient's blood pressure and fluid status)	1-3 (individualize to patient's blood pressure and fluid status)
Fluid	Urine output + 1 L	1-2 L, depending on fluid status	Individualize: Anuric patients may have a fluid restriction of 1-1.2 L
Potassium (g)	2-3 Adjust to serum levels	3-4 Adjust to serum levels	Individualize
Phosphorus (mg)	800-1,200 or 10-12 mg/g protein intake	800-1,200 or 10-12 mg/g protein intake	Individualize
Calcium (g)	<2 g, including calcium from phosphate binders	<2 g, including calcium from phosphate binders	Individualize

Data from National Kidney Foundation: NKF-K/DOQI Clinical practice guidelines for nutrition in chronic renal failure. *Am J Kidney Dis*. 2000;35:S1-S140.

dialysis patient's tolerance of treatment as well as their nutritional status include creatinine, iron studies, PTH, and phosphorus.

The **normalized protein catabolic rate (nPCR)** is a clinical tool used to measure the net protein degradation and protein intake in dialysis patients.[28] This provides a valid indication of protein intake; however, it is limited because it estimates the amount of protein catabolized but not the specific source. Due to the uncertainty of the benefit of using nPCR, **protein equivalent of nitrogen appearance (PNA)** was created to replace it.[28] Protein lost in urine and dialysate are not catabolized and therefore are not quantified. PNA is often normalized to a function of body weight, giving **normalized PNA (nPNA)**. The target nPNA is 1.1 g/kg/day and can acceptably range from 0.8 to 1.4 g/kg/day.[28]

Close monitoring of each patient's current dietary intake and appetite is important to prevent and treat weight loss or malnutrition. Often, patients on dialysis may feel fatigued or generally ill due to nausea, vomiting, or diarrhea, causing them to lose their normal appetite. Food and fluid intake should be evaluated and the diet altered as needed to ensure adequate intake of appropriate foods for CKD.

> **PRACTICE POINT**
>
> Because nPCR and nPNA are normalized to an ideal body weight, compare to the patient's ideal body weight. Multiplying nPCR or nPNA by a patient's actual weight may inadequately report the total daily dietary protein intake in an obese or underweight patient.

Nutrition Support in Kidney Disease

Indications for Nutrition Support

The KDOQI guidelines recommend that nutrition support be initiated in patients who are unable to meet their energy and protein needs through oral intake alone during dialysis treatment.[28]

Enteral Nutrition

Enteral nutrition (EN) should always be used before parenteral nutrition in AKI and hospitalized CKD patients.[21] ESPEN guidelines on EN in adult renal failure recommend 20 to 30 kcal/kg/day and 1.5 g protein/kg/per day, although both energy and protein should be individualized to the patient's needs.[97] Caution should be taken not to overfeed

> ## ⚠ Clinical Controversy
>
> ### Intradialytic Parenteral Nutrition
>
> Due to the high risk of malnutrition associated with long-term HD, it is imperative to find a method of nutrient administration to replace those nutrients lost during HD that has been clinically proven to improve outcomes. Intradialytic parenteral nutrition (IDPN) has been proposed as a way to prevent the development of malnutrition during long-term hemodialysis in stage 5D CKD patients, with an advantage being ease-of-use. The infusion can occur simultaneously with HD because it is possible to use the same venous access for both therapies. Studies such as that by Marsen et al. demonstrate that IDPN improves nutritional status in long-term HD stage 5D CKD patients. However, other studies such as by Cano et al. present conflicting evidence, suggesting that IDPN does not improve nutritional status or long-term outcomes such as survival.
>
> ### Questions
>
> 1. Based upon this research, discuss how you would proceed with a patient on long-term HD showing signs of malnutrition in whom enteral nutrition is contraindicated.
> 2. How would you balance the risks associated with PN with the patient's need for adequate nutrition?
>
> ### References
>
> 1. Marsen TA, Beer J, Mann H. Intradialytic parenteral nutrition in maintenance hemodialysis patients suffering from protein-energy wasting. Results of a multicenter, open, prospective, randomized trial. *Clin Nutr.* 2017;36(1):107-117.
> 2. Cano N, Foque D, Roth H, et al. Intradialytic parenteral nutrition does not improve survival in malnourished hemodialysis patients: a 2-year multicenter, prospective, randomized study. *J Am Soc Nephrol.* 2007;18:2583-2592.

patients on EN, because overfeeding can lead to complications such as hyperglycemia. It was found that patients receiving 40 kcal/kg/day did not have an improved nitrogen balance compared to patients fed 30 kcal/kg/day, but did demonstrate an increased risk of metabolic issues like hyperglycemia.[24]

Parenteral Nutrition

If a patient with AKI or CKD is unable to be fed enterally, parenteral nutrition (PN) may be used to maintain nutritional status. ESPEN guidelines on PN in adult renal failure recommend 30 to 35 kcal/kg/day for stable CKD patients.[97] When a patient is receiving hemodialysis and needs to be fed parenterally, a peripheral or central intravenous catheter may be used. Central access is preferred, because it allows a more concentrated delivery of nutrients for patients with fluid restrictions, which many end-stage renal disease patients require. If central PN is contraindicated, peripheral PN (PPN) may be an option. PPN presents a challenge due to the fact that peripheral veins only accommodate a lower osmotic load. This limitation requires a higher volume in order to administer appropriate calories, making it difficult for patients with fluid restrictions to meet their nutrient needs through PPN. In some cases, **intradialytic parenteral nutrition (IDPN)** can be used to provide supplemental nutrition. An advantage of IDPN over other PN therapies is that the vascular access device used for HD treatments can be concurrently used to provide PN, foregoing the need to place another device. IDPN may provide up to approximately 1,000 calories during each HD treatment, which may only be 3 days per week. The unique infusion method of IDPN, which infuses via HD tubing (unlike standard PN which is infused directly into the patient), raises concern about absorption of the IDPN solution due to potential from rapid clearance from the blood. ESPEN recognizes the evidence that IDPN improves nutritional parameters, but there is insufficient evidence to support its net benefit.[98] A.S.P.E.N. guidelines state that IDPN should not be used for the malnourished stage 5D CKD population due to lack of evidence demonstrating a significant benefit to its use, which costs approximately $30,000 per patient each year.[21] Intraperitoneal PN (IPPN) can be used as a PN route for stage 5D CKD patients receiving CAPD.[97] This method of feeding has been poorly studied and little evidence exists to support its efficacy, although it is an option if patients receiving CAPD are unable to meet their nutritional requirements orally or enterally.

Nephrotic Syndrome

Nephrotic syndrome is a loss of protein through the glomerular membrane.[99] It is a relatively rare disease, with an incidence of 3 cases per 100,000 adults each year.[100] Nephrotic syndrome is defined as proteinuria of greater than or equal to 3.5 g/day and hypoalbuminemia, with serum albumin 3 g/dL or less.[97] The disease leads to edema, dyslipidemia, abnormal blood coagulation, abnormal bone metabolism, and reduced renal function.[99] Most nephrotic syndrome is caused by diabetes, systemic lupus erythematosus, amyloidosis, or renal vein thrombosis. Other causes can be preexisting kidney diseases of any kind, including minimal

TABLE 14.13 NUTRITIONAL GUIDELINES FOR NEPHROTIC SYNDROME

Category	Recommendation	Notes
Energy	35 kcal/kg	Energy should be sufficient to prevent protein utilization for fuel
Protein	0.8-1.0 g/day	Soy protein has been shown to decrease urinary protein excretion and blood lipid levels
Fluid	Restriction may be indicated based on presence or absence of edema	Individualize to patients
Sodium	1-2 g/day	To prevent or manage edema common in nephrotic syndrome
Fat	<30% total calories <200 mg cholesterol/day 10% fat from polyunsaturated fatty acids	Nephrotic syndrome is characterized by increased synthesis and decreased catabolism of lipids
Carbohydrate	High in complex carbohydrates	
Phosphorus	<12 mg/kg/day	
Calcium	1,000-1,500 mg/day, no more than 2,000 mg/day with supplementation or phosphate binders	Calcium is bound to albumin in the blood, so loss of albumin in the urine puts the patient at risk for hypocalcemia. Decreased active vitamin D also decreases calcium absorption.

Data from Academy of Nutrition and Dietetics. Nutrition Care Manual: Nephrotic Syndrome. Accessed 06/22/17.

change disease common in children and focal segmental glomerulosclerosis or scarring of the glomeruli.[101] Medical treatment of nephrotic syndrome often involves the use of steroids, which have a number of nutritional implications such as weight gain and hyperglycemia.

Medical Nutrition Therapy for Nephrotic Syndrome

Nutritional assessment for nephrotic syndrome should include a diet history, weight history with emphasis on recent rapid weight gain due to edema, biochemical assessment to monitor for hypoalbuminemia and electrolytes, and evaluation of the medical history. Medical nutrition therapy for nephrotic syndrome includes a protein intake of 0.8 to 1.0 g/kg/day, and a calorie intake of 35 kcal/kg/day has been shown to promote a positive nitrogen balance (Table 14.13).[100,102] The Japanese Society of Nephrology recommends a fat-restricted diet for patients who develop hyperlipidemia during nephrotic syndrome, although no evidence exists to support that fat restriction improves outcomes of nephrotic syndrome.[99] Sodium restriction may help prevent the worsening of edema or ascites, but a severe sodium restriction is not indicated for all patients with nephrotic syndrome. The patient's diet should be customized based on their fluid status, serum albumin levels, and any underlying diseases such as diabetes, cardiovascular disease, or hypertension.

Chapter Summary

Medical nutrition therapy is a necessary component in the management of kidney disease. MNT plays a key role in the prevention and delay of CKD through management of underlying conditions, such as obesity, hypertension, and diabetes, as well as contributing to improved outcomes by preventing malnutrition. Due to the evolving nature of kidney disease and its treatments, it is critical to provide individualized dietary recommendations to ensure patients maintain a balanced, palatable diet with adequate energy and appropriate protein. The work of the RD in modifying a patient's diet to best suit their needs can make a crucial difference in their health, disease progression, and quality of life.

Key Terms

nephrons, glomerulus, Bowman's capsule, ultrafiltrate, tubules, ureters, glomerular filtration rate (GFR), adaptive hyperfiltration, antidiuretic hormone (ADH), nitrogenous waste, erythropoietin (EPO), oliguria, azotemia, acute kidney injury (AKI), chronic kidney disease (CKD), kidney disease improving global outcomes (KDIGO), estimated glomerular filtration rate (eGFR), renal replacement therapy (RRT), prerenal AKI, intrinsic AKI, postrenal AKI, continuous renal replacement therapy (CRRT), high biological value

(HBV), anuria, end-stage renal disease (ESRD), polycystic kidney disease (PKD), microalbuminuria, standard body weight (SBW), adjusted edema-free body weight (aBW$_{ef}$), renal osteodystrophy, fibroblast growth factor 23 (FGF23), phosphate binders, erythropoietin stimulating agent (ESA), hemodialysis (HD), kinetic modeling, urea reduction ratio (URR), continuous ambulatory peritoneal dialysis (CAPD), continuous cycling peritoneal dialysis (CCPD), normalized protein catabolic rate (nPCR), protein equivalent of Nitrogen Appearance (PNA), normalized PNA (nPNA), intradialytic parenteral nutrition (IDPN), nephrotic syndrome

References

1. Chronic kidney disease. Centers for Disease Control and Prevention. https://www.cdc.gov/diabetes/programs/initiatives/kidney.html. Updated September 13, 2017. Accessed September 27, 2017.
2. Coresh J, Astor BC, Greene T, Eknoyan G, Levey AS. Prevalence of chronic kidney disease and decreased kidney function in the adult US population: Third National Health and Nutrition Examination Survey. *Am J Kidney Dis*. 2003;41(1):1-12.
3. United States Renal Data System. CKD in the United States. *USRDS Annual Data Report*. 2016;1:20.
4. Maarten Taal GC, Marsden P, Skorecki K, Yu A, Brenner B. *Brenner and Rector's the kidney*. 10th ed. Philadelphia, PA: Elsevier; 2011.
5. Metcalf W. How does early chronic kidney disease progress? A Background Paper prepared for the UK Consensus Conference on Early Chronic Kidney Disease Nephrol Dial Transplant 2007;22(9):26-30. doi:10.1093/ndt/gfm446.
6. Remuzzi G, Perico N, Macia M, Ruggenenti P. The role of renin-angiotensin-aldosterone system in the progression of chronic kidney disease. *Kidney Int Suppl*. 2005;(99):S57-65.
7. Helal I, Fick-Brosnahan GM, Reed-Gitomer B, Schrier RW. Glomerular hyperfiltration: Definitions, mechanisms and clinical implications. *Nat Rev Nephrol*. 2012;8(5):293-300.
8. Fogo AB. Mechanisms of progression of chronic kidney disease. *Pediatr Nephrol*. 2007;22(12):2011-2022.
9. Sands JM, Layton HE. The physiology of urinary concentration: an update. *Semin Nephrol*. 2009;29(3):178-195.
10. Leading Causes of Death, 2016. Centers for Disease Control and Prevention. https://www.cdc.gov/nchs/fastats/leading-causes-of-death.htm. Updated March 17, 2017. Accessed September 27, 2017.
11. De Sousa A. Psychiatric issues in renal failure and dialysis. *Indian J Nephrol*. 2008;18(2):47-50.
12. Kidney Disease: Improving Global Outcomes (KDIGO) Acute Kidney Injury Work Group. KDIGO Clinical Practice Guideline for Acute Kidney Injury. *Kidney Int Suppl*. 2012;2:1-138.
13. Kasiske BL, Wheeler DC. Kidney Disease: Improving Global Outcomes-an update. *Nephrol Dial Transplant*. 2014;29(4):763-769.
14. Levey AS, Coresh J, Greene T, et al. Using standardized serum creatinine values in the modification of diet in renal disease study equation for estimating glomerular filtration rate. *Ann Intern Med*. 2006;145(4):247-254.
15. Peralta CA, Shlipak MG, Judd S, et al. Detection of chronic kidney disease with creatinine, cystatin C, and urine albumin-to-creatinine ratio and association with progression to end-stage renal disease and mortality. *JAMA*. 2011;305(15):1545-1552.
16. Inker LA, Schmid CH, Tighiouart H, et al. Estimating glomerular filtration rate from serum creatinine and cystatin C. *N Engl J Med*. 2012;367:20-29.
17. Mehta RL, Kellum JA, Shah SV, et al. Acute Kidney Injury Network: report of an initiative to improve outcomes in acute kidney injury. *Crit Care*. 2007;11(2):R31.
18. Macedo E, Zanetta DM, Abdulkader RC. Long-term follow-up of patients after acute kidney injury: patterns of renal functional recovery. *PLoS One*. 2012;7(5):e36388.
19. Pannu N, James M, Hemmelgarn B, Klarenbach S, Alberta Kidney Disease N. Association between AKI, recovery of renal function, and long-term outcomes after hospital discharge. *Clin J Am Soc Nephrol*. 2013;8(2):194-202.
20. Awdishu L, Wu SE. Acute Kidney Injury. *Medication Administration/Critical Care Research*. Lenexa, KS: American College of Clinical Pharmacy; 2016.
21. Brown RO, Compher C. American Society for Parenteral and Enteral Nutrition Board of Directors. ASPEN clinical guidelines: nutrition support in adult acute and chronic renal failure. *JPEN J Parenter Enteral Nutr*. 2010;34(4):366-377.
22. Bellomo R, Ronco C, Kellum JA, et al. Acute renal failure— definition, outcome measures, animal models, fluid therapy and information technology needs: the Second International Consensus Conference of the Acute Dialysis Quality Initiative (ADQI) Group. *Crit Care*. 2004;8:R204. https://doi.org/10.1016/S1470-2045(07)70246-2
23. Jeremy Levy EB, Christine Daley. *Oxford handbook of dialysis*. New York, NY: Oxford University Press; 2009.
24. Fiaccadori E, Maggiore U, Rotelli C, et al. Effects of different energy intakes on nitrogen balance in patients with acute renal failure: a pilot study. *Nephrol Dial Transplant*. 2005;20(9):1976-1980.
25. Pannu N, Gibney RN. Renal replacement therapy in the intensive care unit. *Ther Clin Risk Manag*. 2005;1(2):141-150.
26. ASPEN Board of Directors and Clinical Guidelines Task Force. Guidelines for the use of parenteral and enteral nutrition in adult and pediatric patients. *JPEN J Parenter Enteral Nutr*. 2002;26(1 suppl):1SA-138S.
27. National Kidney Foundation. Kidney Disease Outcomes Quality Initiative NKF-K/DOQI clinical practice guidelines for chronic kidney disease: evaluation, classification, and stratification. *Am J Kidney Dis*. 2002;39:S1-S266.
28. National Kidney Foundation: NKF-K/DOQI Clinical practice guidelines for nutrition in chronic renal failure. *Am J Kidney Dis*. 2000;35:S1-S140.
29. National Kidney Foundation. KDIGO 2012 Clinical practice guideline for the evaluation and management of chronic kidney disease. *Kidney Int Suppl*. 2013;1(3):1-163.
30. Toto RD. Treatment of hypertension in chronic kidney disease. *Semin Nephrol*. 2005;25(6):435-439.
31. About Chronic Kidney Disease. National Kidney Foundation. https://www.kidney.org/atoz/content/about-chronic-kidney-disease-causes. Reviewed February 15, 2017. Accessed June 15, 2017.
32. Chronic Kidney Disease and Diet: Assessment, Management, and Treatment. Treating CKD patients who are not on dialysis. National Kidney Disease Education Program. https://www.niddk.nih.gov/health-information/health-communication-programs/nkdep/a-z/Documents/ckd-diet-assess-manage-treat-508.pdf. Revised April 2015. Accessed Octover 8, 2017.
33. Vupputuri S, Soucie JM, McClellan W, Sandler DP. History of kidney stones as a possible risk factor for chronic kidney disease. *Ann Epidemiol*. 2004;14(3):222-228.
34. Rule AD, Krambeck AE, Lieske JC. Chronic kidney disease in kidney stone formers. *Clin J Am Soc Nephrol*. 2011;6(8):2069-2075.

35. Ikizler TA, Hakim RM. Nutrition in end-stage renal disease. *Kidney Int.* 1996;50(2):343-357.
36. Harvey KS. Methods for determining healthy body weight in end-stage renal disease. *J Ren Nutr.* 2006;16(3):269-276.
37. Detsky AS, McLaughlin JR, Baker JP, et al. What is subjective global assessment of nutritional status? *JPEN J Parenter Enteral Nutr.* 1987;11(1):8-13.
38. Peterson JC, Adler S, Burkart JM, et al. Blood pressure control, proteinuria, and the progression of renal disease. The Modification of Diet in Renal Disease Study. *Ann Intern Med.* 1995;123(10):754-762.
39. Heimburger O, Qureshi AR, Blaner WS, Berglund L, Stenvinkel P. Handgrip muscle strength, lean body mass, and plasma proteins as markers of nutritional status in patients with chronic renal failure close to start of dialysis therapy. *Am J Kidney Dis.* 2000;36(6):1213-1225.
40. Kaysen GA, Johansen KL, Cheng SC, Jin C, Chertow GM. Trends and outcomes associated with serum albumin concentration among incident dialysis patients in the United States. *J Ren Nutr.* 2008;18(4):323-331.
41. Academy of Nutrition and Dietetics Evidence Analysis Library. Chronic Kidney Disease Energy Requirements. 2009. https://www.andeal.org/topic.cfm?menu=4484&cat=4807. Accessed September 27, 2017.
42. James PA, Oparil S, Carter BL, et al. 2014 evidence-based guideline for the management of high blood pressure in adults: report from the panel members appointed to the Eighth Joint National Committee (JNC 8). *JAMA.* 2014;311(5):507-520.
43. Agarwal R, Sinha AD. Thiazide diuretics in advanced chronic kidney disease. *J Am Soc Hypertens.* 2012;6(5):299-308.
44. CKD Recommendations Summary: Sodium. Academy of Nutrition and Dietetics Web site. https://www.andeal.org/topic.cfm?menu=4484&cat=4807 Published 2010. Accessed May 30, 2017.
45. Sacks FM, Svetkey LP, Vollmer WM, et al. Effects on blood pressure of reduced dietary sodium and the Dietary Approaches to Stop Hypertension (DASH) diet. DASH-Sodium Collaborative Research Group. *N Engl J Med.* 2001;344(1):3-10.
46. Haewook H SA, Seiffer JL, Dwyer JT. Nutrition management of kidney stones. *Clin Nutr Res.* 2015;4:137-152.
47. Kalantar-Zadeh K, Gutekunst L, Mehrotra R, et al. Understanding sources of dietary phosphorus in the treatment of patients with chronic kidney disease. *Clin J Am Soc Nephrol.* 2010;5(3):519-530.
48. Bacchetta J. FGF23 in chronic kidney disease: are we lost in translation? *BoneKEy Reports.* 2016;770(5);1-3.
49. National Kidney Foundation. K/DOQI clinical practice guidelines for bone metabolism and disease in chronic kidney disease. *Am J Kidney Dis.* 2003;42(4 suppl 3):S1-201.
50. Jamal SA, Vandermeer B, Raggi P, et al. Effect of calcium-based versus non-calcium-based phosphate binders on mortality in patients with chronic kidney disease: an updated systematic review and meta-analysis. *Lancet.* 2013;382(9900):1268-1277.
51. Wuthrich RP, Chonchol M, Covic A, Gaillard S, Chong E, Tumlin JA. Randomized clinical trial of the iron-based phosphate binder PA21 in hemodialysis patients. *Clin J Am Soc Nephrol.* 2013;8(2):280-289.
52. Kandula P, Dobre M, Schold JD, Schreiber MJ Jr, Mehrotra R, Navaneethan SD. Vitamin D supplementation in chronic kidney disease: a systematic review and meta-analysis of observational studies and randomized controlled trials. *Clin J Am Soc Nephrol.* 2011;6(1):50-62.
53. Drueke TB, Ritz E. Treatment of secondary hyperparathyroidism in CKD patients with cinacalcet and/or vitamin D derivatives. *Clin J Am Soc Nephrol.* 2009;4(1):234-241.
54. Fukagawa M, Iwasaki Y, Kazama JJ. Skeletal resistance to parathyroid hormone as a background abnormality in uremia. *Nephrology (Carlton).* 2003;8 suppl:S50-52.
55. Levey AS, Beto JA, Coronado BE, et al. Controlling the epidemic of cardiovascular disease in chronic renal disease: what do we know? What do we need to learn? Where do we go from here? National Kidney Foundation Task Force on Cardiovascular Disease. *Am J Kidney Dis.* 1998;32(5):853-906.
56. Collins AJ, Foley RN, Herzog C, et al. United States Renal Data System 2008 Annual Data Report. *Am J Kidney Dis.* 2009;53(1 suppl):S1-374.
57. Weiner DE, Sarnak MJ. Managing dyslipidemia in chronic kidney disease. *J Gen Intern Med.* 2004;19(10):1045-1052.
58. Trevisan R, Dodesini AR, Lepore G. Lipids and renal disease. *J Am Soc Nephrol.* 2006;17(4 Suppl 2):S145-147.
59. National Kidney Foundation. KDOQI clinical practice guidelines and clinical practice recommendations for diabetes and chronic kidney disease. *Am J Kidney Dis.* 2007;49(2 Suppl):S1-S180.
60. Kaysen GA. New insights into lipid metabolism in chronic kidney disease: what are the practical implications? *Blood Purif.* 2009;27(1):86-91.
61. Chmielewski M, Carrero JJ, Nordfors L, Lindholm B, Stenvinkel P. Lipid disorders in chronic kidney disease: reverse epidemiology and therapeutic approach. *J Nephrol.* 2008;21(5):635-644.
62. Babitt JL, Lin HY. Mechanisms of anemia in CKD. *J Am Soc Nephrol.* 2012;23(10):1631-1634.
63. KDIGO. Chapter 2: Use of iron to treat anemia in CKD. *Kidney Int Suppl (2011).* 2012;2(4):292-298.
64. Drueke TB, Parfrey PS. Summary of the KDIGO guideline on anemia and comment: reading between the (guide)line(s). *Kidney Int.* 2012;82(9):952-960.
65. Kalantar-Zadeh K, Rodriguez RA, Humphreys MH. Association between serum ferritin and measures of inflammation, nutrition and iron in haemodialysis patients. *Nephrol Dial Transplant.* 2004;19(1):141-149.
66. Costs of End-Stage Renal Disease. United States Renal Data Systems. https://www.usrds.org/2013/view/v2_11.aspx Published 2013. Accessed July 25, 2017.
67. Thomas LK, Othersen, JB, eds. *Nutrition therapy for chronic kidney disease.* Boca Raton, FL: CRC Press; 2012:82.
68. O'Connor NR, Dougherty M, Harris PS, Casarett DJ. Survival after dialysis discontinuation and hospice enrollment for ESRD. *Clin J Am Soc Nephrol.* 2013;8(12):2117-2122.
69. United States Renal Data System. 2015 USRDS annual data report: Epidemiology of Kidney Disease in the United States. National Institutes of Health, National Institute of Diabetes and Digestive and Kidney Diseases, Bethesda, MD; 2015. https://www.usrds.org/2015/download/vol2_USRDS_ESRD_15.pdf
70. Sprenger KBG, Kratz W, Lewis AE, Stadtmüller U. Kinetic modeling of hemodialysis, hemofiltration, and hemodiafiltration. *Kidney Int.* 1983;24(2):143-151.
71. National Institutes of Health. Hemodialysis Dose and Adequacy Fact Sheet. Bethesda, MD: National Kidney and Urologic Diseases Information Clearinghouse; February 2009.
72. National Institutes of Health. Peritoneal Dialysis Dose and Adequacy Fact Sheet. Bethesda, MD: National Kidney and Urologic Diseases Information Clearinghouse; 2010.
73. Piraino B. Insights on peritoneal dialysis-related infections. *Contrib Nephrol.* 2009;163:161-168.
74. Kerschbaum J, Konig P, Rudnicki M. Risk factors associated with peritoneal-dialysis-related peritonitis. *Int J Nephrol.* 2012;2012:483250.
75. Aparicio M, Cano N, Chauveau P, et al. Nutritional status of haemodialysis patients: a French national cooperative study. French Study Group for Nutrition in Dialysis. *Nephrol Dial Transplant.* 1999;14(7):1679-1686.

76. Combe C, Chauveau P, Laville M, et al. Influence of nutritional factors and hemodialysis adequacy on the survival of 1,610 French patients. *Am J Kidney Dis.* 2001;37(1):S81-S88.

77. Dombros NV. Pathogenesis and management of malnutrition in chronic peritoneal dialysis patients. *Nephrol Dial Transplant.* 2001;16(suppl 6):111-113.

78. Correia MI, Waitzberg DL. The impact of malnutrition on morbidity, mortality, length of hospital stay and costs evaluated through a multivariate model analysis. *Clin Nutr.* 2003;22(3):235-239.

79. Neyra R, Chen KY, Sun M, Shyr Y, Hakim RM, Ikizler TA. Increased resting energy expenditure in patients with end-stage renal disease. *JPEN J Parenter Enteral Nutr.* 2003;27(1):36-42.

80. Briony TJB, ed. *Manual of Dietetic Practice.* 4th ed. Oxford, UK: Blackwell Publishing Ltd; 2007.

81. McCarthy MS, Phipps SC. Special nutrition challenges: current approach to acute kidney injury. *Nutr Clin Pract.* 2014;29(1):56-62.

82. Wooley JA, Btaiche IF, Good KL. Metabolic and nutritional aspects of acute renal failure in critically ill patients requiring continuous renal replacement therapy. *Nutr Clin Pract.* 2005;20(2):176-191.

83. Blumenkrantz MJ, Kopple JD, Moran JK, Coburn JW. Metabolic balance studies and dietary protein requirements in patients undergoing continuous ambulatory peritoneal dialysis. *Kidney Int.* 1982;21(6):849-861.

84. Singh A. Protein restriction and progression of chronic kidney disease. *Wolters Kluwer Health Up to Date.* 2011.

85. Ihle BU, Becker GJ, Whitworth JA, Charlwood RA, Kincaid-Smith PS. The effect of protein restriction on the progression of renal insufficiency. *N Engl J Med.* 1989;321(26):1773-1777.

86. Walser M, Hill S. Can renal replacement be deferred by a supplemented very low protein diet? *J Am Soc Nephrol.* 1999;10(1):110-116.

87. Walser M, Hill SB, Ward L, Magder L. A crossover comparison of progression of chronic renal failure: ketoacids versus amino acids. *Kidney Int.* 1993;43(4):933-939.

88. Levey AS, Greene T, Sarnak MJ, et al. Effect of dietary protein restriction on the progression of kidney disease: long-term follow-up of the Modification of Diet in Renal Disease (MDRD) Study. *Am J Kidney Dis.* 2006;48(6):879-888.

89. Stephenson TJ, Setchell KD, Kendall CW, Jenkins DJ, Anderson JW, Fanti P. Effect of soy protein-rich diet on renal function in young adults with insulin-dependent diabetes mellitus. *Clin Nephrol.* 2005;64(1):1-11.

90. Teixeira SR, Tappenden KA, Carson L, et al. Isolated soy protein consumption reduces urinary albumin excretion and improves the serum lipid profile in men with type 2 diabetes mellitus and nephropathy. *J Nutr.* 2004;134(8):1874-1880.

91. Byham-Gray L SJ, Stover J, Wiesen K (eds.). *A Clinical Guide to Nutrition Care in Kidney Disease.* 2nd ed. Renal Dietetic Practice Group of the Academy of Nutrition and Dietetics and the Council on Renal Nutrition of the National Kidney Foundation; 2013.

92. National Kidney Foundation. Clinical Update on Hyperkalemia. New York, NY: National Kidney Foundation; 2014.

93. Druml W, Kierdorf HP. Working group for developing the guidelines for parenteral nutrition of The German Association for Nutritional M. Parenteral nutrition in patients with renal failure—Guidelines on Parenteral Nutrition, Chapter 17. *Ger Med Sci.* 2009;7:Doc11.

94. Makoff R. Vitamin replacement therapy in renal failure patients. *Miner Electrolyte Metab.* 1999;25(4-6):349-351.

95. Tarng DC, Wei YH, Huang TP, Kuo BI, Yang WC. Intravenous ascorbic acid as an adjuvant therapy for recombinant erythropoietin in hemodialysis patients with hyperferritinemia. *Kidney Int.* 1999;55(6):2477-2486.

96. McCann L. Pocket guide to nutrition assessment of the patient with chronic kidney disease. *National Kidney Foundation.* 2009.

97. Cano NJ, Aparicio M, Brunori G, et al. ESPEN Guidelines on Parenteral Nutrition: adult renal failure. *Clin Nutr.* 2009;28(4):401-414.

98. Cano NJ, Fouque D, Roth H, et al. Intradialytic parenteral nutrition does not improve survival in malnourished hemodialysis patients: a 2-year multicenter, prospective, randomized study. *J Am Soc Nephrol.* 2007;18(9):2583-2591.

99. Nishi S, Ubara Y, Utsunomiya Y, et al. Evidence-based clinical practice guidelines for nephrotic syndrome. *Clin Exp Nephrol* 2016;20:342-370.

100. Hull RP, Goldsmith DJA. Nephrotic syndrome in adults. *BMJ.* 2008;336(7654):1185-1189. doi: 10.1136/bmj.39576.709711.80

101. Nephrotic Syndrome. Mayo Clinic, http://www.mayoclinic.org/diseases-conditions/nephrotic-syndrome/basics/causes/con-20033385?p=1. Reviewed December 18, 2014. Accessed June 15, 2017.

102. Beto JA, Ramirez WE, Bansal VK. Medical nutrition therapy in adults with chronic kidney disease: integrating evidence and consensus into practice for the generalist registered dietitian nutritionist. *J Acad Nutr Diet.* 2014;114(7):1077-1087.

Chapter 15

Nutrition in Liver Disease

Molly Uebele

Chapter Outline

Core Concepts
Introduction to the Liver
Acute Liver Disease
Chronic Liver Disease
Alterations in Metabolism
Nutrition Assessment
Nutrition Therapy for Cirrhosis

CORE CONCEPTS

1. Significant liver cell damage (approximately 80%-90% of liver cells) must occur before physiologic function is impaired. Frank liver failure is incompatible with life and can only be treated with a liver transplant.

2. Malnutrition correlates with severity of liver disease and is nearly universal in patients with end-stage liver disease.

3. Many over-the-counter herbal products can be hepatotoxic including, but not limited to, germander, green tea extracts, kava, skullcap, chaparral, and some Chinese and Ayurvedic herbal medicines.

4. Patients with acute liver failure often need parenteral glucose administration to prevent hypoglycemia related to the liver's failure to release glucose and metabolize insulin. Metabolic and nutrition support should be provided according to the patient's clinical condition and severity of illness.

5. Patients with severe acute alcoholic hepatitis who are unable to take oral nutrition should be given enteral nutrition as soon as feasible.

6. Lifestyle modification through diet and exercise is the primary treatment for nonalcoholic fatty liver disease.

7. Patients with cirrhosis should be monitored for malabsorption of fat and deficiency of fat-soluble vitamins.

8. Muscle and adipose tissue wasting in patients with liver disease is an independent predictor of mortality. Muscle loss is also associated with hepatic encephalopathy.

9. Nutrition status should be determined using the Subjective Global Assessment, with special focus on identification of muscle wasting through physical exam and functional capacity. Traditional methods using weight, BMI, and serum hepatic proteins should be abandoned.

10. Indirect calorimetry should be used to determine energy needs for cirrhotic patients.

11. Protein should not be restricted in patients with liver disease with or without hepatic encephalopathy. Patients should be given 1.2 g/kg or more depending on the severity of their condition.

12. Patients with cirrhosis should be monitored and treated for signs of zinc deficiency, especially if they are malnourished, alcoholic, or on diuretic therapy.

13. Patients with cirrhosis should eat small, frequent meals and a bedtime snack to avoid the accelerated proteolysis and lipid oxidation that occurs after a short period of fasting.

14. Patients with ascites should follow a low-sodium diet. A free water restriction is only indicated in the setting of severe hyponatremia (serum sodium <125 mEq/L).

Learning Objectives

1. Differentiate among acute hepatitis, chronic liver disease, acute liver failure, and fulminant liver failure.
2. Describe the progression of liver disease from hepatitis to cirrhosis and end-stage liver disease.
3. Define and briefly explain the pathogenesis (or theories thereof) of hepatic encephalopathy, coagulopathy, portal hypertension, ascites, and varices.
4. Describe the relationship between malnutrition and complications of liver disease.
5. Explain how alterations in metabolism during liver disease lead to deterioration of lean body mass, hypoglycemia, hyperglycemia, and hypoalbuminemia.
6. Assess the nutrition status of patients with liver disease.
7. Rationalize medical and nutritional treatment options for patients with hepatic encephalopathy.
8. Identify micronutrients that should be monitored for deficiency in patients with various types of chronic liver disease.
9. Recommend lifestyle changes aimed at reversing nonalcoholic liver disease related to metabolic syndrome.
10. Recommend the timing and route of nutrition support for patients unable to take nutrition by mouth.

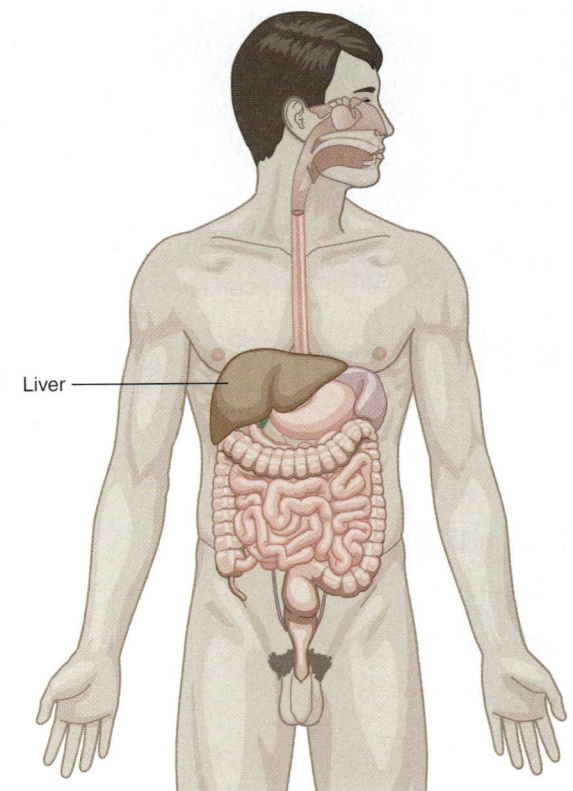

FIGURE 15.1 The Liver

Introduction to the Liver

The liver is often considered the nutritional gatekeeper of the body (**Figure 15.1**). It is the only organ capable of all major metabolic pathways in protein, carbohydrate, and lipid metabolism. Through careful regulation, it maintains a constant supply of energy for the body to do work, whether fed, fasted, or starving. It synthesizes important proteins, such as albumin, clotting factors, and transaminases, just to name a few. It is involved in vitamin and mineral metabolism, including vitamins B_{12} and D, pantothenic acid, and iron. Finally, it metabolizes drugs and clears chemicals such as alcohol and ammonia from the blood. The liver's failure to carry out these functions has a detrimental effect on the body's homeostasis.

Liver Structure and Functions

The liver weighs 1 to 1.5 kg, making it the second-largest organ of the body. Whereas dialysis can replace renal function and mechanical ventilation can stand in for the lungs, the liver's functions are so vital and complex that there is currently no effective medical or surgical substitute. Frank liver failure is incompatible with life and can only be treated with a liver transplant.

The liver is comprised of hepatocytes, Kupffer cells, stellate cells, endothelial cells, and bile ductular cells. Two-thirds of liver cells are hepatocytes, which perform numerous functions including synthesis of serum proteins, production of bile and its carriers, regulation of nutrients, and metabolism and conjugation of compounds (drugs, bilirubin) for excretion via bile or urine. The **Kupffer cells** are macrophages dedicated to the liver. They protect against pathogens arising from the gut, called endotoxin, by releasing pro-inflammatory cytokines such as tumor necrosis factor-alpha (TNF-α). **Stellate cells** are hepatic cells responsible for collagen formation and hold 90% of the body's vitamin A stores (**Figure 15.2**). About 80% to 90% of liver cells must be damaged before a physiologic function is impaired.[1]

CORE CONCEPT 1

Significant liver cell damage (approximately 80%–90% of liver cells) must occur before physiologic function is impaired. Frank liver failure is incompatible with life and can only be treated with a liver transplant.

CASE STUDY INTRODUCTION

Mark is a 38-year-old male, with no past medical history other than obesity, who returns to a primary care physician to establish care following the finding of a slightly elevated hemoglobin A1C and abnormal liver function tests at his last well visit 1 month ago. After reviewing his labs, the doctor confirms that nonalcoholic fatty liver disease (NAFLD) is the cause of Mark's elevated transaminases. She explains to Mark that both NAFLD and prediabetes can be reversed with exercise and weight loss. The doctor refers him to receive diet counseling with the outpatient registered dietitian (RD). Mark lives alone and works 40 hours per week as a mechanic.

Anthropometric Data:
Height: 183 cm (72")
Weight: 134 kg (295 lbs)
BMI: 40 kg/m² (class 3 obesity)
Waist circumference: 114 cm (45")

Biochemical Data:
Hemoglobin A1C 5.9% (<5.7%)
Alanine aminotransferase 60 (4-36 units/L)
Aspartate aminotransferase 40 (10-35 units/L)
Alkaline phosphatase 90 (30-120 units/L)
Bilirubin 0.7 (0.3-1.9 mg/dL)

Clinical Data:
Past Medical History: None
Medications: None
Vital Signs: Blood pressure 150/90 mm Hg, Temperature 97.3°F, Heart rate 85 beats/min
Nutrition-focused Physical Exam: Class 3 obese, apple-shaped body type

Dietary Data:
Dietary History: Mark has a good appetite. He typically has two meals per day, usually at 12 pm and 9 pm. He rarely cooks at home. He drinks 2 to 3 servings of alcohol per week socially.
24-hour Diet Recall:
Lunch (12 pm): Complete meal (burger or chicken sandwich, fries, shake) at a local fast food restaurant.
Dinner (9 pm): Pizza or submarine sandwich (take out)
Snacks: Sweets and baked goods
Fluids: Water and 4 to 5 regular sodas

Questions
1. Is there a common link between prediabetes and NAFLD?
2. Evaluate Mark's liver function tests. What do the elevated values mean with respect to hepatocellular function?
3. Given his conditions, what are the risks that Mark faces? What other labs would you request?
3. Assess Mark's food patterns and intake and determine whether he has a positive or negative energy balance.
4. What are the priorities for Mark? What initial goals and recommendations might you set for him?
5. Is there a medication he can be taking to improve his liver function tests?

The liver has dual blood supply; about 20% is oxygen-rich blood from the hepatic artery, and about 80% is nutrient-rich blood carried by the portal vein from the stomach, intestines, pancreas, and spleen.[1] Because the liver "sees" most of what we put in our mouth, nutrition affects liver function, and vice versa. The intricate relationship between liver and intestines is referred to as the **gut–liver axis**.[2,3]

Overview and Pathophysiology of Liver Disease

With so many different etiologies and pathophysiologies that are not yet fully established, liver disease can be confusing. Before looking in depth at nutrition research and recommendations regarding specific types and causes of liver disease, it is key to understand the basic categories, terminology, progression of disease, and physiologic complications.

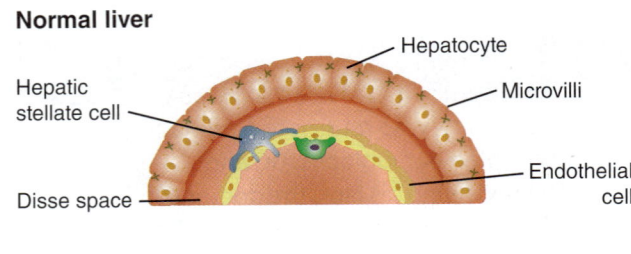

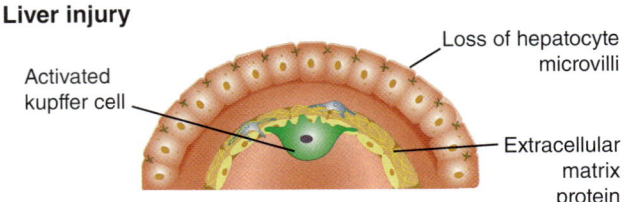

FIGURE 15.2 Cellular Components of the Liver

Hepatocellular versus Cholestatic

Liver disease can be described as either hepatocellular, cholestatic, or mixed. **Hepatocellular liver disease** is caused by liver cell injury. **Cholestatic liver disease** is caused by inhibition of bile flow.[1] Serum tests help to differentiate between hepatocellular and cholestatic damage. Within each category, there are several possible etiologies (see Table 15.1).[4]

Acute versus Chronic Liver Disease

Liver disease is also categorized by duration and severity of injury. **Acute hepatitis** is liver inflammation lasting up to 6 months. However, some cases of acute hepatitis do not completely resolve, progressing to chronic hepatitis. **Acute liver failure** describes massive hepatic necrosis with the onset of hepatic encephalopathy and coagulopathy (described later in the chapter) within 6 months of known liver disease. Acute hepatitis and liver failure are most often caused by a viral infection or hepatotoxic drugs, resulting in hepatic necrosis. **Chronic hepatitis** describes liver inflammation lasting longer than 6 months. It is categorized by etiology, grade of inflammation (minimal, mild, moderate, severe), and stage of fibrosis (none, mild, moderate, severe, cirrhosis); these are determined by liver biopsy. There are many possible causes of chronic hepatitis, both inherited and acquired. These include viral hepatitis, alcoholic and nonalcoholic steatohepatitis, and

TABLE 15.1 LIVER FUNCTION TESTS AND THEIR INTERPRETATION

Lab Measure[4]	Description	Possible Diagnosis with Elevated Values
Alanine Aminotransferase (ALT) (4-36 units/L)	Enzyme present primarily in the liver	Hepatocellular damage
Aspartate Aminotransferase (AST) (10-35 units/L)	Enzyme present primarily in the liver, but also in cardiac muscle, skeletal muscle and other cells	Hepatocellular damage Myocardial infarction
Alkaline Phosphatase (ALP) (30-120 units/L)	Enzyme in the bile canalicular membrane of hepatocytes, but also in the bone, placenta, and small intestine.	Interference with bile flow (cholestasis) Rapid bone growth
Gamma-glutamyl transpeptidase (GGT) (9-48 units/L)	Enzyme in the bile duct epithelial cells	Interference with bile flow (cholestasis)
Total Bilirubin (0.3-1.9 mg/dL)	A breakdown product of heme-containing proteins	Cholestasis or hepatocellular damage
Direct Bilirubin (<0.3 mg/dL)	The fraction of bilirubin that is conjugated, meaning it is water soluble	Cholestasis or hepatocellular damage
Prothrombin Time (PT) (11-13.5 seconds)	Measures clotting factors 2, 5, 7, and 10	Decreased synthetic function vitamin K deficiency (needed for synthesis of clotting factors 2, 7, 9, and 10)
International Normalized Ratio (INR) (0.8-1.1)	A measure that standardizes PT by using the International Sensitivity Index, which is validated only in patients on warfarin therapy	Increased degree of anticoagulation

Data from Pratt DS, Kaplan MM. Chapter 302. Evaluation of liver function. In: Longo DL, et al., eds. *Harrison's Principles of Internal Medicine.* 18th ed. New York: McGraw-Hill; 2012.

autoimmune and metabolic disorders. If the etiology is detected early, appropriate treatment can sometimes delay or reverse the progression of hepatic fibrosis. **Fibrosis** is a buildup of connective tissue, or scar tissue, as a result of hepatocyte regeneration after injury. Unfortunately, chronic hepatitis is often asymptomatic and goes unnoticed until the regenerated tissue forms nodules that permanently alter the structure of the liver. This final stage of fibrosis is **cirrhosis**.[5]

Cirrhosis

Cirrhosis is the 12th leading cause of death in the United States.[6] It progresses clinically in three stages: compensated (asymptomatic), compensated with varices, and decompensated. Extensive fibrosis and tissue scarring obstructs blood flow through the liver (**Figure 15.3**).

This scarring causes increased blood pressure in the portal vein. This **portal hypertension**, technically defined as venous pressure greater than 10 mm Hg (normal 5–10 mm Hg), causes a cascade of imbalances in the body that contributes to fluid retention and ascites, formation of varices, and progressive kidney disease.[5,7,8]

When the pressure in the portal vein is high, blood is redirected to veins in the esophagus, stomach, and rectum, which have lower venous pressure. This is called **porto-systemic shunting**. Increased circulation in those veins causes **varices**, or extremely dilated submucosal veins, which are easily susceptible to rupture. Patients are advised to follow a soft diet to prevent rupture of esophageal varices, and to avoid constipation (through adequate fiber and fluid intake, or use of stool softeners) to prevent straining that might rupture rectal varices (**Figure 15.4**).

Changes in circulation also cause peripheral arteriolar vasodilation, which triggers the renin-angiotensin-aldosterone system, telling the kidneys to increase blood volume by retaining sodium and water. Furthermore,

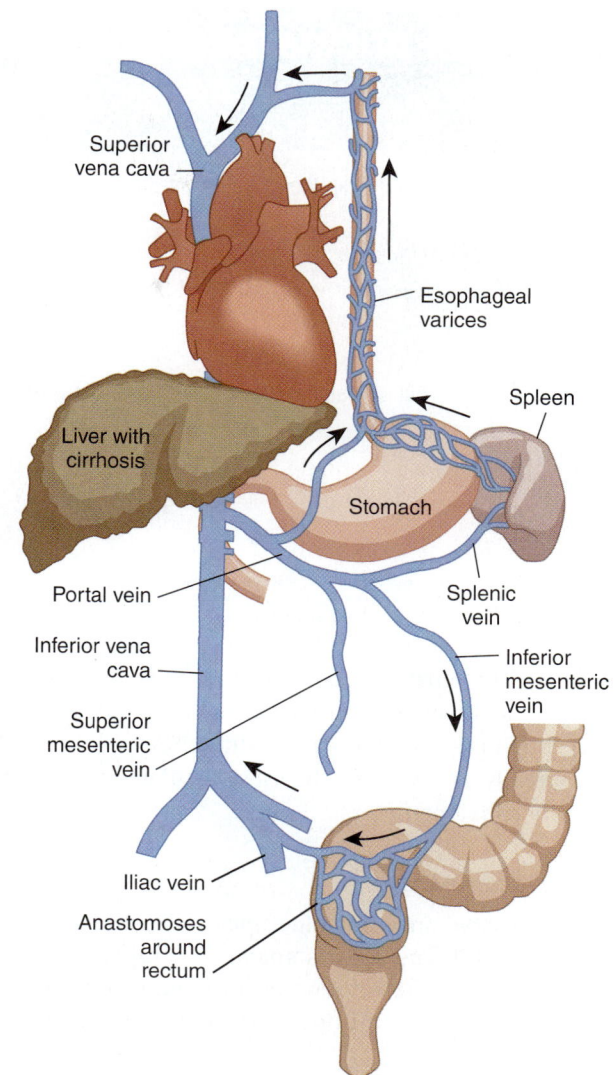

FIGURE 15.4 High Pressure in the Hepatic Portal Vein Causes an Increase in Varices

splanchnic vasodilation increases lymph production so much that fluid accumulates into the peritoneal cavity and exceeds 25 mL in volume. This describes one theory, called the **underfill hypothesis**, for the pathogenesis of **ascites** related to liver disease, although there are other unrelated causes of ascites, such as malignancy, tuberculosis, or abdominal trauma. About 50% of patients with cirrhosis develop ascites within 10 years; it is associated with a poor prognosis and decreased quality of life.[9]

The most complex and nutritionally relevant complication of cirrhosis is **hepatic encephalopathy (HE)**, which is a neuropsychiatric disorder characterized by personality changes, altered levels of consciousness, and cognitive impairment. **Table 15.2** shows how hepatic encephalopathy is classified and staged.[10] HE is associated with porto-systemic shunting and deranged amino acid metabolism caused by liver cirrhosis. The exact pathogenesis is still unclear, but the most popular theories that direct therapies focus on are the increase in chemicals that are neurotoxic, such as aromatic amino acids (AAA), ammonia, and TNF-α. Both ammonia and TNF-α levels are positively correlated

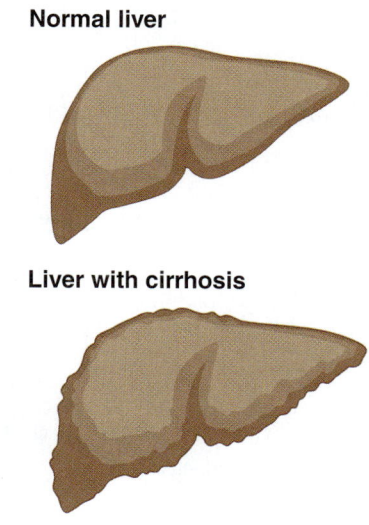

FIGURE 15.3 Scarring Associated with Cirrhosis

TABLE 15.2 CLASSIFICATIONS AND RELATED STAGING OF HEPATIC ENCEPHALOPATHY[10]

Classification		West Haven Stages	
Minimal (MHE)	Subclinical (West Haven Stage 0)	0	Normal consciousness and behavior, impaired psychomotor ability
Persistent	Chronic Never free of overt HE (West Haven Stage 1-4)	1	Mild lack of awareness, shortened attention span, mild asterixis
Episodic	Acute Clinically undetectable (West Haven Stage 0) between overt episodes	2	Lethargic, disoriented, inappropriate behavior, asterixis, slurred speech
		3	Somnolent but arousable, gross disorientation, incoherent speech, bizarre behavior, hyper-reflexia, muscular rigidity
		4	Comatose, decerebrate posturing

Data from Bajaj JS. Review article: The modern management of hepatic encephalopathy. *Aliment Pharmacol Ther.* 2010;31(5):537-547.

with severity of hepatic encephalopathy.[11,12] Hepatic encephalopathy is not associated with a particular etiology of cirrhosis,[13] but it is associated with malnutrition.[13] Table 15.3 gives a brief overview of the theories postulated to lead to hepatic encephalopathy.

Hepatic Decompensation

In **decompensated cirrhosis**, sometimes called **end-stage liver disease (ESLD)**, the body is unable to compensate for the functional deterioration of the liver, resulting in life-threatening complications.[8,14] Patients with acute liver failure without cirrhosis will experience some of the following complications as well:

- Bleeding varices: Patients may present with hematemesis or melena secondary to bleeding varices, which can be treated by endoscopic band ligation. **Transjugular intrahepatic portosystemic shunt (TIPS)** placement helps alleviate portal hypertension to prevent recurrent variceal bleeds.
- Coagulopathy: The liver's inability to synthesize clotting proteins, along with possible vitamin K deficiency, causes coagulopathy, defined by a serum

TABLE 15.3 THEORIES ON THE PATHOGENESIS OF HEPATIC ENCEPHALOPATHY

Ammonia	Increased circulating levels of ammonia, derived primarily from the gut; accumulation due to decreased urea cycle function; result depletes glutamate (an excitatory neurotransmitter) and increases glutamine in astrocytes (causing swelling)
Gamma-aminobutyric acid (GABA)-ergic	Increased circulating levels of GABA, the principal neurotransmitter in the brain, derived from the gut result in inhibition of neuronal function
Benzodiazepene	Increased circulating levels of endogenous benzodiazepine-like compounds enhance central GABAergic inhibition of neuronal function
Manganese	Increased circulating levels of manganese lead to manganese deposition in the brain, causing dopaminergic dysfunction, neuronal loss, and astrocytic changes
False neurotransmitter/aromatic amino acid (AAA)	Increased circulating levels of AAA and decreased circulating levels of branched chain amino acid allow enhanced AAA uptake by brain neurotransmitters
Tumor necrosis factor-alpha (TNF-α)[14]	Circulating levels correlate with severity of encephalopathy in acute and chronic liver disease, which may be neurotoxic. TNF-α is produced in response to intestinal translocation of endotoxin, among other things.

Data from Kalaitzakis E, Josefsson A, Bjornsson E. Type and etiology of liver cirrhosis are not related to the presence of hepatic encephalopathy or health-related quality of life: A cross-sectional study. *BMC Gastroenterol.* 2008;8:46-230X-8-46.; and Bacon BR. Chapter 309: Genetic, metabolic, and infiltrative diseases affecting the liver. In: Longo DL, et al., eds. *Harrison's Principles of Internal Medicine.* 18th ed. New York: McGraw-Hill; 2012.

TABLE 15.4 POTENTIAL THERAPIES FOR HEPATIC ENCEPHALOPATHY[3,10,17,18]

Lactulose	Nonabsorbable disaccharide that promotes elimination of ammonia from the colon
Rifaximin	Nonabsorbable antibiotic that eliminates aerobic and anaerobic gram-positive and gram-negative bacteria.
Metronidazole	Antibiotic that eliminates anaerobic gram-negative bacteria that synthesize ammonia and cause elevation of TNF-α when absorbed into circulation
Neomycin	Antibiotic that selectively eliminates gram-negative bacteria that synthesize ammonia and cause elevation of TNF-α when absorbed into circulation
Probiotic	Bacteria that decrease bacterial urease activity in the intestinal lumen, decrease ammonia absorption, and decrease intestinal permeability
Branched Chain Amino Acids	May inhibit AAA uptake in the brain; provides glutamate, which combines with ammonia to make glutamine in the muscle
Zinc	Cofactor for enzymes involved in ammonia elimination (glutamine synthetase, ornithine transcarbamylase). If deficient, supplementing improves enzyme activity and decreases ammonia.

Data from: Bajaj JS. Review article: The modern management of hepatic encephalopathy. *Aliment Pharmacol Ther*. 2010;31(5):537-547; Sharma V, Garg S, Aggarwal S. Probiotics and liver disease. *Perm J*. 2013;17(4):62-67.; Mouzaki M, Ng V, Kamath BM, Selzner N, Pencharz P, Ling SC. Enteral energy and macronutrients in end-stage liver disease. *JPEN J Parenter Enteral Nutr*. 2014;38(6)673-681; Dienstag JL. Chapter 304: Acute viral hepatitis. In: Longo DL, et al., eds. *Harrison's Principles of Internal Medicine*. 18th ed. New York: McGraw-Hill; 2012.

INR >1.5, which makes it difficult to stop a gastrointestinal bleed. Subcutaneous vitamin K and fresh frozen plasma may be given in an effort to improve blood clotting.
- Refractory ascites: Patients may have respiratory distress, early satiety, and abdominal pain due to severe ascites. This can be treated with **paracentesis** (aspiration of fluid from peritoneal cavity) and parenteral albumin administration. TIPS placement can alleviate refractory ascites as well.
- **Spontaneous bacterial peritonitis (SBP)**: Patients may have fevers and abdominal pain due to SBP, a complication of ascites and paracentesis. This is treated with antibiotics after analysis of peritoneal fluid.
- Jaundice: Patients may notice a yellowing of the skin and eyes, called jaundice or icterus, due to hyperbilirubinemia.
- **Hepatorenal syndrome (HRS)**: Patients may require hemodialysis due to HRS. There are two types of HRS. Type 1 HRS is a rapidly progressive form often triggered by infections. If left untreated, patients with HRS type 1 have a median survival of 2 weeks. HRS type 2 is a stable or slowly progressive renal impairment caused by portal hypertension–induced vasoconstriction of the kidney; median survival is about 6 months without treatment.[15] HRS is only reversed by liver transplant.
- Hepatic encephalopathy: Patients may present with episodic hepatic encephalopathy; stages 3 and 4 usually require admission to an intensive care unit. Hepatic encephalopathy can be precipitated by gastrointestinal bleeding, sepsis, dehydration, hyponatremia, surgery, TIPS, constipation, infection (including SBP), paracentesis, and medication noncompliance. Treatment includes identifying and treating the precipitant and giving medications that alter the gut microbiota to reduce synthesis and absorption of ammonia. Lactulose is a nonabsorbable polysaccharide that acidifies the colon and promotes elimination of ammonia and the bacteria that synthesize ammonia. Rifaximin is a nonabsorbable antibiotic that also eliminates a wide range of colonic bacteria.[10] Other therapies or potential therapies for HE are listed in **Table 15.4**.

The **Child-Pugh classification** is used to classify the severity of disease and predict patient prognosis. It scores severity using serum bilirubin, albumin, INR, and prothrombin time along with severity of ascites and hepatic encephalopathy. Severity is noted as Child-Pugh class A, B, or C, with class C being the most severe. See **Table 15.5**.

Malnutrition in Liver Disease

Multiple factors contribute to poor oral intake and subsequent malnutrition in patients with liver disease (see **Table 15.6**). They may have anorexia and taste changes related to anorexigenic cytokines, zinc deficiency, or elevated brain serotonin levels. Dietary salt and protein

TABLE 15.5 CHILD-PUGH CLASSIFICATION

	1 point	2 points	3 points
Encephalopathy Stage	0	1-2	3-4
Ascites	None	Slight	Moderate
Bilirubin	<2	2-3	>3
Albumin	>3.5	2.-3.5	<2.8
PT	1-4	4-5	>6
INR	<1.7	1.8-2.3	>2.3

Child's A = 5 to 6 points; Child's B = 7 to 9 points; Child's C = 10 to 15 points.
Modified from Pugh RN, Murray-Lyon IM, Dawson JL, et al. Transection of the oesophagus for bleeding oesophageal varices. Br J Surg. 1973;60:646.

Patients with cholestasis have impaired bile secretion, leading to fat and fat-soluble vitamin malabsorption. Patients with alcoholic liver disease tend to ingest most of their calories in the form of alcohol and have impaired absorption of thiamine and folic acid. Altered metabolism, and sometimes hypermetabolism, in liver disease leads to accelerated loss of adipose and muscle tissue. As liver disease progresses, not only are the aforementioned issues compounded, but patients are frequently hospitalized, where they are often incapable of eating or kept nil per os (NPO) for procedures. The severity of malnutrition correlates with the severity of liver disease, and is especially prevalent in alcoholic liver disease patients.[16] Protein calorie malnutrition is present in up to 80% of decompensated liver failure patients.

Malnutrition predicts complications, patient survival, and outcomes following liver transplant. It is associated with increased risk of bacterial infections, encephalopathy, posttransplant mortality, and longer hospital stays. Muscle and adipose tissue wasting is an independent predictor of mortality. Although nearly all ESLD patients are malnourished, it is important to note that up to 70% of Child-Pugh Class A patients have some degree of malnutrition as well. Thus, preventing and treating malnutrition early should be of utmost importance in this population.[17]

restrictions make food options limited and less desirable. If ascites is present, early satiety and abdominal discomfort can severely limit intake. Malabsorption also contributes to malnutrition for patients with liver disease.

TABLE 15.6 CAUSES OF MALNUTRITION IN LIVER DISEASE

Factors Contributing to Malnutrition		Etiology
Impaired intake	Anorexia Abnormal taste	Cytokine mediated, zinc deficiency
	Early satiety	Ascites
	Altered mental status	Severe hepatic encephalopathy with dysphagia
	Frequent hospitalization	Frequent NPO status for procedures
	Dietary restrictions	Inappropriate diet orders
Metabolic alterations	Hypermetabolism	Cytokine mediated
	Early starvation metabolism	Decreased hepatic glycogen content
	Protein deficiency	Decreased synthesis of protein/increased protein needs for gluconeogenesis
	Micronutrient deficiency	Impaired nutrient storage
Increased nutrient losses	Treatment related	Diuretic therapy, paracentesis
	Malabsorption	Alcohol abuse, decreased bile flow

Modified from Saunders J, Brian A, Wright M, et al. Malnutrition and nutrition support in patients with liver disease Frontline Gastroenterol. 2010;1:105-111.

> **CORE CONCEPT 2**
> Malnutrition correlates with severity of liver disease and is nearly universal in patients with end-stage liver disease.

Acute Liver Disease

Acute Viral Hepatitis

Viral hepatitis is a systemic infection that damages the liver, and is almost always caused by one of five viral agents (A, B, C, D, or E) (**Figure 15.5**). Patients present with elevated liver function tests (LFTs), normal or low white blood cell count, malaise, anorexia, nausea, vomiting, fever, jaundice, and tender hepatomegaly. The virus is diagnosed by detecting antibodies and viral nucleic acid in serum. **Table 15.7** describes the different types of hepatitis.[18,19]

Acute Drug-Induced Hepatitis

There are a multitude of pharmacologic and chemical agents that can be hepatotoxic when inhaled, ingested, or given intravenously, either alone or in combination with

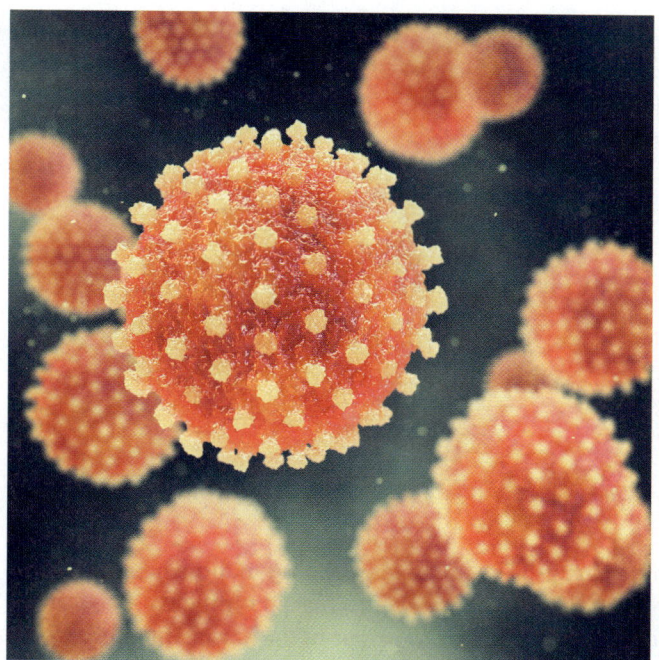

FIGURE 15.5 Viral Hepatitis Infection
© nobeastsofierce/Shutterstock.

TABLE 15.7 CATEGORIES OF ACUTE VIRAL HEPATITIS

Type	Transmission	Risk Factors	Prognosis
Hepatitis A	Fecal–oral	Travel in underdeveloped countries or regions; exposure to international travelers	Recovery from acute illness within 2-3 weeks, with complete recovery within 3 months. Does not lead to chronic hepatitis A. <0.6% mortality rate
Hepatitis B	Inoculation of infected blood, sexual contact, maternal–neonatal	Sexual exposure, history of IV drug use, received a blood transfusion before 1986, exposure to infected individuals in health care (needle sticks), incarceration	Overall 0.1%-1% mortality rate. Greater than 90% recovery within 3-6 months, with fewer than 1% developing acute liver failure (60% mortality rate). Between 1% and 2% of immunocompetent adults and 90% of infected infants (maternal–neonatal transmission) develop chronic hepatitis; 40% of patients with chronic HBV develop cirrhosis.
Hepatitis C	Inoculation of infected blood, sexual contact (low risk), maternal–neonatal (low risk)	IV drug use (most common), received a blood transfusion before 1992, tattooing and body piercing, incarceration, multiple sexual partners	Less than 1% mortality rate; 50%-85% develop chronic hepatitis, and 30% of those with chronic hepatitis C develop cirrhosis.
Hepatitis D	Must have hepatitis B to contract; blood and body fluids	Rare in the United States (mostly in South America, West Africa, Russia, Pacific Islands, Central Asia, the Mediterranean)	
Hepatitis E	Waterborne, swine	Exposure to endemic regions (mostly in Central and Southeast Asia, the Middle East, or North Africa)	In endemic regions, 10%-20% mortality rate in pregnant women

Data from Centers for Disease Control and Prevention (CDC). Viral Hepatitis. https://www.cdc.gov/hepatitis/index.htm. Accessed December 21, 2017.

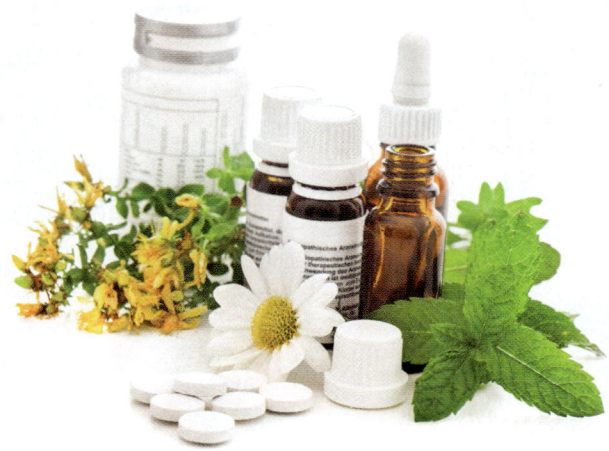

other drugs. These can lead to **drug-induced hepatitis**. The National Institutes of Health has an online database of all possible hepatotoxic drugs or herbal supplements.[20] Nonsteroidal anti-inflammatory drugs and antibiotics are the most common causes because of their widespread use. Presentation is often similar to that of viral hepatitis or biliary tract obstruction. Hepatotoxic drugs can be classified as direct or idiosyncratic. Direct hepatotoxic agents are dose-dependent and have a predictable injury. Examples include acetaminophen, alcohol, carbon tetrachloride, niacin, phosphorus, valproic acid, heavy metals, and vitamin A, to name a few. Most drug-induced hepatotoxicity is considered idiosyncratic, meaning it is sporadic and not related to dose, varying in onset and clinical presentation. These include isoniazid, phenytoin, carbamazepine, fluoroquinolones, and many more.[21]

Many over-the-counter herbal products can be hepatotoxic, including, but not limited to germander, green tea extracts, kava, skull cap, chaparral, and some Chinese and Ayurvedic herbal medicines (**Table 15.8**).[22] If an herb is the suspected cause of liver injury, physicians should apply the Council for International Organizations of Medical Sciences scale to determine causality.[23] In November 2013, the Food and Drug Administration required a recall of OxyElite Pro, a product advertised to aid in weight loss and building muscle that is believed to have caused over 50 cases of acute hepatitis, some even leading to acute liver failure and death.[24]

CORE CONCEPT 3

Many over-the-counter herbal products can be hepatotoxic including, but not limited to, germander, green tea extracts, kava, skullcap, chaparral, and some Chinese and Ayurvedic herbal medicines.

PRACTICE POINT

Ask all patients about their usage of herbal supplements, reviewing the safety of each one with the pharmacist and physician.

TABLE 15.8 HEPATOTOXIC HERBAL SUPPLEMENTS[23]

Aloe vera
Black cohosh
Chinese medicines:
    Ba Jiao Lian
    Chi R Yun
    Ephedra
    Jin Bu Huan
    Sho Saiko To
Fenugreek
Germander
Ginkgo
Ginseng
Glucosamine
Greater celandine
Green tea
Horse chestnut
Kava
Milk thistle
Pennyroyal
St. John's Wort
Saw palmetto
Senna
Skullcap

Data from Teschke R, Frenzel C, Schulze J, Eickhoff A. Herbal hepatotoxicity: Challenges and pitfalls of causality assessment methods. *World J Gastroenterol*. 2013;19(19):2864-2882.

Acute Liver Failure[8,9]

Acute liver failure is a rare critical illness characterized by hepatic necrosis (**Figure 15.6**) and the onset of impaired hepatic synthetic function (coagulopathy, hypoalbuminemia) and hepatic encephalopathy within 6 months of known hepatic disease. The term **fulminant liver failure** is commonly used to describe onset within 8 weeks of known liver disease. Acute liver failure occurs most often in previ-

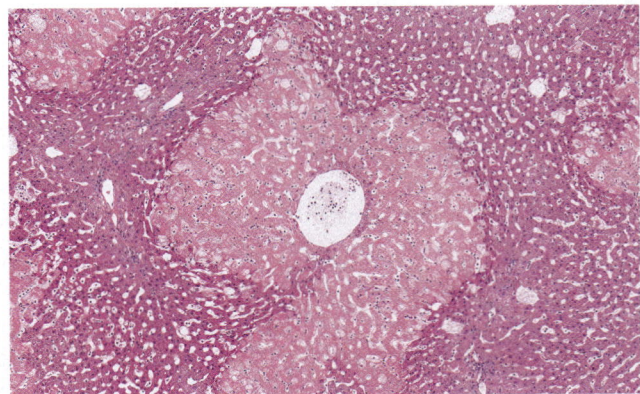

FIGURE 15.6 Acute Necrosis of Liver Cells can be seen in the necrotic pink cells as opposed to the healthy darker cells.

ously healthy adults in their 30s and carries a poor prognosis, with multi-organ failure and death occurring in up to one-half of cases. Treatment depends on the underlying cause, but is primarily supportive and requires hospitalization, preferably at a facility capable of liver transplantation. Identifying candidates for transplant early is key, because the severity of illness and multi-organ failure progresses rapidly. Only 10% of liver transplants are performed in patients with acute liver failure.

In the United States, drug-induced liver injury is responsible for 50% of all cases of acute liver failure, with acetaminophen toxicity being the number one cause overall. Acute liver failure can occur from ingestion of a single 10-g to 15-g dose of acetaminophen, but more often occurs when patients are taking substantial amounts for symptom relief without any intention of self-poisoning. Individuals with malnutrition and alcohol abuse are at increased risk of this due to a decreased threshold for toxicity. Although viral hepatitis causes only 12% of cases of acute liver failure in the United States, hepatitis A and E are probably the most common causes in the developing world, where vaccines are less accessible and sanitation can be poor.

Acute liver failure can be a result of ischemic hepatocellular injury, also called **shock liver**. This occurs in critically ill patients with cardiac, circulatory, or respiratory failure when the liver receives inadequate oxygen perfusion. Other causes of acute liver failure include Budd-Chiari syndrome; heat stroke; mushroom ingestion; undiagnosed Wilson's disease; and, rarely, herpes simplex virus and cytomegalovirus.[1,25]

Nutrition Management

There are no data to support nutrition therapy recommendations specifically for patients with acute hepatitis or acute liver failure. Treatment for these patients is primarily supportive, which includes ensuring adequate nutritional and metabolic support. Patients with acute liver failure may be unable to maintain adequate intake by mouth due to hepatic encephalopathy and critical illness. Appropriate nutrition should be provided in accordance with the patient's clinical condition and severity of illness. In fulminant liver failure, patients may require parenteral dextrose administration to treat hypoglycemia, caused by the liver's failure to metabolize insulin and release glucose via gluconeogenesis.[26] Energy expenditure is increased and should be measured by indirect calorimetry.[27,28] These patients experience some of the same complications as patients with decompensated chronic liver disease, including hepatic encephalopathy, which will be discussed later in the chapter.

> **CORE CONCEPT 4**
>
> Patients with acute liver failure often need parenteral glucose administration to prevent hypoglycemia related to the liver's failure to release glucose and metabolize insulin. Metabolic and nutrition support should be provided according to the patient's clinical condition and severity of illness.

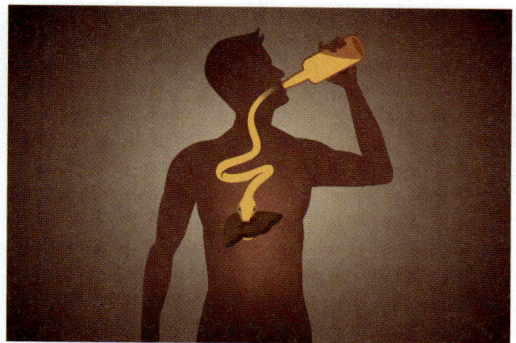
© solar22/Shutterstock.

Chronic Liver Disease

Chronic hepatitis is often asymptomatic, evident only by persistently elevated LFTs. As the disease progresses, people with chronic hepatitis may develop malaise, fatigue, anorexia, nausea, jaundice, dark urine, light stools, itching, abdominal pain, and bloating. The most common causes of chronic hepatitis are viral hepatitis B or C, as discussed earlier, and steatohepatitis caused by alcoholic liver disease (ALD) or NAFLD.[29] Of note, patients with chronic viral or alcoholic hepatitis can have acute symptomatic exacerbations, referred to as **acute-on-chronic hepatitis**.[21]

Alcoholic Liver Disease[30]

Because alcohol intake inhibits fatty acid oxidation and increases lipogenesis, more than 90% of people who consume >40 g of alcohol (three standard servings) per day have fat accumulation in >5% of hepatocytes, which is called **steatosis**, the first stage of **alcoholic liver disease**. This is benign and can be reversed through abstinence from alcohol. However, approximately 30% of patients with chronic heavy alcohol intake (>10 years) can develop **steatohepatitis** of varying severity, characterized by necro-inflammation of the liver.[31] In ALD, steatohepatitis is typically referred to as **alcoholic hepatitis (AH)**. Treatment is complete abstinence from alcohol. The risk of developing cirrhosis is positively correlated with the amount of alcohol intake, but can still occur despite abstinence. About 10% to 20% of patients will develop cirrhosis, and 1% to 2% of cirrhotic patients develop hepatocellular carcinoma.[31]

One key mechanism in the progression of steatosis to steatohepatitis involves the gut–liver axis. Chronic alcohol intake changes the intestinal epithelial barrier and increases gut permeability. This allows bacteria to translocate across the intestinal barrier into portal circulation. Alcohol also promotes the growth of gram-negative bacteria in the intestine; these bacteria have lipopolysaccharide (LPS), called **endotoxin**, in the cell wall. When endotoxin translocates into portal circulation, it stimulates Kupffer cells in the liver to secrete pro-inflammatory cytokines, such as **tumor necrosis factor**-alpha (TNF-α), and generate oxidative stress. This added inflammation might provide enough insult to the liver for progression to AH to occur. Additionally, these cytokines also contribute to fever,

TABLE 15.9 TRENDS IN LIVER FUNCTION TESTS IN LIVER DISEASE

Laboratory Value	Notable Trends[4]
Alkaline phosphatase	• Less than 3x normal: Any type of liver disease • Greater than 4x normal: Cholestatic liver disease, bone disease • Isolated elevation: Early cholestasis, hepatic infiltration by tumor, Hodgkin's disease, diabetes, hyperthyroidism, congestive heart failure, amyloidosis, inflammatory bowel disease
Alanine aminotransferase & aspartate aminotransferase	• Greater than 1000: Indicates severe injury, likely viral, ischemic, or drug-induced hepatitis • AST:ALT ratio <1 Chronic viral hepatitis or NAFLD. As cirrhosis develops, this ratio rises to >1. • AST:ALT ratio >2:1 or 3:1 = ALD (AST is rarely >300, and the ALT is often normal due to pyridoxal phosphate deficiency)
Bilirubin	• The higher the bilirubin, the greater the hepatocellular damage

Data from Pratt DS, Kaplan MM. Chapter 302. Evaluation of liver function. In: Longo DL, et al., eds. *Harrison's Principles of Internal Medicine*. 18th ed. New York: McGraw-Hill; 2012.

anorexia, and muscle wasting, thereby contributing to poor nutrition. Methods of preventing intestinal permeability to endotoxin in ALD are being investigated, including glutamine, oats, or zinc supplementation.[32,33]

At any point in the spectrum of ALD, patients can develop severe acute AH. These patients will present with jaundice and may have systemic inflammatory response syndrome, fever, hypotension, leukocytosis (elevated white blood cells), and skin alterations such as spider angiomata and palmar erythema. AH can be distinguished from acute viral or autoimmune hepatitis by a serum AST to ALT ratio (called the **de ritis ratio**) >2:1 (**Table 15.9**). The suppressed elevation of ALT in comparison to AST is likely secondary to alcohol-induced hepatic mitochondrial damage and deficiency of pyridoxine (vitamin B_6).[34,35] Severe AH may include complications of decompensated liver failure and increases the risk of developing cirrhosis if not already present.[31]

Nearly all patients with severe AH have some degree of malnutrition,[36] and the severity of malnutrition closely correlates with development of all serious complications, mortality, and response to treatment[16,37]; thus, nutrition therapy has become a mainstay of treatment.[38] Pharmacologic therapies include use of corticosteroids, N-acetylcysteine and TNF-α antagonists to attenuate inflammation. In a trial comparing provision of enteral nutrition support (2,000 kcal/day) or steroid therapy (prednisolone) for 28 days, enteral nutrition was shown to be as effective as steroids, with no difference in mortality during the 4-week treatment period. Furthermore, mortality was significantly higher in the steroid group after treatment; 70% died in the first 1.5 months after treatment, and 90% of deaths were related to infections.[39] Enteral nutrition should be started as soon as feasible in all patients with severe AH who are unable to take adequate oral intake. If enteral nutrition is not feasible, early parenteral nutrition (PN) is indicated in a malnourished patient, and a patient with severe AH is most likely malnourished. A meta-analysis on nutritional supplementation (including oral, enteral, and parenteral support) for hospitalized patients with AH found that supplementation provided no benefit in mortality or ascites, but significantly alleviated hepatic encephalopathy.[40]

CORE CONCEPT 5

Patients with severe acute alcoholic hepatitis who are unable to take oral nutrition should be given enteral nutrition as soon as feasible.

CASE STUDY REVISITED

In the nutrition appointment, Mark tells the RD that obesity runs in his family and he has been overweight his whole life. He states that he wants to manage his NAFLD through medications, and would like to take a vitamin E and cinnamon supplement.

Questions

1. How might you respond to Mark's suggestion for taking supplements to improve his NAFLD?
2. What are the current recommendations for the treatment of NAFLD?
3. Create an intervention plan for the RD to use when responding to Mark.

Nonalcoholic Fatty Liver Disease

Nonalcoholic fatty liver disease (NAFLD) is simply hepatic steatosis from a cause other than alcohol; it is the most common liver disease in the world. Diagnosis requires steatosis by histology (biopsy) or imaging, no significant alcohol consumption (<30 g/day in men, <20 g/day in women), and exclusion of other causes of chronic liver disease.[41] NAFLD is often referred to as the hepatic manifestation of metabolic syndrome. It is closely associated with type 2 diabetes, insulin resistance, and visceral obesity. Roughly 80% of these patients are obese,[42] but other causes of NAFLD include several drugs, certain endocrine and metabolic diseases, kwashiorkor, rapid weight loss, refeeding syndrome, excess fructose consumption, and long-term PN. The etiology of NAFLD is not completely understood (Table 15.10).

NAFLD is relatively benign; is called "silent liver disease" because it progresses slowly, if at all; and can be reversed by addressing the cause. However, 10% to 25% of patients with fatty liver develop **nonalcoholic steatohepatitis (NASH)** within 5 years.[43] This progression may involve a second inflammatory insult to the liver, as in ALD, secondary to pro-inflammatory cytokines and adipokines secreted by visceral adipose tissue. However, several factors play a role, including age, gender, and ethnicity.[42,44] With NASH, fibrosis can progress rapidly[45]; after 10 years, approximately 20% of patients with NASH develop cirrhosis. Cirrhosis caused by NAFLD is now the third most common indication for liver transplant in the United States.[46] NAFLD/NASH is also a leading risk factor for the development of hepatocellular carcinoma (HCC).[47]

Treatment of NAFLD aims to improve insulin sensitivity and ameliorate inflammation through diet and lifestyle modification.[48] There is no effective drug therapy. Current evidence supports the recommendation that overweight or obese patients lose 5% to 10% of their weight over 6 months to 1 year through exercise and a reduced-calorie diet.[49,50] Patients enrolled in an intensive lifestyle modification program are more successful than those who receive counseling alone.[50] For those unable to lose weight through lifestyle modification, bariatric surgery can be considered

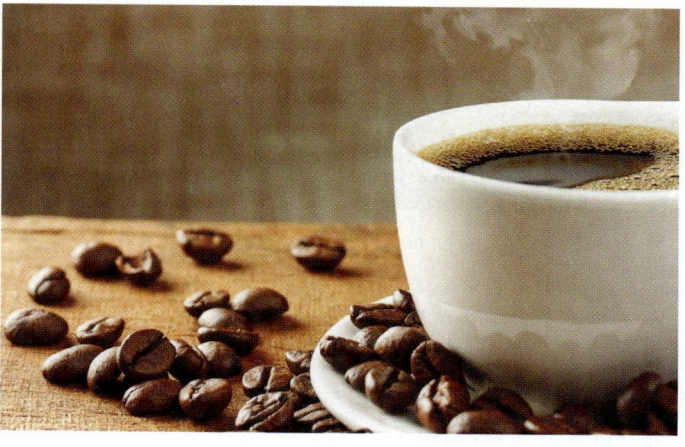
© portumen/Shutterstock.

for treatment.[51] However, rapid weight loss after bariatric surgery has resulted in hepatic decompensation, requiring transplant in some cases.[52]

> **CORE CONCEPT 6**
>
> Lifestyle modification through diet and exercise is the primary treatment for nonalcoholic fatty liver disease. A dietitian should work with the patient alongside an interprofessional team.

Patients should replace sugar-sweetened beverages with regular consumption of unsweetened black coffee. Although the mechanism is unclear, regular filtered coffee has been shown to be beneficial and is recommended for patients with NAFLD according to a recent meta-analysis. In patients with NAFLD, higher coffee consumption—but not espresso or tea—has been associated with a significant decrease in hepatic fibrosis.[53-56] On the other hand, NAFLD is associated with soft drink consumption, even in people without metabolic syndrome. In two studies, 80% of people with NAFLD consumed, on average, >50 g added sugar from soft drinks daily. Their intake was five times more than the intake of healthy controls.[57,58] This may be explained by high intake of fructose, which is metabolized in an unregulated fashion by the liver, unlike glucose. Beverages are sweetened by sugar or high fructose corn syrup, which are 50% and 55% fructose, respectively, and are the primary dietary sources of fructose. Excess consumption may contribute to NAFLD by increasing visceral fat stores, insulin resistance, and postprandial serum triglycerides.[59]

Many nutrients have potential as complementary alternative medicines for NAFLD. Vitamin E may be useful for its antioxidant ability; patients without diabetes who took 800 IU of vitamin E daily for 96 weeks had significantly improved hepatic ballooning and lobular inflammation.[60] However, vitamin E supplements are associated with increased risk of prostate cancer and a slight increase in mortality,[61] so caution is advised until further studies are done.[62,63] Omega-3 fatty acids inhibit pro-inflammatory cytokines and may improve NAFLD; however, while adequate intake is needed from food sources such as oily fish or walnuts, no data are available to support specific

TABLE 15.10 PREVALENCE OF NONALCOHOLIC FATTY LIVER DISEASE AND STEATOHEPATITIS

Prevalance[50]	NAFLD	NASH
Morbidly obese	Up to 91%	Up to 37%
Diabetics	60%-76%	22%
General U.S. Population	32%	2.7%-12.2%

Data from Promrat K, Kleiner DE, Niemeier HM, et al. Randomized controlled trial testing the effects of weight loss on nonalcoholic steatohepatitis. *Hepatology*. 2010;51(1):121-129.

TABLE 15.11 SUMMARY OF RECOMMENDATIONS FOR NONALCOHOLIC FATTY LIVER DISEASE

- Achieve a 5%-10% weight loss over 6 months
- Avoid juice and sugar-sweetened beverages
- Engage in moderate to vigorous physical activity (200 min/week)
- Drink black coffee regularly

recommendations for supplemental doses.[54,64] In recent trials, taking a symbiotic supplement for 28 weeks and taking cinnamon capsules for 12 weeks were both individually shown to improve LFTs more than lifestyle changes alone.[65,66] More studies are needed before any recommendations can be made. **Table 15.11** shows the current recommendations for nonalcoholic fatty liver disease.

Parenteral nutrition–related liver disease (PNALD) is a form of NAFLD that occurs with long-term PN; the etiology is not completely understood. Several factors are likely to contribute, including overfeeding calories and dextrose, resulting in hepatic de novo lipogenesis; inadequate choline intake, inhibiting the liver's ability to make lipoproteins to export triglycerides from the liver; and excess soybean oil–based lipid provision, which promotes inflammation. A pro-inflammatory "second hit" to the liver, such as a central line infection, can cause steatosis to progress to steatohepatitis. Intestinal failure can also result in biliary sludge and cholestatic liver disease due to lack of enteral stimulation with nutrients; this occurs more often in children and neonates.[67]

Inherited Diseases[14]

Hereditary conditions that cause chronic hepatitis include autoimmune hepatitis; cholestatic diseases, such as primary sclerosing cholangitis and primary biliary cirrhosis; and metabolic disorders, such as hemochromatosis, Wilson's disease, and alpha antitrypsin deficiency. Patients with chronic right heart failure can develop "hepatic congestion," called cardiac cirrhosis.

Hemochromatosis is an autosomal recessive disease characterized by accumulation of iron in the liver, pancreas, heart, adrenals, testes, pituitary, and kidneys. Hemochromatosis is caused by an inability to downregulate intestinal iron absorption when iron stores are adequate. Most patients are asymptomatic for four to five decades, but elevated LFTs and ferritin may lead to a diagnosis much earlier. Patients may develop arthropathy, hepatomegaly, altered skin pigmentation (slate-gray or bronze), cardiac enlargement, or erectile dysfunction (in men). Five percent of patients also have cirrhosis at the time of diagnosis, and 15% to 20% of cirrhotic patients develop HCC. Treatment is phlebotomy, which is very effective. Dietary modifications to decrease bioavailability or amount of iron intake may affect iron accumulation and reduce the amount of required phlebotomies, but evidence on whether this affects clinical outcomes is lacking. If patients want to be active in their treatment by modifying their diet, they should be monitored to ensure adequate intake of other nutrients typically in an iron-rich diet (zinc, vitamin B_{12}).[68] Patients should avoid excessive alcohol intake, which increases likelihood of developing cirrhosis. They should also avoid raw shellfish and practice meticulous food safety due to increased risk of infection from siderophilic organisms (bacteria that require free iron) such as *Vibrio vulnificus*, *Listeria monocytogenes*, and *Salmonella enterica*.

> **PRACTICE POINT**
>
> Advise patients with hemochromatosis that if they are to consume alcohol, to not to exceed the recommended daily amount of one serving for women and two servings for men. A strict avoidance of dietary iron is not essential; ensure that patients do not develop deficiencies of other nutrients typically in iron-rich foods if they do follow a modified diet.

Wilson's disease is another autosomal recessive disorder characterized by excessive deposition of copper in the liver and brain. The cause of Wilson's disease is excessive copper absorption in the small intestine combined with decreased copper excretion in the liver. The majority of patients present this disease before the age of 40 years. Symptoms include hepatitis; a brownish or gray-green ring at the rim of the cornea, called the **Kayser-Fleischer ring** (**Figure 15.7**); and neurologic or psychiatric abnormalities. Labs suggestive of Wilson's disease are a low serum ceruloplasmin and elevated urinary copper excretion. Early treatment with penicillamine, a chelating agent, can remove excess copper via urine before hepatic or neurologic damage is incurred. Pyridoxine must be supplemented (50 mg once a week) for patients taking penicillamine, which is

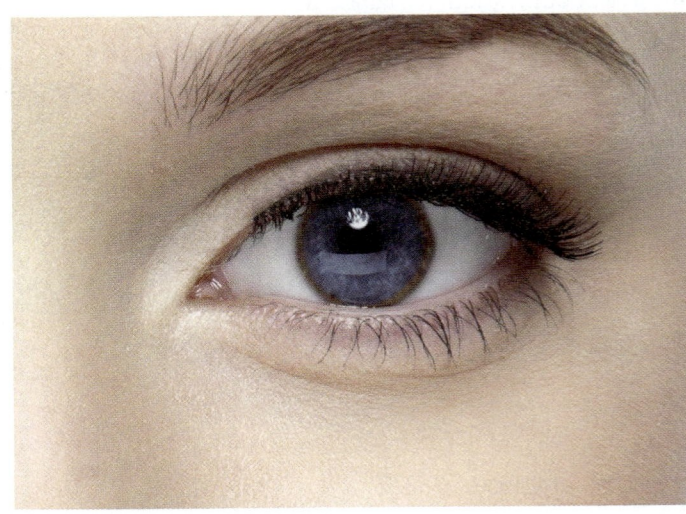

FIGURE 15.7 A Kayser-Fleischer Ring is a Symptom of Wilson's Disease
Courtesy of Wilson Disease Association.

an antimetabolite of the vitamin. Side effects are common, and include **dysgeusia** (altered taste perception), anorexia, vomiting, and diarrhea. Dietary copper restriction may be helpful during early treatment; shellfish, organ foods, nuts, mushrooms, and chocolate are high in copper. Zinc acetate or zinc gluconate (50 mg, three times per day) are also used in presymptomatic patients or as maintenance after chelation therapy. Zinc interferes with intestinal absorption by inducing the expression of intestinal metallothionein. **Metallothionein** binds to copper absorbed into the enterocyte, preventing its absorption. As enterocytes turn over, the copper remains bound to the cell and is excreted along with it in feces.[33] Unfortunately, some patients first present with Wilson's disease in acute liver failure; these patients require a liver transplant.

Alterations in Metabolism

Metabolism is deranged in patients with liver disease, which is not surprising given the prominent role of the liver in regulating nutrient metabolism. Understanding these alterations is key to providing and explaining the rationale of all nutrition recommendations for these patients. Table 15.12 highlights alterations in metabolism of macronutrients.

Carbohydrate Metabolism

A 70-kg, healthy man can store approximately 100 g of glycogen in the liver and 300 to 400 g in skeletal muscle. Thus, without eating, glycogen stores can provide the fuel needed for about one day of normal activity. Glycogen stored in muscle cannot be released into circulation. Therefore, only the liver can release stored glucose into the blood for use by the whole body. Once liver glycogen is depleted, blood glucose is maintained via hepatic gluconeogenesis from amino acids, glycerol, and lactate. During prolonged fasting, the body adapts to spare glucose and amino acids by relying on fatty acid oxidation and ketone synthesis. After 14 days of starvation, adipose tissue provides more than 90% of the body's energy.[69]

Patients with cirrhosis have decreased hepatic glycogen storage and increased insulin resistance.[70] As a result, their metabolism after 12 hours of fasting is similar to that of a healthy person after several days of fasting: They rely primarily on lipid oxidation for energy and proteolysis supplies amino acids for gluconeogenesis. In severe liver failure, inability to metabolize insulin and release glucose via hepatic gluconeogenesis leads to fasting hypoglycemia. Considering these alterations, nutrition therapy focuses on avoiding prolonged fasting through the use of small, frequent meals; late-night, high-carbohydrate snacks; or intravenous glucose administration.[71-73] The goal is to spare lean body mass by preventing early "starvation" metabolism.

Protein Metabolism

A healthy liver is key for protein metabolism as well. The portal vein delivers dietary amino acids to the liver, where they are used to synthesize important transport proteins, such as albumin, prealbumin, transferrin, lipoproteins, fibrinogen, and prothrombin. The breakdown of amino acids (exogenous or endogenous) results in nitrogenous wastes, such as ammonia, which the liver

TABLE 15.12 METABOLIC ALTERATIONS DUE TO CIRRHOSIS

Metabolism	Liver Function	Cirrhotic Liver	Consequences
Carbohydrate	Glycogenolysis Glycogenesis Glycolysis Gluconeogenesis De novo lipogenesis Fructose metabolism	Decreased glycogen stores Impaired gluconeogenesis Insulin resistance	Rapid depletion of glycogen with increased lipolysis and proteolysis while fasting Fasting hypoglycemia Hyperglycemia
Protein	Transamination Urea cycle Synthesis of serum proteins, clotting factors	Increased utilization of BCAA Decreased synthetic function Decreased urea cycle function	Hypoalbuminemia Coagulopathy Hyperammonemia Elevated AAA-to-BCAA ratio
Lipid	Synthesize bile, cholesterol, lipoproteins, phospholipid, ketones Beta oxidation of fatty acid Lipogenesis	Decreased ability to export triglycerides from liver Decreased excretion of bile (derived from cholesterol) Increased reliance on lipid oxidation after short periods of fasting	Steatosis Hyperlipidemia Fat and fat-soluble vitamin malabsorption Adipose and muscle tissue wasting (sarcopenia)

detoxifies via the urea cycle and excretes in urine. Ammonia can also be taken up by skeletal muscle and react with glutamate to form glutamine via glutamine synthetase. Glutamate is supplied by the catabolism of **branched chain amino acids (BCAA)** in muscle. The BCAAs, leucine, isoleucine, and valine, account for 40% of the essential amino acids and are primarily catabolized by skeletal muscle, rather than being taken up by the liver.[74,75]

In liver disease, defects in protein metabolism and synthesis are responsible for major complications of decompensated liver failure. Decreased synthesis of albumin leads to edema and exacerbates ascites. Decreased synthesis of clotting proteins leads to coagulopathy, which then increases the risk of a gastrointestinal hemorrhage. Decreased breakdown of AAAs by the liver, increased breakdown of BCAA by muscle, and failure to excrete nitrogenous wastes may all contribute to hepatic encephalopathy. When BCAA are low, there is increased uptake of the AAAs in the brain; one of these, tryptophan, is a precursor for 5-hydroxytryptamine, which is a neurotransmitter that causes lethargy. With low BCAA, there is also less capacity to detoxify ammonia in the muscle. As liver function fails, the body relies more heavily on muscle to remove ammonia. In cirrhotic patients, muscle depletion or decreased muscle strength was shown to be an independent risk factor of having HE (overt or minimal) and higher serum ammonia.[76,77] These alterations explain why nutrition therapy focuses on appropriate protein provision and possible use of BCAA, aiming to prevent skeletal muscle catabolism and treat or prevent exacerbation of hepatic encephalopathy.

CASE STUDY REVISITED

Mark does not follow up with his dietitian. Five years later, he returns to clinic with complaints of general malaise and fatigue. His doctor refers him back to a dietitian and also sends him to a gastroenterologist for a possible liver biopsy. Upon interview, Mark states that he is feeling motivated to make changes. He has already started working with a personal trainer on an exercise regimen.

Anthropometrics Data:
Height: 183 cm (72")
Weight: 135 kg (298 lbs)
BMI: 40 kg/m² (class 3 obesity)
Waist circumference: 107 cm (42")

Biochemical Data:
Cholesterol 220 mg/dL (Desirable<200 mg/dL)
Hemoglobin A1C 6.1% (4.3-5.8%)
Alanine aminotransferase 58 (4-36 units/L)
Aspartate aminotransferase 45 IU/L (10-35 units/L)
Alkaline phosphatase 100 (30-120 units/L)

Bilirubin 1 (0.3-1.9 mg/dL)
Albumin 3.9 (3.5-5.0 g/dL)
INR 1.4 (0.8-1.1)
PT 3 (11-13.5 seconds)

Clinical Data:
Past Medical History: NAFLD, prediabetic.
Medications: Pioglitazone (30 mg), atorvastatin (50 mg), vitamin E (800 IU)
Vital Sign: Blood pressure 155/90 mm Hg, Temperature 97.8°F, Heart rate 87 beats/min
Nutrition-focused Physical Exam: Class 3 Obese, good appetite, and an apple-shaped body type.

Dietary Data:
Dietary History: Mark eats two meals per day, usually at 12 pm and 7:30 pm. Due to Mark's demanding job, he generally buys at least one meal per day at a fast food restaurant. Recently, Mark has been interested in eating healthier and is trying to consume more fruits and vegetables during his day.
Fluids: Water, 3 sodas per day, and 2 coffees with cream and sugar.

Questions

1. Mark consents for a liver biopsy, which is consistent with cirrhosis from NASH. What is his Child-Pugh Score?
2. How would you evaluate his INR and PT levels?
3. What measures do you need to assess his nutritional status?

Fat Metabolism

The liver is involved in digestion, metabolism, and transport of fat. It synthesizes and excretes bile, which is required for digestion and absorption of long chain fatty acids in the lumen of the intestine. About 8% to 12% of dietary lipid ends up in the liver after a meal,[78] where it can be oxidized for energy or used to create cholesterol, phospholipids, lipoproteins, and ketones. The liver also converts excess dietary carbohydrate into triglycerides via de novo lipogenesis.

Due to decreased ability to store hepatic glycogen, cirrhotic patients rely heavily on lipid oxidation for energy after brief periods of fasting. This has been demonstrated by measuring fasting respiratory quotient (RQ) through indirect calorimetry. Generally speaking, an RQ of 1 indicates carbohydrate as the primary substrate, 0.85 indicates protein or mixed substrate metabolism, and 0.7 indicates lipid metabolism. Both stable and hospitalized patients with cirrhosis have significantly lower RQs than healthy controls, averaging an RQ of 0.78 and sometimes presenting with RQs lower than what is generally considered compatible with life (0.69). Lower RQ correlated with lower skeletal muscle mass and lower visceral and subcutaneous fat mass.[79] Sarcopenia, or loss of muscle mass, is associated with mortality in patients with cirrhosis and HCC.[80,81]

In cirrhosis, lipid digestion and absorption is impaired by the inability of adequate bile to reach the intestinal lumen.[82] Therefore, these patients can have all the consequences of fat malabsorption, including steatorrhea, essential fatty acid and fat-soluble vitamin deficiency, and malnutrition. While the common belief is that patients with cholestatic liver disease are at increased risk of fat-soluble vitamin deficiencies, patients with hepatocellular liver disease are equally at risk. Vitamin A deficiency is actually more common in hepatocellular liver disease, likely because of decreased storage capacity. Deficiencies in vitamins A, D, E, and K are positively correlated with serum bilirubin and severity of disease, regardless of the underlying etiology.[83] In critically ill patients with severely elevated bilirubin, a semi-elemental formula high in medium chain triglycerides should be used if the patient has fat malabsorption (positive fecal fat stain).

> **CORE CONCEPT 7**
>
> Patients with cirrhosis should be monitored for malabsorption of fat and deficiency of fat-soluble vitamins.

Nutrition Assessment

Traditional methods of assessing nutrition status, such as weight changes and hepatic proteins, are of no use in this population. It is impossible to interpret whether a change in serum albumin or prealbumin is secondary to nutrition status or liver function. Similarly, weight changes do not reflect lean body mass in a patient who has edema or ascites. BMI cut-off values of <22 kg/m^2 in patients without ascites and <25 kg/m^2 in patients with tense ascites have been validated for identifying malnutrition,[84] but more studies are needed to adopt this into practice. Therefore, a clinical assessment (medical history and nutrition-focused physical exam) identifies malnutrition more accurately than anthropometric or biochemical measures.

Subjective Global Assessment (SGA) should be used for assessing nutrition status of patients with liver disease.[26] SGA is a clinical evaluation including the patient's weight history, dietary intake, gastrointestinal symptoms, and functional capacity, along with a physical exam of subcutaneous fat, muscle wasting, edema, and ascites.

Body Composition

Sarcopenia, or muscle wasting, is independently associated with mortality in cirrhosis.[85] Significant muscle depletion is more common in men, while women experience more adipose tissue loss.[86] Weight cannot capture these changes. Mid-arm muscle circumference (MAMC) measures lean tissue stores (**Figure 15.8**) and triceps skinfold thickness (TST) measures adipose reserve. These correlate with severity of disease and are not affected by nonnutritional factors, such as fluid retention.[87] MAMC and TST can be compared to reference values, with a value lower than the fifth percentile considered diagnostic of malnutrition. However, they may be more valuable in the outpatient setting to monitor changes in body composition in the same patient over time. Other measures of body composition are the dual-energy x-ray absorptiometry scan or bioelectrical impedance analysis, but these are not always practical in a clinical setting.

As part of SGA, the clinician examines the patient for muscle wasting in the temple, clavicle, shoulder, calf, knee, and scapula, and in between the thumb and forefinger (the interosseous muscle). Examining the fat pads under the eyes and pinching the skin over the triceps and biceps is done to evaluate subcutaneous fat stores. Fluid retention is noted by the presence of edema and ascites.

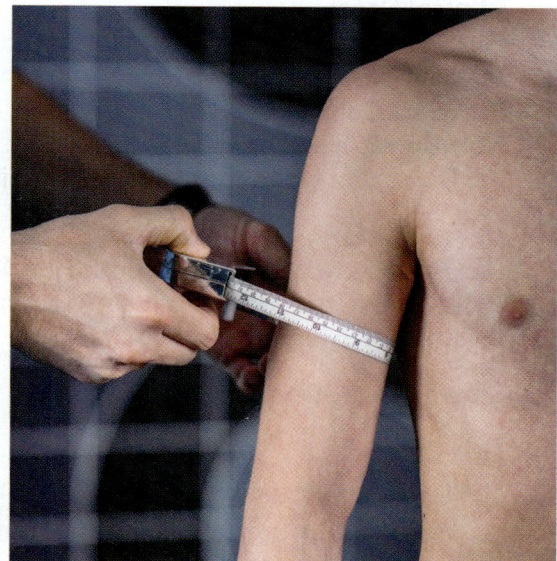

FIGURE 15.8 Mid-Arm Muscle Circumference (MAMC) which Measures Lean Tissue Stores May Be a Useful Indicator of Nutritional Status in Patients with Liver Disease
© Microgen/Shutterstock.

> **CORE CONCEPT 8**
>
> Muscle and adipose tissue wasting in patients with liver disease is an independent predictor of mortality. Muscle loss is also associated with hepatic encephalopathy.

Functional Capacity

Asking the patient about their ability to stand, walk, and engage in normal activities may be as valuable as actual measures of lean body mass. Reduced muscle function correlates with depletion of lean body mass and protein calorie malnutrition.[86]

Handgrip strength measured by a handgrip dynamometer, is an inexpensive, simple tool for objectively measuring functional capacity and identifying malnutrition. In a study of patients with compensated liver disease (88% were Child-Pugh A), handgrip dynamometry identified malnutrition (handgrip strength below mean +/–2 standard deviations) in 63% of patients, and these patients had a significantly higher morbidity and mortality in the following year than those who were adequately nourished. SGA only identified 28% of those patients as malnourished and did not predict morbidity and mortality.[88] Therefore, handgrip strength is useful for identifying undernourished cirrhotic patients in the early stages of disease. Although it is unclear whether early nutrition intervention would affect outcomes, efforts to prevent further nutrition depletion are warranted.

> **CORE CONCEPT 9**
>
> Nutrition status should be determined using the Subjective Global Assessment, with special focus on identification of muscle wasting through physical exam and functional capacity (handgrip dynamometry). Traditional methods using weight, BMI, and serum hepatic proteins should be abandoned.

CASE STUDY REVISITED

A year later, at a follow up visit, the RD sees from Mark's medical record that he has developed mild ascites and is in the early stages of cirrhosis.

Anthropometrics:
Height: 183 cm (72")
Weight: 127 kg (280 lbs)
BMI: 38 kg/m² (class 2 obesity)
Waist circumference: 104 cm (41")

Biochemical Data:
Cholesterol 215 mg/dL (Desirable<200 mg/dL)
Hemoglobin A1C 6.0% (4.3-5.8%)
Alanine aminotransferase 58 (4-36 units/L)
Aspartate aminotransferase 45 (10-35 units/L)
Alkaline phosphatase 100 (30-120 units/L)
Bilirubin 1 (0.3-1.9 mg/dL)
Albumin 3.9 (3.5-5.0 g/dL)

Clinical Data:
Past Medical History: NAFLD, prediabetic, mild ascites
Medications: Pioglitazone (30 mg), atorvastatin (50 mg), vitamin E (800 IU)
Vital Signs: Blood pressure 160/95 mm Hg, Temperature 97.8°F, Heart rate 87 beats/min
Nutrition-focused Physical Exam: MAMC: value lower than the 5%; handgrip strength: two standard deviations below the reference normal. Obese, apple-shaped body type.

Dietary History:
Due to his decreased appetite and fatigue, Mark only manages to eat two meals per day, one of them usually being fast food. He has been avoiding meat because he read online that protein was bad for his liver.

Diet Prescription: per RD

Questions
1. What do you interpret his weight? What confounding factors might be influencing his weight status?
2. What is your diet prescription for this patient?
3. Are there any micronutrients that you would like to supplement?

Nutrition Therapy for Cirrhosis

Energy Requirements

Cirrhotic patients are not necessarily hypermetabolic; in fact, one study found that only 15% to 18% of patients were hypermetabolic, while up to 31% were hypometabolic.[89,90] There is no clinical or biochemical way to predict which patients are hypermetabolic; therefore, indirect calorimetry should be used to measure resting energy expenditure in critically ill patients or in stable patients who experience muscle wasting despite seemingly adequate nutritional intake.[91] Handheld calorimeters are a valid and less-expensive alternative to the metabolic cart in hospitalized patients.[92,93] Although predicted equations are not accurate in this population,[72] if indirect calorimetry is not available or feasible, the Harris–Benedict Equation with a stress factor of 1.3 or 25 to 40 kcal/kg is recommended for cirrhotic patients.[26] If significant edema or ascites are present, A.S.P.E.N. recommends that the patient's estimated dry weight or usual body weight should be used to estimate needs.[91]

> **CORE CONCEPT 10**
>
> Indirect calorimetry should be used to determine energy needs for cirrhotic patients.

Protein Requirements

The practice of protein restriction to prevent hyperammonemia in patients with liver disease is still commonly practiced despite widespread recommendation against it. Guidelines from ESPEN recommend providing 1.2 to 1.5 g/kg of protein for compensated and decompensated cirrhosis, respectively.[26,38,73] A.S.P.E.N. recommends estimating protein requirements similarly to a general intensive care unit patient: 1.2 to 2 g/kg for BMI <30, 2 g/kg ideal body weight for BMI 30 to 40, and 2.5 g/kg ideal body weight for BMI >40. Protein should not be restricted as a strategy to reduce risk of hepatic encephalopathy.[91] A temporary protein restriction (0.6-0.8 g/kg/day) is reasonable in patients with acute episodes of hepatic encephalopathy until the precipitating factor is determined. If no improvement is noted with protein restriction, a high-protein diet or formula should be resumed within a few days to prevent muscle catabolism.[26,94] A prospective study at Veterans Affairs Medical Centers in the 1990s evaluated HE and dietary protein intake in patients with AH. They found that low protein intake was independently associated with worsening HE, whereas those that were less malnourished and had higher protein intake had improved HE.[95] A key trial by Cordoba et al.[96] in 2004 compared a low-protein diet (0.5 g/kg/day) to a normal protein diet (1.2 g/kg/day) for cirrhotic patients admitted with an episode of HE. There was no difference in outcomes and higher endogenous protein breakdown in the low-protein diet compared to the normal protein diet. Therefore, providing adequate protein is safe and preserves lean body mass in patients with HE.[97] There has been some suggestion that a diet high in vegetable and dairy protein is better tolerated than other animal protein and improves HE,[98,99] but there are very few studies to support this and certainly not enough evidence to discourage a diet high in animal protein.

> **CORE CONCEPT 11**
>
> Protein should not be restricted in patients with liver disease with or without hepatic encephalopathy. Patients should be given 1.2 g/kg or more depending on the severity of their condition.

Vitamin D

Vitamin D deficiency is associated with chronic liver disease. Furthermore, people with cirrhosis often have osteoporosis, called hepatic osteodystrophy, although this is not well understood.[100] In one study, severe deficiency (25-hydroxyvitamin D [25(OH)D] <7 ng/mL) was present in about one-third of patients and 92% had 25(OH)D levels less than 30 ng/dL, which is the recommended threshold for vitamin D sufficiency.[101,102] Patients with NAFLD were shown to have lower 25(OH)D levels than healthy controls,

Clinical Roundtable

Background: Protein restriction for patients with HE continues to be debated. Best practice is obscured by the fact that some patients are more tolerant to protein than others. Furthermore, the type of protein seems to be of importance in determining outcome. While BCAA routinely provided to HE patients, diets high in vegetable and dairy protein have also been suggested. Plant-based proteins may be better tolerated than animal protein, improving hepatic encephalopathy. Given that animal protein is often of high biological value, its restriction may impair lean body mass stores.

Roundtable Discussion

What factors should be considered when prescribing protein for patients with hepatic encephalopathy? What are the advantages and disadvantages of a low-protein diet? How might a vegetable protein improve hepatic encephalopathy?

References

1. Nguyen DL, Morgan T. Protein restriction in hepatic encephalopathy is appropriate for selected patients: a point of view. *Hepatol Int.* 2014;8(2):447-451. doi:10.1007/s12072-013-9497-1.

and those with NASH to have lower vitamin D levels than those with NAFLD.[103] Vitamin D deficiency is also associated with presence of NAFLD in nonobese adults.[104] In ALD patients, 25(OH)D levels <10 ng/mL have been associated with increased liver damage and mortality.[105] Finally, vitamin D levels <6 ng/mL were identified as a significant predictor of death in patients with advanced liver cirrhosis (Child-Pugh C).[106] There are many reasons patients with liver disease may become vitamin D deficient. Inadequate intake and sun exposure, fat malabsorption, and decreased hepatic hydroxylation of vitamin D to 25 (OH)D as the first step in converting it to its active form are all reasonable explanations. Although there is no evidence that vitamin D supplementation improves outcomes, oral vitamin D supplementation improves 25(OH)D levels[107] and it is prudent to monitor and replete low levels in patients with all forms of chronic liver disease. The recommended dose for repletion is 50,000 IU of vitamin D_2 or D_3 once a week or the equivalent 6,000 IU daily for 8 weeks followed by a maintenance dose of 1,500 to 2,000 IU daily. Patients who are obese, who have malabsorption syndromes, or are on medications affecting vitamin D metabolism (including steroids) may need even higher doses to maintain sufficient vitamin D status.[102]

> **PRACTICE POINT**
>
> Provide vitamin D supplementation to all liver disease patients as needed to maintain normal serum 25 (OH) vitamin D levels.

Zinc

Zinc deficiency is a common complication in cirrhotic patients and may exacerbate malnutrition and HE related to hyperammonemia. Zinc has a key role in ammonia metabolism in the liver and in skeletal muscle. In the muscle, it inhibits AMP deaminase, which releases ammonia from aspartic acid into circulation. It is also a coenzyme for **glutamine synthetase**, which removes ammonia from the blood to combine with glutamate to make glutamine.[108] In the liver, zinc is a coenzyme for **ornithine transcarbamylase (OTC)**, a key enzyme for ammonia detoxification via the urea cycle. Rats fed a zinc-deficient diet developed significantly decreased hepatic OTC activity and significantly increased plasma ammonia levels compared to those fed a diet adequate in zinc.[109] Similarly, rats with cirrhosis developed lower serum and hepatic zinc levels, reduced OTC activity, and increased ammonia levels compared to those that were supplemented with zinc.[110] Humans fed a low-zinc diet developed higher ammonia levels even with mild zinc deficiency.[111] On a similar note, zinc concentration has also been shown to be lower in the patients with HE compared to those without.[112,113] However, a recent meta-analysis found that there is no clear evidence that zinc supplementation improves HE based on the four randomized controlled trials available, all with small sample sizes.[114-118]

Zinc supplementation may provide benefit in viral hepatitis due to its role in immunologic reactions and as an antioxidant.[119] In patients with chronic hepatitis C, blood zinc concentrations decrease with progression to cirrhosis and HCC. Supplementing with zinc has been shown to significantly decrease AST and ALT levels and decrease incidence of HCC in patients whose serum zinc level increases after supplementation.[120] However, there is insufficient data to recommend zinc supplementation in hepatitis C patients who are not deficient.

Many clinical manifestations of zinc deficiency overlap with symptoms of chronic liver disease (**Table 15.13**). If zinc deficiency is the cause of anorexia, taste abnormalities, weight loss, impaired wound healing, increased susceptibility to infection, mental lethargy and emotional disorders, or hyperammonemia, these can be reversed with supplementation.[121] There are several reasons patients may develop a deficiency. These include inadequate oral intake due to low-protein diets, decreased absorption, and increased urinary excretion. Those taking diuretics or abusing alcohol have especially high urinary excretion and subsequently have higher risk of zinc deficiency.[112,122-124]

TABLE 15.13 SIGNS AND SYMPTOMS OF ZINC DEFICIENCY

Zinc Deficiency[107,117,1]	Mild	Moderate	Severe
Symptoms	Oligospermia	Growth retardation	Alopecia
	Decreased lean body mass	Delayed puberty	Diarrhea
	Hyperammonemia	Hypogonadism	Emotional disorders
	Hypogeusia	Rough skin	Weight loss
	Decreased dark adaptation	Poor appetite	Intercurrent infections
		Mental lethargy	Hypogonadism
		Delayed wound healing	Bullous-pustular dermatitis
		Taste abnormalities	Death

Data from Rode A, Fourlanos S, Nicoll A. Oral vitamin D replacement is effective in chronic liver disease. *Gastroenterol Clin Biol*. 2010;34(11):618-620; Hayashi M, Ikezawa K, Ono A, et al. Evaluation of the effects of combination therapy with branched-chain amino acid and zinc supplements on nitrogen metabolism in liver cirrhosis. *Hepatol Res*. 2007;37(8):615-619.; and Ghany M, Hoofnagle JH. Chapter 301. Approach to the patient with liver disease. Harrison's Principles of Internal Medicine, 18e;2012. In: Longo DL, et al., eds. *Harrison's Principles of Internal Medicine*. 18th ed. New York: McGraw-Hill; 2012.

Because zinc is bound to albumin in the blood, serum zinc level is a not reliable indicator of zinc status in a patient with low albumin. However, it may be prudent to empirically supplement a patient who has symptoms of zinc deficiency, especially those with severe malnutrition, alcoholism, or refractory hyperammonemia, or in those taking diuretics. One concern with zinc supplementation is that it may induce a copper deficiency; however, patients with cirrhosis may have increased copper levels due to decreased excretion via bile.[112] Therefore, it is considered safe to give supplementation of 50 mg elemental zinc (220 mg zinc sulfate) orally per day. It should be taken with a meal to avoid potential side effects of nausea or gastrointestinal distress.[33]

CORE CONCEPT 12

Patients with cirrhosis should be monitored and treated for signs of zinc deficiency, especially if they are malnourished, alcoholic, or on diuretic therapy.

PRACTICE POINT

For patients with signs of zinc deficiency, it is safe and reasonable to empirically give a 2-week course of zinc sulfate (220 mg twice daily).

Oral Nutrition

As described earlier, patients with cirrhosis have accelerated starvation, entering a catabolic state with a very low RQ overnight. For this reason, patients should be instructed to eat regular meals and a bedtime snack to avoid prolonged fasting. Having a late evening snack decreases lipid oxidation and proteolysis (increases fasting RQ), improves nitrogen balance, and significantly increases total body protein compared to not having a snack or having the equivalent snack during the day.[72,125-128] Most studies use a high carbohydrate food containing roughly 200 kcal, but an isocaloric BCAA mixture has been shown to be equally efficacious at ameliorating fasting catabolism.[129] Furthermore, a BCAA-fortified snack increased serum albumin and RQ more than a nonfortified snack after being given for 3 months.[130] Oral nutrition supplements (ONS) are recommended for patients who do not meet their nutrition needs with normal food.[26] Along with dietary advice, use of ONS, particularly in the late evening, improves intake and may improve body composition,[72,131] although there is no clear evidence that it will improve overall outcomes.[40]

CORE CONCEPT 13

Patients with cirrhosis should eat small, frequent meals and a bedtime snack to avoid the accelerated proteolysis and lipid oxidation that occurs after a short period of fasting.

Patients with ascites or edema should follow a 2-g sodium diet restriction. If they have concurrent severe hyponatremia (serum sodium <125 mEq/L), an oral fluid restriction of 1.5 L/day is indicated. Fluid restriction is not recommended for patients with ascites who only have mild to moderate hyponatremia or have hypovolemic hyponatremia. Hyponatremia (serum sodium <135 mEq/L) is associated with greater frequency of HE and increased risk of mortality.[94,132-134] Patients with ascites have early satiety, which is another reason to recommend small, frequent meals and snacks for improved overall intake.

CORE CONCEPT 14

Patients with ascites should follow a low-sodium diet. A free water restriction is only indicated in the setting of severe hyponatremia (serum sodium <125 mEq/L).

Long-term use of oral BCAA supplements have been shown to improve quality of life, reduce the risk for HCC, and prolong survival in patients with cirrhosis.[74,135-137] The first trial to successfully demonstrate this was in Japan, where a BCAA supplement in the form of small granules is approved for use. Other formulations are not palatable, thus patients in prior studies were not compliant with taking them. The BCAA supplemented group had significantly reduced occurrence of hepatic failure, variceal bleeding, development of HCC, and death from any cause compared to the control group. These findings were so significant that the study was discontinued 10 months early out of concern for the control group. Japan now recommends BCAA supplementation for all patients with cirrhosis.[136]

PRACTICE POINT

Long-term oral BCAA supplements are beneficial for patients with cirrhosis, but not yet readily accessible in the United States. For patients that are intolerant to dietary protein, encourage trying vegetable and dairy protein sources, which are higher in BCAA.

Enteral Nutrition

Enteral nutrition support is indicated for patients with a functional gastrointestinal tract who are unable to meet their nutrition needs orally. Although there may be benefit from giving long-term BCAA for chronic liver disease, there is no evidence that a formula high in BCAA provides benefit for acute episodic hepatic encephalopathy or critically ill patients. Therefore, A.S.P.E.N. recommends a standard polymeric protein formula.[91] Patients with severe hyponatremia may need a free water–restricted formula.

Nonbleeding esophageal varices are not a contraindication for nasoenteric tube placement or enteral nutrition. In patients with a variceal bleed, it is recommended to wait 48 hours after endoscopic treatment of the bleed before initiating enteral (or oral) nutrition.[138] If the patient is encephalopathic or withdrawing from alcohol, both oral and enteral nutrition carry a high risk of aspiration. The risk of aspiration must be weighed against the risks associated with PN; there are no studies evaluating

CASE STUDY REVISITED

Another 2 years later, Mark's wife brings him to the emergency department with complaints of bloody emesis and mental status changes. On presentation, Mark is barely arousable and unable to answer questions appropriately. His wife reports that he stayed home with the flu for the past 5 days and recently started having bright-red blood in his vomit. Since then he has become confused and progressively more lethargic. The doctor diagnosed Mark with tense ascites and has requested a nutrition consultation for nutrition assessment and feeding recommendations.

Anthropometrics:
Height: 183 cm (72")
Weight: 114 kg (252 lbs)
BMI: 34 kg/m² (obese)
Waist circumference: 96 cm (38")

Biochemical Data:
Cholesterol 215 (Desirable<200 mg/dL)
Alanine aminotransferase 58 (4-36 units/L)
Aspartate aminotransferase 45 (10-35 units/L)
Alkaline phosphatase 100 (30-120 units/L)
Bilirubin 2.6 (0.3-1.9 mg/dL)

Albumin 2.9 (3.5-5.0 g/dL)
INR 2.6 (0.8-1.1)
PT: 9 (11-13.5 seconds)
Hemoglobin 11.2 (13.5-17.5 g/dL)
Hematocrit 35 (42%-52% in males)

Clinical Data:
Past Medical History: NAFLD, prediabetic, mild ascites
Medications: Pioglitazone (30 mg), atorvastatin (50 mg), vitamin E (800 IU)
Vital Signs: Blood pressure 150/90 mm Hg, Temperature 97.6°F, Heart rate 86 beats/min

Dietary Data:
Diet History: Per Mark's wife, Mark has had minimal oral intake for the last week, but he has not lost any weight recently.

Questions

1. Would you advocate for Mark to be placed on nutrition support? Which formula would you recommend for Mark given his symptoms and lab values?
2. What might be the cause of the blood in Mark's emesis? Can this factor cause a delay in starting Mark on nutrition support?
3. Which signs and symptoms indicate that Mark has developed HE?
4. Which lab values do you think are important to monitor during his stay? What are the risks that he may face? Given his conditions, what other labs would you request?

---

this. Percutaneous gastrostomy and jejunostomy feeding tubes are generally contraindicated in patients with ascites, because leakage of gastric contents into the peritoneum can lead to peritonitis.[26]

> **PRACTICE POINT**
>
> In a patient at high risk of aspirating oral feeding due to altered mental status, consider bolus enteral feeding to prevent aspiration on a continuous infusion that may occur if the feeding tube is dislodged.

Parenteral Nutrition

PN is indicated for patients who are unable to meet their nutrition needs orally or enterally. For such patients who are malnourished, PN should be started immediately. The 2009 European guidelines recommend starting PN for patients who will require fasting for procedures, especially if fasting for more than 3 days is expected. If a patient requires to be fasted >12 hours, they recommend providing continuous intravenous fluid with 5% of 10% dextrose, providing a glucose infusion rate of 2 to 3 mg/kg/min.[73,139] The latter recommendation is based on evidence that late

⚠ Clinical Controversy

Malnutrition that accompanies end-stage liver failure may prompt clinicians to prescribe nutrition support strategies. However, meta-analysis reveals that nutrition supplementation by enteral, parenteral, or oral solution does not consistently improve nutritional status and outcome in patients with end-stage liver disease. Recently Maharshi et al., in a randomized controlled trial, demonstrated improved nutritional status and hospital-related quality of life and reduced symptoms of HE. Findings such as these encourage the use of oral supplementation for improving nutritional status and outcome in advanced stages of liver disease. In contrast, Seguin et al., in their randomized controlled trial, could not demonstrate a benefit of perioperative oral supplementation in patients undergoing hepatic surgery.

How do you interpret the differences in these findings? How might differences in study design impact your results (consider intervention used, sample population, outcomes measured). Would you use either of these supplement strategies for your patients?

References

1. Seguin P, Locher C, Bellissant E, et al. Effect of a perioperative nutritional supplementation with Oral Impact in patients undergoing hepatic surgery for liver cancer: A prospective, placebo-controlled, randomized, double-blind study. *Nutr Cancer*. 2016;68(3):464-472.
2. Maharshi S, Sharma BC, Sachdeva S, Srivastava S, Sharma P. Efficacy of nutritional therapy for patients with cirrhosis and minimal hepatic encephalopathy in a randomized trial. *Clin Gastroenterol Hepatol*. 2016;14:454-460.

---

evening meals ameliorate catabolism during an overnight fast, as described earlier. Certainly, patients with fasting hypoglycemia unable to eat should be given intravenous dextrose infusions. However, many cirrhotic patients are insulin resistant, and it is unclear whether the benefit of providing short-term IV dextrose outweighs the risk of hyperglycemia.[129] Caution against overfeeding via PN is important, because excess dextrose and lipid calories lead to hepatic accumulation of triglycerides, or steatosis, especially in a liver that is incapable of adequately exporting triglycerides in lipoproteins.

A parenteral amino acid solution containing a higher amount of BCAA and lower amount of AAA was developed in the 1980s when studies associated low plasma BCAA and concurrent high plasma AAA with HE and ESLD. European guidelines recommend the use of parenteral BCAA amino acid formulations for patients with severe (Stage 3 and 4) HE based on studies that show improvement in mental status, but not in survival.[73] The evidence for parenteral BCAA provision is not convincing, and at best inconclusive.[140-143]

Patients with cirrhosis have elevated serum copper and manganese, thus they should have copper and manganese decreased or removed from their PN to avoid toxicity.[112] Manganese toxicity is associated with motor and psychiatric disturbances, and may also be a factor in the pathogenesis of HE.[144] Intravenous thiamine should be supplemented to all malnourished patients, especially those with ALD, to prevent deficiency. These patients should also be closely monitored for refeeding syndrome with the initiation of PN. For patients with severe hyponatremia, parenteral nutrients should be mixed in normal saline (154 mEq/L or 0.9% NaCl) to restrict free water. However, an overall fluid restriction is not always indicated, because patients with ascites can still be intravascularly dry.

PRACTICE POINT

In patients with ALD, provide 200 mg intravenous or intramuscular thiamine prior to initiation of nutrition support and daily thereafter for 3 days. In any malnourished patient with liver disease, provide 100 mg oral thiamine for 5 to 7 days. Thereafter, recommend a B complex if the patient is not able to take adequate food on a daily basis.

PRACTICE POINT

Work with the healthcare team to avoid prolonged periods of fasting the patient for procedures. If it will be necessary for more than 3 days, consider starting PN for malnourished patients.

Summary

Although there are many different types of liver disease, all are affected by malnutrition and its associated complications. The liver has a prominent role in metabolism of nutrients; understanding the derangements in metabolism during liver disease and failure is central to providing medical nutrition therapy. The RD is an essential part of the patient's team, not only to provide assessment and counseling of the patient, but to guide and educate physicians on what nutrition interventions can or cannot benefit the patient. Nutrition is as important, if not more important, for the outpatient in the early stages of disease, as it is for the patient with decompensated failure. There is much yet to be understood about therapies for NAFLD, ascites, and HE, as well as the role of probiotics, zinc, BCAA, and other nutrients.

Key Terms

kupffer cells, stellate cells, gut–liver axis, hepatocellular liver disease, cholestatic liver disease, acute hepatitis, acute liver failure, chronic hepatitis, fibrosis, cirrhosis, portal hypertension, porto-systemic shunting, varices, underfill hypothesis, ascites, hepatic encephalopathy (HE), decompensated cirrhosis/end-stage liver disease (ESLD), transjugular intrahepatic portosystemic shunt (TIPS), coagulopathy, paracentesis, spontaneous bacterial peritonitis (SBP), hepatorenal syndrome (HRS), child-pugh classification, viral hepatitis, drug-induced hepatitis, fulminant liver failure, shock liver, acute-on-chronic hepatitis, steatosis, alcoholic liver disease, steatohepatitis, alcoholic hepatitis (AH), endotoxin, tumor necrosis factor (TNF), de ritis ratio, nonalcoholic fatty liver disease (NAFLD), nonalcoholic steatohepatitis (NASH), parenteral nutrition related liver disease (PNALD), hemochromatosis, Wilson's disease, kayser-fleischer ring, dysgeusia, metallothionein, branched chain amino acids (BCAA), subjective global assessment (SGA), glutamine synthetase, ornithine transcarbamylase (OTC)

References

1. Ghany M, Hoofnagle JH. Chapter 301. Approach to the patient with liver disease. In: Longo DL, Fauci AS, Kasper DL, Hauser SL, Jameson JL, Loscalzo J, eds. Harrison's Principles of Internal Medicine, 18th ed;New York: McGraw-Hill;2012. Available from. <http://www.accessmedicine.com/content.aspx?aID=9132925>
2. Zeuzem S. Gut-liver axis. Int J Colorectal Dis. 2000;15(2):59-82.
3. Sharma V, Garg S, Aggarwal S. Probiotics and liver disease. Perm J. 2013;17(4):62-67.
4. Pratt DS, Kaplan MM. Chapter 302. Evaluation of Liver Function. In: Longo DL, Fauci AS, Kasper DL, Hauser SL, Jameson JL, Loscalzo J, eds. Harrison's Principles of Internal Medicine, 18th ed. New York, NY: McGraw-Hill;2012. http://accessmedicine.mhmedical.com/Content.aspx?bookid=331&sectionid=40727097.
5. Friedman LS. Chapter 16. Liver, Biliary Tract,& Pancreas Disorders. In: Papadakis MA, McPhee SJ. eds. Current Medical Diagnosis & Treatment 2014; New York: McGraw-Hill;2014.
6. Murphy S, Xu J, Kochanek K. Deaths: Final data for 2010. Center for Disease Control and Prevention Website. www.cdc.gov/nchs/data/nvsr/nvsr61/nvsr61_04.pdf. Accessed December 20, 2017.
7. Bosch J, Garcia-Pagan JC. Complications of cirrhosis. I. Portal hypertension. J Hepatol. 2000;32(1 Suppl):141-156.
8. Bacon BR. Chapter 308: Cirrhosis and Its Complications. Longo DL, et al. Harrison's Principles of Internal Medicine. 18th ed. New York: McGraw-Hill; 2012.
9. Kashani A, Landaverde C, Medici V, Rossaro L. Fluid retention in cirrhosis: Pathophysiology and management. QJM. 2008;101(2):71-85.
10. Bajaj JS. Review article: The modern management of hepatic encephalopathy. Aliment Pharmacol Ther. 2010;31(5):537-547.
11. Qureshi MO, Khokhar N, Shafqat F. Ammonia levels and the severity of hepatic encephalopathy. J Coll Physicians Surg Pak. 2014;24(3):160-163.
12. Odeh M, Sabo E, Srugo I, Oliven A. Serum levels of tumor necrosis factor-alpha correlate with severity of hepatic encephalopathy due to chronic liver failure. Liver Int. 2004;24(2):110-116.
13. Kalaitzakis E, Josefsson A, Bjornsson E. Type and etiology of liver cirrhosis are not related to the presence of hepatic encephalopathy or health-related quality of life: A cross-sectional study. BMC Gastroenterol. 2008;8:46.
14. Bacon BR. Chapter 309. Genetic, Metabolic, and Infiltrative Diseases Affecting the Liver. In: Longo DL, Fauci AS, Kasper DL, Hauser SL, Jameson JL, Loscalzo J., eds. New York, NY: McGraw-Hill, 2012. Harrison's Principles of Internal Medicine,18th ed. New York, NY: McGraw-Hill; 2012. http://accesspharmacy.mhmedical.com/Content.aspx?bookid=331&sectionid=40727105.
15. Salerno F, Gerbes A, Gines P, Wong F, Arroyo V. Diagnosis, prevention and treatment of hepatorenal syndrome in cirrhosis. Postgrad Med J. 2008;84(998):662-670.
16. Mendenhall C, Roselle GA, Gartside P, Moritz T. Relationship of protein calorie malnutrition to alcoholic liver disease: A reexamination of data from two veterans administration cooperative studies. Alcohol Clin Exp Res. 1995;19(3):635-641.
17. Mouzaki M, Ng V, Kamath BM, Selzner N, Pencharz P, Ling SC. Enteral energy and macronutrients in end-stage liver disease. JPEN J Parenter Enteral Nutr. 2014;38(6)673-681.
18. Dienstag JL. Chapter 304. Acute Viral Hepatitis. In: Longo DL, Fauci AS, Kasper DL, Hauser SL, Jameson JL, Loscalzo J. eds. Harrison's Principles of Internal Medicine,18th ed. New York, NY: McGraw-Hill; 2012.
19. Friedman LS. Chapter 16. Liver, Biliary Tract,& Pancreas Disorders. In: Papadakis MA, McPhee SJ. Rabow MW. eds. Current Medical Diagnosis & Treatment 2016; New York: McGraw-Hill. Available from http://accessmedicine.mhmedical.com/book.aspx?bookid=1585.
20. National Institute of Health. LiverTox: Clinical research information on drug-induced liver injury. https://livertox.nih.gov/Last updated October 16, 2017. Accessed December 20, 2017.
21. Benedict M, Zhang X. Non-alcoholic fatty liver disease: an expanded review. World J Hepatol 2017; 9(16):715-732. DOI://dx.doi.org/10.4254/wjh.v9.i16.715.
22. Bunchorntavakul C, Reddy KR. Review article: Herbal and dietary supplement hepatotoxicity. Aliment Pharmacol Ther. 2013;37(1):3-17.
23. Teschke R, Frenzel C, Schulze J, Eickhoff A. Herbal hepatotoxicity: Challenges and pitfalls of causality assessment methods. World J Gastroenterol. 2013;19(19):2864-2882.
24. Food and Drug Administration. OxyElite pro supplements recalled - food and drug administration. http://www.fda.gov/forconsumers/consumerupdates/ucm374742.htm. Accessed August 8, 2014.
25. Bernal W, Wendon J. Acute liver failure. N Engl J Med. 2013;369(26): 2525-2534.
26. Plauth M, Cabre E, Riggio O, et al. ESPEN guidelines on enteral nutrition: Liver disease. Clin Nutr. 2006;25(2):285-294.
27. Schneeweiss B, Pammer J, Ratheiser K, et al. Energy metabolism in acute hepatic failure. Gastroenterology. 1993;105(5):1515-1521.
28. Walsh TS, Wigmore SJ, Hopton P, Richardson R, Lee A. Energy expenditure in acetaminophen-induced fulminant hepatic failure. Crit Care Med. 2000;28(3):649-654.
29. Dienstag JL Chapter 306. Chronic Hepatitis. In: Longo DL, Fauci AS, Kasper DL, Hauser SL, Jameson J, Loscalzo J. eds. Harrison's Principles of Internal Medicine,18th ed. New York, NY: McGraw-Hill; 2012.
30. Mailliard ME, Sorrell MF, "Chapter 307: Alcoholic Liver Disease." Harrison's Principles of Internal Medicine, 18e Longo DL, Fauci AS,

Kasper DL, Hauser SL, Jameson J, Loscalzo J. eds. New York, NY: McGraw-Hill, 2012.

31. Stickel F, Seitz HK. Update on the management of alcoholic steatohepatitis. *J Gastrointestin Liver Dis*. 2013;22(2):189-197.
32. Purohit V, Bode JC, Bode C, et al. Alcohol, intestinal bacterial growth, intestinal permeability to endotoxin, and medical consequences: Summary of a symposium. *Alcohol*. 2008;42(5):349-361.
33. Mohammad MK, Zhou Z, Cave M, Barve A, McClain CJ. Zinc and liver disease. *Nutr Clin Pract*. 2012;27(1):8-20.
34. Torkadi PP, Apte IC, Bhute AK. Biochemical evaluation of patients of alcoholic liver disease and non-alcoholic liver disease. *Indian J Clin Biochem*. 2014;29(1):79-83.
35. Botros M, Sikaris KA. The de ritis ratio: The test of time. *Clin Biochem Rev*. 2013;34(3):117-130.
36. Mendenhall CL, Moritz TE, Roselle GA, et al. Protein energy malnutrition in severe alcoholic hepatitis: Diagnosis and response to treatment. The VA cooperative study group #275. *JPEN J Parenter Enteral Nutr*. 1995;19(4):258-265.
37. Mendenhall CL, Moritz TE, Roselle GA, et al. A study of oral nutritional support with oxandrolone in malnourished patients with alcoholic hepatitis: Results of a department of veterans affairs cooperative study. *Hepatology*. 1993;17(4):564-576.
38. Jaurigue MM, Cappell MS. Therapy for alcoholic liver disease. *World J Gastroenterol*. 2014;20(9):2143-2158.
39. Cabre E, Rodriguez-Iglesias P, Caballeria J, et al. Short- and long-term outcome of severe alcohol-induced hepatitis treated with steroids or enteral nutrition: A multicenter randomized trial. *Hepatology*. 2000;32(1):36-42.
40. Antar R, Wong P, Ghali P. A meta-analysis of nutritional supplementation for management of hospitalized alcoholic hepatitis. *Can J Gastroenterol*. 2012;26(7):463-467.
41. Hashimoto E, Taniai M, Tokushige K. Characteristics and diagnosis of NAFLD/NASH. *J Gastroenterol Hepatol*. 2013;28 Suppl 4:64-70.
42. Milic S, Lulic D, Stimac D. Non-alcoholic fatty liver disease and obesity: Biochemical, metabolic and clinical presentations. *World J Gastroenterol*. 2014;20(28):9330-9337.
43. Wong VW, Wong GL, Choi PC, et al. Disease progression of non-alcoholic fatty liver disease: A prospective study with paired liver biopsies at 3 years. *Gut*. 2010;59(7):969-974.
44. Rinella ME, Loomba R, Caldwell SH, et al. Controversies in the diagnosis and management of NAFLD and NASH. *Gastroenterol Hepatol (N Y)*. 2014;10(4):219-227.
45. Chan WK, Hilmi IN, Cheah PL, Goh KL. Progression of liver disease in non-alcoholic fatty liver disease—a prospective clinicopathological follow-up study. *J Dig Dis*. 2014;15(10)545-552.
46. Charlton MR, Burns JM, Pedersen RA, Watt KD, Heimbach JK, Dierkhising RA. Frequency and outcomes of liver transplantation for nonalcoholic steatohepatitis in the United States. *Gastroenterology*. 2011;141(4):1249-1253.
47. Sanyal A, Poklepovic A, Moyneur E, Barghout V. Population-based risk factors and resource utilization for HCC: US perspective. *Curr Med Res Opin*. 2010;26(9):2183-2191.
48. Nseir W, Hellou E, Assy N. Role of diet and lifestyle changes in nonalcoholic fatty liver disease. *World J Gastroenterol*. 2014;20(28):9338-9344.
49. Ghaemi A, Taleban FA, Hekmatdoost A, et al. How much weight loss is effective on nonalcoholic fatty liver disease? *Hepat Mon*. 2013;13(12):e15227.
50. Promrat K, Kleiner DE, Niemeier HM, et al. Randomized controlled trial testing the effects of weight loss on nonalcoholic steatohepatitis. *Hepatology*. 2010;51(1):121-129.
51. de Freitas AC, Campos AC, Coelho JC. The impact of bariatric surgery on nonalcoholic fatty liver disease. *Curr Opin Clin Nutr Metab Care*. 2008;11(3):267-274.
52. D'Albuquerque LA, Gonzalez AM, Wahle RC, de Oliveira Souza E, Mancero JM, de Oliveira e Silva A. Liver transplantation for subacute hepatocellular failure due to massive steatohepatitis after bariatric surgery. *Liver Transpl*. 2008;14(6):881-885.
53. Molloy JW, Calcagno CJ, Williams CD, Jones FJ, Torres DM, Harrison SA. Association of coffee and caffeine consumption with fatty liver disease, nonalcoholic steatohepatitis, and degree of hepatic fibrosis. *Hepatology*. 2012;55(2):429-436.
54. Gupta V, Mah XJ, Garcia MC, Antonypillai C, van der Poorten D. Oily fish, coffee and walnuts: Dietary treatment for nonalcoholic fatty liver disease. *World J Gastroenterol*. 2015;21(37):10621-10635.
55. Shen H, Rodriguez AC, Shiani A, et al. Association between caffeine consumption and nonalcoholic fatty liver disease: A systemic review and meta-analysis. *Therap Adv Gastroenterol*. 2016;9(1):113-120.
56. Yesil A, Yilmaz Y. Review article: Coffee consumption, the metabolic syndrome and non-alcoholic fatty liver disease. *Aliment Pharmacol Ther*. 2013;38(9):1038-1044.
57. Abid A, Taha O, Nseir W, Farah R, Grosovski M, Assy N. Soft drink consumption is associated with fatty liver disease independent of metabolic syndrome. *J Hepatol*. 2009;51(5):918-924.
58. Assy N, Nasser G, Kamayse I, et al. Soft drink consumption linked with fatty liver in the absence of traditional risk factors. *Can J Gastroenterol*. 2008;22(10):811-816.
59. Vos MB, Lavine JE. Dietary fructose in nonalcoholic fatty liver disease. *Hepatology*. 2013;57(6):2525-2531.
60. Sanyal AJ, Chalasani N, Kowdley KV, et al. Pioglitazone, vitamin E, or placebo for nonalcoholic steatohepatitis. *N Engl J Med*. 2010;362(18):1675-1685.
61. Miller 3rd ER, Pastor-Barriuso R, Dalal D, Riemersma RA, Appel LJ, Guallar E. Meta-analysis: High-dosage vitamin E supplementation may increase all-cause mortality. *Ann Intern Med*. 2005;142(1):37-46.
62. Pacana T, Sanyal AJ. Vitamin E and nonalcoholic fatty liver disease. *Curr Opin Clin Nutr Metab Care*. 2012;15(6):641-648.
63. Rahimi RS, Landaverde C. Nonalcoholic fatty liver disease and the metabolic syndrome: Clinical implications and treatment. *Nutr Clin Pract*. 2013;28(1):40-51.
64. Di Minno MN, Russolillo A, Lupoli R, Ambrosino P, Di Minno A, Tarantino G. Omega-3 fatty acids for the treatment of non-alcoholic fatty liver disease. *World J Gastroenterol*. 2012;18(41):5839-5847.
65. Askari F, Rashidkhani B, Hekmatdoost A. Cinnamon may have therapeutic benefits on lipid profile, liver enzymes, insulin resistance, and high-sensitivity C-reactive protein in nonalcoholic fatty liver disease patients. *Nutr Res*. 2014;34(2):143-148.
66. Eslamparast T, Poustchi H, Zamani F, Sharafkhah M, Malekzadeh R, Hekmatdoost A. Synbiotic supplementation in nonalcoholic fatty liver disease: A randomized, double-blind, placebo-controlled pilot study. *Am J Clin Nutr*. 2014;99(3):535-542.
67. Tillman EM. Review and clinical update on parenteral nutrition-associated liver disease. *Nutr Clin Pract*. 2013;28(1):30-39.
68. Moretti D, van Doorn GM, Swinkels DW, Melse-Boonstra A. Relevance of dietary iron intake and bioavailability in the management of HFE hemochromatosis: A systematic review. *Am J Clin Nutr*. 2013;98(2):468-479.
69. Ling P, McCowen K. Carbohydrates: Carbohydrate metabolism. In: McClave S, Mueller C, eds. *The A.S.P.E.N. adult nutrition support core curriculum*. 2nd ed. Silver Springs, MD: The American Society of Enteral and Parenteral Nutrition; 2012:43-46.

70. Muller MJ, Willmann O, Rieger A, et al. Mechanism of insulin resistance associated with liver cirrhosis. *Gastroenterology*. 1992;102(6):2033-2041.
71. Verboeket-van de Venne WP, Westerterp KR, van Hoek B, Swart GR. Energy expenditure and substrate metabolism in patients with cirrhosis of the liver: Effects of the pattern of food intake. *Gut*. 1995;36(1):110-116.
72. Plank LD, Gane EJ, Peng S, et al. Nocturnal nutritional supplementation improves total body protein status of patients with liver cirrhosis: A randomized 12-month trial. *Hepatology*. 2008;48(2):557-566.
73. Plauth M, Cabre E, Campillo B, et al. ESPEN guidelines on parenteral nutrition: Hepatology. *Clin Nutr*. 2009;28(4):436-444.
74. Kawaguchi T, Izumi N, Charlton MR, Sata M. Branched-chain amino acids as pharmacological nutrients in chronic liver disease. *Hepatology*. 2011;54(3):1063-1070.
75. Young L, Kearns L, Schoefel S, Canon Clark N. Protein. In: McClave S, Mueller C, eds. *The A.S.P.E.N. adult nutrition support core curriculum*. 2nd ed. Silver Springs, MD: American Society for Parenteral and Enteral Nutrition; 2012:92.
76. Merli M, Giusto M, Lucidi C, et al. Muscle depletion increases the risk of overt and minimal hepatic encephalopathy: Results of a prospective study. *Metab Brain Dis*. 2013;28(2):281-284.
77. Kalaitzakis E, Josefsson A, Castedal M, et al. Hepatic encephalopathy is related to anemia and fat-free mass depletion in liver transplant candidates with cirrhosis. *Scand J Gastroenterol*. 2013;48(5):577-584.
78. Lambert JE, Parks EJ. Postprandial metabolism of meal triglyceride in humans. *Biochim Biophys Acta*. 2012;1821(5):721-726.
79. Glass C, Hipskind P, Tsien C, et al. Sarcopenia and a physiologically low respiratory quotient in patients with cirrhosis: A prospective controlled study. *J Appl Physiol*. 2013;114(5):559-565.
80. Montano-Loza AJ, Meza-Junco J, Prado CM, et al. Muscle wasting is associated with mortality in patients with cirrhosis. *Clin Gastroenterol Hepatol*. 2012;10(2):166-73, 173.e1.
81. Meza-Junco J, Montano-Loza AJ, Baracos VE, et al. Sarcopenia as a prognostic index of nutritional status in concurrent cirrhosis and hepatocellular carcinoma. *J Clin Gastroenterol*. 2013;47(10):861-870.
82. Vlahcevic ZR, Buhac I, Farrar JT, Bell CC,Jr, Swell L. Bile acid metabolism in patients with cirrhosis. I. kinetic aspects of cholic acid metabolism. *Gastroenterology*. 1971;60(4):491-498.
83. Abbott-Johnson W, Kerlin P, Clague A, Johnson H, Cuneo R. Relationships between blood levels of fat soluble vitamins and disease etiology and severity in adults awaiting liver transplantation. *J Gastroenterol Hepatol*. 2011;26(9):1402-1410.
84. Campillo B, Richardet JP, Bories PN. Validation of body mass index for the diagnosis of malnutrition in patients with liver cirrhosis. *Gastroenterol Clin Biol*. 2006;30(10):1137-1143.
85. Montano-Loza AJ, Meza-Junco J, Prado CM, et al. Muscle wasting is associated with mortality in patients with cirrhosis. *Clin Gastroenterol Hepatol*. 2012;10(2):166-73, 173.e1.
86. Peng S, Plank LD, McCall JL, Gillanders LK, McIlroy K, Gane EJ. Body composition, muscle function, and energy expenditure in patients with liver cirrhosis: A comprehensive study. *Am J Clin Nutr*. 2007;85(5):1257-1266.
87. Teiusanu A, Andrei M, Arbanas T, Nicolaie T, Diculescu M. Nutritional status in cirrhotic patients. *Maedica (Buchar)*. 2012;7(4):284-289.
88. Alvares-da-Silva MR, Reverbel da Silveira T. Comparison between handgrip strength, subjective global assessment, and prognostic nutritional index in assessing malnutrition and predicting clinical outcome in cirrhotic outpatients. *Nutrition*. 2005;21(2):113-117.
89. Muller MJ, Lautz HU, Plogmann B, Burger M, Korber J, Schmidt FW. Energy expenditure and substrate oxidation in patients with cirrhosis: The impact of cause, clinical staging and nutritional state. *Hepatology*. 1992;15(5):782-794.
90. Muller MJ, Bottcher J, Selberg O, et al. Hypermetabolism in clinically stable patients with liver cirrhosis. *Am J Clin Nutr*. 1999;69(6):1194-1201.
91. McClave SA, Taylor BE, Martindale RG, et al. Guidelines for the provision and assessment of nutrition support therapy in the adult critically ill patient: Society of Critical Care Medicine (SCCM) and American Society for Parenteral and Enteral Nutrition (A.S.P.E.N.). *JPEN J Parenter Enteral Nutr*. 2016;40(2):159-211.
92. Glass C, Hipskind P, Cole D, Lopez R, Dasarathy S. Handheld calorimeter is a valid instrument to quantify resting energy expenditure in hospitalized cirrhotic patients: A prospective study. *Nutr Clin Pract*. 2012;27(5):677-688.
93. Hipskind P, Glass C, Charlton D, Nowak D, Dasarathy S. Do handheld calorimeters have a role in assessment of nutrition needs in hospitalized patients? A systematic review of literature. *Nutr Clin Pract*. 2011;26(4):426-433.
94. Johnson TM, Overgard EB, Cohen AE, DiBaise JK. Nutrition assessment and management in advanced liver disease. *Nutr Clin Pract*. 2013;28(1):15-29.
95. Morgan TR, Moritz TE, Mendenhall CL, Haas R. Protein consumption and hepatic encephalopathy in alcoholic hepatitis. VA cooperative study group #275. *J Am Coll Nutr*. 1995;14(2):152-158.
96. Cordoba J, Lopez-Hellin J, Planas M, et al. Normal protein diet for episodic hepatic encephalopathy: Results of a randomized study. *J Hepatol*. 2004;41(1):38-43.
97. Cabral CM, Burns DL. Low-protein diets for hepatic encephalopathy debunked: Let them eat steak. *Nutr Clin Pract*. 2011;26(2):155-159.
98. Bianchi GP, Marchesini G, Fabbri A, et al. Vegetable versus animal protein diet in cirrhotic patients with chronic encephalopathy. A randomized cross-over comparison. *J Intern Med*. 1993;233(5):385-392.
99. Gheorghe L, Iacob R, Vadan R, Iacob S, Gheorghe C. Improvement of hepatic encephalopathy using a modified high-calorie high-protein diet. *Rom J Gastroenterol*. 2005;14(3):231-238.
100. Yadav A, Carey EJ. Osteoporosis in chronic liver disease. *Nutr Clin Pract*. 2013;28(1):52-64.
101. Arteh J, Narra S, Nair S. Prevalence of vitamin D deficiency in chronic liver disease. *Dig Dis Sci*. 2010;55(9):2624-2628.
102. Holick MF, Binkley NC, Bischoff-Ferrari HA, et al. Evaluation, treatment, and prevention of vitamin D deficiency: An endocrine society clinical practice guideline. *J Clin Endocrinol Metab*. 2011;96(7):1911-1930.
103. Targher G, Bertolini L, Scala L, et al. Associations between serum 25-hydroxyvitamin D3 concentrations and liver histology in patients with non-alcoholic fatty liver disease. *Nutrition, Metabolism and Cardiovascular Diseases*. 2007;17(7):517-524.
104. Kasapoglu B, Turkay C, Yalcin KS, Carlioglu A, Sozen M, Koktener A. Low vitamin D levels are associated with increased risk for fatty liver disease among non-obese adults. *Clin Med*. 2013;13(6):576-579.
105. Trépo E, Ouziel R, Pradat P, et al. Marked 25-hydroxyvitamin D deficiency is associated with poor prognosis in patients with alcoholic liver disease. *J Hepatol*. 2013;59(2):344-350.
106. Stokes CS, Krawczyk M, Reichel C, Lammert F, Grunhage F. Vitamin D deficiency is associated with mortality in patients with advanced liver cirrhosis. *Eur J Clin Invest*. 2013.
107. Rode A, Fourlanos S, Nicoll A. Oral vitamin D replacement is effective in chronic liver disease. *Gastroenterol Clin Biol*. 2010;34(11):618-620.
108. Yoshida Y, Higashi T, Nouso K, et al. Effects of zinc deficiency/zinc supplementation on ammonia metabolism in patients with decompensated liver cirrhosis. *Acta Med Okayama*. 2001;55(6):349-355.

109. Rabbani P, Prasad AS. Plasma ammonia and liver ornithine transcarbamoylase activity in zinc-deficient rats. *Am J Physiol*. 1978;235(2):E203-6.

110. Riggio O, Merli M, Capocaccia L, et al. Zinc supplementation reduces blood ammonia and increases liver ornithine transcarbamylase activity in experimental cirrhosis. *Hepatology*. 1992;16(3):785-789.

111. Prasad AS, Rabbani P, Abbasii A, Bowersox E, Fox MR. Experimental zinc deficiency in humans. *Ann Intern Med*. 1978;89(4):483-490.

112. Rahelic D, Kujundzic M, Romic Z, Brkic K, Petrovecki M. Serum concentration of zinc, copper, manganese and magnesium in patients with liver cirrhosis. *Coll Antropol*. 2006;30(3):523-528.

113. Chetri K, Choudhuri G. Role of trace elements in hepatic encephalopathy: Zinc and manganese. *Indian J Gastroenterol*. 2003;22 Suppl 2:S28-30.

114. Chavez-Tapia NC, Cesar-Arce A, Barrientos-Gutierrez T, Villegas-Lopez FA, Mendez-Sanchez N, Uribe M. A systematic review and meta-analysis of the use of oral zinc in the treatment of hepatic encephalopathy. *Nutr J*. 2013;12:74-2891-12-74.

115. Reding P, Duchateau J, Bataille C. Oral zinc supplementation improves hepatic encephalopathy. results of a randomised controlled trial. *Lancet*. 1984;2(8401):493-495.

116. Hayashi M, Ikezawa K, Ono A, et al. Evaluation of the effects of combination therapy with branched-chain amino acid and zinc supplements on nitrogen metabolism in liver cirrhosis. *Hepatol Res*. 2007;37(8):615-619.

117. Bresci G, Parisi G, Banti S. Management of hepatic encephalopathy with oral zinc supplementation: A long-term treatment. *Eur J Med*. 1993;2(7):414-416.

118. Takuma Y, Nouso K, Makino Y, Hayashi M, Takahashi H. Clinical trial: Oral zinc in hepatic encephalopathy. *Aliment Pharmacol Ther*. 2010;32(9):1080-1090.

119. Prasad AS. Zinc: Role in immunity, oxidative stress and chronic inflammation. *Curr Opin Clin Nutr Metab Care*. 2009;12(6):646-652.

120. Matsumura H, Nirei K, Nakamura H, et al. Zinc supplementation therapy improves the outcome of patients with chronic hepatitis C. *J Clin Biochem Nutr*. 2012;51(3):178-184.

121. Prasad AS. Clinical manifestations of zinc deficiency. *Annu Rev Nutr*. 1985;5:341-363.

122. Allan JG, Fell GS, Russell RI. Urinary zinc in hepatic cirrhosis. *Scott Med J*. 1975;20(3):109-111.

123. Chiba M, Katayama K, Takeda R, et al. Diuretics aggravate zinc deficiency in patients with liver cirrhosis by increasing zinc excretion in urine. *Hepatol Res*. 2013;43(4):365-373.

124. Zarski JP, Arnaud J, Dumolard L, Favier A, Rachail M. Trace elements (zinc, copper, manganese) in alcoholic cirrhosis: Effect of chronic alcoholism. *Gastroenterol Clin Biol*. 1985;9(10):664-669.

125. Tsien CD, McCullough AJ, Dasarathy S. Late evening snack: Exploiting a period of anabolic opportunity in cirrhosis. *J Gastroenterol Hepatol*. 2012;27(3):430-441.

126. Chang WK, Chao YC, Tang HS, Lang HF, Hsu CT. Effects of extra-carbohydrate supplementation in the late evening on energy expenditure and substrate oxidation in patients with liver cirrhosis. *JPEN J Parenter Enteral Nutr*. 1997;21(2):96-99.

127. Yamanaka-Okumura H, Nakamura T, Takeuchi H, et al. Effect of late evening snack with rice ball on energy metabolism in liver cirrhosis. *Eur J Clin Nutr*. 2006;60(9):1067-1072.

128. Hou W, Li J, Lu J, et al. Effect of a carbohydrate-containing late-evening snack on energy metabolism and fasting substrate utilization in adults with acute-on-chronic liver failure due to hepatitis B. *Eur J Clin Nutr*. 2013;67(12):1251-1256.

129. Nakaya Y, Harada N, Kakui S, et al. Severe catabolic state after prolonged fasting in cirrhotic patients: Effect of oral branched-chain amino-acid-enriched nutrient mixture. *J Gastroenterol*. 2002;37(7):531-536.

130. Nakaya Y, Okita K, Suzuki K, et al. BCAA-enriched snack improves nutritional state of cirrhosis. *Nutrition*. 2007;23(2):113-120.

131. Baldwin C, Weekes CE. Dietary advice with or without oral nutritional supplements for disease-related malnutrition in adults. *Cochrane Database Syst Rev*. 2011;(9):CD002008. doi(9):CD002008.

132. Qureshi MO, Khokhar N, Saleem A, Niazi TK. Correlation of hyponatremia with hepatic encephalopathy and severity of liver disease. *J Coll Physicians Surg Pak*. 2014;24(2):135-137.

133. Umemura T, Shibata S, Sekiguchi T, et al. Serum sodium concentration is associated with increased risk of mortality in patients with compensated liver cirrhosis. *Hepatol Res*. 2015;45(7):739-744

134. Heuman DM, Abou-Assi SG, Habib A, et al. Persistent ascites and low serum sodium identify patients with cirrhosis and low MELD scores who are at high risk for early death. *Hepatology*. 2004;40(4):802-810.

135. Hayaishi S, Chung H, Kudo M, et al. Oral branched-chain amino acid granules reduce the incidence of hepatocellular carcinoma and improve event-free survival in patients with liver cirrhosis. *Dig Dis*. 2011;29(3):326-332.

136. Muto Y, Sato S, Watanabe A, et al. Effects of oral branched-chain amino acid granules on event-free survival in patients with liver cirrhosis. *Clin Gastroenterol Hepatol*. 2005;3(7):705-713.

137. Norman K, Valentini L, Lochs H, Pirlich M. Protein catabolism and malnutrition in liver cirrhosis - impact of oral nutritional therapy. *Z Gastroenterol*. 2010;48(7):763-770.

138. Hebuterne X, Vanbiervliet G. Feeding the patients with upper gastrointestinal bleeding. *Curr Opin Clin Nutr Metab Care*. 2011;14(2):197-201.

139. Plauth M, Schuetz T. Working group for developing the guidelines for parenteral nutrition of The German Association for Nutritional Medicine. Hepatology - guidelines on parenteral nutrition, chapter 16. *Ger Med Sci*. 2009;7:Doc12.

140. Minicucci MF, Azevedo PS, Paiva SA. Parenteral branched-chain amino acids for hepatic encephalopathy. what is the grade of recommendation? *Clin Nutr*. 2011;30(1):131; author reply 132.

141. Naylor CD, O'Rourke K, Detsky AS, Baker JP. Parenteral nutrition with branched-chain amino acids in hepatic encephalopathy. A meta-analysis. *Gastroenterology*. 1989;97(4):1033-1042.

142. Als-Nielsen B, Koretz RL, Kjaergard LL, Gluud C. Branched-chain amino acids for hepatic encephalopathy. *Cochrane Database Syst Rev*. 2003;(2)(2):CD001939.

143. Yarandi SS, Zhao VM, Hebbar G, Ziegler TR. Amino acid composition in parenteral nutrition: What is the evidence? *Curr Opin Clin Nutr Metab Care*. 2011;14(1):75-82.

144. Rivera-Mancia S, Rios C, Montes S. Manganese accumulation in the CNS and associated pathologies. *Biometals*. 2011;24(5):811-825.

Chapter 16

Nutrition in Pulmonary Disease

Grace Phelan

Chapter Outline

Core Concepts
Introduction
Pulmonary Physiology in Health and Disease
Acute Respiratory Distress Syndrome
Nutrition Support and Pulmonary Disease
Immunonutrition
Micronutrients
Quality of Life and Psychosocial Support

CORE CONCEPTS

1. In chronic obstructive pulmonary disease (COPD), weight status correlates with hospital outcomes.
2. Prolonged mechanical ventilation in conjunction with the inflammatory cascade cast by acute respiratory distress syndrome (ARDS) puts patients at risk for lean body mass (LBM) catabolism, including that of the diaphragm and other respiratory muscles.
3. Oxidant-antioxidant imbalance is ubiquitous in many pulmonary diseases, emphasizing the importance of an antioxidant-rich diet.
4. Malnourished individuals have described greater levels of fatigue and scored higher on depression scales.

Learning Objectives

1. Describe the metabolic changes caused by pulmonary disease and cachexia.
2. Recognize the factors that influence the nutritional risk and impact the nutrition status in a patient with chronic obstructive pulmonary disease.
3. Explain the integral role nutrition plays on quality of life in people with pulmonary disease.
4. Identify strategies for weight maintenance in end-stage chronic obstructive pulmonary disease.
5. Formulate appropriate enteral and parenteral nutrition recommendations in the setting of pulmonary disease.
6. Identify specialty enteral nutrition and micronutrients in patients with acute respiratory distress syndrome.

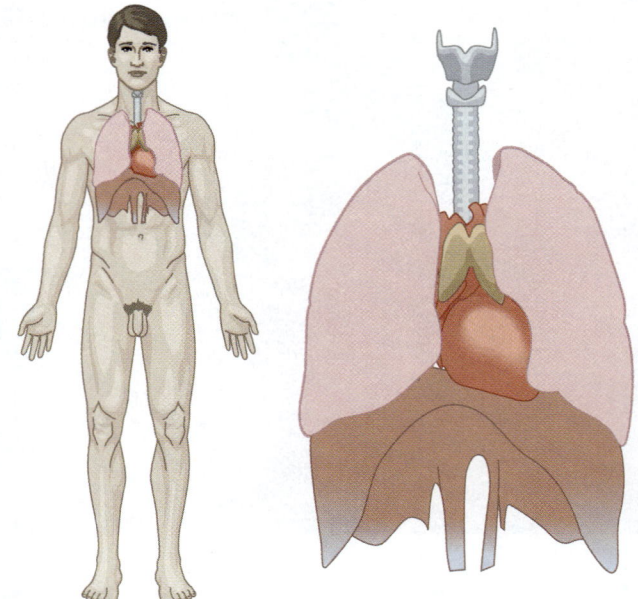

FIGURE 16.1 Respiratory System

Introduction

Pulmonary diseases, such as asthma and chronic obstructive pulmonary disease, are the third leading cause of death in the United States, with approximately 13% of the adult population carrying a diagnosis of chronic bronchitis, emphysema, or asthma.[1,2] Early nutrition intervention is essential for optimal health in the presence of pulmonary disease. Nutrition strategies play an important role in the treatment of certain pulmonary diseases and conditions.

Pulmonary Physiology in Health and Disease

The pulmonary system's primary role is gas exchange, delivering oxygen to the bloodstream and ridding the body of excess carbon dioxide. Air travels through the trachea, bronchi, and bronchioles to the lungs during inspiration (**Figure 16.1**). Oxygen is then delivered to the heart via pulmonary circulation, and excess carbon dioxide later returns to the lungs for expiration. In health, these organs are supported primarily by the diaphragm and intercostal muscles. In the presence of pulmonary disease, accessory muscles, namely the sternocleidomastoid, scalene and abdominal muscles, may be recruited for sufficient gas exchange.[3]

Asthma

Asthma is a chronic inflammatory disease of the lungs characterized by periods of reversible airflow limitation and airway hyperresponsiveness. Symptoms commonly include shortness of breath, wheezing, coughing, and chest tightness. There is no cure for asthma, so treatment targets symptom management (**Figure 16.2**). Overweight and obesity are modifiable risk factors for asthma, with a dose-response effect as body mass index (BMI) increases.[4] No change in diet composition or quality has consistently improved clinical outcomes. Energy restriction leading to weight loss of at least 7.5% in subjects with excess fat mass may improve lung function, quality of life, and disease morbidity.[5-7] Consequently, it is recommended that lifestyle change aimed at healthy weight reduction be considered for overweight and obese individuals with asthma.

Chronic Obstructive Pulmonary Disease

Chronic obstructive pulmonary disease (COPD) is a progressive, systemic disease marked by airflow obstruction. Generally, the term COPD encompasses

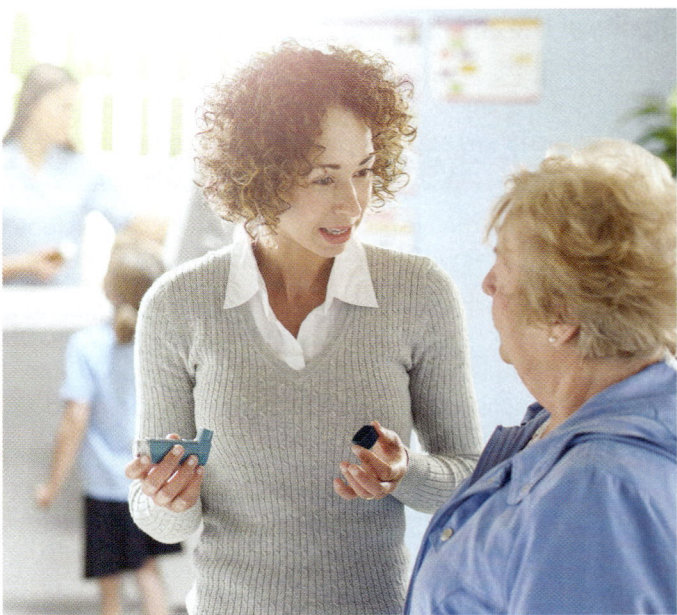

FIGURE 16.2 Patient Learning to Use an Inhaler
© sturti/ E+/Getty Images.

CASE STUDY INTRODUCTION

Leigh is a 79-year-old woman with end-stage chronic obstructive pulmonary disease (COPD) who presents to nutrition clinic with complaints of a 15-pound unintentional weight loss over 3 months due to decreased oral intake over that time period. She is widowed with two adult children. Her daughter and son-in-law live across town and her son lives out of state. She has a history of smoking but quit during her first pregnancy. She denies alcohol use. She appears dyspneic and is unable to speak in complete sentences.

Anthropometric Data:
Weight: 63.6 kg (140 lbs)
Height: 170 cm (67")
BMI: 22 kg/m^2
Weight History
Usual body weight: 71 kg (155 lbs) 3 months ago
Weight at diagnosis 3 years ago: 89 kg (195 lbs)
Leigh has sustained a gradual decline in weight over the last several years since diagnosis.

Biochemical Data:
Sodium 142 (135-145 mEq/L)
Potassium 4.4 (3.6-5.0 mEq/L)
Chloride 96 (98-110 mEq/L)
Carbon dioxide 33 (20-30 mEq/L)
Blood urea nitrogen 18 (6-24 mg/dL)
Creatinine 1.1 (0.4-1.3 mg/dL)
Glucose 117 (70-99 mg/dL)

Arterial blood gases (ABG)
pH 7.09 (7.35-7.45)
$PaCO_2$ 97 (35-45 mm Hg)
PaO_2 72 (85-105 mm Hg)
HCO_3^- 35 (21-28 mEq/L)

Clinical Data:
Past Medical History: COPD, hypertension
Medications: budesonide/formoterol inhaled daily, ipratropium/albuterol as needed
Vital Signs: Blood pressure 170/88 mm Hg, Temperature 98.6 °F, Heart rate 60 beats/min
Nutrition-focused Physical Exam: Leigh appears pale with mild peripheral muscle wasting, including temporal muscle wasting, and loose skin noted on arms. Oral exam notable for dry oral mucosa and cracked lips, good dentition, and normal tongue. Skin appears dry. Significant shortness of breath at rest and exacerbated with conversation and activity noted.

Dietary Data:
Dietary History: Leigh follows a low-sodium diet but often relies on prepackaged meals due to her decreased functional capacity.
Diet Prescription: Low sodium, small frequent meals, limit fluid to between meals

Questions
1. What are Leigh's nutritional risk factors?
2. Does Leigh have malnutrition? What factors explain her weight loss?
3. What additional information would you like to obtain?
4. How would you interpret Leigh's labs, specifically her ABG labs?

---

chronic bronchitis, emphysema, and small airways disease, though not all cases of these diseases fit the specific diagnostic criteria outlined by the Global Initiative for Chronic Obstructive Lung Disease, which requires confirmation by **spirometry**, a pulmonary function test that measures how well lungs work by quantifying the amount of air inhaled and exhaled.[8] Chronic inflammation of the airways, parenchyma, and pulmonary vasculature is characteristic of COPD and leads to tissue damage. Symptoms commonly include chronic cough, sputum production, and **dyspnea**, or difficulty breathing on exertion. Patients tend to experience shortness of breath during basic activities of daily living at advanced stages of the disease. In particular, activities engaging upper extremities pose a greater respiratory challenge than those involving lower extremities.[9]

Oxidative stress has been implicated in the respiratory muscle dysfunction characteristic of severe COPD.[10] Cigarette smoking is the predominant risk factor for the development of COPD, although genetic predisposition accounts for a small percentage of cases. Occupational exposure and air pollution have also been identified as risk factors.[11] Patients with COPD are more likely than those without COPD to have comorbid conditions such as hypertension, cardiovascular disease, diabetes mellitus, osteoporosis, and metabolic syndrome.[12-14] Cognitive dysfunction frequently parallels COPD and is likely multifactorial in nature owing to poor sleep, increased fatigue, depression, and other factors.[15]

Treatment goals are to improve symptoms, slow progression of disease, and improve physical endurance. Strategies to achieve these goals include smoking cessation for smokers and oxygen therapy for hypoxemic individuals. Lung volume reduction surgery is an option in select cases of emphysema. Pharmacologic therapies are commonly used to alleviate symptoms and are shown in **Table 16.1**. Pulmonary rehabilitation is an effective strategy to improve symptoms and decrease disease exacerbations and hospital admissions.

Particularly in advanced stages of disease, and during disease exacerbations, patients with COPD demonstrate a marked increase in basal energy expenditure and

TABLE 16.1 CLASSES OF DRUGS USED IN THE TREATMENT OF CHRONIC OBSTRUCTIVE PULMONARY DISEASE[16]

Drug Class	Mechanism of Action	Nutritional Considerations
Antimuscarinics (anticholinergic agents) Examples • Short-acting: ipratropium bromide • Long-acting: tiotropium	Block the bronchoconstricting effects of acetylcholine on M3 muscarinic receptors in airway smooth muscle	• Tiotropium contains lactose, may contain milk proteins • May cause constipation, taste changes, nausea, vomiting, dyspepsia, xerostomia, or hypokalemia • Caffeine may result in tremor or mild heart rate elevation in those taking albuterol
Bronchodilators (β-2 adrenergic agents [agonists]) Examples: • Short-acting: albuterol • Long-acting: salmeterol	Increase FEV_1 and/or change other spirometric variables; relax airway smooth muscle	• Albuterol and salmeterol contain lactose, may contain milk proteins • Caffeine may result in tremor or mild heart rate elevation • May influence appetite • May cause taste changes, nausea, or dyspepsia
Inhaled corticosteroids Examples: budesonide, fluticasone		• Budesonide and fluticasone contain lactose, may contain milk proteins • May cause taste changes or nausea • Calcium supplements, milk, magnesium hydroxide, or antacids may interfere with enteric coated products due to the influence on pH • Sodium or potassium salts may cause hypernatremia or fluid retention • Echinacea may interact adversely with steroids
Methylxanthines Examples: aminophylline, theophylline	Mechanism of action is controversial	• Some theophylline may be manufactured using corn or corn products • Caffeine may increase symptoms of nausea, irritability, and nervousness • May cause diarrhea, gastroesophageal reflux, hypercalcemia, hypokalemia, and vomiting • Charcoal may decrease drug effectiveness • St. John's Wort may increase metabolism of drug

catabolism.[17] On average resting energy expenditure (REE) is elevated by 15% to 25% in the setting of pulmonary disease,[18-20] but has been quoted to increase REE by up to 45%.[21] Hypermetabolism is consistently greater in COPD patients with weight loss as compared with those of stable weight.[22-25] In healthy subjects, energy expenditure of respiration usually amounts to <3% of resting energy needs.[26] The increased work of breathing exhibited by patients with COPD can increase the total amount of energy used for respiration. Nevertheless increased work of breathing does not appear to be solely responsible for the elevation in energy expenditure.[27] Plasma cytokines and other inflammatory markers have been positively associated with REE independent of airway obstruction or work of breathing, suggesting inflammation as an etiology of hypermetabolism.[28-30] Given the wide variation of REE related to disease stage and individual body composition, indirect calorimetry is the recommended energy assessment tool when available. Though REE is elevated with pulmonary disease, one study found that total daily energy expenditure (TEE) remained similar to that of healthy controls.[31] Total daily energy expenditure was also similar between COPD patients with and without elevated REE.[32] The likely explanation for these findings is a reduction in physical activity resulting from increased fatigue and decreased endurance.

PRACTICE POINT

Resting energy expenditure (REE) is elevated by 15% to 25% in the setting of pulmonary disease.

Body Composition

Weight status correlates with hospital outcomes. Patients with COPD and malnutrition have an increased risk of hospital readmission and in-hospital mortality, whereas obese patients with COPD are less likely to be readmitted or die compared to their normal weight counterparts.[33,34] While these data are interesting, it is unlikely that weight has a linear relationship on COPD mortality. Copenhagen City Heart Study data found improved outcomes in patients with severe COPD as BMI increased. However, a nonsignificant U-shaped curve was found in patients with mild to moderate COPD.

CORE CONCEPT 1

In chronic obstructive pulmonary disease (COPD), weight status correlates with hospital outcomes.

The protective effect of obesity demonstrated in some studies should be interpreted with caution. Obesity plays a role in the development of several comorbidities including, but not limited to, cardiovascular disease, diabetes, certain malignancies, and functional and respiratory impairments.[35] Weight gain has been shown to worsen overall health status in obese smokers,[36] and there are clear data associating obesity and dyspnea.[37] National Health and Nutrition Examination Survey (NHANES) data have linked extreme obesity with an increased risk of death from a respiratory condition.[38] Similarly, excess abdominal visceral fat has been associated with an increase in all-cause mortality stemming from increased interleukin-6 (IL-6).[39] There are no specific recommendations regarding intentional weight loss in overweight or obese subpopulations with COPD.

PRACTICE POINT

Given the substantial body of evidence in support of achieving a healthy weight to prevent chronic disease, nutritional management of individuals with mild to moderate COPD should be centered on achieving a healthy weight.

In contrast, individuals with advanced COPD may lose lean body mass (LBM) over time and experience muscle wasting with or without weight loss. Metabolically there is

CASE STUDY REVISITED

After a few minutes, Leigh catches her breath and manages to report the following diet information:

24-hour Diet Recall:
10am Breakfast: 12 oz coffee with milk and 1-2 pieces of dry wheat toast, occasionally a banana
1pm Lunch: 16 oz water and a frozen dinner, usually baked ziti or pasta primavera
7pm Dinner: 16 oz water and a frozen dinner, usually lasagna or chicken stir fry

Questions
1. How would you assess Leigh's current intake?
2. How does Leigh's weight status impact her COPD outcome?
3. What strategies can you offer Leigh to prevent further weight loss?

a tendency to lose LBM preferentially, a syndrome called cachexia. This is noteworthy, because LBM is independently prognostic of mortality, regardless of fat mass.[40] In a study of 101 patients with COPD, those patients with COPD were noted to have greater visceral fat area than 62 control patients. Excess fat mass did not decline with greater severity of disease.[41] Furthermore, respiratory muscle strength has been correlated with weight and lean body mass.[42,43]

Pharmacologic options to increase weight and LBM have been investigated. Megestrol acetate effectively increases weight, but as additional fat mass.[44] Patients with COPD provided with anabolic steroids (oxandrolone, nandrolone, and testosterone) gain weight and lean body mass.[45-49] Further study should seek to evaluate the target population of patients that benefit, the potential adverse effects, and what duration and dosing regimen will provide the greatest yield on desired parameters.[50] Preliminary data support the use of β-hydroxy β-methylbutyrate (HMB), a metabolite of the branched chain amino acid leucine, to preserve strength and muscle mass in a variety of populations, including elderly, critically ill, HIV-positive, and cancer patients.[51-55] This research provides a framework for use of HMB in pulmonary disease. One short-term study conducted in COPD patients in the intensive care unit achieved anti-inflammatory and anticatabolic effects and improved pulmonary function in subjects provided HMB.[56] Further study is needed to substantiate efficacy and clinical significance in patients with pulmonary disease.

Nutrition Intervention

In the past, studies providing oral nutrition-supplement drinks to patients with COPD have shown mixed results. However, recent data have resolved in support of nutrition supplementation to improve outcomes such as increased respiratory and limb muscle strength and weight gain, with greater benefits realized by malnourished subjects.[57,58] Dietary counseling by a registered dietitian improves intake and maintains body composition in subjects with COPD.[59] COPD patients who are physically active generally have greater LBM than those who are not physically active.[60] Nutrition supplementation in conjunction with a rehabilitation program promotes greater gain of weight and fat-free mass and can offset the increase in energy expenditure due to increased physical activity.[61,62]

There are a number of barriers preventing adequate dietary intake for people with compromised respiratory performance. Frequently these cause early satiety or physical exhaustion. For example, use of continuous positive airway pressure, eating too quickly, and consumption of carbonated beverages can cause **aerophagia**, or excessive swallowing of air. This can create the sensation of fullness, which ultimately lessens appetite and overall food intake. Likewise, any exertion at or around mealtimes by individuals with low pulmonary reserve will affect overall consumption. There are many strategies that can improve intake under these circumstances. Adequate fluid intake is useful to thin mucus produced in COPD. It is also important to note that, for some, liquids ingested with meals can preclude adequate energy and protein intake. In this case, drinking water or other fluids between meals may be helpful. Small frequent meals, four to six times daily, can support those who feel full with larger volumes. This tactic may also reduce mealtime exhaustion. Resting prior to mealtimes is another option to boost mealtime endurance. Consuming more food earlier in the day may be a useful approach for people who find themselves too tired to eat later in the day. Some individuals find softer foods and liquids less demanding than foods requiring a lot of chewing, so modified consistencies and/or oral nutrition-supplement drinks may be merited.

For some patients, the ability to procure groceries and prepare meals can be an obstacle. Community food programs and social support systems are valuable resources to help narrow the nutrition gap caused by impaired functional status and endurance. Services and qualifications (e.g., age, income) will vary by state and community.

Clinical Roundtable

Topic: Weight status in COPD

Background: The role of obesity in COPD is complex. The correlation between weight and hospital outcomes in these patients is well established. In the early stages of COPD, obesity increases risk of comorbidities such as diabetes and cardiovascular disease. In the later stages of the disease, obese patients have better outcomes such as lower rates of hospital readmissions and death. Despite this, there are no recommendations for weight loss in obese individuals with COPD. When treating patients with COPD, clinicians are tasked with the weighing the advantages and disadvantages of current weight status.

Roundtable Discussion

Consider the relationship of weight in COPD.

1. What would be the advantages and disadvantages of recommending weight loss in the COPD patient?
2. What factors would you consider when deciding to prioritize weight management in this population?
3. How might you monitor a COPD patient who is losing weight?

References

1. Zapatero A, Barba R, Ruiz J, et al. Malnutrition and obesity: Influence in mortality and readmissions in chronic obstructive pulmonary disease patients. *J Hum Nutr Diet*. 2013;26:16-22

Acute Respiratory Distress Syndrome

Acute respiratory distress syndrome (ARDS) is a type of hypoxemic respiratory failure accounting for at least 10% of inpatient admissions to the intensive care unit and carrying a high in-hospital mortality rate.[63] ARDS is characterized by acute development of bilateral lung infiltrates that are visible on chest x-ray (**Figures 16.3** and **16.4**), an arterial oxygen tension to fraction of inspired oxygen ratio (PaO_2/FiO_2) less than 300 mm Hg, and a systemic inflammatory response.[64] Diagnosis can also be supported by a pulmonary artery wedge pressure less than 18 mm Hg. Common causes of ARDS are listed in **Table 16.2**. Severity of disease is stratified into mild, moderate, and severe, with PaO_2/FiO_2 ranges of 200 to ≤300 mm Hg, 100 to ≤200 mg Hg, and ≤100 mm Hg, respectively.[65] Treatment for ARDS includes mechanical ventilation and oxygenation strategies to address **hypoxemia**, or low blood oxygen; fluid restriction and diuretic therapy to control edema; and management of acidosis.

Attention to the nutritional status of patients with ARDS is paramount to achieve successful clinical outcomes. Because nutrition is integral to optimal pulmonary function,[66] timely nutrient provision plays a vital role in the management of the patient with ARDS. The critically ill ARDS patient often suffers from other comorbidities and organ failures. Secondary diagnoses, along with medications used to treat these conditions, make it difficult to estimate energy needs. Indirect calorimetry should be used to measure energy expenditure when available; however, respiratory instability often limits the

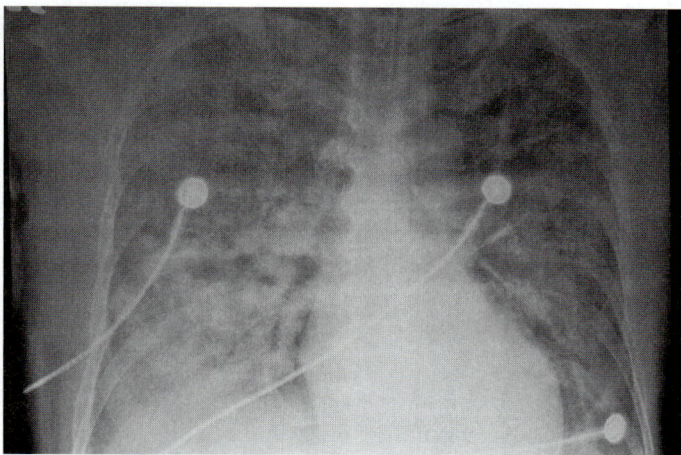

FIGURE 16.3 Chest X-ray of a Patient with ARDS

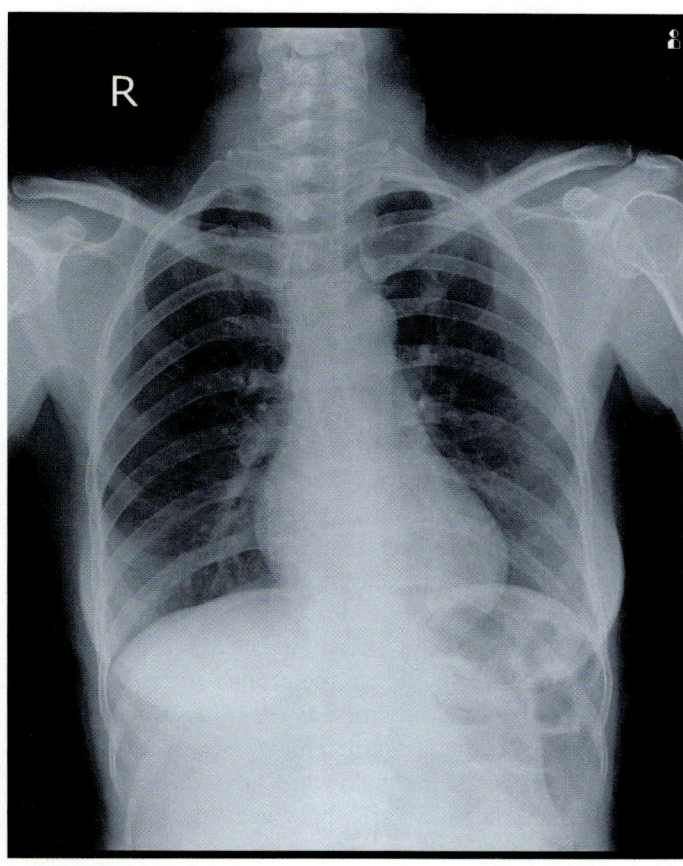

FIGURE 16.4 Normal Chest X-ray

TABLE 16.2 CAUSES OF ACUTE RESPIRATORY DISTRESS SYNDROME

Direct Lung Injury
Aspiration of gastric contents
Inhalation of toxic substances
Near drowning
Pneumonia
Pulmonary contusion
Indirect Lung Injury
Cardiopulmonary bypass
Drug overdose
Pancreatitis
Repeated blood transfusions
Sepsis
Severe trauma

> ### CASE STUDY REVISITED
>
> Leigh is admitted to the hospital 6 months later with a COPD exacerbation. Upon admission, she reports that her weight has been stable for the past 6 months. After a brief stay, she is discharged home only to be readmitted a month later with another COPD exacerbation. During this admission, she is intubated for respiratory failure requiring ventilator support and transferred to the intensive care unit. A nasoenteric tube is placed and the medical team requests enteral nutrition recommendations.
>
> **Anthropometrics:**
> Weight: 60.2 kg (132.4 lbs)
> Last admission weight (6 months ago): 63.6 kg (140 lbs)
>
> #### Questions
> 1. How would you address Leigh's nutrition status?
> 2. How would you assess her energy needs?
> 3. What type of formula would you recommend for Leigh while she is intubated?
> 4. What data would you consider in making this decision?

feasibility of obtaining good quality studies. Mechanical ventilation set to a FiO_2 greater than 60% and/or positive end expiratory pressure (PEEP) greater than 12 cm H_2O will reduce study accuracy.[67] Additionally, hyper- and hypoventilation will prevent attainment of a "steady state," thereby yielding indeterminable results. The Penn State Equation has been validated for use in critically ill mechanically ventilated patients and is an appropriate substitution when indirect calorimetry cannot be performed. Recommended protein intakes for critically ill patients with a BMI <30 kg/m² is between 1.2 g/kg and 2.0 g/kg actual body weight.[68]

> ### CORE CONCEPT 2
> Prolonged mechanical ventilation in conjunction with the inflammatory cascade cast by ARDS puts patients at risk for lean body mass (LBM) catabolism, including that of the diaphragm and other respiratory muscles.

> ### PRACTICE POINT
> Indirect calorimetry is the gold standard for determining energy requirements. When unavailable, the Penn State Equation should be used.

Nutrition Support and Pulmonary Disease

The American Society for Parenteral and Enteral Nutrition 2016 Clinical Guidelines advise the use of a concentrated enteral formula for patients with acute respiratory failure requiring nutrition support that would benefit from fluid restriction.[68] Fluid buildup and pulmonary edema in this population are common and associated with poor clinical outcomes. Accumulation of carbon dioxide in diseased lungs can further impair pulmonary function. Attention has been placed previously on carbohydrate intake because its metabolism generates more carbon dioxide relative to protein and fat. Carbohydrate restriction has not been demonstrated to improve ventilation when compared to provision of a normal distribution of macronutrients within calorie needs. Because carbon dioxide is a byproduct of energy substrate metabolism, it is important to avoid overfeeding, evidence of which can include unexplained hyperglycemia and an ABG revealing an elevated $PaCO_2$.[67]

> ### PRACTICE POINT
> Because carbon dioxide is a byproduct of energy substrate metabolism, it is important to avoid overfeeding.

Customarily, patients rest supine and are fed enterally in conjunction with standard aspiration precautions, including head of bed elevation, confirmation of tube placement, and monitoring for respiratory and abdominal signs of intolerance. ARDS treatment may incorporate prone positioning—lying face down—in select cases to alleviate pressure put on the dorsal lungs by ventral organs to improve gas exchange.[69] Though data are limited, enteral nutrition appears to be safe in the prone patient. It does not appear to significantly increase vomiting, pneumonia, or gastric residuals compared to supine feeding.[70,71] Elevating the head of bed by reverse Trendelenberg positioning, where the body is flat but the head is 15 degrees to 30 degrees higher than the feet; prokinetic agents; and postpyloric feeding with or without gastric decompression may be used to optimize success of enteral nutrition (**Figure 16.5**). Institutional protocols may be helpful to

⚠ Clinical Controversy

Optimal Macronutrient Content of Enteral Feeding in COPD

Manipulation of macronutrients in the management of pulmonary disease has been a topic of discussion for several years. Pulmonary-specific enteral formulas have been designed to provide a higher fat and lower carbohydrate ratio due to the potential impact of carbon dioxide generation by carbohydrate. In one study of mechanically ventilated patients, a high fat, low carbohydrate diet resulted in decreased arterial carbon dioxide tension, improved minute volume and fewer days on ventilation. However, this result is not a consistent finding, and research exists showing no clear benefit to use of disease specific enteral formula in critically ill patients with hyperglycemia. Excessive fat intake can have implications for gastrointestinal tolerance, inflammation and cell dynamics. In addition, critically ill patients may also be receiving lipid-based sedatives, such as propofol, which further increases fat intake. These factors should be weighed against the strength of evidence in support of a high fat, low carbohydrate.

1. Based upon this research, discuss the potential risks and benefits of providing a high-fat, low-carbohydrate enteral formula to pulmonary patients.
2. What factors might you consider in determining if a patient would benefit from a higher-fat diet?

References

1. Faramawy MA, Allah AA, Batrawy SL, Amer H. Impact of high fat low carbohydrate enteral feeding on weaning from mechanical ventilation. *Egyptian Journal of Chest Diseases and Tuberculosis*. 2014;63:931-938.
2. Mesejo A, Acosta JA, Ortega C, et al. Comparison of a high-protein disease-specific enteral formula with a high-protein enteral formula in hyperglycemic critically ill patients. *Clin Nutr*. 2003;22(3):295-305).

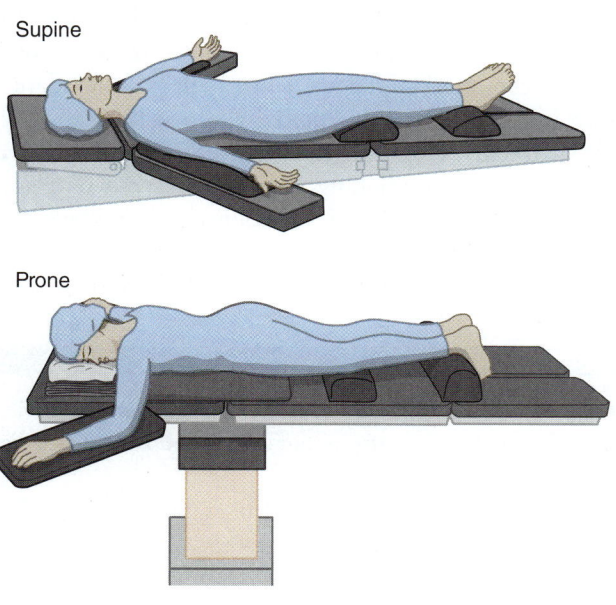

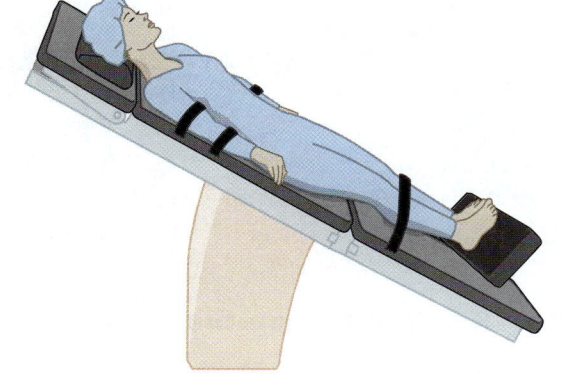

FIGURE 16.5 Supine Position/Prone Position/Reverse Trendelenburg Position

standardize provision and monitoring of enteral nutrition support of patients in the prone position.

Immunonutrition

Because ARDS is characterized by a profound inflammatory response, it theoretically makes sense to consider anti-inflammatory interventions, such as omega-3 polyunsaturated fatty acids, to modulate this process. Several research groups have evaluated the role of enteral formula enriched with eicosapentaenoic acid (EPA), γ-linolenic acid (GLA), and elevated amounts of antioxidants on respiratory outcomes in patients with ARDS.[72-74] This formula improved oxygenation and reduced ventilator days, ICU length of stay, and mortality compared to a control formula.[75] Other studies produced improvements in markers of pulmonary inflammation and oxygenation when patients received EPA and GLA.[76] Enteral diets were only different in fatty acid profile and antioxidant content in these studies.

Despite several studies in support of immune-modulating enteral nutrition, controversy exists. The macronutrient breakdown of the high-fat, low-carbohydrate control formula was comparable to that of the study formula; however, the amount of fat in these formulas exceeds that of a standard polymeric formula. This may be clinically significant because the type of fat in the control formula was predominantly omega-6 in contrast to the high-omega-3 formula provided to the study group. The omega-6 fatty acid arachidonic acid (ARA) is known to generate pro-inflammatory lipid mediators, whereas omega-3 fatty acids may help to reduce inflammation. The omega-3 fatty acids EPA and docosohexaenoic produce resolvins and protectins, which are lipid mediators that work to resolve the inflammatory response. The degree of benefit produced by the high omega-3 formula may be exaggerated by comparison to a formula with greater potential to produce more ARA.

Bolus feeding a supplement containing omega-3s, GLA, and antioxidants has not demonstrated a benefit on clinical outcomes either.[77] In fact, unexpectedly, one trial was terminated early for futility when an interim analysis found significantly better outcomes in the control group. Another failed to influence inflammatory biomarkers compared to a saline placebo, though it was not clear if enteral diets were comparable in each group.[78] It may be that modern day lung-protective ventilator strategies mask any benefit of immune-modulating nutrients.

Optimal dosing, timing, method of administration, and duration of enteral supplementation, or efficacy at all, remain unclear. Interventions have historically contained multiple nutrients, so it is undetermined which, if any, nutrient or nutrient combination influences each clinical outcome. No recommendation can be made at this time on the use of enteral formulas containing an anti-inflammatory lipid profile in patients with ARDS.[68]

Investigation into the role of various parenteral lipid emulsions on pulmonary variables in patients with ARDS has produced inconsistent results. Higher omega-6 fatty acid intakes generate more pro-inflammatory prostaglandins, leukotrienes, and thromboxanes, so they conceivably could have a negative effect on oxygenation. Alterations in various pulmonary parameters have been demonstrated in patients with ARDS receiving a 20% intravenous fat emulsion.[79] Some,[80,81] but not all,[82] studies displacing half of the long chain triglycerides (LCT) with medium chain triglycerides (MCT) did in fact result in improvements in various respiratory parameters, including oxygenation and mean pulmonary artery pressure. Other reports found no difference when comparing LCTs with a mixed LCT:MCT lipid emulsion. Intravenous infusion of omega-3 fatty acids did not improve outcomes in one study,[83] and in general there is no consensus on the use of intravenous omega-3 fatty acids due to limited and conflicting evidence.

One prospective trial reported anti-inflammatory effects and improved exercise tolerance in subjects who consumed an oral supplement rich in omega-3 fatty acids.[84] Epidemiologic evidence investigating the role of fish consumption on COPD has yielded inconsistent results.[85-87] Further evidence is required to make a definitive conclusion.

Micronutrients

Antioxidants

Cigarette smoking increases oxidative damage, thereby increasing the demand for vitamin C. As such, the Dietary Reference Intake for vitamin C is set at an additional 35 mg/day for smokers.[88] It is well-established that people with COPD have low blood levels of antioxidants.[89-91] Higher blood levels of vitamin C have been observed to have a protective effect on **forced expiratory volume (FEV$_1$)**, or the amount of air a person can exhale during forced breathing, in some,[92-95] but not all,[96] studies. Evidence in support of vitamin E to preserve FEV$_1$ is less, with higher vitamin E levels positively associated in one study,[96] but not others.[93,95,97] Vitamin A and several carotenoids also have been shown to protect FEV$_1$.[96-98]

Recognizing that an oxidant–antioxidant imbalance is ubiquitous in a number of pulmonary diseases, the hypothesis that antioxidant supplementation can influence respiratory outcomes is an area of interest for researchers. Various vitamins, carotenoids, and compounds have been studied in COPD and asthma, but intervention trials have rendered less-than-compelling results. A few small trials found positive effects of vitamins A, C, and/or E,[89,99,100] while others have not.[101-106] More study is needed to determine whether supplementation of a particular antioxidant or combination of nutrients at a certain dose and duration can positively affect clinically relevant respiratory parameters.

The importance of high-quality diets to pulmonary health cannot be understated (**Figure 16.6**). Even though intensive supplementation does not appear to prevent or improve respiratory outcomes, a diet high in antioxidants improves levels of vitamin E and β-carotene[99] and may be associated with better lung function.[107] Considering that oxidative damage from smoking and environmental exposures occurs over time, the significance of healthful dietary patterns over the course of a lifetime may produce more meaningful benefit, though this has yet to be investigated.

> **CORE CONCEPT 3**
>
> Oxidant–antioxidant imbalance is ubiquitous in many pulmonary diseases, emphasizing the importance of antioxidant-rich diet.

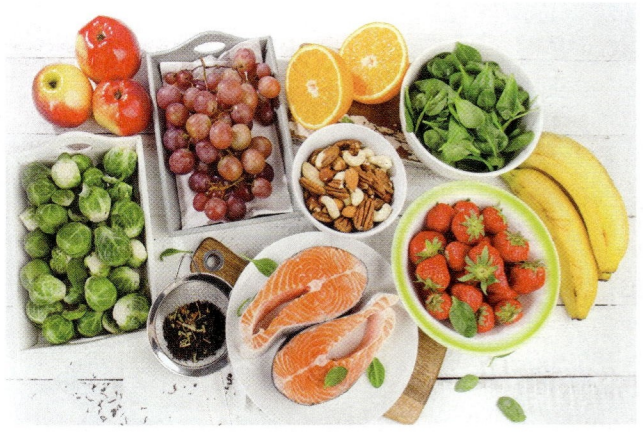

FIGURE 16.6 Foods High in Antioxidants are Beneficial to Pulmonary Health
© bitt24/Shutterstock.

Vitamins and Minerals

Maintenance of blood mineral concentrations is advisable in the patient with pulmonary compromise. Malnourished patients at risk for refeeding syndrome will require additional potassium, magnesium, and phosphate to sustain normal blood levels in the presence of nutrition support.

Phosphorus

Phosphorus is of particular significance to the patient with pulmonary disease due to its role in the production of adenosine triphosphate (ATP) and 2,3-diphosphoglycerate (2,3-DPG). Severe hypophosphatemia diminishes contractility of the diaphragm and leads to subnormal pulmonary function.[108]

Magnesium

Like phosphorus, magnesium is required for ATP. Magnesium also plays a direct role in the relaxation of bronchial smooth muscle—bronchodilation—and has anticholinergic effects. Given these functions, deficiency of magnesium may result in bronchoconstriction. Hypomagnesemia has also been associated with low vitamin D levels given the role magnesium plays on calcium ion transport and cell signaling. Low magnesium levels have been observed in patients with asthma in some,[109-111] but not all, studies.[112-114] Further study is required to inform magnesium supplementation, but patients with magnesium-poor diets may benefit from consumption of high-magnesium foods.

Vitamin D

According to epidemiologic data, it is common for vitamin D deficiency to parallel COPD[115-117]; however, intervention trials have yet to find a link with mortality or frequency of disease exacerbation in patients who are vitamin D replete.[118-120] Supplementation in people with vitamin D deficiency, however, may produce a reduction in COPD exacerbation.[121,122]

Poor vitamin D status has been implicated in the development of osteoporosis due to the role vitamin D plays in bone mineralization. Poor oral intake, underweight, and malnutrition all play a role in the development of bone disease associated with vitamin D deficiency. Some individuals with COPD specifically avoid milk, a significant source of calcium and vitamin D in the American diet, due to the belief that it enhances mucus production; however, this has not been scientifically proven.[123] Medication and lifestyle factors such as glucocorticoid use, immobility, and smoking are also contributors to poor vitamin D status. In addition to maintaining calcium homeostasis, the role of vitamin D in maintaining serotonin levels and reducing inflammation has been proposed to influence the development of depression in deficient persons.[124] There is no recommendation for routine supplementation of vitamin D in this at-risk population, but correction of deficiency may mitigate or prevent some of the comorbidities commonly associated with COPD.

Quality of Life and Psychosocial Support

Chronic obstructive pulmonary disease negatively impacts quality of life. Low FEV_1 has been associated with impaired ability to conduct activities of daily living. People with low FEV_1 display greater impairments relating to energy, physical mobility, and social isolation, marking a significant decline in quality of life with worsening lung function.[125] Underweight respondents in one study reported compromised physical function, emotional status, bodily pain, and general health parameters, which again highlights the significance of weight maintenance in this vulnerable population.[126] Malnourished individuals have described greater levels of fatigue and scored higher on depression scales.[127] Factors most influencing BMI include lung diffusion capacity, early satiety, and active cigarette smoking.

> **CORE CONCEPT 4**
>
> Malnourished individuals have described greater levels of fatigue and scored higher on depression scales.

Chapter Summary

Medical nutrition therapy for patients with pulmonary disease is an integral component of disease management. The influence that adequate nutrient intake and weight management have on the progression of COPD and its response to therapies and patient quality of life cannot be overemphasized. Early interventions that target a combination of healthful diet and exercise strategies provide a therapeutic benefit to COPD patients. Adequate provision of energy in the setting of ARDS, possibly with addition of key micronutrients, optimizes patient and hospital outcomes. Future research is essential to more clearly delineate the unique roles that individual nutrients and/or their combinations can play in the successful treatment of pulmonary disease.

Key Terms

chronic obstructive pulmonary disease (COPD), spirometry, dyspnea, aerophagia, acute respiratory distress syndrome (ARDS), hypoxemia, forced expiratory volume (FEV_1)

References

1. Chronic obstructive pulmonary disease (COPD) includes: Chronic bronchitis and emphysema. National Center for Health Statistics. http://www.cdc.gov/nchs/fastats/copd.htm. Updated 2017. Accessed July 6, 2017.
2. Asthma. National Center for Health Statistics. http://www.cdc.gov/nchs/fastats/asthma.htm. Updated March 31, 2017. Accessed July 6, 2017.
3. Albertine K. Anatomy of the lungs. In: Mason R, Broaddus V, Martin T, et al., eds. *Murray and Nadel's Textbook of Respiratory Medicine*. Fifth ed. Philadelphia, PA: Saunders; 2010:3-25.
4. Beuther DA, Sutherland ER. Overweight, obesity, and incident asthma: a meta-analysis of prospective epidemiologic studies. *Am J Respir Crit Care Med*. 2007;175(7):661-666.
5. Scott HA, Gibson PG, Garg ML, et al. Dietary restriction and exercise improve airway inflammation and clinical outcomes in overweight and obese asthma: a randomized trial. *Clin Exp Allergy*. 2013;43(1):36-49.
6. Dias-Junior SA, Reis M, de Carvalho-Pinto RM, Stelmach R, Halpern A, Cukier A. Effects of weight loss on asthma control in obese patients with severe asthma. *Eur Respir J*. 2014;43(5):1368-1377.
7. Stenius-Aarniala B, Poussa T, Kvarnstrom J, Gronlund EL, Ylikahri M, Mustajoki P. Immediate and long term effects of weight reduction in obese people with asthma: Randomised controlled study. *BMJ*. 2000;320(7238):827-832.
8. *Global strategy for the diagnosis, management and prevention of COPD*. Global initiative for chronic obstructive lung disease (GOLD). 2014. available from: http://goldcopd.org/gold-2017-global-strategy-diagnosis-management-prevention-copd/. Accessed October 1, 2017.
9. Castagna O, Boussuges A, Vallier JM, Prefaut C, Brisswalter J. Is impairment similar between arm and leg cranking exercise in COPD patients? *Respir Med*. 2007;101(3):547-553.
10. Barreiro E, de la Puente B, Minguella J, et al. Oxidative stress and respiratory muscle dysfunction in severe chronic obstructive pulmonary disease. *Am J Respir Crit Care Med*. 2005;171(10):1116-1124.
11. Shapiro S, Reilly J, Rennard S. Chronic bronchitis and emphysema. In: Mason R, Broaddus V, Martin T, et al., eds. *Murray and nadel's textbook of respiratory medicine*. 5th ed. Philadelphia, PA: Saunders Elsevier; 2010:919-967.
12. Mannino DM, Thorn D, Swensen A, Holguin F. Prevalence and outcomes of diabetes, hypertension and cardiovascular disease in COPD. *Eur Respir J*. 2008;32(4):962-969.
13. Watz H, Waschki B, Kirsten A, et al. The metabolic syndrome in patients with chronic bronchitis and COPD: Frequency and associated consequences for systemic inflammation and physical inactivity. *Chest*. 2009;136(4):1039-1046.
14. Ferguson GT, Calverley PMA, Anderson JA, et al. Prevalence and progression of osteoporosis in patients with copd: Results from the towards a revolution in copd health study. *Chest*. 2009;136(6):1456-1465.
15. Dodd JW, Getov SV, Jones PW. Cognitive function in COPD. *Eur Respir J*. 2010;35(4):913-922.
16. Clinical pharmacology [database online]. Tampa, FL: Gold standard; inc.; 2006. http://www.clinicalpharmacology.com. Updated 2017. Accessed April 7, 2017.
17. Creutzberg EC, Schols AM, Bothmer-Quaedvlieg FC, Wouters EF. Prevalence of an elevated resting energy expenditure in patients with chronic obstructive pulmonary disease in relation to body composition and lung function. *Eur J Clin Nutr*. 1998;52(6):396-401.
18. Kao CC, Hsu JW, Bandi V, Hanania NA, Kheradmand F, Jahoor F. Resting energy expenditure and protein turnover are increased in patients with severe chronic obstructive pulmonary disease. *Metab Clin Exp*. 2011;60(10):1449-1455.
19. Donahoe M, Rogers RM, Wilson DO, Pennock BE. Oxygen consumption of the respiratory muscles in normal and in malnourished patients with chronic obstructive pulmonary disease. *Am Rev Respir Dis*. 1989;140(2):385-391.
20. Goldstein SA, Thomashow BM, Kvetan V, Askanazi J, Kinney JM, Elwyn DH. Nitrogen and energy relationships in malnourished patients with emphysema. *Am Rev Respir Dis*. 1988;138(3):636-644.
21. Rao Z, Wu X, Wang M, Hu W. Comparison between measured and predicted resting energy expenditure in mechanically ventilated patients with COPD. *Asia Pac J Clin Nutr*. 2012;21(3):338-346.
22. Schols A, Soeters P, Mostert R, Saris W, Wouters E. Energy balance in chronic obstructive pulmonary disease. *Am Rev Respir Dis*. 1991;143(6):1248-1252.
23. Schols AM, Fredrix EW, Soeters PB, Westerterp KR, Wouters EF. Resting energy expenditure in patients with chronic obstructive pulmonary disease. *Am J Clin Nutr*. 1991;54(6):983-987.
24. Wilson D, Donahoe M, Rogers R, Pennock B. Metabolic rate and weight loss in chronic obstructive lung disease. *JPEN J Parenter Enteral Nutr*. 1990;14(1):7-11.
25. Sahebjami H, Sathianpitayakul E. Influence of body weight on the severity of dyspnea in chronic obstructive pulmonary disease. *Am J Respir Crit Care Med*. 2000;161:886-890.
26. Barrett KE, Barman SM, Boitano S, Brooks H, eds. Introduction to pulmonary structure and mechanics. Ganong's Review of Medical Physiology. 25th ed. New York, NY: McGraw-Hill; 2016:634-652.
27. Nguyen LT, Bedu M, Caillaud D, et al. Increased resting energy expenditure is related to plasmaTNF-α concentration in stable COPD patients. *Clin Nutr*. 1999;18(5):269-274.
28. Cohen RI, Marzouk K, Berkoski P, O'Donnell CP, Polotsky VY, Scharf SM. BOdy composition and resting energy expenditure in clinically stable, non–weight-losing patients with severe emphysema. *Chest*. 2003;124(4):1365-1372.
29. Broekhuizen R, Wouters EFM, Creutzberg EC, Schols AMWJ. Raised CRP levels mark metabolic and functional impairment in advanced COPD. *Thorax*. 2006;61(1):17-22.
30. Schols AM, Buurman WA, Staal van den Brekel AJ, Dentener MA, Wouters EF. Evidence for a relation between metabolic derangements and increased levels of inflammatory mediators in a subgroup of patients with chronic obstructive pulmonary disease. *Thorax*. 1996;51(8):819-824.
31. Hugli O, Schutz Y, Fitting J. The daily energy expenditure in stable chronic obstructive pulmonary disease. *Am J Respir Crit Care Med*. 1996;153(1):294-300.
32. Baarends EM, Schols AM, Westerterp KR, Wouters EF. Total daily energy expenditure relative to resting energy expenditure in clinically stable patients with COPD. *Thorax*. 1997;52(9):780-785.
33. Cao C, Wang R, Wang J, Bunjhoo H, Xu Y, Xiong W. Body mass index and mortality in chronic obstructive pulmonary disease: A meta-analysis. *PLoS One*. 2012;7(8):e43892.
34. Zapatero A, Barba R, Ruiz J, et al. Malnutrition and obesity: Influence in mortality and readmissions in chronic obstructive pulmonary disease patients. *J Hum Nutr Diet*. 2013;26:16-22.
35. Schelbert KB. Comorbidities of obesity. *Primary Care: Clinics in Office Practice*. 2009;36(2):271-285.
36. Sood A, Petersen H, Meek P, Tesfaigzi Y. Spirometry and health status worsen with weight gain in obese smokers but improve in normal-weight smokers. *Am J Respir Crit Care Med*. 2014;189(3):274-281.

37. Sin DD, Jones RL, Man SF. Obesity is a risk factor for dyspnea but not for airflow obstruction. *Arch Intern Med*. 2002;162(13):1477-1481.
38. Jordan JG,Jr, Mann JR. Obesity and mortality in persons with obstructive lung disease using data from the NHANES III. *South Med J*. 2010;103(4):323-330.
39. van den Borst B, Gosker HR, Koster A, et al. The influence of abdominal visceral fat on inflammatory pathways and mortality risk in obstructive lung disease. *Am J Clin Nutr*. 2012;96(3):516-526.
40. Schols AM, Broekhuizen R, Weling-Scheepers CA, Wouters EF. Body composition and mortality in chronic obstructive pulmonary disease. *Am J Clin Nutr*. 2005;82(1):53-59.
41. Furutate R, Ishii T, Wakabayashi R, et al. Excessive visceral fat accumulation in advanced chronic obstructive pulmonary disease. *Int J Chron Obstruct Pulmon Dis*. 2011;6:423-430.
42. Nishimura Y, Tsutsumi M, Nakata H, Tsunenari T, Maeda H, Yokoyama M. Relationship between respiratory muscle strength and lean body mass in men with copd. *Chest*. 1995;107(5):1232-1236.
43. Vermeeren MAP, Creutzberg EC, Schols AMWJ, et al. Prevalence of nutritional depletion in a large out-patient population of patients with COPD. *Respir Med*. 2006;100(8):1349-1355.
44. Weisberg J, Wanger J, Olson J, et al. Megestrol acetate stimulates weight gain and ventilation in underweight COPD patients. *Chest*. 2002;121(4):1070-1078.
45. Daga MK, Khan NA, Malhotra V, Kumar S, Mawari G, Hira HS. Study of body composition, lung function, and quality of life following use of anabolic steroids in patients with chronic obstructive pulmonary disease. *Nutr Clin Pract*. 2014.
46. Yeh S, DeGuzman B, Kramer T. Reversal of COPD-associated weight loss using the anabolic agent oxandrolone. *Chest*. 2002;122(2):421-428.
47. Schols A, Soeters P, Mostert R, Pluymers R, Wouters E. Physiologic effects of nutritional support and anabolic steroids in patients with chronic obstructive pulmonary disease: a placebo-controlled randomized trial. *Am J Respir Crit Care Med*. 1995;152(4 pt 1):1268-1274.
48. Creutzberg EC, Wouters EFM, Mostert R, Pluymers RJ, Schols AMWJ. A role for anabolic steroids in the rehabilitation of patients with copd: a double-blind, placebo-controlled, randomized trial. *Chest*. 2003;124(5):1733-1742.
49. Pison C, Cano N, Chérion C, et al. Multimodal nutritional rehabilitation improves clinical outcomes of malnourished patientswith chronic respiratory failure: a randomised controlled trial. *Thorax*. 2011;66(11):953-960.
50. Pan L, Wang M, Xie X, Du C, Guo Y. Effects of anabolic steroids on chronic obstructive pulmonary disease: A meta-analysis of randomised controlled trials. - *PLoS ONE*. (- 1):- e84855.
51. Molfino A, Gioia G, Rossi Fanelli F, Muscaritoli M. Beta-hydroxy-beta-methylbutyrate supplementation in health and disease: A systematic review of randomized trials. *Amino Acids*. 2013;45(6):1273-1292.
52. Kuhls DA, Rathmacher JA, Musngi MD, et al. Beta-hydroxy-beta-methylbutyrate supplementation in critically ill trauma patients. *J Trauma*. 2007;62(1):125-31; discussion 131-2.
53. May PE, Barber A, D'Olimpio JT, Hourihane A, Abumrad NN. Reversal of cancer-related wasting using oral supplementation with a combination of beta-hydroxy-beta-methylbutyrate, arginine, and glutamine. *Am J Surg*. 2002;183(4):471-479.
54. Clark RH, Feleke G, Din M, et al. Nutritional treatment for acquired immunodeficiency virus-associated wasting using beta-hydroxy beta-methylbutyrate, glutamine, and arginine: A randomized, double-blind, placebo-controlled study. *JPEN J Parenter Enteral Nutr*. 2000;24(3):133-139.
55. Rathmacher JA, Nissen S, Panton L, et al. Supplementation with a combination of beta-hydroxy-beta-methylbutyrate (HMB), arginine, and glutamine is safe and could improve hematological parameters. *JPEN J Parenter Enteral Nutr*. 2004;28(2):65-75.
56. Hsieh LC, Chien SL, Huang MS, Tseng HF, Chang CK. Anti-inflammatory and anticatabolic effects of short-term beta-hydroxy-beta-methylbutyrate supplementation on chronic obstructive pulmonary disease patients in intensive care unit. *Asia Pac J Clin Nutr*. 2006;15(4):544-550.
57. Collins PF, Elia M, Stratton RJ. Nutritional support and functional capacity in chronic obstructive pulmonary disease: A systematic review and meta-analysis. *Respirology*. 2013;18(4):616-629.
58. Ferreira IM, Brooks D, White J, Goldstein R. Nutritional supplementation for stable chronic obstructive pulmonary disease. *Cochrane Database Syst Rev*. 2012;12:CD000998.
59. Weekes CE, Emery PW, Elia M. Dietary counselling and food fortification in stable COPD: A randomised trial. *Thorax*. 2009;64(4):326-331.
60. Monteiro F, Camillo CA, Vitorasso R, et al. Obesity and physical activity in the daily life of patients with COPD. *Lung*. 2012;190(4):403-410.
61. Sugawara K, Takahashi H, Kasai C, et al. Effects of nutritional supplementation combined with low-intensity exercise in malnourished patients with COPD. *Respir Med*. 2010;104(12):1883-1889.
62. Gurgun A, Deniz S, Arg?n M, Karapolat H. Effects of nutritional supplementation combined with conventional pulmonary rehabilitation in muscle-wasted chronic obstructive pulmonary disease: A prospective, randomized and controlled study. *Respirology*. 2013;18(3):495-500.
63. Bellani G, Laffey JG, Pham T, et al. Epidemiology, patterns of care, and mortality for patients with acute respiratory distress syndrome in intensive care units in 50 countries. *JAMA*. 2016;315(8):788-800.
64. Lee W, Slutsky A. Acute respiratory distress syndrome. In: Mason R, Broaddus V, Martin T, et al., eds. *Murray and nadel's textbook of respiratory medicine*. 5th ed. Philadelphia, PA: Saunders; 2010:2104-2129.
65. ARDS Definition Task Force, Ranieri VM, Rubenfeld GD, et al. Acute respiratory distress syndrome: the berlin definition. *JAMA*. 2012;307(23):2526-2533.
66. Rothkopf MM, Stanislaus G, Haverstick L, Kvetan V, Askanazi J. Invited review: Nutritional support in respiratory failure. *Nutr Clin Pract*. 1989;4(5):166-172.
67. Wooley J, Frankenfield D. Energy. In: Mueller C, ed. *The A.S.P.E.N. Adult Nutrition Support Core Curriculum*. 2nd ed.;2012:23-35.
68. McClave SA, Taylor BE, Martindale RG, et al. Guidelines for the provision and assessment of nutrition support therapy in the adult critically ill patient: Society of Critical Care Medicine (SCCM) and Amerian Society for Parenteral and Enteral Nutrition (A.S.P.E.N.). *JPEN J Parenter Enteral Nutr*. 2016;40(2):159-211.
69. Scholten EL, Beitler JR, Prisk GK, Malhotra A. Treatment of ARDS with prone positioning. *Chest*. 2017;151(1):215-224.
70. Saez de la Fuente I, Saez de la Fuente J, Quintana Estelles MD, et al. Enteral nutrition in patients receiving mechanical ventilation in a prone position. *JPEN J Parenter Enteral Nutr*. 2016;40(2):250-255.
71. Linn DD, Beckett RD, Foellinger K. Administration of enteral nutrition to adult patients in the prone position. *Intensive Crit Care Nurs*. 2015;31(1):38-43.
72. Gadek J, DeMichele S, Karlstad M, et al. Effect of enteral feeding with eicosapentaenoic acid, gamma linolenic acid, and antioxidants in patients with acute respiratory distress syndrome. *Crit Care Med*. 1999;27(8):1409-1420.
73. Singer P, Theilla M, Fisher H, Gibstein L, Grozovski E, Cohen J. Benefit of an enteral diet enriched with eicosapentaenoic acid and gamma-linolenic acid in ventilated patients with acute lung injury. *Crit Care Med*. 2006;34(4):1033-1038.
74. Pontes-Arruda A, Aragão A, Albuquerque J. Effects of enteral feeding with eicosapentanoic acid, gamma-linolenic acid, and antioxidants in

mechanically ventilated patients with severe sepsis and septic shock. *Crit Care Med.* 2006;34(9):2325-2333.
75. Pontes-Arruda A, DeMichele S, Seth A, Singer P. The use of an inflammation-modulating diet in patients with acute lung injury or acute respiratory distress syndrome: A meta-analysis of outcome data. *JPEN J Parenter Enteral Nutr.* 2008;32(6):596-605.
76. Pacht E, DeMichele S, Nelson J, Hart J, Wennberg A, Gadek J. Enteral nutrition with eicosapentaenoic acid, gamma-linolenic acid, and antioxidants reduces alveolar inflammatory mediators and protein influx in patients with acute respiratory distress syndrome. *Crit Care Med.* 2003;31:491-500.
77. Rice TW, Wheeler AP, Thompson B, et al. Enteral omega-3 fatty acid, γ-linolenic acid, and antioxidant supplementation in acute lung injury. *JAMA.* 2011;306(14):1574-1581.
78. Stapleton R, Martin T, Weiss N, et al. A phase II randomized placebo-controlled trial of omega-3 fatty acids for the treatment of acute lung injury. *Crit Care Med.* 2011;39(7):1655-1662.
79. Venus B, Smith RA, Patel C, Sandoval E. Hemodynamic and gas exchange alterations during intralipid infusion in patients with adult respiratory distress syndrome. *Chest.* 1989;95(6):1278-1281.
80. Faucher M, Bregeon F, Gainnier M, Thirion X, Auffray JP, Papazian L. Cardiopulmonary effects of lipid emulsions in patients with ARDS. *Chest.* 2003;124(1):285-291.
81. Smirniotis V, Kostopanagiotou G, Vassiliou J, et al. Long chain versus medium chain lipids in patients with ARDS: Effects on pulmonary haemodynamics and gas exchange. *Intensive Care Med.* 1998;24(10):1029-1033.
82. Masclans JR, Iglesia R, Bermejo B, Pico M, Rodriguez-Roisin R, Planas M. Gas exchange and pulmonary haemodynamic responses to fat emulsions in acute respiratory distress syndrome. *Intensive Care Med.* 1998;24(9):918-923.
83. Gupta A, Govil D, Bhatnagar S, et al. Efficacy and safety of parenteral omega 3 fatty acids in ventilated patients with acute lung injury. *Indian J Crit Care Med.* 2011;15(2):108-113.
84. Matsuyama W, Mitsuyama H, Watanabe M, et al. Effects of omega-3 polyunsaturated fatty acids on inflammatory markers in COPD. *Chest.* 2005;128(6):3817-3827.
85. Walda IC, Tabak C, Smit HA, et al. Diet and 20-year chronic obstructive pulmonary disease mortality in middle-aged men from three european countries. *Eur J Clin Nutr.* 2002;56(7):638-643.
86. Tabak C, Smit HA, Heederik D, Ocke MC, Kromhout D. Diet and chronic obstructive pulmonary disease: Independent beneficial effects of fruits, whole grains, and alcohol (the MORGEN study). *Clin Exp Allergy.* 2001;31(5):747-755.
87. Tabak C, Smit HA, Rasanen L, et al. Dietary factors and pulmonary function: A cross sectional study in middle aged men from three european countries. *Thorax.* 1999;54(11):1021-1026.
88. Vitamin C. In: *Dietary reference intakes for vitamin C, vitamin E, selenium, and carotenoids.* Washington, D.C.: The National Academies Press; 2000:95-185.
89. Agacdiken A, Basyigit I, Özden M, et al. The effects of antioxidants on exercise-induced lipid peroxidation in patients with COPD. *Respirology.* 2004;9(1):38-42.
90. Nicks ME, O'Brien MM, Bowler RP. Plasma antioxidants are associated with impaired lung function and COPD exacerbations in smokers. *COPD.* 2011;8(4):264-269.
91. Ahmad A, Shameem M, Husain Q. Altered oxidant-antioxidant levels in the disease prognosis of chronic obstructive pulmonary disease. *Int J Tuberc Lung Dis.* 2013;17(8):1104-1109.
92. McKeever T, Lewis S, Smit H, Burney P, Cassano P, Britton J. A multivariate analysis of serum nutrient levels and lung function. *Respir Res.* 2008;9:67.
93. Kelly Y, Sacker A, Marmot M. Nutrition and respiratory health in adults: Findings from the health survey for Scotland. *Eur Respir J.* 2003;21(4):664-671.
94. Hu G, Zhang X, Chen J, Peto R, Campbell TC, Cassano PA. Dietary vitamin C intake and lung function in rural China. *Am J Epidemiol.* 1998;148(6):594-599.
95. Pearson P, Britton J, McKeever T, et al. Lung function and blood levels of copper, selenium, vitamin C and vitamin E in the general population. *Eur J Clin Nutr.* 2005;59(9):1043-1048.
96. Schünemann HJ, Freudenheim JL, Grant BJB. Epidemiologic evidence linking antioxidant vitamins to pulmonary function and airway obstruction. *Epidemiol Rev.* 2001;23(2):248-267.
97. Grievink, L, de Waart, FG, Schouten E, Kok F. Serum carotenoids, α-tocopherol, and lung function among Dutch elderly. *Am J Respir Crit Care Med.* 2000;161(3 pt 1):790-795.
98. Chuwers P, Barnhart S, Blanc P, et al. The protective effect of beta-carotene and retinol on ventilatory function in an asbestos-exposed cohort. *Am J Respir Crit Care Med.* 1997;155(3):1066-1071.
99. Paiva SA, Godoy I, Vannucchi H, Fávaro RM, Geraldo RR, Campana AO. Assessment of vitamin A status in chronic obstructive pulmonary disease patients and healthy smokers. *Am J Clin Nutr.* 1996;64(6):928-934.
100. Tecklenburg SL, Mickleborough TD, Fly AD, Bai Y, Stager JM. Ascorbic acid supplementation attenuates exercise-induced bronchoconstriction in patients with asthma. *Respir Med.* 2007;101(8):1770-1778.
101. Rautalahti J, Virtamo J, Haukka J, et al. The effect of alpha-tocopherol and beta-carotene supplementation on COPD symptoms. *Am J Respir Crit Care Med.* 1997;156(5):1447-1452.
102. MRC/BHF heart protection study of antioxidant vitamin supplementation in 20 536 high-risk individuals: A randomised placebo-controlled trial. *The Lancet.* 2002;360(9326):23-33.
103. Nadi E, Tavakoli F, Zeraati F, Goodarzi MT, Hashemi SH. Effect of vitamin C administration on leukocyte vitamin C level and severity of bronchial asthma. *Acta Med Iran.* 2012;50(4):233-238.
104. Fogarty A, Lewis SA, Scrivener SL, et al. Corticosteroid sparing effects of vitamin C and magnesium in asthma: A randomised trial. *Respir Med.* 2006;100(1):174-179.
105. Fogarty A, Lewis SA, Scrivener SL, et al. Oral magnesium and vitamin C supplements in asthma: A parallel group randomized placebo-controlled trial. *Clin Exp Allergy.* 2003;33(10):1355-1359.
106. Pearson PJ, Lewis SA, Britton J, Fogarty A. Vitamin E supplements in asthma: A parallel group randomised placebo controlled trial. *Thorax.* 2004;59(8):652-656.
107. Keranis E, Makris D, Rodopoulou P, et al. Impact of dietary shift to higher-antioxidant foods in COPD: A randomised trial. *Egypt J Chest Dis Tuberc.* 2010;36(4):774-780.
108. Aubier M, Murciano D, Lecocguic Y, et al. Effect of hypophosphatemia on diaphragmatic contractility in patients with acute respiratory failure. *N Engl J Med.* 1985;313(7):420-424.
109. Ali AA, Bakr RM, Yousif M, Foad RE. Assessment of serum magnesium level in patients with bronchial asthma. *Egypt J Chest Dis Tuberc.* 2015;64(3):535-539.
110. Alamoudi OS. Hypomagnesaemia in chronic, stable asthmatics: Prevalence, correlation with severity and hospitalization. *Eur Respir J.* 2000;16(3):427-431.
111. Oladipo OO, Chukwu CC, Ajala MO, Adewole TA, Afonja OA. Plasma magnesium in adult asthmatics at the Lagos University Teaching Hospital, Nigeria. *East Afr Med J.* 2003;80(9):488-491.
112. de Valk HW, Kok PT, Struyvenberg A, et al. Extracellular and intracellular magnesium concentrations in asthmatic patients. *Eur Respir J.* 1993;6(8):1122-1125.

113. Fantidis P, Ruiz Cacho J, Marin M, Madero Jarabo R, Solera J, Herrero E. Intracellular (polymorphonuclear) magnesium content in patients with bronchial asthma between attacks. *J R Soc Med*. 1995;88(8):441-445.
114. Kazaks AG, Uriu-Adams JY, Albertson TE, Stern JS. Multiple measures of magnesium status are comparable in mild asthma and control subjects. *J Asthma*. 2006;43(10):783-788.
115. Black PN, Scragg R. RElationship between serum 25-hydroxyvitamin d and pulmonary function in the third national health and nutrition examination survey. *Chest*. 2005;128(6):3792-3798.
116. Persson LJ, Aanerud M, Hiemstra PS, Hardie JA, Bakke PS, Eagan TM. Chronic obstructive pulmonary disease is associated with low levels of vitamin D. *PLoS ONE*. 7(6):e38934.
117. Janssens W, Bouillon R, Claes B, et al. Vitamin D deficiency is highly prevalent in COPD and correlates with variants in the vitamin D-binding gene. *Thorax*. 2010;65(3):215-220.
118. Holmgaard DB, Mygind LH, Titlestad IL, et al. Serum vitamin D in patients with chronic obstructive lung disease does not correlate with mortality: Results from a 10-year prospective cohort study. *PLoS ONE*. 8(1):e53670.
119. Berg I, Hanson C, Sayles H, et al. Vitamin D, vitamin D binding protein, lung function and structure in COPD. *Respir Med*. 2013;107(10):1578-1588.
120. Puhan MA, Siebeling L, Frei A, Zoller M, Bischoff-Ferrari H, ter Riet G. No association of 25-hydroxyvitamin d with exacerbations in primary care patients with COPD. *Chest*. 2014;145(1):37-43.
121. Martineau AR, James WY, Hooper RL, et al. Vitamin D3 supplementation in patients with chronic obstructive pulmonary disease (ViDiCO): A multicentre, double-blind, randomised controlled trial. *Lancet Respir Med*. 2015;3(2):120-130.
122. Lehouck A, Mathieu C, Carremans C, et al. High doses of vitamin D to reduce exacerbations in chronic obstructive pulmonary Disease: A randomized trial. *Ann Intern Med*. 2012;156(2):105-114.
123. Wüthrich B, Schmid A, Walther B, Sieber R. Milk consumption does not lead to mucus production or occurrence of asthma. *J Am Coll Nutr*. 2005;24:547S-555S.
124. Berridge MJ. Vitamin D and depression: Cellular and regulatory mechanisms. *Pharmacol Rev*. 2017;69(2):80-92.
125. Monsó E, Fiz JM, Izquierdo J, et al. Quality of life in severe chronic obstructive pulmonary disease: Correlation with lung and muscle function. *Respir Med*. 1998;92(2):221-227.
126. Katsura H, Yamada K, Kida K. Both generic and disease specific health-related quality of life are deteriorated in patients with underweight COPD. *Respir Med*. 2005;99(5):624-630.
127. Cochrane WJ, Afolabi OA. Investigation into the nutritional status, dietary intake and smoking habits of patients with chronic obstructive pulmonary disease. *J Hum Nutr Diet*. 2004;17(1):3-11; quiz 13-15.

Chapter 17

Nutrition in Cystic Fibrosis

Laura Grande

Chapter Outline

Core Concepts
Introduction
Cystic Fibrosis
Diagnosis
Clinical Manifestations of CF
CF and the Lungs

Relationship between Lung Function and Nutritional Status
Nutrition Assessment
Pancreatic Insufficiency
Nutrition Management in Patients with Cystic Fibrosis
Nutrition-related Complications of Cystic Fibrosis

CORE CONCEPTS

1. Cystic fibrosis is a disease in which nutrition is of utmost importance and routine nutrition screening and assessments are essential in the care of every patient.

2. Energy needs are high in a patient with cystic fibrosis due to an increased metabolic demand associated with breathing and malabsorption of fat due to pancreatic insufficiency.

3. Pancreatic insufficiency affects the majority of patients with cystic fibrosis. It results in malabsorption of fat without proper treatment with pancreatic enzyme replacement therapy.

4. Treatment for pancreatic insufficiency is to provide porcine-derived pancreatic enzymes, taken by mouth with meals and snacks, to substitute for the enzymes the pancreas is not endogenously creating. These enzymes contain lipase, protease, and amylase for the digestion of fat, protein, and carbohydrates.

5. Patients with cystic fibrosis and pancreatic insufficiency require supplementation of vitamins and minerals due to risk for malabsorption-related deficiencies. All fat-soluble vitamins should be assessed annually, because they are the primary nutrients at risk for deficiency.

6. Patients with cystic fibrosis have higher sodium needs than those of the general population due to increased sweat-related losses. All patients with CF are prescribed a high-salt diet to compensate for the additional losses.

7. If an adequate BMI-for-age cannot be maintained with diet alone, oral supplements, and often enteral nutrition support, are recommended to promote weight gain.

8. All patients with cystic fibrosis are at risk for developing CF-related diabetes (CFRD) due to a shortage of insulin and some insulin resistance.

Learning Objectives

1. Identify the etiology of cystic fibrosis and the importance of good nutrition in maintaining good lung health.
2. Explain the specific nutrition needs of a patient with cystic fibrosis.
3. Describe pancreatic insufficiency and its treatment in patients with cystic fibrosis.
4. Recognize specific vitamin and mineral deficiencies associated with cystic fibrosis.
5. Discuss the nutrition-related disease complications that may be associated with cystic fibrosis.

Introduction

This chapter will review cystic fibrosis and its associated nutritional complications. The importance of proper nutrition and strategies to improve the nutritional status of patients with cystic fibrosis will be discussed.

Cystic fibrosis (CF) is a life-threatening, autosomal recessive genetic disorder. It is the most common genetic disorder among Caucasians and affects approximately 30,000 people in the United States. Approximately 1,000 new cases are diagnosed every year; more than 65% of individuals are diagnosed by age 1 year, and 29% before 1 month of age.[1] CF is characterized by an abnormal **CF transmembrane conductance regulator (CFTR) protein** (**Figure 17.1**), which results in abnormal transport of sodium, chloride, and water throughout the cells of the body. This results in abnormally thick mucus that causes damage to many organs, specifically the lungs and the pancreas. The mucus obstructs the airways, causing damage to the lungs promoting bacterial infections that lead to progressive lung disease. The mucus also clogs the ducts of the pancreas, preventing digestive enzymes from being secreted into the small intestine and leading to **pancreatic insufficiency**. Treatment for those with CF aims to promote normal lung function, support normal growth throughout childhood and adolescence, and maintain optimal nutrition in adulthood. It is recommended that all patients with CF in the United States be treated under the care of a Cystic Fibrosis Foundation–accredited center. These centers include a interprofessional team, usually comprising a doctor, registered nurse, registered dietitian, social worker, physical therapist, and respiratory therapist, to help care for the complex needs of a patient with CF.

Diagnosis

Newborn screening for CF is now available in all 50 states. Prior to the development of newborn screening, patients were diagnosed with CF after showing signs and symptoms of the disease, which may have included chronic cough, pneumonia, malnutrition, rectal prolapse, or steatorrhea. Presently, most patients in the United States initially present to a CF center as a result of an abnormal newborn screen. A **sweat test** is ordered to measure the amount of chloride in sweat. If elevated above 60 mmol/L, a diagnosis of cystic fibrosis can be made. If the sweat test is borderline, a blood sample will be sent out to determine whether the patient has any CFTR mutations.[2]

Clinical Manifestations of CF

CF can present with various signs and symptoms and in varying degrees of severity. The disease-causing genetic mutations, if known, often can predict the pancreatic status of the individual. However, patients with the same two CF genotypes can present with very different disease courses throughout the lifespan. The most common respiratory manifestations of the disease include chronic cough, chronic sinusitis, and repeated lung infections, along with **digital clubbing** (focal enlargement of the terminal ends of the fingers). The most common gastrointestinal (GI) manifestations of the disease are malabsorption, steatorrhea, rectal prolapse, and fat-soluble vitamin deficiencies. Some infants may present within 24 hours of birth with meconium ileus, an intestinal obstruction in the early newborn period.

CF and the Lungs

The lungs can be visualized like an upside-down tree. The trunk represents the trachea, the main branches are the **bronchi**, **bronchioles** are the smaller branches, and finally the **alveoli** are the smallest twigs and branches (**Figure 17.2**). **Cilia** are hair-like structures within the lungs that normally remove bacteria.

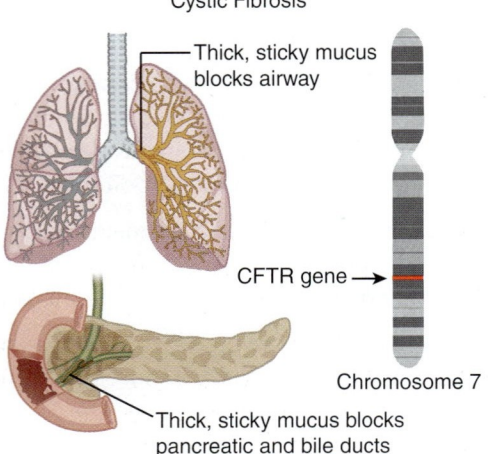

FIGURE 17.1 A Defect in the CFTR Gene Results in Thick Mucus Production in the Lungs and Pancreas

CASE STUDY INTRODUCTION

Lucy is a 4-month-old female with no significant medical history, seen by you for the first time for poor growth. Lucy was breastfed exclusively until 4 months of age and then maintained on a combination of breast milk and infant formula. Her parents report that Lucy is very eager to feed and appears interested; however, she fails to gain weight. They notice that she sweats a significant amount. They are also concerned with her increasing stool pattern, which is foul smelling and appears greasy. Mom and Dad both work. Lucy has an older brother age 3 years. They have support from extended family. Lucy's grandmother takes care of Lucy and is also present for the visit. Lucy's grandmother mentions that when she kisses Lucy, she has a salty taste to her skin.

Anthropometrics:
Length 59.5 cm (23.4)
Weight 5.0 kg (11 lbs)

Weight History

Age (months)	Weight kg (lbs)	Length cm (in)
Birth	3.4 (7)	52 (20.5)
1 month	4 (8.8)	55 (21.7)
2 months	4.8 (10.6)	57 (22.4)
3 months	5.0 (11)	58 (22.8)

Biochemical Data:
Sodium 123 (135-145 mEq/L)
Potassium 2.9 (3.6-5.0 mEq/L)
Chloride 73 (98-110 mEq/L)
Carbon dioxide 22 (20-30 mEq/L)
Blood urea nitrogen 25 (6-24 mg/dL)
Creatinine 1.8 (0.4-1.3 mg/dL)
Glucose 78 (70-139 mg/dL)

Clinical Data:
Past Medical History: None
Medications: None
Vitals Signs: Normal
Nutrition-focused Physical Exams: Lucy is alert but appears distressed. When you observe her, she has a productive cough during the visit.

Questions
1. Describe Lucy's growth pattern.
2. How would you assess her nutritional status?
3. What additional biochemical measures would you request?

Thick mucus in CF prevents the cilia from performing this function. Microorganisms become trapped in the mucus, leading to infection. An inflammatory immune response ensues, increasing white cell production. Tissue damage caused by infection and the immune response itself further contribute to thickened mucus. Inflammation, which constricts the passageways, makes it more difficult to clear mucus secretions. A cycle of inflammation, weakened immunity, and recurrent infections occurs (**Figure 17.3**).

The mainstay of medical management in CF includes a series of interventions aimed at airway clearance, fighting

490 SECTION 2 NUTRITION IN DISEASE STATES

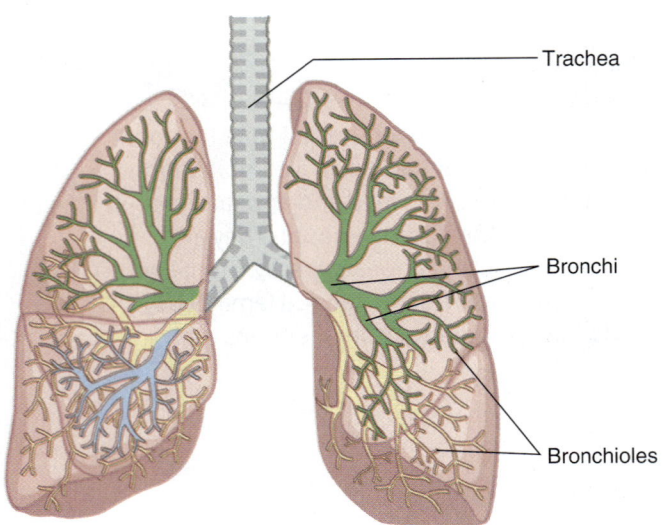

FIGURE 17.2 The Lungs

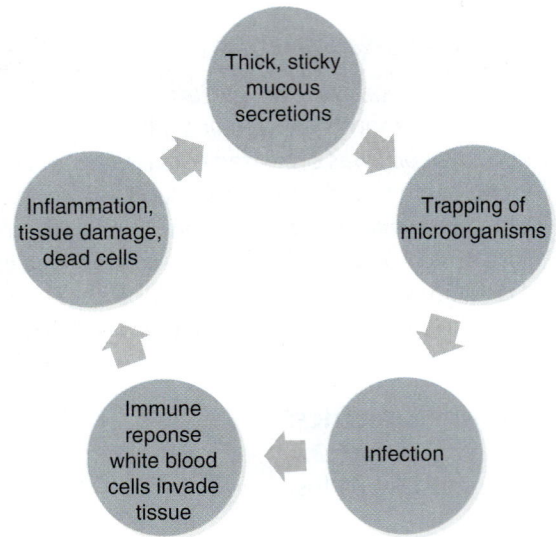

FIGURE 17.3 Cycle of Increased Mucus Production, Inflammation, and Recurrent Infections

respiratory infections, and preserving lung function. **Bronchiodilators** are oral and inhaled medications used to expand constricted passageways and improve breathing. **Mucolytics** help mobilize mucus and decrease sputum thickness. **Nebulizers**, which turn liquid medication into a mist, are commonly used (**Figure 17.4**). Airway clearance techniques also include chest physical therapy; use of a **percussor** (a hand-held device that helps mobilize bronchial secretions); use of therapeutic vests that provide high-frequency chest compression to remove mucus; and intrapulmonary percussive ventilation, a technique that uses compressed gas to deliver medications and loosen secretions. Anti-inflammatory medications are given to decrease lung inflammation. Finally, antibiotics are given to treat infection. **Table 17.1** shows commonly used medications in CF.

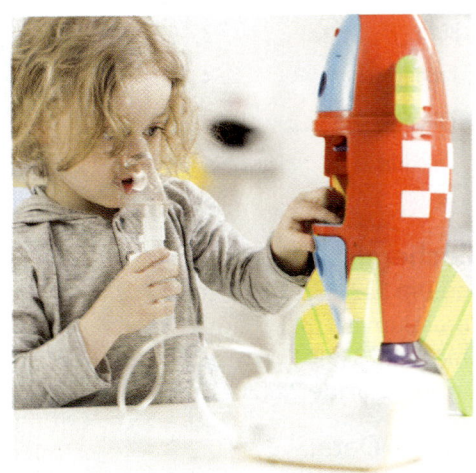

FIGURE 17.4 Use of a Nebulizer in a Child with CF
© Photographee.eu/Shutterstock.

TABLE 17.1 CATEGORIES OF MEDICATIONS USED TO TREAT PULMONARY COMPLICATIONS OF CF

Treatment Category	Purpose	Administration	Examples of Common Medications
Bronchodilators	Open airway passages in the lungs by relaxing smooth muscle	Inhaler Oral Aerosol	Albuterol, theophylline, ipratropium
Mucolytics	Thin mucus, increase sputum secretion	Nebulizer	DNase (Pulmozyme), hypertonic saline (Hypersal)
Anti-inflammatories	Decrease lung inflammation	Inhaler Oral Intravenous	Triamcinolone, flunisolide, prednisone
Antibiotics*	Treat bacterial infection	Oral Aerosol Sinus Intravenous	Ciprofloxin, co-trimoxazole, tobramycin

* Antibiotics are prescribed according to infection type.
Data from https://www.cff.org/Life-With-CF/Treatments-and-Therapies/Medications/.

Relationship between Lung Function and Nutritional Status

CF is a disease in which nutrition is of utmost importance, and routine nutrition screening and assessments are essential in the care of every patient. Studies have been conducted to show a strong association between lung function and nutritional status, specifically body mass index (BMI).[3,4] According to data from the CF Foundation registry database, there is a direct correlation of **forced expiratory volume at 1 second (FEV$_1$)** and body mass index.[1] In patients ages 6 to 20 years, the FEV$_1$ is optimized when the BMI/age reaches the 50th percentile (**Figure 17.5**). Similarly, the same trend is seen in adult patients, in which lung function is optimized at a BMI-for-age 22 kg/m^2 for females and 23 kg/m^2 for males (**Figure 17.6**). As a result of these findings, the CF Foundation emphasizes the importance of optimizing nutrition status in the patient with CF to delay the progressive lung damage that results from the disease.

CORE CONCEPT 1

CF is a disease in which nutrition is of utmost importance, and routine nutrition screening and assessments are essential in the care of every patient.

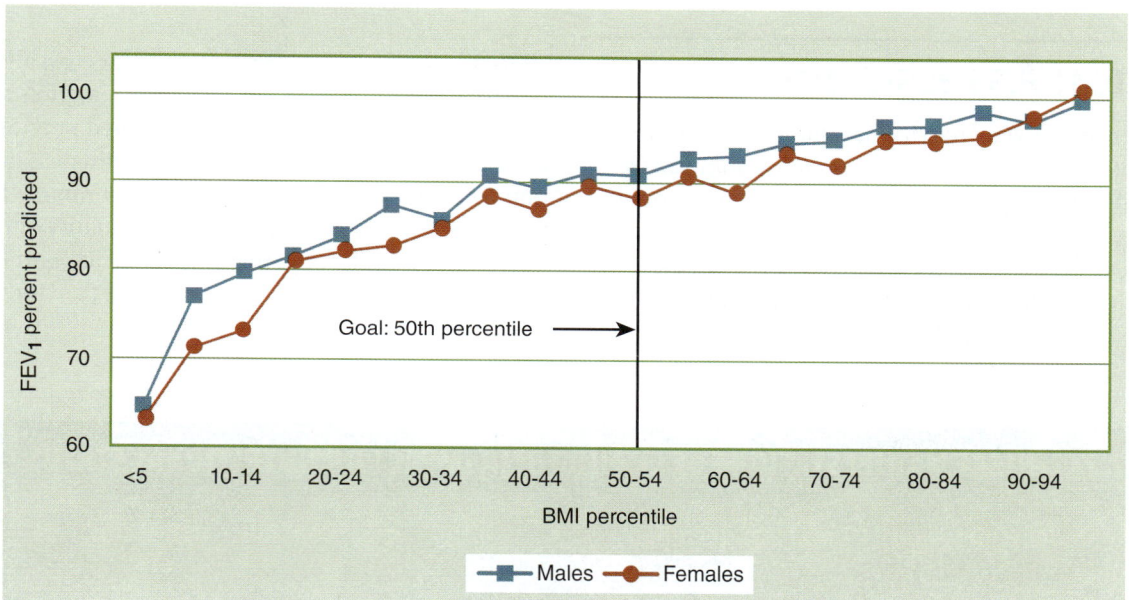

FIGURE 17.5 Positive Relationship between FEV$_1$ Percentage Predicted and BMI/Age in Children
Reproduced from Cystic Fibrosis Foundation Patient Registry, 2016 Annual Data Report, Bethesda, Maryland. ©2017 Cystic Fibrosis Foundation.

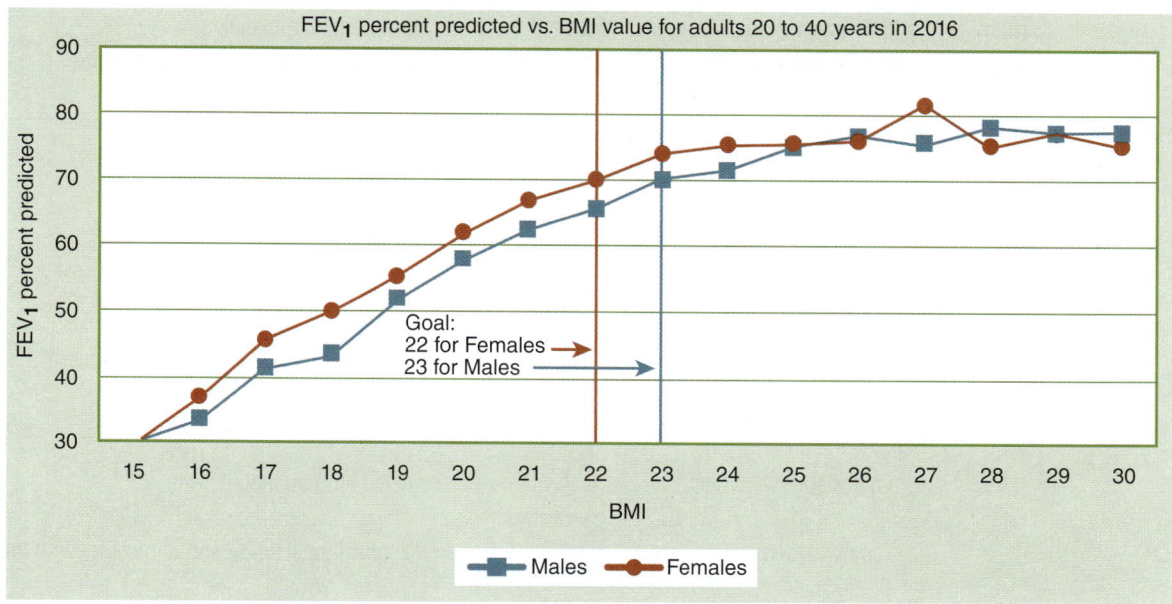

FIGURE 17.6 Positive Association between FEV$_1$ Percentage Predicted and BMI in Adults
Reproduced from Cystic Fibrosis Foundation Patient Registry, 2016 Annual Data Report, Bethesda, Maryland. ©2017 Cystic Fibrosis Foundation.

> ### CASE STUDY REVISITED
> Following Lucy's diagnosis of CF, you are asked to provide energy and protein goals for Lucy.
>
> #### Questions
> 1. What factors should be considered in determining energy and protein requirements?
> 2. What are Lucy's nutritional risk factors? What nutritional indices will you monitor routinely? What goals will you set?
> 3. In addition, suggestions for micronutrient supplementation are requested. Provide your recommendations with appropriate rationale.

Nutrition Assessment

The relationship between nutritional status and trajectory of CF cannot be overstated. Clinical manifestations of the disease itself impart significant risk factors to nutritional status and growth (**Table 17.2**). While the increased work of breathing and pancreatic insufficiency are the most-prominent determinants of nutritional status, inflammation associated with recurrent infections, other GI disturbances, altered appetite, and psychosocial factors can all influence nutritional adequacy. Conversely, malnutrition negatively impacts clinical outcome in CF. As stated previously, a low BMI-for-age is associated with diminished lung function. Diminished fat-free mass impairs immune function, reduces exercise capacity, and lowers quality of life.[5] These factors make ongoing nutritional assessment and aggressive diet therapy a cornerstone of care for the CF patient.

TABLE 17.2 CLINICAL MANIFESTATIONS OF CF AND THEIR IMPACT ON NUTRITIONAL STATUS

CF-related Pathophysiology or Disturbance	Clinical Manifestation	Impact on Nutritional Status
Diminished pulmonary function	Increased work of breathing	Increased resting energy expenditure Weight loss
Recurrent respiratory infections	Pulmonary exacerbations and frequent hospitalizations	Systemic inflammation Interruption in normal nutritional intake
Gastrointestinal abnormalities	Pancreatic insufficiency	Steatorrhea and malabsorption Micronutrient deficiencies • Essential fatty acids • Fat-soluble vitamins Bone demineralization CF-related diabetes
	Gastrointestinal reflux, esophagitis, intestinal obstruction, nausea	Impaired nutrient intake
	Cholestatic liver disease	Altered nutrient metabolism
Psychosocial	Family stressors Depression	Poor nutritional intake and compliance with therapy

Energy and Protein Needs

Children with CF are expected to gain weight and grow at the same rate as a child without CF. Additionally, adults with CF are expected to maintain a weight and BMI comparable to a healthy adult. As energy needs in the patient with CF are much higher than in one without CF, maintenance of good nutritional status requires extra effort on the part of the patient and family. Energy expenditure is higher due to the higher metabolic demand required to breathe. Chronic pulmonary infections can cause an increased work of breathing, and therefore an increased metabolic rate. Additionally, in spite of pancreatic enzyme replacement therapy aimed to treat pancreatic insufficiency, there continue to be some losses of fat in the stool, contributing to a loss of calories. Although the mechanism is unknown, measured resting energy expenditure (REE) is increased with pancreatic insufficiency. Research shows that CF children with pancreatic insufficiency had higher REEs than their pancreatic-sufficient CF counterparts. A negative linear relationship between pulmonary function, as measured by FEV_1, and REE exists with pancreatic insufficiency.[6] Most patients with CF require 110% to 200% of the energy needs of a healthy individual of similar age, sex, and size.[4] Calorie needs are often estimated using REE multiplied by a factor to accommodate physiologic impact of the disease and an activity factor. Equations for energy needs are not precise in CF given the variability in disease and symptom severity. Clinicians must evaluate the extent of diminished lung function, pancreatic insufficiency, physical activity, and current nutritional status when determining the proper factor to use. Energy needs and appropriateness of set targets are based on clinical outcomes of weight gain and growth.[7]

There are no specific recommendations for protein intake, and it is usually assumed that protein intake is adequate as long as energy needs are met. However, recognizing the importance of promoting anabolism and fat-free mass in CF patients is advocated. Patients with low fat-free mass have reduced lung function, bone mineral loss, altered muscle function, and a high frequency of pulmonary exacerbations requiring hospitalization.[5] Anabolism can be induced in CF with increasing levels of protein intake. This dose–response association between protein intake and protein synthesis prompts consideration of protein and amino acid supplements, particularly in patients with diminished fat-free mass. Because higher amounts of protein are needed for this effect, the optimal provision of protein must be considered to minimize the colonic effects of undigested protein. Amino acid supplements may be useful in this respect.[5]

⚠ Clinical Controversy

Use of BMI-for-age to Classify Nutritional Failure

The CF Foundation, based on consensus report for children with CF, recommends that patients ages 2 to 20 years achieve a BMI-for-age at or above the 50th percentile. This classification, while useful for standardizing nutritional assessment and guidelines for initiation nutrition based interventions, has a number of shortcomings.

Konstan et al. showed that many children, despite BMI-for-age between the 25th and 50th percentiles, had weights and heights that were below the 10th percentile for age. The researchers emphasize that BMI-for-age fails to identify poor nutritional status in stunted children.

There are other patient subgroups that may not benefit from the standard BMI-for-age recommendation. Stephenson et al. showed that the benefit of increasing BMI on lung function was only clinically significant in underweight patients. The effect was much less in overweight patients. They conclude that the greatest benefit of improving BMI was in underweight, pancreatic-insufficient patients. The authors caution that given the risk of obesity, standard recommendations for increasing BMI, which do not make a distinction between under- and overweight patients, may have implications for overweight CF patients.

Similarly, Engelgen et al. emphasize that with the increasing numbers of patients who are overweight and obese and who may still have diminished fat-free mass, use of BMI-for-age may not be sensitive enough to identify sarcopenic obesity in CF patients.

Questions

1. Using the reports referenced above, discuss the implications of relying on BMI-for-age alone to assess nutritional risk and dietary intervention for all CF patients.

References

1. Borowitz D, Baker RD, Stalling VD. Consensus report on nutrition for pediatric patients with cystic fibrosis. *J Pediatr Gastroenterol Nutr*. 2002; 35(3):246-59.
2. Konstan MW, Pasta DJ, Wagener JS, VanDevanter DR, Morgan WJ. BMI fails to identify nutritional risk in stunted children. *J Cystic Fibr*. 2017 (16):158-160.
3. Stephenson AL, Mannik LA, Walsh S, Brotherwood M, Robert R, Darling PB, Nisenbaum R, Moerman J, Stanojevic S. Longitudinal trends in nutritional status and the relation between lung function and BMI in cystic fibrosis: a population based cohort study, *AM J Clin Nutr*. 2013;97(4):872-877.

> **CORE CONCEPT 2**
>
> Energy needs are high in a patient with cystic fibrosis due to an increased metabolic demand associated with breathing and malabsorption of fat due to pancreatic insufficiency.

> **PRACTICE POINT**
>
> Patients with CF may have energy requirements equivalent to 110% to 200% of the energy needs of a healthy individual of similar age, gender, and size.

Anthropometrics

Weight and height should be measured and BMI calculated at every visit. For children, all anthropometrics should be plotted on the growth chart appropriate for age and sex. The CF Foundation, based on consensus reports, recommends that all children ages 2 to 20 years achieve a BMI-for-age at or above the 50th percentile. For children and infants younger than 2 years of age, a zero standard deviation (50th percentile) of weight-and-height/length for age is recommended. In this context, is also important to ensure that children with CF are growing within their genetic height potential, because chronic malnutrition can result in stunting.[7]

Biochemical Assessment

As part of the nutrition assessment, routine labs should be monitored annually per the recommendations of the CF Foundation.[7] At approximately 2 months after starting vitamin supplementation and annually thereafter, serum vitamin A (retinol), vitamin E (alpha-tocopherol), and 25-hydroxy vitamin D levels should be measured to assess vitamin status.[8] **PIVKA-II** is the laboratory test of choice to assess vitamin K status. If this test is unavailable, prothrombin time can be used in the setting of a patient without liver dysfunction. Hemoglobin and hematocrit should be measured yearly to evaluate iron status. Serum electrolytes, particularly sodium levels, should also be measured annually to ensure adequate sodium intake to compensate for increased losses in the sweat. Liver function tests are also monitored to follow for any signs of CF-related liver disease. All patients with CF, starting at the age of 10 years, should complete a 2-hour oral glucose tolerance test in conjunction with their annual labs to monitor for the development of CF-related diabetes.[9] In special circumstances, other laboratory tests may be completed. Additionally, for patients with concern for poor bone health, a dual energy x-ray absorptiometry (DXA) scan can be completed starting at age 8 years to monitor bone status.[10]

> **PRACTICE POINT**
>
> At approximately 2 months after starting vitamin supplementation and annually thereafter, serum vitamin A (retinol), vitamin E (alpha-tocopherol), 25-hydroxy vitamin D, and vitamin K via either PIVKA-II or prothrombin time should be measured to assess vitamin status.

Diet Assessment

Every patient with CF should be evaluated by a registered dietitian (RD) at least once per year. In patients who are struggling to maintain normal nutrition status, more frequent nutrition assessment should be completed. It is important to evaluate fluid, calorie, sodium, and calcium intake to ensure the diet is meeting the needs of the patient. A 24-hour diet recall or a 3-day food record can be used to better evaluate the patient's normal dietary intake. The nutrition assessment should also include any oral supplements, tube feeds, and vitamin supplements that the patient may be taking to augment their dietary consumption. Laboratory values should be reviewed and adjustments to the vitamin regimen should be made based on results. Stool pattern should also be evaluated to assess for any signs or symptoms of malabsorption. The RD should also note any medications that the patient may be taking that may have drug–nutrient interactions.

> **PRACTICE POINT**
>
> Patients with CF should be evaluated by an RD at least once per year. In patients who are struggling to maintain normal nutrition status, more frequent nutrition assessment should be completed.

Pancreatic Insufficiency

Approximately 90% of all patients with CF have pancreatic insufficiency, a loss of the exocrine function of the pancreas.[1] Some patients may present initially with normal function of the pancreas and may convert to pancreatic insufficiency over time. Pancreatic status can often determined by reviewing the mutations causing the CF, because many mutations are associated with pancreatic disease. All patients presenting with CF should have a stool test to measure pancreatic elastase-1 (**Figure 17.7**). Pancreatic elastase-1, a digestive enzyme secreted exclusively by the pancreas, is a fecal marker used to assess exocrine pancreatic function. If the result is <200 mcg/g stool, **pancreatic enzyme replacement therapy (PERT)** should be initiated.[7] Additionally, the CF Foundation recommends initiating PERT before the results of a stool test in a patient with two

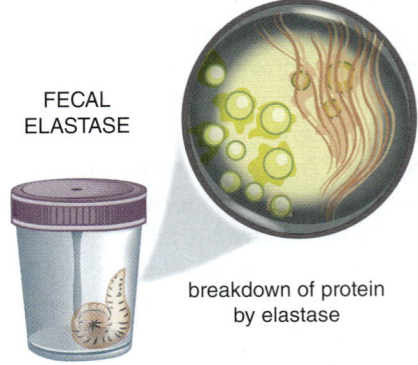

FIGURE 17.7 Fecal Elastase Test Is Used to Assess Pancreatic Insufficiency in Children Presenting with CF

CASE STUDY REVISITED

Lucy is now 3 years old. Her weight is 12 kg and her height is 91 cm. Her steatorrhea has improved with PERT; however, she remains substantially underweight. Her mother gives her enzymes immediately following all meals and snacks. Her enzyme dose has not been adjusted recently, and she is currently receiving 500 units lipase/kg/meal. She has not been given the prescribed proton pump inhibitor (PPI) because it is felt that Lucy is taking too many pills already.

Questions

1. Assess the adequacy of her dosing amount and schedule.
2. What is the purpose for prescribing PPIs for Lucy?
3. How might you improve Lucy's nutritional status and symptoms?

---

known CFTR mutations that are known to cause pancreatic insufficiency or in a patient showing signs and symptoms of malabsorption upon diagnosis.[7]

CORE CONCEPT 3

Pancreatic insufficiency affects the majority of patients with cystic fibrosis; it results in malabsorption of fat without proper treatment with pancreatic enzyme replacement therapy.

Pancreatic insufficiency results in the pancreas's inability to secrete lipase, protease, and amylase, the digestive enzymes needed to break down and utilize the calories from food. Untreated pancreatic insufficiency results in malabsorption of these nutrients and can contribute to poor nutritional status and fat-soluble vitamin deficiencies. Treatment for pancreatic insufficiency is to give **porcine-derived pancreatic enzymes**, taken by mouth with meals and snacks to substitute for the enzymes the pancreas is not endogenously making. These enzymes contain lipase, protease, and amylase for the digestion of fat, protein, and carbohydrates.

Most pancreatic enzymes on the market currently are in capsule form and contain small microspheres or microtablets that are each enterically coated to protect them from the acidic environment of the stomach. The enteric coating is designed to dissolve in the alkaline pH of the duodenum, where absorption of nutrients occurs. Often, acid blockers in the form of H_2 antagonists or proton pump inhibitors (PPIs) are prescribed to assist in decreasing the acidity of the duodenum to possibly aid in enzyme efficacy.[11] All brands and dosages of pancreatic enzymes, generically known as pancrelipase, on the market today are approved by the U.S. Food and Drug Administration (FDA) and no generic forms should be used.[12] Additionally, there is one nonenteric-coated product in tablet form normally prescribed for patients with chronic pancreatitis that can be used off-label in patients with CF who are receiving enteral feeds.[12]

CORE CONCEPT 4

Treatment for pancreatic insufficiency is to provide porcine-derived pancreatic enzymes, taken by mouth with meals and snacks to substitute for the enzymes the pancreas is not endogenously creating. These enzymes contain lipase, protease, and amylase for the digestion of fat, protein, and carbohydrates.

Recommendations for weight-based dosing of PERT are available from the CF Foundation; however, dosages must be individualized to the patient. It is important to closely monitor the dose of pancreatic enzymes, because extremely high lipase doses have been associated with fibrosing colonopathy or bowel wall thickening. For infants, the recommended starting dose is 2,000 to 5,000 units lipase per 120-mL feeding.[7] In patients who are diagnosed after infancy, enzymes can be dosed based upon weight, with a starting dose of 1,000 units lipase/kg/meal for patients younger than 4 years of age and 500 units lipase/kg/meal for those older than age 4 years.[13] Enzyme doses for snacks are generally half of the usual meal dose. Enzyme doses can be adjusted upward based on clinical assessment of stools, weight gain, and growth. The maximum recommended dose is 2,500 units lipase/kg/meal, with a maximum daily dose of 10,000 units lipase/kg/day.[13] If signs of malabsorption are still present after the maximum enzyme dose has been reached, the method of administration, adherence to the enzyme regimen, timing of enzymes with meals, and the method of enzyme storage should be assessed.

PRACTICE POINT

For infants, the recommended starting dose is 2,000 to 5,000 units lipase per 120-mL feeding. In patients who are diagnosed outside of the period of infancy, enzymes can be dosed based upon weight, with a starting dose of 1,000 units lipase/kg/meal for patients younger than 4 years of age and 500 units lipase/kg/meal for those older than age 4 years.

Clinical Roundtable

Topic: Pancreatic enzyme replacement therapy in tube-fed patients

Background: Many CF patients rely on enteral tube feedings to maintain their nutritional status. Elemental or peptide-based enteral feedings provide free amino acids and carbohydrate sources in simpler form, which may be easier to digest. However, due to instability of hydrolyzed fat, the fat component of enteral feeding products is intact. Therefore, omission of enzymes, even with hydrolyzed feedings, is not an option. This poses a challenge to the clinician regarding the optimal method for administration of pancreatic enzymes per feeding tube. Improper preparation and administration of enzymes can lead to clogged feeding tubes, intolerance of feedings by the patient, and malabsorption.

Several options have been proposed as discussed in this section. Nonenteric-coated enzymes such as Viokace may be crushed, diluted, and added directly to the enteral feeding bag. Although enteric-coated enzymes cannot be added to the enteral feedings directly, a number of techniques are described. The fluid diluent and method of administration is of great importance and can have implications for clogging and enzyme function. Ferrie et al. provide instruction on provision of a slurry containing enzyme microspheres mixed with an acidic, thickened juice via a syringe. Another option, posed by Nicolo et al., involves mixing the granules with sodium bicarbonate and adding it to the tube feeding every 4 hours. Recently emerged is Relizorb (Alcresta Therapeutics, Inc, Newton, MA), a cartridge containing digestive enzymes that connects in-line with the enteral feeding set. With this novel approach, the fat in the enteral feeding is hydrolyzed as it comes into contact with the cartridge. Freedman et al. have shown Relizorb to be safe and effective in increasing fat absorption.

Roundtable Discussion

1. Discuss the available methods for administering pancreatic enzymes. What recommendations or guidelines would you provide for patients requiring enteral support?
2. Describe preparation and administration techniques. How might location of the feeding tube (gastric versus postpyloric) and schedule of feeding (intermittent continuous) influence your decision?

References

1. Freedman S, Orenstein D, Black P, Brown P, McCoy K, Stevens J, Grujic D, Clayton R. Increased fat absorption from enteral formula through an in-line digestive cartridge in patients with cystic fibrosis. *J Pediatr Gastroenterol Nutr*. 2017;65:97–101.
2. Ferrie S, Graham C, Hoyle M. *Pancreatic enzyme supplementation for patients receiving enteral feeds*. Nutr Clin Pract. 2011;26:349–351.
3. Nicolo M, Stratton KW, Rooney W, Boullata J. Pancreatic enzyme replacement therapy for enterally fed patients with cystic fibrosis. *Nutr Clin Pract*. 2013;28(4):485–489.

Pancreatic enzymes should be taken immediately prior to any meal containing fat or protein so that the enzymes reach the duodenum before any food. For infants and small children unable to swallow pills, the capsules should be opened up and the beads mixed with a small amount of acidic, pureed food, such as applesauce, and given via spoon. As soon as the patient is able, the capsules can be swallowed whole.

> **PRACTICE POINT**
>
> Pancreatic enzymes should be taken immediately before any meal containing fat or protein so that the enzymes reach the duodenum before any food.

When patients are receiving enteral feeds, they require enzymes for proper absorption. The most common method to provide enzymes for these feeds is to provide a meal dose of enzymes by mouth before and after overnight feeds or a meal dose prior to a bolus feed. However, in some instances, patients with CF are physically unable to take their enzymes by mouth. Examples include intubation during critical illness or oral aversion. There are currently no pancreatic enzymes on the market that are FDA approved for administration through an enteral tube. Many CF centers have developed methods by which to give enzymes through a tube. The most common method is to use a nonenteric-coated enzyme called Viokace. To use this method, Viokace tablets are crushed into a fine powder and the powder is added directly to the enteral formula.[12] This method allows the macronutrients in the enteral formula to be predigested prior to administration of the enteral feed. Other methods have also been described. One is to dissolve the enteric-coated enzyme beads into a bicarbonate solution and add the enzyme/bicarbonate solution to the enteral formula or bolus directly prior to formula administration.[14] Another described method is to mix the enteric-coated enzyme beads into nectar-thick fruit juice and administer into a 10 French or larger feeding tube prior to administering formula.[15] Enteric-coated beads should not be administered directly via feeding tube due to the risk of clogging the tube. When using any of the above methods, enzyme

> ### CASE STUDY REVISITED
>
> Lucy is now 9 years old. She is doing well with minimal steatorrhea. Her BMI-for-age is still below recommended CF standards. The medical team advises that if she cannot improve her weight gain from the oral route, then a feeding tube would be recommended.
>
> **Anthropometric Data:**
> Height: 129 cm (4'2")
> Weight: 25 kg (55 lbs)
>
> **Biochemical Data:**
> Prealbumin 13 (17 – 36 g/dL)
>
> **Clinical Data:**
> **Meds:** Albuterol, Pulmozyme, Flovent, Creon, AquaDEKs
>
> **Dietary Data:**
> **Dietary Recall:**
> Breakfast (7:30 am): Orange juice, Shredded wheat (1 cup) with 6 oz skim milk, 1 slice toast with jelly
> Lunch (11:30 am): Apple juice, garden salad with hard-boiled egg, and tuna with low-fat dressing or a turkey sandwich with mustard
> Dinner (5 pm): Spaghetti with marinara sauce
> Dessert (5:30 pm): Frozen yogurt
>
> ### Questions
> 1. How might Lucy improve the caloric density of her diet?
> 2. What macronutrient would you emphasize? Why?

dosing should be calculated by the grams of fat that the formula contains. Usual dosing ranges from 500 to 4,000 units lipase/g fat, with usual dosing approximately 2,000 units lipase/g fat.[13]

The stool pattern of the patient should be assessed at every visit to determine adequacy of the enzyme dose. Signs and symptoms of malabsorption may include increased frequency of stools, bulky stools, foul-smelling stools, stool that floats in the toilet, presence of oil in diaper or toilet, increased gassiness, or frequent rectal prolapse.

Nutrition Management in Patients with Cystic Fibrosis

Macronutrients

In general, patients with CF require a high-calorie diet for proper weight gain and growth. Historically, it was recommended to restrict fat in the diet to avoid the symptoms of fat malabsorption. Now, with adequate PERT, the diet of patients with CF should be liberal in fat because it is more calorie-dense than carbohydrates and protein. Typically, patients with CF require a diet with approximately 35% to 40% of calories derived from fat to meet their increased energy needs.[6]

> ### PRACTICE POINT
> When given adequate PERT, fat restriction is not indicated and a high-fat diet should be promoted to meet elevated calorie needs.

Infants

As a result of newborn screening, infants are commonly diagnosed with CF in the first few months of life. Human milk is recommended as the CF infant's primary source of nutrition due to its widely recognized benefits. If human milk is not available, standard infant formula should be used.[7] Hydrolyzed protein formulas have not shown a benefit over standard formulas when proper pancreatic enzyme replacement is used.[16] Introduction of solid foods should be initiated per standard recommendations by the American Academy of Pediatrics. Some infants may require fortified human milk or calorie-dense infant formulas due to the high metabolic demands of CF. Once solids are introduced to the infant's diet, purees and table foods can be made more energy dense with the addition of oils or butter. These adjustments in diet should be done only in infants who are demonstrating poor weight gain and growth.[7]

Micronutrients

Patients with CF and pancreatic insufficiency require supplementation of vitamins and minerals due to risk for deficiencies as a result of malabsorption. Fat-soluble vitamin (vitamins A, E, D, and K) deficiencies are usually present in infancy at diagnosis and are normally corrected once PERT and vitamin supplements are initiated.[17] There are many vitamin supplements on the market today that are specifically designed for patients with CF. These supplements contain higher amounts of fat-soluble vitamins in addition to water-soluble vitamins and zinc. Infants are started on these vitamins upon diagnosis of CF and pancreatic insufficiency.[7] Dosages of CF-specific vitamins are adjusted based on results of vitamin levels drawn annually as part of routine CF care. Some patients require single-nutrient supplementation of vitamins A, E, D, or K if deficiency of a particular vitamin persists despite supplementation with a CF-specific multivitamin. The CF Foundation has published consensus guidelines specifically on the treatment of vitamin D deficiency. In summary, the CF Foundation recommends all patients maintain a 25-OH vitamin D level greater than 30 ng/mL and that all low levels be treated with vitamin D_3 (cholecalciferol).[18] These guidelines should be referred to when treating a CF patient with a low vitamin D level because they differ based on the patient's age and vitamin D level. All patients should be counseled that their vitamins should be taken with a fat-containing food or beverage in conjunction with PERT to ensure adequate absorption.

> **CORE CONCEPT 5**
>
> Patients with cystic fibrosis and pancreatic insufficiency require supplementation of vitamins and minerals due to risk for malabsorption-related deficiencies. All fat-soluble vitamins should be assessed annually, because they are the primary nutrients at risk for deficiency.

In addition to fat-soluble vitamins, there are some mineral deficiencies that may be present in CF. Zinc losses occur in the stool prior to initiation of enzyme therapy or in patients whose enzyme regimen is not optimized.[19] Zinc deficiency is difficult to diagnose because the lab measure is not a good predictor of zinc stores in the body. In patients in whom a zinc deficiency is suspected, 1 mg elemental zinc/kg weight can be prescribed for 6 months in addition to a regular CF-specific multivitamin.[6]

Dietary intake of calcium should be assessed regularly due to higher risk for bone disease in CF. With risk for vitamin D deficiency apparent, it is essential that calcium intake is adequate in the diet.[20] If dietary intake of calcium is poor, calcium supplements should be recommended.

Sodium Chloride

Patients with CF have higher sodium needs than those of the general population. This is due to increased sodium losses in their sweat.[21] All patients with CF are prescribed a high-salt diet. For infants, the CF Foundation guidelines recommend 1/8 teaspoon of salt daily upon diagnosis and through 6 months of age.[7] The salt should be added in small, frequent amounts throughout the day in bottles or in the applesauce used to administer enzymes. At 6 months, ¼ teaspoon salt should be given daily.[7] After the child is eating a variety of table foods, salt should be added liberally to foods. Special attention should be made in months where the temperature is very warm or when the patient is participating in strenuous activity.

> **CORE CONCEPT 6**
>
> Patients with cystic fibrosis have higher sodium needs than those of the general population due to increased sweat-related losses. All patients with CF are prescribed a high-salt diet to compensate for the additional losses.

> **PRACTICE POINT**
>
> CF Foundation guidelines recommend 1/8 teaspoon of salt daily upon diagnosis and through 6 months of age. The salt should be added in small, frequent amounts throughout the day in bottles or in the applesauce used to administer enzymes. At 6 months, ¼ teaspoon salt should be given daily.

Nutrition Support

Adequate nutrition status and BMI-for-age are essential to maintaining normal lung function in CF. If an adequate BMI-for-age cannot be maintained with a high-calorie diet alone, high-calorie oral supplements are often prescribed. These supplements may range from 30 to 60 calories per ounce and are usually given in conjunction with meals to boost calorie intake. Patients and families may also choose to make their own high-calorie shakes due to the high cost of commercial supplements or due to taste preference.

Oral supplements are sometimes not sufficient in promoting weight gain and normal growth, so enteral feeds are often recommended.[4] Enteral feeds are typically given at a continuous rate overnight during sleep. The patient eats and drinks normally throughout the day and receives additional calories overnight. Most patients choose to have a gastrostomy tube inserted; however, nasogastric feeds can be used if the feeds are thought to be only needed on a short-term basis. Both intact protein and semi-elemental formulas can be used, but both formulas require PERT for proper absorption.[22] Postpyloric feeds are rarely needed, although they may be beneficial in patients with severe reflux or those who are intubated and ventilated. Parenteral nutrition is not routinely used in CF but may be required in circumstances where the GI tract cannot be used or when enteral feeds are not tolerated.

Prior to prescribing enteral feeds, a trial of appetite stimulants may be indicated. If oral supplements are not sufficient or are not tolerated by the patient and inadequate calories

> ## CASE STUDY REVISITED
>
> Lucy is 18 years of age. She is admitted to evaluate new-onset CF-related diabetes. She also experienced a wrist fracture last summer while playing softball. Her clinical information is as follows:
>
> **Anthropometrics:**
> Height: 162 cm (5'4")
> Weight: 56 kg (123 lbs)
>
> **Biochemical Data:**
> Electrolytes Normal
> 2-hour glucose on glucose tolerance test 204 (<200 mg/dL)
> HbA1c 8.9 (4.3-5.8%)
> Vitamin D 14 (20-100 ng/mL)
>
> **Questions**
> 1. What is Lucy's BMI-for-age How would you describe her nutritional status at this point?
> 2. What concerns might you have given her biochemical data at this visit?
> 3. How might this relate to her CF?

are suspected, appetite stimulants may stimulate hunger enough to promote adequate weight gain.[23] Other causes of poor weight gain, such as malabsorption or increased energy expenditure due to respiratory illness, should be ruled out before appetite stimulants are prescribed. Cyproheptadine hydrochloride (Periactin™) is a common appetite stimulant used in CF.[24] It is an antihistamine with a secondary effect of appetite stimulation. It is often used due to its low side effect profile, but it may cause fatigue initially in some patients. Megestrol acetate (Megace™) is successful in promoting weight gain; however, it must be used with caution due to its risk of causing adrenal suppression and diabetes.[25,26] Dronabinol (Marinol™) has also been described as helpful in patients with severe lung disease, as the medication can improve appetite and nausea.[27]

> **CORE CONCEPT 7**
>
> If an adequate BMI-for-age cannot be maintained with diet alone, oral supplements, and often enteral nutrition support, are recommended to promote weight gain.

Nutrition-related Complications of Cystic Fibrosis

Gastrointestinal Complications

Gastroesophageal reflux is more common in patients with CF and it must be treated effectively to prevent additional damage to the lungs.[28] Untreated reflux can result in inadequate oral intake and poor weight gain and can also exacerbate lung disease.[29] Constipation is also a very common complication of CF. This is a result of poor CFTR function in the GI tract, causing the stool to become dehydrated and difficult to pass.[30] Untreated constipation can result in distal intestinal obstruction syndrome that may require surgical intervention if left untreated.[31] It is important to prevent constipation in CF with adequate hydration and salt intake. Often, stool softeners such as polyethylene glycol are used as a maintenance medication to prevent constipation.[31]

Patients with CF who remain pancreatic sufficient are at risk for developing pancreatitis. These particular patients may go on to become pancreatic insufficient and should be closely monitored with an annual pancreatic elastase. Patients with CF are also at risk to develop CF-related liver disease. This may progress to end-stage liver disease, in which a liver transplant may be indicated. Liver function tests are recommended on an annual basis in conjunction with annual lab studies to monitor the liver.[32]

CF-related Diabetes

All patients with CF are at risk for developing **CF-related diabetes (CFRD)**. CFRD is its own entity with similarities to both type 1 and type 2 diabetes.[33] The major problem is shortage of insulin, but insulin resistance can also play a role in hyperglycemia.[33] The risk of developing CFRD increases with age.[34-36] Hyperglycemia can also occur without a diagnosis of CFRD during times of illness or when patients are receiving corticosteroid therapy. CFRD is usually diagnosed by a 2-hour oral glucose tolerance test completed annually starting at age 10 years.[33] A 2-hour value >200 mg/dL is diagnostic for CFRD. Other diagnostic criteria include a fasting glucose ≥126 mg/dL, a HbA1c ≥6.5, or a random glucose ≥200 mg/dL. HbA1c should not be used exclusively as a screening tool for CFRD due to increased red blood cell turnover in patients with CF.[33]

> **CORE CONCEPT 8**
>
> All patients with cystic fibrosis are at risk for developing CF-related diabetes (CFRD) due to a shortage of insulin and some insulin resistance.

Treatment for CFRD is usually insulin, and oral hypoglycemic medications are typically not used. Insulin regimens should be individualized for every patient by an endocrinologist who is familiar with CFRD. A high-calorie diet should continue to be recommended and carbohydrates should not be restricted.[33] Proper treatment with insulin and normal blood sugar control is vital to maintaining adequate nutrition status.

CF-related Bone Disease

Patients with CF are at a greater risk for developing bone disease.[37] Mainly, malabsorption of fat results in fat-soluble vitamin deficiencies, specifically vitamin D. Additionally, chronic malnutrition and frequent use of corticosteroids may contribute to poor bone health. By the age of 18 years, all patients with CF should have a DXA scan. Based on the results, patients should have a repeat scan every 1 to 5 years. It is recommended that children with CF who have strong risk factors for bone disease should receive a DXA scan prior to age 18 years.[38] For abnormal DXA scans, it is important that calcium, vitamin D, and vitamin K are optimized in the diet and/or supplements are used.

> **CORE CONCEPT 9**
>
> Patients with cystic fibrosis are at a greater risk for developing bone disease due to fat-soluble vitamin deficiencies, specifically vitamin D, and often chronic malnutrition.

> **PRACTICE POINT**
>
> All patients with CF should have a dual energy x-ray absorptiometry (DXA) scan by age 18 years. Children at high risk may need to receive one prior to 18 years of age.

Summary

Cystic fibrosis is a genetic disease associated with the abnormal transport of sodium, chloride, and water at the cellular level resulting in abnormally thick mucus leading to organ damage. Nutritional management of CF involves promoting normal growth during childhood and adolescence and maintaining optimal nutrition in adulthood. CF is associated with high energy needs related to an increased work of breathing and consumption of a calorically dense high fat, increased sodium diet is often recommended. Malabsorption due to pancreatic insufficiency occurs in the majority of individuals with CF. Treatment of pancreatic insufficiency involves the use of pancreatic enzyme replacement therapy to provide exogenous lipase, protease, and amylase to assist in macronutrient digestion. Due to the prevalence of malabsorption, individuals with CF should be monitored for fat soluble vitamin status and receive supplementation as appropriate. If an adequate BMI cannot be achieved or maintained in those with CF, oral supplements or enteral nutrition support is recommended. Management of CF-related conditions such as gastroesophageal reflux, constipation, CF-related diabetes, and CF-related bone disease is important to maintain optimal health and nutritional status.

Key Terms

CF transmembrane conductance regulator (CFTR) protein, pancreatic insufficiency, sweat test, digital clubbing, bronchi, bronchioles, alveoli, cilia, bronchodilators, mucolytics, nebulizers, percussor, forced expiratory volume at 1 second (FEV_1), PIVKA-II, pancreatic enzyme replacement therapy (PERT), CF-related diabetes (CFRD).

References

1. Cystic Fibrosis Foundation. Cystic fibrosis foundation patient registry. [2015 Annual Data Report to the Center Directors]. 2016.
2. Farrell PM, Rosenstein BJ, White TB, et al. Guidelines for diagnosis of cystic fibrosis in newborns through older adults: Cystic fibrosis foundation consensus report. *J Pediatr*. 2008;153(2): S4-S14.
3. Yen EH, Quinton H, Borowitz D. Better nutritional status in early childhood is associated with improved clinical outcomes and survival in patients with cystic fibrosis. *J Pediatr*. 2013;162(3):530-535.e1.
4. Stallings VA, Stark LJ, Robinson KA, Feranchak AP, Quinton H. Evidence-based practice recommendations for nutrition-related management of children and adults with cystic fibrosis and pancreatic insufficiency: Results of a systematic review. *J Am Diet Assoc*. 2008;108(5):832-839.
5. Engelen,MP, Com G, Deutz NE. Protein is an important but undervalued macronutrient in the nutritional care of patients with Cystic Fibrosis. *Curr Opin Nutr Metab Care*. 2014; 17(6):515-520.
6. Moudiau T, Galli-Tsinopoulou, Vamvakoudis E, Nousia-Arvanitakis S. Resting energy expenditure in cystic fibrosis as an indicator of disease severity. *J Cystic Fibr*. 2007;6:131-136.
7. Borowitz D, Baker RD, Stalling VD. Consensus report on nutrition for pediatric patients with cystic fibrosis. *J Pediatr Gastroenterol Nutr*. 2002;35(3):246-259.
8. Borowitz D, Robinson KA, Rosenfeld M, et al. Cystic fibrosis foundation evidence-based guidelines for management of infants with cystic fibrosis. *J Pediatr*. 2009;155(6):S73-S93.
9. Moran A, Brunzell C, Cohen RC, et al. Clinical care guidelines for cystic fibrosis-related diabetes: A position statement of the American Diabetes Association and a clinical practice guideline of the cystic fibrosis foundation, endorsed by the pediatric endocrine society. *Diabetes Care*. 2010;33(12):2697-2708.

10. Aris RM, Merkel PA, Bachrach LK, et al. Guide to bone health and disease in cystic fibrosis. *J Clin Endocrinol Metab.* 2005;90(3):1888-1896.

11. O'Brien CE, Harden H, Com G. A survey of nutrition practices for patients with cystic fibrosis. *Nutr Clin Pract.* 2013;28(2):237-241.

12. Berry AJ. Pancreatic enzyme replacement therapy during pancreatic insufficiency. *Nutr Clin Pract.* 2014;29(3):312-321.

13. Borowitz DS, Grand RJ, Durie PR. Use of pancreatic enzyme supplements for patients with cystic fibrosis in the context of fibrosing colonopathy. *J Pediatr.* 1995;127(5):681-684.

14. Nicolo M, Stratton KW, Rooney W, Boullata J. Pancreatic enzyme replacement therapy for enterally fed patients with cystic fibrosis. *Nutr Clin Pract.* 2013;28(4):485-489.

15. Ferrie S, Graham C, Hoyle M. Pancreatic enzyme supplementation for patients receiving enteral feeds. *Nutr Clin Pract.* 2011;26(3):349-351.

16. Ellis L, Kalnins D, Corey M, Brennan J, Pencharz P, Durie P. Do infants with cystic fibrosis need a protein hydrolysate formula? A prospective, randomized, comparative study. *J Pediatr.* 1998;132(2):270-276.

17. Feranchak AP, Sontag MK, Wagener JS, Hammond KB, Accurso FJ, Sokol RJ. Prospective, long-term study of fat-soluble vitamin status in children with cystic fibrosis identified by newborn screen. *J Pediatr.* 1999;135(5):601-610.

18. Tangpricha V, Kelly A, Stephenson A, et al. An update on the screening, diagnosis, management, and treatment of vitamin D deficiency in individuals with cystic fibrosis: Evidence-based recommendations from the cystic fibrosis foundation. *J Clin Endocrinol Metab.* 2012;97(4):1082-1093.

19. Easley D, Krebs N, Jefferson M, et al. Effect of pancreatic enzymes on zinc absorption in cystic fibrosis. *J Pediatr Gastroenterol Nutr.* 1998;26(2):136-139.

20. Ross AC, Manson JE, Abrams SA, et al. The 2011 report on dietary reference intakes for calcium and vitamin D from the institute of medicine: What clinicians need to know. *J Clin Endocrinol Metab.* 2011;96(1):53-58.

21. Arvanitakis S, Lobeck C. Metabolic alkalosis and salt depletion in cystic fibrosis. *J Pediatr.* 1973;82(3):535-536.

22. Durie P, Newth C, Forstner G, Gall D. Malabsorption of medium-chain triglycerides in infants with cystic fibrosis: Correction with pancreatic enzyme supplements. *J Pediatr.* 1980;96(5):862-864.

23. Nasr SZ, Drury D. Appetite stimulants use in cystic fibrosis. *Pediatr Pulmonol.* 2008;43(3):209-219.

24. Homnick DN, Homnick BD, Reeves AJ, Marks JH, Pimentel RS, Bonnema SK. Cyproheptadine is an effective appetite stimulant in cystic fibrosis. *Pediatr Pulmonol.* 2004;38(2):129-134.

25. Eubanks V, Koppersmith N, Wooldridge N, et al. Effects of megestrol acetate on weight gain, body composition, and pulmonary function in patients with cystic fibrosis. *J Pediatr.* 2002;140(4):439-444.

26. Marchand V, Baker SS, Stark TJ, Baker RD. Randomized, double-blind, placebo-controlled pilot trial of megestrol acetate in malnourished children with cystic fibrosis. *J Pediatr Gastroenterol Nutr.* 2000;31(3):264-269.

27. Anstead M, Kuhn R, Martyn D, Craigmyle L, Kanga J. Dronabinol, an effective and safe appetite stimulant in cystic fibrosis. *Pediatr Pulmonol.* 2003;36:343.

28. Mousa HM, Woodley FW. Gastroesophageal reflux in cystic fibrosis: Current understandings of mechanisms and management. *Curr Gastroenterol Rep.* 2012;14(3):226-235.

29. Cucchiara S, Santamaria F, Andreotti MR, et al. Mechanisms of gastro-oesophageal reflux in cystic fibrosis. *Arch Dis Child.* 1991;66(5):617-622.

30. van der Doef, Hubert PJ, Kokke FT, van der Ent, Cornelis K, Houwen RH. Intestinal obstruction syndromes in cystic fibrosis: Meconium ileus, distal intestinal obstruction syndrome, and constipation. *Curr Gastroenterol Rep.* 2011;13(3):265-270.

31. Colombo C, Ellemunter H, Houwen R, Munck A, Taylor C, Wilschanski M. Guidelines for the diagnosis and management of distal intestinal obstruction syndrome in cystic fibrosis patients. *J Cystic Fibrosis.* 2011;10(Suppl 2):S24-S28.

32. Debray D, Kelly D, Houwen R, Strandvik B, Colombo C. Best practice guidance for the diagnosis and management of cystic fibrosis-associated liver disease. *J Cystic Fibrosis.* 2011;10(Suppl 2):S29-S36.

33. Moran A, Brunzell C, Cohen RC, et al. Clinical care guidelines for cystic fibrosis-related diabetes: A position statement of the American Diabetes Association and a clinical practice guideline of the Cystic Fibrosis Foundation, endorsed by the Pediatric Endocrine Society. *Diabetes Care.* 2010;33(12):2697-2708.

34. Moran A, Dunitz J, Nathan B, Saeed A, Holme B, Thomas W. Cystic fibrosis-related diabetes: Current trends in prevalence, incidence, and mortality. *Diabetes Care.* 2009;32(9):1626-1631.

35. Solomon MP, Wilson DC, Corey M, et al. Glucose intolerance in children with cystic fibrosis. *J Pediatr.* 2003;142(2):128-132.

36. Lanng S, Hansen A, Thorsteinsson B, Nerup J, Koch C. Glucose tolerance in patients with cystic fibrosis: Five year prospective study. *BMJ.* 1995;311(7006):655-659.

37. Stalvey MS, Clines GA. Cystic fibrosis-related bone disease: Insights into a growing problem. *Curr Opin Endocrinol Diabetes Obes.* 2013;20(6):547-552.

38. Aris RM, Merkel PA, Bachrach LK, et al. Guide to bone health and disease in cystic fibrosis. *J Clin Endocrinol Metab.* 2005;90(3):1888-1896.

Chapter 18

Nutrition in Solid Organ Transplantation

Lauren Parsly
Jenna Stefin

Chapter Outline

Core Concepts
Introduction
Background
Indications and Contraindications for Transplantation
Medical Treatment
Nutritional Management

CORE CONCEPTS

1. Medical advances have made solid organ transplants a viable option for many people with end-stage organ failure.

2. Organ transplant recipients are those who are deemed as able to survive the rigors of surgery and recovery and go on to lead productive, higher quality lives for many years following the transplant.

3. As organ transplant recipients live longer, there is increased risk of chronic issues from long-term use of immunosuppressants.

4. Postoperative nutritional management should be individualized according to the patient's nutritional status, the organ being transplanted, and any complications that may arise during or after surgery.

Learning Objectives

1. Describe indications and contraindications for solid organ transplants.
2. Recognize complications that can arise from solid organ transplantation.
3. Identify immunosuppressant medications and their nutritional implications.
4. Estimate short-term and long-term needs for patients who have undergone solid organ transplants.

Introduction

The number of solid organ transplants, which includes kidney, heart, liver, lung, pancreas, and small-bowel transplantation, has been increasing over the last decade. Organ transplantation is considered life-saving surgery or a last stage intervention to improve one's quality of life. Medical nutrition therapy has an important role throughout all phases of the transplantation process. Early preoperative nutrition intervention is essential to optimize surgery outcomes, while long-term postoperative monitoring is vital to prevent the development of chronic disease.

Background

The act of transplanting one part of the body, or part of someone else's body, onto another has been around for several millennia. Hindu texts dating from 2500 BC to 3000 BC describe skin grafts that were taken from the buttocks and chin and molded to make new noses on criminals who had lost theirs to punishment.[1] A **graft** is any tissue or organ used for implantation or transplantation, while a **host** is the recipient of the organ or tissue. There has been evidence from the Bronze Age of both autograft transplantation and allograft transplantation of bone, skin, and teeth.[1] **Autograft transplantation**, also known as autotransplantation, is defined as transplantation of a tissue or an organ from one site onto another one or in the body of the same individual. **Allograft transplantation**, also known as allotransplantation or allogenic transplantation, describes a graft of tissue transplanted between individuals of the same species but of disparate genotype; types of donors are cadaveric, living related, and living unrelated. Some solid organ transplants are characterized as **orthotopic**, which describes something that occurs in the normal or usual place in the body, such as tissue or an organ that is transplanted into its normal place in the body.

It was not until the early 1900s that advances in surgical and clinical skills allowed solid organ transplantation experimentation to garner attention. In 1902, French surgeon Alexis Carrel wrote a paper detailing successful kidney reimplantation in the neck of the same dog and later, between two dogs.[1] Through his experiments, Dr. Carrel noted that unsuccessful organ transplants were due to host rejection of the transplant.[1] **Rejection** is an immune reaction against grafted tissue that results in failure of the graft to survive. In 1954, successful kidney transplants were achieved in monozygotic twins.[1] The surgeries were performed by Dr. Joseph Murray and Dr. John Merrill at the Peter Bent Brigham Hospital and identified that genetic matching of the allograft transplantation donor and recipient was necessary.

In lieu of genetic matching, it was soon discovered that **immunosuppression**, or suppression of the immune response by drugs or radiation, could decrease the rate of host rejection of the transplanted organ.[1] By suppressing the immune system, the organ recipient has a decreased risk of immune cells identifying the transplanted organ as an invading body and attacking it. Blunt irradiation of the organ recipient led to premature deaths, not from host rejection, but from the effects of the radiation.[1] The discovery of using a combination of immunosuppressive drugs to eliminate organ rejection from nongenetically matched donors opened the door to organ transplantation with both live and deceased donors as a viable option to save lives.[1] Today, many immunosuppressive drugs such as cyclosporine and tacrolimus are widely used in organ transplantation. They are so effective in suppressing the immune system that 90% to 95% of kidney and 85% of heart transplant recipients survive 1 year after their surgery.[2,3]

As organ transplant recipients live longer, additional problems occur due to the effects of the immunosuppressive medications. Organ recipients face increased risk of viral, bacterial, and other pathogenic infections that their bodies are no longer able to resist. As organ transplantation moves into the 21st century and antibiotic development advances, organ transplantation and immunosuppression have the highest success rate thus far. Doctors can successfully transplant hearts, kidneys, lungs, livers, intestines, and pancreata. According to the Organ Procurement and Transplantation Network, more than 115,000 candidates on the U.S. organ transplant waiting list await one or more solid organ(s).[4] An individual's placement on the organ waitlist varies by organ, but allocation involves many factors, including degree of illness and medical urgency, waiting time, donor/recipient immune system compatibility, and distance from donor hospital.[5]

In 2016, there were more than 33,500 organ transplants in the United States.[4] There has been a 20% increase in transplants over the last 5 years, although current demand for organs exceeds supply.[4] Survival rates vary according to recipient gender, age, diagnosis, organ, blood type, age, and vital status (deceased versus living) of the donor. For example, the median survival period for heart transplant recipients ranges from 11 to 14 years.[3]

> **CORE CONCEPT 1**
>
> Medical advances have made solid organ transplants a viable option for many people with end-stage organ failure.

CASE STUDY INTRODUCTION

George is a 59-year-old male with ischemic cardiomyopathy, an ejection fraction (EF) of 15%, type 2 diabetes, and hypertension (HTN). He presents for a nutrition assessment as part of a multidisciplinary pretransplant evaluation for a heart transplant. His cardiovascular history includes a myocardial infarction 5 years ago, requiring percutaneous coronary intervention (PCI); a cardiac arrest 2 years ago; and an implantable cardioverter defibrillator (ICD) placement last year. George has had several hospital admissions over the last year due to decompensated heart failure and recently started on home milrinone. George had been working in construction but has been unable to work over the last few months due to progressive shortness of breath (SOB) and fatigue. He is divorced and currently lives alone.

Anthropometric Data:
Weight: 115 kg (253 lbs)
Height: 178 cm (70")
Body mass index (BMI): 36 kg/m^2
Weight History
Usual body weight (UBW): 126 kg (277 lbs) 6 months ago
Recent highest weight: 132 kg (290 lbs) 3 months ago, in the setting of volume overload
Estimated dry weight: 113 kg (249 lbs)

Biochemical Data:
Sodium 132 (135-145 mEq/L)
Potassium 4.2 (3.6-5.0 mEq/L)
Blood urea nitrogen 23 (6-24 mg/dL)
Creatinine 1.0 (0.4-1.3 mg/dL)
Blood glucose 169 (70-139 mg/dL)

Total cholesterol 140 (Desirable <200 mg/dL)
Low-density lipoprotein 69 (Desirable <100 mg/dL)
High-density lipoprotein 19 (Desirable ≥40 mg/dL)
Triglycerides: 200 (Desirable <150 mg/dL)
HbA1C 7.5% (4.3-5.8%)

Clinical Data:
Past Medical History: Ischemic cardiomyopathy with EF 15%, MI s/p PCI, ICD placement, Type 2 DM, left leg deep vein thrombosis, obstructive sleep apnea, obesity, hypertension, dyslipidemia, and depression
Medications: Atorvastatin, Carvedilol, potassium chloride 20 meq, Lantus 18 units at bedtime, Lispro 8 units 3 times daily, Lasix 20 mg daily, Losartan, milrinone, warfarin
Vital Signs: Blood pressure: 98/70 mm Hg; Temperature 98.6°F; Heart rate 100 beats/min
Nutrition-focused Physical Exam: Appears obese with central adiposity. Skin feels warm to touch, appears slightly dry. There is evidence of pitting edema on legs bilaterally. Good dentition noted with normal mouth and tongue. No wounds or skin breakdown noted. No obvious SOB noted when in conversation.

Dietary Data:
Dietary History: George reports decreased appetite in comparison to baseline over the last 1 to 2 months. He continues to eat three meals/day but portion sizes are smaller than he usually eats. He does not count carbohydrates but has been trying to follow a low-sodium diet by not adding salt to foods. Due to SOB and fatigue, he has been eating more prepared/take out foods lately.
Diet Prescription: low sodium, 1.5 liter fluid restriction, consistent carbohydrate

Questions
1. What is George's nutritional status and nutritional risk factors?
2. What are the nutrition priorities for George?
3. What additional information would you like to obtain?
4. Is George an appropriate candidate for heart transplant? Why or why not?
5. Should weight loss be encouraged?
6. Does he have any nutrition-related contraindications to transplant?

Indications and Contraindications for Transplantation

Who is a candidate for organ transplant? Individuals with decompensated end-stage organ failure are eligible to be placed on the organ waitlist. This is a life-saving surgery for individuals who need heart, liver, and lung transplants. While dialysis, insulin therapy, and parenteral nutrition (PN) are alternative treatments for patients with renal, pancreatic, and intestinal failure, respectively, life-threatening complications may lead to loss of intravenous (IV) access for PN or dialysis, necessitating alternative options. The benefits of transplantation must outweigh the risks associated with major surgery and long-term immunosuppression.

Kidney Transplant Indications

There are a number of diseases and etiologies leading to end-stage renal disease (ESRD), such as glomerulonephritis, hypertension, diabetes, congenital abnormalities, polycystic kidney disease, or urinary tract obstruction.[6] Diabetic nephropathy and hypertensive nephrosclerosis are the most common causes of ESRD.[7] In the absence of contraindications, kidney transplantation is indicated when a patient reaches ESRD, which is demonstrated by either requiring dialysis or having a GFR of ≤20 mg/dL.[8]

Pancreas Transplant Indications

The most common indication for pancreas transplantation is type 1 diabetes, to produce independence from injected insulin. Pancreas transplants are typically done in conjunction with a kidney transplant due to the underlying etiology of diabetes-related ESRD. It is not a life-saving surgery, but rather completed as a means of improving quality of life. A very small percentage of pancreas transplants are done for other reasons, such as after a pancreatectomy in the setting of chronic pancreatitis.[9]

Liver Transplant Indications

Hepatitis C virus–related chronic liver disease is the most common indication for liver transplantation in the United States.[10] Hepatitis B virus–related chronic disease, alcoholic liver disease, and hepatic malignancy are other common etiologies for liver transplant, followed by primary biliary cirrhosis and metabolic diseases, such as Wilson's disease.[2,10] Patients with alcoholic liver disease must abstain from drinking alcohol for at least 6 months prior to placement on the waiting list.[2]

Heart Transplant Indications

Chronic heart failure from cardiomyopathy of various etiologies and ischemic heart disease are the most common reasons for a heart transplant (**Figure 18.1**).[2] Critically ill heart failure patients may require placement of a ventricular assist device, a surgically implanted mechanical pump that supports heart function by pumping blood to circulate

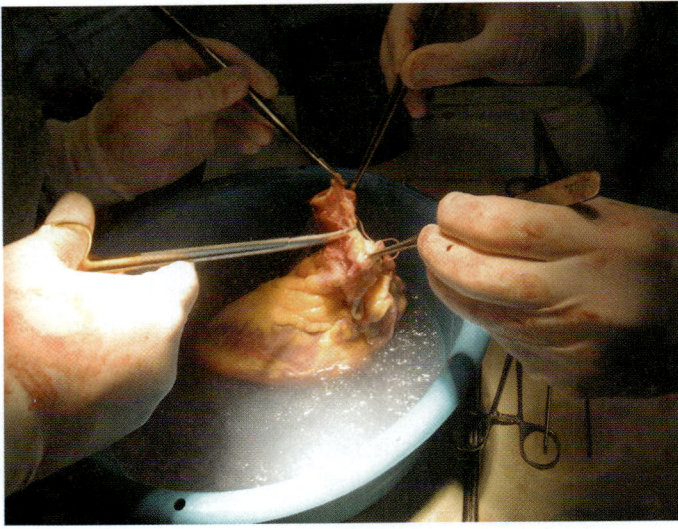

FIGURE 18.1 Heart Being Prepared for Transplantation
© kalewa/Shutterstock.

oxygen-rich blood throughout the body until a donor heart is available.

Lung Transplant Indications

The most common diseases requiring lung transplantation are cystic fibrosis, chronic obstructive pulmonary disease (COPD), pulmonary fibrosis, and pulmonary hypertension.[2] Bilateral lung transplants tend to take place more frequently than unilateral lung transplants. Some patients may require both heart and lung transplantation if the lung failure precipitated heart failure.[2]

Small-bowel Transplant Indications

Short bowel syndrome, dysmotility syndrome, impaired enterocyte absorption, and failure of parenteral nutrition (PN) are common reasons for small-bowel transplantation.[11] Currently, Medicare approves intestinal transplantation in patients with irreversible intestinal failure who have failed PN. Failure of PN is defined as one or more of the following: liver failure caused by PN, thrombosis of major central venous access of two or more vessels, frequent line infections or sepsis defined as two or more episodes of systemic sepsis per year or one episode of line fungemia, septic shock, acute respiratory distress syndrome, and/or frequent episodes of severe dehydration.[11]

Contraindications to Transplantation

Contraindications for an organ transplant include advanced age; poor posttransplant prognosis; sepsis; malignancies; infections (both active or latent); poor social support; active substance abuse; multisystem organ failure; active psychiatric or psychological pathologies; or inability to adhere to a complex medical regimen, which may be demonstrated by lack of insight or medication noncompliance.[12] Proper evaluation for transplant candidacy requires a multidisciplinary approach. Dietitians, pharmacists, social workers, medical doctors, surgeons, and financial coordinators collaborate to bring their unique expertise to produce a thorough assessment of participants. Nutritionally, malnutrition and obesity may be contraindications to transplant due to risk for poor surgical outcomes and significantly higher morbidity and mortality compared with other groups.[13] While not an absolute contraindication, obesity has been shown to increase a patient's risk of wound complications.[14,15] Patients with morbid obesity must be evaluated by the transplant team for associated comorbidities such as infection, uncontrolled diabetes, uncontrolled blood pressure, or other organ dysfunction to determine transplant recipient candidate suitability.[14]

CORE CONCEPT 2

Organ transplant recipients are those who are deemed as able to survive the rigors of surgery and recovery and go on to lead productive, higher quality lives for many years following the transplant.

In simultaneous pancreas/kidney transplants, obesity (BMI 30-40 kg/m^2) has been shown to delay kidney graft function and increase rates of 1-year acute kidney rejection, pancreas graft thrombosis, and patient death.[16] **Graft thrombosis**, or obstruction of blood flow to a graft, can lead to graft rejection. A BMI of >27 has been associated with increased pancreas and kidney graft loss.[16,17] Obesity has also been associated with a greater risk of graft dysfunction and decreased short- and long-term survival in lung transplant recipients.[14,18]

Studies have demonstrated an obesity paradox in the heart failure population.[19] The best heart failure outcomes occurred in overweight patients followed by obese patients, while the worst outcomes occurred in underweight heart failure patients followed by normal BMI.[19] Obese patients who undergo open heart surgery have higher risk for poor wound healing, infection, pulmonary complications, and lower extremity thrombosis. Specifically, BMI <18.5 kg/m^2 and BMI of >35 kg/m^2 have been shown to increase morbidity and mortality.[13] Despite the uncertainties regarding the obesity survival paradox in heart failure, there are several potential benefits of weight loss, such as improvement in insulin sensitivity, blood pressure, and lipid profile, for example. It is important to keep in mind that meaningful weight loss may be challenging for patients with limited exercise capacity due to their end-stage organ failure.

The obesity survival paradox is not evident in the kidney transplant recipients because both extremes of pretransplant BMI are linked to higher mortality in this population. In 2011, more than one-third of the U.S. kidney transplant recipients were categorized as obese.[20] Of these, 23% had a BMI of 30 to 34.9, 9.4% had BMI 35 to 39.9 and 2.1% had BMI ≥40 kg/m^2.[20] A retrospective review of all recipients in the United Network of Organ Sharing (UNOS) database from 2004 to 2009 revealed a significantly increased risk for delayed graft function among obese patients, with odds ratios rising in parallel with degree of obesity.[20] Overall, the risk of surgical site complications, delayed graft function, and increased hospital length of stay is associated with obesity in kidney transplant recipients. Recipients with an underweight BMI have poorer graft survival as well as poorer overall survival. While studies appear to support a neutral impact of obesity on long-term graft and patient survival, there is an increased risk of new-onset diabetes.[20] A study that reviewed the U.S. Renal Data System database from 1995 to 1999 found that the survival benefit of kidney transplantation versus remaining on dialysis was lost above a BMI of 41 kg/m^2.[21]

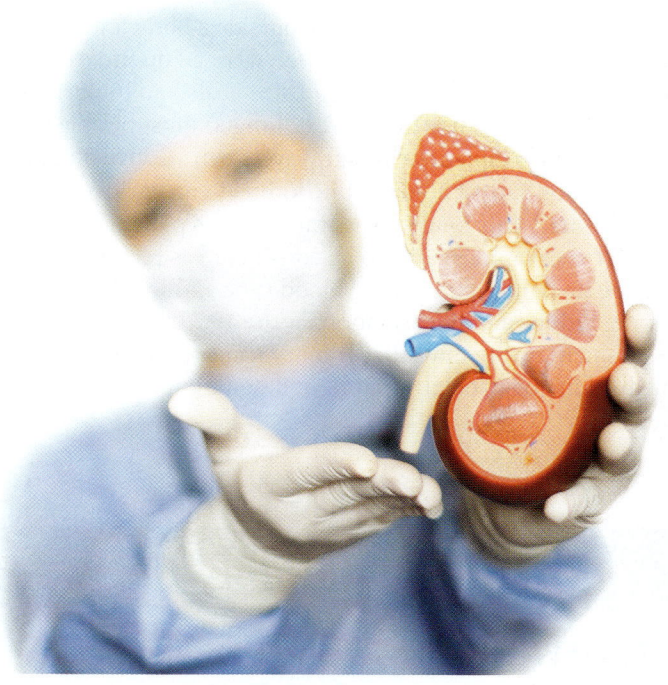
© yezry/Shutterstock.

The 2013 American Association for the Study of Liver Disease practice guidelines state that morbid obesity (BMI ≥40 kg/m^2) is a relative contraindication in liver transplantation.[22] This guideline is based on a 2002 Nair et al. study that reported that 1, 2, and 3-year mortality rates were significantly higher in patients with BMI >40 kg/m^2.[14,23] Underweight status is associated with higher perioperative mortality and poorer patient and graft survival among liver transplant patients as well.[24]

Although current literature regarding weight loss prior to transplantation is limited, it is generally recommended to encourage weight loss in the obese patient before they are transplanted.[12] Some studies suggest that bariatric surgery may be a safe and symptomatically beneficial procedure for obese heart failure or renal failure patients at experienced centers.[25,26] Overall BMI cutoffs may vary depending on the organ and transplant center.

Medical Treatment

Organ Donation and Matching

Once an organ donor has been evaluated for **brain death**, where irreversible cessation of all brain activity over a period of time has been acknowledged, organs are then evaluated for possible donation. In order to meet the increasing demand for donated organs, additional avenues are explored to increase organ donation among deceased donors. Donation of organs can also occur after a patient is deceased by means of cardiac death, referred to as **donation after cardiac death (DCD)**. When a deceased organ donor is identified, the UNOS system creates a ranked list of candidates who are appropriate to receive each organ based on blood type, tissue type, body size, medical urgency, waiting time, and geography, as well as other criteria.[5] Heart and lung organs can only survive outside a body for 4 to 6 hours, so these organs are first offered based on proximity to the donor's hospital.[5] Organ size is also an important consideration because the heart or lung(s) must be able to fit inside the recipient's rib cage. Livers can survive outside the body for 8 to 12 hours, while kidneys can survive for 24 to 36 hours.[5] This longer time frame allows patients from a wider geographical area to be considered as recipients of the organ, pending matching blood type and waitlist time. Living kidney and liver donors (**Figure 18.2**) require an assessment by the multidisciplinary transplant team. Past medical history, social support, and donation intentions are reviewed. Many centers have BMI cutoffs for living donors to minimize surgical complications and infection postoperatively. It has been found that obesity significantly increases the risk of end-stage renal disease among living kidney donors.[27]

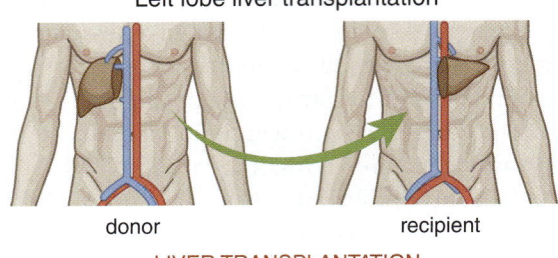

FIGURE 18.2 Liver Transplantation from Living Donor

Complicating Factors

Graft Versus Host Disease

Mostly observed after allogeneic stem cell transplants, graft-versus-host disease (GVHD) is a rare but potentially fatal complication following solid organ transplant.[28,29] There are two forms of GVHD; in the more common form, the host will have the A, B, or AB blood type but receive a solid organ from a donor with blood type O. In this case, the antibodies in the graft view the host as a foreign body and begin attacking the recipient's red cell antigens, which

---

Clinical Roundtable

Topic: Weight Loss Prior to Transplantation

Background: The current literature regarding weight loss in end-stage organ failure, especially prior to transplantation, is limited. There is evidence to support that having overweight and obese BMIs may be protective for heart failure patients and for patients requiring renal replacement therapy. Conversely, there are significant data demonstrating that obesity can increase risk of complications like wound infections or delayed graft function among all transplant candidates. Many patients struggle and often fail to achieve the requested weight loss. Achieving a BMI <30 kg/m² is usually the recommended weight loss goal for the general population. It has also been demonstrated that modest weight loss of 5% to 10% can help with insulin resistance, cholesterol, and blood pressure in healthy individuals. One study has shown that <10% of potential kidney recipients lose weight when recommended for listing, while <5% reach the goal BMI of <30 kg/m². Moreover, many of the patients who lost weight to become eligible on the waiting list had a high risk for quickly regaining weight in the early posttransplant period without significant benefit to transplant outcomes (i.e., survival or graft outcomes). The long-term sustainability of weight maintenance is also a common issue.

Roundtable Discussion

1. Should BMI cutoffs be an absolute contraindication to transplant?
2. Should weight loss be recommended in patients with end-stage organ failure who are overweight or obese despite their compromised medical condition? Why or why not?
3. Should bariatric surgery be considered and, if so, when?

References

1. Chan G, Garneau P, Hajjar R. The impact and treatment of obesity in kidney transplant candidates and recipients. *Can J Kidney Health Dis*. 2015;2:26. doi:10.1186/s40697-015-0059-4.

can lead to a mild and temporary form of hemolytic anemia. In the cellular type of GVHD, the antibodies in the graft will attack the host's skin, gastrointestinal tract, liver, and bone marrow. In order for GVHD to occur, the graft must contain immunologically competent cells that trigger host's antibodies.[29] GVHD will usually manifest between 1 and 12 weeks after transplantation; however, there have been cases of kidney transplant recipients developing GVHD as late as 9 months posttransplant.[28,29]

Malnutrition

Malnutrition can be a complicating factor in solid organ transplantation and has been shown to compromise posttransplant survival as well as increase length of hospital stay and wound healing times.[30-34] It is common for individuals with end-stage organ failure to have a degree of malnutrition; for example, 70% to 79% of patients undergoing liver transplantation are malnourished.[9] Patients must be assessed carefully for signs of deficiencies related to weight loss or malabsorption caused by their end-stage organ disease. Efforts must be made to reverse the malnutrition before the patient undergoes transplant surgery to decrease risks of posttransplant complications and comorbidities. Oral nutrition therapy is the preferred method of correcting malnutrition, but enteral nutrition may be considered to increase caloric intake for patients who are unable to meet their needs orally.

Immunosuppression

Although patients need to be adequately immunosuppressed for rejection prevention, a balance needs to be maintained to avoid other life-threatening infections and complications. Suppression of the natural immune system of the organ recipient increases the vulnerability of organ recipients to infection, GVHD, and malignancies as they are less able to resist bacteria and viruses or destroy rogue cells that have the potential to turn malignant.[2] Induction immunosuppression, an intense prophylactic therapy, is usually administered as a short course during the immediate pre- and postoperative periods of transplant to prevent or delay the onset of rejection. This is followed by a long-term immunosuppression regimen, which usually consists of two or more medications from different drug classes with varying mechanisms of action (**Figure 18.3**). Most patients will require a calcineurin inhibitor, such as tacrolimus or cyclosporine, and DNA synthesis inhibitor, such as mycophenolate mofetil, and some will also require steroids, such as prednisone. Patients will need to be on immunosuppressive drugs for the rest of their lives, as long as the transplanted organ is still functioning.[2] The amount of immunosuppression may be tapered to a lower maintenance level 3 to 6 months after the transplant. The immune system must always be kept in check to avoid rejection of the graft, even years later. Different organs may require varying amounts and combinations of immunosuppressive drugs.[2] Immunosuppressive medications come with a variety of side effects that can have nutritional consequences. **Table 18.1**

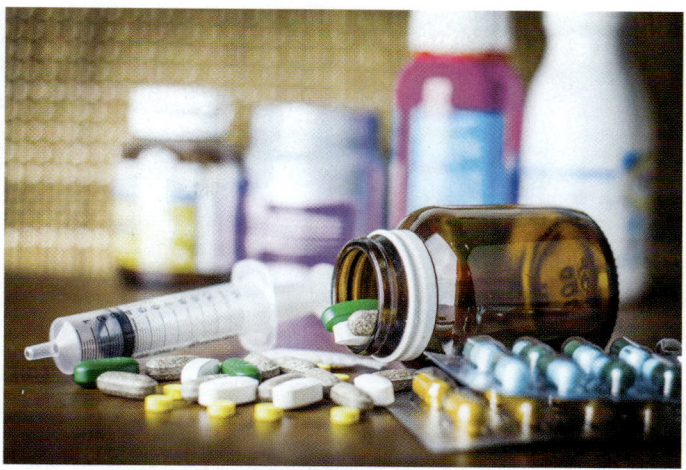

FIGURE 18.3 There Is a Complex Medication Regimen after Transplantation
© Adul10/Shutterstock.

details common side effects and nutrition interventions for immunosuppressive medications.

CORE CONCEPT 3

As organ transplant recipients live longer, there is increased risk of chronic issues from long-term use of immunosuppressants.

Nutritional Management

Pretransplant Phase

Before a patient can be placed on the organ transplant waiting list, they must be assessed to ensure an optimal nutritional status to allow for adequate healing after surgery. Both subjective and objective nutrition status measures can be used. Objective measures include a weight history based on past medical records; patient's current weight, height, BMI, and percentage weight loss; and laboratory values. It may be difficult to obtain accurate weights on pretransplant patients due to fluid shifts and retention. Body composition is important to evaluate because standard calculations like BMI do not take frame size or lean body mass into consideration. The waist-to-hip ratio (WHR), which is calculated by dividing the waist circumference by the hip (or gluteal) circumference, can be a helpful tool that assesses the proportion of fat stored on the waist and hips.[35] It is preferred that the waist circumference is less than the hip circumference; therefore, a WHR <1 is ideal.[35] There is an increased risk of diabetes, heart disease, and hypertension with increased abdominal fat.[35] A full subjective global assessment should be performed and a diet recall/history should be completed to assess adequacy of calorie, fluid, protein, and micronutrient intake.[36] As there are advantages and drawbacks to a variety of methods, it is important to use a combination of objective and subjective measures when assessing a patient's nutritional status.[12]

TABLE 18.1 TRANSPLANT IMMUNOSUPPRESSIVE MEDICATIONS, SIDE EFFECTS, AND INTERVENTIONS

Common Drug Brands and Class	Potential Nutrition Side Effects	Nutrition Intervention
Azathioprine (Imuran) • Antimetabolite	• Nausea, vomiting, diarrhea, steatorrhea • Stomatitis, esophagitis • Anorexia	• Monitor for adequate nutrient intake. Encourage small, frequent bland meals; consider antiemetic agents; ensure adequate fluid intake; decrease fat in diet for steatorrhea • Avoid spicy and acidic foods; consider soft food diet • Monitor oral intake; consider appetite stimulants
Cyclosporine (Neoral, Sandimmune, Gengraf) • Calcineurin inhibitors (Avoid grapefruit products)	• Anorexia • Gum hyperplasia • Hyperglycemia • Hyperkalemia • Hyperlipidemia • Hypertension • Hypomagnesemia	• Monitor oral intake; consider appetite stimulants • Emphasize good oral hygiene; consider soft diet • Monitor blood sugar and need for carbohydrate-controlled diet • Restrict high-potassium foods • Encourage a heart-healthy diet* and maintenance of healthy weight • Avoid high-sodium foods and maintain healthy weight • Increase high-magnesium foods or consider magnesium supplements
Mycophenolate mofetil (Cellcept), mycophenolic acid (Myfortic) • Antimetabolite/DNA synthesis inhibitor	• Nausea, vomiting, constipation, diarrhea • Dyspepsia • Oral candidiasis, stomatitis • Hypomagnesemia • Hypercholesterolemia	• Monitor for adequate nutrient intake. Encourage small, frequent bland meals; consider antiemetic agents; ensure adequate fluid intake; add more fiber and fluid for constipation. Consider nutrition support if oral intake remains suboptimal • Avoid caffeine, acidic foods, carbonated beverages • Monitor oral intake; emphasize good oral hygiene; consider soft food diet • Increase high-magnesium foods or consider magnesium supplements (supplementation should be taken separately from drug) • Encourage heart-healthy diet* and maintenance of healthy weight
Prednisone (deltasone), methylprednisolone (solumedrol) • Corticosteroid	• Increased appetite, weight gain • Slow wound healing, increased protein catabolism • Hyperglycemia • Osteoporosis due to calcium wasting • Altered fluid and sodium retention, hypertension	• Educate on balanced meals, portion control, and mindful eating behaviors • Ensure adequate protein intake; maintain good blood glucose control; consider need for vitamin/mineral supplements • Monitor blood sugar and need for carbohydrate-controlled diet • Ensure adequate calcium and vitamin D intake; consider need for bone-building medications • Avoid high-sodium foods, maintain a healthy weight
Sirolimus (Rapamune), everolimus (Zortress) • mTOR inhibitors	• Nausea, vomiting, diarrhea, constipation • Hyperlipidemia	• Monitor for adequate nutrient intake. Encourage small, frequent bland meals; consider antiemetic agents; ensure adequate fluid intake; add fiber and fluid for constipation • Encourage heart-healthy diet* and maintenance of healthy weight
Tacrolimus (Prograf) • Calcineurin inhibitor (Avoid grapefruit products)	• GI adverse effects such as abdominal pain, dyspepsia, nausea, vomiting, diarrhea, constipation, gastritis • Hyperglycemia • Hypertension • Oral candidiasis, stomatitis, dysphagia • Hyperkalemia • Hypomagnesemia	• Monitor for adequate nutrient intake. Encourage small, frequent bland meals; consider antiemetic agents; ensure adequate fluid intake; add fiber and fluid for constipation. Avoid caffeine, acidic foods, and carbonated beverages with gastritis • Monitor blood sugars and need for long-term carbohydrate-controlled diet • Avoid high-sodium foods and maintain healthy weight • Emphasize good oral hygiene; consider soft diet • Avoid high-potassium foods • Increase high-magnesium foods or consider magnesium supplements

* A heart-healthy diet is characterized as a diet low in saturated fat and added sugars and high in fiber from whole grains, fruits, and vegetables.
Data from Pronsky ZM, Elbe D, Ayoob K. *Food-Medication Interactions*, 18th ed. Birchrunville, PA: Food-Medication Interactions; 2015.

> ### CASE STUDY REVISITED
>
> George has been approved and placed on the waiting list for a heart transplant. After 9 months on the list, George receives a heart transplant and is now postoperative day (POD) #3. His transplant was uncomplicated. He has been extubated and no longer requires ventilatory support, but remains in the ICU for volume overload and hyperglycemia requiring an insulin drip.
>
> **Anthropometric Data:**
> Preoperative weight: 115 kg (253 lbs)
> Current weight: 118 kg (260 lbs)
>
> **Biochemical Data:**
> Sodium 139 (135-145 mEq/L)
> Potassium 4.1 (3.6-5.0 mEq/L)
> Blood urea nitrogen 26 (6-24 mg/dL)
> Creatinine 1.6 (0.4-1.3 mg/dL)
> Glucose 112 (70-139 mg/dL)
>
> **Dietary Data:**
> **Diet Prescription:** Low microbial, carbohydrate controlled
>
> ### Questions
> 1. What factors should you consider when developing a nutrition plan?
> 2. What are his acute postop nutrition requirements?
> 3. What nutrition relevant labs would you monitor? What electrolyte complications might you encounter?

Acute Posttransplant Phase

The acute posttransplant period is usually defined as the first 2 months after surgery.[11] Posttransplant nutrition goals focus on achieving adequate nutrient intake for the patient, providing increased nutrition during the process of healing, and preventing infection and complications of acute rejection. Proper nutrition can help the body resist infections, heal surgical wounds, and enhance strength to participate in physical therapy.[12] Depending on the organ being transplanted and any other comorbidities, the patient may be able to start eating within a few days of surgery. For example, following orthotopic heart transplantation, most patients are able to start an oral diet within the first 2 to 5 days if there are no complications. If the patient is unable to eat an oral diet by this duration, enteral or parenteral nutrition may be considered based on the patient's diagnosis. Many medications used to prevent or treat rejection and infection, including antibiotics and antifungal drugs, can cause nausea, vomiting, diarrhea, and changes in taste, and ultimately can impact dietary intake.[37] The side effects of mycophenolate mofetil, a common immunosuppressive agent, are primarily gastrointestinal issues such as nausea, esophageal reflux, and diarrhea, which can be reduced by decreasing the dosage or substituting with a different medication.[9]

Energy

The stress of surgery and side effects from immunosuppressive medications can cause changes in the posttransplant patient's metabolism.[12] If no secondary conditions such as sepsis are present, the posttransplant patient is unlikely to be significantly hypermetabolic, so caloric needs are similar to other surgical patients.[9,12] It is necessary to consider factors such as pretransplant nutritional status and other medical conditions when estimating needs. Studies assessing energy needs among liver transplant patients during the first posttransplant month found that resting energy expenditure (REE) was 7% to 42% above predicted values, based on indirect calorimetry results.[12]

Protein

Although not necessarily hypermetabolic, posttransplant patients will have increased protein catabolism, protein losses, and protein oxidation, which will acutely increase protein requirements after surgery.[12,38] Surgical stress and high corticosteroid use in addition to losses from wounds, surgical drains, stomas, dialysis, malnutrition, infection, or acute rejection can contribute to elevated protein needs.[5,38,39] It has been demonstrated in liver transplant recipients that protein catabolism is increased postoperatively as evidenced by excretion of large quantities of urinary nitrogen.[39] The use of steroids is a main cause of increased protein oxidation; higher doses of steroids are given during the acute phase, which leads to increased protein needs.[12,38] As the steroid dose is tapered, protein needs will also likely decrease.[12]

Fluid

Fluid losses may be increased due to losses from diarrhea, wounds, surgical drains, and urine and ostomy output. Fluid status must be monitored closely because excess fluid administration and/or decreased urine output can lead to fluid overload. Adequate hydration is usually encouraged to avoid nephrotoxic effects of some medications, such as tacrolimus.

Additional Metabolic Abnormalities

It is common to observe electrolyte abnormalities after transplantation. In the acute setting, serum potassium, phosphorus, and magnesium levels may be depleted due to diuretic use or refeeding syndrome and require close monitoring.[39] In liver transplantation, many of these electrolyte shifts are attributed to gastrointestinal losses from abdominal drains and other sources, as well as fluid overload.[39] Hyperkalemia is a frequent side effect of the immunosuppressive agent tacrolimus, often requiring a low-potassium diet restricting potassium to 1 to 3 g/day.[40] Hypophosphatemia has been documented to occur in up to 90% of renal transplant recipients during the acute posttransplant phase, which has been attributed to renal phosphate wasting.[41] Hypomagnesemia is another common electrolyte abnormality observed due to calcineurin inhibitors, such as tacrolimus or cyclosporine, often requiring additional magnesium supplementation to maintain levels.[11,40] Because high doses of magnesium oxide may exacerbate diarrhea, the provision of magnesium-rich foods may be a better choice to mitigate low serum levels.

Hyperglycemia is common immediately posttransplant, with a frequency reported at 80% or more for kidney recipients in the first days to week following transplant.[42] Research has indicated that hyperglycemia postoperatively can lead to an increased risk of kidney transplant rejection.[12] There is also an increased risk for infection with uncontrolled hyperglycemia.[42] Even in patients with no history of diabetes mellitus, it may be prudent to use insulin to control blood glucose after a transplant until serum glucose levels improve. If PN is warranted, an intravenous insulin infusion or insulin in the PN may be needed to tightly manage blood glucose levels. For patients who were obese before transplantation, it is important to consider strategies to safely lower the amount of corticosteroids if possible to help reduce weight gain after surgery.[12] See **Tables 18.2** to **18.6** for additional nutritional recommendations for patients recovering from organ transplantation.

> ### CORE CONCEPT 4
> Postoperative nutritional management should be individualized according to the patient's nutritional status, the organ being transplanted, and any complications that may arise during or after surgery.

TABLE 18.2 NUTRIENT RECOMMENDATIONS POST-KIDNEY TRANSPLANT

	Acute Postoperative Nutrition	Long-Term Nutrition
Calories	REE x 1.3-1.5 or 30-35 kcal/day	25-30 kcal/kg BW or enough to reach/maintain IBW vs. BEE x 1.2-1.3
Protein	1.3-2 g/kg	0.8-1 g/kg
Fat	30%-35% of total kcals	25%-35% total calories (emphasis on mono- and polyunsaturated fats)
Fluids	30-35 mL/kg; in renal graft dysfunction: 1000 mL + urine output	30-35 mL/kg vs ≥2 L/day
All phases posttransplant	**Recommendation**	
Carbohydrate	50% of total calories	
Fiber	25-35 g	
Sodium	3-4 g; restricted to 1-3 g for hypertension, fluid retention, or oliguria	
Phosphorus	1200-1500 mg; 800 mg in chronic rejection	

Data from Martins C, Pecoits-Filho R, Riella MC. Nutrition for the post–renal transplant recipients. Transplant. Proc. 2004;36(6):1651 and Blue LS. Adult kidney transplantation. In: Hasse JM, Blue LS, eds. *Comprehensive Guide to Transplant Nutrition*. Chicago, Illinois: American Dietetic Association; 2002:47,51.

TABLE 18.3 NUTRIENT RECOMMENDATIONS POST-LIVER TRANSPLANT

	Acute Postoperative Nutrition	Long-Term Nutrition
Calories	REE × 1.3 or 30-35 kcal/kg	REE × 1.2-1.3 or 30-35 kcal/kg
Protein	1.3-2 g/kg	0.8-1 g/kg
Carbohydrate	50%-70% of calories	50%-60% of calories
Fat	30% of calories	25%-35% of calories (limit saturated fat)
Vitamins and minerals	According to RDA levels	According to RDA levels

Data from Martins C, Pecoits-Filho R, Riella MC. Nutrition for the post–renal transplant recipients. Transplant. Proc. 2004;36(6):1651 and Blue LS. Adult kidney transplantation. In: Hasse JM, Blue LS, eds. *Comprehensive Guide to Transplant Nutrition*. Chicago, Illinois: American Dietetic Association; 2002:47,51.

TABLE 18.4 NUTRIENT RECOMMENDATIONS POST-HEART AND LUNG TRANSPLANT

	Acute Postoperative Nutrition	Long-Term Nutrition
Calories	REE × 1.3-1.5 or 30-35 kcal/kg	REE × 1.2-1.3
Protein	1.3-2 g/kg up to 2.5 g/kg	1 g/kg
Fat	30% of calories	~30% of calories (limit saturated fat)
Carbohydrate	50%-70% of calories	50%-60% of calories
Fluid	No restriction unless hyponatremia present	
All phases posttransplant	**Recommendation**	
Sodium	2-4 g if edema or hypertension present	
Vitamins	Lung: Monitor for hypervitaminosis A and E[37]	

Data from Pahwa N, Hedberg A-M. Adult heart and lung transplantation. In: Hasse JM, Blue LS, eds. *Comprehensive Guide to Transplant Nutrition*. Chicago, Illinois: American Dietetic Association; 2002:35,38.

> **PRACTICE POINT**
>
> Organ recipients should be encouraged to limit added sugar and sodium, choose heart-healthy fats and oils and lean proteins, and increase fiber.

Nutrition Support Nutrition support following transplant surgery is rarely necessary. Most patients will be able to eat following the return of bowel function after surgery, which can be as early as 1 or 2 days postoperatively.[43] If the patient requires ventilation for a prolonged period of time, enteral nutrition (EN) via an orogastric or nasogastric tube may be indicated (**Figure 18.4**).[43] Other indications for EN include the inability of a patient to tolerate an oral diet due to chewing and/or swallowing issues or the inability of the patient to meet their nutrient needs orally, possibly related to extended sedation after surgery. In liver transplant patients, EN has been associated with decreased postoperative infection rates and fewer metabolic complications in comparison to PN.[39] PN may be indicated in cases with prolonged gastrointestinal bleeding, ileus, or high-output intestinal fistula.[12]

Patients who have undergone a small-bowel transplant have unique nutritional concerns. The main role of nutrition support in this population depends on recovery of intestinal motility. Although each transplant center's protocol may vary, PN is usually reinitiated posttransplant, but with a lower volume needed to maintain adequate hydration.[12] Parenteral nutrition may be provided for the first 4 weeks, transitioning to EN as tolerated after the first few

TABLE 18.5 NUTRIENT RECOMMENDATIONS POST-PANCREAS TRANSPLANT

	Acute Postoperative Nutrition	Long-term Nutrition
Calories	REE × 1.3-1.4 or 30-35 kcal/kg (+500 kcal if underweight)	REE × 1.2-1.3 or as necessary to maintain weight
Protein	1.3-2 g/kg	0.8-1 g/kg
Fat	30%-50% of nonprotein calories	<30% of calories (limit saturated fat)
Carbohydrate	50%-70% of nonprotein calories	45%-50% of calories
Fluid	30-50 mL/kg or to keep up with output if bladder drainage; 35 mL/kg if enteric drainage	30-50 mL/kg or greater if bladder drainage to keep up with output
Minerals	Sodium and bicarbonate replacement if bladder drainage	

Data from Obayashi PAC. Adult pancreas transplantation. In: Hasse JM, Blue LS, eds. *Comprehensive Guide to Transplant Nutrition*. Chicago, Illinois: American Dietetic Association; 2002:94, 101.

TABLE 18.6 NUTRIENT RECOMMENDATIONS POST–SMALL-BOWEL TRANSPLANT

	Acute Postoperative Nutrition	Long-term Nutrition
Calories	REE × 1.5 or 35-40 kcal/kg	REE × 1.3-1.5 or as necessary to maintain weight
Protein	1.5-2 g/kg	1-1.5 g/kg
Fat	Provide medium-chain triglycerides (MCT oil), limit long-chain triglycerides	Reintroduce long-chain triglycerides as tolerated; limit saturated fat
Carbohydrate	50%-70% of calories; limit lactose if possible	50%-60% of calories; allow lactose as tolerated
Fluid	Replace high ostomy output (>1 L/day) with 1 mL for every mL of output over 1 L/day	Monitor for long-term requirement of IV fluid replacement
Minerals	Monitor zinc	Monitor sodium, chloride, and potassium for replacement as needed

Data from Obayashi PAC. Adult pancreas transplantation. In: Hasse JM, Blue LS, eds. *Comprehensive Guide to Transplant Nutrition*. Chicago, Illinois: American Dietetic Association; 2002:94, 101.

weeks, depending on observation of allograft motility.[44] Some centers may start EN at a rate of 5 to 10 mL/hr and slowly taper PN as EN tolerance improves and the rate increases.[12] Since lacteals and lymphatics of the small intestines are impacted by the surgery, there may be fat malabsorption in the initial postoperative period.[11] Limiting dietary fat may be warranted to prevent chylous ascites, but long-chain fatty acid absorption should improve within 2 to 6 weeks postoperatively as lacteals and lymphatics are regenerated.[11] Medium-chain triglycerides can be provided as an alternative during this period. Some practitioners do not recommend restricting fat after the transplant due to limited evidence of significant malabsorption; therefore, the type of EN formula will vary by center.[12,44] When an oral diet is advanced as tolerated, sometimes within the first 2 weeks, a clear, lactose-free, low-fiber, sugar-free diet is often provided.[12] There may also be carbohydrate malabsorption with secondary lactase deficiency that may increase ostomy output, so lactose should be limited during the acute posttransplant phase. Concentrated sweets should be limited as the hyperosmolar quality of sugar may cause osmotic diarrhea and increase ostomy output.[11] Due to high intestinal output, oral rehydration solution or IV fluid replacement may be needed.[11]

For patients who may have had a gastrostomy tube prior to surgery, especially those with a history of cystic fibrosis, it is recommended to delay the removal of the tube until BMI >19 is achieved and maintained for 3 months without supplementary nutrition.[37]

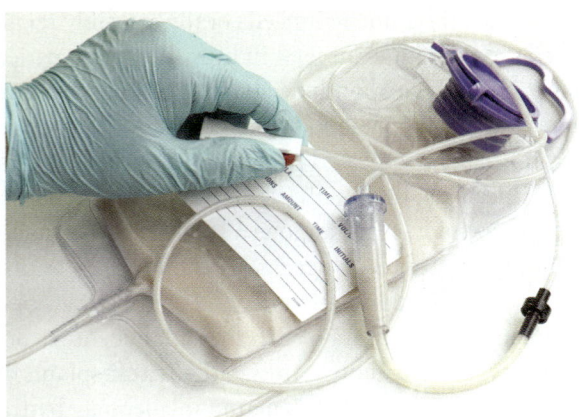

FIGURE 18.4 Enteral Nutrition May Be Warranted Postoperatively
© Sherry Yates Young/Shutterstock.

Dietary Therapy

General diet education should focus on adequacy of oral intake and importance of meeting increased protein needs for wound healing and infection prevention. The use of oral supplements may be indicated to help meet energy and protein requirements. Many recipients follow a much more restricted diet prior to the transplant, so it is necessary to review changes for short-term and long-term dietary goals.

Food Safety Guidelines

Transplant patients receive high doses of immunosuppressive medications that minimize rejection of the new organ(s), but also increase infection risk due to reduced immunity. **Neutropenia** is defined as an abnormally low level of neutrophils in the blood. Neutrophils are white blood cells produced in the bone marrow that protect the body against infectious disease or foreign invaders by engulfing bacteria. Neutropenia is a serious disorder because it makes the body vulnerable to bacterial and fungal infections. A low-microbial diet, also known as low-bacteria or neutropenic diet, is designed to prevent foodborne illnesses in immunocompromised patients (**Figure 18.5**). There are no published guidelines constituting what should be considered a low-bacteria diet, and published studies have determined no benefit of this diet.[45] Many institutions independently determine which foods may or may not be given to patients following a transplant as well as the length of time the patient must comply with the low-bacteria diet. Some institutions may recommend a patient follow the low-bacteria diet for

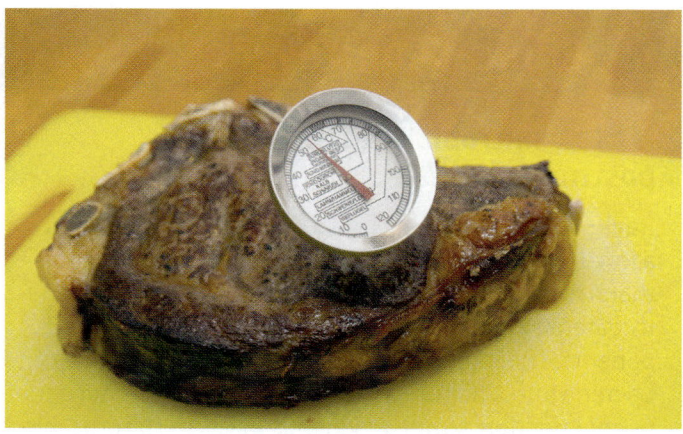

FIGURE 18.5 Transplant Recipients Are at High Risk for Foodborne Illnesses
© 1eyeshut/Shutterstock.

CASE STUDY REVISITED

George's condition improves and he is transferred out of the ICU. His appetite is slow to return, so oral nutrition supplements are recommended. On POD #7, George's appetite has improved significantly and he continues to drink high-calorie/high-protein supplements with all of his meals. The medical team is worried about his hyperkalemia and hyperglycemia.

Anthropometric Data:
Current weight: 114.5 kg (252 lbs)

Biochemical Data:
Sodium 141 (135-145 mEq/L)
Potassium 5.2 (3.6-5.0 mEq/L)
Blood urea nitrogen 24 (6-24mg/dL)
Creatinine 1.3 (0.4-1.3 mg/dL)
Glucose 296 (70-139 mg/dL)

Clinical Data:
Medications (include): Cyclosporine, Prednisone, Tacrolimus, insulin

Dietary Data:
Diet Order: Low bacteria, diabetic + high-calorie/protein oral supplement three times daily with meals (provides 360 kcal, 14 g protein, 45 g CHO, 460 mg K+ per 8 oz bottle)

Questions
1. What adjustment could be made to his diet order?
2. How might his medication regimen influence his nutritional status and diet prescription?
3. What diet education could be provided for the acute phase as well with consideration for the chronic (long-term) phase?

> ## ⚠ Clinical Controversy
>
> ### Is a low microbial diet beneficial posttransplant?
>
> **Background**: A low-microbial diet, also referred to as a low-bacteria or neutropenic diet, is one intervention that has been used to reduce the risk of developing life-threatening infections among immunocompromised patients. The intended purpose is to limit the intake of bacteria into a host's gastrointestinal tract to reduce the risk of infection. Limited evidence exists to support this cause-and-effect relationship or determine whether a restricted diet is beneficial. One group of researchers conducted a study that evaluated 46 patients undergoing allogenic stem cell transplants and found that there were no significant differences between infection rates or nutritional status among patients who received the neutropenic diet or an unrestricted diet.
>
> Another study assessed the outcomes of patients undergoing induction for acute myeloid leukemia who were randomly assigned to a diet containing raw fresh fruits and vegetables (raw diet, n = 75) or one that excluded raw fresh fruits and vegetables (cooked diet, n = 78). There appeared to be a trend toward fewer fevers of unknown origin in the cooked-diet group, while the incidence of bacteremia was higher in the raw-diet group.
>
> ### Questions
> 1. What are potential advantages and disadvantages of the low-microbial diet in the transplant population?
> 2. Can the results of the two studies referenced above, which were conducted with oncology patients, be applied to solid organ transplant recipients?
> 3. Would you recommend a low-microbial diet to a solid organ transplant recipient?
>
> ### References
> 1. Lassiter M, Schneider SM. A pilot study comparing the neutropenic diet to a non-neutropenic diet in the allogeneic hematopoietic stem cell transplantation population. *Clin J Oncol Nurs*. 2015;19(3):273-278
> 2. Gardner A, Mattiuzzi G, Faderl S, et al. Randomized comparison of cooked and noncooked diets in patients undergoing remission induction therapy for acute myeloid leukemia. *J Clin Oncol*. 2008;26:5684-5688

as long as they are taking immunosuppressants (which may be the entire duration of the patient's life) or they may allow a patient to follow a regular diet after discharge.

A low-microbial diet follows food safety basics and emphasizes the importance of hand washing before touching food, avoiding cross-contamination of raw food, sanitizing cooking areas, washing fruits and vegetables, heating foods to the proper temperature, and cooling foods to the proper temperature in a timely manner.[46] **Cross-contamination** is the passage of pathogens indirectly from one source to another due to the improper use of sterilization procedures, unclean instruments, or recycling of products. In general, most patients are advised to avoid higher risk foods, which include unpasteurized dairy products, undercooked or raw meats, poultry, eggs, seafood, soft or moldy cheeses, leftovers or deli meats that have not been heated to the proper temperature, water from a well, and buffets or salad bars.[46]

> **PRACTICE POINT**
>
> Following basic food safety rules and guidelines can prevent immunosuppressed patients from contracting foodborne illnesses.

Chronic Posttransplant Phase

Prevention of chronic disease is the main long-term goal of nutrition therapy in the chronic posttransplant phase. There are currently no guidelines and research is limited on long-term dietary intervention posttransplant.[47] Emphasizing and reinforcing dietary compliance to recommended diets, particularly those treating comorbidities such as diabetes or hypertension that led to the original organ failure, is of utmost importance. A transplant is not eradicating the preexisting condition. A healthy diet such as a heart-healthy diet, Mediterranean diet, and the American Heart Association (AHA) Step 1 diet will likely benefit the transplant recipient and can help with some of the common chronic posttransplant metabolic conditions, such as diabetes mellitus, obesity, hypertension, and dyslipidemia.[12,47] Surgical complications or infections, particularly those that prompt multiple hospitalizations or procedures, may compromise a recipient's nutritional status, requiring more aggressive nutrition intervention to prevent or reverse malnutrition or replete losses. Individualized diet recommendations continue to benefit the patient and can help to manage nutritional issues that arise over time.

Food–Drug Interactions and Supplement Use

There are significant drug–nutrient interactions observed with grapefruit and grapefruit products. Cyclosporine and tacrolimus, as well as other medications, are metabolized by the cytochrome P450 system in the gastrointestinal tract.[9] Research suggests that flavonoids and other substances in grapefruit juice act by inhibiting the cytochrome P450 enzymes, which can increase the bloodstream concentration, activity, and potential toxicity of these drugs.[9]

It is recommended that grapefruit products be avoided.[9] Most herbal and alternative supplements are discouraged due to concern for interactions with immunosuppressive medications or the potential to damage organs.[11]

There are increasing reports of probiotic-associated infections, calling into question the safety of using these products. One case study looked at a cardiothoracic transplant recipient who received *Lactobacillus rhamnosus* GG and developed an empyema.[48] The same strain of lactobacillus that the patient was taking in supplement form was found in the pleural fluid. Special caution should be exercised when using these supplements in immunocompromised patients.[48,49]

Long-term Metabolic and Nutritional Consequences

Organ transplantation is designed to help people lead longer, healthier lives. The screening process for organ recipients helps ensure that those who receive an organ will be healthy enough not only to survive the transplant, but to continue to live many productive years. By correctly matching organ donors to recipients and using immunosuppressive medication, organ recipients are living longer than ever. Acknowledgement of nutrition-related impacts of specific immunosuppression regimens is vital for appropriate posttransplant management.

Weight Gain Posttransplant weight gain is common among recipients. Weight gain after transplantation has been associated with increased postoperative complications, worsening of metabolic syndromes, increased graft loss, and reduced patient and graft survival (**Figure 18.6**).[21] Corticosteroids may play a significant role in weight gain, but other factors may include a less-restricted diet and overall improved appetite and well-being. It has been shown that the greatest weight gain occurs 6 months after liver transplantation,[39] possibly related to a reduction in energy expenditure following liver transplantation that can lead to increased fat mass and obesity.[50-52] Another study found that for each 5 kg/m² increment increase in BMI during the first year after kidney transplantation, there was 1.23 additional relative risk for death.[20]

Diabetes Transplant recipients may require long-term management of blood glucose. New-onset diabetes after transplantation (NODAT) has been reported to occur in 4% to 25% of renal transplant recipients, 4% to 40% of heart transplant recipients, 2.5% to 25% of liver transplant recipients, and 30% to 35% of lung transplant recipients.[53] Immunosuppression regimens contribute to hyperglycemia. About 5% of patients on long-term cyclosporine will develop diabetes, despite careful monitoring of blood levels.[2] Tacrolimus has an even higher incidence of neurotoxicity and diabetes.[2] Corticosteroid dose reduction has been shown to improve glucose tolerance during the first year after transplant.[53] Studies assessing the impact of NODAT on patient and allograft outcomes have generated a variety of results, yet substantial research suggests that renal transplant recipients who develop NODAT are at two- to three-fold increased risk of cardiovascular events compared to nondiabetic patients.[53] The development of NODAT is also associated with an increased risk for graft rejection and infectious complications. Nutrition intervention for NODAT includes diabetes diet education, modest weight loss of 5% to 10% of total body weight if overweight, and physical activity.[53] Additional pharmacological management, such as insulin, may be needed if hyperglycemia persists. Increased risk of NODAT appears to be associated with increased age, BMI, and waist circumference among kidney recipients.[20] Early detection and routine monitoring for hyperglycemia is very important in both acute and chronic postoperative phases.

Hypertension The prevalence of hypertension also remains an issue among renal transplant recipients, affecting up to 90% of recipients.[54] Immunosuppressive medications like corticosteroids and calcineurin inhibitors contribute to high blood pressure through vasoconstriction, sodium retention, and vasodilation inhibition.[54] A study completed in Japan found that short-term dietary counseling on sodium intake among renal transplant recipients can be effective in reducing blood pressure and perhaps the quantity of antihypertensive medications needed.[54]

Hyperlipidemia Impaired lipid metabolism, which has been observed among many transplant recipients, is associated with some immunosuppressive medication. Up to 45% of liver transplant recipients develop hyperlipidemia.[55] Cyclosporine and steroids are associated with hyperlipidemia.[9] Cyclosporine can bind to the low-density lipoprotein (LDL) cholesterol receptor and can inhibit hepatic clearance of LDL, leading to an increase of circulating LDL.[55] Dietary restrictions and modifications, such as following a Mediterranean diet or the AHA Step 1 diet, have been shown to help improve dyslipidemia in patients after renal transplants.[47] Reducing saturated fats, balancing

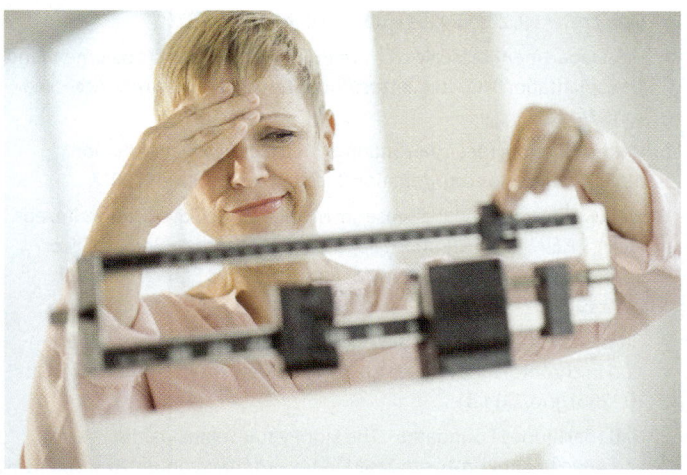

FIGURE 18.6 Weight Gain Can Be a Complicating Factor Posttransplant
© tmcphotos/Shutterstock.

carbohydrates at 50% to 60% of calories, and increasing plant sterols have been shown to be effective diet therapies for posttransplant kidney and heart recipients with dyslipidemia or uncontrolled weight gain.[47] Some studies have found that hyperlipidemia may persist despite dietary modifications and weight reduction, so more aggressive pharmacological interventions, such as a statin, may also be necessary in conjunction with diet modification.[55]

Cancer The success of immunosuppression in transplant recipients has led to an increased rate of malignancy in this population. There is a three-fold increased risk for cancer in those who have received an organ compared to the general population.[56] Most of the cancer types that tend to afflict organ recipients have a known or suspected infectious cause, such as Kaposi sarcoma; Hodgkin's lymphoma; hepatobiliary and liver cancer; melanoma; colorectal cancer; and cancers of the cervix, anus, vulva, penis, oral cavity, and pharynx.[56-59] The higher incidence of cancers among the transplant population may be the result of years on immune suppression therapy, with a smaller percentage stemming from prior disease risk from their end-stage organ failure.[56]

Bone Health and Osteoporosis Osteoporosis can arise from both pretransplant bone disease and immunosuppressive agent use after transplantation.[60] **Osteodystrophy**, or abnormal development of bone, is frequently observed. Specifically, renal osteodystrophy from kidney disease, decreased bone mineral density in end-stage heart disease, hepatic osteodystrophy and malabsorption in liver disease, and the use of steroids in COPD can all lead to osteoporosis and increased risk of fractures before transplant occurs.[60,61] After transplant, the reported prevalence of vitamin D insufficiency ranges from 51% to 97% and severe deficiency can range from 26% to 33%.[61] Transplant recipients are at risk for vitamin D deficiency due to compromised health status postoperatively, which may lead to reduced dietary intake of vitamin D–containing foods. There is also an increased risk of skin cancer in this population, leading to a decrease in intentional sun exposure.[61] Some studies demonstrate that glucocorticoids can increase catabolism of 25-hydroxyvitamin D.[61] Impaired absorption or increased excretion of calcium is also observed in the setting of corticosteroids.[11] It has been reported that bone loss can occur within the first 3 to 6 months after liver transplantation, but then becomes more stable over the next 12 months.[39] Vitamin D deficiency should be corrected whenever possible, and patients should be encouraged to take at least the recommended daily allowance for both calcium and vitamin D before and after their transplant to counteract the bone mineral–depleting effects of their medications.[60] Based on the 2017 American College of Rheumatology guidelines for the prevention and treatment of glucocorticoid-induced osteoporosis, calcium intake of 1000 to 1200 mg/day, vitamin D intake of 600 to 900 IU/day, and serum vitamin D levels ≥20 ng/mL are recommended.[62] Weight-bearing activities are also encouraged.

> **PRACTICE POINT**
>
> Long-term nutrition therapy is recommended to manage long-term side effects from medications such as diabetes, hyperlipidemia, hypertension, and weight gain.

Chapter Summary

Solid organ transplantation has evolved since the beginning of the 20th century. As medical technology improves, an increase in both organ donation and survival of recipients is evident. Advances in immunosuppressive medications have improved the health and longevity of organ recipients. Medical nutrition therapy plays an important role both pre- and posttransplant to reverse malnutrition and assist with weight loss for obese potential transplant candidates. Postoperative medical nutrition therapy is critical to optimize outcomes by supporting wound healing and managing nutritional consequences and/or side effects of immunosuppressive medications. Long-term medical nutrition therapy can optimize the health and productivity of transplant recipients, decrease the risk of foodborne illness, and promote a well-balanced diet and lifestyle.

Key Terms

graft, host, autograft transplantation, allograft transplantation, orthotopic, rejection, immunosuppression, graft thrombosis, brain death, donation after cardiac death (DCD), neutropenia, cross-contamination, new-onset diabetes after transplant (NODAT), osteodystrophy

References

1. Linden PK. History of solid organ transplantation and organ donation. *Crit Care Clin*. 2009;25(1):165-184.
2. Watson CJ, Dark JH. Organ transplantation: historical perspective and current practice. *Br J Anaesth*. 2012;108 Suppl 1:29-42.
3. Anand J, Singh SK, Antoun DG, et al. Durable mechanical circulatory support versus organ transplantation: past, present, and future. *Biomed Res Int*. 2015:849571. doi:10.1155/2015/849571.
4. U.S. Department of Health & Human Services. Organ Procurement and Transplantation Network. https://optn.transplant.hrsa.gov. Accessed June 14, 2017.
5. United Network for Organ Sharing. Facts about organ donation. https://www.unos.org/donation/facts. Accessed June 9, 2017.
6. Wolk R, Foulks C. Renal disease. In: Mueller C, McClave S, Kuhn JM, eds. *The A.S.P.E.N. Adult Nutrition Support Core Curriculum*. 2nd ed. Silver Spring, MD: American Society for Parenteral and Enteral Nutrition; 2012:491-510.
7. Ghaderian SB, Beladi-Mousavi SS. The role of diabetes and hypertension in chronic kidney disease. *J Renal Inj Prev*. 2014;3(4):109-110. DOI: 10.12861/jrip.2014.31
8. National Kidney Foundation. The kidney transplant waitlist—what you need to know. https://www.kidney.org/atoz/content/transplant-waitlist. Last reviewed February 10, 2017. Accessed August 2, 2017.
9. Hasse JM, Blue LS. *Comprehensive Guide to Transplant Nutrition*. Chicago, IL: American Dietetic Association; 2002.

10. Varma V, Mehta N, Kumara V, Nundy S. Indications and contraindications for liver transplantation. *Int J Hepatol.* 2011. doi:10.4061/2011/121862

11. Academy of Nutrition and Dietetics. Nutrition Care Manual. https://www.nutritioncaremanual.org. Accessed June 14, 2017.

12. Hasse JM, Matarese LE. Solid organ transplantation. In: Mueller C, McClave S, Kuhn JM, eds. *The A.S.P.E.N. Adult Nutrition Support Core Curriculum.* 2nd ed. Silver Spring, MD: American Society for Parenteral and Enteral Nutrition; 2012:523-535.

13. Russo MJ, Hong KN, Davies RR, et al. The effect of body mass index on survival following heart transplantation: do outcomes support consensus guidelines? *Ann Surg.* 2010;251(1):144-152.

14. Hasse J. Pretransplant obesity: A weighty issue affecting transplant candidacy and outcomes. *Nutr Clin Pract.* 2007;22(5):494-504.

15. Potluri K, Hou S. Obesity in kidney transplant recipients and candidates. *Am J Kidney Dis.* 2010;56(1):143-156.

16. Sampaio MS, Reddy PN, Kuo HT, et al. Obesity was associated with inferior outcomes in simultaneous pancreas kidney transplant. *Transplantation.*2010;89(9):1117-1125.

17. Bumgardner GL, Henry ML, Elkhammas E, et al. Obesity as a risk factor after combined pancreas/kidney transplantation. *Transplantation.*1995;60(12):1426-1430.

18. Lederer DJ, Kawut SM, Wickersham N, et al. Obesity and primary graft dysfunction after lung transplantation: the lung transplant outcomes group obesity study. *Am J Respir Crit Care Med.* 2011;184(9):1055-1061.

19. Lavie CJ, Milani RV, Ventura HO. Obesity and cardiovascular disease: risk factor, paradox, and impact of weight loss. *J Am Coll Cardiol.* 2009;53:1925-1932.

20. Tran M-H, Foster CE, Kalantar-Zadeh K, Ichii H. Kidney transplantation in obese patients. *World J Transplant.* 2016; 6(1):135-143. doi:10.5500/wtj.v6.i1.135

21. Chan G, Garneau P, Hajjar R. The impact and treatment of obesity in kidney transplant candidates and recipients. *Can J Kidney Health Dis.* 2015;2:26. doi:10.1186/s40697-015-0059-4.

22. Martin P, DiMartini A, Feng S, Robert Brown J, Fallon M. Evaluation for Liver Transplantation in Adults: 2013 Practice Guideline by the AASLD and the American Society of Transplantation. *Hepatology.* 2014;l59:3.

23. Nair S, Verma S, Thuluvath PJ. Obesity and its effect on survival in patients undergoing orthotopic liver transplantation in the United States. *Hepatology.* 2002;35(1):105-109.

24. Ayloo S, Hurton S, Cwinn M, Molinari M. Impact of body mass index on outcomes of 48281 patients undergoing first time cadaveric liver transplantation. *World J Transplant.* 2016;6(2):356-369. doi:10.5500/wjt.v6.i2.356.

25. Vest AR, Patel P, Schauer PR, et al. Clinical and echocardiographic outcomes after bariatric surgery in obese patients with left ventricular systolic dysfunction. *Circulation: Heart Failure.* 2016;9:e002260. DOI: 10.1161/circheartfailure.115.002260.

26. Shimada YJ, Tsugawa Y, Brown DFM, Hasegawa K. Bariatric surgery and emergency department visits and hospitalizations for heart failure exacerbation: population-based, self-controlled series. *J Am Coll Cardiol.* 2015;67:895-903.

27. Locke JE, Reed RD, Massie A, et al. Obesity increases the risk of end-stage renal disease among living kidney donors. *Kidney Int.* 2017;91(3):699-703

28. Assi MA, Pulido JS, Peters SG, McCannel CA, Razonable RR. Graft-vs.-host disease in lung and other solid organ transplant recipients. *Clin. Transplant.* 2007;21(1):1-6.

29. Gulbahce HE, Brown CA, Wick M, Segall M, Jessurun J. Graft-vs-host disease after solid organ transplant. *Am J Clin Pathol.* 2003;119(4):568-573.

30. Hasse JM. Nutrition assessment and support of organ transplant recipients. *JPEN J. Parenter Enteral Nutr.* 2001;25(3):120-131.

31. Lowell JA. Nutritional assessment and therapy in patients requiring liver transplantation. *Liver Transpl Surg.* 1996;2(5 Suppl 1):79-88.

32. Molnar MZ, Kovesdy CP, Bunnapradist S, et al. Associations of pretransplant serum albumin with post-transplant outcomes in kidney transplant recipients. *Am. J. Transplant.* 2011;11(5):1006-1015.

33. ter Wee PM. Protein energy wasting and transplantation. *J Ren Nutr.* 2013;23(3):246-249. doi: 10.1053/j.jrn.2013.02.004

34. Merli M, Giusto M, Gentili F, et al. Nutritional status: its influence on the outcome of patients undergoing liver transplantation. *Liver Int.* 2010;30(2):208-214.

35. Lee RD, Nieman DC. *Nutritional Assessment.* 6th ed. New York, NY: McGraw-Hill Education; 2013.

36. Hammad A, Kaido T, Uemoto S. Perioperative nutritional therapy in liver transplantation. *Surg Today.* 2015;45(3):271-283.

37. Hirche TO, Knoop C, Hebestreit H, et al. Practical guidelines: lung transplantation in patients with cystic fibrosis. *Pulm Med.* 2014;2014:621342. doi:10.1155/2014/621342.

38. Martins C, Pecoits-Filho R, Riella MC. Nutrition for the post–renal transplant recipients. *Transplant. Proc.*2004;36(6):1650-1654.

39. Sanchez AJ, Aranda-Michel J. Nutrition for the liver transplant patient. *Liver Transpl.* 2006;12(9):1310-1316.

40. Pronsky ZM, Elbe D, Ayoob K. *Food-Medication Interactions.* 18th ed. Birchrunville, PA: Food-Medication Interactions; 2015.

41. Kanaan N, Claes K, Devogelaer J-P, et al. Fibroblast growth factor-23 and parathyroid hormone are associated with post-transplant bone mineral density loss. *Clin J Am Soc Nephrol.* 2010;5(10):1887-1892. doi: 10.2215/CJN.00950110 .

42. Boerner B, Shivaswamy V, Goldner W, Larsen J. Management of the hospitalized transplant patient. *Curr Diab Rep.* 2015;15(4):19. doi:10.1007/s11892-015-0585-6.

43. Cresci, G, ed. *Nutrition Support for the Critically Ill Patient. A Guide to Practice.* Boca Raton: Taylor & Francis Group; CRC Press; 2005.

44. Weseman RA, Gilroy R. Nutrition management of small bowel transplant patients. *Nutr Clin Pract.* 2005; 20:509-516.

45. Jubelirer SJ. The benefit of the neutropenic diet: fact or fiction? *Oncologist.* 2011;16(5):704-707.

46. U.S. Food and Drug Administration. Food safety for transplant recipients. https://www.fda.gov/food/foodborneillnesscontaminants/peopleatrisk/ucm312570.htm Published 2006. Updated 2011. Accessed on June 21, 2017.

47. Zeltzer SM, Taylor DO, Tang WH. Long-term dietary habits and interventions in solid-organ transplantation. *J. Heart Lung Transplant.* 2015;34(11):1357-1365.

48. Luong M-L, Sareyyupoglu B, Nguyen MH, et al. Lactobacillus probiotic use in cardiothoracic transplant recipients: a link to invasive Lactobacillus infection? *Transpl Infect Dis.* 2010;12:561–564

49. Twombley KE, Seikaly MG. New paradigms for the use of prebiotics, probiotics, and synbiotics in renal disease. *Dial Transplant.* 2011;40:200-204. doi:10.1002/dat.20568.

50. Richardson RA, Garden OJ, Davidson HI. Reduction in energy expenditure after liver transplantation. *Nutrition.* 2001;17(7-8):585-589.

51. Ferreira LG, Santos LF, Anastacio LR, Lima AS, Correia MI. Resting energy expenditure, body composition, and dietary intake: a longitudinal study before and after liver transplantation. *Transplantation.* 2013;96(6):579-585.

52. Giusto M, Lattanzi B, Di Gregorio V, Giannelli V, Lucidi C, Merli M. Changes in nutritional status after liver transplantation. *World J Gastroenterol*. 2014;20(31):10682-10690.
53. Pham P-TT, Pham P-MT, Pham SV, Pham P-AT, Pham P-CT. New onset diabetes after transplantation (NODAT): an overview. *Diabetes Metab Syndr Obes*. 2011;4:175-186. doi:10.2147/DMSO.S19027.
54. Asai K, Kobayashi T, Miyata H, et al. The short-term impact of dietary counseling on sodium intake and blood pressure in renal allograft recipients. *Prog Transplant*. 2016;26(4)365-371.
55. Charlton M. Obesity, hyperlipidemia, and metabolic syndrome. *Liver Transpl*. 2009;15(S2): S83-S89. doi:10.1002/lt.21914.
56. Vajdic CM, van Leeuwen MT. Cancer incidence and risk factors after solid organ transplantation. *Int J Cancer*. 2009;125(8):1747-1754.
57. Safaeian M, Robbins HA, Berndt SI, Lynch CF, Fraumeni JF, Jr., Engels EA. Risk of colorectal cancer after solid organ transplantation in the United States. *Am J Transplant*. 2016;16(3):960–967. doi:10.1111/ajt.13549.
58. Robbins HA, Clarke CA, Arron ST, et al. Melanoma risk and survival among organ transplant recipients. *J Invest Dermatol*. 2015;135(11):2657-2665.
59. Koshiol J, Pawlish K, Goodman MT, McGlynn KA, Engels EA. Risk of hepatobiliary cancer after solid organ transplant in the United States. *Clin Gastroenterol Hepatol*. 2014;12(9):1541-1549.e1543.
60. Lan G-b, Xie X-b, Peng L-k, Liu L, Song L, Dai H-l. Current status of research on osteoporosis after solid organ transplantation: pathogenesis and management. *BioMed Res Int*. 2015;2015:10.
61. Stein EM, Shane E. Vitamin D in organ transplantation. *Osteoporosis Int*. 2011;22(7):2107-2118. doi:10.1007/s00198-010-1523-8.
62. Buckley L, Guyatt G, Fink HA, et al. 2017 American College of Rheumatology guideline for the prevention and treatment of glucocorticoid-induced osteoporosis. *Arthritis Care Res*. 2017;69(8):1095-1110. doi:10.1002/acr.23279.

Chapter 19

Nutrition in Oncology and Hematopoietic Stem Cell Transplant

Alicia Romano
Jennifer Mayer
Deena Altschwager

Chapter Outline

Core Concepts
Background/Etiology
Epidemiology
Cancer Staging
Medical Treatment of Cancer
Nutrition Screening and Assessment in Cancer Patients
Cancer Cachexia and Metabolic Changes Associated with Cancer
Overview of Nutritional Support in the Cancer Patient
Nutritional Management of Specific Solid Tumors
Nutritional Management of Hematological Cancers Undergoing Hematopoietic Stem Cell Transplant
Nutrition Support in the Advanced Cancer Patient
Complementary and Alternative Medicine, Integrative Medicine, and the Cancer Patient

CORE CONCEPTS

1. One-third of cancer deaths are caused by preventable lifestyle choices, including obesity, poor nutrition, physical inactivity, tobacco use, and heavy alcohol consumption.
2. Cancer is the second most common cause of death in the United States, exceeded only by heart disease.
3. Medical treatment of cancer can lead to nutrition impact symptoms that may impair a patient's nutritional status.
4. Weight loss and malnutrition are well documented in cancer patients and may influence disease prognosis, treatment tolerance, quality of life, and be predictive of early mortality.
5. Dietary counseling by a registered dietitian (RD) results in improved outcomes, including fewer treatment-related side effects, improved quality of life, and better dietary intake.
6. Nutrition impact symptoms and energy requirements differ based on the specific solid tumor present.
7. Cancer cachexia can lead to progressive functional impairment in advanced cancers. Pro-inflammatory cytokines may play a role in mediating alterations in metabolism seen in cancer cachexia and may also affect other gastrointestinal processes.

8. Cancer cachexia results in preferential loss of skeletal muscle mass and may contribute to an increase in resting energy expenditure.
9. Because no evidence-based treatments are available for cancer cachexia, focus should be placed on early nutrition interventions to prevent the onset and acceleration of cancer cachexia.
10. Head and neck cancer patients have the highest risk for malnutrition compared to other malignancies.
11. The allogeneic hematopoietic stem cell transplant (HSCT) is considered one of the most intense treatments in the oncology population and puts patients at nutritional risk due to prolonged neutropenia, gastrointestinal side effects, and risk of graft versus host disease (GVHD).
12. Patients undergoing HSCT have increased energy needs due to increased catabolism and treatment-related complications.
13. Nutrition is critical following HSCT because impaired nutritional status can lead to longer engraftment time and a greater likelihood of developing infection.
14. Graft versus host disease can occur following allogeneic HSCT and places patients at nutritional risk due to impaired function of the gastrointestinal tract, including the oral mucosa.
15. Nutrition support in the advanced cancer patient should be assessed on a case-by-case basis with consideration of goals of care.

Learning Objectives

1. Describe the magnitude and etiology of cancer today.
2. Explain the medical treatment of cancer, including the nutrition impact symptoms related to the treatment.
3. Describe the prevalence of malnutrition among the cancer population and the types of tools used to screen for malnutrition.
4. Assess the nutrition status and develop nutrition care plans for people with cancer diagnoses.
5. Describe cancer cachexia, including the changes in metabolism associated with cachexia, and appropriate nutritional management.
6. Determine optimal enteral and parenteral feeding practices for the cancer patient.
7. Identify high-risk cancer types based on tumor sites and their associated nutritional management.
8. Assess the unique nutritional needs of patients with hematological cancers undergoing hematopoietic stem cell transplant.
9. Develop care plans for patients undergoing hematopoietic stem cell transplants, including management and treatment of graft versus host disease.
10. Compare appropriate diet recommendations for immunosuppressed patients versus nonimmunosuppressed patients.
11. Select optimal nutritional support practices for the advanced cancer patient.

Background/Etiology

Cancer is a term used to describe a group of more than 100 diseases characterized by uncontrolled growth of abnormal cells, with the ability to invade other tissues.[1]

All cancer starts as a single cell that has lost control of its normal growth and replication process. Cancer is caused by both external factors (such as tobacco, alcohol, and chemicals) and internal factors (such as inherited mutations and immune conditions). These factors may act together or in sequence to imitate or promote the development of cancer.[1] Only about 5% to 10% of cancers are strongly hereditary, as most cancers result from the damage to genes occurring during a person's lifetime.[2] Inherited factors are known to play a larger role in determining risk for some cancers, including colorectal, breast, and prostate cancers.[3]

A substantial portion of cancers can be prevented (Table 19.1). According to the National Cancer Institute (NCI) and American Cancer Society (ACS), the cause of 1 in every 3 cancer deaths is preventable, related in part to obesity, poor nutrition, or physical inactivity.[1,4] Additionally,

TABLE 19.1 EXOGENOUS CANCER RISK FACTORS

Risk Factor	Cancers with Increased Risk
Tobacco	Gastrointestinal, lung, pancreatic, cervical, renal
Alcohol	Gastrointestinal, liver
Obesity	Pancreatic, colorectal, prostate, gynecologic, renal, biliary, gallbladder
Low fruit/vegetable intake	Most cancers
High fat intake	Prostate, lymphoma

CASE STUDY INTRODUCTION

Seth is a 65-year-old male with newly diagnosed acute myelogenous leukemia (AML). He has completed two cycles of high-dose chemotherapy complicated by weight loss, nausea, anorexia, mucositis, and febrile neutropenia. He will eventually require an allogeneic hematopoietic stem cell transplant. Seth is a retired banker; he currently is married and lives with his wife.

Anthropometric Data:
Height: 178 cm (70")
Weight: 86 kg (189 lbs)
BMI: 27.2 kg/m²
Weight history
Usual body weight (UBW): 95.5 kg (210 lbs) 6 months ago
Weight 1 month ago: 92 kg (202 lbs)

Biochemical Data:
Sodium 137 (135-145 mEq/L)
Potassium 3.7 (3.6-5.0 mEq/L)
Chloride 103 (98-110 mEq/L)
Carbon dioxide 25 (20-30 mEq/L)
Blood urea nitrogen 20 (6-24 mg/dL)

Creatinine 0.9 (0.4-1.3 mg/dL)
Glucose 134 (70-99 mg/dL)
Phosphorus 3.1 (2.7-4.5 mg/dL)
Magnesium 1.8 (1.8-2.1 mEq/L)
Albumin 3.0 (3.5-5.0 g/dL)

Clinical Data:
Past Medical History: AML s/p two cycles of high dose chemotherapy, hypertension, pre-diabetes, obesity
Medications: Metoprolol, Pravastatin, multivitamin with minerals
Vital Signs: Blood pressure: 130/85 mm Hg; Temperature 99°F; Heart rate 80 beats/min
Nutrition-focused Physical Exam: Appears tired. Central adiposity noted. Skin intact, no edema or wounds noted. Evident muscle loss of upper extremities. Oral exam notable for dry mucosa, intact dentition, normal tongue.

Dietary Data:
Dietary History: Seth follows a low-sodium, low–saturated fat diet. Prior to starting chemotherapy, he had decreased intake due to fatigue and poor appetite. Since starting chemotherapy, Seth's oral intake and appetite have decreased even more significantly to 50% of his typical intake due to treatment-related side effects. He has intermittently relied on a soft-solid/full-liquid diet due to pain with eating. He is not currently supplementing his diet with a commercial liquid beverage.
Usual Diet Recall:
Breakfast (9 am): 12 oz coffee, ½ cup oatmeal
Lunch (12 pm): chicken sandwich with 3 oz chicken and fat-free mayonnaise, 12 oz diet ginger ale
Dinner (5 pm): 1 cup pasta with tomato sauce, ½ cup green beans, 12 oz water
Diet Prescription: Regular diet with high calorie high protein liquid supplements

Questions:
1. Describe Seth's weight status and rate of weight loss.
2. How would you describe Seth's nutritional status? What are Seth's nutrition priorities?
3. How would you interpret Seth's labs?
4. How would you assess Seth's current intake? What are Seth's nutritional priorities? What are Seth's nutritional priorities?
5. What nutritional interventions can you make to aid Seth's nutritional management of treatment-related side effects?
6. What strategies can you offer Seth to prevent further weight loss?

all cancers caused by tobacco use and heavy alcohol consumption could be prevented. In 2015, almost 171,000 of estimated 589,430 cancer deaths in the United States were caused by tobacco smoking.[4] Certain cancers caused by infectious agents (such as human papillomavirus, hepatitis B and C virus, and HIV) could be avoided by preventing infection through behavioral changes, vaccination, or treatment of infection. Greater than three million skin cancer cases that are diagnosed annually could be prevented by protecting skin from excessive sun exposure and avoiding indoor tanning.[4]

Endogenous causes can occur through inherited germ line mutations, oxidative stress from reactive oxygen species, and inflammation. Chronic inflammation can produce cytokines, growth factors, reactive oxygen, and nitrogen species, which can increase proliferation and differentiation, inhibit apoptosis (programmed cell death), and induce angiogenesis.[5] In addition to inflammation and stress, lifetime exposure to estrogen has been shown to raise the risk of breast, ovarian, and endometrial cancers.[5]

> **CORE CONCEPT 1**
>
> One-third of cancer deaths are caused by preventable lifestyle choices, including obesity, poor nutrition, physical inactivity, tobacco use, and heavy alcohol consumption.

Epidemiology

According to the ACS, lifetime risk of cancer development is 1 in 2 for men and 1 in 3 for women; however, risk changes with exposure and genetic susceptibility. Cancer risk is known to increase with age, with 77% of cancer diagnosed in people 55 years or older.[4] In addition, more than 500,000 Americans are expected to die of cancer annually (about 1,620 people per day), making cancer the second most common cause of death in the United States, exceeded only by heart disease.[4]

More than 100 types of cancer exist; they occur as a solid or hematologic malignancy and are named primarily for the organ or type of cell in which they originate. Solid malignancies present as an abnormal mass of tissue that is typically not cystic or liquid. Types of solid malignancies include **carcinomas** (beginning in the skin or tissues that line or cover internal organs) and **sarcomas** (cancers that begin in the bone, cartilage, fat, muscle, blood vessels, or connective or supportive tissue). **Hematologic malignancies** are defined as cancers that begin in the blood-forming tissue, such as bone marrow (leukemias) or in the cells of the immune system (lymphomas and myelomas), and can be classified as acute or chronic in nature.

> **CORE CONCEPT 2**
>
> Cancer is the second most common cause of death in the United States, exceeded only by heart disease.

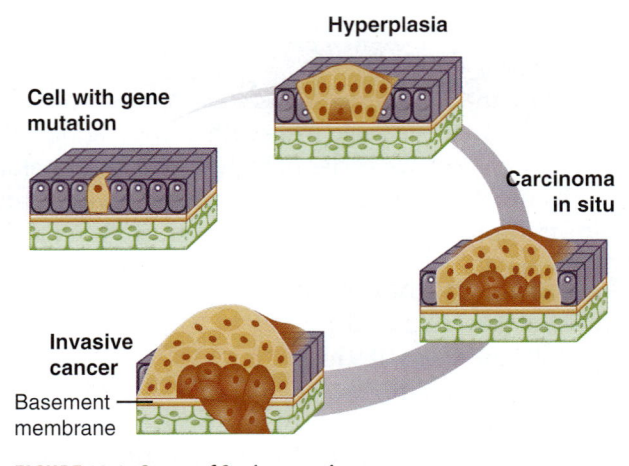

FIGURE 19.1 Stages of Carcinogenesis

Cancer Staging

When cancer is diagnosed, it must be staged to determine the most effective treatment plan and offer prognosis (**Figure 19.1**). Staging describes the severity of a cancer based on the extent of disease and whether the primary tumor has spread to other areas of the body.[6] There are four different types of cancer staging, according to the American Joint Commission on Cancer (AJCC)[6]:

- Clinical staging: Based on physical exam, image testing, and biopsies
- Pathologic staging: For patients who have had surgery to remove a tumor or explore the extent of cancer
- Posttherapy or Post-neoadjuvant therapy staging: Determines how much cancer remains after a patient is first treated with systemic and/or radiation therapy; assessed by clinical and/or pathologic staging guidelines
- Restaging: Used to determine the extent of disease after cancer comes back after treatment

The Tumor, Lymph Node, and Metastasis (TNM) Staging System was developed and is maintained by the AJCC and the Union for International Cancer Control[6] and is a tool for staging different types of cancers based on standardized criteria (**Table 19.2**). This is the most widely used staging tool among physicians.

Restaging may be done after completion of treatment to determine the extent to which the cancer responded to treatment. Restaging may also be done when a cancer has recurred and may require further treatments.

Medical Treatment of Cancer

Once the medical team determines the stage of cancer, the patient and team decide on a treatment plan, which may include radiation therapy, chemotherapy, surgery,

TABLE 19.2 CANCER STAGING VIA THE TMN STAGING SYSTEM

TNM Category	Description
T: Describes the original (primary) **tumor**	**Tx:** Primary tumor cannot be evaluated **T0:** No evidence of primary tumor **Tis:** Carcinoma in situ (early cancer that has not spread to neighboring tissue) **T1-T4:** Size and/or extent of primary tumor
N: Describes whether or not the cancer has reached nearby lymph **nodes**	**Nx:** Nearby lymph nodes not assessed (number and/or extent of spread) **N0:** No regional lymph node involvement (no cancer found in the lymph nodes) **N1-N3:** Involvement of regional lymph nodes (number and/or extent of spread)
M: Tells whether there are distant **metastases** (spread of cancer to other parts of the body)	**M0:** No distant metastasis (cancer has not spread to other parts of the body) **M1:** Distant metastasis (cancer has spread to distant parts of the body)

Used with the permission of the American Joint Committee on Cancer (AJCC), Chicago, Illinois. The original source for this material is the *AJCC Cancer Staging Manual*, Eighth Edition (2017) published by Springer Science and Business Media LLC, www.springer.com.

or a combination of therapies. Anticancer treatments may impact the cancer patient's appetite and ability to ingest/digest food, placing patients at nutritional risk. Each cancer has its own unique set of nutrition-related side effects called **nutrition impact symptoms**. Table 19.3 outlines typical nutrition impact symptoms related to specific cancers and anticancer treatments and their management.

Radiation Therapy

Radiation therapy is the use of high-energy radiation from x-rays, gamma rays, or other sources used to kill cancer cells and shrink tumors (**Figure 19.2**). It can be external or systemic, which uses a radioactive substance that circulates throughout the body. Side effects of radiation therapy typically start 2 weeks after the beginning of treatment, with the type and severity dependent on the location of the radiation treatment. Common side effects include fatigue, skin changes, nausea, and anorexia. **Odynophagia**, or pain with swallowing; dysphagia; and pneumonitis are more commonly seen in head and neck

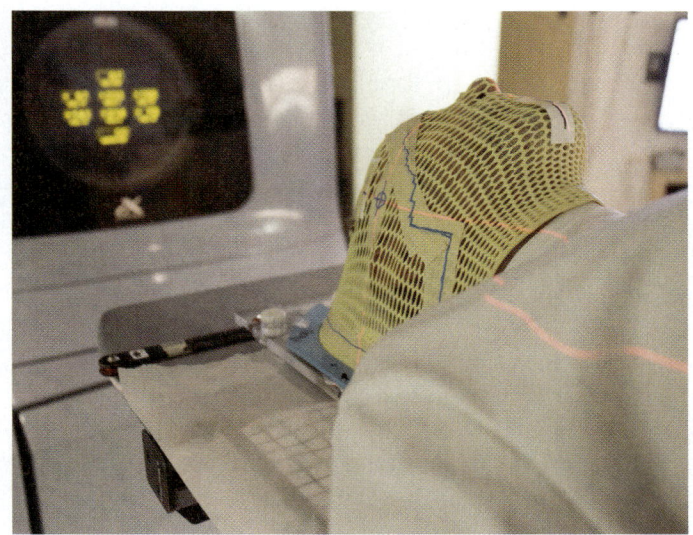

FIGURE 19.2 Patient Receiving Radiation Therapy
©John Panella/Shutterstock.

TABLE 19.3 NUTRITION IMPACT SYMPTOMS AND THEIR NUTRITIONAL MANAGEMENT

Nutrition Impact Symptom	Description	Associated Cancers	Nutritional Management
Dysphagia	Difficulty swallowing	Head and neck, esophageal, gastric, lung	Change textures of foods based on level of dysphagia Thickening agents may be indicated for fluids
Mucositis (**Figure 19.3**)/stomatitis	Inflammation of mucosal membranes, often in oral cavity	Head and neck, esophageal, gastric, lung	Consume soft, nonfibrous, nonacidic foods Avoid hot foods and beverages
Xerostomia	Diminished or loss of saliva production	Head and neck, esophageal, gastric, lung	Chew sugar-free gum or suck on tart candies Use sauces and gravies to moisten foods

(continues)

TABLE 19.3 NUTRITION IMPACT SYMPTOMS AND THEIR NUTRITIONAL MANAGEMENT (continued)

Nutrition Impact Symptom	Description	Associated Cancers	Nutritional Management
Dysgeusia	Alterations in taste	Head and neck, esophageal, gastric, lung	*Metallic taste*: Use plastic utensils; eat nuts, cheese, and poultry for protein as red meats are often not tolerated *Sweet sensitivity*: Drink flavorless supplements or diluted juices *Impaired taste*: Use spiced or very flavorful foods
Esophagitis/gastritis	Inflammation of the esophageal and gastric mucosa	Esophageal, gastric, lung	Eat bland, pureed, or soft foods Avoid alcohol, coffee, or spicy and acidic foods
Radiation enteritis	Inflammation of the small and/or large intestine caused by radiation	Intestinal, pancreatic	Follow a lactose-free and low-fat diet Drink electrolyte-fortified beverages for hydration
Dumping syndrome	Rapid influx of food, especially sugar, into the small bowel that results in cramps, diarrhea, and hypoglycemia	Esophageal, gastric, intestinal, pancreatic	Avoid drinking beverages with meals Consume soluble fiber Follow a lactose-free diet
Nausea	Uneasiness or queasiness of the stomach	All	Avoid noxious odors by using microwaves or opening windows when cooking
Vomiting	Emptying of stomach contents through the mouth	All	Avoid greasy foods the day of treatment Drink electrolyte-fortified beverages after vomiting
Constipation	Infrequent or hard-to-pass bowel movements	All	Ensure adequate fiber and fluid intake
Diarrhea	Frequent, loose, and watery stools	All; especially intestinal, pancreatic	Avoid highly concentrated sweets, sip electrolyte-fortified beverages, eat soluble fiber
Steatorrhea	Frequent, loose, and watery stools that contain excess fat	All; especially intestinal, pancreatic	Take pancreatic replacement enzymes, follow a low-fat diet, supplement with medium-chain triglyceride oil
Anorexia	Lack of appetite, possibly due to delayed gastric emptying	All	Maximize intake when appetite is present Limit fluid with meals to avoid feeling of fullness Eat small, frequent meals

cancer patients. Radiation enteritis and diarrhea are more common in cancers of the lower gastrointestinal (GI) tract and pelvic region.

Chemotherapy

Chemotherapy involves the use of antineoplastic drugs, used as a single agent or in combination with other agents, that disrupt the reproductive cycle of cancer cells. The goal of chemotherapy is to shrink cancer cells, control tumor growth, and palliate symptoms related to cancer, such as pain. Chemotherapy is utilized as a primary treatment for hematological cancers, as an adjuvant treatment after surgery, as a neo-adjuvant treatment before surgery, or as a concurrent treatment with radiation therapy. Chemotherapy acts by targeting rapidly dividing cells such as cancer cells, but it may also attack

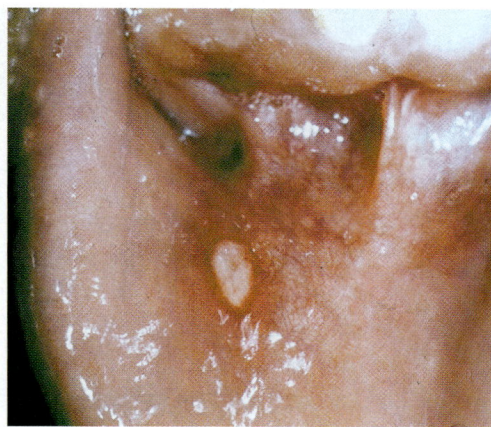

FIGURE 19.3 Mucositis
Courtesy of Department of Pathology and Laboratory Medicine, University of North Carolina at Chapel Hill.

healthy cells, such as those that line the GI tract, resulting in unwanted GI side effects such as nausea, vomiting, diarrhea, and mucositis that may place patients at nutritional risk.

Surgery

Surgery is used in solid tumors as both a palliative and curative regimen with a goal to remove a localized tumor or limit the local regional spread by removal of cancer cells. It may be used as a primary, adjuvant, or combination treatment or as a salvage therapy, which is an extensive surgery to treat local recurrence after a less-extensive primary approach has been implemented. When resection cannot be performed, other treatment modalities may be used in an attempt to reduce the size of the cancer and allow for future surgical removal. The nutritional status of patients should be monitored both pre- and postoperatively because surgical interventions can lead to nutritional deterioration due to changes in metabolism, tissue function, and body composition.

Biotherapy

Biotherapy, also known as biological therapy, is a cancer therapy that may stimulate or suppress the body's immune system to kill cancer cells. It is used in the treatment of many types of cancer to prevent or slow tumor growth and spread with fewer side effects than other cancer treatments. Biotherapy works by either inducing the immune system to attack cancer cells or making cancer cells easier for your immune system to recognize. Biotherapy is a very active area of cancer research and predominantly available in clinical trials.

Hormone Therapy

Hormone therapy is a treatment aimed at slowing or stopping the growth of certain cancers (such as breast and prostate) through synthetic hormones. These hormones may be given to block the body's natural hormones.

> **CORE CONCEPT 3**
>
> Medical treatment of cancer can lead to nutrition impact symptoms that may impair a patient's nutritional status.

Nutrition Screening and Assessment in Cancer Patients

Oncology patients are at high risk of malnutrition given disease burden, treatment-related side effects, and metabolic and physiological side effects related to cancer. Weight loss and malnutrition have been documented in more than 30% to 90% of patients, often at the time of diagnosis, depending on disease severity, treatment regimen, and associated side effects and is the single most common secondary diagnosis for patients with advanced cancer.[7-9] As many as 20% of patients with cancer die from the effects of malnutrition rather than malignancy.[9] Nutritional status may influence disease prognosis, treatment tolerance, and quality of life (QOL) and may hasten the onset of cancer cachexia. Weight loss as little as 5% before initiation of chemotherapy is predictive of early mortality and predicts a reduction in response to treatment, survival, and QOL.[10] Weight loss associated with cancer treatments can be highly distressing to the patient and caregiver and may further impair QOL.

> **CORE CONCEPT 4**
>
> Weight loss and malnutrition are well documented in cancer patients and may influence disease prognosis, treatment tolerance, and quality of life and be predictive of early mortality.

Nutrition Screening

Screening patients newly diagnosed with cancer and those undergoing therapy is key to preventing and identifying malnutrition at the earliest phase in an attempt to prevent or halt negative outcomes. According to the Academy of Nutrition and Dietetic Evidence Analysis Library, "all adult patients should be screened for malnutrition risk on entry into oncology services; early identification and management of malnutrition risk improves and protects nutrition status and QOL, which leads to improved outcomes. Rescreening should be repeated routinely throughout treatment to facilitate referral as needed."[11]

A variety of nutrition screening tools are recommended for use in ambulatory cancer centers; unfortunately, there is a lack of implementation of consistent screening, triage, and assessment tools that are evidence based in the oncology population.[12] Appropriate screening tools should be validated for use in the oncology population and be able to identify malnutrition risk in oncology patients. The current screening tools validated for use in the oncology population include the Patient Generated Subjective Global Assessment (PG-SGA), the Malnutrition Screening Tool (MST), the Malnutrition Screening Tool for Cancer Patients (MSTC), and the Malnutrition Universal Screening Tool (MUST).[6] **Table 19.4** provides a summary of the validated screening tools along with their advantages and disadvantages.

TABLE 19.4 NUTRITION SCREENING TOOLS VALIDATED IN THE ONCOLOGY POPULATION[13-17]

Tool	Oncology Population	Summary	Advantages/Disadvantages
Patient Generated SGA (PG-SGA)	Oncology inpatients and outpatients	• Screening tool adapted from the SGA that assesses nutritional risk based on anthropometrics, intake, symptoms, activity, age and metabolic stress • Highlights nutrition impact symptoms • Includes nutrition triage recommendations	• Includes section with GI symptoms, highlighting nutrition impact symptoms • Incorporates nutrition triage recommendations • Can predict direction and magnitude of change in QOL • Associated with large costs in terms of time and manpower • Reliability influenced by experience of facilitator
Malnutrition Screening Tool (MST)	Oncology outpatients	Short-form screening tool that assesses recent weight loss and recent poor intake	• Suitable screening tool for both radiation and chemotherapy outpatients • Quick and easy calculations with no additional tables, which may increase compliance • Good sensitivity in outpatient setting • Poor sensitivity for oncology inpatients • Does not include times frame for weight loss • Does not include triage recommendations
Malnutrition Screening Tool for Cancer Patients (MSTC)	Oncology inpatients	Uses intake change, weight loss, BMI, and Eastern Cooperative Oncology Group performance status	High validity compared with other available screening tools
Malnutrition Universal Screening Tool (MUST)	Oncology inpatients	Uses BMI, weight loss percentage, and acute disease effect score (acute disease effect as well as potential for no oral intake)	• Consistent and reliable screening tool • Presence of obesity is noted • Management guidelines for care plan included

Patients identified as malnourished or at nutritional risk should be referred to an RD for evaluation, nutritional assessment, and, if indicated, medical nutrition therapy to manage nutrition risk.

> **PRACTICE POINT**
>
> All cancer patients should be screened for nutrition because early identification and management of malnutrition risk can lead to improved outcomes. Patients identified at nutritional risk should be referred to a Registered Dietitian for nutrition assessment.

Nutrition Assessment

Nutritional assessment of the oncology patient should include a thorough assessment of the patient's oral food and fluid intake, including the addition of medical food supplements, vitamin/mineral and herbal supplements, and enteral nutrition (EN) and parenteral nutrition (PN). The patient's current treatment regimen with assessment of current and predicted nutrition impact symptoms should be included in the nutritional assessment. Weight trends, including degree of unintentional weight loss, should be assessed in conjunction with a physical assessment of fluid retention/edema, muscle wasting, and decline in functional status. A nutrition care plan is then developed by the RD and shared with the interprofessional care team. During active cancer treatment, the overall goals of nutrition care that guide the care plan are to prevent or reverse nutritional deficiencies, to preserve lean body mass, to minimize nutrition-related side effects, and to maximize QOL. Studies suggest that there is a tremendous benefit of dietary counseling during cancer treatment for improving outcomes, such as fewer treatment-related side effects, improved QOL, and better dietary intake.[18]

> **CORE CONCEPT 5**
>
> Dietary counseling by a registered dietitian (RD) results in improved outcomes, including fewer treatment-related side effects, improved quality of life, and better dietary intake.

Estimating Nutrition Needs in Cancer Patients

The individual nutrition needs of cancer patients vary greatly and are based on tumor type, treatment regimen, presence of stressors (such as infection), and need for weight gain. A universal resting energy expenditure (REE) of cancer patients has been deemed inconsistent in research as **hypermetabolism**, or the physiological state of increased rate of metabolic activity characterized by an abnormal increase in the body's basal metabolic rate, and is not uniformly present in cancer patients. Indirect calorimetry remains the ideal method of determining energy expenditure in this patient population; however, it is not always accessible. Estimated energy requirements should use predictive equations and should be individualized and based on clinical judgment; needs should be reassessed based on weight trends and changes in the patient's clinical picture. The Harris–Benedict Equation (HBE), along with a stress factor, has been utilized in practice as an estimation equation in this population, but it has been shown to both over- and underestimate calorie needs in the cancer population. Weight loss of >10% is associated with an increased REE when compared to weight-stable cancer patients.[19] Additionally, the metabolic effects of the tumor and pro-inflammatory cytokines may alter energy expenditure as a result of altered macronutrient metabolism and the progressive syndrome of cancer cachexia.

Energy requirements differ depending on the type of tumor present. Normal resting energy expenditure has been reported in patients with gastric or colorectal cancers, while those with pancreatic cancer usually have higher energy expenditures. The current recommendation for all cancer patients is 30 to 35 kcal/kg and 1.2 to 2.0 grams protein/kg body weight.[20]

> **PRACTICE POINT**
>
> Energy needs assessment should be individualized and based on clinical judgment, as hypermetabolism is not uniformly present in cancer patients.

> **PRACTICE POINT**
>
> Weight loss of >10% is associated with increased energy expenditure.

> **CORE CONCEPT 6**
>
> Nutrition impact symptoms and energy requirements differ based on the specific solid tumor present.

Cancer Cachexia and Metabolic Changes Associated with Cancer

Cancer Cachexia

The term *cachexia* comes from the Greek word for "poor condition" and is a clinical syndrome of debilitation and weight loss associated with the end stage of numerous chronic conditions. **Cancer cachexia** is a multifactorial syndrome characterized by an ongoing loss of skeletal muscle mass that cannot be fully reversed by conventional nutritional support.[21-25] It reduces cardiac mass and influences cardiac muscle contraction and may subsequently lead to progressive functional impairment in up to 80% of progressive cancers.[22,26] The degree of cachexia can vary according to tumor type, site, mass, and anatomical position. Clinical characteristics can include anorexia, early satiety, weakness, and weight loss. The mechanisms of cancer cachexia are poorly understood, but are thought to be tumor induced and driven by pro-inflammatory **cytokines**. Cytokines are cell-signaling molecules that aid in cell-to-cell communication in immune responses and stimulate the movement of cells toward sites of inflammation, infection, and trauma and include tumor necrosis factor, interleukin-1, and interleukin-6. Pro-inflammatory cytokines play a large role in alterations in metabolism, as seen in advanced cancer and cancer cachexia, and also can affect other physiologic processes, including altered gastric emptying, decreases in intestinal blood flow, and changes in bowel motility. The tumor-induced factors are further confounded by the effects of cancer treatment, such as GI side effects, reduced appetite, and reduced or loss of taste, which may further impair nutritional intake.

> **CORE CONCEPT 7**
>
> Cancer cachexia can lead to progressive functional impairment in advanced cancers. Pro-inflammatory cytokines may play a role in mediating alterations in metabolism seen in cancer cachexia and may also affect other GI processes.

The metabolic effect of cancer cachexia has been shown to be similar to that of severe sepsis or injury, in that nutrients move from the periphery to the liver, resulting in increased gluconeogenesis and breakdown in fat stores.[24] In contrast to severe sepsis, there is a preferential loss of skeletal muscle associated with decreased protein synthesis and increased protein degradation in the presence of pro-inflammatory cytokines (**Table 19.5**).[26,27] Unlike the mechanisms of starvation, where REE is conserved, it is unclear whether cancer patients have elevated energy expenditure. The proposed mechanism of presumed hypermetabolism in cachectic patients seems to be due to systemic inflammation, high rates of glycolysis, and the result of adrenergic state, not reversed by feeding alone.[21,22] Studies indicate that overall glucose fluctuation between gluconeogenesis and glycogenolysis increases in weight-losing cancer patients, which contributes up to 40% of increased REE in metastatic cancer.[19]

> **CORE CONCEPT 8**
>
> Cancer cachexia results in preferential loss of skeletal muscle mass and may contribute to an increase in resting energy expenditure.

TABLE 19.5 CHANGES IN MACRONUTRIENT METABOLISM ASSOCIATED WITH CANCER/CANCER CACHEXIA

Macronutrient	Metabolism in Cancer/Cachexia	Proposed Mechanism
Protein	Increased protein degradation and skeletal muscle breakdown Amino acids diverted to synthesis of acute phase reactants, resulting in muscle degradation and decreased muscle protein synthesis Increased turnover of whole body protein and amino acids	Presence of pro-inflammatory cytokines Increased metabolic demands by tumor
Carbohydrates	Increased rate of anaerobic glycolysis leading to increased consumption rate of glucose, resulting in lactate production Elevated Cori cycle activity converting lactate back to glucose via gluconeogenesis, resulting in net consumption of adenosine triphosphate	Presence of pro-inflammatory cytokines High rate of anaerobic glycolysis in malignant cells
Lipids	Enhanced lipolysis via pro-inflammatory cytokines further induced by hyperlipidemia Decreased/inhibited lipogenesis Increased mobilization of lipids, specifically triglycerides hydrolyzed to free fatty acids resulting in fat atrophy	Effect of pro-inflammatory cytokines, adrenergic activation, and tumor-related lipolytic factor

Approaches to Management in Cancer Cachexia

No evidence-based treatments are available for the treatment of cancer cachexia, and standard nutritional support may not necessarily improve outcomes in this group. Early identification of patients at risk of cachexia would be ideal in preventing the onset of this syndrome, but this remains limited as the mechanisms of cancer cachexia remain poorly understood. Early nutrition intervention plays a large role in delaying the progression of weight loss, which may further delay the onset and acceleration of cancer cachexia.[28] Research has been conducted on multiple drugs and feeding strategies to mitigate the effects of cancer cachexia. Current treatment strategies remain inadequate and fail to improve clinical outcomes. An overview of researched medical treatment strategies for cancer cachexia can be found in **Table 19.6**.

TABLE 19.6 MEDICAL MANAGEMENT OF CANCER CACHEXIA[29-42]

Medical Treatment	Proposed Benefit	Risk
Progesterones (megasterol acetate)	Associated with increased appetite and weight gain	Weight gain remains largely fat mass and edema with limited improvements in lean body mass, performance status, or QOL Insufficient evidence to define optimal dose Efficacy set at 400-800 mg/day
Glucocorticoids	Associated with increased appetite and improved quality of life	Inconclusive effects on lean body mass Adverse side effects associated with long-term use, including insulin resistance, water retention, adrenal insufficiency Can be used to improve appetite and QOL in a short-term setting
Omega-3 fatty acids	Associated with profound anti-inflammatory effects and potential to stabilize weight loss and attenuate lean tissue wasting in cancer patients	Lack of consistent data supporting the dose, duration, timing, and route of administration Larger randomized controlled trials have not demonstrated a clear benefit in maintaining weight, lean body mass, survival, or QOL

(continues)

TABLE 19.6 MEDICAL MANAGEMENT OF CANCER CACHEXIA[29-42] (continued)

Medical Treatment	Proposed Benefit	Risk
Branch chain amino acids (BCAA)	Associated with increased protein synthesis and decreased protein degradation due to integral role in skeletal muscle proteins	Results have only been demonstrated in cachectic rats and not replicated in human studies using leucine and valine Supplements also contained fish oil/omega-3 fatty acids, which may confound the results More clinical trials needed to show a clear benefit
β-hydroxy-β-methylbutryate (HMB)	Leucine metabolite thought to preserve lean muscle mass	Supplements studied were enriched with arginine and glutamine, which may confound results Exact reason HMB may promote fat-free mass gain remains unknown Larger randomized trials needed to clarify benefit

The use of hypercaloric feeding via nutrition support in the form of oral supplements and/or EN and PN is often encouraged in the cachectic cancer patient, but may not be associated with a measureable clinical benefit. Studies have failed to show that there are improvements in lean body mass when providing patients with a hypercaloric feeding regimen; in fact, loss of lean body mass persists and weight gain is seen in the form of fat mass.[22,25,28] Feeding regimens do not come without risk, and the use of PN support in particular is associated with increased risk of catheter-related sepsis and is not associated with a measurable clinical benefit.[22] The timing of nutritional support in the cancer population remains controversial due to lack of rigorous randomized controlled trials.

> **PRACTICE POINT**
>
> Nutritional support and hypercaloric feeding in cachectic cancer patients is not associated with a measureable clinical benefit.

> **CORE CONCEPT 9**
>
> Because no evidence-based treatments are available for cancer cachexia, focus should be placed on early nutrition interventions to prevent the onset and acceleration of the condition.

Overview of Nutritional Support in the Cancer Patient

Although nutrition support may not provide clinical benefit to the cachectic cancer patient, nutrition support interventions with EN or PN may be important in optimizing the patient's nutritional status to achieve best possible outcomes. Nutrition support should be initiated if it is expected that a patient will be unable to eat for a minimum of 7 days. Patients with severe nutrition risk (>10% weight loss in 6 months or BMI <18.5 kg/m^2) benefit from nutrition support 10 to 14 days prior to major surgery, even if the surgery has to be delayed. PN should only be initiated when patients cannot be fed through the enteral route, possibly from severe GI disturbances.[20]

> **PRACTICE POINT**
>
> Nutrition support is important for malnourished cancer patients or those who may not be able to eat for 7 days. Patients with severe nutrition risk benefit from nutrition support 10 to 14 days prior to major surgery.

Standard formulas are generally recommended for EN; however, **immunonutrition** (IN) formulas are becoming increasingly used in GI cancers. Immunonutrition is the effect of nutrients, including macronutrients, vitamins, minerals, and trace elements, on inflammation, the formation of antibodies, and the resistance to disease. Common immune-modulating formulas contain higher amounts of omega-3 fatty acids, arginine, nucleic acids, glutamine, and antioxidants, which may improve GI mucosal integrity and enhance cell-mediated immune response. Some controversy exists regarding use of glutamine in cancer patients given in vitro evidence of glutamine being a primary fuel source for tumor cells. However, clinical studies show that glutamine benefits host metabolism, mucosal integrity, and immune function without enhancing tumor cell growth.[41] ESPEN guidelines recommend using IN in GI and head and neck cancer patients for 5 to 7 days prior to abdominal surgery, independent of their nutritional status.[20]

> **PRACTICE POINT**
>
> Immune-modulating formulas may provide clinical benefit to GI and head and neck cancer patients when used for 5 to 7 days prior to abdominal surgery, independent of nutritional status.

Nutritional Management of Specific Solid Tumors

Head and Neck Cancers

Head and neck cancers (HNC) make up 3% to 5% of all cancer cases in the United States.[42,43] HNC include those of the sinus cavity and oropharyngeal region (**Figure 19.4**).[42] New cases occur most frequently in African American men, aged 50 years or older, who have a history of alcohol and tobacco use. Other risk factors are poor oral hygiene and history of human papillomavirus infection.[44] Those with early, localized HNC are managed by surgery and/or radiation. If the cancer is more advanced, aggressive multimodal therapies including surgery, chemotherapy, and radiation may be indicated.[45]

HNC patients are the most at risk for malnutrition compared to any other malignancy. Dysphagia secondary to the physical obstruction of the tumor and a history of alcohol and tobacco use are the biggest predictors of malnutrition observed in this population.[43,46] Nutrition intake is often limited during treatment. Food textures may have to be modified depending on the severity of dysphagia present.

Surgical interventions in HNC usually demand nutrition support. Both nasogastric tubes (NGT) and percutaneous endoscopic gastrostomy (PEG) tubes are equal in maintaining body weight 6 months after treatment; however, each route poses its own unique benefits and risks.[47] NGTs are placed for the short term (<30 days), while PEG tubes are for longer use (>30 days).[5] A PEG tube may have decreased chance of tube displacement compared to an NGT, but the cancer may metastasize to the gastrostomy itself. If a patient is suffering from ulcerative mucositis, the presence of an NGT may exacerbate irritation, and thus a PEG may be a more ideal choice.[44] Prophylactic PEG placement is an acceptable practice with HNC patients to reduce treatment-induced

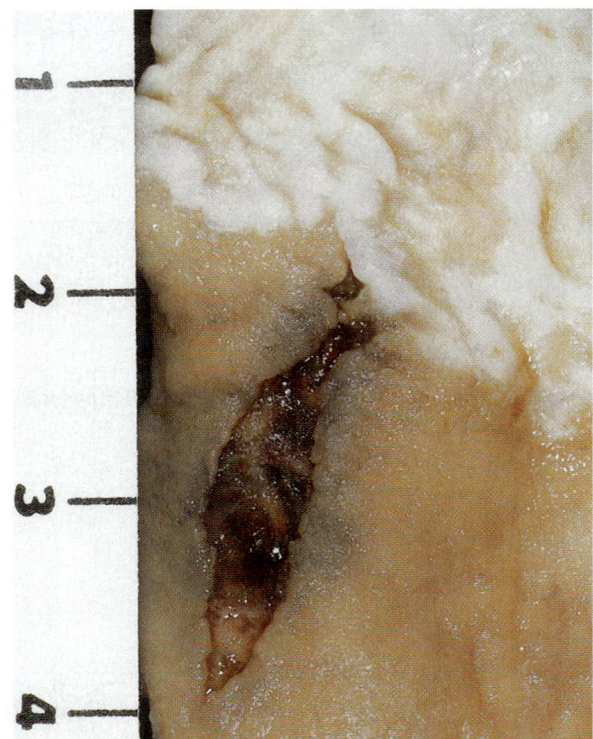

FIGURE 19.4 Cancer of Oral Mucosa
Courtesy of Leonard V. Crowley, MD, Century College.

⚠ Clinical Controversy

Do head and neck cancer (HNC) patients benefit from prophylactic percutaneous endoscopic gastrostomy (PEG) placement?

HNC patients are at increased risk of malnutrition due to impaired swallowing function and odynophagia impacting their ability to eat and drink. Inadequate intake can lead to weight loss, malnutrition, dehydration, increased risk of hospitalization, poor treatment tolerance, lower quality of life, and increased mortality. Silander et al. randomized 134 patients with advanced HNC to receive a PEG tube or no PEG tube. The results of the study revealed that there was no difference in hospital stay between the two groups. The healthcare-related quality of life was significantly better and weight loss was significantly less in the PEG group. Madhoun et al. evaluated characteristics of 143 HNC patients with prophylactic PEGs and concluded that there was a high rate of unnecessary PEG placement when done prophylactically in HNC due to the fact that almost half of the patients never used the PEG or used it for less than 2 weeks.

1. What are the potential advantages and disadvantages of prophylactic PEG placement in HNC patients?

2. How would you assess a HNC patient for a prophylactic PEG placement?

3. Would you recommend a prophylactic PEG for your HNC patient?

References

1. Silander E, Nyman J, Bove M, Johansson L, Larrson, S, Hammerlid E. Impact of prophylactic percutaneous endoscopic gastrostomy on malnutrition and quality of life in patients with head and neck cancer – a randomized study. *Head Neck*. 2012;34(1):1–9

2. Madhoun MF, Blakenship MM, Blankenship DM, Krempl GA, Tierney WM. Prophylactic PEG placement in head and neck cancer: How many feeding tubes are unused (and unnecessary)? *World J Gastroenterol*. 2011;17(8): 1004-1008

weight loss, although there is little evidence to support that they actually increase body weight.[43]

> **PRACTICE POINT**
>
> Food textures may have to be modified if dysphagia is present. NGT and PEG tubes are commonly used in malnourished patients; prophylactic PEG placement is an accepted practice with HNC patients to reduce treatment-induced weight loss.

> **CORE CONCEPT 10**
>
> Head and neck cancer patients have the highest risk for malnutrition compared to other malignancies.

Esophageal Cancer

Esophageal cancer (EC) (**Figure 19.5**) is relatively uncommon in the United States, with only 18,170 new cases in 2014.[48] Most patients are often asymptomatic until late in the disease process, thus a poor long-term survival rate remains.[41] History of tobacco/alcohol use and Barrett's esophagus, a complication of long-term gastroesophageal reflux, are the major risk factors for EC. Some attribute the obesity epidemic, a risk factor of reflux, to a rise in incidence of esophageal cancers.[48]

Esophageal resection is the treatment of choice if the cancer is detected early. Surgical options include esophagectomy (resection of part of the esophagus) and esophagogastrectomy (a procedure where the stomach is used to replace the resected esophagus; **Figure 19.6**). For advanced stages, multimodal therapy including radiation, chemotherapy, and surgery is utilized.[48]

As with HNC patients, those with EC may benefit from modifying food textures if dysphasia is present. If the stomach was used to reconstruct the esophagus, patients may experience dumping syndrome. Dumping syndrome results from rapid delivery of nutrients into the proximal small

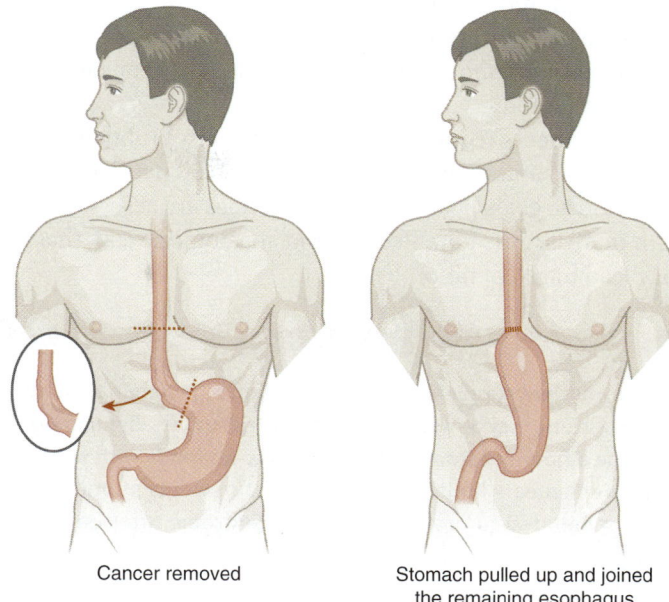

Surgery for esophageal cancer

Cancer removed | Stomach pulled up and joined the remaining esophagus

FIGURE 19.6 Surgery for Treatment of Esophageal Cancer

bowel characterized by sweating, tachycardia, GI symptoms, and hypoglycemia. In order to avoid dumping syndrome, patients should limit concentrated sweets, lactose, and high-fat foods. Patients should also avoid drinking beverages until 30 to 60 minutes postprandially to minimize rapid gastric emptying during meal times.[49] For patients who require nutrition support, jejunostomy tubes (J tubes) are the preferred enteral route to bypass the fresh anastomoses in the esophagus or stomach.[41] Most patients are able to tolerate jejunal feeding as early as 48 to 72 hours postoperatively.[49,51]

> **PRACTICE POINT**
>
> Food textures may have to be modified if dysphagia is present in patients with esophageal cancer. Jejunostomy tubes are often used and can be tolerated early after surgery.

Gastric Cancer

About 22,000 new cases of gastric cancer (GC) are diagnosed annually.[52] Common risk factors include *Heliobacter pylori* infection and male gender. If caught early, GC maintains about a 50% cure rate; the five-year survival rate for localized gastric cancer is 67%.[42] The primary treatment for GC is surgery, either a total or subtotal gastrectomy (80% to 85% removal of the stomach). Chemotherapy and radiation are adjuvant therapies.[53]

Postgastrectomy syndrome predisposes the GC patient to micronutrient deficiencies, fat malabsorption, and dumping syndrome. Decreased gastric acid and intrinsic factor production may result in iron, calcium, and vitamin B_{12} deficiencies. Patients are encouraged to take a daily multivitamin, 1,000 mcg sublingual vitamin B_{12} daily (or 1,000 mcg intramuscular shot once monthly), and 500 mg calcium citrate twice daily to prevent such deficiencies. If fat malabsorption occurs, at least 1,000 units

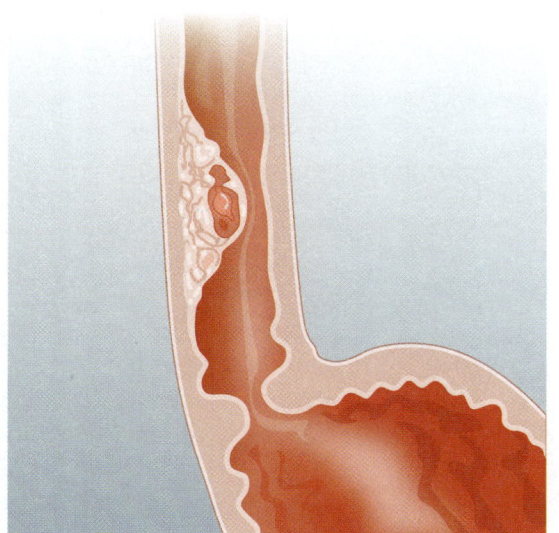

FIGURE 19.5 Esophageal Cancer

of vitamin D should be supplemented daily and fat-soluble vitamins should be monitored routinely.[54] Because postgastrectomy patients are also at risk for dumping syndrome, patients should limit concentrated sweets, lactose, and high-fat foods.

For patients requiring nutrition support, J tubes are often placed at the time of the surgery to help patients reach their caloric goals postgastrectomy. J tubes are associated with increased risk of infection and anastomotic leak that may lead to re-operation.[52]

> **PRACTICE POINT**
>
> Micronutrient supplementation, including B_{12}, vitamin D, iron, and calcium, may be necessary after gastric surgery, depending on the amount of stomach resected. Low-fat foods with small, frequent meals limited in concentrated sweets should be recommended to prevent dumping syndrome after gastric surgery.

Intestinal Cancers

Small bowel malignancies are rare, about 0.5% of all malignancies, and the most common are carcinoid tumors. Conversely, colorectal cancer (CRC) is the third most common cancer diagnosed in the United States. Age is the main risk factor for CRC, with 90% of new cases occurring after age 50 years. Screening for CRC by fecal occult blood testing or routine colonoscopy beginning at 50 years has significantly decreased the mortality rates.[55] Surgical intervention is the initial mode of treatment for intestinal cancers, with radiation to the abdomen or pelvis serving as a standard adjuvant therapy.

Abdominal and pelvic radiation may induce enteritis accompanied by diarrhea and malabsorption of fat, electrolytes, and lactose.[56] Nutritional management data for radiation enteritis is limited; however, a low-residue, low-fat, and lactose-free diet with emphasis on hydration is tolerated well in most patients.[57] After bowel resection, a low-residue diet with progression to a regular diet as tolerated is recommended. Those who require colostomies or ileostomies after surgery should eat foods with soluble fiber to thicken stool (such as bananas and applesauce) and avoid gas- and odor-producing foods (such as broccoli and beans). If massive resection of the bowel should take place, the patient is at risk for short bowel syndrome, a malabsorptive state of macro- and micronutrients. Most of these patients often require nutrition support. If an oral diet is tolerated, then small, frequent meals high in protein and low in fat, fiber, and lactose are encouraged. Micronutrient supplementation depends on what portion of the bowel remains, but most require additional vitamin B_{12} supplements.[58]

For patients requiring nutrition support, continuous nasogastric feedings of intact protein formulas increase absorption of macronutrients and reduce osmotic diarrhea compared to elemental formulas in patients with short bowel syndrome.[59] PN may be indicated after bowel resection if obstructions, fistulae, or anastomotic leaks should occur.[58]

> **PRACTICE POINT**
>
> Bowel resection after intestinal surgery requires a diet progression from low residue with advancement to regular diet. If short bowel syndrome should occur, nutrition support is often indicated to maintain nutrition and hydration.

Pancreatic Cancer

Pancreatic cancer is an extremely aggressive malignancy. Despite being the 12th most common cancer in the United States, it is the 4th leading cause of cancer death.[60] The etiology of pancreatic cancer is poorly understood, but some risk factors include cigarette smoking, increased BMI, and high dietary fat intake.[42] Local surgical resection of the tumor is the mainstay treatment, despite that only 15% to 20% of patients present with resectable disease.[61] Pancreaticoduodenectomy (Whipple procedure; **Figure 19.7**) and distal or total pancreatectomy are the most commonly performed procedures. Chemotherapy and radiation may be used as well.

Pancreatic exocrine insufficiency after resection can lead to extreme weight loss secondary to fat malabsorption. Pancreatic enzymes can ease steatorrhea, or stool that contains excess fat, and weight loss.[60] Delayed gastric emptying due to the attenuation of the exocrine hormones motilin and cholecystokinin is another common morbidity. The use of small, frequent, low-fat meals helps aid digestion and absorption. Total pancreatectomy, although a rare procedure, results in new-onset diabetes and requires consistent carbohydrate intake in addition to exogenous insulin therapy to achieve glycemic control.[60] Fat-soluble vitamins should be monitored routinely and supplemented as indicated due to increased risk of deficiency with fat malabsoption.

For patients requiring nutrition support, elemental nasojejunal feeds may be warranted in this population

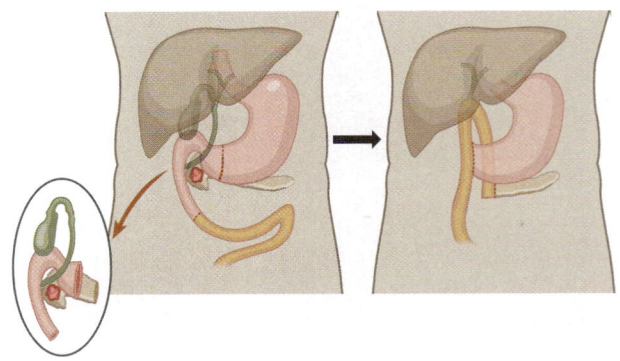

FIGURE 19.7 Whipple Procedure or Pancreaticoduodenectomy is a Treatment of Cancer in the Head of the Pancreas

CASE STUDY REVISITED

Seth was readmitted to the hospital 2 months after his initial chemotherapy for a matched unrelated donor allogeneic HSCT (allo-HSCT). His conditioning regimen for transplant includes high-dose chemotherapy and radiation therapy.

Anthropometric Data:
Weight: 82 kg (180 lbs)

Biochemical Data:
Sodium 145 (135-145 mEq/L)
Potassium 5.0 (3.6-5.0 mEq/L)
Blood urea nitrogen 29 (6-24 mg/dL)
Creatinine 1.0 (0.4-1.3 mg/dL)
Glucose 95 (70-139 mg/dL)
Albumin 2.8 (3.5-5.0 g/dL)

Dietary Data:
Dietary History: Reports poor appetite.
Diet Prescription: High-calorie/high protein diet.

Questions:
1. What do you think Seth's nutritional status and risks are as he prepares for an allo-HSCT?
2. How would you assess Seth's nutritional needs during allo-HSCT? What calorie and protein goals would you set for Seth?
3. If you had all available resources, how would you monitor Seth's nutritional status during transplant?
4. Would Seth benefit from a hypercaloric diet?

---

if a patient is refractory to pancreatic enzymes. The development of a pancreatic fistula may require the use of PN.[61]

> **PRACTICE POINT**
>
> Pancreatic enzyme supplementation and low-fat meals are usually indicated after pancreatic surgery to prevent weight loss secondary to fat malabsorption due to pancreatic exocrine insufficiency. Fat-soluble vitamins should be monitored routinely and supplemented as indicated.

Lung Cancer

Lung cancer (LC) is the leading cause of death from cancer for both men and women, with the most common diagnosis being nonsmall cell lung cancer.[42] Cigarette smoking remains the primary risk cancer for LC, accounting for 90% of all cases. Common symptoms include coughing with or without blood, shortness of breath, and weight loss.[62] Many present at advanced stages of the disease, which means the tumors typically cannot be resected. If it is caught early, patients may have a segmentectomy, lobectomy, or pneumonectomy.[63] The majority of patients undergo radiation and chemotherapy.

Limited evidence exists on effective lung cancer–specific nutrition interventions, despite their significant nutrition risk.[64] Individuals with lung cancer often have increased energy needs secondary to increased work of breathing and have decreased intake from becoming easily fatigued during mealtimes. There is no evidence to support the routine use of nutrition support in patients with lung cancer. Appropriate utilization should be evaluated on an individual basis.

> **PRACTICE POINT**
>
> Small, frequent meals may help patients who easily tire during meal times due to increased work of breathing.

Nutritional Management of Hematological Cancers Undergoing Hematopoietic Stem Cell Transplant

Patients with hematological cancers such as leukemia and lymphoma may undergo an autologous or allogeneic **hematopoietic stem cell transplant (HSCT)** in hopes of causing an antitumor effect.[65,66] The stem cells for this treatment are collected from bone marrow, peripheral blood, or umbilical cord blood from the patient's own stem cells, known as an **autologous HSCT**, or from a related or matched unrelated donor, known as an **allogeneic HSCT** (**Figure 19.8**). Prior to transplantation, patients undergo various high-dose chemotherapy and radiation regimens, placing patients at nutrition risk due to treatment-related side effects including nausea, vomiting, anorexia, malabsorption, and increased metabolic requirements.[67]

Generally, patients undergoing autologous HSCT have shorter periods of **neutropenia**, or a low neutrophil count, resulting in quicker resolution of GI side effects and less frequent use of nutritional support.[68] Patients undergoing an allogeneic HSCT are at increased nutritional risk due to prolonged periods of neutropenia and the risk of developing graft versus host disease (GVHD). During allogeneic HSCT, a patient's immune system is eroded to prevent graft rejection, which may result in prolonged GI side effects necessitating nutritional support. The allogeneic HSCT is considered to be one of the most intense regimens in oncology treatment.[69] Studies indicate that higher body mass index (BMI >30 kg/m²) in well-nourished patients may have a protective effect on survival as patients in this category may be more prepared to withstand catabolic stages following transplant than other weight groups.[70]

> **CORE CONCEPT 11**
>
> The allogeneic hematopoietic stem cell transplant (HSCT) is considered one of the most intense treatments in the oncology population and puts patients at nutritional risk due to prolonged neutropenia, gastrointestinal side effects, and risk of graft versus host disease.

Estimating Energy Needs

Energy needs in patients undergoing HSCT transplants are increased due to the catabolic stress associated with radiation and chemotherapy prior to transplant, graft versus host disease, and the need for blood count reconstitution.[67] A well-nourished patient with mild complications requires approximately 30 kcals/kg of body weight and 1.5 to 1.8 g protein/kg body weight.[71] For a malnourished patient with severe side effects following transplant, 35 to 45 kcals/kg may be needed along with 1.8 to 2.5 g protein/kg.[71] It is important to continuously monitor these patients and adjust their needs accordingly based on any complications that may develop.

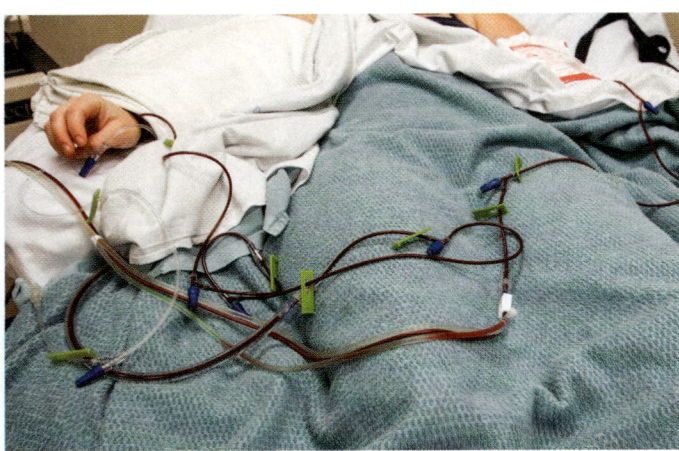

FIGURE 19.8 Bone Marrow Donation
©Dani Blanchette/EyeEm/Getty Images.

CASE STUDY REVISITED

Seth has completed his conditioning regimen and has received his allogeneic HSCT today. He has been in the hospital for 1 week with continued poor appetite and now mucositis and vomiting. He is receiving intravenous (IV) fluids and multiple IV medications.

Anthropometric Data:
Current weight: 78 kg (172 lbs)

Biochemical Data:
Albumin 2.1 g/dL (3.5-5.0 g/dL)

Clinical Data:
Nutrition-focused Physical Exam: Appears pale, tired; hollow appearance under eyes, prominent clavical bone, depressed interosseous muscle

Questions:
1. How would you describe Seth's nutritional status?
2. Would you provide Seth with nutrition support?
3. If so, what type and why?

Malnutrition can be difficult to estimate in these patients because body weight may not be reflective of nutritional status. Many patients experience edema in the month following transplant due to the use of corticosteroids, nephrotoxic drugs, and intravenous hydration, along with the presence of hypoalbuminemia.[65] Additionally, serum markers of albumin and prealbumin are negative acute phase proteins and may be falsely low in the presence of inflammation during transplant. Midarm circumference and handgrip strength may be better tools to assess changes to nutritional or functional status.

> **CORE CONCEPT 12**
>
> Patients undergoing HSCT have increased energy needs due to increased catabolism and treatment-related complications.

> **PRACTICE POINT**
>
> Body weight and serum albumin and prealbumin are not reliable markers of nutritional status in the immediate post-transplant period.

Nutritional Support During Acute Phase of HSCT

Nutrition support is often needed for patients during the acute, hospital phase of transplant, but this remains controversial. The American Society for Parenteral and Enteral Nutrition states that nutrition support therapy is appropriate for malnourished patients undergoing HSCT or those who are anticipated to be unable to ingest or absorb nutrients for at least 7 days.[69] Today, acute nutrition support is more routine in treatment centers for patients following an allogeneic HSCT due to increased nutritional needs and treatment associated complications that affect nutritional status.[72] Nutrition is critical following transplant, as impaired nutritional status can lead to longer engraftment time and a greater likelihood of developing infection.[73]

Historically, giving PN to patients undergoing HSCT was preferred due to availability of central venous access, reluctance to use perceived aggressive and hazardous NGT for enteral feedings, and the high risk of mucositis and enterocolitis in these patients.[65,69] Early studies also demonstrated prolonged survival, decreased incidence of relapse, and longer relapse free survival with PN use in this population.[74]

EN has been associated with improved nitrogen balance and weight gain with a lower risk of infection than PN (**Figure 19.9**).[69,75] After HSCT, EN has been shown to limit gut atrophy and bacterial translocation, which may decrease the risk of sepsis and acute graft versus host disease.[65] However, nausea, vomiting, GI mucositis, and the increased risk of bleeding after tube placement in patients with thrombocytopenia may make EN difficult to implement.[71,73] Patients with continuous GI side effects, such as

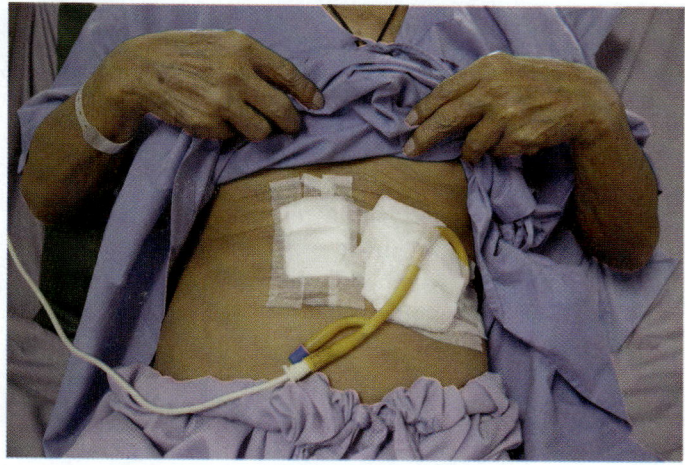

FIGURE 19.9 Patient Receiving Enteral Nutrition
©stockphoto mania/Shutterstock.

vomiting, should not receive EN due to the increased risk of aspiration.[76]

Patients who are unable to utilize EN should have PN if they require nutrition support. Many patients will require PN for nutrition repletion due to rapid nitrogen losses from diarrhea and rapid fluid shifts induced by chemotherapy.[74] As patients are able to increase oral intake, PN should be tapered down in accordance with the amount they can consume orally. When patients are able to consistently consume 50% to 70% of their needs orally, nutrition support can be discontinued.[67,71,76]

While nutrition support is beneficial in the acute care setting, patients may still have difficulty maintaining adequate nutrition in the long term. The majority of patients are unable to return to their pretransplant weight 1 year posttransplant due to impaired oral intake.[77]

> **PRACTICE POINT**
>
> Nutrition support during HSCT is indicated in malnourished patients and patients unable to ingest or absorb nutrition for 7 days.

> **CORE CONCEPT 13**
>
> Nutrition is critical following transplant as impaired nutritional status can lead to longer engraftment time and a greater likelihood of developing infection.

Graft Versus Host Disease

Graft versus host disease (GVHD) is a condition that can occur after allogeneic HSCT, when the donor's cells recognize the host's cells as foreign, causing an immune response designed to eliminate the foreign tissue in the recipient. Organs become vulnerable to infections and their functions are disrupted. Donor compatibility, the age of the patient, and immunosuppressive therapy are a few of the factors that influence GVHD development.[78] Despite advances in medicine, the incidence of GVHD remains high, likely related to the increased use of allogeneic HSCT.[69] There are

Clinical Roundtable

Topic: Use of Enteral Nutrition in Allogeneic HSCT

Parenteral nutrition (PN) is often the first choice of nutrition support in clinical practice post-allogeneic HSCT despite studies that show the feasibility and tolerance of enteral nutrition (EN). Preference for PN may be related to the prevalence of GI side effects such as nausea, vomiting, and mucositis potentially impacting EN tolerance, as well as the concern with placing a nasogastric tube in patients with thrombocytopenia due to increased risk of bleeding. There are no guidelines for the specific use of EN in the allogeneic HSCT population, although it is well understood that EN is more physiologic, safer, easier to use, and less costly than PN. EN has been found to significantly improve patient outcomes by reducing early posttransplant mortality and GVHD incidence and has been associated with a lower risk of infection.

Roundtable Discussion

1. How do you balance the potential risks of administering EN with the outcome benefits of using EN in the HSCT population?
2. What parameters would you use in determining the suitability of and to monitor tolerance to EN?
3. Would you recommend using EN in clinical practice when caring for your HSCT patient?

References:

1. Guieze R, Lemal R, Cabrespine A, et al. Enteral versus parenteral nutrition support in allogenic haematopoietic stem-cell transplantation. *Clin Nutr.* 2014;33(3):533-538. doi: 10.1016/j.clnu.2013.07.012.
2. Seguy D, Duhmael A, Rejeb MB, et al. Better outcomes of patients undergoing enteral tube feeding after myeloablative conditioning for allogeneic stem cell transplantation. *Transplantation.* 2012;94(3):287-294. doi: 10.1097/TP.0b013e3182558f60.

---

two kinds of GVHD: acute, which occurs within 100 days of transplant, and chronic, which occurs after 100 days posttransplant. Acute GVHD affects approximately 50% of allogeneic HSCT patients, targeting the skin, liver, and GI tract.[65,69] One-third of the patients with acute GVHD will develop chronic GVHD that can involve the skin, oral mucosa, GI tract, eyes, musculoskeletal system, liver, lungs, and vagina.[65,69]

Patients with GVHD may have increased energy and protein needs related to hypermetabolism, infections, protein losses from skin and GI involvement, and use of high-dose corticosteroids.[71,78] Energy needs may increase by 10% in chronic GVHD, requiring 35 to 45 kcal/kg and 1.8 to 2.5 g protein/kg/day.[71,78,79] Research suggests that increased serum concentrations of norepinephrine and glucagon in patients with chronic GVHD may also be responsible for this increase in REE.[79]

PRACTICE POINT

Energy and protein needs are increased in patients with GVHD due to hypermetabolism, protein loss, and use of high-dose corticosteroids.

The metabolic and physiologic burden of GVHD results in a high rate of malnutrition, impacting nearly one-half of patients with GVHD.[80] Patients with oral mucosa and GI involvement may experience weight loss due to malabsorption and/or inability to ingest adequate nutrition from odynophagia, mucositis, nausea, and vomiting. Medical and nutrition management is key in maintaining the nutritional status of these patients.

More than half of patients who develop GVHD will experience symptoms in their GI tract that impair oral intake, such as dysphagia, anorexia, nausea, mucositis,

---

CASE STUDY REVISITED

Seth has developed acute GI GVHD resulting in large volumes of diarrhea (approximately 2 L/day). He is now receiving high-dose steroids and is NPO (*nil per os* or nothing by mouth).

Questions

1. How would Seth's diagnosis of GI GVHD change your nutritional management?
2. How would GI GVHD change Seth's nutritional needs?
3. How would you provide Seth nutrition support while he is NPO?
4. What additional biochemical markers would you closely monitor?
5. Should you provide Seth with glutamine?

and diarrhea, leading to weight loss and progressive cachexia.[71,81] Diminished oral intake and nutrient malabsorption in patients with GVHD places patients at risk for multiple micronutrient deficiencies, including folic acid, zinc, and vitamin B_{12}. A multivitamin supplement (without iron) can be considered for patients with chronic poor oral intake to prevent deficiencies.[78] Rapid decline in bone mineral density is seen within 1 year following HSCT as a result of steroid use, and decreased oral intake, and additional calcium and vitamin D supplementation is often required.[82]

Nutritional support is often indicated in patients with GVHD when oral intake is impaired. The type of nutritional support for patients with oral and GI GVHD is decided on a case-by-case basis. In cases of GI dysfunction and severe diarrhea (>1 L per day), bowel rest is indicated with initiation of PN for full nutritional support until stool volume and frequency is controlled and diet is able to be advanced.[83]

> **CORE CONCEPT 14**
>
> Graft versus host disease can occur following allogeneic HSCT and places patients at nutritional risk due to impaired function of the gastrointestinal tract, including the oral mucosa.

> **PRACTICE POINT**
>
> Nutrition support is indicated due to interruption of normal GI function. PN is utilized in cases of severe GI GVHD necessitating bowel rest until stool volume and frequency decrease.

Glutamine and Nutrition Support

Glutamine is the most abundant nonessential amino acid in the body and has been researched in the acute HSCT population for its role in fueling immune and GI cells and reducing the severity of mucositis and GVHD. Despite its status as a nonessential amino acid, needs for glutamine are increased during critical illness and catabolism.[84]

Research related to glutamine in the HSCT population shows conflicting results. Some studies suggest that administration of parenteral glutamine to HSCT patients may preserve nitrogen loss following transplant, reduce rates of infection, and reduce duration of diarrhea compared to patients given a standard PN formula. Use of parenteral glutamine has also been associated with longer duration of opioid use, longer hospital stays, higher rates of relapse, and death.[85] Glutamine is not included in standard PN formulas because it is nonessential, has a shorter shelf-life than other amino acids, and is a costly intervention.[86]

Due to conflicting research and potential for poor outcomes, there is not a standard practice for the use of glutamine supplementation in the HSCT population. More randomized controlled trials are needed to learn about the effects of glutamine on clinical outcomes following HSCT.

> **PRACTICE POINT**
>
> Research related to glutamine supplementation in the HSCT population remains controversial. There is no standard practice for use of glutamine supplementation and more randomized controlled trials are needed.

Low-Microbial Diets

Patients who are able to maintain an oral diet status post-HSCT have historically followed a low-microbial diet, also referred to as the low-bacteria or neutropenic diet. This diet emerged and gained popularity due to concerns that ingesting foodborne pathogens could increase infection rates in HSCT patients. There is no evidence to show the benefit of the low-bacteria diet in this population. In fact, research has demonstrated that patients who followed a low-microbial diet after HSCT had no difference in infection rates as compared to patients with no diet restrictions after HSCT.[87,88]

The low-microbial diet lacks consistent dietary definition and implementation parameters, creating variability among institutions that continue to use it.[88] The significant dietary limitations of the low-microbial diet may further limit adequate caloric intake in a population at high nutritional risk. Despite the lack of evidence and consistency in this diet, many institutions continue to utilize the low-microbial diet in their HSCT patients. Rather than following the low-microbial diet, patients should focus on food safety by utilizing the Food and Drug Administration's published guidelines for patients who have undergone transplants.[89]

CASE STUDY REVISITED

Seth's diarrhea has become more manageable, with less than 500 mL of stool output per day. The plan is to send Seth home within the next week.

Questions

1. What type of diet should Seth follow at home?
2. Should Seth adhere to a low microbial diet?

> **PRACTICE POINT**
>
> The low-microbial diet lacks consistent definition and implementation parameters and has no evidence-based benefit for use after HSCT. Individuals should follow food safety guidelines for transplant patients published by the Food and Drug Administration.

Nutrition Support in the Advanced Cancer Patient

The role of nutritional support in the advanced cancer patient remains controversial as the timeline for initiating, withholding, and/or withdrawing nutritional support in the terminally ill patient remains unclear. The notion that providing nutritional support will provide comfort and reduce suffering is not evidence based. Evidence suggests the provision of nutrition support in terminally ill patients may not enhance a patient's QOL and may in fact increase suffering.[69,90-94] There are instances along the spectrum of advanced disease where nutrition support may provide benefit, including improving fluid status and nutrient intake and improving QOL. It is important to remember that nutrition and hydration are considered life-sustaining measures and should be in line with the patient's wishes. Nutritional support should be considered on a case-by-case basis, with the patient's best interest in mind and assessment of multiple factors, including the patient's wishes, goals of care (palliation versus end-of-life care), treatment plan, estimated need for nutritional support, estimated lifespan, ability of patient and/or caregiver to perform tasks to infuse nutrition support, and a safe and clean home environment.[95,96] The assessment of potential risks, including the need for routine blood work; risk of infection; mobility limitations during feeding; bladder and bowel incontinence; edema; and negative GI symptoms, such as nausea, vomiting, and diarrhea, as well as the therapy's perceived futility should also be considered in this decision.[93]

> **CORE CONCEPT 15**
>
> Nutrition support in the advanced cancer patient should be assessed on a case-by-case basis with consideration of goals of care.

Complementary and Alternative Medicine, Integrative Medicine, and the Cancer Patient

Complementary and alternative medicine (CAM) refers to medical products and practices that are not part of standard medical care (**Figure 19.10**). **Complementary medicine**

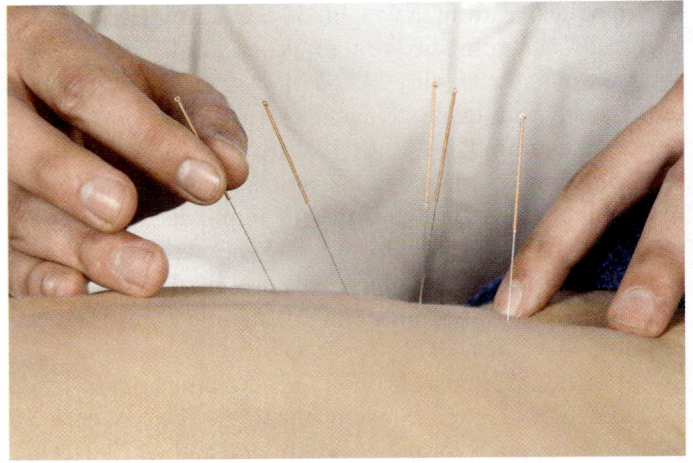

FIGURE 19.10 Acupuncture is a Type of Complementary Medicine that can be Used in Oncology Treatment
©Nanette Grebe/Shutterstock.

is used along with standard medicine (such as acupuncture), **alternative medicine** is used instead of standard medicine treatment (such as botanicals/herbals used to treat cancer instead of prescribed anticancer drugs), and **integrative medicine** is a total approach to medicine that combines standard medicine with CAM practices. Integrative medicine has been shown to be a safe and effective practice and is aimed at treating the patient's mind, body, and spirit. A national survey conducted in 2007 showed that 4 out of 10 adults use a CAM therapy, with nearly 50% of patients most commonly using prayer and spiritual practice, relaxation, faith and spiritual healing, and nutritional supplements and vitamins.[97,98] While many CAM therapies have been evaluated and found to be safe and effective, some have been found to be potentially harmful for the patient. Less in known about many CAM therapies as a result of limitations in research due to lack of careful research practices such as those used in standard cancer treatments. The RD should be aware of any botanicals and nutritional products, including dietary supplements, herbal supplements, and vitamins, that a patient is using, as they may be harmful to the patient or interact with the patient's current treatment. Patients are recommended to inform their clinician if they are using or considering using any CAM therapy to evaluate the safety and efficacy of the product. Reliable organizations to find out more about CAM therapies include the National Center for Complementary and Integrative Health, the NCI Office of Cancer Complementary and Alternative Medicine, and the Office of Dietary Supplements.

Chapter Summary

Cancer is a complex disease caused by environmental, genetic, and lifestyle factors that is the second most common cause of death in the United States. Medical management of cancer can lead to significant nutrition impact symptoms that may lead to weight loss and malnutrition. Symptoms and their nutritional management can vary greatly based on cancer type and tumor location. Head and neck as well as GI cancers are associated with high rates of malnutrition due to their negative impact on the ability of the patient to ingest and absorb food. Cancer cachexia, a complicating factor in advanced cancer, leads to a loss of lean body mass and can contribute to increased resting energy expenditure. Hematopoietic stem cell transplants, a treatment for hematological cancers, are considered one of the most intense medical treatments and can have significant nutrition implications including increased energy needs and GI side effects. Nutrition interventions during and after cancer treatments can improve nutritional status influencing treatment tolerance, quality of life, prognosis, and mortality.

Key Terms

carcinomas, sarcomas, hematologic malignancies, nutrition impact symptoms, radiation therapy, odynophagia, biotherapy, chemotherapy, hypermetabolism, cancer cachexia, cytokines, immunonutrition, hematopoietic stem cell transplant (HSCT), autologous HSCT, allogeneic HSCT, glutamine, graft versus host disease (GVHD), complementary medicine, alternative medicine, integrative medicine.

References

1. Understanding Cancer. National Institutes of Health (US); Biological Sciences Curriculum Study. Bethesda (MD): National Institutes of Health (US); 2007.
2. Anand P, Kunnumakara AB, Sundaram C, et al. Cancer is a preventable disease that requires major lifestyle changes. *Pharm Res.* 2008;25(9):2097–2116. doi: 10.1007/s11095-008-9661-9
3. Genetics and Cancer. American Cancer Society Web site. http://www.cancer.org/cancer/cancercauses/geneticsandcancer/heredity-and-cancer. Updated April 19, 2017. Accessed September 10, 2017.
4. American Cancer Society. *Cancer Facts and Figures 2015*. Atlanta, GA: American Cancer Society; 2015. http://www.cancer.org/acs/groups/content/@editorial/documents/document/acspc-044552.pdf
5. Reuter S, Gupta SC, Chaturvedi MM, Aggarwal BB. Oxidative stress, inflammation, and cancer: How are they linked? *Free Radic Biol Med.* 2010;49(11):1603-1616. 10.1016/j.freeradbiomed.2010.09.006
6. What is cancer staging? The American Joint Committee on Cancer. https://cancerstaging.org/references-tools/Pages/What-is-Cancer-Staging.aspx. Accessed November 4, 2017.
7. Nitenberg G, Raynard B. Nutritional support of the cancer patient: issues and dilemmas. *Crit Rev Oncol Hematol.* 2000;(34):137-168.
8. Hebuterne X, Lemarie E, Michallet M, et al. Prevalence of malnutrition and current use of nutrition support in patients with cancer. *J Parenter Enteral Nutr.* 2014;38(2):196-204. doi: 10.1177/0148607113502674.
9. Bauer JD, Capra S. Nutrition intervention improves outcomes in patients with cancer cachexia receiving chemotherapy: pilot study. *Support Care Cancer.* 2005;13:270-274. doi: 10.1007/s00520-004-0746-7
10. Dewys WD, Begg C Lavin PT, et al. Prognostic effect of weight loss prior to chemotherapy in cancer patients. *Am J Med.* 1980;69:491-497.
11. Academy of Nutrition and Dietetics Evidence Analysis Library. Oncology: Executive Summary of Recommendations (2013). https://www.andeal.org/topic.cfm?menu=5291&cat=5067. Accessed: October 10, 2015.
12. Kim JY, Wie G-A, Cho Y-A, et al. Development and validation of screening tool for adult hospitalized cancer patients. *Clin Nutr.* 2011;30:724-729. http://www.cancer.be/sites/default/files/1-article-original-Clinical-Nutrition-2011.pdf
13. Bauer J, Capra S, Ferguson M. Use of the scored patient-generated subjective global assessment (PG-SGA) as a nutrition assessment tool in patients with cancer. *Eur J Clin Nutr.* 2002;56(8):779-785.
14. Isenring E, Bauer J, Capra S. The scored patient-generated subjective global assessment (PG-SGA) and its association with quality of life in ambulatory patients receiving radiotherapy. *Eur J Clin Nutr.* 2003;57(2):305-309.
15. Shaw C, Fleuret C, Pickard M, et al. Comparison of Novel Screening Tools for Adult oncology Patients. *Support Care Cancer.* 2015;23:47-54. doi: 10.1007/s00520-041-2319-8.
16. Boléo-Tomé C, Monteiro-Grillo I, Camilo M, et al. Validation of the Malnutrition Universal Screening Tool (MUST) in cancer. *Br J Nutr.* 2012;108(2):343-348. doi: 10.1017/S000711451100571X. Epub 2011 Dec 6.
17. Chao P, Chuang H, Tsao L, et al. The Malnutrition Universal Screening Tool (MUST) and a nutrition education program for high risk cancer patients: strategies to improve dietary intake in cancer patients. *Biomedicine* (Taipei). 2015;5(3):17. doi: 10.7603/s40681-015-0017-6
18. Isenring EA, Bauer JD, Capra S. Nutrition support using the American Dietetic Association medical nutrition therapy protocol for radiation oncology patients improves dietary intake compared with standard practice. *J Am Diet Assoc.* 2007;107(3):404-412.
19. Mattox TW. Treatment of unintentional weight loss in patients with cancer. *Nutr Clin Prac.* 2005;20(4):400-410.
20. Arends J, Bodoky G, Bozzetti F, et al. ESPEN Guidelines on enteral nutrition: non-surgical oncology. *Clin Nutr.* 2006;25:245-259.
21. Fearon K C.H., Glass DJ, Guttridge DC. Cancer cachexia: mediators, signaling, and metabolic Pathways. *Cell Metab.* 2012;16(2)153-166.
22. Gullett NP, Mazurak V, Hebbar G, Ziegler TR. Nutritional interventions for cancer-induced cachexia. *Curr Probl Cancer.* 2011;35(2)58-90. doi: 10.1016/j.currproblcancer.2011.01.001.
23. Baracos VE. Regulation of skeletal muscle protein turnover in cancer associated cachexia *Nutrition.* 2000;16(10):1015-1018.
24. Tisdale M. J. Tisdale. Mechanisms of cancer cachexia. *Physio Rev.* 2009; 89(2):381-410.
25. McCreery E, ACostello J. Providing nutritional support for patients with cancer cachexia. *Int J Palliat Nurs.* 2013;19(1):32-37.
26. Donohue CL, Ryan AM, Reynolds JV. Cancer cachexia: mechanisms and clinical implications. *Gastroenterol Res Prac.* 2011:601434.
27. Matthews C M. Cancer cachexia: Athophysiology and approaches to management. *Support Line.* 2010;32(4):5-8.
28. Aapro M, Arends J, Bozzetti F, et al. Early recognition of malnutrition and cachexia in the cancer patient: a position paper of a European School of Oncology Task Force. *Ann Oncol.* 2014;25(8):1492-1499. doi: 10.1093/annonc/mdu085.
29. Loprinzi CL, Ellison NM, Schaid DJ, Krook JE, Athmann LM, Dose AM, et al. Controlled trial of megestrol acetate for the treatment of cancer anorexia and cachexia. *J Natl Cancer Inst.* 1998;82:1127-1132.
30. Loprinzi CL, Kugler JW, Sloan JA, et al. Randomized comparison of megestrol acetate versus dexamethasone versus fluoxymesterone for the treatment of cancer anorexia/cachexia. *J Clin Oncol.* 1999;17:32993306.

31. Jatoi A, Windschitl HE, Loprinzi CL, et al. Dronabinol versus megestrol acetate versus combination therapy for cancer associated anorexia: A North Central Cancer Treatment Group study. *J Clin Oncol.* 2002;20:567-573.

32. Loprinzi CL, Kugler JW, Sloan JA, et al. Randomized comparison of megestrol acetate versus dexamethasone versus fluoxymesterone for the treatment of cancer anorexia/cachexia. *J Clin Oncol.* 1999;17:3299-3306.

33. Moertel CG, Schutt AJ, Reitemeier RJ, Hahn RG. Corticosteroid therapy of preterminal gastrointestinal cancer. *Cancer.* 1974;33:1607-1609.

34. Willox JC, Corr J, Shaw J, et al. Prednisolone as an appetite stimulant in patients with cancer. *Br Med J (Clin Res Ed).* 1984;288:27.

35. Fearon KC, Von Meyenfeldt MF, Moses AG, et al. Effect of a protein and energy dense N–3 fatty acid enriched oral supplement on loss of weight and lean tissue in cancer cachexia: A randomised double blind trial. *Gut.* 2003;52:1479-1486.

36. Jatoi A, Rowland K, Loprinzi CL, et al. An eicosapentaenoic acid supplement versus megestrol acetate versus both for patients with cancer-associated wasting: A North Central Cancer Treatment Group and National Cancer Institute of Canada collaborative effort. *J Clin Oncol.* 2004;22:2469-2476.

37. Fearon KC, Barber MD, Moses AG, et al. Double-blind, placebo-controlled, randomized study of eicosapentaenoic acid diester in patients with cancer cachexia. *J Clin Oncol.* 2006;24:3401-3407.

38. Dewey A, Baughan C, Dean T, Higgins B, Johnson I. Eicosapentaenoic acid (EPA, an omega-3 fatty acid from fish oils) for the treatment of cancer cachexia. *Cochrane Database Syst Rev.* 2007:CD004597.

39. Laviano A, Muscaritoli M, Cascino A, et al. Branched-chain amino acids: The best compromise to achieve anabolism? *Curr Opin Clin Nutr Metab Care.* 2005;8:408-414.

40. Eley HL, Russell ST, Tisdale MJ. Effect of branched-chain amino acids on muscle atrophy in cancer cachexia. *Biochem J.* 2007;407:113-120

41. Kuhn KS, Muscaritoli M, Wischmeyer P, Stehle P. Glutamine as indispensable nutrient in oncology: experimental and clinical evidence. *Eur J Nutr.* 2010 Jun;49(4):197-210. doi: 10.1007/s00394-009-0082-2. Epub 2009 Nov 21. Review

42. National Cancer Institute. Surveillance, Epidemiology, and End Results Program. https://seer.cancer.gov/statfacts/. Accessed November 4, 2017.

43. Languis JA, Zandbergen MC, Eerenstein SE, et al. Effect of nutritional interventions on nutritional status, quality of life and mortality in patients with head and neck cancer receiving chemoradiotherapy: a systematic review. *Clin Nutr.* 2013(32):671-678.

44. Nugent B, Lewis S, O'Sullivan JM. Enteral feeding methods for nutritional management in patients with head and neck cancers being treated with radiotherapy and/or chemotherapy (review). *Cochrane Database Syst Rev.* 2013;CD007904.

45. Furness S, Glenny AM, Worthington HV, et al. Interventions for the treatment of oral cavity and oropharyngeal cancer: chemotherapy. *Cochrane Database Syst Rev.* 2010;CD006386.

46. Dechaphunkul T, Martin L, Alberda C, Olson K, Baracos V, Gramlich L. Malnutrition assessment in patients with cancers of the head and neck: A call to action and consensus. *Onc Hem.* 2013;88:459-476.

47. Corry J, Poon W, McPhee N, Milner AD, et al. Randomized study of percutaneous endoscopic gastrostomy versus nasogastric tubes for enteral feeding in head and neck cancer patients receiving chemoradiation. *J Med Imaging Radiat Oncol.* 2008;52:503-510.

48. Rubenstein JH, Shaheen NJ, Epidemiology, diagnosis, and management of esophageal adenocarcinoma. *Gastroenterology.* 2015;149:302-317.

49. Ukleja A. Dumping syndrome: pathophysiology and treatment. *Nutr Clin Pract.* 2005;20(5):517-525.

50. Gupta V. Benefits versus risks: a prospective audit. Feeding jejunostomy during esophagectomy. *World J Surg.* 2009;33:1432-1438.

51. Ryan AM, Rowley SP, Healy LA, et al. Post-oesophagectomy early enteral nutrition via a needle catheter jejunostomy: 8-year experience at a spleacialist unit. *Clin Nutr.* 2006;25:386-393.

52. Dann GC, Squires MH, Postlewait LM, et al. An assessment of feeding jejunostomy tube placement at the time of resection for gastric adenocarcinoma: a seven-institution analysis of 837 patients from the U.S. gastric cancer collaborative. *J Surg Onc.* 2015;112:195-202.

53. Allum WH, Blazeby JM, Griffin M, Cunningham D, Jankowski JA, Wong R. Guidelines for the management of oesophageal and gastric cancer. *Gut.* 2011;60:1449-1472.

54. Brolin RE, Gorman RC, Milgrim LM, Kenler HA. Multivitamin prophylaxis in prevention of post-gastric bypass vitamin and mineral deficiencies. *Int J Obes.* 1991;15(10):661-667.

55. Siegel RL, Miller DK, Jemal A. Cancer statistics, 2016. *Can J Clin.* 2016;66-7.

56. Hauer-Jensen M, Wang J, Denham J. Bowel injury: current and evolving management strategies. *Semin Radiat Oncol.* 2013;13:357-371.

57. Andreyev HJ. Gastrointestinal problems after pelvic radiotherapy: the past, the present and the future. *Clin Oncol.* 2007;19:790-799.

58. Wall EA. An overview of short bowel syndrome management: adherence, adaptation, and practical recommendations. *J Acad Nutr Diet.* 2013;113:1200-1208.

59. Joly F, Dray X, Corcos O, et al. Tube feeding improves intestinal absorption in short bowel syndrome patients. *Gastroenterology.* 2009;136:824.

60. Berry AJ. Pancreatic surgery: indications, complications, and implications for nutrition intervention. *Nut Clin Prac.* 2013;28:330-357.

61. Afaneh C, Gerszber D, Slatter E, Seres DS, Chabot JA, Kluger MD. Pancreatic cancer surgery and nutrition management: a review of the current literature. *HepatoBiliary Surg Nutr.* 2015;4(1):59-71.

62. Gift A, Stommel M, Jablonski A, Given W. A cluster of symptoms over time in patients with lung cancer. *Nurs Res.* 2003;52:393-400.

63. Jagoe RT, Goodship THJ, Gibson GJ. The influence of nutritional status on complications after operations for lung cancer. *Ann Thorac Surg.* 2001;71:936-943.

64. Kiss NKK, Krishnasamy M, Isenring EA. The effect of nutrition intervention in lung cancer patients undergoing chemotherapy and/or radiotherapy: a systematic review. *Nutr Canc.* 2014;66(1):45-56.

65. Buhl ND, Seguy D. Nutritional support in adult patients undergoing allogeneic stem cell transplantation following myeloablative conditioning. In: Rajendram, Rajkumar, Preedy, Victor R., Patel, Vinood (Eds.). *Diet and Nutrition in Critical Care.* New York, NY: Springer Science+Business Media; 2015:593-605. doi: 10.1007/978-1-4614-7836-2.

66. Lemal R, Cabrespine A, Pereira B, et al. Could enteral nutrition improve the outcome of patients with haematological malignancies undergoing allogeneic haematopoietic stem cell transplantation? A study protocol for a randomized controlled trial (the NEPHA study). *Trials.* 2015;16(136):1-9. doi: 10.1186/s13063-015-0663-8.

67. Zatarain L, Savani BN. The role of nutrition and effects on the cytokine milieu in allogeneic hematopoietic stem cell transplantation. *Cell Immunol.* 2012;276:6-9. doi: 10.1016/j.cellimm.2012.05.003.

68. Andersen S, Brown T, Kennedy G, Banks M. Implementation of an evidenced based nutrition support pathway for haematopoietic progenitor cell transplant patients. *Clin Nutr.* 2015;34:536-540. doi: 10.1016/j.clnu.2014.06.006.

69. August DA, Huhmann MB, American Society of Parenteral and Enteral Nutrition Board of Directors. A.S.P.E.N. clinical guidelines: nutrition support therapy during adult anticancer treatment and in hematopoietic cell transplantation. *JPEN J Parenter Enteral Nutr.* 2009;33(5):472-500. doi: 10.1177/0148607109341804.

70. Jaime-Pérez JC, Colunga-Pedraza PR, Gutiérrez-Gurrola B, et al. Obesity is associated with higher overall survival in patients undergoing an outpatient reduced-intensity conditioning hematopoietic stem cell transplant. *Blood Cells Mol Dis.* 2013;51:61-65. doi: 10.1016/j.bcmd.2013.01.010.

71. Martin-Salces M, de Paz R, Canales MA, Mesejo A, Hernandez-Navarro F. Nutritional recommendations in hematopoietic stem cell transplantation. *Nutrition.* 2008;24:769-775. doi: 10.1016/j.nut.2008.02.021.

72. Muscaritoli M, Conversano L, Torelli GF, et al. Clinical and metabolic effects of different parenteral nutrition regimens in patients undergoing allogeneic bone marrow transplantation. *Transplantation.* 1998;66(5):610-616. ht

73. Wilson S, Kohli-Seth R, Aldeguer Y, et al. Parenteral nutrition utilization in bone marrow transplant recipients. *J Nutr Heal Sci.* 2014;1(1):1-4. doi: 10.15744/2393-9060.1.102.

74. Weisdorf S, Lysne J, Wind D, et al. Positive effect of prophylactic total parenteral nutrition on long-term outcome of bone marrow transplantation. *Transplantation.* 1987;43(6):276-279.

75. Guieze R, Lemal R, Cabrespine A, et al. Enteral versus parenteral nutritional support in allogeneic haematopoietic stem-cell transplantation. *Clin Nutr.* 2014;33:533-538. doi: 10.1016/j.clnu.2013.07.012.

76. Williams-Hooker R, Adams M, Havrilla D, Leung W, Roach R, Mosby T. Caregiver and health care provider preferences of nutritional support in a hematopoietic stem cell transplant unit. *Pediatr Blood Cancer.* 2015;62:1473-1476. doi: 10.1002/pbc.

77. Iestra JA, Fibbe WE, Zwinderman AH, van Staveren WA, Kromhout D. Body weight recovery, eating difficulties and compliance with dietary advice in the first year after stem cell transplantation: a prospective study. *Bone Marrow Transplant.* 2002;29(5):417-424. doi: 10.1038/sj.bmt.1703375.

78. Roberts S, Thompson J. Clinical observations graft-vs-host disease: nutrition therapy in a challenging condition. *Nutr Clin Pract.* 2005;20:440-450.

79. Zauner C, Rabitsch W, Schneeweiss B, et al. Energy and substrate metabolism in patients with chronic extensive graft-versus-host disease. *Transplantation.* 2001;71:524-528.

80. Jacobsohn D, Margolis J, Doherty J, Anders V, Vogelsang G. Weight loss and malnutrition in patients with chronic graft-versus-host disease. *Bone Marrow Transplant.* 2002;29:231-236.

81. Akpek G, Chinratanalab W, Lee LA, et al. Gastrointestinal involvement in chronic graft-versus-host disease: A clinicopathologic study. *Biol Blood Marrow Transplant.* 2003;9(1):46-51. doi: 10.1053/bbmt.2003.49999.

82. Schulte CMS, Beelen DW. Bone loss following hematopoietic stem cell transplantation : a long-term follow-up. *Blood.* 2004;103(10): 3635-3643. doi: 10.1182/blood-2003-09-3081.An.

83. Szeluga DJ, Stuart RK, Brookmeyer R, Szeluga DJ, Utermohlen V, Santos GW. Nutritional support of bone marrow transplant recipients: a prospective, randomized clinical trial comparing total parenteral nutrition to an enteral feeding program nutritional support of bone marrow transplant recipients. *Cancer Res.* 1987;47:3309-3316.

84. Oudemans-van Straaten HM, Bosman RJ, Treskes M, Van der Spoel HJI, Zandstra DF. Plasma glutamine depletion and patient outcome in acute ICU admissions. *Intensive Care Med.* 2001;27(1):84-90. doi: 10.1007/s001340000703.

85. Pytlík R, Benes P, Patorková M, et al. Standardized parenteral alanyl-glutamine dipeptide supplementation is not beneficial in autologous transplant patients: a randomized, double-blind, placebo controlled study. *Bone Marrow Transplant.* 2002;30(12):953-961. doi: 10.1038/sj.bmt.1703759.

86. Zeigler T, Young L, Benfell K, et al. Clinical and metabolic efficacy of glutamine supplemented parenteral nutrition after bone marrow transplantation. *Ann Intern Med.* 1992;116:821-828.

87. van Dalen EC, Mank A, Leclercq E, et al. Low bacterial diet versus control diet to prevent infection in cancer patients treated with chemotherapy causing episodes of neutropenia. *Cochrane Database Syst Rev.* 2012;(9):CD006247. doi: 10.1002/14651858.CD006247.pub2.

88. Lassiter M, Schneider SM. A pilot study comparing the neutropenic diet to a non-neutropenic diet in the allogeneic hematopoietic stem cell transplantation population. *Clin J Oncol Nurs.* 2015;19(3):273-278. doi:10.1188/15.CJON.19-03AP.

89. Laird K. New and emerging bacterial food pathogens. In Ricke SC, Donaldson JR, Phillips C, eds. *Food Safety.* Academic Press, Amsterdam; 2015: 309-316. doi: 10.1016/B978-0-12-800245-2.00014-9.

90. Easson AM, Hinshaw DB, Johnson DL. The role of tube feeding and total parenteral nutrition in advanced illness. *J Am Coll Surg.* 2002;194(2):225-229. doi: 10.1016/S1072-7515(01)01154-1.

91. A.S.P.E.N. Board of Directors and the Clinical Guidelines Task Force. Guidelines for the Use of Parenteral and Enteral Nutrition in Adult and Pediatric Patients. Section I : Introduction. *JPEN J Parenter Enteral Nutr.* 2001;26(1):1SA-138 SA.

92. Nitenberg G, Raynard B. Nutritional support of the cancer patient: issues and dilemmas. *Crit Rev Oncol Hematol.* 2000;34(3):137-168. doi: 10.1016/S1040-8428(00)00048-2.

93. Care H. Bridging the Continuum: nutrition support in palliative and hospice care medical ethics: should vs could. *Curr Oncol.* 2006:134-141.

94. Klein S, Koretz RL. Nutrition support in patients with cancer: What do the data really show? *Nutr Clin Pract.* 1994;9(3):91-100.

95. Mirhosseini N, Fainsinger RL, Baracos V. Parenteral nutrition in advanced cancer: Indications and clinical practice guidelines. *J Palliat Care.* 2005;8(5):914-918.

96. Gavrin JR. Ethical considerations at the end of life in the intensive care unit. *Crit Care Med.* 2007;35(2 Suppl):S85-S94.

97. Barnes PM, Bloom B, Nahin RL. Complementary and alternative medicine use among adults and children: United States, 2007. *Natl Health Stat Report.* 2009;12:1-23.

98. Gansler T, Kaw C, Crammer C, et al. A population-based study of prevalence of complementary methods use by cancer survivors: a report from the American Cancer Society's studies of cancer survivors. *Cancer.* 2008;113(5):1048-1057.

Chapter 20

Nutrition in HIV/AIDS

June N. Pierre-Louis

Chapter Outline

Core Concepts
Introduction
HIV Infection
Epidemiology
Medical Management
Food Insecurity

Pathophysiology and Alterations in Physical State
Gastrointestinal Function, Inflammation, and Micronutrient Deficiencies
Breastfeeding
Nutritional Management

CORE CONCEPTS

1. The CD4 cell count is a marker of immune function and disease progression.
2. Viral load is a marker of infection status and treatment efficacy. When antiretroviral drug treatment adherence is good, viral load is undetectable/suppressed in most cases.
3. Food security is correlated with HIV care, treatment adherence, and viral suppression.
4. Energy requirements are increased in untreated and treated HIV infection.
5. Preservation of lean body mass should be the main focus of metabolic support during unintentional weight loss in HIV infection. HIV wasting is characterized by advanced loss of body fat and lean body mass.
6. HIV-associated lipodystrophy is a syndrome that includes body fat redistribution, visceral fat deposition, blood lipid abnormalities, and insulin resistance.
7. Bone mineral density is significantly lower in people living with HIV infection.
8. In countries where infant formula feeding is universally affordable, feasible, acceptable, safe, and sustainable, postpartum women living with HIV are advised to avoid all breastfeeding.
9. Opportunistic infections occur when the CD4 count falls below 200 cells/mm^3.
10. HIV infection is a life-long chronic disease for which self-management is key.

SECTION 2 NUTRITION IN DISEASE STATES

Learning Objectives

1. Describe the etiology and epidemiology of HIV infection.
2. Identify the classes of HIV antiretroviral drugs and potential nutritional side effects of specific HIV medications.
3. Assess major nutritional problems and formulate nutrition recommendations for individuals with HIV infection.
4. State the benefits and risks of breastfeeding by women living with HIV who are adherent to antiretroviral drug treatment.
5. Identify the impact of food insecurity on the health and nutritional status of people living with HIV.

Introduction

Metabolic alterations in human immunodeficiency virus (HIV) infection include wasting, unintentional weight loss, lipodystrophy, and bone loss. Medical nutrition therapy is an important component of the management of the acute and chronic nutritional issues in HIV infection. Knowledge of the metabolic alterations and the body composition and shape changes that occur in HIV infection and HIV disease progression is vital in the treatment of this condition.

HIV Infection

Human immunodeficiency virus (HIV) is the virus that causes HIV infection and **acquired immune deficiency syndrome (AIDS)**. The first cases of HIV infection were recognized in 1981, and the virus was identified in 1983.[1] AIDS is diagnosed when HIV infection has progressed to the point that the T lymphocyte CD4 cell count falls below 200 cells/mm^3 and/or one or more of the following AIDS-defining conditions is present: wasting syndrome; dementia; certain types of cancers (Kaposi's sarcoma, invasive cervical cancer); and certain types infections caused by viruses (cytomegalovirus), fungi (*Candida*, *Pneumocystis*), or bacteria (tuberculosis).[2] Once a patient has been diagnosed with AIDS, this diagnosis never changes. While AIDS was universal early in the HIV epidemic, its incidence and the mortality rate have declined dramatically since new classes of antiretroviral drugs became available in 1995. **Figure 20.1** depicts the AIDS memorial quilt which is celebrates the lives of people who have died of AIDS related causes.[1]

The HIV virus infects the CD4 T lymphocyte. The CD4 T-cell test, simply called the CD4 count, is a blood test that measures the number of T lymphocyte CD4 cells,

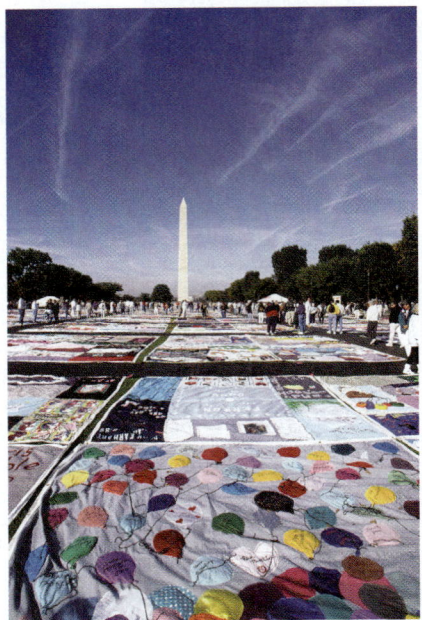

FIGURE 20.1 AIDS Memorial Quilt, Washington, DC
© Hisham Ibrahim/Getty Images.

which is one type of immune cell, in the blood (**Table 20.1**). The **CD4 cell count** is a marker of immune function that establishes the risk of developing infections, determines the need for prophylaxis against opportunistic infections, and determines the need for and response to antiretroviral therapy. **Opportunistic infections** are secondary infections, such as thrush, that are typical of HIV infection and occur when the CD4 count falls below 200 cells/mm^3. As the CD4 count decreases, one's risk of developing secondary opportunistic infections increases.

> **CORE CONCEPT 1**
>
> The CD4 cell count is a marker of immune function and disease progression.

Viral load refers to the amount of virus in the blood. Determination of the viral load provides a baseline to measure and monitor response to therapy and is used to assess prognosis. It is also an indicator of treatment adherence. Viral suppression is generally considered to be successful when viral load is <50 copies/mL. Low level viremia is <200 copies/mL.

> **CORE CONCEPT 2**
>
> Viral load is a marker of infection status and treatment effectiveness. When antiretroviral drug treatment adherence is good, viral load is undetectable/suppressed in most cases.

TABLE 20.1 CD4 T-CELL LYMPHOCYTE SUBSET TEST

	Normal range	Unit measure
Total CD4 T-cells	590 to 1120	Cells per mm^3
CD4 T-cell percentage	28 to 58	Percentage of total number of lymphocytes

> ## CASE STUDY INTRODUCTION
>
> Case #23 is a 55-year-old male living with HIV who discloses his HIV status only to his HIV providers and partners. His identity is protected by state HIV confidentiality laws. He was seen by a dietitian at a congregate meal and food pantry program for people living with HIV. The following information was obtained by the dietitian.
>
> **Anthropometric Data:**
> Weight: 82 kg (180 lbs)
> Height: 178 cm (60")
> BMI: 26 kg/m^2
> Mid-upper arm circumference: 24 cm (<5th percentile)
> Waist circumference: 88 cm (5th-95th percentile)
> *Weight History*
> Stable weight for the past 6 months
>
> **Biochemical Data:**
> Glucose: 153 (70-99 mg/dL)
> Total cholesterol: 220 (Desirable: <200 mg/dL)
> Triglycerides: 175 (Desirable: <150mg/dL)
> CD4 count: 600 (590-1120 cells/mm^3)
> Viral load: 100 (<50 copies/mL)
>
> **Clinical Data:**
> **Past Medical History:** HIV diagnosis 11 years ago, type 2 diabetes
> Last HIV primary care visit was 3 months ago.
> **Medications:** Patient reports he is on medications for HIV but unable to state which medications.
> **Nutrition-focused Physical Exam:** The patient presents with notable facial muscle wasting and thin extremities. Appears well hydrated. Poor dentition noted with missing teeth. No wounds or skin breakdown evident.
>
> **Dietary Data:**
> **Dietary History:** The patient has been going to a weekly community congregate meal and food pantry nutrition program, receiving take-home pantry bags for the past 6 months. He does not follow a special diet because his food choices are limited, in part to what he is provided in the congregate meal and food pantry program. He consumes 3 to 4 meals daily and will have a bedtime snack if food is available.
>
> **Questions**
> 1. How would you describe the patient's nutritional status?
> 2. Describe his nutritional risk factors.
> 3. What are his short-term and long-term nutrition goals?

Epidemiology

HIV infection is transmitted through anal, vaginal, and oral intercourse; sharing intravenous needles; occupational or medical exposure to infected blood; and from mother to infant during labor, delivery, pregnancy, and breastfeeding. There are 1.1 million people in the United States who are living with HIV.[3] In 2010, about 56,000 people in the United States were newly infected with HIV. The state of New York has the largest number of HIV cases in the United States. Globally, in 2016, there were an estimated 36.7 million people living with HIV; more than half of HIV-positive individuals live in southern and eastern Africa.[4] An estimated 3.2 million children under the age of 15 were living with HIV in 2015[5].

Ryan White, a hemophiliac boy who received a contaminated blood transfusion and was diagnosed in 1984, advocated for humane and fair treatment of persons living with HIV and AIDS (**Figure 20.2**). The Ryan White Care Act, first enacted in 1990, is named for him. He died in 1990 at the age of 18 before most antiretroviral drugs became available.

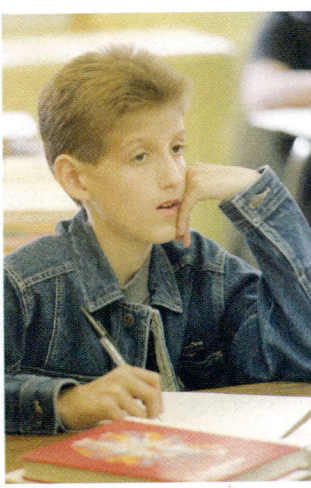

FIGURE 20.2 Ryan White
© Bettmann / Contributor/Getty Images.

The African American, Latino, homosexual, and bisexual male communities in the United States, all medically underserved populations, have higher rates of HIV infection. Women, mainly African American women, make up a quarter of all HIV infections in the United States, while globally, women account for about half of the people living with HIV.[3,6] With fewer complications and increased survival, people living with HIV are living longer.[7] People aged 50 years and older living with HIV represent about one-quarter of all cases in the United States, and this percentage is increasing.

Medical Management

Antiretroviral Treatment

Azidothymidine, or AZT, the first effective drug against HIV infection, became available for use in 1987. HIV quickly developed resistance to AZT because of the virus's propensity to replicate and mutate rapidly, making any single drug unlikely to hold it in check.[1] Beginning in 1995, new classes of antiretroviral drugs became available for use.[1] The new drugs, used in combination, were initially called highly active antiretroviral therapy and are now simply called antiretroviral therapy or treatment. **Antiretroviral treatment (ART)** refers to the use of pharmacologic agents that have specific inhibitory effects on HIV replication. Antiretroviral treatment is effective in keeping viral loads of HIV in the blood at low or undetectable levels in the majority of cases, and in maintaining or improving CD4 counts. The CD4 cell count and viral load are used as markers of immune function/disease progression and infection status, respectively. Clinical guidelines are to treat patients with three drugs at the same time.[8] Antiretroviral treatment is life long because of the ability of HIV to hide within cells in the body.[1]

HIV drugs are classified depending on how they work to inhibit HIV replication. The main drug classes are nucleoside and nucleotide reverse transcriptase inhibitors (NRTIs), nonnucleoside reverse transcriptase inhibitors (NNRTIs), protease inhibitors (PIs), and fusion inhibitors. Classes of HIV drugs and specific HIV drugs within a class may have nutrition-related side effects for individuals, which affect treatment adherence and metabolism. Treatment adherence, or taking medications on time and not missing doses, greatly affects the effectiveness of antiretroviral treatment and the development of drug resistance. Examples of NRTI drugs are AZT and tenofovir; efavirenz is an NNRTI; and lopinavir is a PI. Two or three HIV medications combined into one tablet are available.

Historically, clinical guidelines allowed for delay of initiation of treatment until CD4 counts were below the threshold of 350 to 500 cells/mm^3. Guidelines now recommend initiation of antiretroviral treatment regardless of CD4 count in all cases of HIV infection based on evidence that all patients benefit from antiretroviral treatment and the transmission risk is reduced among individuals on antiretroviral treatment.[9] Certain conditions increase the urgency of initiation of antiretroviral treatment in patients, including an AIDS diagnosis, two successive CD4 counts below 500, hepatitis B infection, hepatitis C infection, and age of 50 years or older.[8]

Linkage to and retention in HIV care is of great importance to HIV outcomes, contributing to higher CD4 count, suppressed viral load, fewer hospital and emergency room visits, and reduced transmission of HIV. Retention in care may be defined as at least two CD4 counts/viral loads reported in the last calendar year. Viral suppression significantly reduces transmission from the infected person to HIV-negative partners.[9] The cascade of HIV care shown in **Figure 20.3**, depicts the declining percentages of the HIV-infected population who are diagnosed and know their HIV status, linked to HIV care, engaged/retained in HIV care, and virally suppressed. The majority of HIV-infected individuals in the United States are not retained in care and are not virally suppressed.[6]

Food Insecurity

Food insecurity is anxiety and uncertainty about one's food supply, along with insufficient food intake with or without physical hunger. Food insecurity is higher among people living with HIV than in the general population.[10,11] Among people living with HIV, food insecurity has been shown to be higher among women and individuals who have less education, a history of substance use, or unstable housing. In the New York City metropolitan area, 80% of a representative sample of people living with HIV participated in the Supplemental Nutrition Assistance Program and more than half received some form of additional food assistance, such as pantry bags, congregate meals, home-delivered meals, and/or food vouchers (**Figure 20.4**) during the period 2008-2010. Forty percent of the sample did not have enough money for food and went at least one day without anything to eat in the previous 30 days.[12]

People living with HIV who are food insecure miss more HIV primary care appointments, make more

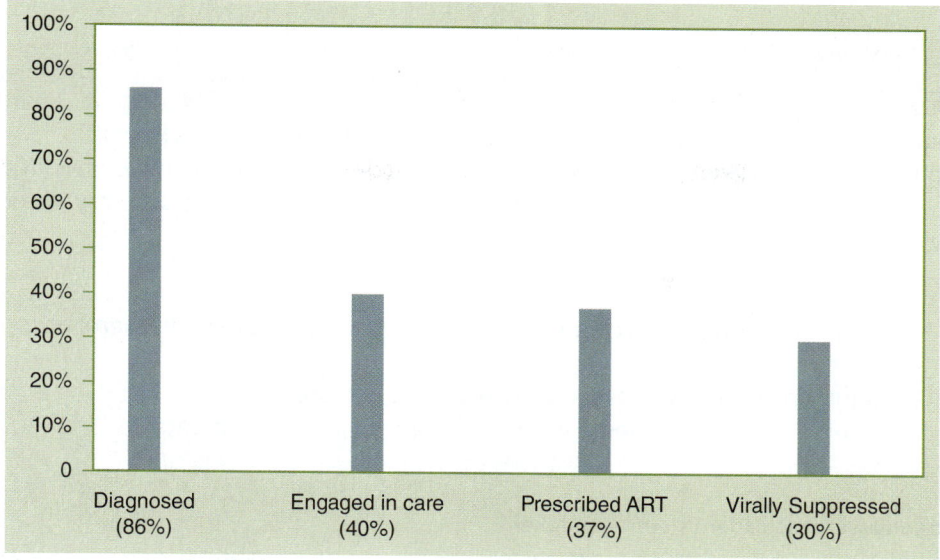

FIGURE 20.3 HIV Care Cascade in the United States, 2011
Centers for Disease Control and Prevention (CDC). Vital Signs: HIV Diagnosis, Care, and Treatment Among Persons Living with HIV—United States, 2011. (2014, November 28). Retrieved from https://www.cdc.gov/mmwr/preview/mmwrhtml/mm6347a5.htm.

emergency room visits, and are less likely to be retained in HIV care.[12-15] Food insecurity is associated with depression, substance use, incomplete viral suppression, and a higher probability of disease progression and AIDS-defining illness (**Figure 20.5**).[12]

> **CORE CONCEPT 3**
>
> Food insecurity is associated with linkage to and retention in HIV care, treatment adherence, and viral suppression.

Primary Care

The major cause of death for people living with HIV today is not HIV infection; the major causes are liver disease, cardiovascular disease, cancer, and renal disease, which are all nevertheless related to HIV infection.[16] **Chronic inflammation**, an immune response of the body to ongoing HIV infection, is believed to cause premature aging and contribute to the risk for these diseases, which increases over time. Because HIV infection is no longer the sole or a direct cause of death or morbidity in most HIV cases, primary care and treatment of metabolic comorbidities including cardiovascular disease, hepatitis C, diabetes, hyperlipidemia, and osteoporosis is the new HIV treatment focus. Increasingly, treatment of HIV infection benefits the course of non-AIDS diseases, such as cardiovascular disease and bone disease.[17]

At the same time, with fewer complications and increased survival, people living with HIV are increasingly developing prevalent health problems affecting the general population, such as hyperlipidemia, obesity/overweight, hypertension, and diabetes. Substance use, such as tobacco use, alcohol use, and illicit drug use, also contributes to higher rates of comorbidities in HIV patients.[18]

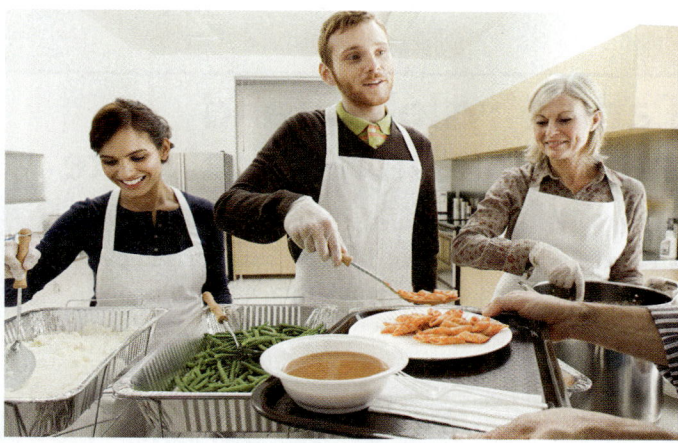

FIGURE 20.4 Food Pantries and Congregate Meal Programs Provide Food Assistance for Food-insecure Individuals
© Image Source/Getty Images.

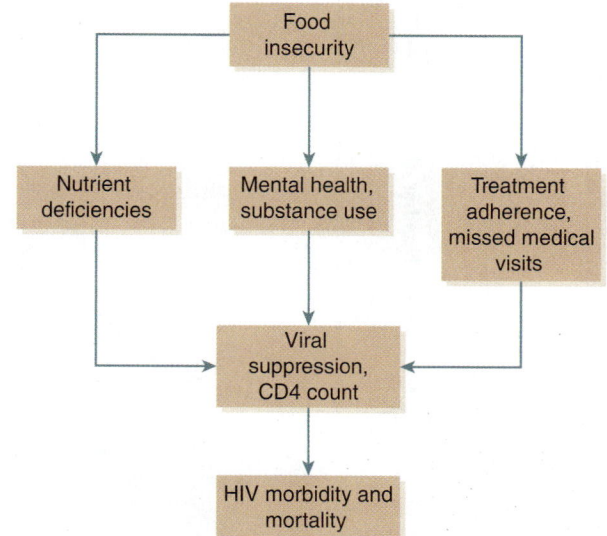

FIGURE 20.5 Conceptual Framework of Relationships Between Food Insecurity and HIV Infection

CASE STUDY REVISITED

You ask the patient about his appetite and intake. He reports that he sometimes has difficulty chewing tough foods and purposely chooses soft foods at the food pantry. He denies any difficulty swallowing. He reports that he has been feeling more fatigued lately and has less energy to complete his daily activities.

24-hr Diet Recall:
8 am   Breakfast: 8 oz instant coffee with cream and sugar, 1 packaged muffin (blueberry or corn), 1 pat butter
12 pm Lunch: 2 peanut butter sandwiches on white bread, 12 oz water
5 pm Dinner: 1 bowl of macaroni and cheese (prepared from package), 12 oz water

Questions

1. How would you assess the patient's current intake?
2. Considering his current laboratory values, what dietary suggestions do you have for him to address his short-term nutrition concerns?
3. What might you suggest to address his long-term nutrition risk?

Pathophysiology and Alterations in Physical State

Energy and Protein Metabolism

HIV infection is a chronic disease characterized by immune dysfunction, inflammation, and acute infections. Studies have consistently shown that resting energy expenditure (REE), largely determined by lean body mass, is about 10% higher in HIV-infected persons compared to uninfected controls.[19,20] While REE is increased by about 10% in both untreated and treated asymptomatic HIV infections, REE may be increased by 20% to 30% in symptomatic HIV infections.[19] Most people with HIV infection in the United States appear to maintain their weight by increasing energy intake or decreasing physical activity.[21]

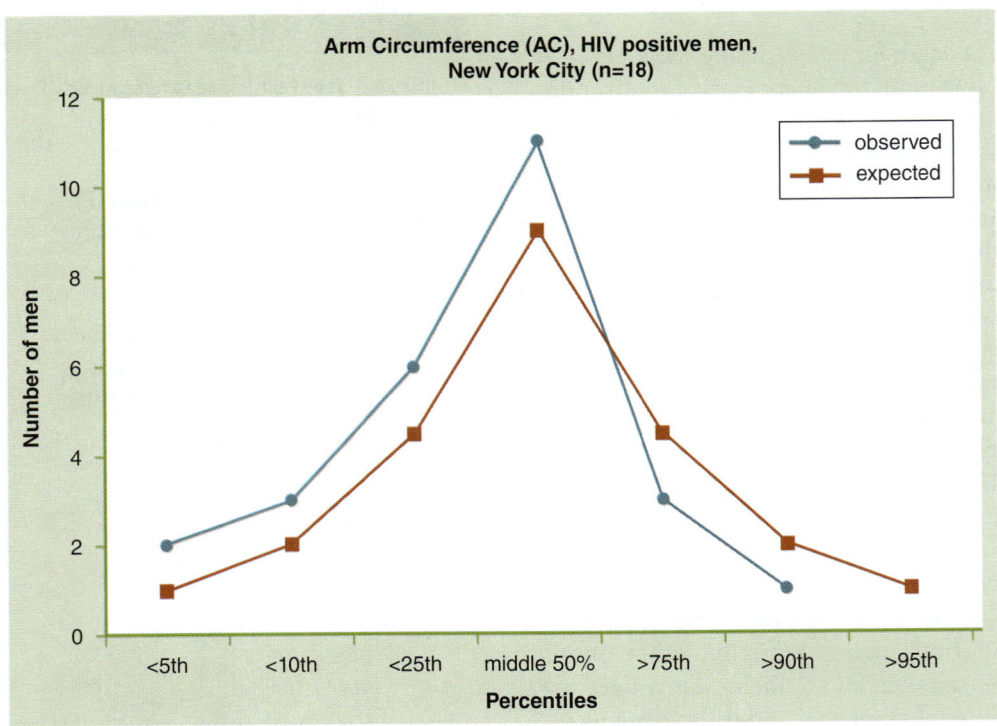

FIGURE 20.6 Upper Arm Circumference Adjusted for Age and Ethnicity of HIV-positive Males Enrolled in a Congregate Meal Program Showing Distribution Shift Left (Downward) Compared to the Normal Distribution

> **CORE CONCEPT 4**
>
> Energy expenditure is increased in untreated and treated HIV infection.

HIV wasting syndrome is an AIDS-defining condition and is diagnosed when there is weight loss of at least 10% of body weight, with symptoms of chronic fever, weakness, or diarrhea in the absence of other related illnesses that could contribute to the weight loss. HIV wasting syndrome was one of the most prevalent AIDS-defining conditions before the advent of antiretroviral drug treatment. It has been greatly reduced by antiretroviral treatment, but still exists in cases of nonadherence to treatment, medication resistance, and end-of-life situations.[7,22] HIV-associated unintentional weight loss is still prevalent; it occurs in untreated persons, patients on antiretroviral treatment, and in cases where there is no secondary infection.[11] In a prospective study of 633 individuals with HIV infection, the prevalence of weight loss was 38%.[11] In a prospective study of HIV clients receiving home-delivered meals in New York City, 50% of clients had weight loss at intake.[23] Preservation of lean body mass should be the main focus of metabolic support during unintentional weight loss in HIV infection.

HIV wasting is characterized by the advanced loss of body fat and lean body mass and is due to metabolic derangement and/or other causes of weight loss. Cachexia is the most severe form of wasting, with loss of fat and muscle mass.[9] Loss of lean body mass is associated with increased risk of mortality. In a study of HIV patients with CD4 counts <200 cells/mm^3 and opportunistic infections, such as pneumonia, oral thrush, or pulmonary tuberculosis, weight changes at 1 month after initiation of ART were significantly associated with mortality and varied by baseline BMI.[24] Being overweight, with a BMI greater than 25, at HIV diagnosis has been shown to be protective against weight loss and mortality in HIV infection, but not when fat-free mass is depleted.[11,25] Total daily energy expenditure, including REE, diet-induced thermogenesis, and physical activity, may be decreased in HIV wasting and as a result of secondary infections because physical activity levels decrease during wasting and illness.[21]

There is no clear evidence to support increased protein intake in HIV infection.[19] In a study of protein supplementation of HIV patients with a history of weight loss, a whey protein supplement did not increase lean body mass and weight compared to controls, but did increase CD4 counts.[26] Study subjects receiving the protein supplement experienced more gastrointestinal (GI) symptoms.

Lipid Metabolism

While the benefits of antiretroviral treatment outweigh the long-term health risks, long-term exposure to antiretroviral drugs can lead to major metabolic complications, including cardiovascular disease and serum lipid abnormalities, altered glucose metabolism and insulin resistance, and bone loss.[19] HIV-associated **lipodystrophy** is a syndrome that includes body fat redistribution and/or metabolic abnormalities.[27] It occurs to some extent in the majority of individuals on antiretroviral treatment.[28] Energy requirements are increased in lipodystrophy due to the body's inability to store triacylglycerol in a normal manner.[11,21,29]

Body fat redistribution involves subcutaneous fat loss (atrophy) at peripheral body sites (arms, legs, face, and buttocks) and/or fat deposition at central body sites (trunk/abdomen, upper back, and breasts of both men and women).[30,31] Fat loss and fat deposition may occur together or separately. Abdominal fat deposition associated with HIV infection is an abnormal accumulation of visceral adipose tissue surrounding the abdominal organs; it differs from obesity, in which adipose tissue is subcutaneous. Low baseline CD4 counts, high viral loads, and low energy intakes predict extremity fat loss in men.[30] Predictive factors for trunk fat gain are increased baseline body fat and high BMI.

Metabolic abnormalities include elevated triglyceride, total cholesterol, and low-density lipoprotein (LDL) levels; decreased high-density lipoprotein (HDL) levels; and/or insulin resistance.[18,31] These may or may not occur at the same time as body fat redistribution. Hypertriglyceridemia is hypothesized to result from the recycling of peripheral free fatty acids and re-esterification of triglycerides instead of oxidation in the liver. Fat deposition in the viscera of the abdomen in lipodystrophy is linked to altered energy metabolism, including impaired glucose tolerance and insulin resistance.

Men with long-term HIV infections are more likely than uninfected men to develop plaque in their coronary arteries, controlling for high cholesterol, smoking, and high blood pressure. Coronary stenosis is also associated with more advanced HIV and longer antiretroviral treatment.[32] The HIV infection itself may contribute to the development of noncalcified lesions, which are more prone to rupture.[32] Immune dysfunction and related inflammation is the postulated mechanism by which HIV infection increases the risk of cardiovascular disease. Cardiovascular risk is lower for patients on antiretroviral treatment and virally suppressed groups compared to untreated persons. Early antiretroviral treatment is least likely to produce the lipid abnormalities that increase cardiovascular risk.

> **CORE CONCEPT 5**
>
> Preservation of lean body mass should be the main focus of metabolic support during unintentional weight loss in HIV infection.

> **CORE CONCEPT 6**
>
> HIV-associated lipodystrophy is a syndrome that includes body fat redistribution, visceral fat deposition, blood lipid abnormalities, and insulin resistance.

Changes in ART may be effective in reducing body fat redistribution and/or lipid levels. Body fat redistribution secondary to HIV infection was first described in 1998 after antiretroviral medications, in particular protease inhibitors, were first used, but discontinuation of protease inhibitors has not been consistently observed to result in reversal or improvement of fat redistribution in patients. Some nucleoside and nucleotide reverse transcriptase inhibitor drugs have also been associated with fat loss.

Body fat distribution in perinatally HIV-infected children follows a pattern associated with cardiovascular disease risk.[33] Specifically, perinatally infected children tend to have greater trunk fat, lower extremity fat, and lower body fat compared to uninfected children. Analysis of the growth and body fat distribution of children in the Pediatric HIV/AIDS Cohort Study shows that HIV-infected children have lower mean heights, BMI z-scores, and percentages of total body fat and extremity fat, and higher mean percentages of trunk fat and trunk-to-extremity fat ratios.

Bone Loss

HIV infection has a direct effect on bone mineral density and accelerates the normal bone turnover that occurs with age. HIV patients have lower bone mineral density than uninfected controls and bone loss is seen disproportionately among untreated persons with HIV infection as well as patients receiving HIV medications.[17,34] Bone loss is associated with duration of HIV infection. HIV patients are at higher risk of hip and spine fractures compared to controls; bone fractures occur at a higher rate in both men and women.[17]

> **CORE CONCEPT 7**
>
> Bone mineral density is significantly lower in people living with HIV infection.

Gastrointestinal Function, Inflammation, and Micronutrient Deficiencies

An estimated 75% of the body's CD4 T cells are located in the gut and function to prevent pathogens from entering the bloodstream. HIV infection is characterized by chronic inflammation and immune activation. Immune activation is postulated to occur as a result of the destruction of the CD4 T cells in the gut, allowing intestinal bacteria to leak into the bloodstream and leading to an overstimulated and overworked immune system. Chronic inflammation in HIV infection is hypothesized to produce mitochondrial toxicity and oxidative stress.

Micronutrient deficiencies frequently occur in untreated HIV infection and are associated with low CD4 counts and disease progression.[19,35] Deficiencies of thiamin; riboflavin; vitamins B_6, B_{12}, A, C, D, and E; selenium; iron; and zinc have been reported.[17,18,35] Concentrations of selenium, an antioxidant that plays a key role in immunity, are low in untreated HIV infections and decline as HIV infection progresses.[36] Some micronutrient concentrations, such as selenium, iron, carotene, tocopherol, vitamin B_{12}, and folate, become replete after initiation of antiretroviral treatment.

Breastfeeding

Antiretroviral treatment is recommended for all pregnant and breastfeeding women to prevent maternal-to-child transmission of HIV infection during pregnancy, delivery, and the breastfeeding period. Globally, most mother-to-child-transmission now occurs during the breastfeeding period, when retention in care and treatment adherence falter. Programs to increase coverage of antiretroviral treatment during pregnancy and delivery have greatly decreased transmission during pregnancy and delivery.

In untreated infections, there is a risk of HIV transmission during breastfeeding.[37] The site of infection is not known; hypotheses include the mouth, tonsils, immune tissue in the gut (Peyer's patches), enterocytes, or perforations in the immature gut mucosa. National recommendations for HIV and infant feeding are based on the local epidemiology of maternal and child undernutrition and mortality, quality of health services, and local prevalence of HIV. Postpartum women living with HIV in the United States are advised to avoid all breastfeeding. In low- and middle-income countries with a high HIV burden, optimal breastfeeding practices (exclusive breastfeeding for the first 6 months of life, introduction of appropriate complementary foods thereafter, and continued breastfeeding until a nutritionally adequate and safe diet without breast milk can be provided) are generally recommended because of the risk of infant mortality due to formula feeding has been shown to outweigh the risk of HIV transmission. Modeling studies and programmatic experience strongly suggest that the risk of transmission during breastfeeding by women receiving antiretroviral treatment is very low. Women who are adherent to antiretroviral treatment from early pregnancy through the breastfeeding period have very low risk (<5%) of transmitting HIV to their breastfed infants.

> **CORE CONCEPT 8**
>
> In countries where infant formula feeding is universally affordable, feasible, acceptable, safe, and sustainable, postpartum women living with HIV are advised to avoid all breastfeeding.

Nutritional Management

Modifiable risks in HIV infection are antiretroviral treatment, inflammation, lipid levels, glucose intolerance, insulin resistance, and lifestyle behaviors. The goals of nutritional management of HIV infection are to achieve a healthy body weight; minimize loss of lean body mass and body fat redistribution; optimize the effectiveness of antiretroviral treatment; prevent the development of specific nutrient deficiencies; and minimize the long-term metabolic complications of HIV, including cardiovascular disease, diabetes, and bone loss.[36]

Medical History and Antiretroviral Treatment Adherence

The dietitian should review the patient's medical history, including viral load, CD4 count, history of opportunistic infections, HIV medications, HIV treatment adherence, and comorbidities. Opportunistic infections tend to occur when the CD4 count falls below 200 cells/mm^3 and are associated with wasting. Having had more than one opportunistic infection in the past increases the risk of underweight, weight loss, and wasting. However, opportunistic infections do not explain the etiology of weight loss in many cases.[11]

> **CORE CONCEPT 9**
>
> Opportunistic infections occur when the CD4 count falls below 200 cells/mm^3.

Classes of HIV drugs and specific HIV drugs within a class may have nutrition-related side effects that affect treatment adherence and metabolism. In addition to potentially impacting treatment adherence, the pharmacokinetics of HIV medications are postulated to mediate the relationship between food insecurity and incomplete viral suppression.[13] Many HIV medications cause gastrointestinal symptoms (**Table 20.2**).[18] Some can be taken with or without food; some should taken with a meal or snack or on an empty stomach (**Table 20.3**).[38] Refer to **Table 20.4** for a summary of HIV comorbidities and implications and **Table 20.5** for a review of common oral problems associated with HIV infection.

> **PRACTICE POINT**
>
> Review of a patient's HIV medications for potential side effects and treatment adherence is important to optimize compliance.

Nutritional Assessment

Anthropometric Assessment

The anthropometric assessment of individuals with HIV infection should evaluate the patient for weight loss (**Table 20.6**), underweight status, and body fat redistribution in lipodystrophy. Weight history should be

TABLE 20.2 POTENTIAL NUTRITION-RELATED SIDE EFFECTS AND HOW TO TAKE HIV MEDICATIONS

HIV Medication	Potential Side Effects	Administration Guidelines
Atripla	GI symptoms	Take on empty stomach before bed
Complera	GI symptoms	Take with meals
Efavirenz	Bone loss	Take on empty stomach before bed
Indinavir	Kidney stones	Take on empty stomach or with low-fat snack/water
Lamivudine	GI symptoms	No food restrictions
Lopinavir/ritonavir	GI symptoms	Take with food
Nelfinavir	GI symptoms	Take with meal or snack
Ritonavir	Vitamin D deficiency	Take with food
Stavudine	Impaired glucose metabolism	No food restrictions
Tenofovir	Bone loss	No food restrictions
Truvada	GI symptoms	No food restrictions
Zidovudine (AZT)	Anemia, vitamin B_{12} deficiency	No food restrictions

Data from International Association of Providers of AIDS Care. Taking Current Antiretroviral Drugs Fact Sheet 401B and Branch, 2013.

TABLE 20.3 POTENTIAL INTERACTIONS BETWEEN FOOD INTAKE AND HIV DRUGS

Pharmacokinetic Process	Potential Interaction
Absorption	Protease inhibitors (nelfinavir and ritonavir) require food for maximal absorption.
Metabolism	Enzymes found in the liver and GI tract (the cytochrome P450 group and, in particular, CYP3A4) are involved in the metabolism of HIV drugs, nutrients, and food. For example, grapefruit juice inhibits CYP3A4, leading to HIV drug toxicity. Certain HIV drugs may interfere with the enzymatic activity of vitamin D metabolism, increasing the risk of vitamin D deficiency.
Distribution	Distribution depends on tissue integrity and infection (acute phase response and inflammation). For persons on ART, wasting and weight loss are associated with higher viral loads.
Elimination	Drugs and nutrients can act synergistically and competitively to increase or decrease excretion.

Data from Raiten DJ. Nutrition and pharmacology: general principles and implications for HIV. *Am J Clin Nutr*. 2011;94(suppl):1697S-702S and Kress K. Role of Cytochrome P450 in the Management of HIV Infection. Positive Communication. A Newsletter of the Infectious Disease Nutrition Dietetic Practice Group, American Dietetic Association. 2010;15(1):1.

TABLE 20.4 HIV COMORBIDITIES AND IMPLICATIONS

HIV Comorbidities	Implications
Cardiovascular disease and diabetes	• A history of cardiovascular disease or diabetes may be related to or exacerbate metabolic abnormalities of lipodystrophy. • Lipodystrophy may adversely affect existing comorbidities of diabetes and cardiovascular disease.
Hepatitis C infection and liver disease	• Hepatitis C co-infection, which occurs in 15% to 30% of HIV patients, leads to higher rates of liver disease than mono-infected patients.[39] • Liver injury is prognostic of HIV disease progression.[40]
Kidney disease	• HIV infects cells of the kidney; kidney function is abnormal in up to 30% of HIV-infected patients. • HIV-associated nephropathy is a cause of end-stage renal disease in HIV infection.[41,42]
Obesity	• Obesity is as prevalent among people living with HIV as in the general population. Waist–hip ratio does not differentiate the accumulation of subcutaneous fat in obesity and visceral fat in lipodystrophy.
Depression and substance abuse	• Depression and substance use are prevalent among people living with HIV in the United States. Both depression and substance use are associated with food insecurity.
Gastrointestinal problems	• Gastrointestinal problems may lead to weight loss.
Mouth/dental problems	• Oral problems may lead to weight loss
Swallowing problems	• Swallowing problems may lead to weight loss.
Anorexia	• Anorexia may lead to weight loss.

(continues)

TABLE 20.4 HIV COMORBIDITIES AND IMPLICATIONS (continued)

HIV Comorbidities	Implications
Cognitive impairment • Slowing of thought processes • Poor coordination • Memory loss • Loss of executive function • Learning, verbal, and attention deficits	• HIV-associated dementia is an advanced form of cognitive impairment and is associated with a high viral load in the central nervous system • Neuropsychological deficits in HIV infection affect the ability to shop, to cook, and to manage finances and medications.[43,44] • Cognitive impairment can negatively affect food security, food shopping and preparation and/or medication and treatment adherence.
Anemia	• HIV infection is hypothesized to affect hematopoiesis.[45] • Specific HIV medications (zidovudine), hepatitis C medications (ribavirin), opportunistic infections, G6PD deficiency, and HIV-associated cancers may suppress bone marrow red cell production.[45] • Hemoglobin concentration and clinical anemia improve after initiation of antiretroviral treatment.[16,35,45]

TABLE 20.5 ORAL PROBLEMS IN HIV INFECTION

Caries: Tooth decay caused by bacteria

Oral thrush: An opportunistic infection in the mouth due to *Candida*

Apthous stomatitis (canker sores): Red sores, usually found on tongue, inside cheek, and on lips. Herpes simplex: A viral infection that causes red sores on roof of mouth or lips

Human papilloma virus: A virus associated with genital warts

Linear gingival erythema: Inflammation of the gingiva, unique to immunocompromised patients

Kaposi's sarcoma: A cancer that causes red or purple patches of abnormal tissue in the lining of the mouth, nose, throat, or other organs

Necrotizing ulcerative periodontitis: A severe form of periodontal disease in which gums pull away from teeth and form pockets

Data from Lavigne H. New York State Department of Health HIV Oral Health Regional Resource Center.

TABLE 20.6 CATEGORIES OF WEIGHT LOSS IN HIV INFECTION

Significant weight loss	>10% of body weight
Acute or rapid weight loss	>5% of body weight in less than 6 months
Advanced weight loss (HIV wasting)	BMI < 20

Gerrior JL. Unintentional weight loss and wasting in HIV infection. In: *Nutritional Management of HIV and AIDS*. Hendricks, KM, Dong KR, Gerrior JL, eds. American Dietetic Association. Chicago, IL;2009.

taken and actual weight can be compared to usual body weight or recent weights. The time period over which any unintentional weight loss occurred should be reported to document any rapid weight loss (e.g., >5% body weight loss in less than 6 months).

The assessment of weight loss in HIV infection should determine the etiology of the weight loss. Inadequate food intake may be a result of anorexia, mouth sores, dental

CASE STUDY REVISITED

The patient complains about his loss of facial fat and his thin arms.

Questions

1. Does the patient have lipodystrophy? Which parameters suggest this?
2. What related comorbidities may he develop?
3. What lifestyle changes can he make to help regain normal body shape?
4. What nutrition relevant labs would you monitor?

problems, oral thrush, swallowing problems, nausea, depression, substance use, food insecurity, diarrhea, malabsorption, opportunistic infections, cancer, hormonal changes, or the HIV infection itself.[36]

While a BMI <20 suggests HIV wasting syndrome, a patient's weight may remain in the normal or overweight range even when there is significant or rapid weight loss with loss of lean body mass and wasting. Body composition must also be evaluated to assess HIV wasting.

Standard anthropometric measures of weight, height, and BMI as well as changes to these measures will not detect fat redistribution in HIV infection, a hallmark sign of lipodystrophy. BMI can be within the healthy or overweight range at the same time that, for example, one's limbs are abnormally thin. BMI and weight are also not substantially changed by visceral fat accumulation. Mid-upper arm circumference (MUAC) and waist-to-hip ratio (WHR) have been used to screen for fat atrophy of the arms and fat deposition in the abdomen, respectively. Limitations include the fact that MUAC does not differentiate loss of subcutaneous tissue from wasting and loss of muscle, and that WHR does not differentiate subcutaneous fat and visceral fat. Alternatively, skinfold measurements may be used to evaluate body fat redistribution. Triceps skinfolds differentiate loss of subcutaneous tissue from muscle mass and wasting. Suprailiac skinfolds differentiate subcutaneous fat gain in obesity from visceral fat deposition in lipodystrophy. Mid-thigh skinfolds can be used to assess fat atrophy of the thighs and subscapular skinfolds can assess fat deposition on the upper back.

Measures of MUAC, waist and hip circumferences, and of skinfolds may be compared to reference standards by age group, gender, and race/ethnic group. Measures that fall below the 5th percentile indicate fat loss. Measures greater than the 95th percentile indicate fat deposition. For men, WHR >0.95 or for waist circumference >102 cm (40 inches) are high; for women, >0.85 for WHR or >88 cm (>35 inches) for waist circumference are high.[18,31]

> **PRACTICE POINT**
>
> Screen for body fat redistribution by asking the patient about any changes in body shape and by measuring waist and upper arm circumferences.

Nutrition-focused Physical Assessment

The patient may present with complaints of and should be evaluated for body shape changes and HIV wasting. Body shape changes may be self-reported and/or observed. Patients may report that their waist has gotten bigger or report pain associated with breast enlargement. Other body shape changes reported by patients include fat loss in the cheeks and buttocks. Patients may also complain of discomfort when sitting when there is atrophy of the buttocks. Physical examination should include examination of the abdomen, legs, back, breasts, and face for body shape changes, as well as assessment of temporal muscles and extremities for muscle wasting and fat loss. In abdominal fat deposition, the belly feels hard to the touch. Prominent venous markings on legs suggest subcutaneous fat atrophy.[18] Body shape changes and HIV wasting may be associated with loss of self-esteem and social stigma.

Body Composition

Assessment of wasting is essential to differentiate weight loss due to wasting from other causes of weight loss. In addition, fat mass and fat-free mass/lean body mass are altered over time in most cases of HIV infection. In clinical settings, bioelectrical impedance analysis (BIA) is used to measure fat-free mass. Use of BIA to track lean body mass improves the specificity of the nutrition assessment and monitoring of weight changes, guides the nutritional care plan, and serves as a tool for patient education.[22]

BIA is based on the principle that fat tissue and fat-free tissue impede electrical current differently. Electrodes are placed on the patient's hand and foot and a weak electrical current is transmitted through the body. Adequate hydration is essential for accurate measurement.[18] The resulting measurement is the phase angle, which is used to estimate fat-free mass (FFM) and fat mass according to height, weight, age, and sex. Phase angle has been shown to be associated with serum albumin, hemoglobin level, and energy intake in asymptomatic untreated patients and to be prognostic of HIV disease progression and mortality.[46] FFM values are compared to age-, sex-, and race-specific reference values. Cutoff values for low FFM are 17.4 for men and 15.0 for women. Population phase angle reference values by age and sex are also available.[47]

> **PRACTICE POINT**
>
> Bioelectrical impedance analysis (BIA) is a useful method to assess and monitor lean body mass in HIV-infected individuals.

BIA does not measure regional fat distribution and so cannot be used to assess body fat redistribution in lipodystrophy. Dual energy x-ray absorptiometry (DXA) can be used to measure fat mass and FFM in the trunk and limbs but cannot differentiate between subcutaneous and visceral fat in the abdomen.[30] Computed tomography (CT) scans can differentiate subcutaneous and visceral fat. Both DXA and CT scans are expensive, used primarily in research settings, and generally not recommended for clinical practice.

Dietary Assessment

The dietary assessment should pay particular attention to fat, saturated fat, and fiber intakes, which are linked to cardiovascular disease and insulin resistance; adequacy of energy intake and the patient's level of physical activity, including the frequency of any exercise; intake of micronutrients which are common deficiencies in untreated infections; and food security (Table 20.7).[48]

TABLE 20.7 QUESTIONS USED BY THE USDA TO ASSESS HOUSEHOLD FOOD SECURITY

During the last 12 months:

Did you worry that your food would run out before you got money to buy more?

Did the food you bought not last and you didn't have money to get more?

Could you afford to eat balanced meals?

Did you ever cut the size of meals or skip meals because there wasn't enough money for food?

Did you eat less than you felt you should because there wasn't enough money for food?

Were you ever hungry, but didn't eat, because there wasn't enough money for food?

Did you lose weight because there wasn't enough money for food?

Did you ever not eat for a whole day because there wasn't enough money for food?

Data from USDA, www.ers.usda.gov/topics/food-nutrition-assistance/food-security-in-the-us/measurement.aspx.

> **PRACTICE POINT**
>
> Evaluation for the need for food assistance is an important component of nutrition assessment for HIV-infected individuals.

Biochemical Assessment

> **PRACTICE POINT**
>
> Monitor the patient's CD4 count and viral load for viral suppression.

The CD4 count generally improves as nutritional status improves. Current medical guidelines are to monitor the CD4 count and viral load every 6 months for disease progression and viral suppression. Opportunistic infections occur when the CD4 count falls below 200 cells/mm^3. The CD4 count predicts cardiovascular disease as well as liver failure, cancers, and mortality from all causes.[17]

Lipid Profile Lipid abnormalities may be present as part of the metabolic abnormalities of HIV lipodystrophy syndrome.[39] A fasting lipid profile should be done every 6 to 12 months in all patients. Antiretroviral treatment, the HIV infection itself, and host factors are independently associated with elevated total cholesterol and triglyceride levels and low HDL levels. Fasting lipid levels should be checked prior to starting antiretroviral treatment and again 4 to 6 weeks later.

Insulin Resistance and Glucose Intolerance Fasting glucose level should be completed to screen for glucose intolerance every 6 to 12 months in all patients. Insulin resistance may be present as part of the metabolic abnormalities of HIV lipodystrophy syndrome. Fasting glucose should be monitored prior to and 4 to 6 weeks after starting ART. Patients with diabetes should have hemoglobin A1C measured every 6 months.[41]

Gastrointestinal Function Abnormalities of GI function, including diarrhea, abnormal D-xylose absorption as a marker for intestinal absorption, and fat malabsorption, are frequently seen in HIV infection.[11] For diarrhea, investigation into the etiology of the diarrhea and integrity of intestinal absorption may be warranted. Diarrhea is sometimes a side effect of antiretroviral drugs.

Iron Deficiency Iron deficiency anemia in HIV has features of anemia of inflammation and with chronic disease and is generally normochromic and normocytic.[45] Similar to other chronic diseases, HIV patients typically have a low hemoglobin concentration, low reticulocyte count but normal mean corpuscular volume, low serum iron level and iron binding capacity, and normal to elevated ferritin level and stores in the bone marrow. The rate of iron deficiency anemia increases from 1% to 10% in asymptomatic infections and among patients on effective ART, to 10% to 25% in symptomatic infections and to 30% to 60% in AIDS. Higher rates of anemia and severe anemia are seen in women and African Americans.[45] Vitamin B_{12} deficiency also occurs in up to 30% of patients, whereas folate deficiency is uncommon. Hemoglobin concentration should be routinely monitored.

Bone Loss The bone density of all patients older than 50 years of age should be evaluated using DXA following the guidelines of the National Osteoporosis Foundation and risk should be evaluated by the World Health Organization fracture risk assessment tool. All risk factors should be assessed, including HIV infection, smoking, sun exposure, vitamin D intake, calcium intake, weight-bearing exercise, age, and history of fracture.[34]

Renal and Liver Function Kidney injury and the glomular filtration rate should be routinely monitored because of the increased risk for nephropathy in HIV infection, particularly among African Americans. Renal function should be tested before and after initiation of treatment with tenofovir or indinavir. Liver injury/liver fibrosis and hepatitis C status should also be routinely monitored.[16]

Serum Albumin Cachexia is associated with excess cytokines and with low albumin and anemia. HIV infection also produces chronic inflammation, which also lowers serum albumin.

Micronutrient Deficiencies Vitamin A, B_1, B_3, B_6, B_{12}, C, D, and E; zinc; and selenium serum concentrations should be determined before and after initiation of antiretroviral treatment.

⚠ Clinical Controversy

Should care guidelines for non-AIDS conditions be adapted for those living with HIV infection?

Most deaths among persons living with HIV infection in the United States are non-AIDS deaths, such as those from cardiovascular disease, cancer, liver disease, and renal disease.[14] As those living with HIV survive longer, clinicians are tasked to determine how to best approach providing care to this unique aging population. Should established guidelines set forth for the general population be used for those with HIV? This question can be explored in cardiovascular disease (CVD). Individuals with HIV have a high incidence of CVD, even with low viral load and high CD4 counts.[1] The benefit of statin medications on survival, cardiovascular outcomes, and lowering of inflammatory biomarkers in HIV-free subjects is well known. It is unclear whether statins can elicit the same benefit in HIV infected individuals. A study by Lo et al.[2] found that statin therapy seems to have similar effects in those with HIV as in those without it, specifically reducing non-calcified plaque volume and high risk coronary plaque features. However, Krask et al.[3] in a retrospective cohort analysis of 438 HIV infected individuals, did not find a significant benefit of statin therapy on the incidence of myocardial infarction, stroke, and all-cause mortality.

1. How might the differences in study design impact how you interpret these conflicting findings?
2. Discuss how evaluation of plaque features (in the Lo study) versus hard clinical endpoints (in the Krsak study) influence your interpretation of the studies?
3. What are some risks of statin therapy in the HIV population?
4. Based on this information, would you recommend a statin for aging individuals with HIV?

References:

1. Justice A, Freiberg MS, Lo Re V. Should everyone ageing with HIV take a statin? *Lancet HIV*. 2015;2(2):e36-e37.

2. Lo J, Lu MT, Ihenachor EJ, et al. Effects of statin therapy on coronary artery plaque volume and high risk-plaque morphology in HIV-infected patients with subclinical atherosclerosis: a randomized, double-blind, placebo-controlled trial. *Lancet HIV*. 2015;2(2):e36-e37

3. Krsak M, Kent DM, Terrin N, Holcroft C, Skinner SK, Wanke C. Myocardial infarction, stroke, and mortality in cART-Treated HIV patients on statins. *AIDS Patient Care and STDs*. 2015;29(6):307-313,

---

CORE CONCEPT 10

HIV infection is a life-long chronic disease for which self-management is key.

Nutritional Management of HIV Wasting

Underweight adults with HIV infection are frequently wasted and early nutritional management of weight loss has been shown to be critical for underweight adults. In cases of HIV wasting, the goal is to stop catabolism and regain lean body mass and to identify and treat any secondary infections. Energy requirements are high (30-40 kcal/kg body weight) and protein requirements are often greater than the Recommended Daily Allowance for healthy individuals (1.2-2.0 g/kg body weight).[18] Liquid supplemental foods for weight losses ≥5% or BMI <18.5 are appropriate. Body composition should be monitored.

PRACTICE POINT

Liquid energy supplements may be useful for patients who have limited access to kitchen facilities and cooked meals.

In cases of severe weight loss (>10% within 6 months or >5% within 1 month) and serious comorbidities, including poorly controlled diabetes, end-stage renal disease, chronic diarrhea, liver disease, or central nervous system disease, enteral or parenteral nutrition support may be indicated.[18]

Nutritional Management of Unintentional Weight Loss

The clinician should ensure that HIV patients with unintentional weight loss are receiving effective antiretroviral treatment. Nutritional management of weight loss depends on the etiology of weight loss. The nutrition assessment may find inadequate food intake as a result of mouth sores, oral thrush, dental problems, swallowing problems, anorexia, nausea, diarrhea, malabsorption, depression, substance use, food insecurity, opportunistic infections, cancer, hormonal changes, or the HIV infection itself.[36]

Once the cause of weight loss is addressed, most patients with HIV-associated weight loss increase food intake and regain weight. For nausea and anorexia, nutrition guidance should be provided to eat small, nutrient-dense meals and snacks every 2 to 3 hours throughout the day.[36,38] For constipation, noncaffeinated fluids, high-fiber foods, and light exercise are recommended.[36] For swallowing problems, soft foods are advised.[38] For cases of diarrhea, food sources of soluble fiber and electrolyte-repleting fluids are recommended. Avoidance of foods high in fat, caffeinated beverages, and alcohol is recommended.[36,38]

Nutritional Management of Lipodystrophy

High-fiber diets are associated with less central fat deposition.[49] In a study of HIV male patients (excluding patients with low MUAC in order to eliminate cases with fat atrophy), patients without central fat gain (WHR <0.95) had higher intakes of energy, protein, soluble fiber, insoluble fiber, and pectin; tended to do more resistance training; and were less likely to smoke than patients with fat gain. Endurance and resistance exercise can reduce visceral adipose tissue.[31]

The National Cholesterol Education Program guidelines should be used to treat lipid abnormalities in HIV infection.[18,31] Consumption of fish and fish oils and avoidance of simple sugars and alcohol can decrease triglyceride levels. Exercise, substituting monounsaturated oils, and increasing fiber intake may lead to improvements in HDL and LDL levels. For insulin resistance, increased intake of fiber-rich foods may benefit patients; exercise and weight reduction can reduce insulin resistance and progression to diabetes.[18,31]

Nutritional Management of Bone Loss

HIV medications initially accelerate bone turnover, but eventually stabilize bone loss and are protective against fracture risk.[34] Bone disease in HIV infection should be managed by assessment of all risk factors for bone loss, including HIV infection, smoking, sun exposure, vitamin D intake, calcium intake, weight-bearing exercise, age, and history of fracture.[34] Patients should be educated about the benefits of regular exercise and adequate calcium and vitamin D intake through the consumption of fortified and dairy foods and the adverse effect of cigarette smoking. A supplement that contains 100% of the Daily Recommended Intakes for calcium and vitamin D may be recommended as needed. Secondary causes of decreased bone density such as vitamin D deficiency and hypogonadism should be treated.

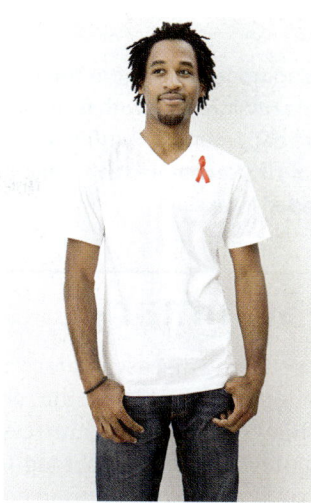

The AIDS Awareness Ribbon Reduces Social Stigma and Raises Awareness of HIV and AIDS
© Image Source/DigitalVision/Getty Images.

Micronutrient Supplementation

Evidence for the benefits of micronutrient supplementation in patients on antiretroviral treatment is inconclusive. Micronutrient supplementation of patients on antiretroviral treatment may have several benefits, including reduction in mitochondrial toxicity and oxidative stress and improved immune reconstitution. In untreated infections, high-dose micronutrient supplementation with B, C, and E vitamins and selenium has been shown to slow the decline in CD4 levels.[50] However, high-dose micronutrient supplementation may in fact be harmful in HIV infection; vitamin C and calcium supplementation, for example, can affect the pharmacology of indivanir and nelfinavir. The World Health Organization recommends micronutrient intakes at recommended levels through the consumption of diversified diets, fortified foods, and micronutrient supplements as needed.[19]

Clinical Roundtable

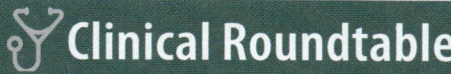

Topic: Use of Probiotics in HIV Infection

Background: In HIV infection, the gastrointestinal tract and gut-associated lymphoid tissue often deteriorates, leading to alterations in intestinal epithelium. This compromised intestinal status is thought to lead to microbial translocation, which can contribute to chronic immune activation and worsen disease progression. Probiotics may have a beneficial effect on reducing intestinal permeability and HIV chronic inflammation. A double blind study of 44 patients with HIV infection showed a significant decrease in markers of microbial translocation and inflammation after 12 weeks of treatment with the probiotic *Saccharomyces boulardii*.[50] However, there is no clinical guidance on the use of probiotics to improve gut function in HIV infection.

Roundtable Discussion

1. Would you recommend using probiotic supplements in HIV-infected individuals?
2. What are potential risks in this population?
3. How would you monitor outcomes?

References

1. Villar-Garcia J, Hernandez JJ, Guerri-Fernandez R, et al. Effect of probiotics (*Saccharomyces boulardii*) on microbial translocation and inflammation in HIV-treated patients: A double-blind, randomized, placebo-controlled trial. *JAIDS*. 2015;68:256-263

> **PRACTICE POINT**
>
> A commonsense approach to micronutrient supplementation for clinically stable HIV infection with no apparent deficiencies is to recommend a daily multivitamin/mineral supplement that provides 100% of the Recommended Daily Allowance (RDA) Daily Recommended Intakes.

Chapter Summary

HIV infection is a chronic disease characterized by immune dysfunction, inflammation, and acute opportunistic infections. While the benefits of antiretroviral treatment outweigh the long-term health risks, long-term exposure to antiretroviral treatment can lead to major metabolic complications, including cardiovascular disease and serum lipid abnormalities, altered glucose metabolism and insulin resistance, and bone loss. HIV wasting is characterized by the advanced loss of body fat and lean body mass and is associated with increased mortality risk. HIV-associated lipodystrophy is a syndrome that includes body fat redistribution and/or metabolic abnormalities and occurs in the majority of cases. Micronutrient deficiencies occur in untreated HIV infection and are associated with low CD4 counts and disease progression. Modifiable risks in HIV infection are antiretroviral treatment, inflammation, lipid levels, glucose intolerance, insulin resistance, and lifestyle behaviors. Medical nutrition therapy is an important component of HIV care. Evaluation for body fat redistribution in lipodystrophy, underweight, and weight loss and monitoring of weight changes guides the nutritional care plan and serves as a tool for patient education.

Key Terms

acquired immune deficiency syndrome (AIDS), CD4 count, opportunistic infections, viral load, viral suppression, antiretroviral treatment (ART), food insecurity, chronic inflammation, HIV wasting syndrome, lipodystrophy

References

1. Fauci AS. 25 years of HIV. *Nature*. 2008;453:289-290.
2. Council of State and Territorial Epidemiologists; AIDS Program, Center for Infectious Diseases. Revision of the CDC surveillance case definition for acquired immunodeficiency syndrome. *MMWR*. 1987;36 (suppl 1):1-15.
3. Centers for Disease Control and Prevention. Subpopulation estimates from the HIV incidence surveillance system – United States, 2006. *MMWR*. 2008; 57(36):985-989.
4. UNAIDS. UNAIDS Fact Sheet July 2017. http://www.unaids.org/en/resources/fact-sheet. Accessed November 14, 2017.
5. UNICEF. The State of the World's Children 2016. https://www.unicef.org/sowc2016/. Accessed November 14, 2107.
6. Centers for Disease Control and Prevention. Diagnoses of HIV in the United States and Dependent Areas, 2011. *HIV Surveillance Report*. February 2013.
7. Gross J. AIDS patients face downside of living longer. *The New York Times*. Jan 6, 2008.
8. New York State Department of Health AIDS Institute. Antiretroviral therapy. www.hivguidelines.org. Accessed August 25, 2017.
9. National Institutes of Health. Treating HIV-infected people with antiretrovirals significantly reduces transmission to partners. *NIH Press Release*. May 12, 2011.
10. Normén L, Chan K, Braitstein P, et al. Food insecurity and hunger are prevalent among HIV-positive individuals in British Columbia, Canada. *J Nutr*. 2005;135(4):820-825.
11. Mangili A, Murman DH, Zampini AM, Wanke CA. Nutrition and HIV infection: review of weight loss and wasting in the era of highly active antiretroviral therapy from the Nutrition for Healthy Living cohort. *CID*. 2006;42:836-842.
12. Aidala AA. HIV/AIDS, food & nutrition service needs. Community Health Advisory and Information Network, Mailman School of Public Health, Columbia University, 2011.
13. Weiser SD, Frongillo EA, Ragland K, et al. Food insecurity is associated with incomplete HIV RNA suppression among homeless and marginally housed HIV-infected individuals in San Francisco. *J Gen Intern Med*. 2008;24:14-20.
14. Weiser SD, Young SL, Cohen CR, et al. Conceptual framework for understanding the bidirectional links between food insecurity and HIV/AIDS. *Am J Clin Nutr*. 2011;94:1729S-1739S.
15. Institute of Medicine. Monitoring HIV care in the United States – Indicators and data systems, 2012. www.iom.edu/monitoringhivcare. Accessed August 25, 2017.
16. Justice AC, Freiberg MS, Tracy R, et al. Does an index composed of clinical data reflect effects of inflammation, coagulation, and monocyte activation on mortality among those aging with HIV? *Clin Infect Dis*. 2012;54(7):984-994. doi: 10.1093/cid/cir989
17. Fitch K, Grinspoon S. Nutritional and metabolic correlates of cardiovascular and bone disease in HIV-infected patients. *Am J Clin Nutr*. 2011;94:1721S-1728S.
18. Gerrior JL, Neff LM. Nutrition assessment in HIV infection. *Nutr Clin Care*. 2005;8(1); 6-15.
19. WHO. Nutrition and HIV/AIDS Report by the Secretariat. Executive Board 116th Session, 12 May 2005.
20. Mittelsteadt AL, Hileman CO, Harris SR, et al. Effects of HIV and antiretroviral therapy on resting energy expenditure in adult HIV-infected women. *J Acad Nutr Diet*. 2013;113:1037-1042.
21. Kosmiski L. Energy expenditure in HIV infection. *Am J Clin Nutr*. 2011;94:1677S-1682S.
22. Pinault L, Mittelsteadt A. Measuring body composition of HIV patients using Bioelectrical Impedance Analysis. Positive Communication Newsletter of the Infectious Diseases Nutrition Dietetic Practice Group. Academy of Dietetics and Nutrition, Fall 2010.
23. Pierre-Louis J, Zullig L. Changes in nutrition related conditions among HIV positive men and women receiving home-delivered meals for six months. Ryan White Grantee Meeting, U.S. Department of Health and Human Services, Washington, DC, 2010.
24. Sudfeld CR, Isanaka S, Mugusi FM, et al. Weight change at 1 mo of antiretroviral therapy and its association with subsequent mortality, morbidity, and CD4 T cell reconstitution in a Tanzanian HIV-infected adult cohort. *Am J Clin Nutr*. 2013;97:1278-1287.
25. Gonzalez MC, Pastore CA, Orlandi SP, Heymsfeld SB. Obesity paradox in cancer: new insights provided by body composition. *Am J Clin Nutr*. 2014;99:999-1005.
26. Sattler FR, Rajicic N, Mulligan, K, et al. Evaluation of high-protein supplementation in weight-stable HIV-positive subjects with a history

26. of weight loss: a randomized, double-blind, multicenter trial. *Am J Clin Nutr.* 2008;88:131-132.
27. Tien PC, Benson C, Zolopa AR, et al. The Study of Fat Redistribution and Metabolic Change in HIV Infection (FRAM): Methods, design, and sample characteristics. *Am J Epidemiol.* 2006;163:860-869.
28. Carr A, Samaras K, Thorisdottir A, Kaufmann GR, et al. Diagnosis, prediction, and natural course of HIV-1 protease-inhibitor-associated lipodystrophy, hyperlipidemia, and diabetes mellitus: a cohort study. *Lancet.* 1999;353:2093-2099.
29. Kosmiski LA, Nessesen DH, Stotz S, et al. Short-term overfeeding increases resting energy expenditure in patients with HIV lipodystrophy. *Am J Clin Nutr.* 2007;86:1009-1015.
30. McDermott AY, Terrin N, Wanke C, et al. CD4+ Cell count, viral load, and highly active antiretroviral therapy use are independent predictors of body composition alterations in HIV-infected adults: A longitudinal study. *CID.* 2005;41:1662-1670.
31. Wohl DA, McComsey G, Tebas P, et al. Current concepts in the diagnosis and management of metabolic complications of HIV infection and its therapy. *CID.* 2006;43:645-653.
32. Post WS, Budoff M, Kingsley L, et al. Associations between HIV infection and subclinical coronary atherosclerosis. *Ann Intern Med.* 2014;160(7):458-467.
33. Jacobson DL, Patel K, Siberry GK, et al. Body fat distribution in perinatally HIV-infected and HIV-exposed but uninfected children in the era of highly active antiretroviral therapy. *Am J Clin Nutr.* 2011;94(6):1485-1495.
34. Mondy K, Yarasheski K, Powderly WG, Whyte M, et al. Longitudinal evolution of bone mineral density and bone markers in human immunodeficiency virus-infected individuals. *Clin Infect Dis.* 2003;36:482-490.
35. Drain PK, Kupka R, Mugusi F, Fawzi WW. Micronutrients in HIV-positive persons receiving highly active antiretroviral therapy. *Am J Clin Nutr.* 2007;85:333-345.
36. Wanke, C, Dong K. The future of HIV nutrition. Food and Nutrition Conference & Expo, Academy of Nutrition and Dietetics, Boston, MA, 2010.
37. Guideline Updates on HIV and Infant Feeding. World Health Organization and UNICEF. World Health Organization Website. Published 2016. http://apps.who.int/iris/bitstream/10665/246260/1/9789241549707-eng.pdf?ua=1. Accessed November 15, 2017.
38. Trepal EM, Zullig LM, eds. *Eating tips: A nutrition guide for people living with HIV/AIDS.* New York, NY: God's Love We Deliver; 2010.
39. Sherman KE, Rouster SD, Chung RT. Hepatitis C virus prevalence among patients infected with HIV: a cross-sectional analysis of the U.S. Adult AIDS Clinical Trials Group. *Clin Infect Dis.* 2002;34:731-837.
40. Lo Re V, Kallan MJ, Tate JP, et al. Hepatic decompensation in antiretroviral-treated patients co-infected with HIV and hepatitis C virus compared with hepatitis C virus-monoinfected patients. *Ann Intern Med.* 2014:160(6):369-382.
41. Aberg JA, Kaplan JE, Libman H, et al. Primary care guidelines for the management of persons infected with Human Immunodeficiency Virus: 2009 update by the HIV Medicine Association of the Infectious Diseases Society of America. *Clin Infect Dis.* 2009;49:651-681.
42. Canaud G. The kidney as a reservoir for HIV-1 after renal transplantation. *J Am Soc Nephrol.* 2013;25:212-215.
43. Schouten J, Cinque P, Gisslen M, Reiss P, Portegies P. HIV-1 infection and cognitive impairment in the cART era. *AIDS.* 2011;25:561-575.
44. Heaton RK, Marcotte TD, Mindt MR, et al. The impact of HIV-associated neuropsychological. *J Int Neuropsychol Soc.* 2004;10:317-331.
45. Volberding PA, Levine AM, Dieterich D, et al. Anemia in HIV infection: clinical impact and evidence-based management strategies. *Clin Infect Dis.* 2004;38:1454-1463.
46. Sales S, Tsalaile L, Dusara P, et al. Phase angle from bioimpedance measures is an indicator of nutritional status in HIV disease. XVII International AIDS Conference, Mexico City, Mexico, 2008.
47. Barbosa-Silva MCG, Barros AJD, Wang J, et al. Bioelectrical impedance analysis: population reference values for phase angle by age and sex. *Am J Clin Nutr.* 2005;82:49-52.
48. Hendricks KM, Willis K, Houser R, Jones CY. Obesity in HIV infection: dietary correlates. *J Am College Nutr.* 2006; 25:321-331.
49. Hendricks KM, KR Dong, AM Rang, et al. High-fiber diet in HIV-positive men is associated with lower risk of developing fat deposition. *Am J Clin Nutr.* 2003;78:790-795.
50. Baum MR, Campa A, Lai S, et al. Effect of micronutrient supplementation on disease progression in asymptomatic, antiretroviral-naïve, HIV-infected adults in Botswana. *JAMA.* 2013;310(20):2154-2163.
51. Villar-Garcia J, Hernandez JJ, Guerri-Fernandez R, et al. Effect of probiotics *(Saccharomyces boulardii)* on microbial translocation and inflammation in HIV-treated patients: A double-blind, randomized, placebo-controlled trial. *JAIDS.* 2015;68:256-263.

Section 3

Nutrition in the Lifecycle

Chapter 21 Nutrition in Pregnancy and Lactation
Chapter 22 Nutrition in Neonatology
Chapter 23 Nutrition in Pediatrics
Chapter 24 Nutritional Management of Childhood Obesity
Chapter 25 Nutrition in Eating Disorders
Chapter 26 Nutrition in Developmental Disabilities
Chapter 27 Nutrition in Geriatrics

Chapter 21

Nutrition in Pregnancy and Lactation

Sarah Trautman
Emily Trussler

Chapter Outline

Core Concepts
Introduction: Nutrition in Pregnancy
Nutrition Therapy Throughout Pregnancy
Nutritional Management of Preexisting Diseases in Pregnancy
Nutrition Support in Pregnancy
Summary: Nutrition in Pregnancy
Introduction: Nutrition in Lactation
The Lactating Mother: Nutritional Considerations
The Registered Dietitian's Role in Breastfeeding Promotion
Summary: Nutrition in Lactation

CORE CONCEPTS

1. Pregnancy is a complex stage of the lifecycle in which the mother must be the sole source of nutrients and functional compounds for her fetus.

2. Maternal behavior, health, diet, and pre-pregnancy weight can have major impacts for mother and fetus during gestation. Interventions should center on these factors to ensure a healthy pregnancy and a strong start for the infant.

3. The 40% to 50% increase in maternal blood volume is mediated by the renin-angiotensin system. Increased plasma volume will allow adequate hydration, perfusion, and fluid conservation during pregnancy and delivery.

4. As progesterone levels rise, the muscles of the gastrointestinal tract relax, decreasing gastric motility and leading to symptoms of heartburn, reflux, constipation, and nausea.

5. When maternal glucose supply to the fetus is elevated, fetal insulin production is increased. This may lead to detrimental hypoglycemia at delivery, as insulin secretions remain elevated while the glucose load from the mother ceases rapidly.

6. The basal metabolic rate of overweight and obese pregnant women, who have excess fat reserves, increases during pregnancy to prevent further deposition of adipose tissue. Undernourished pregnant women seem to conserve energy to accommodate for additional demands of fetal growth and development.

7. It is recommended by the United States Public Health Service, the Institute of Medicine, and the United States Preventive Services Task Force that all women of childbearing age consume 400 micrograms of folic acid during the preconception period.

8. A minimum weight loss of 10% can improve fertility, as well as symptoms of insulin resistance in gestational diabetes, abnormal lipid profiles, and elevated blood pressure.

9. Energy needs during the first trimester of pregnancy are no different from that of the nonpregnant female population.

10. An extra 340 kcal/day in the second trimester and an extra 452 kcal/day in the third trimester are sufficient to support metabolic changes and fetal growth.

11. Maternal protein needs increase to 1.1 g/kg/day from the standard 0.8 g/kg/day for nonpregnant women.

12. Avoidance or strict limitation of trans-fatty acids during pregnancy is strongly recommended.

13. It is unlikely that iron needs during pregnancy will be met through diet alone, and iron supplementation should be taken to meet the recommendations and enhance fetal growth.

14. Key nutrients of concern during pregnancy, and those for which needs are increased, include folate, calcium, and iron.

15. During a multiple pregnancy, there is an even greater increase in maternal tissue mass required, which further increases fetal demands on maternal nutrition resources and reserves.

16. Although bariatric surgery's induction of weight loss decreases the risk of the adverse fetal outcomes associated with obesity, it is highly recommended that pregnancy be prevented until weight stabilizes, usually around 12 to 18 months postsurgery.

17. Avoiding episodes of hypoglycemia (<60 mg/dL) is critical to maintaining adequate supply of glucose to the fetus.

18. During pregnancy, a hemoglobin level of <11 g/dL is defined as moderate anemia, while a hemoglobin level <7 g/dL is defined as severe anemia.

19. In the presence of starvation, severe malnutrition, or severe vomiting or diarrhea, thiamine stores may deplete, insulin levels drop, and gluconeogenesis stops, so that amino acids and adipose tissue become primary sources of energy.

20. The overall goal of treatment for hyperemesis gravidarum (HG) is fluid maintenance, electrolyte balance, adequate caloric intake, and symptom control.

21. Gestational diabetes mellitus (GDM) is defined as increased glucose intolerance that is first discovered during the second or third trimester; such symptoms in the first trimester are now considered to be due to standard type 2 diabetes mellitus.

22. Up to 50% of women who develop gestational hypertension will be diagnosed with preeclampsia between weeks 24 and 35.

23. Preeclampsia is a serious complication and must be dealt with promptly, because any degree can cause IUGR due to an altered blood supply in the placenta and umbilical cord.

24. HELLP syndrome is a variant of severe preeclampsia characterized by hemolysis, elevated liver enzymes, and low platelet count; common symptoms are right upper quadrant or epigastric pain, nausea, and vomiting.

25. When indicated, providing nutrition support can play a pivotal role in preventing complications and adverse effects of nutritional deficit during pregnancy. The benefits and risk of providing this therapy should be weighed.

26. Lactogenesis involves five major stages: embryogenesis, pubertal development, development in pregnancy, lactation, and involution. This means that the breasts actually cannot produce milk until after pregnancy, and once breastfeeding has ceased, mammary gland tissue returns to inactivity (involution).

27. The nutrient content of mature milk is influenced by preterm delivery, maternal BMI, dietary proteins, whether the mother is primi- or multiparous, and how often she breastfeeds. In general, it will contain 65 to 70 kcal/dL, 3.2 to 3.6 g/dL of fat, 0.9 to 1.2 g/dL of protein, 6.7 to 7.8 g/dL of carbohydrates (as lactose), and sufficient amounts of all micronutrients except vitamins D and K.

28. The proteins and "good bacteria" in breast milk have been found to modulate the infant immune system, leading to fewer cases of respiratory tract infections, pneumonia, otitis media, severity of respiratory syncytial virus bronchiolitis, gastrointestinal tract infections, necrotizing enterocolitis, asthma, sudden infant death, celiac disease, inflammatory bowel disease, diabetes, acute lymphocytic leukemia, and acute myeloid leukemia during infancy.

29. Maternal diet and stores of various nutrients will determine the exact levels of macro- and micronutrients in mature breast milk.

Chapter 21 Nutrition in Pregnancy and Lactation

Learning Objectives

1. Describe the physiologic and metabolic changes that occur during pregnancy and lactation, and how they affect maternal nutritional status.
2. Understand the associations between maternal pre-pregnancy and gestational health and the health of the infant.
3. Decide appropriate nutritional interventions for pregnancy-related symptoms and conditions.
4. Identify appropriate nutritional biomarkers for assessing health during pregnancy and lactation.
5. Note the impact of weight status, particularly obesity, on pregnancy and lactation.
6. Discuss common nutritional concerns before, during, and after pregnancy.
7. Explain the physiology and benefits of breastfeeding for mother and child.
8. Suggest interventions for lactation-related issues in order to promote longer breastfeeding duration.

Introduction: Nutrition in Pregnancy

Pregnancy is a complex stage of life during which a mother serves as the sole source of nourishment to support fetal growth and development. Within 40 weeks, a fertilized egg develops into a human being, and the mother supports this process through the nutrients and functional compounds she provides. This chapter will explain how the choices made before, during, and after pregnancy will impact both mother and child in all stages of the lifecycle. Throughout this chapter, we will focus on the optimal prenatal health, the demands of pregnancy on the mother, the dietary needs throughout the various stages of gestation, and the consequential effects of maternal health on the fetus. As we conclude the 9 months of pregnancy, we will discuss the next stage, breastfeeding and lactation: the physiologic processes, the maternal demands, and the overwhelming benefits to the mother and infant. It is the goal of this chapter to develop an independent pathway of thinking to prevent complications throughout this stage of the lifecycle and to provide solutions should those complications arise.

> **CORE CONCEPT 1**
>
> Pregnancy is a complex stage of the lifecycle in which the mother must be the sole source of nutrients and functional compounds for her fetus.

Maternal Health and Birth Outcome

From the time of conception until 40 weeks of gestation, a fetus is fully dependent on its mother for nourishment. Maternal factors such as pre-pregnancy nutritional status, pre-pregnancy weight status, gestational weight gain, the presence of comorbidities, **gravida** (number of pregnancies a woman has experienced) and **parity** (number of births a woman has given in her lifetime), smoking status, and maternal behavior can therefore directly influence birth weight, health, and outcomes.[1] In fact, pre-pregnancy weight alone has been shown to significantly impact the mother's health and weight gain during pregnancy, as well as the health of her child at birth.[2] These maternal behaviors, along with the provision of adequate, under-, or overnutrition throughout **gestation** (the time between conception and birth), can affect the genetic and metabolic components of the fetus and may result in epigenetic changes in the infant.[3,4] In addition to the adverse birth outcomes that occur secondary to less-than-ideal pregnancy circumstances, including **small-for-gestational-age (SGA)** birth weight (when an infant is small given their number of weeks gestation, usually at the 10th percentile), **large-for-gestational-age (LGA)** birth weight (which is when an infant's weight is greater than the 90th percentile for their gestational age), infantile hypoglycemia, and extended length of hospital stay, there are long-term health implications for the mother and fetus. These may include stunted growth, delayed development, increased risk of diabetes, and increased risk of overweight/obesity.[5,6] Education and lifestyle interventions during the prenatal, periconceptional, and postnatal periods ensure that the mother will be able to support her fetus throughout gestation, and provide a strong foundation for a lifetime of healthy maturation (**Figure 21.1**).

> **CORE CONCEPT 2**
>
> Maternal behavior, health, diet, and pre-pregnancy weight can have major impacts for mother and fetus during gestation. Interventions should center on these factors to ensure a healthy pregnancy and a strong start for the infant.

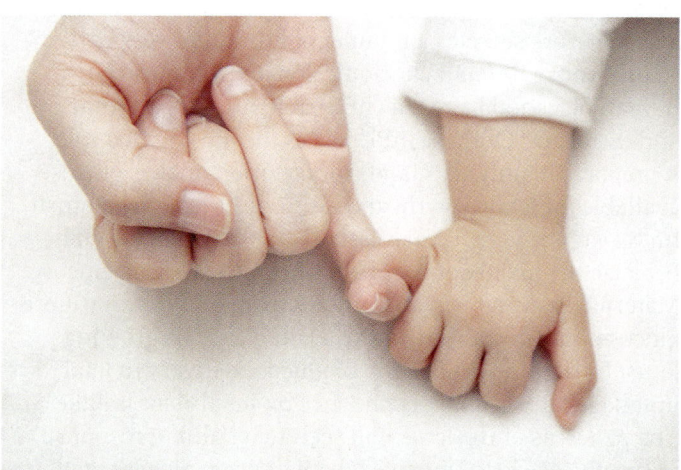
©DONOT6_STUDIO/Shutterstock.

CASE STUDY INTRODUCTION

Meg is a 32-year-old para 1 gravida 0 female (G1P0) who is now 14 weeks pregnant. At her check-up with her obstetrician, Meg presents with mild confusion, and reports nausea and vomiting for the past 6 weeks. She initially experienced this nausea over the first month of pregnancy. It then subsided and did not return until 8 weeks' gestation. Meg lives with her husband and works in a corporate office.

Anthropometric Data:
Height: 167 cm (66")
Current Weight: 66.8 kg (147 lbs)
Prepregnancy BMI: 24.5 kg/m^2
Weight History
Pre-pregnancy weight 68.2 kg (150 lbs)
Eight weeks' gestation 69.5 kg (153 lbs)

Biochemical Data: None

Clinical Data:
Past Medical History: none
Medications: Prenatal vitamin daily
Vital Signs: Blood pressure 142/90 mm Hg
Nutrition-focused Physical Findings: Appears tired and pale, no temporal wasting or obvious muscle loss

Dietary Data:
Dietary History: Meg reports that, over the past 3 weeks, she has been able to drink only ginger ale and has struggled to keep down any solid food. She has also noticed some weight loss due to persistent vomiting and her lack of appetite. Usually Meg is a very picky eater.

Questions
1. What are your initial concerns for Meg? Is Meg experiencing morning sickness?
2. What nutritional markers will you evaluate to assess Meg's nutritional status and risk?

Physiological Alterations Throughout Pregnancy

During pregnancy, an abundance of physiologic changes begin as early as 4 weeks after conception (**Figure 21.2**). These prepare the mother's body for the growth and delivery of a child.

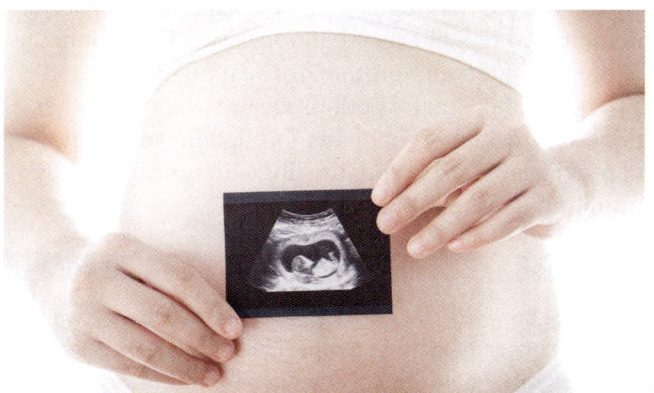

FIGURE 21.1 During Pregnancy, an Abundance of Physiological Changes Prepare the Mother's Body for the Growth and Delivery of a Child
© Bunwit Unseree/Shutterstock.

Placenta

The **placenta** is a blood-rich structure that develops in the uterus and is responsible for transferring nutrients and gasses from the mother to the fetus via the umbilical vein.[7] It begins to form on the 8th day after conception, and therefore secretes a number of hormones very early in pregnancy: human chorionic gonadotropin (hCG), human placental lactogen (hPL), relaxin, progesterone, and estrogen.[8] Of these, hPL serves the most varied role: it prepares mammary glands for lactation, makes glucose available for fetal growth, and also causes a degree of insulin resistance in maternal tissue.[8] This last effect is vital, because the major source of energy for the fetus is glucose. Maternal insulin resistance allows the blood to carry more glucose, thereby making more available to the growing fetus. In fact, the proportion of glucose delivery to fetal uptake is 1:1, with no dependence on insulin for uptake. The pancreas of the fetus will secrete insulin in response to the glucose load transported.[9] If oxygen, glucose, and amino acid transport through the umbilical vein is hindered (known as **placental insufficiency**), metabolic processes

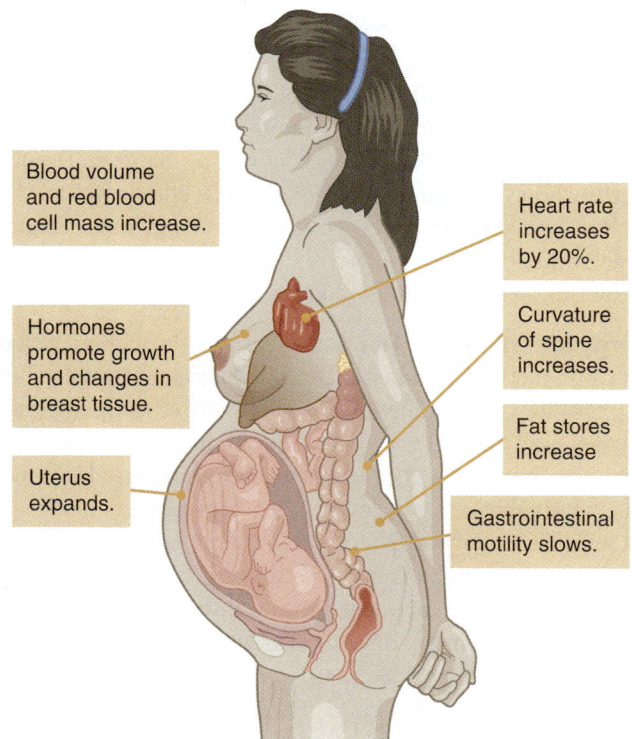

FIGURE 21.2 Pregnancy Requires Numerous Adaptations Within Most of the Mother's Organ Systems, such as Increased Blood Volume and the Growth of a New Organ, the Placenta

compensate for decreased substrate utilization and fetal growth will suffer. In the presence of hypoglycemia (i.e., decreased glucose supply), fetal growth of the spleen, liver, pancreas, and lungs is reduced.[10] Placental insufficiency also increases the risk of **intrauterine growth restriction (IUGR)**, in which the fetus is unable to grow and develop normally, putting it at high risk of serious consequences after birth.[11] IUGR may be precipitated by maternal malnutrition, advanced maternal diabetes, hypertension and **preeclampsia** (a condition during pregnancy characterized primarily by high blood pressure and protein in the urine), local uterine factors, or other placental pathologies.[11-13]

Blood Volume

In order to provide adequate hydration to the fetal and maternal tissues, perfuse the growing uterus, and conserve fluid to compensate for that which will be lost during birth, maternal blood volume begins to increase around weeks 10 to 12 until weeks 32 to 34.[8] This increase, generally of 40% to 50%, is the result of water retention.[14] As progesterone and estrogen levels rise, the kidneys are triggered to release renin, which in turn activates the aldosterone-renin-angiotensin mechanism. This causes the kidneys to reabsorb sodium and fluid, increasing total body water and leading to a greater plasma volume.[15]

> **CORE CONCEPT 3**
>
> The 40% to 50% increase in maternal blood volume is mediated by the renin-angiotensin system. Increased plasma volume will allow adequate hydration, perfusion, and fluid conservation during pregnancy and delivery.

Cardiovascular and Pulmonary

As blood volume increases, several physiologic changes must occur in the mother's cardiovascular and pulmonary systems. To account for increased maternal blood volume during pregnancy, the heart enlarges slightly, stroke volume and heart rate increase, and cardiac output rises by 30% to 50%.[8,14,16] Mild hypertension during pregnancy is diagnosed at a blood pressure of 140/90 mm Hg.[17] However, blood pressure decreases overall throughout pregnancy as a result of peripheral vasodilation caused by progesterone, and any increase in blood pressure should be assessed.[8]

As blood volume increases, plasma and red blood cell volume also increase. Due to the greater increase in plasma compared to red blood cells (hemodilution), mothers may experience physiologic anemia of pregnancy.[14] Practitioners should remember, however, that iron- and folate-deficiency anemias are also common in pregnancy and require treatment; as such, any mother displaying pallor, fatigue, dizziness, and shortness of breath should be examined.[18] Expectant mothers may also experience **orthostatic hypotension**, a fall in blood pressure associated with a change in position from recumbent to sitting to standing. In pregnancy, orthostatic hypotension occurs secondary to the compression of the inferior vena cava by the uterus during the last trimester.[16] To prevent these symptoms, the mother should position herself in a side-lying position when lying down. Because hypotension can also be a sign of anemia, any patient experiencing low blood pressure should be thoroughly examined.[18]

Gastrointestinal

Throughout pregnancy, the gastrointestinal tract is affected by various hormonal and physical factors. As progesterone levels rise, the gastrointestinal muscles are relaxed, often leading to symptoms of gastroesophageal reflux, heartburn, and even decreased gastric motility. The increased transit time through the colon can then lead to a higher reabsorption of fluid, exacerbating the effect of increased urination during pregnancy.[8] Constipation may also be a side effect of reduced motility, but can also be due to low-fiber food choices, reduced fluid intake, iron supplements, decreased activity, and intestinal displacement secondary to a growing uterus.[8] "Morning sickness" describes the symptoms of nausea and vomiting that may occur in the morning or persist all day. This is thought to be a result of the high levels of hCG and estrogen, reduced stomach acidity, and lowered tone and motility of the digestive tract.[8]

> **CORE CONCEPT 4**
>
> As progesterone levels rise, the muscles of the gastrointestinal tract relax, decreasing gastric motility and leading to symptoms of heartburn, reflux, constipation, and nausea.

Renal

As mentioned, the kidneys play a major role during pregnancy by increasing maternal blood volume through water and sodium resorption. This increase in plasma necessitates a 50% to 85% increase in glomerular filtration rate

(GFR) and kidney, renal pelvis, and ureter diameter in order to maintain normal kidney function, including stabilizing blood pressure and electrolyte balance.[8,16] Increased GFR, while necessary, does also increase glucose and protein losses in the urine, although these losses should not be great enough to cause concern.[16] Mothers may experience frequent urination during pregnancy as a result of high progesterone levels and the pressure of the growing uterus, both of which act upon the enlarged kidneys, ureters, and bladder.[8,14] These factors, which often lead to pooling of urine within the ureters, may also put mothers at higher risk for contracting urinary tract infections.[14,16] During pregnancy, serum creatinine is the best biomarker of kidney function, with a value over 0.8 mg/dL considered abnormal; serum sodium and osmolarity are less reliable as, like red blood cells, they will appear low due to the hemodilution effect discussed earlier.[14]

Endocrine

While there are abundant changes throughout the endocrine system during pregnancy, changes in thyroid hormones and pancreatic hormones relate most closely to nutrient metabolism. The thyroid gland enlarges and becomes more active during pregnancy due to changing levels of hCG from the placenta, resulting in elevated secretions of thyroid stimulating hormone and a 25% increase in maternal basal metabolic rate.[8,16] It is important to note that these changes in thyroid activity, as well as the growth of the fetus, necessitate a greater iodine intake of 150 to 200 micrograms per day (see the Micronutrients section for further information on iodine needs during pregnancy).[16]

As pregnancy progresses, placental hormones such as human placental lactogen and progesterone modulate the insulin receptor function of maternal cells, causing increased insulin resistance. The pancreas is increasingly active and physically creates more beta cells to meet this increased demand for insulin.[16] Unlike glucose, amino acids, and lipids, maternal insulin cannot cross the **placental barrier** (a semi-permeable barrier that limits the amount and type of material exchange between the mother and fetus); therefore, the fetus is responsible for producing its own insulin. Given this increased insulin resistance, the mother is at increased risk of hyperglycemia.[8] When maternal glucose supply to the fetus is elevated, fetal insulin production is increased. This may lead to detrimental hypoglycemia at delivery, because insulin secretions remain elevated while the glucose load from the mother ceases rapidly.[15] This risk to the fetus means that clinicians will be very strict in managing the maternal blood glucose throughout pregnancy, even if gestational diabetes is diagnosed late (see the Gestational Diabetes section).[19]

CORE CONCEPT 5

When maternal glucose supply to the fetus is elevated, fetal insulin production is increased. This may lead to detrimental hypoglycemia at birth due to elevated insulin secretions when the glucose load from the mother ceases rapidly.

Metabolic Alterations throughout Pregnancy

Maternal weight gain during pregnancy occurs to accommodate the nutritional and physiologic demands of the fetus. Of this weight gain, 40% is attributable to the fetus, placenta, and amniotic fluid, while 60% accounts for maternal tissues (uterine, breast, blood, adipose, and extracellular fluids).[20] Maternal metabolism adapts quickly to further support fetal growth and development, as a result of placental hormone production, fetal nutrient demands, and maternal stores.[21]

Energy metabolism Hormonal changes throughout gestation cause metabolic and circulatory adjustments in the maternal physiology. These alterations allow more efficient utilization of energy for fetal growth and development. As compared to all other mammals, the human fetal growth period is slow and extends across 40 weeks. This requires a lower energy cost for the mother per maternal kilogram of weight.[22]

Energy consumed is utilized through three different mechanisms: energy deposited in the embryo as new tissue (4,780 kcal), energy deposited as fat in well-nourished women (35,800 kcal), and energy required to maintain new maternal tissue (35,800 kcal).[22] The amount of this energy deposited as fat is dependent upon maternal energy reserves upon conception.[22] As the mass of metabolically active tissue and the work of maternal cardiovascular, renal, and respiratory systems increase, energy metabolism changes.[23] Towards the end of pregnancy, when the fetus is preparing for birth, fetal growth demands are dramatically increased.[22]

In general, physiologic and metabolic adjustments occur within the mother based on her pre-pregnancy body composition. The basal metabolic rate of overweight and obese pregnant women, who have excess fat reserves, increases during pregnancy to prevent further deposition of adipose tissue. Undernourished pregnant women seem to conserve energy to accommodate for additional demands of fetal growth and development.[22] Inadequate energy consumption during pregnancy may lead to reduced birth weight of the child so clinicians should monitor mothers carefully for signs of an eating disorder.[23]

CORE CONCEPT 6

The basal metabolic rate of overweight and obese pregnant women, who have excess fat reserves, increases during pregnancy to prevent further deposition of adipose tissue. Undernourished pregnant women seem to conserve energy to accommodate for additional demands of fetal growth and development.

Carbohydrate Metabolism As mentioned previously, the main source of fuel for the fetus is glucose, which requires a certain level of insulin resistance (mediated by placental hormones) in the mother throughout pregnancy. This insulin resistance naturally requires some adaptations in normal carbohydrate metabolism. Following a meal, for example, maternal glucose intolerance allows blood glucose levels to remain elevated for longer periods of time.[22] Utilization of glucose supply for maternal energy is limited in order to provide sufficient glucose to the fetus, so the mother will rely mainly upon her own fat stores.[16] This state of glucose intolerance is exacerbated in obese pregnant women, and further increases the risk of fetal hyperglycemia. With a decrease in insulin sensitivity, fat breakdown increases and hypertriglyceridemia occurs, increasing the risk of birthing an LGA infant. This is in part due to the unbalanced supply of glucose, free fatty acids, ketones, and amino acids to the fetus, as well as the production of glucose and triglycerides by the liver.[16,22]

Fat Metabolism   Maternal fat reserves exist as a source of energy to minimize protein breakdown and preserve glucose and amino acid supply for fetal demands.[22] There is an increased maternal fat utilization secondary to the increased insulin resistance.[16] When these are metabolized, free fatty acids and glycerol are released. The liver converts these free fatty acids to triglycerides, which are released into the bloodstream as very-low-density lipoproteins (VLDLs; one cause of gestational dyslipidemia). Triglycerides are not able to cross the placental barrier, but lipases convert them into fatty acids that can move through the placenta. The essential fatty acids (α-linolenic acid and linoleic acid) consumed by the mother provide a major source of nutrition for the fetus, providing it with building blocks for growth and neurologic development.[22,24]

Pregnant women are also at increased risk for ketosis. After transport across the placenta, free fatty acids in the bloodstream are oxidized by the liver into ketones, which may be used as fuel by the mother or fetus.[22] New research studies suggest that ketone production is intensified due to a protein, DLK1, that is only produced during pregnancy. The purpose of the protein appears to be activating the "accelerated starvation response," essentially ensuring that the mother's body has a consistent energy source (in the form of ketones) between meals, when her blood glucose is being sequestered for the fetus.[25]

Protein Metabolism   In normal physiology, protein can be either oxidized or used for tissue synthesis. However, throughout pregnancy, there is a 10% reduction in protein oxidation and a 15% to 25% increase in protein synthesis during the second and third trimesters. Overall, women experience a positive nitrogen balance during pregnancy due to decreased protein oxidation and therefore decreased urinary urea nitrogen levels.[22] This is, in part, attributable to the increased use of adipose tissue for energy.[16]

Nutrition Therapy Throughout Pregnancy

The numerous physiologic changes outlined above can lead to a number of issues requiring medical nutrition therapy. In this section, a pregnancy-specific assessment will be outlined along with special attention to serum markers to direct interventions.

Nutrition Assessment During Pregnancy

Nutrition Risk Factors

Upon assessment of pregnant women, especially those who are nutritionally at risk (underweight, overweight, or obese), it is important to establish a detailed assessment of the patient's nutritional status and evaluate specific nutrition risk factors as shown in **Table 21.1**.

TABLE 21.1 NUTRITIONAL RISK FACTORS AND THEIR ASSESSMENT DURING PREGNANCY

Risk Factors	Measures
Inappropriate weight gain	Pre-pregnancy weight, weight, height, body mass index (BMI)
Anemia	Hemoglobin, hematocrit, mean corpuscular volume, red cell distribution width Important to determine iron, vitamin B12, and folate status
Diabetes risk	Urine glucose, fasting plasma glucose, and/or oral glucose tolerance test results
Renal compromise	Assess creatinine and protein levels in urine
Vitamin D status	Serum 25-hydroxy vitamin D
Metabolic syndrome (Positive metabolic syndrome diagnosis increases the risk of complications in pregnancy)	This diagnosis requires the presence of three of five of the following criteria[26]: 　Abdominal obesity: a pre-pregnancy waist circumference at or above 35 inches 　Hypertriglyceridemia: at or above 150 mg/dL 　Reduced high-density lipoprotein (HDL) cholesterol: below 50 mg/dL 　Hypertension: above 130/85 mm Hg 　Insulin resistance: fasting glucose above 100 mg/dL
Nutrient deficiencies	Look for soft brittle nails, dry hair, concave nails, poor skin turgor

CASE STUDY REVISITED

On that same day, Meg is admitted to the hospital due to her vomiting, weakness, and confusion. Labs were drawn at admission and she was started on a hydration protocol with 0.9% normal saline at 100 mL/hour. A nutrition consult is ordered.

Biochemical Data:

Sodium 131 (135-145 mEq/L)
Potassium 3.0 (3.6-5.0 mEq/L)
Blood urea nitrogen 21 (6-24 mg/dL)
Creatinine 1.2 (0.4-1.3 mg/dL)
Carbon dioxide 18 (20-30 mEq/L)
Chloride 109 (98-110 mEq/L)
Calcium 9 (8.5-10.5 mEq/L)

Magnesium 2.0 (1.3 to 2.1 mEq/L)
Phosphorus 3.2 (2.7 to 4.5 mg/dL)
Glucose 60 (70-139 mg/dL)
Hemoglobin A1c 6.0% (4.3-5.8%)
Hemoglobin 11.8 (12-15.5 g/dL)
Hematocrit 34.4% (35%-47%)
Urine ketones +1

Clinical Data:
Vital Signs: Blood pressure: 158/80 mm Hg

Questions

1. Which of Meg's labs are abnormal? How might they explain her symptoms?
2. How might pregnancy cause these values to be altered?
3. Given the known common micronutrient deficiencies during pregnancy, what additional laboratory values would you request?

Biochemical Markers

Interpretation of biochemical markers and the risk they indicate is challenging given the physiologic alterations that accompany pregnancy. Use of reference values specific to pregnancy can be used to discern between normal and abnormal states.[27] While many parameters are similar to that of normal females, a number of differences can be expected due to altered physiology during pregnancy. Changes in electrolytes and blood indices may result from expanded fluid and blood volume. For example, hyponatremia and hypokalemia judged by reference standards in non-pregnant women may actually be a normal finding during pregnancy.[27] These changes may be due to activation of aldosterone-renin-angiotensin mechanism by the kidneys to increase total body water to support volume expansion, resulting in a dilution effect. Alterations in glucose and fat metabolism are reflected by increased fasting glucose and random glucose levels, ketonuria, increased hemoglobin A1c (HbA1c) and hyperlipidemia. These alterations in metabolism are to support glucose supply to the fetus by allowing the mother to rely on fatty acids for energy and ketones for obligatory glucose. Increased need for iron and nutrients by the fetus may result in alterations in iron, vitamin B_{12}, folate and vitamin D circulating levels, which can often diminish over time with pregnancy.[27] Evaluating biochemical indices against normal values requires a critical understanding of changes in physiology, homeostasis, and metabolism during pregnancy. Values should usually be interpreted in the context of other aspects of assessment including presenting symptoms, dietary intake, and nutrition-focused physical exam.

Preconception/Prenatal Care

Preconception health concerns the physical and nutritional health of both men and women in relation to reproduction.[28] Paying close attention to the Recommended Dietary Allowances (RDAs) for important prenatal nutrients is a key way to improve preconception health (**Figure 21.3**).[1]

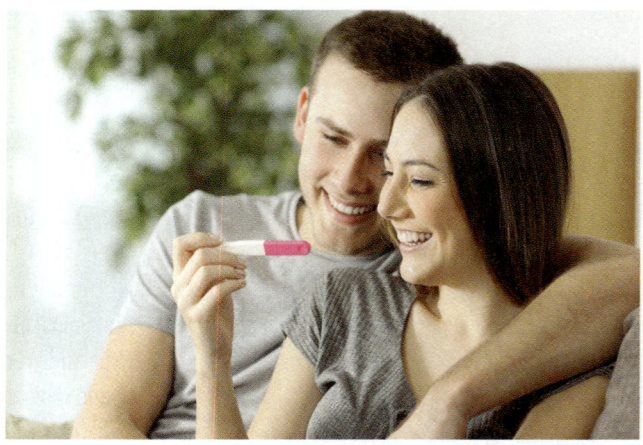

FIGURE 21.3 Paying Close Attention to the RDAs for Important Prenatal Nutrients is a Key Way to Improve Preconception Health
© Antonio Guillem/Shutterstock.

Any existing chronic undernutrition cannot be overcome by a few months of supplementation during pregnancy; therefore, when plausible, interventions, education, and nutritional guidance should be provided throughout the lifecycle to prevent unnecessary and adverse outcomes.[23]

Other nutrition-related risk factors to target in preconception care include smoking cessation, diabetes control, folic acid supplementation, management of maternal phenylketonuria, weight loss for obesity, and treating alcohol abuse.[29] These factors can be influenced by health behaviors and health status based upon environment and social factors.

> **PRACTICE POINT**
>
> When plausible, interventions, education, and nutritional guidance should be provided throughout the lifecycle to prevent unnecessary and adverse outcomes.

Folic Acid

The **neural tube** is a hollow tube that houses the brain, spinal cord, and other neural tissue and eventually differentiates into the respective organs of the central nervous system. Its development begins in utero within the first 21 days after conception and closes by day 28.[30] Folic acid is critical to new cell differentiation and therefore plays a vital role in the growth and development of the neural tube during the early stages of gestation. Closure of the neural tube will often occur prior to the mother's knowledge of her pregnancy due to its early development. If the neural tube closes prior to full development, birth defects will occur. Most common is **spina bifida**, a defect characterized by vertebrae not properly forming around the spine. Spina bifida can vary from mild to severe in nature. Other defects include **anencephaly** (absence of portions of the brain, skull, and scalp) and craniorachischisis. **Craniorachischisis** is the most severe type of neural tube defect, in which both the brain and spinal cord remain open. Therefore, adequate intake or supplementation of folic acid is critical during the months before and after a missed menstrual cycle.[31] It is recommended by the United States Public Health Service, and the Center for Disease Control and Prevention that all women of childbearing age consume 400 micrograms of folic acid before and during early pregnancy.[30-32] Those with a history of **neural tube defect** (NTD)-affected pregnancy or at high risk of NTD are recommended to consume at least 4 mg of synthetic folic acid supplements daily.[32]

> **CORE CONCEPT 7**
>
> It is recommended by the United States Public Health Service, the Institute of Medicine, and the United States Preventive Services Task Force that all women of childbearing age consume 400 micrograms of folic acid during the preconception period.

Iron Deficiency

Iron deficiency is one of the most common nutrient deficiencies worldwide.[33] Maternal iron deficiency during pregnancy is associated with adverse consequences to the mother and infant, including increased likelihood of excessive postpartum bleeding, mother and child mortality, sepsis, and SGA birth size.[33] As maternal blood volume increases, components of the blood such as hemoglobin decrease in response to a hemodilution effect (plasma:hemoglobin ratio increases), resulting in the clinical symptoms of anemia.[14] To aid in delivery of oxygen to the placenta and fetus, iron needs must dramatically increase during pregnancy. Maintaining adequate iron stores prior to pregnancy can alleviate the dramatic reduction in iron levels and low iron status preconceptually, which will decrease the risk of anemia in the latter gestational period of pregnancy. It is estimated that a woman maintains stores of 300 mg iron prior to conception to meet the additional iron demands during pregnancy.[34] Two methods of increasing iron intake are increasing intake of food high in heme iron, such as red meat, and providing iron supplementation. Increasing dietary iron intake *during* pregnancy will not be sufficient to meet the increased demands of 24 mg/day during the second half of pregnancy.[35] It is important to note, too, that high doses of iron supplementation (greater than 30 mg/day or 120 mg/week) are associated with adverse effects of fetal growth via increased oxidative stress secondary to elevated serum iron and decreased zinc and copper absorption (competitive inhibition).[35] To prevent the occurrence of iron deficiency before the time of conception, thorough screening, management, and monitoring of iron status in women of childbearing years is recommended.

CASE STUDY REVISITED

Refer back to Meg's pre-pregnancy BMI.

Questions

1. Is Meg underweight, normal weight, overweight, or obese?
2. Does this BMI classification put her at risk for complications?
3. What range of weight gain would you recommend throughout pregnancy?

> **PRACTICE POINT**
>
> Maintaining adequate iron stores prior to pregnancy can alleviate the dramatic reduction in iron levels and low iron status preconceptually, which will decrease the risk of anemia in the latter gestational period of pregnancy. Two methods of increasing iron intake are increasing intake of food high in heme iron, such as red meat, and providing iron supplementation. To prevent the occurrence of iron deficiency before the time of conception, thorough screening, management, and monitoring of iron status in women of childbearing years is recommended.

Pre-Pregnancy Weight Status

A major factor in assessing prenatal health and determining weight gain goals during pregnancy is pre-pregnancy BMI. Adverse effects to the mother and fetus can occur with both underweight and overweight/obese mothers. Underweight mothers (BMI <18.5) are at risk for chronic nutritional deficiencies and are more likely to give birth to an SGA infant,[36] while obese mothers are at risk for numerous complications, which will be outlined in this section.

To assess maternal weight status, determine weight reported at last menstrual cycle; maternal pre-pregnancy weight can be classified as follows:[2]

- Pregravid Underweight (Institute of Medicine (IOM) - BMI <19.8; World Health Organization (WHO) - BMI <18.5)
- Pregravid Normal weight (IOM - BMI 19.8-26; WHO - BMI 18.5-24.9)
- Pregravid Overweight (IOM - BMI >26-29; WHO- BMI 25-29.9)
- Pregravid Obese (IOM - BMI >29; WHO - 30-34.9)

Due to the obesity epidemic, much of the current research in prenatal and pregnancy nutrition is focused on the effects of overweight and obesity on birth outcome and maternal health. A recent report for the IOM stated that "Women today are heavier, a greater percentage of them are entering pregnancy overweight or obese, and many are gaining too much weight during pregnancy."[2] According to the National Health and Nutrition Examination Survey (NHANES) 2011-2014, 34.4% of young women (20-39 years), and 38% of all women, are clinically obese.[37] The excess adipose tissue present in obesity is critical in regulating sex hormone availability, which can be linked to insulin resistance and altered lipid metabolism. In the setting of metabolic changes, subclinical inflammation, and vascular dysfunction throughout pregnancy, obesity increases the risk of prenatal, periconceptional, and postpregnancy complications.[38]

As previously noted, risks to an obese mother are numerous and often serious for both mother and infant. These issues begin in the prenatal phase, when overweight and obesity decrease a woman's fertility by between 30% and 40%; a 10% weight loss can mediate this effect.[39] Through assessing the patient's usual intake and activity level, changes can be recommended to increase the nutrient density and decrease the energy density of intake, reach physical activity goals, and establish an appropriate weight-loss target. Visiting an outpatient registered dietitian (RD) would be the recommended route for these patients.

During pregnancy, the complications of obesity include gestational diabetes, gestational hypertension, preeclampsia, cesarean delivery, early spontaneous abortion, postpartum hemorrhage, postpartum weight retention, and risk of type 2 diabetes.[40,41] Obese individuals who are at high risk of gestational diabetes should be screened early in pregnancy to enhance their ability to maintain tight glucose control.[38] While folic acid, as discussed previously, is effective in the prevention of neural tube defects in mothers with a normal weight or even type 2 diabetes, research shows that when supplemented at appropriate levels in obese pregnant women, there is no change in the rate of neural tube defects in the infant.[31] Further consequences for the developing fetus include **fetal macrosomia** (a newborn that is significantly larger than normal), intrauterine fetal death, IUGR, cardiac malformation, fetal distress, asphyxia, stillbirth, prematurity, birth defects (neural tube defects, oral clefts, heart anomalies, hydrocephaly, and abdominal wall abnormalities), postpartum anemia, and childhood obesity.[22,38,42]

> **PRACTICE POINT**
>
> To assess maternal weight status, determine weight reported at last menstrual cycle; maternal pre-pregnancy weight can be classified. Obese individuals who are at high risk of gestational diabetes should be screened early in pregnancy to enhance their ability to maintain tight glucose control.

Interventions for Pre-Pregnancy Overweight and Obesity

To mitigate the adverse effects of obesity on pregnancy, weight loss is recommended prior to conception. A minimum weight loss of 10% can improve fertility as well as symptoms of insulin resistance in gestational diabetes, abnormal lipid profiles, and elevated blood pressure. Most overweight and obese women will struggle to reach a normal weight range before pregnancy; therefore, clinicians should focus upon emphasizing recommended weight gain goals from the IOM to moderate weight gain during pregnancy (see **Table 21.2**). Keeping a record of the patient's pre-pregnancy height and weight, charting her weight gain throughout pregnancy, and sharing the results are great strategies to maintain communication with patient and keep her focused on the importance of healthy pregnancy behaviors.[2]

> **CORE CONCEPT 8**
>
> A minimum weight loss of 10% can improve fertility as well as symptoms of insulin resistance in gestational diabetes, abnormal lipid profiles, and elevated blood pressure.

> **PRACTICE POINT**
>
> Keeping a record of the patient's pre-pregnancy height and weight, charting weight gain throughout pregnancy, and sharing the results are great strategies to maintain communication with patient and keep focused on the importance of healthy pregnancy behaviors.

TABLE 21.2 GESTATIONAL WEIGHT GAIN RECOMMENDATIONS

Pre-pregnancy Weight Class	BMI (kg/m^2)	Total Weight Gain Range (lbs)	Rates of Weight Gain* in Second and Third Trimester (Mean Range in lbs/week)
Underweight	<18.5	28-40	1 (1-1.3)
Normal Weight	18.5-24.9	25-35	1 (0.8-1)
Overweight	25-29.9	15-25	0.6 (0.5-0.7)
Obese (includes all classes)	>30	11-20	0.5 (0.4-0.6)

*Per National Academy of Medicine (formerly the Institute of Medicine) guidelines
Weight gain rates calculated assuming that 0.5 to 2 kg (1.1-4.4 lb) was gained during first trimester.
Data from Rasmussen KM, Yaktine AL. *Weight Gain During Pregnancy: Reexamining the Guidelines*. 2009.

Gestational Weight Gain

Maternal diet is a key factor in pregnancy outcome and the long-term health of both the mother and infant. Recommendations for gestational weight gain and nutrient intake are provided in order to prevent both pregnancy complications and adverse birth outcomes (**Figure 21.4**).[43] Essentially, gestational weight gain must be sufficient to support the physiologic products of conception: the growth of the fetus, placenta, and amniotic fluid, as well as the expansion of maternal blood volume and extracellular fluid, uterine and mammary glands, and maternal fat stores.[44] However, excessive weight gain can cause or exacerbate pregnancy complications. These include gestational diabetes, hypertension and preeclampsia, birth defects, cesarean delivery, and fetal macrosomia, as well as perinatal death and postpartum anemia.[39]

Throughout the first trimester of the pregnancy, the mother should only gain a total of 1 to 4 pounds. From the beginning of the second semester until birth, gains should average 3 to 4 pounds per month. In sum, this equates with a 25- to 35-lb weight gain for an average, normal weight woman,[36] but weight gain goals will differ depending upon pre-pregnancy BMI.[2] The guidelines established by the World Health Organization (WHO) account for varying pre-pregnancy weight and should be administered with clinical judgment based on the patient's pre-pregnancy BMI and discussed in detail with both physician and patient.[2] Maintaining a record of weight gain can be very helpful for the mother, offering a way to observe her weight gain trend and its relationship to the fetal growth and development. Studies have also suggested that one-on-one interventions, tailored dietary guidance, and physical activity counseling may improve weight gain during pregnancy, which can provide significant benefits to overweight and obese mothers.[32]

Macronutrient Requirements

Calories

Basal energy expenditure is increased in pregnancy to support growth of tissue and increased metabolic demands, such as increased cardiac output and oxygen consumption. However, overall energy needs during the first trimester of pregnancy are no different to those of the nonpregnant female population.[1] In fact, the National Academy of Medicine (formerly the IOM) recommends that energy intake remain the same as pre-pregnancy intake during the first trimester for the general population.[32]

> **CORE CONCEPT 9**
> Energy needs during the first trimester of pregnancy are no different than the nonpregnant female population.

As the mother progresses into the second and third trimesters, energy needs increase due to the increased demand from the growth and development of the fetus and

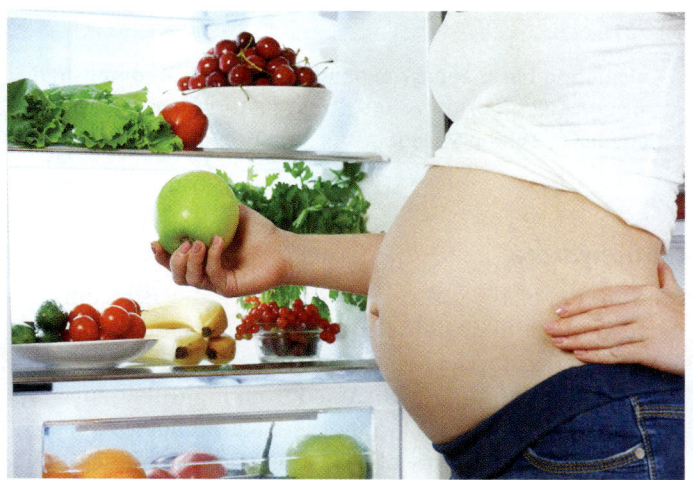

FIGURE 21.4 Maternal Diet is a Key Factor in Pregnancy Outcome and the Long-term Health of both the Mother and Infant
© Evgeny Atamanenko/Shutterstock.

> ## CASE STUDY REVISITED
>
> Meg is stable and ready to be discharged home from the hospital. You see her prior to discharge to provide general nutrition counseling.
>
> **Biochemical Data:**
> Hemoglobin 10 (12-15.5 g/dL)
> Hematocrit 31 (35%-47%)
> Serum iron 40 (50-170 micrograms/dL)
> Vitamin D (20-100 ng/dL)
>
> **Dietary Data:**
> **24-hour Diet Recall (when feeling well):**
> Breakfast: Cereal with low-fat milk, banana, coffee with Splenda
> Midmorning: Six saltine crackers with 2 tablespoons of peanut butter
> Lunch: One cup of soup (usually tomato) and garden salad with ranch dressing, Diet Coke
> Midafternoon: Yogurt
> Dinner: Pasta with marinara sauce, 8 ounces of sweetened iced tea
>
> ### Questions
> 1. Calculate Meg's calorie and macronutrient needs based on her pre-pregnancy weight.
> 2. Provide recommendations related to her laboratory values.
> 3. Assess Meg's diet recall. Can she meet her micronutrient requirements without a supplement?
> 4. How might you adjust her diet to improve her iron intake?

placenta. An extra 340 kcal/day in second trimester and an extra 452 kcal/day in third trimester are predicted estimates of energy to support metabolic changes and fetal growth.[1] The Food and Agriculture Organization (FAO), WHO, and United Nations University (UNU) advise that because some fat is deposited early during pregnancy and given that appetite and work requirements among women are variable, an average daily increase of 285 kcal/day throughout pregnancy is reasonable. Alternatively, 85 kcal/day extra in the first trimester, 285 kcal/day extra in second trimester, and 475 kcal/day extra in third trimester has also been recommended.[23] Calculating basal energy expenditure can be accomplished through the algorithms and stress factors such as Harris–Benedict or Mifflin–St. Jeor. The Academy of Nutrition and Dietetics suggests using the following equations for estimating estimated energy requirement (EER) according to trimester, age, weight, height and physical activity (PA)[1]:

- EER (Pre-Pregnancy/First Trimester):

    $354 - [(6.91 \times age) + (PA \times 9.36 \times weight (kg)) + (726 \times height (m))]$

- EER (Second Trimester):

    First trimester EER + 340

- EER (Third Trimester):

    First trimester EER + 452

With these recommendations at hand, clinicians can evaluate current intake behaviors and advise clients on methods to maintain appropriate weight gain. Patients can reference MyPlate for Pregnancy to receive additional resources for weight gain monitoring.

> ### CORE CONCEPT 10
> An extra 340 kcal/day in the second trimester and an extra 452 kcal/day in the third trimester are predicted estimates of energy to support metabolic changes and fetal growth.

> ### PRACTICE POINT
> Calculating basal energy expenditure can be accomplished through the algorithms and stress factors such as Harris–Benedict or Mifflin–St. Jeor.

Carbohydrate

A minimum of 175 g of carbohydrates per day is recommended to maintain sufficient glucose transport to the fetus as well as to fuel the mother. A goal of 45% to 65% of total calories should be consumed from high-fiber, low-glycemic carbohydrates.[1] In mothers with diabetes during pregnancy, the Academy of Nutrition and Dietetics (AND) recommends that less than 45% of calorie intake be from carbohydrates.[1] Dietary interventions are encouraged even if insulin therapy is deemed necessary, because poorly controlled blood glucose can lead to macrosomia.[1]

Protein

The fetus consumes about 1 kg of protein throughout the entire gestation period, a majority of which is consumed in the last two trimesters.[23] This increases maternal protein needs to 1.1 g/kg/day from the standard 0.8 g/kg/day for nonpregnant women. Additional protein needs for a pregnant woman are based on the amount of protein needed for initial expansion and maintenance of new maternal tissue.[23]

Lysine is one of the primary limiting amino acids in cereals and grains but is found in many high-protein food sources (dairy, meats, beans). During pregnancy, lysine is vital in the process of protein synthesis and is in increased demand.[23] When lysine is added to the diet of lower socioeconomic status mothers, fetal growth rates have been shown to improve.[23] Increasing protein intake by 1 g correlates with 8 to 16 g increase in birth weight.[45,46] This positive effect is compounded with consumption of dairy protein and was associated with a 25 g to 108 g increase in birth weight.[46,47]

CORE CONCEPT 11

Maternal protein needs increase to 1.1 g/kg/day from the standard 0.8 g/kg/day for nonpregnant women.

PRACTICE POINT

In mothers with diabetes during pregnancy, the Academy of Nutrition and Dietetics recommends that less than 45% of calorie intake be from carbohydrates.[1] Dietary interventions are encouraged even if insulin therapy is deemed necessary, because poorly controlled blood glucose can lead to macrosomia. When lysine is added to the diets of lower socioeconomic status mothers, fetal growth rates have been shown to improve.

Fat

Dietary fat consumed during pregnancy will serve as an important structural element for cell membranes and new tissues, construction of which is occurring rapidly during pregnancy. AND recommends that mothers-to-be eat 20% to 35% of their daily calories as fat.[1] The profile of fat intake, mainly in terms of saturated versus unsaturated, greatly influences adverse outcomes. Polyunsaturated fatty acids including linoleic acid (omega-6) and omega-3 (alpha-linolenic acid, eicosapentaenoic acid, and docosahexaenoic acid [DHA]) are essential in human development. They cannot be synthesized by the body, so the fetus must depend on the maternal stores for an adequate supply.[23] Higher intake of the long chain omega-3 fatty acids during pregnancy may increase duration of gestation and improve fetal growth.[23] While research is inconclusive regarding the risks of consuming high levels of omega-3 fatty acids—such as greater likelihood for LGA infants and longer pregnancy—it does suggest some maternal and fetal benefits to consuming an *adequate* amount of omega-3 fatty acids from food sources, including reduced inflammation and better fetal brain development.[24]

There may also be adverse consequences to inappropriate fat consumption. As mentioned, increased consumption of saturated fatty acids increases the risk of gestational diabetes as tissues become more resistant to insulin signals. Recommendations for the general population call for less than 10% of fat intake to come from saturated fat.[48] Trans fatty acids should be limited, because they are transported across the placenta proportional to maternal intake, and may cause adverse fetal side effects. This is potentially due to interference with essential fatty acid metabolism, effects on membrane structures or metabolism, or replacement of maternal intake of *cis* essential fatty acids. It is strongly recommended and supported by research that mothers-to-be strictly limit or avoid intake of trans fatty acids.

CORE CONCEPT 12

Avoidance or strict limitation of trans fatty acid during pregnancy is strongly recommended.

PRACTICE POINT

The Academy of Nutrition and Dietetics recommends that mothers-to-be eat 20% to 35% of their daily calories as fat. While research is inconclusive regarding the risks of consuming high levels of omega-3 fatty acids—such as greater likelihood of LGA infants and longer pregnancy—it does suggest some maternal and fetal benefits to consuming an **adequate** amount of omega-3 fatty acids from food sources, including reduced inflammation and better fetal brain development.

Vitamin D

Vitamin D is acquired both through diet or synthesized in the epidermis with exposure to ultraviolet-B (UVB) sunlight. During the summer, epidermal synthesis is usually sufficient to meet vitamin D recommendations. Adequate vitamin D may be difficult to meet during winter months, however, especially for women with darkly pigmented skin. During pregnancy, renal, placental, and endometrial synthesis of 1,25-dihydroxyvitamin D_3 ($1,25(OH)_2D_3$ or calcitriol) increases two-fold by the third trimester.[49] This leads to increased intestinal absorption and enhanced accumulation of calcium in the mother, meaning that both calcium and activated vitamin D can cross the placenta at nearly a 1:1 ratio with the mother's blood levels.

While vitamin D plays a major role in calcium absorption and possibly even immune function, vitamin D deficiency is becoming more prevalent. Pre-pregnancy obesity increases the risk of vitamin D deficiency due to the absorption and retention of serum vitamin D in the excess adipose tissue. Decreased sun exposure and inadequate consumption of source foods such as fatty fish are other reasons why deficiency is becoming commonplace.[42] Fetal and neonatal vitamin D status is dependent upon maternal vitamin D status, and poor vitamin D status during pregnancy can adversely affect the mother and fetus. Maternal vitamin D deficiency is associated with increased risks of preeclampsia, gestational diabetes, and recurrent miscarriages.[50] It also leads to fetal hypocalcemia during intrauterine growth and possibly causes adverse effects to neonatal bone metabolism, leading to rickets, growth retardation, skeletal deformities, and increased risk of fractures.[44,49] Inadequate vitamin D status in pregnancy has also been related to increased severity of respiratory tract infections in the first months of infancy and to the prevalence of type 1 diabetes in children.[51] In mothers, low (25-hydroxy vitamin D) ($25(OH)D_3$) status during pregnancy has been associated with early onset preeclampsia and preterm delivery.[51] Nevertheless, there are still limited data to support prophylactic vitamin D supplementation for the prevention of these complications.[49]

Although the prevalence of vitamin D deficiency is rising, exact vitamin D requirements during pregnancy remain inconclusive. As such, healthcare providers should frequently evaluate maternal vitamin D status through serum markers. Because $25(OH)D_3$ can be influenced by other external factors, parathyroid hormone (PTH) and ionized calcium may be measured as indicators of vitamin D status. PTH is a hormone secreted by the parathyroid gland in response to low serum calcium concentrations that stimulates production of ($1,25(OH)_2D_3$) by the kidneys. If vitamin D levels are low, PTH rises.[52] Serum levels of $25(OH)D_3$ are often the best indicators of vitamin D status. Women with one or more risk factors for vitamin D deficiency (residing in northern latitudes, having limited sun exposure, using sunscreen regularly, having dark skin, being obese, wearing extensive clothing coverage, or having a malabsorptive syndrome) should have vitamin D status checked at the beginning and middle of pregnancy.[53] If vitamin D supplementation is administered, $25(OH)D_3$ levels should be monitored every 3 months until within normal limits.[54] Current consensus defines serum $25(OH)D_3$ levels <30 nmol/L as insufficient and possibly deficient, 40 to 50 nmol/L as meeting average requirements, and ≥50 nmol/L as sufficient.[49] While there are no pregnancy-specific supplementation recommendations, these guidelines support daily intake of 400 international units (IU) or 10 micrograms vitamin D to achieve average serum requirements, although some mothers may need to increase their intake to 2,000 IU per day if deficient.[55]

> **PRACTICE POINT**
>
> Serum levels of $25(OH)D_3$, are often the best indicators of vitamin D status. While there are no pregnancy-specific supplementation recommendations, these guidelines support daily intake of 400 international units (IU) or 10 micrograms vitamin D to achieve average serum requirements, although some mothers may need to increase their intake to 2,000 IU per day if deficient.

Folate

The demand for folic acid increases during periods of rapid tissue growth, such as pregnancy. Insufficient intake is associated with low birth weight, IUGR, NTDs, and preterm birth.[23] All women of childbearing age are encouraged to consume 400 micrograms of folic acid supplements before, during, and after pregnancy to reduce the risk of NTDs like spina bifida.[30] Women with a history of NTDs in their family, or those with risk factors for NTDs such as pregestational diabetes or obesity, need an extra 4 mg of synthetic folic acid supplementation daily.[32,56]

Folate deficiency during pregnancy may present with signs of anemia, hyperpigmentation, and/or low-grade fever. If occurring simultaneously with a vitamin B_{12} deficiency, symptoms may include depression, dementia, and peripheral neuropathy.[34] If folate deficiency is suspected, diagnostic parameters are as follows[34]:

- Serum folate <2 micrograms/L
- Red blood cell folate <160 micrograms/L
- Homocysteine >15 micromoles/L

Low serum folate levels are indicative of folate deficiency, while high serum folate levels may indicate a risk of B_{12} deficiency. Low red blood cell folate concentration indicates depletion of the body's folate stores and, in the absence of B_{12} deficiency, suggests severe folate deficiency.[34]

> **PRACTICE POINT**
>
> If folate deficiency is suspected, diagnostic parameters are as follows:
>
> - Serum folate <2 micrograms/L
> - Red blood cell folate <160 micrograms/L
> - Homocysteine ≥15 micromoles/L

Vitamin B_{12}

Vitamin B_{12} is found exclusively in animal-derived products and plays an important part in red blood cell formation, DNA synthesis, and neurologic development.[34] During pregnancy, as vitamin B_{12} is transported to the placenta, serum levels of vitamin B_{12} steadily decrease until delivery, after which they rise to pre-pregnancy levels.[34] Signs of vitamin B_{12} deficiency during pregnancy include mental slowness, memory defects, hallucinations, and numbness or tingling in the extremities.[34] Maternal deficiency may adversely affect fetal growth and is associated with complications such as NTDs and delayed myelination or demyelination.[48]

It is estimated that the fetus requires 50 micrograms of vitamin B_{12} throughout pregnancy. Pre-pregnant women consuming a mixed diet containing animal products have stores >1000 micrograms.[57] Those following a vegan or strict vegetarian diet must supplement B_{12} during pregnancy and lactation to ensure adequate transfer to the fetus to reduce the risk of developmental delays.[32,44,56] However, vitamin B_{12} stores in women with a less-restrictive diet would not benefit from supplementation.[34] Prior to providing folate supplementation, vitamin B_{12} levels should be evaluated to

Clinical Roundtable

Vitamin D Supplementation during Pregnancy

Background: Knowledge of vitamin D's function in bone metabolism and cardiovascular, oncologic, endocrine, and immune health has expanded significantly. While vitamin D status is dependent upon geographical location, dietary intake, and genetic characteristics, insufficient vitamin D stores prior to pregnancy may lead to adverse outcomes in fetal growth, bone metabolism, and immune system development. In addition, further information regarding altered vitamin D metabolism during pregnancy is warranted, because this affects vitamin D requirements.

In general, vitamin D requirements throughout pregnancy are unknown. While the literature emphasizes the importance of maintaining adequate vitamin D status pre-pregnancy for fetal bone development, other potential benefits for the mother and fetus include prevention of gestational hypertension, preeclampsia, low birth weight, and preterm delivery.

The thresholds to monitor vitamin D status are varied. It is recommended that a serum value of 25(OH)D$_3$, vitamin D less than 30 nmol/L be used as the threshold for vitamin D deficiency. However, higher serum values are likely more beneficial during pregnancy. Serum values of 50 nmol/L are considered a sufficient cutoff. While supplementation of 400 IU (10 micrograms) of vitamin D$_3$ is shown to maintain maternal serum values >30 nmol/L, it is unknown whether it is adequate for fetal vitamin D availability. Cord blood concentrations at the time of delivery are about 60% to 80% of maternavl serum values. Mothers who maintain a serum value of >50 nmol/L with 1,000 IU (25 micrograms) per day of vitamin D$_3$ were able to sustain a serum value for their infant of at least 30 nmol/L. Supplementation above these doses is not strongly supported for preventing adverse pregnancy/birth outcomes.

No pregnancy-specific recommendations have been formulated. More research is needed for further support. The minimum supplementation dose to maintain adequate maternal stores is 400 IU (10 micrograms) of vitamin D$_3$ per day; however, a higher dose is likely warranted to prevent neonatal deficiency.

Discussion: Due to the lack of evidence of vitamin D in this population, vitamin D recommendations vary considerably. How should clinicians monitor vitamin D status and make recommendations for optimizing nutrition status during such a critical developmental period? What considerations might drive recommending minimum versus higher vitamin D supplementation?

References

1. Kiely M, Hemmingway A, O'Callaghan KM. Vitamin D in Pregnancy: Current Perspective and Future Directions. *Adv Musculoskelet Dis*. 2017;9(6):145-154. doi: 10.1177/175972X17706453.

---

avoid masking a vitamin B$_{12}$ deficiency. Activation of folate requires B$_{12}$, and folate supplementation increases the risk of masking signs and symptoms of B$_{12}$ deficiency.[34]

> **PRACTICE POINT**
>
> If vitamin B$_{12}$ deficiency is suspected, diagnostic parameters include the following[27,34,56]:
>
> - Complete blood count: macrocytic anemia
> - Plasma cobalamin: <130 pg/mL
> - Homocysteine >15 micromoles/L
> - Methylmalonic acid >0.56 micromoles/L

Iron

Iron's primary role is to deliver oxygen throughout the body via hemoglobin, but it is also involved in immune and enzyme functions. Females store 2 g of iron in the body on average, with 0.5 to 1.0 g stored as iron and 1.0 to 1.5 g as hemoglobin. Nutritional iron deficiency occurs most often in populations experiencing a peak rate of growth, such as infants, young children, and pregnant women.[23] During pregnancy there is increased production of red blood cells as blood volume expands, increasing iron needs to satisfy the demands of hemoglobin formation and increased needs of the fetus.[8]

In utero, the fetus is completely dependent upon the mother's intake, absorption, and storage of iron for its own metabolism and growth. It is estimated that 300 to 500 mg of iron is lost from the maternal liver as it is transferred across the placenta to the fetus.[58] There is an especially high risk of iron deficiency during pregnancy because iron needs are higher than the average absorption rates.[23] To prevent deficiency, a woman must add extra iron to her diet as well as maintain sufficient iron stores (equal to at least 500 mg) throughout pregnancy.[59] Insufficient intake of iron during pregnancy will result in a woman drawing from her own iron stores to supply the fetus with iron, possibly leading to maternal anemia and increased risk of low birth weight, preterm delivery, perinatal mortality, and impaired maternal–infant interaction.[1,23]

If a woman has iron-deficiency anemia when she conceives, repleting her iron stores during pregnancy will be somewhat difficult.[44,60] Increasing iron intake can be accomplished by consuming foods high in heme iron (such as red meat) or iron-fetal foods (such as some cereals) in combination with iron absorption enhancers like vitamin C–rich fruits and vegetables.[44] It is worth noting that recent research has indicated that even these dietary measures might not be sufficient to raise serum levels if the woman is obese.[61] However, it is unlikely that iron needs for any woman during pregnancy will be met through diet alone, and so iron supplementation should be taken to enhance fetal growth.[44,60] In nonpregnant females of childbearing age, the recommended dietary allowance of iron is 15 to 18 mg/day. The IOM recommends 27 mg/day for women with adequate iron status and the Centers for Disease Control and Prevention recommends 30 mg/day beginning at the first prenatal visit.[32] Anemia during pregnancy (evidenced by a hemoglobin <11 g/dL with hematocrit <33% in the first and third trimesters or less than 32% in the second trimester) has required management with 60 mg/day of oral iron along with consumption of iron-rich foods (red meat, clams, oysters, spinach, lentils, chickpeas, and fortified ready-to-eat cereals) to replete stores.[32] However, iron supplementation should be provided at a low dose without exceeding the upper limit of 45 mg/day.[35] Any increase in dosage should be based on maternal lab values.

> **CORE CONCEPT 13**
>
> It is unlikely that iron needs during pregnancy will be met through diet alone, and so iron supplementation should be taken to meet the recommendations and enhance fetal growth.

> **PRACTICE POINT**
>
> Anemia during pregnancy (evidenced by a hemoglobin <11 g/dL with hematocrit <33% in the first and third trimesters or less than 32% in the second trimester) has required management with 60 mg per day of oral iron along with consumption of iron-rich foods (red meat, clams, oysters, spinach, lentils, chickpeas, and fortified ready-to-eat cereals) to replete stores.

When screening for iron deficiency, serum markers are the best tools, because the patient may be asymptomatic. In a clinical setting, the following lab values will likely be checked routinely; monitoring them for inconsistencies and indicators of iron deficiency, however, can ensure that anemia is caught and treated early in pregnancy. Exact values will vary by hospital lab, but values will trend towards the following[34]:

- Hemoglobin: low
- Hematocrit: low
- Mean corpuscular volume: low
- Red cell distribution width: high

If the initial lab values are consistent with possible iron deficiency, proceed to screen the following lab values. These may also be checked initially if the patient presents with symptoms of clinical iron deficiency such as extreme fatigue, cold hands and feet, shortness of breath, chest pain, and/or headache. Lab values suggesting iron deficiency include the following[34]:

- Serum iron: low
- Serum ferritin: low
- Total iron binding capacity: high
- Transferrin: high

It is important to note that, due to pregnancy itself and iron supplementation, iron-deficiency anemia and folate or B_{12} deficiency lab values may give an unclear picture. In this case, the hematologic parameters above would not be sufficient to diagnose anemia. For example, during the third trimester, lower levels of folate, iron, and B12 are common.[27] Nutrition-focused physical findings that have the potential to detect moderate or severe anemia include pale mucosa under the tongue, palms, and nail bed.[34]

> **PRACTICE POINT**
>
> It is important to note that, due to pregnancy itself and iron supplementation, iron deficiency anemia and folate or B_{12} deficiency lab values may give an unclear picture.

Calcium

Calcium demands increase dramatically during pregnancy; however, the body accommodates these demands through doubling the efficiency of intestinal absorption and withdrawing calcium from maternal bone stores.[56] Calcium supplementation is therefore recommended for women with inadequate dietary calcium intake during pregnancy to maintain maternal bone density. Calcium supplementation in women with inadequate dietary intake may also reduce the risk of preeclampsia by preventing vasoconstriction, which is a possible result of low calcium levels.[62]

> **CORE CONCEPT 14**
>
> Key nutrients of concern during pregnancy, and those for which needs are increased, include folate, calcium, and iron.

Iodine

Iodine is a major component of thyroid hormones; serves a role in the growth, formation, and development of organs and tissues; and is especially important in early embryonic and fetal central nervous system development.[63] During pregnancy, maternal iodine is the only source for synthesis of fetal hormones, so inadequate iodine intake can result in adverse pregnancy outcomes such as spontaneous abortion, perinatal mortality, birth defect, and neurologic disorders.[64,65] It is important to note that altered maternal physiology, increased demand for iodine, and increased renal excretion of iodine all place the mother at an increased risk for deficiency.[63] It is recommended that adequate dietary iodine intake or supplementation of 220 micrograms per day be maintained pre-pregnancy and throughout the first trimester to ensure adequate development throughout the second trimester into the third year of life.[66] Prenatal multivitamins typically provide only 150 micrograms per serving. Additional iodine intake can be acquired through foods such as iodized table salt, milk, eggs, yogurt, cod, shrimp, and haddock.

Other Micronutrients

Practitioners generally recommend daily multivitamin supplementation during pregnancy to prevent inadequate micronutrient intake; however, the evidence to support this practice is not well documented, nor is it supported by research.[67] AND and the IOM recommend supplementation of a multivitamin only for women with iron-deficiency anemia; poor diet quality; vegan diet restrictions; multiple fetuses; or presence of alcohol, cigarette, or drug abuse.[1,67] The daily multivitamin should contain at least 30 mg iron, 250 mg calcium, and 0.6 mg folate. It should also provide enough to supplement and meet needs for vitamins A, B complex, E, C, and D, and zinc.

> **PRACTICE POINT**
>
> The Academy of Nutrition and Dietetics and the Institute of Medicine recommend supplementation of a multivitamin only for women with iron-deficiency anemia; poor diet quality; vegan diet restrictions; multiple fetuses; or presence of alcohol, cigarette, or drug abuse.

Physical Activity Recommendations

Physical activity activates **AMPK (adenosine monophosphate-activated protein kinase)**, an enzyme that increases the transport of glucose into the muscles, upregulates fat oxidation, and reduces insulin resistance and serum levels of inflammatory cytokines. When performed throughout gestation, it has been shown to reduce the risk of gestational diabetes and preeclampsia.[68,69] Physical activity can also decrease the intensity of two main components of metabolic syndrome—subclinical inflammation and insulin resistance—and help the mother to preserve her muscle mass and may even contribute to happiness and relaxation (**Figure 21.5**).[69,70] The American College of Obstetricians and Gynecologists recommends against exercise in the following specific circumstances: heart disease, restrictive respiratory diseases, if likely to give birth preterm, bleeding, placenta previa, premature labor, preeclampsia, hypertension, and clinically significant anemia.[69] Aerobic exercise might need to be modified or substituted if the mother is anemic; has a cardiac arrhythmia, chronic bronchitis, inadequately controlled type 1 diabetes mellitus, or morbid obesity; is very underweight (BMI <12); was very inactive/sedentary before pregnancy; experiences IUGR; has inadequately controlled hypertension, seizure disorder, or hyperthyroidism; is a heavy smoker; or has some kind of

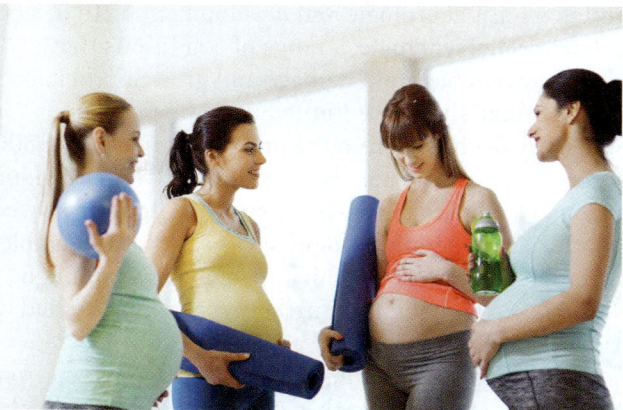

FIGURE 21.5 Low Impact Exercise Throughout Pregnancy is Associated with Reduced Insulin Resistance and Inflammation
© Syda Productions/Shutterstock.

physical disability or injury.[69] Most mothers, however, are able to exercise and will benefit from doing so.

There are limitations to physical activity during pregnancy due to the physical and physiologic changes that take place. For example, yoga and stretching that involves lying on the back or staying still for a long time can cause symptomatic hypotension, and anaerobic exercise will become extremely difficult; any of these exercises are inadvisable.[69] Given these considerations, any exercise regimen should be individually structured with regard to the patient's goals, physical conditioning, and general health, and be modified per a thorough physical examination by a physician.[69] Exercise should begin at a level of intensity, duration, and frequency that does not cause pain, shortness of breath, or excessive fatigue. In total, pregnant women should try to reach a minimum goal of 150 minutes of moderate-intensity, low-impact aerobic exercise every week, although higher intensity workouts are often permissible if the mother was very active prior to pregnancy.[1,69,71] The only forms of physical activity that should not be undertaken at all are sports in which the mother may fall or be hit (such as horseback riding, gymnastics, boxing, and basketball), scuba diving, sky diving, and heated stretching (such as hot yoga or hot Pilates).[69] Instead, activities such as walking, stationary bicycling, swimming, yoga or Pilates (when modified), jogging (depending on mother's fitness level) and strength training are good choices, paying particular attention to warm up, cool down, water intake, and body temperature.[69,71] Wearing light clothes and staying indoors when it is particularly warm or humid outside, as well as avoiding saunas after a workout, will ensure that the mother and fetus stay safe while exercising.[69]

Dietary Restrictions During Pregnancy

Because of the direct relationship between maternal intake and fetal supply, there are some foods that should be limited in the mother's diet during pregnancy. Alcohol, for example, should not be consumed by pregnant women or women who might become pregnant because it is strongly correlated with neurologic and development birth defects like **fetal alcohol syndrome**, a range of conditions that include irreversible brain damage and growth problems.[1] Caffeine intake should be limited to no more than 200 mg/day (a change from the previous guideline of 300 mg), because caffeine metabolism slows during pregnancy, which can lead to maternal discomfort.[1] Alternative sweeteners that are generally recognized as safe are acceptable to consume in moderation during pregnancy, although AND does recommend that further research be carried out for nondiabetic mothers.[1,44]

Other dietary restrictions during pregnancy result from concern for the mother's weakened immune system, which puts her and her fetus at higher risk of developing a food-borne illness.[72] Foods to avoid include soft cheeses made with unpasteurized milk (feta, queso, blanco, brie), cold-smoked fish, cold deli salads, hot dogs, luncheon meats, bologna (unless reheated to steaming hot), raw or unpasteurized milk or milk products, raw or partially cooked eggs, raw or undercooked meat and poultry, unpasteurized juice, raw sprouts, and raw or undercooked fish and shellfish.[32,72] Some fish products contain high levels of mercury, which can be toxic to the fetus, and include shark, marlin, orange roughy, swordfish, king mackerel, bigeye tuna, and tilefish from the Gulf of Mexico.[73] It is important to note that the U.S. Food and Drug Administration recommends eating 2-3 servings weekly from the "best choices" list which includes fish lower in mercury, such as shrimp, canned light tuna, salmon, pollock, and tilapia, among others, which are safe and provide high-quality protein for the mother.[73] Alternatively, one serving per week can be consumed from the "good choices" list which includes Albacore tuna, halibut, and striped bass, among others. These fish should be limited to once weekly due to their higher mercury content.[73]

Food Cravings and Aversions

Food cravings and aversions are commonly reported during pregnancy. In general, food aversions include alcohol, coffee, fried foods, meat, and eggs, while dairy, citrus fruit, pickles, and sweet foods are the most common cravings. It is not proven that these symptoms necessarily have a deleterious effect on the quality of diet during pregnancy.[72] The exception to this rule is **pica**, a condition in which the mother craves clay and dirt (**geophagia**, literally "eat earth"); ice (**pacophagia**); and even soap, chalk, wood ash, cornstarch and baking soda—all of which can be symptoms of nutrient deficiency or pollutants.[72]

Gastroenterologic Symptoms During Pregnancy

As discussed in the section on physiologic changes, there are several gastroenterologic symptoms a mother can experience during pregnancy due to hormonal changes that relax gastrointestinal muscles.

Gastroesophageal reflux

The hormonal changes during pregnancy that relax the gastrointestinal tract musculature in turn cause the loosening of the lower esophageal sphincter. This increases the risk for gastroesophageal reflux, or "heartburn," leading up to 45% of mothers reporting this symptom.[72] Avoiding "trigger foods" to reduce stomach acid production will help to prevent this painful condition. Trigger foods to avoid will differ for every individual, but common items include coffee (caffeinated and decaffeinated), red and black pepper, alcohol, and chocolate. In addition, foods that are high in fat, mint, or carbonation may exacerbate symptoms and should be limited or eliminated. Consuming small, frequent meals throughout the day may also alleviate symptoms, because large meals typically stimulate acid-producing cells as well as delaying gastric emptying. Not lying down after eating, and not eating 3 to 4 hours before going to bed, will also prevent reflux.[72] Other common treatments include non-mint chewing gum to increase saliva, calcium-based antacids, and limiting saturated fat in the diet.

Constipation

The relaxation of gastrointestinal muscles slows the transit time of stool through the colon, which in turn increases fluid losses from the stool, leading to constipation. Regular iron supplementation, which is recommended during pregnancy, can also cause constipation. Maintaining adequate intake of fiber (a recommended 25-35 g/day) and fluid may relieve symptoms, as will light exercise.[72] If it remains unresolved, the patient should discuss options with his or her physician, such as using a laxative or stool softener to aid with bowel movements.[8]

Nausea and Vomiting

Nausea and vomiting are reported by 75% of mothers, although the onset, duration, and extremity of these symptoms differs between women.[72] It is thought to be caused by high levels of hCG from the placenta, estrogen, reduced stomach acidity, and lowered tone and motility of the digestive tract.[8] Strategies to resolve these symptoms are individual to each woman, but are generally similar to those for preventing heartburn: smaller, more frequent meals and avoiding trigger foods. Many women find themselves getting nauseated if they go too long without eating and their stomach remains empty, so keeping small snacks and meals on hand at all times may be a successful solution. Cold foods are also commonly recommended, as are protein-rich snacks.[74]

Nutrition Therapy in Unique Pregnancies

Teenage Pregnancies

Pregnancy during adolescence (ages 13-19 years) has a number of social consequences for the mother, but evidence now suggests that teenage pregnancy also has numerous negative physical effects on the mother and fetus because the mother too is not yet fully developed.[75] Many of these issues, such as SGA size and higher miscarriage and infant mortality rates, can be traced to nutritional inadequacies.[75] As such, it is important to monitor teenage mothers closely for deficiencies in all nutrients as early as possible.

As in adult women, pre-pregnancy weight is important to the success of an adolescent pregnancy. Reducing the risk of low birth weight while simultaneously preventing postpartum weight retention is problematic in overweight, pregnant teenagers. Teenagers who become pregnant should therefore use the adult BMI categories to determine their weight gain range until more research is done to determine whether special categories are needed for them.[2]

Multiple Pregnancy

Multiple pregnancy, or having more than one fetus in the uterus during the same pregnancy, has become more common, as women are delaying pregnancy until age 35 years and must then rely more on in vitro fertilization treatments.[76] During multiple pregnancy, there is an even greater increase in maternal tissue mass required, which further increases fetal demands on maternal nutrition resources and reserves. This can often lead to preterm delivery and a higher risk of postpartum hemorrhage, thereby putting physical stress on both mother and infant.[76] Rates of preeclampsia, gestational diabetes, and infant respiratory distress syndrome are also more common in multiple pregnancy, as are iron deficiency anemia and kidney disease.[77,78]

> **CORE CONCEPT 15**
>
> During a multiple pregnancy, there is an even greater increase in maternal tissue mass required, which further increases fetal demands on maternal nutrition resources and reserves.

Because the majority of multiple pregnancies are delivered early by 4 to 12 weeks, the fetus has less time provided for intrauterine growth.[79] Providing adequate nutritional supply and stores prior to and during pregnancy is important. As in singleton pregnancies, the glycogen utilization increases in multiple pregnancies. However, with multiple pregnancies there is also an increased glycogen store depletion rate, increasing the metabolism of fat stores between meals and during overnight fasts. This could potentially lead to ketonuria, a further risk factor for preterm delivery. Some researchers have found success with intake regimens consisting of 40% low-glycemic carbohydrate foods, 20% protein, and 40% fat to better control serum glucose levels.[79]

As mentioned earlier in this chapter, maternal weight gain during singleton and multiple pregnancies is a strong indicator of birth outcome. These weight gain goals are based upon pre-pregnancy BMI. In the case of pregnancy with twins, the IOM recommends the following weight gain goals for each BMI category[2]:

- Normal: 37 to 54 lbs
- Overweight: 31 to 50 lbs
- Obese: 25 to 42 lbs

In general, the ideal weight gain for twins is 35 to 45 pounds.[80] While there are insufficient data to determine standardized weight gain recommendations for pregnancies of triplets and greater, 50 lbs or more is the typical goal.[78,81]

The rate of weight gain is important in regard to birth outcome. In singleton pregnancies, the majority of gestational weight gain should begin during the second trimester, because first trimester calorie needs are not increased. In multiple pregnancies, however, early weight gain before 20 to 24 weeks is beneficial.[76] This is partly due to the expectation of an overall shorter gestational period and likelihood of preterm delivery. In general, mothers of twins or other multiples should aim to gain up to 3.2 kg (7 lbs) in the first trimester; in the latter half of pregnancy, she should be gaining up to 0.9 kg (about 2 lbs) every week.[78] The peak rate of growth in multiple pregnancies occurs at 31 weeks' gestation, compared to 33 weeks' gestation in singleton pregnancies. Early weight gain is also recommended because the placenta ages more rapidly during multiple pregnancies, which shortens the period of time that it most effectively transfers nutrient to the fetus.[79]

This substantial weight gain in multiple gestations accounts for the increased energy demands of two or more fetuses. An estimated 150 kcal/day over singleton pregnancy energy needs (450 kcal more than a nonpregnant woman) is necessary during this period of gestation.[78] Estimated calorie needs are 3,000 kcal for obese and 4,000 kcal for underweight women carrying more than one fetus.[44] Estimated energy needs are based on pre-pregnancy weight, and follow the trend outlined in **Table 21.3**.[82]

In the case of multiple pregnancies, 500 calories/day should be added to estimated energy needs. As discussed, multiple pregnancies typically deliver preterm, so providing adequate nutrition for maximum growth is the goal.[82] Given that multiple fetuses require a significantly more tissue and DNA synthesis than a single fetus, protein intake should also be increased, adding an additional 50 g/day at the beginning of the second trimester to the singleton pregnancy standard.[83]

Because iron deficiency is common in multiple pregnancy, iron supplementation at 30 mg per day is recommended to maintain iron maternal stores and fetal supply.[84] Folate supplementation is recommended at a level of

TABLE 21.3 ESTIMATED ENERGY NEEDS BASED ON PRE-PREGNANCY WEIGHT IN MULTIPLE PREGNANCIES

Percent Ideal Body Weight	Energy Needs
100-120% (Normal)	30 kcal/kg
>120% (Overweight, Obese)	24 kcal/kg
<90% (Underweight)	36-40 kcal/kg

Data from Marcason W. What Are the Calorie Requirements for Women Having Twins?. *J Am Diet Assoc*. 2006;106(8):1292. doi: http://dx.doi.org.ezproxy.library.tufts.edu/10.1016/j.jada.2006.06.023.

1,000 micrograms (1 mg) of folic acid daily throughout twin pregnancy.[84] Maintaining adequate consumption of essential fatty acids through sources such as sunflower, safflower, corn and soybean oil; fatty fish; egg yolk; and spinach is vital for fetal neurologic and visual development; the recommended level is 300 to 500 mg of omega-3 fatty acids per day.[84,85] In addition to intake of adequate calories, women pregnant with multiple fetuses should ensure that their diet meets the following micronutrient requirements: 14 to 45 mg zinc (15 mg in first trimester, 30 mg in last two trimesters), 2 mg copper, 1,500 to 2,500 mg calcium, 1,000 mg folic acid, 500 to 1,000 mg vitamin C, 400 IU vitamin E, 1,000 IU vitamin D, and 60 mg of iron in the second and third trimesters.[84,85] Supplements may be required.

> **PRACTICE POINT**
>
> In multiple pregnancies, early weight gain before 20 to 24 weeks is beneficial.

Pregnancy Following Bariatric Surgery

With the current obesity epidemic, there have been an increased number of bariatric surgeries performed. Weight loss from surgery can improve fertility, regulate menstrual cycles and hormone levels, and work in favor of pregnancy. However, 80% of individuals receiving bariatric surgery as a treatment for obesity are of childbearing age.[42] Due to the many physiologic changes that occur in the body that affect metabolism, micro- and macronutrient status, and the increased nutritional demand of the mother during gestation, there are concerns about pregnancy following bariatric surgery.

Most weight loss occurs 12 months post–bariatric surgery.[86] Although this weight loss decreases the risk of the adverse fetal outcomes associated with obesity, it is highly recommended to prevent pregnancy until weight stabilizes, usually around 12 to 18 months postsurgery.[87] This is due to the high likelihood of vomiting, malabsorption of nutrients, and inadequate pregnancy weight gain during pregnancy.[42,70,86] Patients who undergo bariatric surgery (sleeve gastrectomy, gastric banding, or roux-en Y gastric bypass) should supplement vitamins and minerals daily due to the altered physiology of their gastrointestinal tract with multivitamins (200% Dietary Reference Intake) containing iron, folic acid, selenium, zinc, vitamin D, calcium citrate, and vitamin B_{12}.[86] These will also serve to build up a good prenatal foundation.

If a woman does conceive postsurgery and intake is inadequate during pregnancy, nutritional deficiencies can ensue and affect maternal and fetal health and birth outcome.[86] Infants of roux-en-Y gastric bypass mothers are already at increased risk for SGA birth weight, possibly due to these common deficiencies and low intake.[88] Anemia is a particularly common complication of the roux-en-Y gastric bypass procedure, with iron deficiency as the most common etiology.[86] With dramatically increased iron needs during pregnancy and a high rate of iron deficiency among pregnant women with no history of bariatric surgery, clinicians must be vigilant in monitoring for iron deficiency during pregnancy post–bariatric surgery. Monitor parameters for nutritional status post-surgery and throughout pregnancy. Appropriate serum markers include iron studies; vitamin B_{12}/methylmalonic acid; folate/red blood cell folate; calcium/ionized calcium; $25(OH)D_3$ vitamin D and vitamins A, E, and K.[87] Patients should also be referred to an obstetrician specializing in high-risk pregnancies.[70]

> **CORE CONCEPT 16**
>
> Although bariatric surgery's induction of weight loss decreases the risk of the adverse fetal outcomes associated with obesity, it is highly recommended that pregnancy be prevented until weight stabilizes, usually around 12 to 18 months postsurgery.

Nutritional Management of Preexisting Diseases in Pregnancy

Eating Disorders During Pregnancy

The most common cause of inadequate energy intake (or indeed energy supply from the body itself) during pregnancy is a maternal eating disorder. According to the National Eating Disorder Association (NEDA), the increased calorie and weight requirements in pregnancy can be a source of anxiety to women with anorexia nervosa or bulimia nervosa, and women in both groups may attempt to offset these requirements by eating too little or purging (vomiting or taking laxatives). Eating disorders during pregnancy can cause numerous other issues aside from insufficient energy to the fetus, including dehydration, electrolyte imbalances, gestational diabetes, cardiac arrhythmias, and severe depression. If the eating disorder cannot be managed and the mother does not intake enough nutrients to supply the fetus there is a high risk of preterm birth, fetal developmental issues, SGA birth weight, and difficulty breathing after delivery. Providers must try to be empathetic when working with mothers with eating disorders by simply listening and providing education or being sensitive to discussions around weight. NEDA suggests weighing mothers backwards (facing away from the scale or digital screen) so that they feel more comfortable, and discussing positive points such as "The baby is growing well" rather than telling the patient her exact weight.[89]

Diabetes (Nongestational)

The presence of type 1 or type 2 diabetes mellitus during the pre-gestational period should be addressed when performing a pregnancy assessment. Poor glucose control or hyperinsulinemia can increase the risk of birth defects and stillbirths.[90] As maternal insulin resistance increases with pregnancy, poor control of blood glucose increases the risk of adverse outcomes in birth weight, infant body composition, and fetal growth. The American Diabetes Association recommends that a diabetic mother check her blood sugar as often as 10 times per day, both before conception and during pregnancy, to ensure she is not hypoglycemic at any time.[90]

Hyperglycemia, however, may be nearly as damaging as hypoglycemia. Elevated serum glucose levels expose the fetus to all major fuel sources—glucose, free fatty acids, ketones, and amino acids—increasing the risk of an LGA infant at birth.[22] As the degree of maternal insulin resistance worsens, the increased fetal glucose supply stimulates fetal insulin release and storage of excess glucose as fat. This phenomenon results in **asymmetric macrosomia**, defined as a high fetal fat relative to fetal length.[22] An elevated HbA1c reflective of persistently high glucose levels, is associated with altered fetal growth patterns by favoring adipogenesis over chondrogenesis (the formation of cartilage). Exposed fetuses demonstrate decreased occipito–frontal diameter, relatively long upper limbs compared to lower limbs, and reduced limb length compared to limb circumference.[22] Many congenital malformations may occur in infants born to mothers with uncontrolled diabetes in the first few weeks of pregnancy.[44]

Dietary management is key for nongestational diabetes mellitus during pregnancy. Medical nutrition therapy provided by an RD and ideally a certified diabetes educator, should be scheduled. Strategies to maintain adequate blood glucose levels include consuming high-fiber, low-glycemic carbohydrates; limiting simple sugars such as cookies and cakes; eliminating sugar-sweetened beverages such as soda and juice; and avoiding concentrated sweets, such as fruit, in the early hours. To reduce the stress on the pancreas (type 2 diabetes mellitus) and improve the control of blood glucose (type 1 diabetes mellitus), maintaining consistent carbohydrate is recommended; diabetic mothers should consume consistent carbohydrate individualized as per their usual intake aiming for 40-55% of total calories from carbohydrates.[91] Keeping daily food records paired with self-monitoring of blood glucose (SMBG) should be encouraged to help determine issue foods that may cause spikes or lows in blood sugar levels. If the mother is experiencing hyperglycemia between 3 am and 5 am (before breakfast), this is likely a result of poor insulin management or high carbohydrate intake before bed. If the mother experiences a normoglycemia between 3 am and 5 am but hyperglycemia before breakfast, this is likely due to a surge of regulatory hormones such as growth hormone that occurs overnight and results in the "dawn phenomenon." In both instances, the protein-to-carbohydrate ratio at dinner can be increased to optimize blood glucose control. If taking insulin, this can be adjusted to attenuate the surge of hormones overnight.[92]

TABLE 21.4 GOALS FOR HbA1c DURING PREGNANCY

HbA1c	Preprandial/Fasting Blood Glucose	Postprandial Blood Glucose
<7	60-99 mg/dL	100-129 mg/dL
≥7	60-79 mg/dL	90-109 mg/dL

Data from Joslin Diabetes Center and Joslin Clinic. Guideline for Detection and Management of Diabetes in Pregnancy. 2010.

For women with preexisting diabetes, SMBG and testing of urine ketones at home should be practiced. This includes checking glucose levels preprandially and 1 hour postprandially, and checking fasting urine ketones daily. Because of the high risk of adverse effects to the fetus, blood glucose control is managed much more tightly during pregnancy than during normal adulthood. The goals of blood glucose management are based upon HbA1c readings; **Table 21.4** shows standard goals for HbA1c during pregnancy.[91]

Avoiding episodes of hypoglycemia (<60 mg/dL) is critical to maintaining adequate supply of glucose to the fetus. In the presence of a blood glucose level <60 mg/dL, utilize the 15-15 rule: provide 15 g of simple carbohydrate and recheck blood glucose levels in 15 minutes. If serum level remains below 60 mg/dL, repeat the 15-15 rule.[91]

> **CORE CONCEPT 17**
>
> Avoiding episodes of hypoglycemia (<60 mg/dL) is critical to maintaining adequate supply of glucose to the fetus.

> **PRACTICE POINT**
>
> The American Diabetes Association recommends that a diabetic mother check her blood sugar as often as 10 times per day, both before conception and during pregnancy, to ensure she is not hypoglycemic at any time. To reduce the stress on the pancreas (type 2 diabetes mellitus) and improve the control of blood glucose (type 1 diabetes mellitus), maintaining a consistent carbohydrate intake is recommended. In the presence of a blood glucose level <60 mg/dL, utilize the 15-15 rule: provide 15 g of simple carbohydrate and recheck blood glucose levels in 15 minutes. If serum level remains below 60 mg/dL, repeat the 15-15 rule.

HIV Infection

During pregnancy, there is a certain degree of normal physiologic immunosuppression that occurs to protect the fetus from maternal antibodies. Pregnancies complicated by human immunodeficiency virus (HIV) infection are defined as high-risk pregnancies because the virus increases this degree of immunosuppression and makes it difficult to treat any infections that occur, as well as increasing the maternal basal metabolic rate and making it more difficult to gain adequate weight.[93,94] Other nutrition-related risk factors such as poor prenatal care, poverty, and poor nutrition increases risk of the infant for IUGR, prematurity, low birth weight, and infection.[8,95] In general, nutrition status can be compromised during illness due to the associated effects of the infection; however, women with HIV are at much higher risk of malnutrition and deficiency and so need to be monitored closely.[95]

Iron is a particularly important micronutrient in HIV-positive pregnancies. The virus causes iron to accumulate in the macrophage cells of the immune system, usually clustering in the bone marrow, and leading either to abnormally high stored iron levels or to anemia.[96] The purpose of this "iron-loading" is to fuel various transcription factors that will help to reproduce and spread the HIV virus throughout the body.[96] As such, it is important to screen and monitor iron status in HIV-positive mothers prior to recommending iron supplementation and to check iron studies frequently throughout pregnancy. In the presence of elevated iron stores, reduction of iron intake can be accomplished through decreasing intake of high-iron foods such as red meat, legumes, dark leafy greens, and oysters and reducing or eliminating iron supplementation.[94]

Vitamin A deficiency is a major cause of xerophthalmia, night blindness, and anemia. This fat-soluble vitamin is essential for immune function and mucosal integrity, and during fetal development it is also involved in organogenesis, limb formation, and body symmetry.[97] The risk of vitamin A deficiency is increased during high-risk pregnancy. In the presence of HIV, vitamin A deficiency is associated with infant mortality, but supplementation has proven beneficial in reducing this adverse outcome and improving birth weight and growth among infants.[56,94] Excess supplementation should be avoided due to the teratogenic effects of vitamin A toxicity, and as such beta carotene is often the preferred supplemental form for pregnant women.[56]

As mentioned, individuals with HIV are at an increased risk of muscle wasting and overall poor nutrition status.[95] Daily prenatal multivitamin or micronutrient supplementation is recommended in all women with HIV during pregnancy to improve maternal and neonatal status. Due to the increased immunosuppression with HIV, these women also have an increased vulnerability to foodborne illness; emphasize avoidance of raw or undercooked foods and following food safety rules.[94] RDs should also be aware that certain medications for HIV can cause gastrointestinal discomfort, so encourage eating patterns that accommodate these symptoms, such as small, frequent meals and avoiding trigger foods.[94]

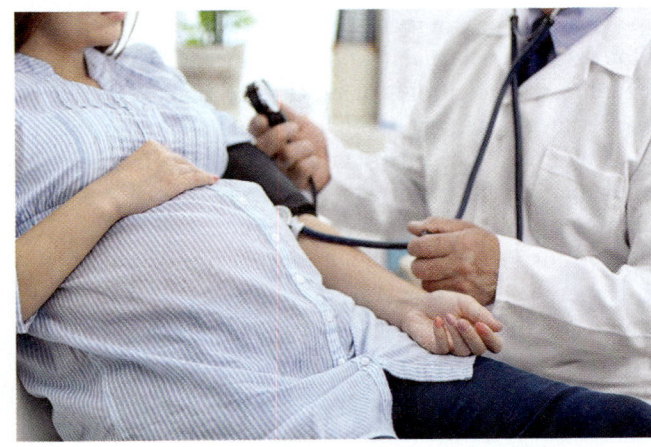

FIGURE 21.6 Due to the Hematological and Physical Changes that Take Place During Pregnancy, Certain Pregnancy-induced Conditions May Develop
© Africa Studio/Shutterstock.

Pregnancy-Induced Diseases

Physiologic Anemia of Pregnancy

Due to the hematologic changes that take place during pregnancy, **physiologic anemia of pregnancy** is likely to develop (**Figure 21.6**).[14] As discussed previously, red blood cell numbers increase during pregnancy to provide adequate oxygenation throughout the body. In turn, there is a greater increase in plasma volume due to fluid and sodium retention, causing a dilution effect. This is reflected in a decrease of serum hemoglobin and hematocrit.[8] The steepest reduction is within the first 20 to 24 weeks of gestation, which may be attributed to physiologic effects of pregnancy.[34,98]

During pregnancy, a hemoglobin level <11 g/dL is defined as moderate anemia, while a hemoglobin <7 g/dL is defined as severe anemia.[34] Both may be associated with increased risk of low birth weight, maternal and child mortality, and infectious diseases.[59] The most common cause of anemia during pregnancy is iron deficiency, although vitamin B_{12} deficiency and folate deficiency are also common anemic conditions.[34]

Factors increasing the risk of physiologic anemia of pregnancy include multiple pregnancy, teenage pregnancy, and high parity.[34] Prior to treating any form of anemia, the underlying cause should be identified.[34] See the Micronutrients section for screening parameters for iron, folate, and vitamin B_{12}.

> **CORE CONCEPT 18**
>
> During pregnancy, a hemoglobin level of <11 g/dL is defined as moderate anemia, while a hemoglobin level <7 g/dL is defined as severe anemia.

Hyperemesis Gravidarum

Nausea and vomiting of pregnancy (NVP) affects nearly 70% to 85% of all pregnancies.[99,100] A more severe form of NVP is termed **hyperemesis gravidarum (HG)**, defined

> **CASE STUDY REVISITED**
>
> Recall Meg's symptoms upon her hospital admission.
>
> ### Questions
> 1. Is Meg's presentation of symptoms consistent with that of HG?
> 2. Do you think that Meg's symptoms of confusion are related to Wernicke's encephalopathy?
> 3. What intervention would you first recommend prior to authorizing nutrition support?

as persistent nausea and vomiting resulting in dehydration, muscle wasting, electrolyte imbalances, ketonuria, nutritional deficiencies, and weight loss of greater than 5% of pre-pregnancy weight.[99,100] The symptoms of HG affect an average of 0.3% to 2.3% of pregnancies; they begin between the 4th and 10th weeks and typically resolve by 20 weeks of gestation, although they may not subside until delivery.[99,101] The effects of HG increase the risk of preterm delivery for the mother and fetus potentially due to inadequate maternal weight gain. Therefore, it is vital to intervene when pregnant women experience these symptoms in order to prevent complications and adverse outcomes.[102] As a result of untreated electrolyte imbalance, malnutrition, and maternal weight loss during pregnancy, infants delivered in a pregnancy complicated by HG may suffer from premature birth, low birth weight, in utero hemorrhage, and failure of the testes to descend.[99,101]

Related Nutritional Issues and Therapy Women suffering from HG are susceptible to a number of serious nutritional side effects. The hypermetabolic state of pregnancy causes increased glucose metabolism and increases the risk of thiamin deficiency in HG.[103] Thiamin, or vitamin B_1, is a key factor in the oxidation of glucose to provide energy; as a water-soluble vitamin stored in the liver, the body can only store up to 30 mg of thiamin.[104] In the presence of starvation, severe malnutrition, or severe vomiting or diarrhea, thiamine stores may deplete, leading insulin levels to drop, gluconeogenesis to stop, and amino acids and adipose tissue to become primary sources of energy.

> **CORE CONCEPT 19**
>
> In the presence of starvation, severe malnutrition, or severe vomiting or diarrhea, thiamin stores may deplete, leading insulin levels to drop, gluconeogenesis to stop, and amino acids and adipose tissue to become primary sources of energy.

> **PRACTICE POINT**
>
> The hypermetabolic state during pregnancy causes increased glucose metabolism and increases the risk of thiamin deficiency in HG.

Once glucose is reintroduced, usually in the form of enteral or parental support in cases of poor intake with HG, insulin levels rise dramatically, resulting in an influx of glucose into the cells and increased utilization of electrolytes and thiamine for metabolic processes. If glucose is introduced too quickly, this will exacerbate symptoms of refeeding syndrome. This presents clinically as a drop in serum values of all electrolytes—calcium, magnesium, sodium, potassium, and phosphorus—and symptoms may be neurologic (confusion, seizures, or coma), urologic (compromised renal function), respiratory (respiratory failure), or cardiovascular (tachyarrhythmias, bradyarrhythmias, or cardiac failure).[105] Feeding of glucose before thiamine repletion will also exacerbate Wernicke's encephalopathy, resulting in neurologic, ocular, and musculoskeletal changes (**Table 21.5**). Magnetic resonance imaging of the brain may reveal complications such as central pontine myelinolysis. Repletion of thiamine is recommended in any pregnant patient with 2 weeks or more of emesis prior to administration of glucose. Thiamine repletion should be initiated prior to administration of glucose at a dose of 200 to 300 mg

TABLE 21.5 SIGNS AND SYMPTOMS OF WERNICKE'S ENCEPHALOPATHY

Ocular Signs	Horizontal nystagmus
	Bilateral paralysis of lateral rectus muscles of the eye
Neurologic	Global confusion
	Inattention
	Disorientation
Musculoskeletal	Ataxia/leg tremors

Data from Kumar D, Geller F, Wang L, Wagner B, Fitz-Gerald MJ, Schwendimann R. Wernicke's encephalopathy in a patient with HG. *Psychosomatics*. 2012;53(2):172-174. doi: 10.1016/j.psym.2011.06.005; 10.1016/j.psym.2011.06.005.

intravenously or enterally daily for the first 10 days of feeding.[106] If Wernicke's encephalopathy is suspected, provide 200 to 300 mg thiamin IV three times daily until there is no further improvement in symptoms.[107,108] Intravenous fluids should be administered to replenish fluid lost and restore electrolyte balance. Normal saline or lactated Ringer's solution may be administered with potassium chloride added as needed.[99]

When assessing patients with HG and determining a management plan, realize that each woman differs in hormone levels and reactions to different foods. Developing an effective management plan for HG may take time and dedication from the patient and RD. The overall goal of treatment for HG is fluid maintenance, electrolyte balance, adequate calorie intake, and symptom control.[110] The patient should be assessed for degree of HG. Assessment of pregnancy weight changes are most effective in identifying the degree of illness, and should be evaluated after the fluid resuscitation needed to treat the increased risk of dehydration from persistent vomiting.[103] Assessing the urine for the presence of ketones is also important, because ketones may cross the placenta and impair fetal neuropsychologic development.[103]

> **CORE CONCEPT 20**
>
> The overall goal of treatment for HG is fluid maintenance, electrolyte balance, adequate calorie intake, and symptom control.

> **PRACTICE POINT**
>
> Assessment of pregnancy weight changes are most effective in identifying the degree of illness, and should be evaluated after the fluid resuscitation needed to treat the increased risk of dehydration from persistent vomiting.[103] Assessing the urine for the presence of ketones is also important, because ketones may cross the placenta and impair fetal neuropsychologic development.

To alleviate symptoms of HG, it may be effective to consume smaller, more frequent meals that are higher in protein and carbohydrates and lower in fat every 1 to 2 hours. This will prevent an empty stomach, feelings of hunger, low blood sugar, and gastric distention, all of which can cause nausea and vomiting during pregnancy. If the mother notices that certain foods trigger symptoms, these foods should be eliminated throughout gestation. Providing liquid nutritional supplements or meal replacement formulas can be an effective strategy to provide adequate nutrient intake for women struggling to consume solid foods. Clinicians should encourage adequate hydration, especially for women who are vomiting frequently. Cold fluids between meals may also be helpful in reducing symptoms.[99,100] These general dietary recommendations should be trialed by each patient experiencing symptoms of HG, due to the individuality of food and odor aversions that occur during pregnancy.

If dietary management is not effective in reducing symptoms, other means of treatment of HG, such as antiemetics, hypnosis, or acupuncture, should be considered. Various antiemetics that may be effective but shown not to cause adverse birth outcomes include vitamin B_6 (up to 200 mg/day), ginger (up to 1,000 mg/day), imenhydrinate (IV), doxylamine succinate, metoclopramide, promethazine, prochlorperazine, chlorpromazine, ondansetron, droperidol, and trimethobenzamide.[99,100] Promethazine is recommended by American Congress of Obstetricians and Gynecologists.[99] Steroids, such as methylprednisolone, may be used after all other causes of vomiting have been excluded, vomiting has continued after the first trimester and is associated with dehydration, and the risks and benefits of the treatment have been explained.[99,100]

If the woman has undergone therapies to manage HG through dietary changes and/or antiemetics that were unsuccessful at relieving symptoms, nutrition support via enteral nutrition (EN) or parenteral nutrition (PN) is indicated to ensure adequate nutrition supply to the fetus. EN is useful for patients whose nausea and vomiting are associated with visual cues, food aromas, and flavors that stimulate salivary and gastric secretions that induce nausea and vomiting.[103] PN via a central catheter or peripherally inserted central catheter (PICC) is useful for patients with severe HG or lack of absorption who are intolerant of oral and enteral feedings. (See Nutrition Support section for further recommendations.)

> **PRACTICE POINT**
>
> To alleviate symptoms of HG, it may be effective to consume smaller, more frequent meals that are higher in protein and carbohydrates and lower in fat every 1 to 2 hours. These general dietary recommendations should be trialed by each patient experiencing symptoms of HG, due to the individuality of food and odor aversions that occur during pregnancy.

Gestational Diabetes

To accommodate the increased glucose demand of the fetus during pregnancy, the mother experiences some insulin resistance to ensure adequate glucose delivery across the placenta. **Gestational diabetes mellitus (GDM)** is defined as increased glucose intolerance that is first discovered during the second or third trimester; such symptoms in the first trimester are now considered to be due to standard type 2 diabetes mellitus.[111] While the exact etiology of GDM is unknown, it is possibly related to the hormonal changes that occur in pregnancy and how each woman's body responds physiologically. Other risk factors for GDM include obesity, a diet high in saturated fat, personal history of GDM, delivery of a previous LGA infant, glycosuria, polycystic ovary syndrome, or strong family history of diabetes.[44,72,111]

> **CORE CONCEPT 21**
>
> Gestational diabetes mellitus (GDM) is defined as increased glucose intolerance that is first discovered during the second or third trimester; such symptoms in the first trimester are now considered to be due to standard type 2 diabetes mellitus.

As insulin sensitivity of peripheral tissues decreases, all pregnant women will experience some degree of insulin resistance and hyperinsulinemia. If the woman's pre-pregnancy weight is considered overweight or obese, a greater degree of hyperinsulinemia will occur to enhance maternal use of fat stores as fuel. This is clinically evident through the dyslipidemia and most notably very elevated low-density lipoprotein levels during pregnancy.[70] Weight loss prior to conception may aid in reducing this risk of gestational diabetes in overweight and obese women.

Blood glucose levels that remain elevated during pregnancy can result in adverse birth outcomes for the mother and fetus. As mentioned, the fetus is completely dependent on the mother for nutrition, so glucose is transported across the placenta to the fetus. With elevated maternal blood glucose, the fetus must produce excess insulin to utilize glucose supply. This results in an LGA infant (also called macrosomia) and severe risk of both hypoglycemia and jaundice as high insulin levels remain after birth.[112] Long-term implications include a significantly higher risk of type 2 diabetes after pregnancy, as well as increased risks for the infant of obesity, diabetes, and hypertension throughout childhood.[111,113]

Testing and Diagnosing GDM The risk of gestational diabetes is present for all women without preexisting diabetes. Some women, however, are at lower risk of developing GDM, including those with the following characteristics[114]:

- Younger than 25 years old
- Normal weight before pregnancy
- Not Hispanic or African American
- No first-degree relatives with known diabetes
- No history of abnormal glucose tolerance
- No history of poor obstetric outcome

Women who are high risk for GDM should be tested for alterations in glucose metabolism by means of a oral glucose tolerance test (OGTT) as soon as possible, usually at 24 to 28 weeks; testing can be completed as a one- or two-step series, as shown in **Table 21.6**.[111]

Women who have had GDM and/or continue to have impaired glucose tolerance after birth are at high risk of developing type 2 diabetes and should be followed up for glucose screening and counseling for diabetes prevention. The American Diabetes Association recommends glucose screening at 6 weeks postpartum for women with GDM and annual testing for women with impaired fasting glucose or impaired glucose tolerance.[44]

Managing Gestational Diabetes Management of gestational diabetes mellitus may be established through lifestyle alterations, medical nutrition therapy, and SMBG. If this means of management is unsuccessful in reaching target blood glucose levels (**Table 21.7**), the next recommended line of therapy is insulin. Oral antihyperglycemia agents, such as metformin and glyburide, are approved by the U.S. Food and Drug Administration for treatment of GDM in pregnancy. However, glyburide is associated with neonatal hypoglycemia and macrosomia, while metformin may increase the risk of prematurity. The long-term effects

TABLE 21.6 TESTING FOR GESTATIONAL DIABETES

	One-Step Diagnosis		
	Fasting	1 hour	2 hours
Step 1. Fasting OGTT (75 g glucose dose)	92 mg/dL or higher	180 mg/dL or higher	153 mg/dL or higher

	Two-Step Diagnosis			
	Fasting	1 hour	2 hours	3 hours
Step 1. Random plasma glucose test (50 g glucose dose)		130 mg/dL or higher		
Step 2. Fasting OGTT (must be repeated twice to confirm diagnosis)	95 mg/dL or higher	180 mg/dL or higher	155 mg/dL or higher	140 mg/dL or higher

Data from American Diabetes Association, Cefalu WT. Standards of Medical Care in Diabetes. *Journal of Clinical and Applied Research and Education.* 2017;40(1):1-142.

TABLE 21.7 TARGET GLUCOSE LEVELS FOR SELF-MONITORING BLOOD GLUCOSE IN GESTATIONAL DIABETES

Target Blood Glucose Levels for Self-Monitoring of Blood Glucose

Parameter	HbA1c <7	HbA1c >7
Fasting plasma glucose	60-95 mg/dL	60-79 mg/dL
1-hour postprandial plasma glucose	100-129 mg/dL	90-109 mg/dL

Data from American Diabetes Association, Cefalu WT. Standards of Medical Care in Diabetes. *Journal of Clinical and Applied Research and Education*. 2017;40(1):1-142.

of these agents on offspring are unknown, so clinicians should weigh the risks to benefits prior to administering pharmacologic therapy.[115]

Medical nutrition therapy provided for gestational diabetes should be individualized to each patient's current dietary habits and lifestyle factors. A carbohydrate-controlled meal plan with adequate calories for weight gain and appropriate blood glucose should be followed to ensure adequate glucose supply for the mother and fetus with a minimum of 175 g of carbohydrates consumed per day.[44,111] Structured meal and snack times with consistent carbohydrate intakes are recommended to prevent peaks and valleys in blood glucose patterns. Three meals per day with 45 g of carbohydrates at each and two to three snacks per day with 15 to 30 g of carbohydrates should be sufficient to maintain appropriate blood glucose serum levels and supply to the fetus.

A low-glycemic, high-fiber diet will also aid in the management of GDM, because fiber slows the release of glucose into the bloodstream. This diet often also means that mothers can avoid insulin injections.[111] An average of 40% to 55% of caloric intake should be from carbohydrate sources, with 25 to 30 g of fiber intake per day.[111] The majority of glucose transfer from the mother to fetus occurs after consumption; therefore, controlling blood glucose postprandially can have the best effect on slowing any accelerated fetal growth.[22] In general, increasing cereal fiber and polyunsaturated fatty acid intake while reducing the glycemic load, refined carbohydrate, and saturated fat content of dietary intake may help reduce risk of glucose intolerance and GDM.[44,70] Clinicians should instruct pregnant women to limit concentrated sweets such as cookies, cakes, pastries, fruit juices, and sweetened beverages throughout pregnancy. Due to hormones secreted early in the morning during pregnancy, avoidance of concentrated sweets and fruit at breakfast will prevent a spike in blood sugar.

In addition to dietary changes, physical activity that utilizes the large skeletal muscles will aid in glucose utilization by activating adenosine monophosphate-activated protein kinase. This enzyme increases glucose transport into the muscle, enhances fat oxidation, and reduces insulin resistance.[70] See the section on Physical Activity for addition recommendations on exercise during pregnancy.

> **PRACTICE POINT**
>
> The majority of glucose transfer from the mother to fetus occurs after consumption; therefore, controlling blood glucose postprandially can have the best effect on slowing any accelerated fetal growth.

Hypertensive Disorders of Pregnancy

Hypertensive disorders, including chronic hypertension, gestational hypertension, and preeclampsia, represent the most common medical complications in pregnancy.[116] Chronic hypertension is defined as blood pressure of 140/90 mm Hg or higher on two occasions before 20 weeks' gestation that persists beyond 12 weeks postpartum; treatment of mild to moderate chronic hypertension does not benefit the mother or fetus and might excessively lower blood pressure, resulting in decreased placental perfusion and adverse perinatal outcomes.[116] **Gestational hypertension** is defined as systolic blood pressure equal to or greater than 140 mm Hg or a diastolic blood pressure equal to or greater than 90 mm Hg that occurs without proteinuria after 20 weeks' gestation.[116] Often, like gestational diabetes, gestational hypertension resolves quickly after delivery; however, up to 50% of women who develop gestational hypertension will be diagnosed with preeclampsia between weeks 24 and 35.[116,117] Preeclampsia is a multi-organ disease with a diagnosis of hypertension and proteinuria after 20 weeks' gestation, with 32 weeks' or earlier considered **early-onset preeclampsia**, and after 34 weeks' considered **late-onset preeclampsia**.[116-118]

> **CORE CONCEPT 22**
>
> Up to 50% of women who develop gestational hypertension are diagnosed with preeclampsia between weeks 24 and 35.

Preeclampsia There are two causes of preeclampsia: placental and maternal. **Maternal preeclampsia** arises in women with a normal placenta, but with low-grade inflammation secondary to obesity, hypertension, or diabetes. In **placental preeclampsia**, the hypoxic state resulting from a poorly developed placenta and maternal supply causes the release of debris into the maternal circulation, eliciting a systemic inflammatory response.[22,44] If not managed properly, any type of preeclampsia can progress to eclampsia, defined as grand mal seizures occurring in women with preeclampsia.[44] Preeclampsia is a serious complication and must be dealt with promptly, as any degree can cause IUGR due to an altered blood supply in the placenta and umbilical cord.[118]

> **CASE STUDY REVISITED**
>
> Unfortunately, one week later, Meg is admitted due to her HG.
>
> **Questions**
> 1. Do you think that enteral nutrition is an appropriate form of therapy for Meg?
> 2. What type of access would you recommend?
> 3. If Meg is unable to tolerate tube feeding, and parenteral nutrition is administered, how many calories from fat would you recommend?

Preeclampsia is characterized as mild or severe based on hypertension; proteinuria; and the presence of symptoms resulting from involvement of kidneys, brain, liver, and cardiovascular system, such as severe headaches, visual disturbances, or hyperreflexia.[116] Risk factors include anti–phospholipid antibody syndrome, chronic hypertension, chronic kidney disease, overweight/obesity, maternal age >40 years, multiple gestation, nulliparity, preeclampsia in previous pregnancy (especially if severe and before 32 weeks' gestation), and history of GDM.[116]

> **CORE CONCEPT 23**
>
> Preeclampsia is a serious complication and must be dealt with promptly, as any degree can cause IUGR due to an altered blood supply in the placenta and umbilical cord.

As poorly managed preeclampsia progresses to severe preeclampsia or eclampsia, HELLP syndrome may develop. **HELLP syndrome** is a variant of severe preeclampsia characterized by **h**emolysis, **e**levated **l**iver enzymes, and **l**ow **p**latelet count.[116] Common symptoms are right upper quadrant or epigastric pain, nausea, and vomiting.[116] Patients with these symptoms must be admitted to hospital, placed on bed rest, and carefully monitored, as treatment goals are seizure prevention, lowering blood pressure to avoid maternal organ damage, and expediting delivery.[116] Delivery is the only cure for preeclampsia. Decisions about the timing of delivery are based upon maternal and fetal factors such as gestational age, evidence of lung maturity, and signs of fetal compromise.[116] Delivery is not recommended for women with mild preeclampsia until 37 to 38 weeks, but should occur by 40 weeks.[116]

> **CORE CONCEPT 24**
>
> HELLP syndrome is a variant of severe preeclampsia characterized by hemolysis, elevated liver enzymes, and low platelet count; common symptoms are right upper quadrant or epigastric pain, nausea, and vomiting.

Preeclampsia is more common in obese women with GDM than in women without GDM.[70] Because of the increased risk of preeclampsia with overweight and obesity, weight loss should be highly encouraged prior to conception to prevent complications. Women who have GDM should maintain tight regulation of blood sugars to reduce their risk of developing preeclampsia.[70] Calcium and magnesium levels tend to be low in women suffering from preeclampsia, and as such are now the focus of many studies.[119] Calcium supplementation has been shown to reduce the risk of preeclampsia in high-risk women and those with low dietary calcium intake. In these high-risk populations, supplementation of 1,500 to 2,000 mg of elemental calcium divided into three doses per day from 20 weeks of gestation to the end of pregnancy may be effective in preventing preeclampsia.[120]

In the setting of a hypertensive emergency, high-dose supplementation of magnesium sulfate helps to prevent maternal seizures by slowing neuromuscular conduction and depressing central nervous system irritability without significant effects on blood pressure.[116] Magnesium levels should be monitored closely as toxicity can lead to respiratory paralysis, central nervous system depression, and cardiac arrest; if this presents, treatment for magnesium toxicity is 1 g calcium gluconate infused intravenously over 2 minutes.[116]

> **PRACTICE POINT**
>
> Because of the increased risk of preeclampsia with overweight and obesity, weight loss should be highly encouraged prior to conception to prevent complications.

Nutrition Support in Pregnancy

With the increased mental, physiologic, and biologic demands of pregnancy, prolonged nutritional deprivation in a pregnant woman increases the risk of nutritional deficiencies, dehydration, electrolyte imbalances, low birth weight infants, and even fetal death.[121] When indicated, providing nutrition support can play a pivotal role in preventing complications and adverse effects of nutritional deficit during pregnancy. With this said, the benefits and risks of providing this therapy should be weighed.

Enteral Nutrition

Indications and Contraindications

HG, as discussed previously, is associated with dehydration, electrolyte imbalance, ketonuria, and weight loss of greater than 5%. As a result, nutrient intake and stores are reduced, increasing the risk of adverse birth or fetal outcomes. Nutrition support is extremely successful in managing this condition.[99] EN is the primary therapy for this population, if tolerated, to avoid the risk of other forms of nutrition therapy.[122] The goal of therapy is to ensure that the mother can retain sufficient calories and nutrients to fuel herself and her fetus given the significant needs of both during pregnancy (see Physiologic Changes of Pregnancy). Studies of HG patients suggest that this treatment is indicated for mothers who are sensitive to smells and tastes, as tube feeding will bypass these signals.[103] It is contraindicated if vomiting or aspiration occurs, or if the mother suffers from a malabsorptive condition such as Crohn's disease, has severe diabetes, or has had any sort of gastrointestinal resection.[99]

Access and Administration

Administration of EN is provided via a nasogastric tube, nasojejunal tube, percutaneous endoscopic gastronomy (PEG) tube, or percutaneous endoscopic gastrojejunostomy (PEG-J) tube. While placing the feeding tube past the pylorus is effective if the patient is at aspiration risk, there seems to be a greater improvement in symptoms of nausea and vomiting with gastric feeding through bypassing the visual, oral, and psychologic response to food.[103,110,123] PEG tubes carry risks with changing anatomy in pregnancy and percutaneously inserted jejunostomy tubes and nasojejunostomy tubes are at increased risk of dislodgement and gastric coiling with ongoing vomiting and retching.[110] For long-term feeding, a PEG tube may be most beneficial because nasogastric tubes may become dislodged or blocked as well.[103,123] If the patient is unable to tolerate gastric feedings, postpyloric feedings via a nasojejunal, PEGJ, or surgical jejunostomy tube should be considered.

Schedule of feeding may be provided as continuous drips over 20 to 24 hours, or as small, frequent feedings during the day with nighttime continuous feeding to meet the daily volume goal.[103,110] When first initiating enteral feeds, the patient can be instructed not to eat until full volume goal is reached.[103] If symptoms of intolerance are experienced, the medical team should distinguish whether the cause is enteral feeds or the supplemental oral feeding. Once the mother is orally consuming at least 75% of her calorie, protein, and fluid needs for pregnancy, enteral feeding may be discontinued.[103] EN for ensuring adequate caloric goals has proven successful in the pregnancy population with inadequate weight gain and even weight loss into the late periods of gestation, resulting in adequate weight gain and positive fetal and maternal birth outcomes.[100,123,124]

> **PRACTICE POINT**
>
> While placing the feeding tube past the pylorus is effective if the patient is at aspiration risk, there seems to be a greater improvement in symptoms of nausea and vomiting with gastric feeding through bypassing the visual, oral, and psychologic response to food.

Complications

Gastric enteral feedings are not guaranteed to alleviate symptoms of nausea and vomiting. Nasogastric tubes are somewhat more likely to dislodge, and so can increase the risk of aspiration (formula entering the lungs).[124] Patients who receive nasojejunal or PEG-J tubes may also experience dislodgement or coiling as a result of repeated retching and vomiting.[124] Aesthetic and comfort factors can be a barrier to nasojejunal and nasogastric tubes and should be assessed and accounted for when determining a nutrition plan.[124]

Monitoring

Because these patients typically experience prolonged episodes of vomiting and are at increased risk of refeeding syndrome, repletion of thiamine should be provided prior to initiation of feeding.[124] Tube feeds should begin at a low rate compared to the goal rate to monitor tolerance of maternal transitioning. During the initial 24 to 48 hours of enteral feeding at the goal rate, it is important to monitor for signs of intolerance of tube feeds, including nausea, vomiting, abdominal discomfort, and abdominal distention (if early in pregnancy). If the patient is experiencing these symptoms, determine what other factors may be causing them. EN may need to be withheld until investigations are complete. As with any tube-fed patient and pregnant woman, weight should be monitored closely.

> **PRACTICE POINT**
>
> During the initial 24 to 48 hours of enteral feeding at the goal rate, it is important to monitor the signs of intolerance of tube feeds including nausea, vomiting, abdominal discomfort, and abdominal distention (if early in pregnancy).

Parenteral Nutrition

Indications and Contraindications

For women who are unable to tolerate EN, PN may be indicated for severe forms of HG, jejunoileal bypass, diabetes, or Crohn's disease to maintain nutritional status.[99] A retrospective study assessed women with single pregnancies and HG and found that those who received PN during the first trimester had a significant decrease in preterm delivery, admission to neonatal intensive care unit, and composite mortality, and an increase in infant birth weight.[102] However, research has not provided a definitive benefit to this therapy compared with regard to the potential complications.[99,102] In the presence of persistent nausea and vomiting that affects intake and hydration of a pregnant woman, however, providing PN is used as a means to supply adequate fluid, fat, essential amino acids, glucose, vitamins, and minerals when EN is not tolerated.

Access

Central vein access is needed for the administration of PN. This can be achieved by inserting a PICC line.

Complications

Due to the invasive nature of PN, potential complications are serious and can include catheter infections and thrombosis.[102] In peripheral PN the most common complication is phlebitis, or inflammation of the vein, which is caused by the insertion technique, size of the vein, pH of the solution, osmolarity, and medications provided.[121] During pregnancy, there are also elevated coagulation factors, which increase the risk of catheter-related thromboembolism.[103,110] Intravenous lipid emulsions have been found to induce uterine muscle contractions, placental fat deposition, and placental infarction and should therefore be limited to no more than 3 g/kg/day or less than 60% of caloric needs.[99]

When intravenous fluid, PN, antibiotics, or medications are needed, PICC lines are recommended due to the ease of insertion and overall lower risk of complications (1%-4%) in the nonpregnant population. However, in the pregnant population, there is roughly a 50% risk of complications from PICC lines such as bacteremia, need for surgery, phlebitis, thrombosis, or catheter malfunction, as the immune system becomes more suppressed during pregnancy.[103,110,125] This, along with the increased cost associated with PN, explain the preference for EN as initial nutrition therapy and PN as a secondary therapy.[103,110]

> **PRACTICE POINT**
>
> In the pregnant population, there is roughly a 50% risk of complications from PICC lines such as bacteremia, need for surgery, phlebitis, thrombosis, or catheter malfunction, as the immune system becomes more suppressed during pregnancy.

Monitoring

With PN, glucose, protein, and fat are infused directly into the bloodstream, increasing the chance of abnormal blood values. Triglycerides should be monitored once a week and maintained <400 mg/dL. Blood glucose levels should be tightly controlled to reduce the risk of hyperglycemia and prevent excess glucose supply to the fetus. Finger sticks taken every 6 hours should be sufficient to assess blood glucose. If glucose readings begin to rise or fall dramatically, finger sticks can be drawn every hour. A daily chemistry panel including sodium, potassium, bicarbonate, chloride, blood urea nitrogen, creatinine, glucose, calcium, magnesium, and phosphorus is necessary for all patients on PN until stable.

Patients on PN must also be checked for signs of intolerance, including catheter infections, which may appear as a fever and positive blood cultures. Monitor fetal growth with fundal height, fetal heart sounds, and ultrasounds when relying on nutrition support for maternal and fetal needs.

> **CORE CONCEPT 25**
>
> When indicated, providing nutrition support can play a pivotal role in preventing complications and adverse effects of nutritional deficit during pregnancy. The benefits and risks of providing this therapy should be weighed.

> **PRACTICE POINT**
>
> Triglycerides should be monitored once a week and maintained <400 mg/dL. Blood glucose levels should be tightly controlled to reduce the risk of hyperglycemia and prevent excess glucose supply to the fetus. Finger sticks taken every 6 hours should be sufficient to assess blood glucose. If glucose readings begin to rise or fall dramatically, finger sticks can be drawn every hour.

Summary: Nutrition in Pregnancy

The entire physiologic process of pregnancy is dependent upon maternal pre-pregnancy nutritional status and nutrition stores and intake during pregnancy. As gestation progresses, energy and protein needs increase and the growth of the fetus is altered by the nutrient supply provided. Supplementation of certain nutrients is highly recommended during pregnancy due to overall increased utilization. These include calcium, iron, folic acid, and vitamin D. Folic acid intake or supplementation should be adequate prior to 21 days of gestation due to the closure of the neural tube. While there are several complications that may occur throughout pregnancy, including GDM, HG, and preeclampsia, there are accepted medical nutrition therapy interventions for each to enhance maternal weight gain and improve birth outcome. Enhancing maternal nutrition status prior to conception is the gold standard to managing a health pregnancy. Maintaining nutritional reserve throughout pregnancy to prepare for lactation is crucial and requires education and dedication by the patient, but can prove helpful, and even life-saving, in both low- and high-risk pregnancies.

Introduction: Nutrition in Lactation

As you learned in the first part of this chapter, the mother's body makes numerous physiologic adjustments in order to supply her fetus with ample material to grow and develop properly over the 9 months of gestation. Throughout the last weeks of gestation and postpartum, the mother's body is still fully adapted to care for and feed her child. This period is called lactation; from birth until the mother chooses to cease breastfeeding, her body will use its nutrient stores to feed her child the optimal blend of antibodies and nutrients. Because of the many benefits to mother and baby, breastfeeding promotion is a key strategy to improve public health of major national organizations, such as the Centers for Disease Control and Prevention (CDC) and Women, Infants, and Children (WIC).[126] The American Academy of Pediatrics (AAP), Academy of Breastfeeding Medicine, American Academy of Family Physicians, American College of Obstetricians and Gynecologists, WHO, UNICEF, and the U.S. Surgeon General all recommend that breastfeeding be the exclusive source of nutrition for all infants until 6 months.[127] At the age of 4 to 6 months, complementary solid foods may be introduced based on infant cues of readiness. Breastfeeding may be continued along with solid food intake until 12 months.[127] RDs play a central role in teaching mothers about the nutritional side of breastfeeding, and as such are main promoters of health in this arena.

In this part of the chapter, we will cover breast milk production, composition, and nutritional and immunologic benefits; successful breastfeeding techniques; common barriers; and major nutrient requirements. We will also review special cases that RDs may encounter, such as mothers with infectious diseases, indications for breast milk fortification, common breastfeeding problems and solutions, and current trends and programs for lactating mothers. By the end of this section, you should have gained the knowledge you need to advise and assist new mothers.

Physiology of Lactation

Mammary Gland Development

In order to produce breast milk, a woman must have fully mature mammary glands (**Figure 21.7**). The maturation of the breast tissue occurs in five definitive stages: embryogenesis, puberty, pregnancy, lactation, and involution.[128] The first stage, embryogenesis, occurs at 18 to 19 weeks of gestation. At this time, the mammary bud, fat-pad precursor, and foundation of the ductal system all develop within the female fetus. While these structures will continue to grow throughout childhood, the next major stage of maturation will not occur until puberty. At that time, development is directed by growth-stimulating hormones such as estrogen and pituitary hormone, as well as progesterone, after menarche. These hormones cause the growth of the lobulo-alveoli, which will eventually store breast milk during lactation. Years of hormonal activity (following the menstrual cycle) also elicit further alveolar and epithelial growth in the breast tissue, but none of these cells is fully mature or functional until pregnancy.

As during puberty, breast and mammary gland development in pregnancy is dictated by the hormones progesterone, lactogenic hormone, prolactin, and human placental lactogen. These hormones finish the final stages of development, yielding functional cells able to produce milk after the infant is born (see Lactogenesis and Human Milk Composition).

Lactogenesis

A woman's mammary glands reach full functionality (i.e., are able to produce breast milk) during pregnancy when a hormonal cascade causes the final maturation of the alveolar and epithelial cells. The complex process of converting inert breast cells to milk-producing cells is called **lactogenesis**, and it begins at 20 weeks of pregnancy.[129] The first change to occur in this process is the

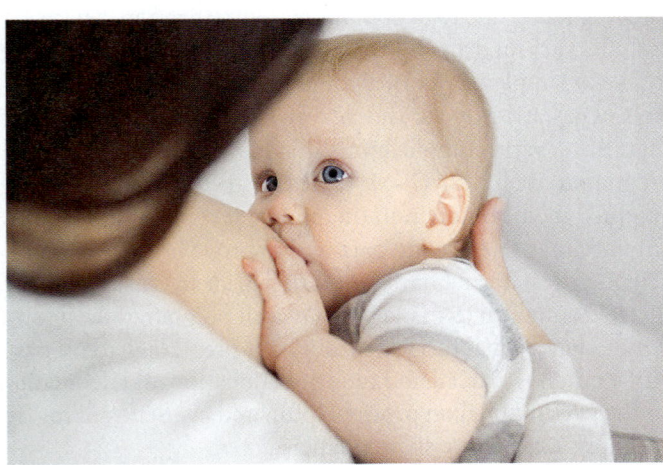

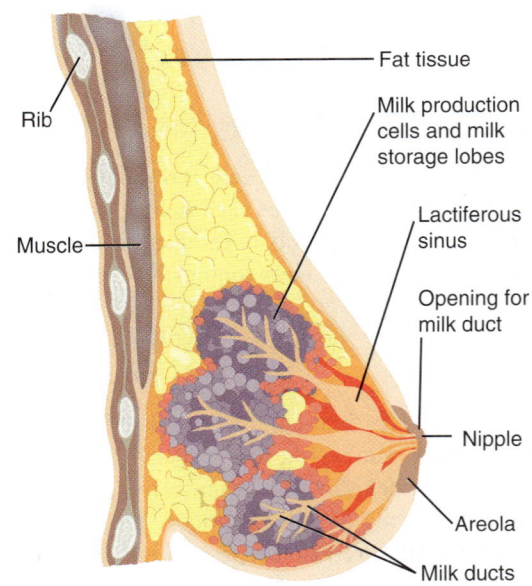

FIGURE 21.7 Breast Tissue and Mammary Glands

CASE STUDY INTRODUCTION

Meg is now 33-years-old para 1 gravida 1 (G1P1) who is 1 month postdelivery. Meg delivered a baby boy, Ryan, at 37 1/7 weeks' gestation at a weight appropriate for gestational age (AGA). At the beginning of her pregnancy, Meg decided that she would exclusively breastfeed her baby. After delivery, Ryan developed mild respiratory distress and was admitted to the neonatal intensive care unit (NICU). During his NICU admission, Meg pumped her breast milk until Ryan was able to breastfeed. After one week, Ryan was discharged home.

At home, Meg reports that she feeds Ryan every 5 to 6 hours for about 30 minutes total. He has about eight wet diapers per day. At his 3-week check-up, Ryan remains at his birthweight.

Overall, Meg is very anxious about her breastfeeding experience and the weight she has gained throughout her pregnancy. She does not feel that she has been able to lose any weight since her delivery because she was under a lot of stress while Ryan was in the NICU, and is still exhausted now. She just wants to lose the weight she gained and regain the energy she once had.

Anthropometric Data:
Height: 167 cm (66")
Weight: 84.1 kg (184 lbs)
BMI: 30.5 kg/m^2
Weight History
Pre-pregnancy weight: 68.2 kg (150.4 lbs)
Postpartum weight: 85 kg (187 lbs)
Total pregnancy weight gain: 20.5 kg (45 lbs)

Biochemical Data: None

Clinical Data:
Past Medical History: None
Medications: Multivitamin daily
Vital Signs: None
Nutrition-focused Physical Exam: Appears tired, teary

Dietary Data:
Dietary History: Meg reports that she has felt extremely fatigued since her baby came home and does not feel that he is getting enough to eat from her breast milk. She is also concerned that she is not consuming enough food or fluid. Per 24-hour recall, you determine that Meg is consuming about 2,400 calories and 74 g of protein per day, with four small meals per day and one snack. The only vegetable she likes is broccoli, which she consumes about once per week. Because of her history of lactose intolerance, she does not eat or drink any dairy products and has never tried other sources of calcium.

Questions

1. Based on Meg's pre-pregnancy BMI, did she gain an appropriate amount of weight during her pregnancy?
2. Based on her current weight, what is her current weight status?
3. According to Meg's diet recall, is she consuming adequate calories? What dietary recommendations might you make?

---

differentiation of mammary cells, which will allow the breast to secrete specific nutrients and compounds into the breast milk, adjusting as the infant grows. The main biomarker of this stage is a small amount of lactose in the mother's blood and urine.[129] Throughout pregnancy, the woman's breasts will continue to be sensitive to the high levels of prolactin and progesterone in her blood, allowing the breasts to completely mature. The mammary glands are then fully functional, although they will not physically secrete milk until after the infant is delivered.[8,128,129]

The second phase of lactogenesis begins upon delivery of both infant and placenta. This event causes a steep decline in progesterone, which elicits the "coming in" of colostrum, the first secretion from the breasts.[8,128-130] This **lactation** is possible after lactogenesis is complete. The infant will "latch" onto the breast, and the sucking stimulus from the infant, along with the hormones prolactin and oxytocin, will cause the production and "**let down**" (release) of breast milk. If production does not begin within 72 hours postpartum, the mother is considered to have **delayed onset lactation**, a diagnosis often correlated with obesity and preterm delivery.[130] Throughout lactation, the amount of milk the infant needs and sucks from the glands each day signals the continuation of this hormonal cycle, and determines the amount of milk produced and secreted during breastfeeding through a supply-and-demand system.[8,128,131]

The final stage of mammary gland development is **involution**. This occurs as the mother begins to wean her infant to solid food and the mammary glands return to their pre-pregnancy, inactive state. Fewer feedings also lead to lower levels of prolactin and tissue involution. At that time, milk production will stop, additional epithelial cells will die, and the breasts will lose their ability to produce milk.[128] Involution and the loss of ability to breastfeed may occur as quickly as 2 days after ceasing breastfeeding.[131] New mothers should be made aware of this effect, as a brief break from regular feedings could prevent them from resuming afterwards.

> **CORE CONCEPT 26**
>
> Lactogenesis involves five major stages: embryogenesis, pubertal development, development in pregnancy, lactation, and involution. This means that the breasts actually cannot produce milk until after pregnancy, and once breastfeeding has ceased, mammary gland tissue returns to inactivity (involution).

Human Milk Composition

Types of Breast Milk

Throughout the lactation period, breast milk composition changes in order to reflect the infant's growth and needs. This special characteristic of breast milk begins at delivery with the secretion of colostrum. **Colostrum** is not technically milk, but rather a yellow liquid that provides immunologic factors, such as secretory IgA (sIgA) white blood cells and lactoferrin, and nutrients to the newborn. The exact proportion of nutrients is highly specific, including high concentrations of sodium, chloride, and magnesium and low concentrations of lactose, calcium, and potassium.[130,131] Colostrum also contains sufficient carbohydrates to prevent hypoglycemia in a healthy, term infant.[132]

As the infant grows, breast milk composition evolves to meet their nutritional needs. In the 2-week liminal stage between colostrum and final mature milk, the epithelial cells in the mammary glands grow closer together, allowing for the production of **transitional milk**. This milk is released in higher quantities than colostrum, as the infant has learned to latch on to the breast, suck, and swallow the smaller amounts of colostrum. The infant is also able to tolerate the higher lactose concentration that transitional milk provides.[130,132]

Beginning at 2 to 4 weeks postpartum and lasting until the mother chooses to stop breastfeeding, the mammary glands produce **mature milk**. Interestingly, the exact nutritional makeup of mature milk can be variable, reacting to the mother's body and intake.[130] The nutrient content of breast milk is influenced by preterm delivery, maternal BMI, dietary protein, whether the mother is primiparous or multiparous, breastfeeding frequency, and the infant's gestational age.[130] In general, however, it will contain 65 to 70 kcal/dL, 3.2 to 3.6 g/dL of fat, 0.9 to 1.2 g/dL of protein, and 6.7 to 7.8 g/dL of carbohydrates (as lactose), as well as sufficient amounts of all micronutrients except vitamins D and K.[130] These latter two vitamins are commonly supplemented during infancy.

> **CORE CONCEPT 27**
>
> The nutrient content of mature milk is influenced by preterm delivery, maternal BMI, dietary proteins, whether the mother is primi- or multiparous, and how often she breastfeeds. In general, it will contain 65 to 70 kcal/dL, 3.2 to 3.6 g/dL of fat, 0.9 to 1.2 g/dL of protein, and 6.7 to 7.8 g/dL of carbohydrates (as lactose) and sufficient amounts of all micronutrients except vitamins D and K.

Nutritional Composition of Breast Milk

Energy (Kilocalories)

While the energy content of breast milk is completely dependent on macronutrient ratios, it is estimated to contain 65 to 70 kcal/dL (19 to 21 kcal/oz).[130] New research shows that calorie content also varies depending upon whether or not the child is preterm, whether the milk is **foremilk** (the first milk released at feeding) or **hindmilk** (the last milk of a feeding), and the time of day of the feeding (nighttime feedings tend to be higher in energy due to a higher fat content).[133]

Protein

Proteins are necessary for the infant's growth, transportation of vitamins and hormones, enzymatic activity, and other vital functions.[134] The main source of protein in breast milk is alpha-lactalbumin, a whey protein. Breast milk also includes lactoferrin, sIgA, lysozyme and serum albumin. With the infant's gastrointestinal tract still developing, alpha-lactalbumin and whey proteins are easiest to digest.[130,135] Overall protein content (except casein) is more influenced by maternal BMI and the gestational age of the infant than maternal intake.[130,136,137] For example, the protein concentration of initial breast milk and breast milk from mothers of preterm infants is higher (15.8 g/L), but total protein content will decrease over the first 6 weeks.

Mature milk contains 0.9 to 1.2 g/dL of protein.[130] The lower protein content is beneficial, as infant kidneys cannot process a high nitrogen load.[135]

Carbohydrates

Lactose is the main source of carbohydrate in breast milk. The prebiotic oligosaccharides (1 g/dL) are the only other carbohydrate present.[130] While the immunologic secretion colostrum has a low concentration of lactose, mature breast milk will contain 6.7 to 7.8 g/dL, or more if more milk is produced.[130]

Fat

Breast milk fat is an ever-changing part of the macronutrient ratio and is made up of mostly triglycerides.[130,134] Mature milk usually contains 3.2 to 3.6 g/dL of fat,[130] but the exact content will vary frequently. Even during a single feeding, foremilk will be lower in fat and hindmilk will be higher in fat.[130] Unlike protein content, fat is subject to maternal intake, particularly the amount of omega-6 fatty acids and omega-3 fatty acids in her diet.[136] To ensure that breast milk is the excellent source of linoleic acid and alpha-linolenic acid that it certainly can be, lactating mothers who eat very little DHA should take a supplement while breastfeeding.[130,134]

Vitamins

While the macronutrients in breast milk are, for the most part, present in guaranteed amounts, vitamin concentrations in breast milk are entirely reliant upon the mother's diet and pregnancy stores. Because the standard American diet lacks nutritional diversity and quality, women should continue to take a prenatal vitamin throughout the lactation period.[130,138] The only two vitamins present in truly insufficient quantities are vitamin D and vitamin K. As such, the AAP suggests both vitamin D supplementation (400 IU per day) in exclusively breastfed infants, and a vitamin K injection at birth to protect the baby against hemorrhagic disease of the newborn.[130,135]

Vitamin D

Vitamin D deficiency in infants is easily prevented with appropriate nutritional therapy. While humans synthesize vitamin D from UVB sunlight, the AAP currently recommends that all infants younger than 6 months old be protected from direct sunlight, due to the risk of skin cancer with early sun exposure.[54] Without supplementation, human milk contains about 25 IU/L or less of vitamin D, dependent upon maternal vitamin D status; as such, the AAP recommends that breastfed infants (exclusively breastfed or with formula supplementation) be given 400 IU of vitamin D per day from first few days of life until weaning.[54] Without this supplementation, infants are at higher risk for vitamin D deficiency and rickets; this will usually occur between the ages of 3 and 18 months, due to chronic deficiency leading to hypocalcemia.[54]

Infant vitamin D supplements, like adult versions, are available in two forms: vitamin D_2 (ergocalciferol) or vitamin D_3 (cholecalciferol). Cholecalciferol is typically more effective in raising $25(OH)D_3$ vitamin D levels, and the liquid form can be easily administered in pumped breast milk or directly into the infant's mouth. A liquid multivitamin containing 400 IU of vitamin D is also suitable if the infant requires supplementation with other vitamins.[54] Higher doses of vitamin D are generally unnecessary, and so must be given only on the advice of the infant's pediatrician, and with close monitoring of vitamin D status. Cases in which high-dose vitamin D could be necessary are fat malabsorption disorders, such as cystic fibrosis, or long-term antiseizure medication administration. Supplementation is not necessary if an infant is consuming at least 1,000 mL of vitamin D–fortified formula, or is being fed vitamin D–fortified cow's milk as a complementary food by age 1 year.[54]

Minerals

Many of the minerals present in breast milk are bound to transport proteins to ensure optimal absorption by the infant.[135] Exact mineral levels will depend predominantly on the maturity of the breast milk. Colostrum, for example, is higher in sodium, chloride, and magnesium, but lower in potassium and calcium than the final, mature milk.[130,135] While some minerals, such as zinc, calcium, and iron, are present in low quantities in breast milk, their bioavailability (due to the protein carriers) guarantees absorption, and therefore their benefit to the infant.[135] For example, calcium and phosphorus are present in a 2:1 ratio to maximize calcium absorption.[135]

It is also important to note the sources of these minerals. While the mother's diet supplies the majority of minerals, copper, iron, and zinc are sourced from the maternal liver stores accumulated during the last trimester of pregnancy.

Iron

The average iron content of human milk is estimated at 0.35 mg/L.[139] For term infants, this provides the adequate intake for iron up until 4 months of age. At this point, exclusively breastfed infants should receive iron supplementation of 1 mg/kg/day until complementary foods containing iron are incorporated into their diet.[139]

Because 80% of iron present in newborn term infants is accrued during the last trimester of pregnancy, premature infants (<37 weeks gestation) will not have access to adequate iron stores and will require supplementation.[134,139] Exclusively breastfed preterm infants are recommended to receive elemental iron at 2 mg/kg/day starting from 1 month of age until 12 months. This can be supplied through iron supplements or iron-fortified complementary foods.[139] All breastfed infants are recommended to receive around 11 mg of iron once they are old enough to be fed complementary foods, from 4 to 6 months through 12 months of age. Dry infant cereal fortified with iron is an excellent iron source at that time.[140,141]

Practice of Lactation

Benefits for the Infant

Breast milk is a very special form of sustenance for an infant. Indeed, the AAP recommends breast milk as the standard for infant feeding and nutrition.[142] Breastfeeding gives the infant perfectly balanced nutrition; allows them the ability to self-regulate intake from birth; and directly provides many immunologic factors that prevent illness, child morbidity and mortality, and possibly childhood obesity.[70,142]

Reduced Infant Morbidity and Mortality: The Gut Microbiome The favorable relationship between breast milk and infant health is based on both its benefits for growth and development and immune modulation. Specific factors, such as sIgA, antibodies from the mother's immune system, anti-inflammatory substances, lactoferrin, growth factors, and white blood cells, in both colostrum and breast milk support the growth of an appropriate microbiome for the maturation of a strong immune system and gut development.[130,143-145] Each of these molecules supports the growth of beneficial bacteria and impart mucosal protection.[144] For example, the protein sIgA prevents pathogen adherence to the gut mucosa and can even fight off toxins.[143] Lactoferrin has anti-inflammatory and antimicrobial aspects, while lysozyme breaks open bacteria for sIgA and lactoferrin to kill the pathogen.[143] The various white blood cells in the breast milk, such as macrophages, stem cells, and cytokines, allow the mother to support the infant's immune system from birth, ensuring that the child can defend itself from pathogenic bacteria and viruses.[130]

The microbiome plays a role in mediating breast milk's effect on infant immunity. Breast milk microorganisms begin to colonize the infant's gut and provide prebiotic "food" for these "good bacteria" in the form of oligosaccharides and lactoferrin, ensuring they can displace pathogenic invaders.[130,144] A recent report found that breastfeeding could create sufficient immune function to prevent over 50% of infant diarrhea cases and about 30% of upper respiratory tract infections.[146] The AAP additionally states that breastfed infants are better protected against pneumonia, otitis media, severe respiratory syncytial virus, bronchiolitis, gastrointestinal tract infections, necrotizing enterocolitis, asthma, sudden infant death, celiac disease, inflammatory bowel disease, diabetes, acute lymphocytic leukemia, and acute myeloid leukemia during infancy.[142] This impressive effect can be attributed to the diverse bacterial composition in each type of breast milk; colostrum, for example, contains the most variety of bacteria, particularly of the *Lactobacillales* genus, although its composition is different in mothers who deliver by cesarean section.[144] As such, exclusively breastfeeding for the first 6 months of life plays a large role in reducing the risk of infant morbidity and mortality, notably reducing hospitalizations among infants.[135]

> **CORE CONCEPT 28**
>
> The proteins and "good bacteria" in breast milk have been found to modulate the infant immune system, leading to fewer cases of respiratory tract infections, pneumonia, otitis media, severity of respiratory syncytial virus bronchiolitis, gastrointestinal tract infections, necrotizing enterocolitis, asthma, sudden infant death, celiac disease, inflammatory bowel disease, diabetes, acute lymphocytic leukemia, and acute myeloid leukemia during infancy.

Long-Term Benefits Breastfeeding offers the infant myriad of benefits throughout the lifecycle. Recent research correlates breastfeeding with normalized blood pressure, lower risk of obesity/overweight, lower total cholesterol, and better intellectual performance in early childhood as compared to formula-fed infants.[135] This is likely related to formula's higher protein content and the elevated insulin response seen in formula-fed infants; both often result in unnecessary adiposity and related metabolic issues.[147] Children who are breastfed have also been shown to be more open to new foods, such as vegetables, which can support an overall healthier lifestyle; this is thought to be due to the slight differences in breast milk flavor due to a varied maternal diet.[148] The decreased risk of obesity/overweight, the lower sodium content of breast milk compared to formula, and breast milk's long-chain polyunsaturated fatty acid content also yield a lower risk of hypertension.[135] Long-chain polyunsaturated fats and maternal-infant bonding are correlate with increased intellectuality.[135]

Maternal Benefits of Breastfeeding

The act of breastfeeding also offers a number of positive outcomes for the mother, ranging from weight loss to reduced economic and environmental expense, and are covered in detail below.

Uterine Contractility A major benefit to the breastfeeding mother is increased uterine contractility, or the involution of the uterus back almost to pre-pregnancy size in a short time frame. A long-accepted benefit of breastfeeding, this particular effect comes from the oxytocin involved in the lactation pathway, a contractile hormone that also prevents excessive bleeding after delivery.[149]

Reduction in Maternal Morbidities Breastfeeding mothers have been found to have a decreased risk of breast cancer and ovarian cancer over time.[135] With each 6-month duration of breastfeeding or each additional child breastfed, there is a further decrease in the risk of breast cancer.[135] Benefits also include a reduced risk of type 2 diabetes mellitus for women with no history of gestational diabetes and a lower risk of hip fracture via improved bone mineral density in postmenopausal women.[135]

> ⚠ **Clinical Controversy**
>
> ### Breastfeeding and Childhood Obesity
>
> There is little debate surrounding the superiority of breast milk in infant feeding. Its nutrient quality and composition, bioavailability of immune factors, and promotion of a healthy microbiome are just a few of the proposed benefits of breastfeeding. Breastfeeding is associated with reduced incidence of a number of chronic disease states. The role that breastfeeding may play in preventing childhood obesity is of great research and public health interest. However, the findings are not without controversy. Gibbs et al. found, in their longitudinal study of 8,030 infants, that formula-fed infants were 2.5 times more likely to be obese at 24 months when compared to breastfed babies. However, in a similar study by Vehapoglu et al., there was no association between duration of breastfeeding incidence of obesity in children aged 2 to 14 years.
>
> Pediatric obesity rates are high and continue to rise in some age categories. A better understanding of the potential role of breastfeeding in curbing obesity rates is sorely needed. After critically reviewing the results of the studies referenced below, explain what factors related to study design and population type may alter the results. Should we be advising our patients that breastfeeding can prevent obesity in their child?
>
> **References**
>
> 1. Gibbs BG, Forste R. Socioeconomic status, infant feeding practices and early childhood obesity. *Pediatr Obes*. 2014 Apr;9(2): 135-146. doi: 10.1111/j.2047-6310.2013.00155.x.
> 2. Vehapoglu A, Yazıcı M, Demir AD, Turkmen S, Nursoy M, Ozkaya E. Early infant feeding practice and childhood obesity: the relation of breast-feeding and timing of solid food introduction with childhood obesity. *J Pediatr Endocrinol Metab*. 2014;27(11-12): 1181-1187. doi: 10.1515/jpem-2014-0138.

Effects on Maternal Fertility Extended breastfeeding suspends ovulation, and therefore helps in the spacing pregnancies by preventing the return of regular menses.[131,135] Continuing lactation halts the secretion of luteinizing and gonadotropin-releasing hormones, which prolongs the period before ovulation resumes. This provides 98% protection from pregnancy during the first 6 months of lactation, also known as the lactational amenorrhea method.[131] Amenorrhea also protects maternal iron stores and decreases the risk of iron-deficiency anemia for at least 6 months postpartum.[150]

Maternal Weight Loss Women who breastfeed will lose more weight in the short-term period than mothers who use formula, because their bodies will use fat stores to supply breast milk.[135] Exclusive breastfeeding for at least 6 months maximizes weight loss. It is important to note that factors such as pre-pregnancy weight, total pregnancy weight changes, and parity greatly impact total weight loss during lactation.[135]

Economic and Environmental Benefits Breastfeeding provides significant economic benefits in the short and the long term. Clinicians counseling women of lower economic status should emphasize the fact that breast milk is free, while formula, bottles, rubber nipples, and sterilizing solution can represent quite a financial and environmental investment. The cost of formula for one infant from birth until weaning is estimated to be a minimum of $800 to $1,200.[151] The Mother and Child Health and Education Trust also points out other environmental savings of breast milk, including its zero-waste nature and lack of a carbon footprint.[151] Likewise, healthcare-related expenses and time off from work to care for a sick infant are greatly reduced for breastfeeding mothers due to the immunologic benefits that breast milk imparts.[135]

Breastfeeding Initiation and Techniques

Education and Preparation

Prenatal education is key to ensuring a positive attitude towards breastfeeding. Because maternal obesity is linked with lower rates of breastfeeding initiation and a lower volume of milk supply to the infant, mothers who are overweight or obese should be encouraged to achieve a healthy weight before they get pregnant.[135] Throughout the 40 weeks of gestation, the clinician can work with the mother to identify possible barriers to breastfeeding (discussed later in this section) and teach the proper techniques to support successful breastfeeding for her and her baby.

Immediately after delivery, the newborn should be held skin-to-skin with their mother, because this practice has been shown to ease the transition of the newborn to the external environment, increase the success of the first breastfeeding session, and lead to more effective breastfeeding overall. Rooming-in (when the infant sleeps in the mother's hospital room after delivery) is another easy-to-implement practice that helps the mother initiate and continue breastfeeding.[127] Breastfeeding soon after delivery increases the volume of milk produced, elicits the earlier passage of meconium (newborn stool), and improves the likelihood of a longer duration of breastfeeding.[127]

Breastfeeding Technique

When initiating breastfeeding, it is important to pay close attention to the infant's feeding cues. A baby's **feeding cues** may include sucking motions, "rooting" motions, sounds, stirring, stretching, or crying; ideally, breast milk is provided before the infant begins to cry. When breastfeeding, an effective latch, good suck, and proper positioning of the infant to the breast will provide the infant with the right amount of milk and keep the mother comfortable.[127] Latching on, or the positioning of the infant's mouth on the nipple, may take several tries to ensure that the baby is able to suck a sufficient amount of milk from the breast. The mother should have the baby get as much of the nipple and areola into their mouth as possible (about 2 to 3 cm of the areola).[127] Many infants will not form a good latch until 48 hours after birth.[127]

Breastfeeding positions should be chosen by the mother to keep her comfortable and give the baby the best opportunity to latch on. These include the cradle hold, across the chest, or belly-to-belly contact on the side.[127] There may be some pain experienced with feeding during the first weeks, particularly when the baby latches on. However, during feeding the mother should only feel pulling, not pain.[127] If she is concerned that the baby is not actually taking in milk, the mother can look for signs that the child is sucking and swallowing. An average breastfeeding session will take around 5 to 20 minutes on each breast; if the baby falls asleep, the mother should wake them and switch them to the other breast. Most babies will release the breast without assistance, but if they remain latched on, the mother can break the suction with her finger.[127]

The physical and mental well-being of the mother, including her sleep, weight status, and stress level, can directly affect her breastfeeding experience. It is important to create a relaxed environment when breastfeeding, because this will ease the production of breast milk and offer a more positive experience for the mother and the infant. Simple actions such as slow deep breaths or thinking of her baby can help. If the mother would like further resources for breastfeeding, the Le Leche League and the International Board Certified Lactation Consultants are helpful.

> **PRACTICE POINT**
>
> The mother should have the baby to get as much of the nipple and areola into their mouth as possible (about 2 to 3 cm of the areola). Many infants will not form a good latch until 48 hours after birth.

Breastfeeding Frequency

Many mothers do not know exactly how many times per day they should be breastfeeding their child. Indeed, some mothers will stop breastfeeding for fear that they cannot possibly be giving their child enough milk.[135] During the first week of life, infants will increase their number of feeds over 24 hours from 4-5 on days 1 and 2, up to 8-12 times by day 7. Correspondingly, urine output and stools will increase to be in the range of 5-8 times daily (for each) by 7 days.

Pumping Breast Milk

If the mother and infant must be separated during the lactation period, whether due to infection, work, or other reasons, the clinician should educate the mother on appropriate techniques for pumping and storing breast milk. Pumping breast milk can be done either by hand or electric breast pumps with polypropylene or glass containers. When expressing milk this way, it is helpful to stimulate the breast with deep breathing, relaxing music, or breast massage to enhance the "let-down" reflex. Looking at a picture of the baby may also increase success in pumping breast milk.[135]

Once pumped, the breast milk must be properly stored and prepared to protect its various immunologic and nutritional components. Storage time for breast milk varies with the method of storage: if at room temperature, breast milk may be left for up to 4 hours, while refrigerated breast milk is safe for 48 to 72 hours and frozen breast milk for 3 months.[152] If frozen, it should be stored in the back of the freezer to prevent defrosting when the freezer door is opened, because this could increase the likelihood of bacterial growth. Mothers should always use the older milk in the refrigerator or freezer first. Defrosting or reheating breast milk should be done through overnight defrosting in the refrigerator, running the bottle under warm water, or setting the bottle in a container of warm water. Mothers should not reheat breast milk in the microwave, because it can result in uneven heating and hot spots that may burn the infant's mouth. Microwaving may also reduce the overall health properties of breast milk. Do not rewarm stored milk to greater than 104°F, because this can denature the proteins in the milk, leading to a loss of enzyme activity.

Common Breastfeeding Barriers

Despite the numerous benefits of breastfeeding, many women see barriers to their ability to breastfeed. Common challenges noted by women who do not initiate breastfeeding, or who breastfeed for less than 3 months, include concerns about their baby's intake or the milk they produce, nipple and breast issues, discomfort, fatigue, embarrassment, work, concerns about weight loss and diet, and anxiety about feeding the infant.[135] These barriers are more prevalent among Medicaid recipients, adolescent mothers, and mothers of preterm or SGA infants.[135] Pre-pregnancy obesity is also tightly correlated with low rates of breastfeeding initiation and continuation.[153] Some cases, however, cause more difficulty than others, and are discussed in the following sections.

Adolescent Parenthood

The rate of breastfeeding among adolescent mothers in the United States is lower than among mature mothers, with an estimated 60% of women younger than 20 years initiating breastfeeding versus 80% of mothers older than 30 years.[154] The stigma and embarrassment of being a "teen mom," not being ready or knowledgeable for parenthood and breastfeeding, peer pressure, and a lack of support for breastfeeding in schools and other systems are all factors that decrease breastfeeding rates among younger mothers.[154] When approaching

CASE STUDY REVISITED

Ryan has not gained weight since birth.

Questions

1. What are some of the struggles that Meg is facing in breastfeeding her baby?
2. What are ways that you can encourage discussion about these struggles?
3. Is Meg's difficulty with breastfeeding due to her weight status?
4. What recommendations do you have for Meg?
5. What additional information or evaluation would you suggest?

---

these patients, the clinician should be sensitive to the stresses of teenagehood, particularly those that are social and school related, in delivering advice about breastfeeding.[155] The clinician should also emphasize benefits such as money savings, birth spacing, and bonding time with the baby.[154]

The Breastfeeding Environment

The prenatal and postpartum environments have a major influence on breastfeeding attitudes and experiences. If hospital protocols, healthcare providers, and feeding regimens do not support breastfeeding, they may in fact hinder initiation of, and attitudes towards, breastfeeding. The CDC found that 22% of infants in 2016 were exclusively breastfed for 6 months, although this is up from 18% in 2014 and 11% in 2007 due to the strong health promotion initiatives.[126] In 1991, WHO and UNICEF began sponsoring the Breastfeeding Hospital Initiative based upon the "Ten Steps to Successful Breastfeeding" (**Figure 21.8**) in order to do their part to combat this particular barrier.

Preterm Births

If an infant is born preterm (34 0/7 weeks to 36 6/7 weeks), their delicate condition might lead to easy fatigue; low stamina; and difficulty with latching, sucking, and swallowing. Growth monitoring is vital for these infants, because they have greater challenges with temperature maintenance, decreased immunity, delayed bilirubin excretion (jaundice), and greater respiratory instability.[156] The first 12 to 24 hours after delivery indicate difficulties a preterm infant is likely to experience, and as such are important for planning a successful breastfeeding experience through appropriate education.[156] The stress of the baby's weakness and need for carefully calculated nutrition, particularly iron, can create anxiety for the mother. It is important that the clinician be proactive in educating the mother about the benefits of breast milk for preterm infants, including that breast milk composition adapts to the preterm baby's special needs.[137]

Weight as a Barrier

Many weight-related factors, such as pre-pregnancy BMI and pregnancy weight gain, will affect the success and adequacy of the breastfeeding experience. Whether the patient is underweight or obese, there is an associated effect with the success and quality of breastfeeding. Postpartum overweight or obesity in particular bring specific challenges, including mechanical difficulties with latching on, improper positioning of the infant for breastfeeding, and inadequate milk production due to reduced levels of prolactin.[70,157] In addition, due to the higher risk of complications during pregnancy, this population has a high cesarean delivery rate, which correlates with later initiation of first suckling. With this, a lower prolactin response may compromise milk production and over time lead to early cessation of lactation.[70] Women with inadequate weight gain during pregnancy and who present with a low/underweight BMI may also be compromised in their ability to

---

Every facility providing maternity services and care for newborn infants should:

1. Have a written breastfeeding policy that is routinely communicated to all healthcare staff.
2. Train all healthcare staff in skills necessary to implement this policy.
3. Inform all pregnant women about the benefits and management of breastfeeding.
4. Help mothers initiate breastfeeding within a half hour of birth.
5. Show mothers how to breastfeed and how to maintain lactation even if they should be separated from their infants.
6. Give newborn infants no food or drink other than breastmilk unless medically indicated.
7. Practice rooming in—allow mothers and infants to remain together 24 hours a day.
8. Encourage breastfeeding in response to feeding cues.
9. Give no artificial teats or pacifiers (also called dummies or soothers) to breastfeeding infants.
10. Foster the establishment of breastfeeding support groups and refer mothers to them on discharge from the hospital or clinic.

FIGURE 21.8 Ten Steps to Successful Breastfeeding.
World Health Organization (WHO/UNICEF). Protecting, Promoting, and Supporting Breastfeeding: A Joint WHO/UNICEF Statement. Geneva, Switzerland, WHO; 1989.

produce quality breast milk. Because some minerals, such as calcium, will be drawn from the bones and other maternal stores, it is important to build and maintain adequate nutritional status throughout all stages of lactation.

Common Problems and Solutions

Despite the many benefits of breastfeeding and a high initiation rate (81%), the most recent CDC Breastfeeding Report Card reports that only 51% of mothers continue breastfeeding until the 6 month benchmark, and only 22% breastfeed exclusively until that time.[126] Women often stop breastfeeding due to discomfort or a breastfeeding issue, but there are plenty of ways to overcome the common complications that might occur.[158] Providing education and encouragement through the complications is important to the success and sustainability of breastfeeding practices. All women should receive education regarding potential complications from breastfeeding and instructions on manually expressing breast milk prior to discharge from the hospital to promote continued breastfeeding until at least the 6-month benchmark.[159]

Engorged Breasts Engorgement typically occurs within the first 3 to 5 days of lactation due to vascular dilation and milk production.[159] It is defined as hard, lumpy, warm, and painful swelling of the breasts due to the incomplete release of breast milk, causing tight skin that also inhibits proper latch-on.[158,160] Techniques such as breast pumping, massage, increasing the number of feeds per day, and cold and/or warm compresses tend to relieve symptoms quickly.[158] If the symptoms of engorgement are still preventing the infant from nursing, provide expressed milk via a bottle.[159]

Sore Nipples Nipple pain is typically a result of improper position, incorrect latch, incorrect suction release, not allowing nipples to dry fully after feeds, or improper breast pump usage.[158] The most effective prevention for this complication is prenatal education and proper breast care.[160] Breastfeeding education should focus on position and correct latch-on technique; proper method for breaking suction; the use of a breast pump; lanolin ointment; and avoiding plastic-backed breast pads, because these trap moisture and block air circulation.[158,160] Mothers should also avoid washing their breasts with soap, because this can aggravate eczema and dry skin that cause nipple pain.[158] Breastfeeding frequently (every 2 hours) will also prevent the infant from sucking too hard out of hunger.[158] Expressed breast milk, rubbed on the nipple, will speed healing.[160]

Before these interventions are introduced, the cause of nipple damage must be determined. Common causes include forceful or disorganized suckling, tight infant frenulum, or a yeast infection (*Candida albicans*). In the presence of disorganized suckling, monitoring and education should focus on improving latch-on or suckling technique; methods such as massaging the infant's jaw may give them a more relaxed latch, preventing pain for the mother.[160] If yeast infection is determined to be the source of the nipple pain, it is important to reduce its spread through good hand washing, using paper towels to dry hands, and boiling any items that will be placed in infant's mouth. Expressed milk is still safe for the infant when the mother has a yeast infection.

Tight Frenulum A tight or short frenulum (**ankyloglossia**) is a very common issue among infants. Because it impedes the infant's ability to move his or her tongue, it is associated with many breastfeeding and swallowing issues.[161] These issues tend to include improper suckling, lack of growth, refusal to feed, and even emotional distress for the infant, as well as nipple and breast pain and engorgement for the mother.[161] The frenulum may need to be stretched or even clipped so that the infant can suck out enough milk.[160]

Inverted (Retracted) and Flat Nipples Inverted or retracted nipples occur most often as a side effect of a separate complication, usually engorgement, but can also be due to skin adhesions beneath the nipple. Inversion makes it difficult for the infant to access the nipple to feed.[158] Simple steps, such as rolling the nipple before feeding or pumping breast milk, will loosen the nipple and separate problematic adhesions.[158,160] Another physiologic complication is flat nipples that may be less stimulated by breastfeeding after delivery. Practices such as pumping briefly before breastfeeding can raise the nipple and allow the infant to latch on properly.[160]

Plugged Ducts Plugged ducts occur secondary to **milk stasis**—the incomplete release of breast milk from the breast—or lactocele cysts that eventually obstruct the ducts and cause tenderness, white spots around the nipple, redness, and/or a tangible lump.[158] While exact causes of this complication are difficult to identify, potential factors include constrictive clothing, fatigue, stress, and inadequate drainage due to changes in feeding frequency or duration.[160] Common treatments include increasing frequency and duration of feedings, maternal rest, moist heat therapy, and massage.[158] If prolonged separation between the mother and infant is required, expressing milk manually will help to prevent milk stasis.[160]

Mastitis Mastitis is defined as inflammation of the breast that generally occurs due to infection after milk stasis or initial issues breastfeeding in the first 6 weeks after delivery.[158,162] Preventing mastitis must begin during pregnancy by making the mother aware of good breastfeeding techniques.

Infrequent or missed feedings are the most common causes of milk stasis that causes mastitis, but poor attachment or weak suckling, maternal or infant illness, oversupply of milk, rapid weaning, pressure on the breast, blocked nipple duct, maternal stress and fatigue, and maternal malnutrition may also be contributors.[162] In the presence of cracks or abrasions near the nipple, disease-producing organisms such as staphylococci, *Escherichia coli*, or streptococci may enter the breast tissue and result in mastitis. Bacterial cellulitis within the connective tissue of the breast and mammary glands also causes breast soreness, fever, and flu-like symptoms.[160] Mastitis should be treated promptly, particularly if a fever is present, because it might indicate progression to an abscess or even to sepsis.[158]

Standard treatments for mastitis are bed rest, increased fluid intake, moist heat to affected area, and antibiotic therapy, as well as continued breastfeeding or pumping to prevent further problems.[158,160] If the mother is having difficulty expressing milk, massaging the breast from the blocked area toward the nipple may be helpful; if she is truly unable to continue breastfeeding, she should still pump her breast milk to avoid an abrupt stop, because this will increase the risk for an abscess.[162] Infants may respond negatively to breast milk produced during mastitis, because it can be higher in sodium and chloride and might taste salty, but this will resolve with frequent feedings.[160]

Special Cases and Contraindications

Under certain rare circumstances, the mother may not be able to breastfeed, or might be advised to adjust her breastfeeding regimen based upon infection or medication. It is important that clinicians are aware of these special cases and empathetically support the mother if she cares for her child with formula.

Maternal Infections

Surprisingly, mothers can breastfeed through the majority of infections. There are a number of viruses, however, that will pass into the breast milk and might infect the baby. As such, appropriate guidelines must be adhered to by new mothers. These are covered in the following sections.

HIV It is possible to transmit HIV infection during breastfeeding, although recommendations for breastfeeding vary based upon geographical location. Developed, first-world countries are often able to provide formula and antiviral treatments to children of HIV-infected mothers; in other areas of the world, however, breast milk and its myriad benefits, especially against diarrheal and upper respiratory tract infections, are too vital to withhold.[142,163] Recommendations from the WHO state that mothers can follow standard breastfeeding guidelines (exclusive breastfeeding for 6 months, then continued breastfeeding with complementary foods for 1 year) as long as they stay on antiretroviral therapy. Even if the mother cannot maintain exclusive breastfeeding, breast milk's benefits still apply.[164]

Herpes Simplex, Tuberculosis, and Other Viruses In the presence of herpes simplex lesions on the breast, brucellosis, T-cell lymphotropic virus, or active/untreated tuberculosis, breastfeeding is not recommended.[142] However, expressed breast milk will not transfer the infections and is a safe option for women with any of these infections. This is particularly true for tuberculosis, when the mother might need to be physically separated from her baby.[165] In the case of tuberculosis, direct breastfeeding should be encouraged after 2 weeks of drug treatment and medical clearance.[142,165]

Other infections are of concern during lactation, but many can be overcome. Varicella, or chickenpox, and H1N1 (swine flu) can infect an infant through skin-to-skin contact and airborne particles; as such, direct breastfeeding should be stopped and pumped breast milk offered instead.[142] Cytomegalovirus (CMV)-positive mothers, however, are now permitted to breastfeed, but antiviral treatments are sometimes recommended to prevent CMV syndrome in the infant, a condition that can lead to symptoms akin to sepsis in preterm or SGA infants.[142]

Lead Poisoning
Initiation of breastfeeding can and should be encouraged for women with a serum lead level <40 micrograms/dL. A breastfeeding woman with a confirmed blood lead level of 40 micrograms/dL or higher should be advised to pump and discard her breast milk until the level has decreased to less than 40 micrograms/dL. If no external cause is identified, and the maternal blood lead level is greater than 20 micrograms/dL and the infant level is 5 micrograms/dL or more, breast milk is likely the source of lead in the infant's blood, and as such breastfeeding should cease until further investigations are carried out.[166]

Metabolic Disorders
In the presence of infant metabolic disorders, including **galactosemia** (intolerance to galactose) or phenylketonuria, breastfeeding is contraindicated and other specially formulated infant formulas should be utilized for primary nutrition. In some cases, combining breastfeeding sessions with feedings of low-protein formula (with frequent blood monitoring) can offer the infant the benefits of breast milk without taxing their organ systems.[142]

Drug Usage
Illicit drug and substance abuse remains a major issue among young women. When these women wish to breastfeed, there are many issues that pose a risk to the infant. For one, drug-user populations are at risk for blood infections such as HIV and hepatitis B and C, as well as malnutrition. Most illicit drugs such as PCP, cocaine, and marijuana can also enter breast milk and affect the infant's brain. As such, the AAP advises against breastfeeding in mothers taking any of these drugs.[142] Throughout the perinatal period, postpartum substance abuse treatment and formula preparation should be discussed frequently, given the recommendation against breastfeeding and the possibility of drug abuse relapse.[167]

Some mothers may also need medications for specific diseases. There are many drugs that might interfere with or enter breast milk. These should be reviewed by the mother's physician. Any current maternal treatment with radioactive isotopes, chemotherapeutic agents, and other specific medications are contraindicated with breastfeeding.[142]

Infant Disease States

Infants born with certain medical conditions might not be able to grow and develop on breast milk alone. These cases tend to occur when babies are born with diseases that cause malabsorption or higher energy needs. Other reasons might be lifestyle related. Examples of these cases include infants who have persistent failure to thrive or weight under 2,000 g, were born preterm, have cystic fibrosis, have been NPO for a medical procedure, must be kept on fluid restrictions, have low bone density, or have a lactase deficiency.[168-171]

Other Indications for Formula Usage

Supplemental feedings may be given in addition to breast milk during the first 6 months of an infant's life and are typically specialized and medically necessary (the infant cannot breastfeed due to a maternal infection or delicate infant condition such as NICU admission, the infant has a metabolic condition such as galactosemia, the infant cannot breastfeed due to a mechanical issue such as cleft lip, or the mother must take a medication that will pass into her breast milk).[132] These feedings usually consist of mixtures of pumped or banked breast milk and formula, with ratios determined by a doctor or RD.[132]

The Lactating Mother: Nutritional Considerations

Nutrition Assessment of a Lactating Mother

While breast milk undeniably provides an excellent and nutritionally balanced source of energy for the infant, the mother must also ensure that she nourishes her own body. The mother's diet and her stores of various nutrients determine the exact macro- and micronutrient levels in mature breast milk.[130] During lactation, the body prioritizes the mammary glands in allotting nutrients, and as such, breast milk often drains maternal nutrient reserves in order to ensure that the baby is properly nourished.[131] This ensures that unless a woman is extremely malnourished, she will be able to produce an adequate amount of nutrient-rich breast milk for her infant. Maternal dietary inadequacies are more likely to reduce the quantity, but not significantly impact the quality, of breast milk. Quality of breast milk is maintained to a certain degree at the expense of maternal stores. When the mother is exclusively breastfeeding her infant, a majority of her energy and nutrient stores, acquired throughout pregnancy, must be utilized to produce enough breast milk to support the high degree of infant growth that occurs in the first 4 to 6 months of life. If a mother's intake of key nutrients, such as vitamin A, vitamin D, and the B vitamins, is suboptimal, less of these nutrients will be produced in the breast milk and her body may struggle with its own numerous metabolic adjustments in lactating and recovering from childbirth.[136,172]

The nutrition status of all patients may affect the quantity of the breast milk produced and may compromise the short- and long-term health of the breastfeeding mother if not managed properly. When assessing the nutritional status of a mother planning to breastfeed, it is important to analyze a number of factors, including pre-pregnancy BMI, pregnancy weight gain, past medical history, comorbidities during pregnancy (i.e., gestational diabetes, preeclampsia, etc.), vitamin and mineral supplementation, and diet recall. In analyzing patient anthropometrics, utilize the National Academy of Medicine weight gain recommendations for pregnancy (Table 21.3) to assess the gestational weight gain of the patient. Breastfeeding will aid in weight loss for all patients, but adequate intake during lactation is vital to ensuring adequate quantity of the breast milk provided to the infant. As such, calorie needs will differ for those patients with inadequate adipose tissues stores acquired during pregnancy compared with overweight and obese mothers. Other nutrient requirements can be determined based on the following information.

> **CORE CONCEPT 29**
>
> Maternal diet and stores of various nutrients will determine the exact levels of macro- and micronutrients in mature breast milk.

> **PRACTICE POINT**
>
> When assessing the nutritional status of a mother planning to breastfeed, it is important to analyze a number of factors, including pre-pregnancy BMI, pregnancy weight gain, past medical history, comorbidities during pregnancy (i.e., gestational diabetes, preeclampsia, etc.), vitamin and mineral supplementation, and diet recall.

CASE STUDY REVISITED

Calculate Meg's calorie and protein needs.

Questions

1. How does her reported intake compare to her needs assessment?

Nutritional Requirements for Lactation

Macronutrient Requirements

Energy (Kilocalories) Breastfeeding an infant requires 20% (about 500 kcal) of a moderately active woman's usual energy output; as such, breastfeeding mothers must mediate their energy balance.[128] The current recommendation is that lactating mothers eat 300 extra calories each day (compared to pre-pregnancy) from nutrient-dense sources such as dairy, fish, nuts, fruits, and vegetables.[172] While this represents only a fraction of the increased metabolic demand of 500 calories, a more substantially increased intake is not necessary because during a healthy pregnancy the mother should have gained extra fat stores to account for lactation.[173] In total, the mother should never eat fewer than 1,800 kcal per day (even in an effort to lose weight), because she will negatively affect her own health.[136]

Carbohydrate Carbohydrate intake is not an area of concern for most lactating women, unless the mother is severely malnourished or her breast milk's lactose content is notably decreased.[136] Overall, the RDA for carbohydrates for a lactating woman is 210 g per day with 25 to 35 g of fiber.[83] Due to the variability of maternal intake, physiology, activity, medical history, and weight loss during lactation, total carbohydrate intake may also be individualized. For example, if the patient has a history of GDM, carbohydrate and fiber intake will need to be closely monitored to prevent the development of type 2 diabetes, a common risk for women who suffered GDM during pregnancy.[111] Adequate fiber enhances blood glucose control, normalizes cholesterol levels, reduces the risk of cardiovascular disease, and increases weight loss by increasing satiety.[83] Fiber for lactating mothers should come from soluble sources such as oats, nuts, beans, and some fruits and vegetables, or insoluble sources such as whole grains and high-cellulose vegetables like celery.

Protein Throughout the first 6 months of lactation, mothers require 71 g of protein per day to maintain adequate nitrogen balance and preserve lean body mass.[172,174] After 6 months of lactation, 62 g (or 1.3 g/kg/day) of protein intake will suffice.[83,174]

Fat Due to the influence that maternal fat intake plays on breast milk composition (see Human Milk Composition), fat is a high-priority nutrient for lactating mother. While lactating women do not need to increase their total fat intake, they should aim to provide 200 to 300 mg of omega-3 long-chain polyunsaturated fatty acids (DHAs) to improve concentration of DHA within breast milk. This amount of DHA is equivalent to one to two portions of fatty fish per week,[136,142] but supplementation with DHA is also an option, particularly for vegetarian or vegan mothers.[142]

Fluid Fluid needs of lactating women increase and it is therefore important for a woman to maintain appropriate fluid consumption. The DRI for this period of development is 3.1 L/day.[83] However, it is important to note that fluid intake does not affect volume of breast milk produced. Women should not be concerned that inadequate volume is due to intake fluid intake.[136]

> **PRACTICE POINT**
>
> The RDA for carbohydrates for a lactating woman is 210 g per day with 25 to 35 g of fiber. Throughout the first 6 months of lactation, mothers require 71 g of protein per day to maintain adequate nitrogen balance and preserve lean body mass. While lactating women do not need to increase their total fat intake, they should aim to provide 200 to 300 mg of omega-3 long-chain polyunsaturated fatty acids (DHAs) to improve concentration of DHA within breast milk.

Micronutrient Requirements

The vitamin and mineral needs of the mother also increase during lactation to account for the loss of nutrients transferred into breast milk. This is important for mothers of one child, but particularly important for mothers of two or more infants, because their bodies will need to produce much more milk, often causing the depletion of vitamin and mineral reserves.[83,128]

Calcium During the postpartum period, before the menstrual cycle has returned to pre-pregnancy status quo, estrogen levels remain low, increasing the amount of calcium drawn from the bones.[128] While dietary calcium will not prevent the loss of calcium from the maternal skeleton during lactation, it has numerous other uses within the mother's body (such as muscle contraction) and for the growing infant. The recommended dietary allowance for calcium to meet 100% of the needs of lactating women ranges from 1,000 mg/day for females 19 to 50 years old to 1,300 mg/day for females 14 to 18 years old, and so mothers should supplement if they cannot meet this level through their diet.[173]

Vitamin B_{12} Supplementation of vitamin B_{12} as synthetic cyanocobalamin form is highly recommended for lactating women who are strict vegetarians, but all women should consume at least 2.8 micrograms per day.[131,173] If the patient is at particularly high risk of vitamin B_{12} deficiency (for example, those following a vegan diet or on specific medications), it is important to evaluate the suitability of folic acid supplementation. Folic acid may mask the symptoms of vitamin B_{12} deficiency. This can lead to serious and often irreversible neurologic, gastrointestinal, and hematologic damage.[83]

Vitamin A The majority of vitamin A in the body (90%) is stored in the liver. Throughout lactation, maternal vitamin A stores are utilized to feed the infant, so dietary needs increase. Vitamin A needs during lactation are 1,200 (18 years old or younger) to 1,300 (19 to 50 years old) micrograms RAE (retinoic acid equivalents) per day, which is based on the daily requirement for age plus the estimated amount of vitamin A excreted in breast milk.[83,173]

Iron Maternal dietary and stored iron has little effect on the iron concentration of breast milk.[173] Iron needs decrease to 10 mg per day for those 18 years or younger and 9 mg per day for women 19 to 50 years old.[173] This decreased RDA is due to the preservation of iron monthly due to the lack of menstrual cycle throughout lactation.[83]

Multivitamin and Multimineral Supplements

Due to the increased nutrient demands of lactation, many women resort to vitamin and mineral supplementation to decrease the risk of deficiencies. However, documentation of benefits from multinutrient supplementation during lactation is not well established. Individual supplementation of micronutrients at risk of deficiency secondary to lifestyle or dietary restrictions, such as vitamin B_{12}, iron, calcium, and vitamin D, can and should be utilized.[67,173] If a mother is particularly concerned, continuing to take her prenatal vitamin can be a good choice.[138]

The Registered Dietitian's Role in Breastfeeding Promotion

Promoting Breastfeeding as an RD

RDs can serve a leading role in educating about and promoting the short- and long-term benefits of breastfeeding. Educational methods such as teaching prenatal classes on breastfeeding within the hospital have had major successes in increasing breastfeeding rates and rates of exclusive breastfeeding for long durations.[135] Classroom education on breastfeeding taught to adolescents is also helpful in fostering positive attitudes towards breastfeeding, leading to firmer intent to breastfeeding their children in the future.[135] Whether counseling patients during pregnancy, prior to a planned pregnancy, or postpartum, RDs are valuable resources to promote and support breastfeeding, providing up-to-date information to the patient. It is important to include close friends and family (as desired by the patient) in these conversations to build a good support system throughout pregnancy and lactation.[135]

During these nutrition counseling sessions, there are various strategies that will ensure success in breastfeeding education. These include maintaining a positive attitude towards breastfeeding, stating the benefits of breastfeeding, teaching listeners how to surmount common barriers and obstacles, and avoiding breastfeeding brochures written by formula manufacturers.[175] Additionally, RDs should promote prenatal weight loss among overweight and obese clients (as it decreases prolactin) and create a friendly environment even for women who decide that they do not wish to breastfeed.[175]

Current Trends and Breastfeeding Assistance Programs

Due the strong educational and promotional efforts by healthcare clinicians, breastfeeding rates are now on the rise. As of 2013, 29 states met the *Healthy People 2020* goal rate for breastfeeding initiation (81.9%).[126] Of these infants, 50% were breastfed until 6 months and 30% for a whole year; these numbers are close to set goals of 60.6% and 34.1%, respectively. Exclusive breastfeeding rates at 3 months (44.4%) and 6 months (22.3%) also demonstrate an uptrend (goals 46.2% and 25.5%).[126] These statistics demonstrate a great success in public health through the educational principles outlined in this chapter and providing support to all mothers.

For some, breastfeeding assistance may be the difference between continuing to breastfeed or switching to formula feeds WIC is the main federal program for low-income mothers and offers free RD services, specialized breastfeeding programs and mentorships, breast pumps/supplies, and food assistance.[176] Local hospitals often provide helpful resources. Boston Children's Hospital, for example, suggests the following websites, accessible to any mother[177]:

- https://massbreastfeeding.org/: The website of the Massachusetts Breastfeeding Coalition, which offers numerous handouts and materials for healthcare practitioners and encourages breastfeeding advocacy.
- http://www.zipmilk.org/: A zip code-based search engine that allows mothers to find local lactation experts and support groups.
- https://toxnet.nlm.nih.gov/newtoxnet/lactmed.htm: LactMed helps mothers to identify medications and compounds that may enter breast milk and do harm to the infant; it also suggests alternatives to discuss with the mother's doctor.
- http://milkbankne.org/: Mother's Milk Bank Northeast is a breast milk bank that gives breast milk to those mothers who cannot breastfeed, delivering its benefits to their children.

Summary: Nutrition in Lactation

Breast milk is unique in that it responds and adapts to infant needs immediately after delivery, when immunologically rich colostrum is produced, until the mother chooses to stop breastfeeding. Due to numerous benefits for the mother and infant, it is recommended that infants be breastfed exclusively until 6 months of age and breastfed with complementary foods until at least 12 months. The success of the breastfeeding experience is dependent upon numerous maternal factors ranging from sleep adequacy and stress level to dietary intake and postpartum nutritional status. Ensuring that a mother completes her pregnancy with an optimal nutritional status will prevent nutrient store depletion that may carry over into lactation and adversely affect breast milk for the infant. Meeting the increased dietary needs during both pregnancy and lactation will give the breastfeeding mother the nutritional support optimal for producing the breast milk that her infant needs. While some mothers will face barriers and complications during breastfeeding, the clinician and the mother's support system can overcome most obstacles and give the infant a solid foundation.

Key Terms

pregnancy, gravida, para/parity, gestation, small for gestational age, large-for-gestational age, placenta, placental insufficiency, preeclampsia, intrauterine growth restriction (IUGR), physiologic anemia of pregnancy, orthostatic hypotension, placental barrier, preconception health, neural tube, spina bifida, anencephaly, craniorachischisis, neural tube defect, fetal macrosomia, AMPK (adenosine monophosphate-activated protein kinase), fetal alcohol syndrome, pica, geophagia, pacophagia, asymmetric macrosomia, nausea and vomiting of pregnancy (NVP), hyperemesis gravidarum (HG), gestational diabetes mellitus (GDM), gestational hypertension, early-onset preeclampsia, late-onset preeclampsia, maternal preeclampsia, placental preeclampsia, HELLP syndrome, lactogenesis, lactation, "let down", delayed onset lactation, involution, colostrum, transitional milk, mature milk, foremilk, hindmilk, feeding cues, engorgement, ankyloglossia, milk stasis, mastitis, galactosemia

References

1. Procter SB, Campbell CG. Position of the Academy of Nutrition and Dietetics: nutrition and lifestyle for a healthy pregnancy outcome. *J Acad Nutr Diet*. 2014;114(7):1099-1103. doi: 10.1016/j.jand.2014.05.005 [doi].
2. Weight Gain During Pregnancy: Reexamining the Guidelines. Institute of Medicine (US) and National Research Council (US) Committee to Reexamine IOM Pregnancy Weight Guidelines; Rasmussen KM, Yaktine AL, eds. Washington (DC): National Academies Press (US); 2009.
3. Lee HS. Impact of maternal diet on the epigenome during in utero life and the developmental programming of diseases in childhood and adulthood. *Nutrients*. 2015;7(11):9492-9507. doi: 10.3390/nu7115467 [doi].
4. Gluckman PD, Hanson MA, Cooper C, Thornburg KL. Effect of in utero and early-life conditions on adult health and disease. *N Engl J Med*. 2008;359(1):61-73. doi: 10.1056/NEJMra0708473; 10.1056/NEJMra0708473.
5. Das JK, Salam RA, Imdad A, Bhutta ZA. Infant and young child growth. In: Black RE, Laxminarayan R, Temmerman M, Walker N, eds. *Reproductive, maternal, newborn, and child health: disease control priorities*. Vol. 2. 3rd ed. Washington, DC: International Bank for Reconstruction and Development/The World Bank; 2016.
6. Lassi ZS, Mansoor T, Salam RA, Das JK, Bhutta ZA. Essential pre-pregnancy and pregnancy interventions for improved maternal, newborn and child health. *Reprod Health*. 2014;11(suppl 1):S2-4755-11-S1-S2. Epub 2014 Aug 21. doi: 10.1186/1742-4755-11-S1-S2 [doi].
7. Glanze WD, Anderson KN, Anderson LE, Urdang L, Swallow HH, eds. *Mosby's medical and nursing dictionary*. 2nd ed. St. Louis, MO: The C.V. Mosby Company; 1986.
8. Ricci SS. *Essentials of maternity, newborn, and women's health nursing*. 2nd ed. Philadelphia, PA: Wolters Kluwer | Lippincott Williams and Wilkins; 2009.
9. Hay WW Jr. Recent observations on the regulation of fetal metabolism by glucose. *J Physiol*. 2006;572(part 1):17-24. doi: jphysiol.2006.105072 [pii].
10. Myers RE, Hill DE, Holt AB, Scott RE, Mellits ED, Cheek DB. Fetal growth retardation produced by experimental placental insufficiency in the rhesus monkey. I. Body weight, organ size. *Biol Neonate*. 1971;18(5):379-394.
11. Unterscheider J, Daly S, Geary MP, et al. Optimizing the definition of intrauterine growth restriction: the multicenter prospective PORTO Study. *Am J Obstet Gynecol*. 2013;208(4):290.e1-290.e6. doi: 10.1016/j.ajog.2013.02.007 [doi].
12. Howarth C, Gazis A, James D. Associations of Type 1 diabetes mellitus, maternal vascular disease and complications of pregnancy. *Diabet Med*. 2007;24(11):1229-1234. doi: DME2254 [pii].
13. Kanaka-Gantenbein C, Mastorakos G, Chrousos GP. Endocrine-related causes and consequences of intrauterine growth retardation. *Ann N Y Acad Sci*. 2003;997:150-157.
14. Costantine MM. Physiologic and pharmacokinetic changes in pregnancy. *Front Pharmacol*. 2014;5:65. doi: 10.3389/fphar.2014.00065 [doi].
15. Heidemann BH, McClure JH. Changes in maternal physiology during pregnancy. *BJA CEPD Reviews*. 2003;3(3):65-68. doi: 10.1093/bjacepd/mkg065.
16. Soma-Pillay P, Nelson-Piercy C, Tolppanen H, Mebazaa A. Physiological changes in pregnancy. *Cardiovasc J Afr*. 2016;27(2):89-94. doi: 10.5830/CVJA-2016-021 [doi].
17. Magee LA, Pels A, Helewa M, Rey E, von Dadelszen P. SOGC Hypertension Guideline Committee. Diagnosis, evaluation, and management of the hypertensive disorders of pregnancy: executive summary. *J Obstet Gynaecol Can*. 2014;36(7):575-576. doi: S1701-2163(15)30533-8 [pii].
18. Friel LA. Merck Manual: Anemia in pregnancy. http://www.merckmanuals.com/professional/gynecology-and-obstetrics/pregnancy-complicated-by-disease/anemia-in-pregnancy. Revised March 2017. Accessed August 18, 2017.
19. Infant of diabetic mother. Children's Hospital of Philadelphia website. http://www.chop.edu/conditions-diseases/infant-diabetic-mother. Accessed August 18, 2017.
20. Kalhan SC. Protein metabolism in pregnancy. *Am J Clin Nutr*. 2000;71(suppl 5):1249S-1255S.
21. King JC. Physiology of pregnancy and nutrient metabolism. *Am J Clin Nutr*. 2000;71(5):1218s-1225s.
22. King JC. Maternal obesity, metabolism, and pregnancy outcomes. *Annu Rev Nutr*. 2006;26:271-291. doi: 10.1146/annurev.nutr.24.012003.132249.
23. Abu-Saad K, Fraser D. Maternal nutrition and birth outcomes. *Epidemiol Rev*. 2010;32(1):5-25. doi: 10.1093/epirev/mxq001; 10.1093/epirev/mxq001.
24. Akerele OA, Cheema SK. A balance of omega-3 and omega-6 polyunsaturated fatty acids is important in pregnancy. *J Nutr Intermediary Metabol*. 2016;5:23-33.
25. Cleaton MA, Dent CL, Howard M, et al. Fetus-derived DLK1 is required for maternal metabolic adaptations to pregnancy and is associated with fetal growth restriction. *Nat Genet*. 2016;48(12):1473-1480. doi: 10.1038/ng.3699 [doi].
26. Wang S. Metabolic Syndrome. http://emedicine.medscape.com/article/165124-overview. Accessed July 10, 2017.
27. Abbassi-Ghanavati M, Greer LG, Cunningham FG. Pregnancy and laboratory studies: a reference table for clinicians. *Obstet Gynecol*. 2009 Dec;114(6):1326-1331. PMID:19935037.

28. Centers for Disease Control and Prevention. Overview: Preconception Health. https://www.cdc.gov/preconception/overview.html. Accessed July 14, 2017.
29. Johnson K, Posner SF, Biermann J, et al. Recommendations to Improve Preconception Health and Health Care—United States: A Report of the CDC/ATSDR Preconception Care Work Group and the Select Panel on Preconception Care. *MMWR Recomm Rep*. 2006;55(RR06):1-23.
30. Folic acid recommendations. Centers for Disease Control and Prevention website. https://www.cdc.gov/ncbddd/folicacid/recommendations.html Updated December 28, 2016. Accessed November 9, 2017.
31. Parker SE, Yazdy MM, Tinker SC, Mitchell AA, Werler MM. The impact of folic acid intake on the association among diabetes mellitus, obesity, and spina bifida. *Am J Obstet Gynecol*. 2013;209(3):239.e1-239.e8. doi: 10.1016/j.ajog.2013.05.047; 10.1016/j.ajog.2013.05.047.
32. Widen E, Siega-Riz AM. Prenatal nutrition: a practical guide for assessment and counseling. *J Midwifery Womens Health*. 2010;55(6):540-549. doi: 10.1016/j.jmwh.2010.06.017; 10.1016/j.jmwh.2010.06.017.
33. Florescu L, Temneanu OR, Nistor N, Mindru DE. Iron deficiency and iron deficiency anemia—A global public health problem. *Romanian J Med Prac*. 2016;11(3):254-303.
34. Goonewardene M, Shehata M, Hamad A. Anaemia in pregnancy. *Best Prac Res Clin Obstetr Gynaecol*. 2012;26(1):3-24.
35. Hwang JY, Lee JY, Kim KN, et al. Maternal iron intake at mid-pregnancy is associated with reduced fetal growth: results from Mothers and Children's Environmental Health (MOCEH) study. *Nutr J*. 2013;12(1):38. doi: 10.1186/1475-2891-12-38. Marcel C. Quick lesson: Nutrition in pregnancy. Accessed July 17, 2017.
36. Marcel C. Quick lesson: Nutrition in pregnancy. Accessed July 17, 2017. Marcel C. Nutrition in Pregnancy. CINAHL Nursing Guide [serial online]. October 21, 2016. Available from: Nursing Reference Center Plus, Ipswich, MA. EBSCOhost, ezproxy.simmons.edu:2048/login?url=https://search-ebscohost-com.ezproxy.simmons.edu/login.aspx?direct=true&db=nup&AN=T706243&site=eds-live&scope=site. Accessed July 17, 2017
37. Ogden CL, Carroll MD, Fryar CD, Flegal KM. Prevalence of obesity among adults and youth: United States, 2011-2014. *NCHS Data Brief*. 2015;(219)(219):1-8.
38. American Society for Parenteral and Enteral Nutrition (A.S.P.E.N.) Board of Directors. Clinical Guidelines for the Use of Parenteral and Enteral Nutrition in Adult and Pediatric Patients, 2009. *JPEN J Parenter Enteral Nutr*. 2009;33(3):255-259. doi: 10.1177/0148607109333115; 10.1177/0148607109333115.
39. Stang J, Huffman LG. Position of the Academy of Nutrition and Dietetics: Obesity, Reproduction, and Pregnancy Outcomes. *J Acad Nutr Dietet*. 2016;116(4):677-691.
40. Schub T, Boling B. CINAHL Nursing Guide [serial online]. April 15, 2016; Available from: Nursing Reference Center Plus, Ipswich, MA. Accessed July 17, 2017.
41. Sharmila G, Sudha M. Maternal body mass index in outcome of pregnancy. *Int J Reprod Contracep Obstet Gynecol*. 2016;5(8):2652-2656. doi: http://dx.doi.org/10.18203/2320-1770.ijrcog20162639.
42. Medeiros M, Saunders C, Chagas CB, Pereira SE, Saboya C, Ramalho A. Vitamin D deficiency in pregnancy after bariatric surgery. *Obes Surg*. 2013;23(10):1679-1684. doi: 10.1007/s11695-013-1045-5; 10.1007/s11695-013-1045-5.
43. Shin D, Bianchi L, Chung H, Weatherspoon L, Song WO. Is gestational weight gain associated with diet quality during pregnancy? *Matern Child Health J*. 2014;18(6)1433-1443. doi: 10.1007/s10995-013-1383-x.
44. Kaiser L, Allen LH, American Dietetic Association. Position of the American Dietetic Association: nutrition and lifestyle for a healthy pregnancy outcome. *J Am Diet Assoc*. 2008;108(3):553-561.
45. Cuco G, Arija V, Iranzo R, Vila J, Prieto MT, Fernandez-Ballart J. Association of maternal protein intake before conception and throughout pregnancy with birth weight. *Acta Obstet Gynecol Scand*. 2006;85(4):413-421. doi: 10.1080/00016340600572228.
46. Moore VM, Davies MJ, Willson KJ, Worsley A, Robinson JS. Dietary composition of pregnant women is related to size of the baby at birth. *J Nutr*. 2004;134(7):1820-1826.
47. Olsen SF, Halldorsson TI, Willett WC, et al. Milk consumption during pregnancy is associated with increased infant size at birth: prospective cohort study. *Am J Clin Nutr*. 2007;86(4):1104-1110.
48. Sacks FM, Lichtenstein AH, Wu JHY, et al. Dietary fats and cardiovascular disease: A Presidential Advisory From the American Heart Association. *Circulation*. 2017;136(3):e1-e23. doi: 10.1161/CIR.0000000000000510 [doi].
49. Kiely M, Hemmingway A, O'Callaghan KM. Vitamin D in pregnancy: Current perspective and future directions. *Ther Adv Musculoskelet Dis*. 2017;9(6):145-154. doi: 10.1177/175972X17706453.
50. Ji J, Muyayalo KP, Zhang Y, Hu X, Liao A. Immunological function of vitamin D during human pregnancy. *Am J Reprod Immunol*. 2017;78(2). doi: 10.1111/aji.12716.
51. Principi N, Bianchini S, Baggi E, Esposito S. Implications of maternal vitamin D deficiency for the fetus, the neonate and the young infant. *Eur J Nutr*. 2013;52(3):859-867. doi: 10.1007/s00394-012-0476-4; 10.1007/s00394-012-0476-4.
52. Nussey S, Whitehead S. Endocrinology: An Integrated Approach. Oxford: BIOS Scientific Publishers; 2001. Chapter 5: The parathyroid glands and vitamin D. Available from: https://www.ncbi.nlm.nih.gov/books/NBK24/
53. Mulligan ML, Felton SK, Riek AE, Bernal-Mizrachi C. Implications of vitamin D deficiency in pregnancy and lactation. *Obstet Gynecol*. 2010;202(5):429.e1-429.e9.
54. Wagner CL, Greer FR, and the Section on Breastfeeding and Committee on Nutrition. Prevention of rickets and vitamin D deficiency in infants, children, and adolescents. *Pediatrics*. 2008;122(5):1142-1152. doi: 10.1542/peds.2008-1862.
55. Holick MF, Binkley NC, Bischoff-Ferrari HA, et al. Evaluation, treatment, and prevention of vitamin D deficiency: an Endocrine Society clinical practice guideline. *J Clin Endocrinol Metab*. 2011;96(7):1911-1930. doi: 10.1210/jc.2011-0385 [doi].
56. Hovdenak N, Haram K. Influence of mineral and vitamin supplements on pregnancy outcome. *Eur J Obstet Gynecol Reprod Biol*. 2012;164(2):127-132. doi: 10.1016/j.ejogrb.2012.06.020; 10.1016/j.ejogrb.2012.06.020.
57. Dror DK, Allen LH. Interventions with vitamins B6, B12 and C in pregnancy. *Paediatr Perinat Epidemiol*. 2012;26:55-74. doi: 10.1111/j.1365-3016.2012.01277.x.
58. McArdle HJ, Gambling L, Kennedy C. Iron deficiency during pregnancy: the consequences for placental function and fetal outcome. *Proc Nutr Soc*. 2013:1-7. doi: 10.1017/S0029665113003637.
59. Pena-Rosas JP, De-Regil LM, Dowswell T, Viteri FE. Intermittent oral iron supplementation during pregnancy. *Cochrane Database Syst Rev*. 2012;7:CD009997. doi: 10.1002/14651858.CD009997; 10.1002/14651858.CD009997.
60. Zhao G, Xu G, Zhou M, et al. Prenatal iron supplementation reduces maternal anemia, iron deficiency, and iron deficiency anemia in a randomized clinical trial in rural China, but iron deficiency remains widespread in mothers and neonates. *J Nutr*. 2015;145(8):1916-1923. doi: 10.3945/jn.114.208678 [doi].

61. Cepeda-Lopez AC, Melse-Boonstra A, Zimmermann MB, Herter-Aeberli I. In overweight and obese women, dietary iron absorption is reduced and the enhancement of iron absorption by ascorbic acid is one-half that in normal-weight women. *Am J Clin Nutr*. 2015;102(6):1389-1397. doi: 10.3945/ajcn.114.099218 [doi].

62. Hofmeyr GJ, Lawrie TA, Atallah AN, Duley L, Torloni MR. Calcium supplementation during pregnancy for preventing hypertensive disorders and related problems. *Cochrane Database Syst Rev*. 2014;(6):CD001059. doi(6):CD001059. doi: 10.1002/14651858.CD001059.pub4 [doi].

63. Torres MT, Francés L, Vila L, et al. Iodine nutritional status of women in their first trimester of pregnancy in Catalonia. *BMC*. 2017;17(1):249. doi: 10.1186/s12884-017-1423-4.

64. Xiao Y, Sun H, Li C, et al. Effect of iodine nutrition on pregnancy outcomes in an iodine-sufficient area in China. *Biol Trace Elem Res*. 2017. doi: 10.1007/s12011-017-1101-4.

65. Marangoni F, Cetin I, Verduci E, et al. Maternal diet and nutrient requirements in pregnancy and breastfeeding. An Italian Consensus Document. *Nutrients*. 2016;8(10):E629.

66. Ghanbari M, Ghasemi A. Maternal hypothyroidism: An overview of current experimental models. *Life Sciences*. 2017;187:1-8.

67. Picciano MF, McGuire MK. Use of dietary supplements by pregnant and lactating women in North America. *Am J Clin Nutr*. 2009;89(2):663S-7S. doi: 10.3945/ajcn.2008.26811B; 10.3945/ajcn.2008.26811B.

68. Russo LM, Nobles C, Ertel KA, Chasan-Taber L, Whitcomb BW. Physical activity interventions in pregnancy and risk of gestational diabetes mellitus: a systematic review and meta-analysis. *Obstet Gynecol*. 2015;125(3):576-582. doi: 10.1097/AOG.0000000000000691 [doi].

69. On Obstetric Practice C. ACOG Committee Opinion No. 650: Physical activity and exercise during pregnancy and the postpartum period. *Obstet Gynecol*. 2015;126(6):e135-42. doi: 10.1097/AOG.0000000000001214 [doi].

70. American Dietetic Association, American Society of Nutrition, Siega-Riz AM, King JC. Position of the American Dietetic Association and American Society for Nutrition: Obesity, Reproduction, and Pregnancy Outcomes. *J Am Diet Assoc*. 2009;109(5):918-927.

71. Evenson KR, Barakat R, Brown WJ, et al. Guidelines for physical activity during pregnancy: comparisons from around the world. *Am J Lifestyle Med*. 2014;8(2):102-121. doi: 10.1177/1559827613498204.

72. Kaiser LL, Campbell CG, Academy Positions Committee Workgroup. Practice paper of the Academy of Nutrition and Dietetics abstract: nutrition and lifestyle for a healthy pregnancy outcome. *J Acad Nutr Diet*. 2014;114(9):1447.

73. Eating Fish: What Pregnant Women and Parents Should Know. U.S. Food and Drug Administration website. https://www.fda.gov/Food/ResourcesForYou/Consumers/ucm393070.htm. Updated November 29, 2017. Accessed December 30, 2017.

74. Ebrahimi N, Maltepe C, Einarson A. Optimal management of nausea and vomiting of pregnancy. *Int J Womens Health*. 2010;2:241-248.

75. Marvin-Dowle K, Burley VJ, Soltani H. Nutrient intakes and nutritional biomarkers in pregnant adolescents: a systematic review of studies in developed countries. *BMC Pregnancy Childbirth*. 2016;16:268-016-1059-9. doi: 10.1186/s12884-016-1059-9 [doi].

76. Bucciarelli A, Chisholm A. Multiple Pregnancies. Health Library: Evidence-Based Information [serial online]. April 2016; Available from: Nursing Reference Center Plus, Ipswich MA. EBSCOhost, ezproxy.simmons.edu:2048/login?url=https://search-ebscohost-com.ezproxy.simmons.edu/login.aspx?direct=true&db=nup&AN=2010368544&site=eds-live&scope=site.Accessed December 2, 2017.

77. Lazarov S, Lazarov L, Lazarov N. Complications of multiple pregnancies. *Trakia J Sci*. 2017;14(1):108-111. doi: 10.15547/tjs.2016.01.016.

78. Brown J. *Nutrition through the lifecycle*. 6th ed. Boston, MA: Cengage Learning; 2017.

79. Luke B. Nutrition and multiple gestation. *Semin Perinatol*. 2005;29(5):349-354. doi: 10.1053/j.semperi.2005.08.004.

80. Escott-Stump S, ed. *Nutrition and diagnosis-related care*. 7th ed. Baltimore, MD and Philadelphia, PA: Lippincott Williams and Wilkins; 2012.

81. Committee on Obstetric Practice. Committee Opinion: Weight Gain During Pregnancy. *Obstet Gynecol*. 2013;121(1):210-212.

82. Marcason W. What are the calorie requirements for women having twins? *J Am Diet Assoc*. 2006;106(8):1292.

83. Otten JJ, Hellwig JP, Meyers LD. *Dietary Reference Intakes: The essential guide to nutrient requirements*. Washington, DC: National Academies Press; 2006.

84. Goodnight W, Newman R, Society of Maternal-Fetal Medicine. Optimal nutrition for improved twin pregnancy outcome. *Obstet Gynecol*. 2009;114(5):1121-1134. doi: 10.1097/AOG.0b013e3181bb14c8 [doi].

85. Klein L. Nutritional recommendations for multiple pregnancy. *J Am Diet Assoc*. 2005;105(7):1050-1052.

86. Kominiarek MA. Preparing for and managing a pregnancy after bariatric surgery. *Semin Perinatol*. 2011;35(6):356-361. doi: 10.1053/j.semperi.2011.05.022; 10.1053/j.semperi.2011.05.022.

87. Mechanick JI, Youdim A, Jones DB, et al. Clinical practice guidelines for the perioperative nutritional, metabolic, and nonsurgical support of the bariatric surgery patient–2013 update: cosponsored by American Association of Clinical Endocrinologists, The Obesity Society, and American Society for Metabolic & Bariatric Surgery. *Obesity (Silver Spring)*. 2013;21(suppl 1):S1-27. doi: 10.1002/oby.20461 [doi].

88. Adams TD, Hammoud AO, Davidson LE, et al. Maternal and neonatal outcomes for pregnancies before and after gastric bypass surgery. *Int J Obes (Lond)*. 2015;39(4):686-694. doi: 10.1038/ijo.2015.9 [doi].

89. Eating Disorder Association N. Pregnancy and eating disorders. https://www.nationaleatingdisorders.org/pregnancy-and-eating-disorders. Accessed August 18, 2017.

90. Chiang JL, Kirkman MS, Laffel LM, Peters AL, Type 1 Diabetes Sourcebook Authors. Type 1 diabetes through the life span: a position statement of the American Diabetes Association. *Diabetes Care*. 2014;37(7):2034-2054. doi: 10.2337/dc14-1140 [doi].

91. Guideline for detection and management of diabetes in pregnancy, Joslin Diabetes Center and Joslin Clinic 11/10/2016 corrected 01/11/17. http://www.joslin.org/Pregnancy-Guidelines_11-13-2016_corrected_1-11-2017.pdf. Accessed 12/31/2017.

92. Greene MF, Bentley-Lewis R, Nathan DM, Berghella V, Barss VA. Pregestational diabetes mellitus: Glycemic control during pregnancy. https://www.uptodate.com/contents/pregestational-diabetes-mellitus-glycemic-control-during-pregnancy?source=search_result&search=Dawn%20phenomenon&selectedTitle=3~3. Accessed August 29, 2017.

93. Morrison JL, Regnault TR. Nutrition in pregnancy: optimising maternal diet and fetal adaptations to altered nutrient supply. *Nutrients*. 2016;8(6):10.3390/nu8060342. doi: 10.3390/nu8060342 [doi].

94. Montgomery KS. Nutrition and HIV-positive pregnancy. *J Perinat Educ*. 2003;12(1):42-47. doi: 10.1624/105812403X106711.

95. Mala J. Effect of dietary intakes on pregnancy outcomes: a comparative study among HIV-infected and uninfected women at Nyanza Provincial General Hospital, Kenya. *African Journal of Food, Agriculture, Nutrition and Development*. 2012;12(6):6776-6793.

96. Drakesmith H, Prentice A. Viral infection and iron metabolism. *Nat Rev Microbiol*. 2008;6(7):541-552. doi: 10.1038/nrmicro1930 [doi].

97. Elmadfa I, Meyer AL. Vitamins for the first 1000 days: preparing for life. *Int J Vitam Nutr Res.* 2012;82(5):342-347. doi: 10.1024/0300-9831/a000129; 10.1024/0300-9831/a000129.

98. Bencaiova G, Burkhardt T, Breymann C. Anemia—prevalence and risk factors in pregnancy. *Eur J Intern Med.* 2012;23(6):529-533.

99. Wegrzyniak LJ, Repke JT, Ural SH. Treatment of HG. *Rev Obstet Gynecol.* 2012;5(2):78-84.

100. Maltepe C, Koren G. The management of nausea and vomiting of pregnancy and HG–a 2013 update. *J Popul Ther Clin Pharmacol.* 2013;20(2):e184-192.

101. Paauw JD, Bierling S, Cook CR, Davis AT. HG and fetal outcome. *JPEN J Parenter Enteral Nutr.* 2005;29(2):93-96.

102. Peled Y, Melamed N, Hiersch L, Pardo J, Wiznitzer A, Yogev Y. The impact of total parenteral nutrition support on pregnancy outcome in women with HG. *J Matern Fetal Neonatal Med.* 2014;27(11):1146-1150. doi: 10.3109/14767058.2013.851187.

103. Parrish CR, Lord LM, Pelletier K. Management of HG with enteral nutrition. *Prac Gastroenterol.* 2008;series #63:15-31.

104. Lonsdale D. A review of the biochemistry, metabolism and clinical benefits of thiamin(e) and its derivatives. *Evid Based Complement Alternat Med.* 2006;3(1):49-59. doi: 10.1093/ecam/nek009.

105. Walmsley RS. Refeeding syndrome: screening, incidence, and treatment during parenteral nutrition. *J Gastroenterol Hepatol.* 2013;28(suppl 4):113-117. doi: 10.1111/jgh.12345; 10.1111/jgh.12345.

106. Frank LL. Thiamin in clinical practice. *JPEN J Parenter Enteral Nutr.* 2015;39(5):503-520. doi: 10.1177/0148607114565245 [doi].

107. Galvin R, Brathen G, Ivashynka A, et al. EFNS guidelines for diagnosis, therapy and prevention of Wernicke encephalopathy. *Eur J Neurol.* 2010;17(12):1408-1418. doi: 10.1111/j.1468-1331.2010.03153.x [doi].

108. Berdai MA, Labib S, Harandou M. Wernicke's encephalopathy complicating hyperemesis during pregnancy. *Case Rep Crit Care.* 2016;2016:8783932. doi: 10.1155/2016/8783932 [doi].

109. Kumar D, Geller F, Wang L, Wagner B, Fitz-Gerald MJ, Schwendimann R. Wernicke's encephalopathy in a patient with HG. *Psychosomatics.* 2012;53(2):172-174. doi: 10.1016/j.psym.2011.06.005; 10.1016/j.psym.2011.06.005.

110. Saha S, Loranger D, Pricolo V, Degli-Esposti S. Feeding jejunostomy for the treatment of severe HG: a case series. *JPEN J Parenter Enteral Nutr.* 2009;33(5):529-534. doi: 10.1177/0148607109333000; 10.1177/0148607109333000.

111. Diabetes Association A, Cefalu WT. Standards of Medical Care in Diabetes. *J Clin Appl Res Ed.* 2017;40(1):1-142.

112. Kc K, Shakya S, Zhang H. Gestational diabetes mellitus and macrosomia: a literature review. *Ann Nutr Metab.* 2015;66(suppl 2):14-20. doi: 10.1159/000371628 [doi].

113. Kleinwechter H, Schafer-Graf U, Buhrer C, et al. Gestational diabetes mellitus (GDM) diagnosis, therapy and follow-up care: Practice Guideline of the German Diabetes Association(DDG) and the German Association for Gynaecologyand Obstetrics (DGGG). *Exp Clin Endocrinol Diabetes.* 2014;122(7):395-405. doi: 10.1055/s-0034-1366412 [doi].

114. American Diabetes Association. Gestational diabetes mellitus. *Diabetes Care.* 2003;26(suppl 1):s103-s105. doi: 10.2337/diacare.26.2007.S103.

115. Diabetes Association A. Management of Diabetes in Pregnancy. *Diabetes Care.* 2017;40(Supplement 1):S114-S119.

116. Leeman L, Fontaine P. Hypertensive disorders of pregnancy. *Am Fam Physician.* 2008;78(1):93-100.

117. American College of Obstetricians and Gynecologists. Frequently asked questions: pregnancy—preeclampsia and high blood pressure during pregnancy. https://www.acog.org/Patients/FAQs/Preeclampsia-and-High-Blood-Pressure-During-Pregnancy. Accessed July 10, 2017.

118. Huppertz B. Placental origins of preeclampsia: challenging the current hypothesis. *Hypertension.* 2008;51(4):970-975. doi: 10.1161/HYPERTENSIONAHA.107.107607 [doi].

119. Patwari M, Talukdar B, Solo N. Estimation of serum calcium and magnesium in pre-eclampsia and eclampsia. *J Evol Med Dental Sci.* 2016;5(58):3985-3987. doi: 10.14260/jemds/2016/912.

120. World Health Organization. Guideline: Calcium supplementation in pregnant women. *WHO Guideline.* 2013:1-35. http://apps.who.int/iris/bitstream/10665/85120/1/9789241505376_eng.pdf.

121. Watson LA, Bommarito AA, Marshall JF. Total peripheral parenteral nutrition in pregnancy. *JPEN J Parenter Enteral Nutr.* 1990;14(5):485-489.

122. Stokke G, Gjelsvik BL, Flaatten KT, Birkeland E, Flaatten H, Trovik J. HG, nutritional treatment by nasogastric tube feeding: a 10-year retrospective cohort study. *Acta Obstet Gynecol Scand.* 2015;94(4):359-367. doi: 10.1111/aogs.12578 [doi].

123. Godil A, Chen YK. Percutaneous endoscopic gastrostomy for nutrition support in pregnancy associated with HG and anorexia nervosa. *JPEN J Parenter Enteral Nutr.* 1998;22(4):238-241.

124. Lee NM, Saha S. Nausea and vomiting of pregnancy. *Gastroenterol Clin North Am.* 2011;40(2):309-334, vii. doi: 10.1016/j.gtc.2011.03.009; 10.1016/j.gtc.2011.03.009.

125. Cape AV, Mogensen KM, Robinson MK, Carusi DA. Peripherally inserted central catheter (PICC) complications during pregnancy. *JPEN J Parenter Enteral Nutr.* 2014;38(5):595-601. doi: 10.1177/0148607113489994.

126. National Center for Chronic Disease Prevention and Healthy Promotion. Breastfeeding Report Card: Progressing Toward National Breastfeeding Goals. *CDC.* 2016:1-8.

127. Holmes AV. Establishing successful breastfeeding in the newborn period. *Pediatr Clin North Am.* 2013;60(1):147-168.

128. Neville MC. Anatomy and physiology of lactation. *Pediatr Clin North Am.* 2001;48(1):13-34.

129. Neville MC, Morton J, Umemura S. Lactogenesis. The transition from pregnancy to lactation. *Pediatr Clin North Am.* 2001;48(1):35-52.

130. Ballard O, Morrow AL. Human milk composition: nutrients and bioactive factors. *Pediatr Clin North Am.* 2013;60(1):49-74. doi: 10.1016/j.pcl.2012.10.002 [doi].

131. Picciano MF. Pregnancy and lactation: physiological adjustments, nutritional requirements and the role of dietary supplements. *J Nutr.* 2003;133(6):1997S-2002S.

132. Academy of Breastfeeding Medicine Protocol Committee. ABM clinical protocol #3: hospital guidelines for the use of supplementary feedings in the healthy term breastfed neonate, revised 2009. *Breastfeed Med.* 2009;4(3):175-182. doi: 10.1089/bfm.2009.9991 [doi].

133. Kociszewska-Najman B, Borek-Dzieciol B, Szpotanska-Sikorska M, Wilkos E, Pietrzak B, Wielgos M. The creamatocrit, fat and energy concentration in human milk produced by mothers of preterm and term infants. *J Matern Fetal Neonatal Med.* 2012;25(9):1599-1602. doi: 10.3109/14767058.2011.648239 [doi].

134. Picciano MF. Nutrient composition of human milk. *Pediatr Clin North Am.* 2001;48(1):53-67.

135. James DC, Lessen R, American Dietetic Association. Position of the American Dietetic Association: promoting and supporting breastfeeding. *J Am Diet Assoc.* 2009;109(11):1926-1942.

136. Ares Segura S, Arena Ansotegui J, Diaz-Gomez NM, en representacion del Comite de Lactancia Materna de la Asociacion Espanola de Pediatria. The importance of maternal nutrition during breastfeeding: Do breastfeeding mothers need nutritional supplements? *An Pediatr (Barc).* 2016;84(6):347.e1-347.e7. doi: 10.1016/j.anpedi.2015.07.024 [doi].

137. Gidrewicz DA, Fenton TR. A systematic review and meta-analysis of the nutrient content of preterm and term breast milk. *BMC Pediatr.* 2014;14:216-2431-14-216. doi: 10.1186/1471-2431-14-216 [doi].
138. American College of Obstetricians and Gynecologists. Frequently Asked Questions: breastfeeding your baby. https://www.acog.org/Patients/FAQs/Breastfeeding-Your-Baby. Accessed August 16, 2017.
139. Baker RD, Greer FR. Diagnosis and prevention of iron deficiency and iron-deficiency anemia in infants and young children (0-3 Years of Age) [- 5]. *Pediatrics.* 2010;126(5):104-119.
140. Johnson D. First AAP recommendations on iron supplementation include directive on universal screening. *AAP News.* 2010. doi: 10.1542/aapnews.20101005-1.
141. Groh-Wargo S, Thompson M, Cox JH. *ADA pocket guide to neonatal nutrition.* Chicago, IL: Academy of Nutrition and Dietetics; 2009.
142. Section on Breastfeeding. Breastfeeding and the use of human milk. *Pediatrics.* 2012;129(3):e827-41. doi: 10.1542/peds.2011-3552; 10.1542/peds.2011-3552.
143. Lovelady CA, Hunter CP, Geigerman C. Effect of exercise on immunologic factors in breast milk. *Pediatrics.* 2003;111(2):E148-52.
144. Cabrera-Rubio R, Collado MC, Laitinen K, Salminen S, Isolauri E, Mira A. The human milk microbiome changes over lactation and is shaped by maternal weight and mode of delivery. *Am J Clin Nutr.* 2012;96(3):544-551. doi: 10.3945/ajcn.112.037382 [doi].
145. Chirico G, Marzollo R, Cortinovis S, Fonte C, Gasparoni A. Antiinfective properties of human milk. *J Nutr.* 2008;138(9):1801S-1806S. doi: 138/9S-II/1801S [pii].
146. Victora CG, Rollins NC, Murch S, Krasevec J, Bahl R. Breastfeeding in the 21st century—Authors' reply. *Lancet.* 2016;387(10033):2089-2090. doi: S0140-6736(16)30538-4 [pii].
147. Weber M, Grote V, Closa-Monasterolo R, et al. Lower protein content in infant formula reduces BMI and obesity risk at school age: follow-up of a randomized trial. *Am J Clin Nutr.* 2014;99(5):1041-1051. doi: 10.3945/ajcn.113.064071 [doi].
148. Harris G, Coulthard H. Early eating behaviours and food acceptance revisited: breastfeeding and introduction of complementary foods as predictive of food acceptance. *Curr Obes Rep.* 2016;5(1):113-120. doi: 10.1007/s13679-016-0202-2 [doi].
149. Blincoe AJ. The health benefits of breastfeeding for mothers. *Br J Midwifery.* 2005;13(6):398-401.
150. Lopez A, Cacoub P, Macdougall IC, Peyrin-Biroulet L. Iron deficiency anaemia. *Lancet.* 2016;387(10021):907-916. doi: 10.1016/S0140-6736(15)60865-0 [doi].
151. Mother and Child Health and Education Trust. Benefits of breastfeeding for the environment and society. http://www.tensteps.org/benefits-of-breastfeeding-for-the-environment-society.shtml. Accessed August 18, 2017.
152. Academy of Breastfeeding Medicine Protocol Committee, Eglash A. ABM clinical protocol #8: human milk storage information for home use for full-term infants (original protocol March 2004; revision #1 March 2010). *Breastfeed Med.* 2010;5(3):127-130. doi: 10.1089/bfm.2010.9988; 10.1089/bfm.2010.9988.
153. Martinez JL, Chapman DJ, Perez-Escamilla R. Prepregnancy obesity class is a risk factor for failure to exclusively breastfeed at hospital discharge among Latinas. *J Hum Lact.* 2016;32(2):258-268. doi: 10.1177/0890334415622638 [doi].
154. Sipsma HL, Magriples U, Divney A, Gordon D, Gabzdyl E, Kershaw T. Breastfeeding behavior among adolescents: initiation, duration, and exclusivity. *J Adolesc Health.* 2013;53(4):394-400. doi: 10.1016/j.jadohealth.2013.04.005 [doi].
155. Smith PH, Coley SL, Labbok MH, Cupito S, Nwokah E. Early breastfeeding experiences of adolescent mothers: a qualitative prospective study. *Int Breastfeed J.* 2012;7(1):13-4358-7-13. doi: 10.1186/1746-4358-7-13; 10.1186/1746-4358-7-13.
156. Academy of Breastfeeding Medicine. ABM clinical protocol #10: breastfeeding the late preterm infant (34(0/7) to 36(6/7) weeks gestation) (first revision June 2011). *Breastfeed Med.* 2011;6(3):151-156. doi: 10.1089/bfm.2011.9990; 10.1089/bfm.2011.9990.
157. Rasmussen KM, Kjolhede CL. Prepregnant overweight and obesity diminish the prolactin response to suckling in the first week postpartum. *Pediatrics.* 2004;113(5):e465-471.
158. White-Guthro M, Schub T. Breastfeeding: Breast and Nipple Problems. CINAHL Nursing Guide [serial online]. April 22, 2016. Available from: Nursing Reference Center Plus, Ipswich, MA. EBSCOhost, ezproxy.simmons.edu:2048/login?url=https://search.ebscohost.com/login.aspx?direct=true&db=nup&AN=T702033&site=eds-live&scope=site Accessed December 2, 2017.
159. Academy of Breastfeeding Medicine Protocol Committee, Berens P. ABM clinical protocol #20: Engorgement. *Breastfeed Med.* 2009;4(2):111-113.
160. Prachniak GK. Common breastfeeding problems. *Obstet Gynecol Clin North Am.* 2002;29(1):77-88.
161. Francis DO, Krishnaswami S, McPheeters M. Treatment of ankyloglossia and breastfeeding outcomes: a systematic review. *Pediatrics.* 2015;135(6):e1458-66. doi: 10.1542/peds.2015-0658 [doi].
162. Academy of Breastfeeding Medicine Protocol Committee. ABM clinical protocol #4: mastitis. Revision, May 2008. *Breastfeed Med.* 2008;3(3):177-180. doi: 10.1089/bfm.2008.9993; 10.1089/bfm.2008.9993.
163. Health Organization H. Guidelines Updates On HIV and Infant Feeding. *WHO/UNICEF.* 2016:1-68. doi: NBK379872
164. Health Organization H. Questions and answers on HIV and infant feeding. http://www.who.int/features/qa/hiv-infant-feeding/en/. Accessed August 26, 2017.
165. Mittal H, Das S, Faridi MM. Management of newborn infant born to mother suffering from tuberculosis: current recommendations & gaps in knowledge. *Indian J Med Res.* 2014;140(1):32-39. doi: IndianJMedRes_2014_140_1_32_139965 [pii].
166. Committee on Obstetric Practice. Lead Screening during pregnancy and lactation [American College of Obstetricians and Gynecologists]. 2012;533. Committee on Obstetric Practice. Lead Screening During Pregnancy and Lactation: Committee Opinion No. 533 [American College of Obstetricians and Gynecologists]. Obstet Gynecol. 2012(120):415-420.
167. Academy of Breastfeeding Medicine Protocol Committee, Jansson LM. ABM clinical protocol #21: Guidelines for breastfeeding and the drug-dependent woman. *Breastfeed Med.* 2009;4(4):225-228. doi: 10.1089/bfm.2009.9987; 10.1089/bfm.2009.9987.
168. Bankhead R, Boullata J, Brantley S, et al. Enteral nutrition practice recommendations. *JPEN J Parenter Enteral Nutr.* 2009;33(2):122-167. doi: 10.1177/0148607108330314 [doi].
169. Fibrosis Foundation C. Nutrition for your infant with cystic fibrosis (Birth to 1 Year). 2011. Cystic Fibrosis Foundation. Nutrition For Your Infant with Cystic Fibrosis (Birth to 1 Year). https://www.cff.org/PDF-Archive/Nutrition-for-Your-Infant-(Birth-to-1-Year).pdf. Accessed August 18, 2017.
170. Carlson S, Wojcik B, Barker A, Klein J. University of Iowa Stead Family Children's Family Hospital: Guidelines for the Use of Human Milk Fortifier in the Neonatal Intensive Care Unit. https://uichildrens.org/health-library/guidelines-use-human-milk-fortifier-neonatal-intensive-care-unit. Accessed August 16, 2017, Internally Peer Reviewed.
171. Academy of Pediatrics Committee on Nutrition, American. Soy Protein-Based Formulas: Recommendations for Use in Infant Feeding. *Pediatrics.* 1998;101:148-153.

172. Valentine CJ, Wagner CL. Nutritional management of the breastfeeding dyad. *Pediatr Clin North Am*. 2013;60(1):261-274. doi: 10.1016/j.pcl.2012.10.008 [doi].

173. Drake VJ, Angelo G, Koletzko BV. Pregnancy and lactation: micronutrient needs during pregnancy and lactation. http://lpi.oregonstate.edu/mic/life-stages/pregnancy-lactation. Accessed July 10, 2017.

174. Academy of Nutrition and Dietetics. Nutrition Care Manual. http://www.nutritioncaremanual.org. Accessed August, 16, 2017.

175. Lessen R, Kavanagh K. Position of the academy of nutrition and dietetics: promoting and supporting breastfeeding. *J Acad Nutr Diet*. 2015;115(3):444-449. doi: 10.1016/j.jand.2014.12.014 [doi].

176. U.S. Department of Agriculture. Women, Infants and Children (WIC): Breastfeeding Is a Priority in the WIC Program. https://www.fns.usda.gov/wic/breastfeeding-priority-wic-program. Accessed August 16, 2017.

177. Boston Children's Hospital. Lactation support program: overview. http://www.childrenshospital.org/centers-and-services/programs/f-_-n/lactation-support-program/overview. Accessed August 16, 2017.

Chapter 22

Nutrition in Neonatology

Antoinette Pert

Chapter Outline

Core Concepts
Introduction
Background
Goals of Growth and Nutrition for Premature Infants
Metabolism and Body Composition in Prematurity
Methods of Feeding
Feeding Selection

CORE CONCEPTS

1. Infants that do not complete their full gestation are more susceptible to many physiologic conditions that can impact their ability to feed, grow, and thrive, putting them at increased nutritional risk.

2. Compared to term infants, premature infants have higher calorie needs.

3. Protein needs of premature infants are nearly 1.5 to 2 times higher than protein needs of term infants.

4. Carbohydrate is a major energy source for infants, accounting for 40% to 50% of their calorie intake.

5. Fat is the primary energy source for preterm infants, with 40% to 50% of their daily calories coming from fat.

6. Neonates born prior to completing their third trimester are born relatively calcium deficient and osteopenic.

7. Parenteral nutrition is a critical element of neonatal care in terms of the survival, development, and prevention of extrauterine growth restriction of premature infants.

8. Carbohydrate in the form of dextrose, providing 3.4 kcal/g, is the major energy source in parenteral nutrition.

9. Provision of amino acids within the first hours of life prevents postnatal growth failure, reduces complications and morbidities, and promotes neurodevelopment, even at low calorie intake.

10. Feeding the gastrointestinal (GI) tract early has been shown to promote endocrine adaptation and to accelerate early motility patterns. Premature infants also have better tolerance of feeds, achieve full feeding volume sooner, and have a reduced risk of feeding aversion when fed early, all of which may lead to decreased length of hospital stay.

11. Human milk is the ideal choice for enterally feeding premature infants.

Learning Objectives

1. Recognize the factors that contribute to the increased nutritional risk of premature infants.
2. Identify and explain the anthropometrics used in assessing a neonate's size at birth.
3. Assess the calorie and protein needs of neonates when receiving enteral and parenteral nutrition.
4. Define the initial, advancement rate, and goal of macronutrient provision for neonatal parenteral nutrition support.
5. Identify the enteral feeding selection options for premature neonates.
6. Explain the benefits of feeding breast milk to premature infants.
7. Describe the ways in which preterm infant formula differs from term infant formula.
8. State the criteria of a neonate necessary for discharge from the hospital.

TABLE 22.1 BIRTH WEIGHT CLASSIFICATIONS

Classification	Acronym	Birthweight
Low Birth Weight	LBW	<2500 g
Very Low Birth Weight	VLBW	<1500 g
Extremely Low Birth Weight	ELBW	<1000 g

Introduction

Preterm neonates are one of the most medically and nutritionally fragile populations. Premature births are the number one cause of mortality in infancy and almost 10% of infants born in the United States are born prematurely.[1] Although technological advances in the care of premature infants have improved outcomes, preterm infants have unique nutritional needs and often require complex interventions. Providing nutrition care to this group is often challenging, but vital to improve survival. Medical nutrition therapy is key to ensuring optimal growth and development.

Background

Neonatology and neonatal nutrition are subspecialties of pediatrics and pediatric nutrition, respectively, that focus primarily on the care of infants born prematurely. Full-term is defined as 40 weeks gestational age (WGA), but a range of 37 to 42 weeks is considered to be term.[2] Term is further delineated into early term (37 0/7 to 38 6/7 weeks), full term (39 0/7 to 40 6/7 weeks), late term (41 0/7 to 41 6/7 weeks), and postterm (42 0/7 weeks and beyond) to reflect the heterogeneity of outcomes within the 5-week span.[2] Any neonate born prior to 37 weeks gestation is considered to be a preterm infant. The earlier an infant is born, the greater the nutrition risk because infants will be smaller and less developed. The weeks and days of gestation that have elapsed when the preterm infant is born become the neonate's gestational age (GA). Each day and week following birth becomes the neonate's chronologic age. The GA plus chronologic age is considered the postmenstrual age (PMA) until the infant reaches 40 0/7 weeks PMA or the mother's previously assigned due date.[3] For example, a neonate born at 30 weeks gestation is considered to have a GA of 30 weeks. One week later, the neonate has a chronologic age of 1 week and is considered to be 31 weeks' PMA.

The immediate nutrition risk of an infant can be assessed just after birth based on weight (Table 22.1). Infants born less than 2,500 g are considered to be **low birth weight (LBW)**, infants born less than 1,500 g are considered to be **very low birth weight (VLBW)**, and infants born less than 1,000 g are considered to be **extremely low birth weight (ELBW)**.[4]

Weight for gestational age is also an important factor to consider when assessing a neonate's nutrition risk. Size for gestational age can be assessed by using premature growth curves for intrauterine and extrauterine growth.[5-9] Infants that are born with weights that chart less than the 10th percentile are **small-for-gestational-age (SGA)**.[5-9] Birth weights that chart greater than the 90th percentile are **large-for-gestational-age (LGA)**.[5-9] All infants with birth weights that chart between the 10th and 90th percentiles are **appropriate-for-gestational-age (AGA)**.[5-9] Neonates are symmetric SGA or LGA if their birth weight, length, and head circumference are all below the 10th percentile for age or above the 90th percentile, respectively.[10] If at least one of those measurements, but not all three, is below the 10th percentile or above the 90th percentile, the infants are considered to be asymmetric SGA or LGA, respectively.[10]

Infants that are born AGA or SGA may be at increased nutritional risk if they experienced **intrauterine growth restriction (IUGR)**. IUGR describes a fetus that had been tracking along a healthy growth curve throughout gestation and then starts to track at least one standard deviation below their curve because of problems *in utero*.[11,12] Because a drop in the standard deviation may still be well above the 10th percentile for age, not all neonates with IUGR are necessarily SGA. IUGR can occur because of problems relating to the mother, the fetus, or the placenta, all of which result in reduced tissue deposition due to a reduced nutritional supply from the utero-placental circulation.[11-13] Some maternal causes of IUGR include malnutrition or being underweight, hypertensive disorders, pre-gestational diabetes, hyperthyroidism, renal disease, autoimmune diseases, cardiac disease, asthma, living at high altitude or in developing countries, low socio-economic status, race,

CASE STUDY INTRODUCTION

A baby girl (Quinn) was born at 30 5/7 weeks gestational age to a 28-year-old mother with 1 other child (G_2P_2). The pregnancy was complicated by preeclampsia, placental insufficiency, and **oligohydramnios** (insufficient amniotic fluid). The mother's obstetrician had been monitoring the pregnancy closely because Quinn was diagnosed with intrauterine growth restriction (IUGR) at 27 weeks gestation. Quinn was born via induced vaginal delivery due to her mother's worsening preeclampsia and Quinn's IUGR status. She admitted to the neonatal intensive care unit (NICU) on her day of birth or day of life 0 (DOL 0).

Anthropometric Data:

Birth Anthropometrics:
Length: 36 cm (9th percentile on Fenton preterm growth chart)
Weight: 965 g (8th percentile on Fenton preterm growth chart)
Head circumference: 27 cm (33rd percentile on Fenton preterm growth chart)

Clinical Data:
Past Medical History: none
Medications: D10W with heparin @ 80 mL/kg/day
Vitals: Blood pressure: 54/33 mmHg, Temperature: 97.7°F, Heart rate: 122 beats/min

Nutrition-focused Physical Exam:
Overall appearance: Infant is in no acute distress, laying supine in an incubator. Continuous positive airway pressure (CPAP) in place (**Figure 22.1**). Moves extremities symmetrically. Palate intact, abdomen soft, not distended. Patent anus. Anterior fontanelles are open, soft, and flat. No dysmorphic features. Alert, active, normal tone for gestational age (GA). Pink skin, no rash, no petechiae noted.

Dietary Data:
Diet Prescription: NPO

Questions
1. What are Quinn's most significant nutrition risk factors?
2. What additional information would you like to obtain about Quinn?
3. What additional information would you like to obtain from Quinn's mom?

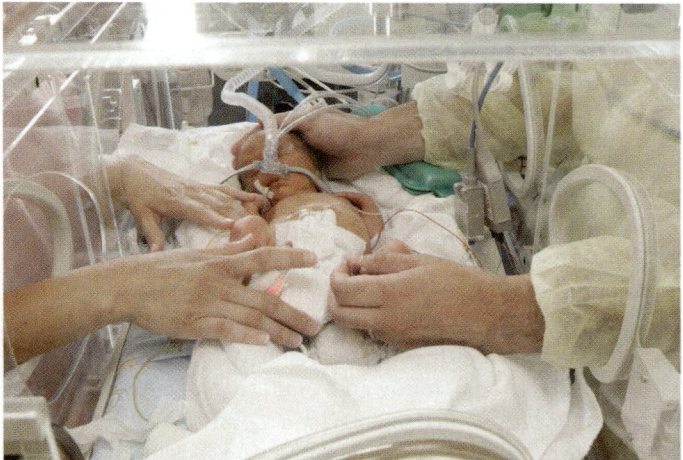

FIGURE 22.1 Preterm Infant on CPAP in an Incubator
© BSIP/UIG/Getty Images.

family history or previous pregnancy with IUGR, extremes of maternal age, short interpregnancy interval, cystic fibrosis, tobacco use, and substance abuse.[13] Placental reasons include placental placement, placental abruption, decreased placental blood flow, or uneven perfusion.[11] Fetal causes include genetic diseases, infection, multiple gestation, and fetal malformations.[13]

Being part of a multiple gestation puts a neonate at increased nutritional risk because abnormal fetal growth is more common in these infants. It is also common for multiples to have a shorter gestational period than singletons, resulting in most multiples being preterm at birth.[14] Multiples are at increased risk of experiencing IUGR and the rate and severity of growth restriction increases as the number of fetuses increases.[13] Because severe IUGR is so common in multiples, multiples are also at increased risk

> **CASE STUDY REVISITED**
>
> 1. How would you assess Quinn's weight at birth? Is she ELBW, VLBW, or LBW?
> 2. How would you describe her growth? Is she SGA, AGA, or LGA?
> 3. Is her growth symmetrical or asymmetrical?
> 4. What prenatal factors could have contributed to Quinn's IUGR?

of being born SGA. Another common risk in multiples is growth discordance, which is a significant size or weight difference between the two fetuses of a twin pregnancy. Birth weight discordance in conjunction with IUGR is associated with increased rates of fetal demise and neonatal morbidity and mortality.[13] Mortality rates of the smaller twin or multiple increases with increasing discordance in the setting of SGA.[13] However, both the smaller and larger subsets of discordant multiples are at increased risk of morbidities and mortalities. Nutritional issues arise because of uneven nutrient deposition potentially leading to malnutrition, blood glucose instability, fluid and electrolyte shifts, and compromised gut perfusion. These issues can result in feeding issues and difficulty in providing adequate nutrition for the infants.

> **CORE CONCEPT 1**
>
> Infants that do not complete their full gestation are more susceptible to many physiologic conditions that can impact their ability to feed, grow, and thrive, putting them at an increased nutritional risk.

Goals of Growth and Nutrition for Premature Infants

> **PRACTICE POINT**
>
> The goal of nutrition management of premature infants is to achieve weight gain, growth, and development potential ex-utero to match in-utero growth potential.

Fetal weight gain is the most rapid rate of growth that humans will experience in their lifetimes. If infants born prematurely do not achieve fetal rate of weight gain, they are at risk of growth failure.[15] Therefore, achieving rapid growth in the immediate postnatal period is essential. This is done through a mixture of parenteral nutrition (PN), breast milk, and specific premature infant enteral nutrition formula products. Weight gain goals of premature infants have been established based on weight and gestational age at birth and change throughout the postnatal course until the infant reaches term PMA.[16,17] Ziegler et al established goals of neonatal weight gain based on fetal weight gain standards.[17] These goals range from 14 to 21 grams per kilogram body weight per day (g/kg/day) and have an inverse relationship to the body weight of the infant.[17]

> **PRACTICE POINT**
>
> It is expected that the smallest neonates will gain the most weight per kilogram at the most rapid rate.

There are several options to assess neonatal anthropometrics at birth and also to track growth and weight gain throughout the neonatal course. Growth charts created by Lubchenco et al and then by Babson and Benda became the standard for assessing fetal growth and weight gain at birth by establishing norms for fetal growth.[7,8,18] These charts have since been updated to include newer data and a larger sample size, especially for the purpose of tracking growth and weight gain over time *ex utero*.[5-9,18] The growth charts that have become the standard to track weight gain and catch-up growth from extreme prematurity (22 weeks GA) through term were published by Fenton in 2013 and by Olsen in 2010 (**Figures 22.2** to **22.7**).[5,6,9]

> **PRACTICE POINT**
>
> The Fenton and the Olsen intrauterine growth charts have become the standards for tracking preterm neonatal growth throughout neonatal intensive care units and special care nurseries internationally.

Metabolism and Body Composition in Prematurity

Energy Requirements

It is estimated that preterm infants need about 105 to 130 kcal/kg/day when being enterally fed to maintain adequate growth and development, compared to 105 to 110 kcal/kg/day for their full-term counterparts. Basal metabolic rate accounts for the majority of calorie demand (40%-45% of needs), followed by calories for growth (20% of needs).[19,20] Intermittent activity accounts for 10% to 15% of needs; metabolic stress of having to regulate and maintain normal body temperature, also known as cold stress, and fecal losses account for 10% each of these needs; and the thermic effect of feeding makes up the final

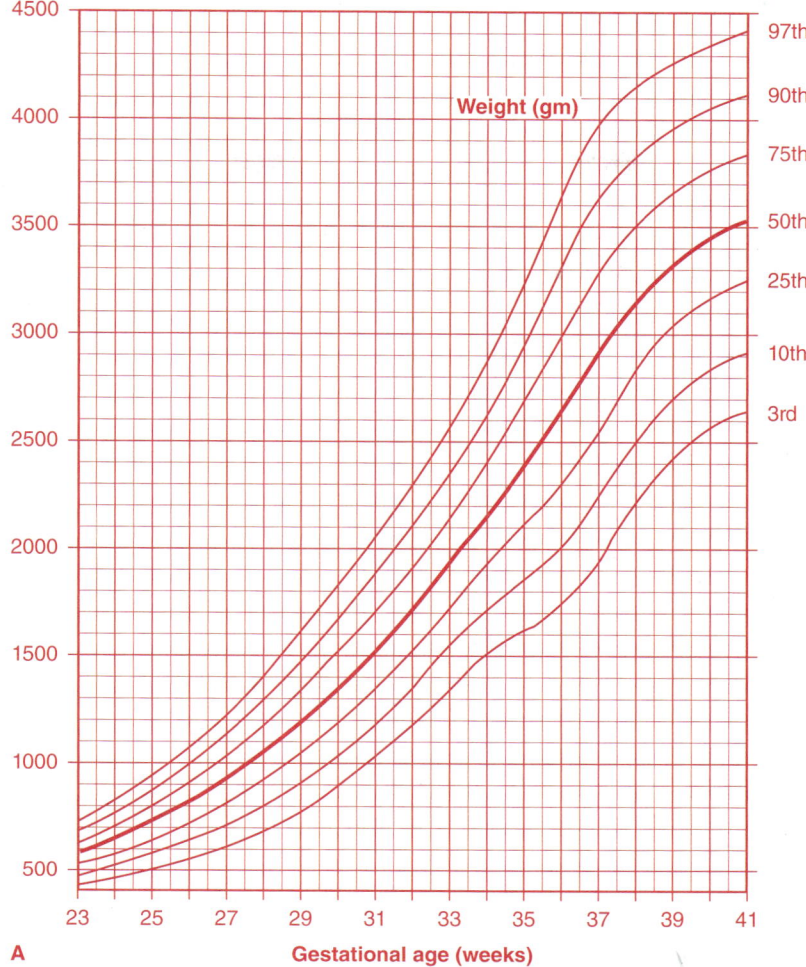

FIGURE 22.2 Olsen Girls' Weight-for-Age Growth Curve
Reproduced with permission from Journal of Pediatrics, 125(2):e214-24, Copyright © 2010 by the AAP.

5% of needs.[19] Placing preterm infants in an incubator will help minimize heat and evaporative water losses, thereby diminishing energy cost of maintaining body core temperature (**Figure 22.8**). When the GI tract is not being fed, there is no longer a calorie demand for fecal losses or the thermic effect of feeding, so the energy needs of parenterally fed neonates are generally lower than those being enterally fed.

> **PRACTICE POINT**
>
> Calorie needs for complete PN are about 15% to 20% less than those of enterally fed infants.

> **CORE CONCEPT 2**
>
> Compared to term infants, premature infants have higher calorie needs.

Protein Requirements

Because premature infants are born with virtually no or minimal energy stores, they are at high risk of becoming catabolic if not provided with adequate calories and protein soon after birth. If infants become catabolic, they will break down whatever limited amount of lean body mass they have to try to meet their energy and protein needs. The smaller and more immature an infant is, the greater risk of accelerated protein losses.[16,21] Without adequate protein provision, preterm infants will lose an average of 0.6 to 1.2 grams protein/kg/day, which amounts to a loss of about 1.5% of total body protein loss per day.[16,21] Three days without adequate protein will result in a 10% loss of total body protein.[16,21] Ideally, premature infants should experience an accumulation of 2% total body protein per day.[16,21] Providing adequate protein for these infants is of extreme importance, but maintaining optimal protein/energy ratio is also crucial for ensuring ideal protein accretion, with the highest ratio being required by the smallest preterm infants.[16]

> **PRACTICE POINT**
>
> Premature infants will need approximately 3.5 to 4.5 g protein/kg/day to achieve optimal growth rates *ex utero*, with an optimal protein/energy ratio of 2.7 to 4.1 g protein per 100 kcals.

> **CORE CONCEPT 3**
>
> Protein needs of premature infants are nearly 1.5 to 2 times higher than protein needs of term infants.

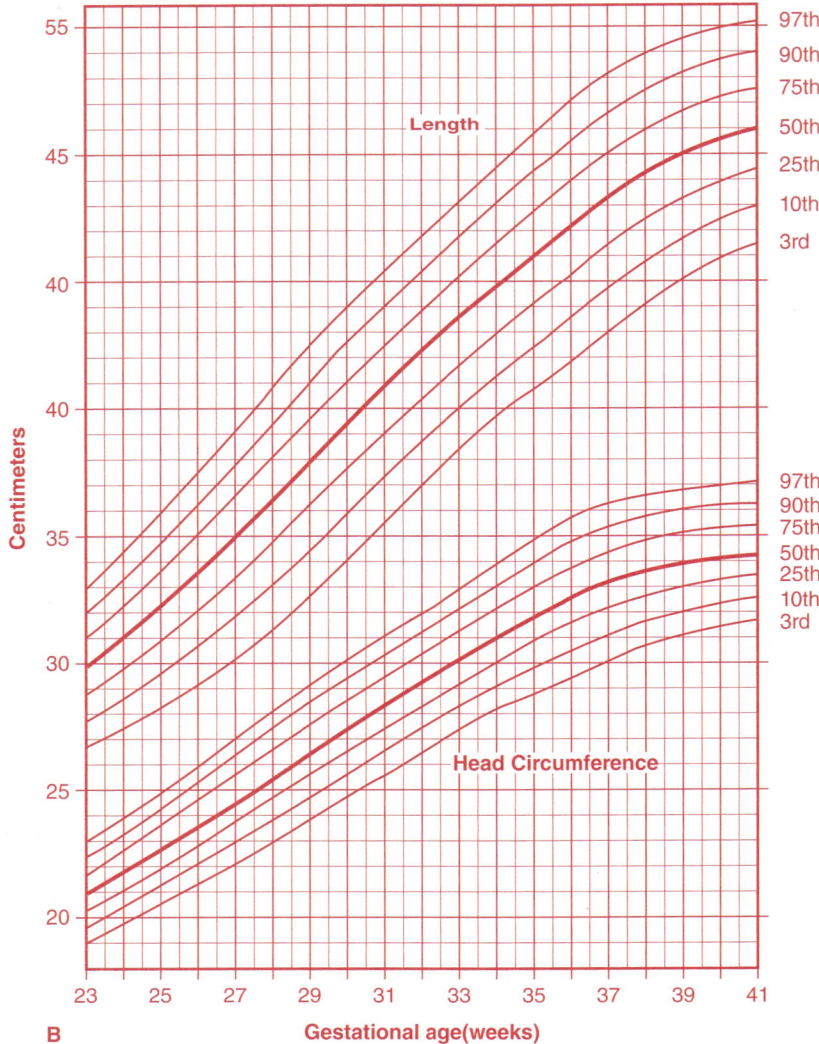

FIGURE 22.3 Olsen Girls' Length- and Head-Circumference-for-Age Growth Curve
Reproduced with permission from Journal of Pediatrics, 125(2):e214-24, Copyright © 2010 by the AAP.

Carbohydrate Requirements

The carbohydrate requirement for preterm infants is approximately 10 to 14 grams carbohydrate per kilogram per day (g/kg/day).[19] Glucose is the primary substrate used by the brain for energy and function. Carbohydrate is also a more effective energy substrate for preventing protein breakdown than fat. Late preterm infants have intestinal lactase activity; however, it is only about 30% as active as in term infants.[22] Despite this, lactose intolerance is rarely seen in premature infants. Lactose is the carbohydrate source in human milk and is typically well tolerated. This may be because premature infants are very efficient at being able to hydrolyze carbohydrates in the small intestines.[23] Glucose polymers are well tolerated in preterm infants, likely because glucosidase enzymes for metabolizing glucose polymers are active in preterm infants.[19] For this reason, commercial preterm infant formulas provide about 50% of the carbohydrate as glucose polymers and about 50% as lactose.[24] The glucose polymers also contribute a lower osmotic load per unit weight than lactose, so this formulation can keep the osmolarity of the premature infant formula relatively low to improve (GI) tolerance.[19] Both the amount of carbohydrate and the balance of carbohydrate with the other macronutrients provided are important to a premature infant's metabolism. It is not uncommon for premature infants to have unstable blood glucose control because of their limited glycogen stores at birth. Providing them with adequate amounts of carbohydrate is essential to avoid hypoglycemia. It is equally as important to avoid excessive carbohydrates. Feeding preterm infants excessive amounts of carbohydrates has been shown to lead to fat deposition in the liver, heart, and subcutaneous adipose tissue.[20] Overall, carbohydrates should be provided in adequate amounts along with adequate calories from fat and protein to help the infant with glucose control and stability.

CORE CONCEPT 4

Carbohydrate is a major energy source for infants, accounting for 40% to 50% of their daily calorie intake.

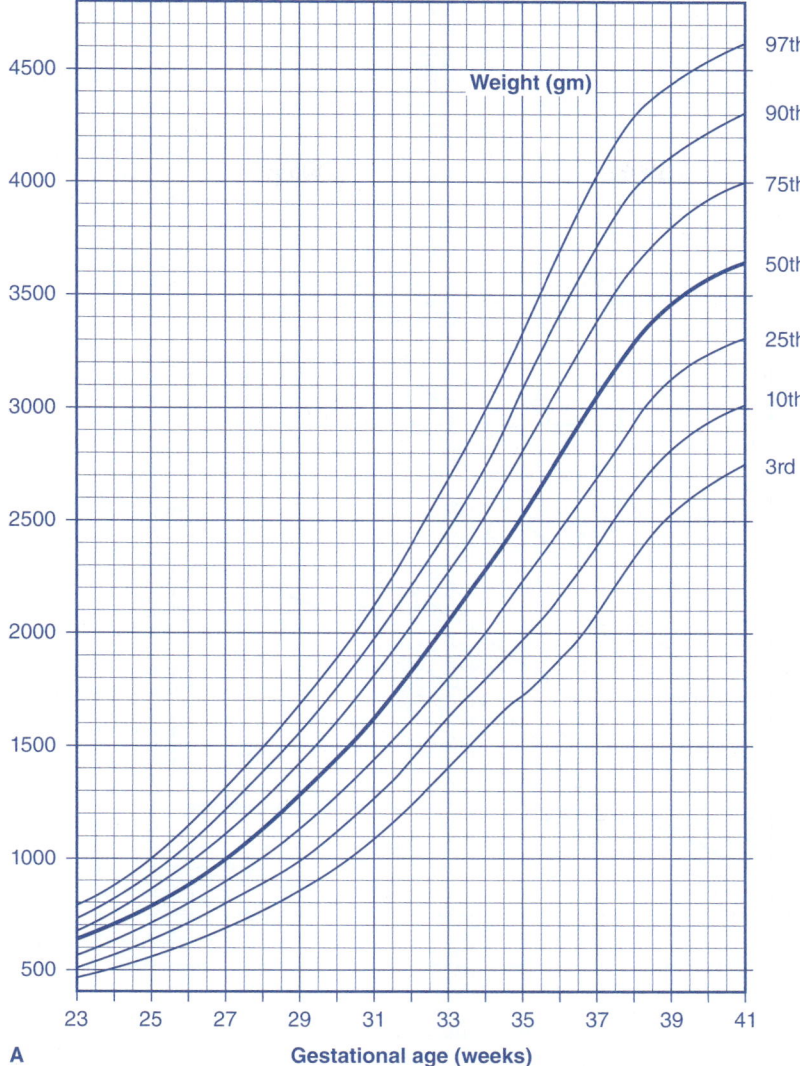

FIGURE 22.4 Olsen Boys' Weight-for-Age Growth Curve
Reproduced with permission from Journal of Pediatrics, 125(2):e214-24, Copyright © 2010 by the AAP.

Fat Requirements

The daily fat requirement is approximately 5 to 7 g/kg.[19] Adequate fat provision is important for protein metabolism because optimal protein retention can be achieved when providing 30% to 40% of nonprotein calories as fat. Saturated fat, primarily triglycerides, is the major fat source of human milk. The saturated fat in human milk is easily digested, absorbed, and tolerated due to the specific fatty acid chemical structure, compared to that of bovine milk, along with the lingual and gastric lipases in the GI tract of the preterm infant and bile salt–activated lipases within the breast milk.[19] These lipase activities compensate for the lack of pancreatic lipase and intraluminal bile salt concentration in preterm infants compared to their full-term counterparts. Because formula-fed infants do not benefit from the bile salt–activated lipases that are found in human milk, premature formulas contain 40% to 50% of their fat content as saturated fat and 40% to 50% as medium chain triglyceride (MCT) oils.[14] The MCT oil is readily absorbed from the GI tract because it is able to bypass the lymphatic system. Infants who receive feeds of preterm formula mixed with human milk have increased fat absorption compared to formula alone.[19] Human milk also contains small, yet well absorbed, amounts of the fatty acids docosahexaenoic acid (DHA) and arachidonic acid (ARA). Because these fatty acids are known to be beneficial for visual function and neurodevelopment, DHA and ARA are routinely added to premature infant formulas. **Table 22.2** summarizes macronutrient requirements for carbohydrate, protein and fat in premature infants.

> **CORE CONCEPT 5**
>
> Fat is the primary energy source for preterm infants with 40% to 50% of their daily calories coming from fat.

Fluid Requirements

Fluid and electrolyte management is a critical part of the medical management of neonates, especially extremely premature infants. At the beginning of the third trimester (24 weeks gestation), the fetus is about 90% total body water (TBW).[15,20] Sixty-five percent of the TBW at this gestation is extracellular fluid (ECF) and 25% is intracellular

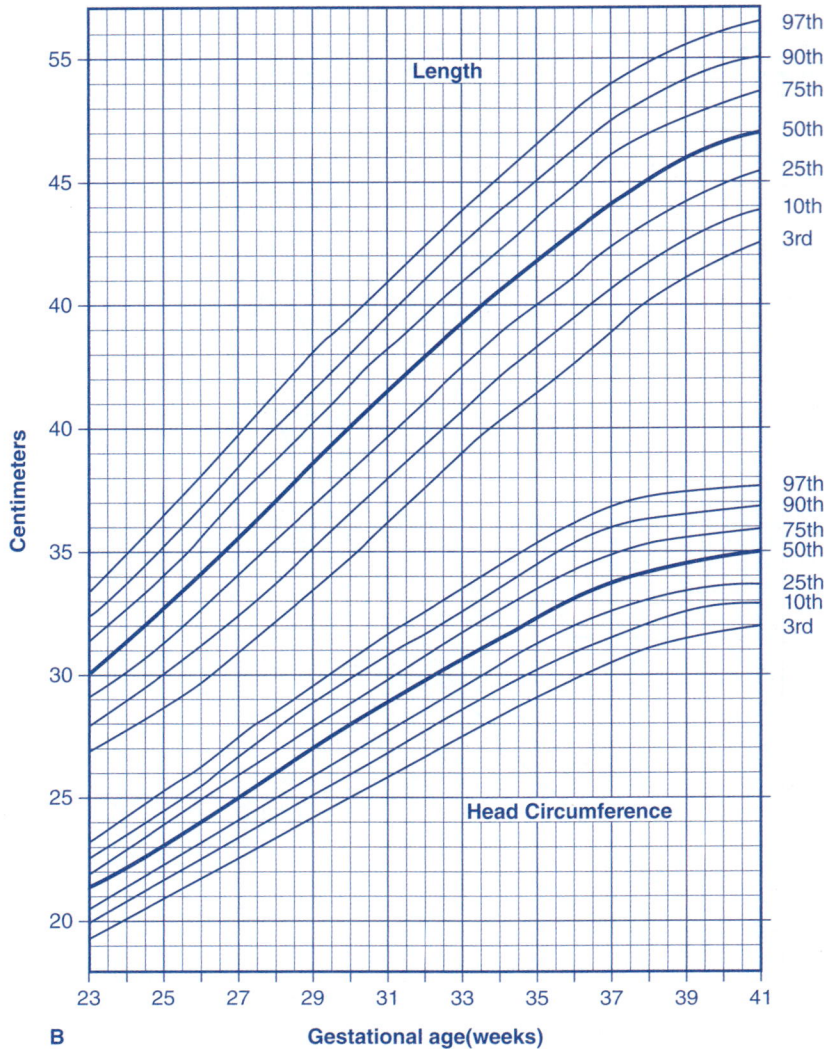

FIGURE 22.5 Olsen Boys' Length- and Head-Circumference-for-Age Growth Curve
Reproduced with permission from Journal of Pediatrics, 125(2):e214-24, Copyright © 2010 by the AAP.

fluid (ICF). As the fetus approaches term, TBW decreases to approximately 75%, with ECF accounting for 40% and ICF accounting for 35%.[15,20] In the days following delivery, the infant undergoes a contraction of ECF and expected physiologic **postnatal diuresis**. This diuresis results in a loss of approximately 10% to 15% of birth weight gradually over the first 10 to 14 days of life for an extremely premature infant.[15] Expected losses are less and occur over a shorter length of time for neonates that are later in gestation and physiologically more mature. Comparatively, a term infant would be expected to experience a diuresis of 5% to 10% during the first week of life and regain birth weight by DOL 7 to 10. The other major reasons for this difference are reduced insensible losses due to more mature skin and respiratory tract and reduced renal losses due to more mature kidneys of the term infant. These fluid losses should be accounted for when estimating fluid needs. Diuresis should not exceed 2% to 3% loss of birth weight per day, equating to a daily urine output of 1 to 3 mL/kg/hour, with a maximum of 5 to 7 mL/kg/hour. Fluid requirements may vary depending on physiologic maturity, clinical conditions, and environmental factors. Generally, initial fluid requirements for neonates born at 24 to 25 weeks gestation will be approximately 100 mL/kg/day, 70 to 90 mL/kg/day for neonates born at 26 to 34 weeks gestation, and 60 mL/kg/day for infants born later than 34 weeks gestation.[25] Fluid needs may be higher for infants with abdominal wall defects or other GI losses, with high-output renal failure, or receiving care under a radiant warmer or receiving phototherapy. Conversely, fluid needs may be lower for infants residing in a humidified incubator, infants with a **patent ductus arteriosus (PDA)**, which is a congenital heart defect causing abnormal blood flow between the arteries connecting to the heart, oliguric renal failure, or brain injury. Indicators of overhydration may be excessive weight gain, edema, increased urine output, and normal or reduced urine output with hyponatremia. Indicators of dehydration may be excessive weight loss, decreased urine output with hypernatremia, hyperkalemia, azotemia, and metabolic acidosis. After the first few days of life, once diuresis rates and electrolyte losses begin to normalize, total fluid volumes may be advanced, typically by 10 to 20 mL/kg/day to a usual goal of 130 to 160 mL/kg/day based on weight, urine output, electrolytes, respiratory status, and cardiovascular status.[25] Infants with severe respiratory disease or a hemodynamically

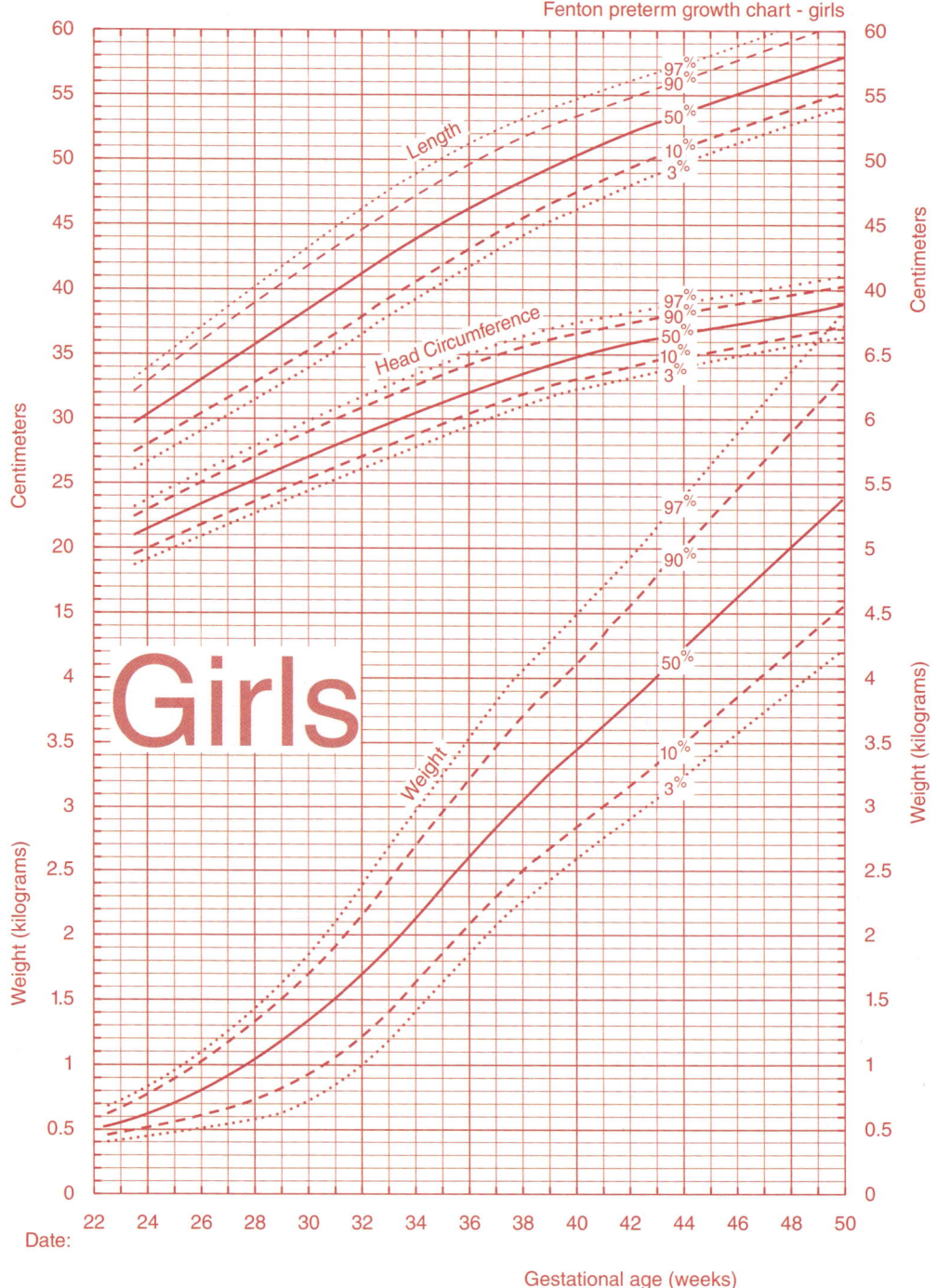

FIGURE 22.6 Fenton Preterm Growth Chart: Girls
Reproduced from Fenton TR, Kim JH. A systematic review and meta-analysis to revise the fenton growth chart for preterm infants. *BMC Pediatr*. 2013;13:59-2431-13-59.

significant PDA may need their fluids restricted to 120 to 140 mL/kg/day.[25]

Electrolyte Requirements

During the diuresis period, electrolyte homeostasis should be maintained. This may be done with electrolyte supplementation in intravenous fluid, but, most commonly, electrolyte requirements are managed in PN solution for infants weighing less than 1,800 g. Maintaining electrolyte homeostasis may be challenging due to increased urinary losses of electrolytes via premature kidneys. In preterm kidneys, glomerular and tubular function is immature, resulting in reduced glomerular filtration rate and reduced capacity to resorb sodium, potassium, and bicarbonate. Immature kidneys also have decreased ability to concentrate and dilute urine, leading to serum sodium, potassium, and bicarbonate abnormalities, most readily seen in ELBW infants. Thus, ELBW infants often receive PN solutions that minimize sodium and potassium and/or maximize acetate in the first few days of life during postnatal diuresis.

Sodium

In the first 24 to 72 hours of life, a premature neonate requires very little to no exogenous sodium. Sodium

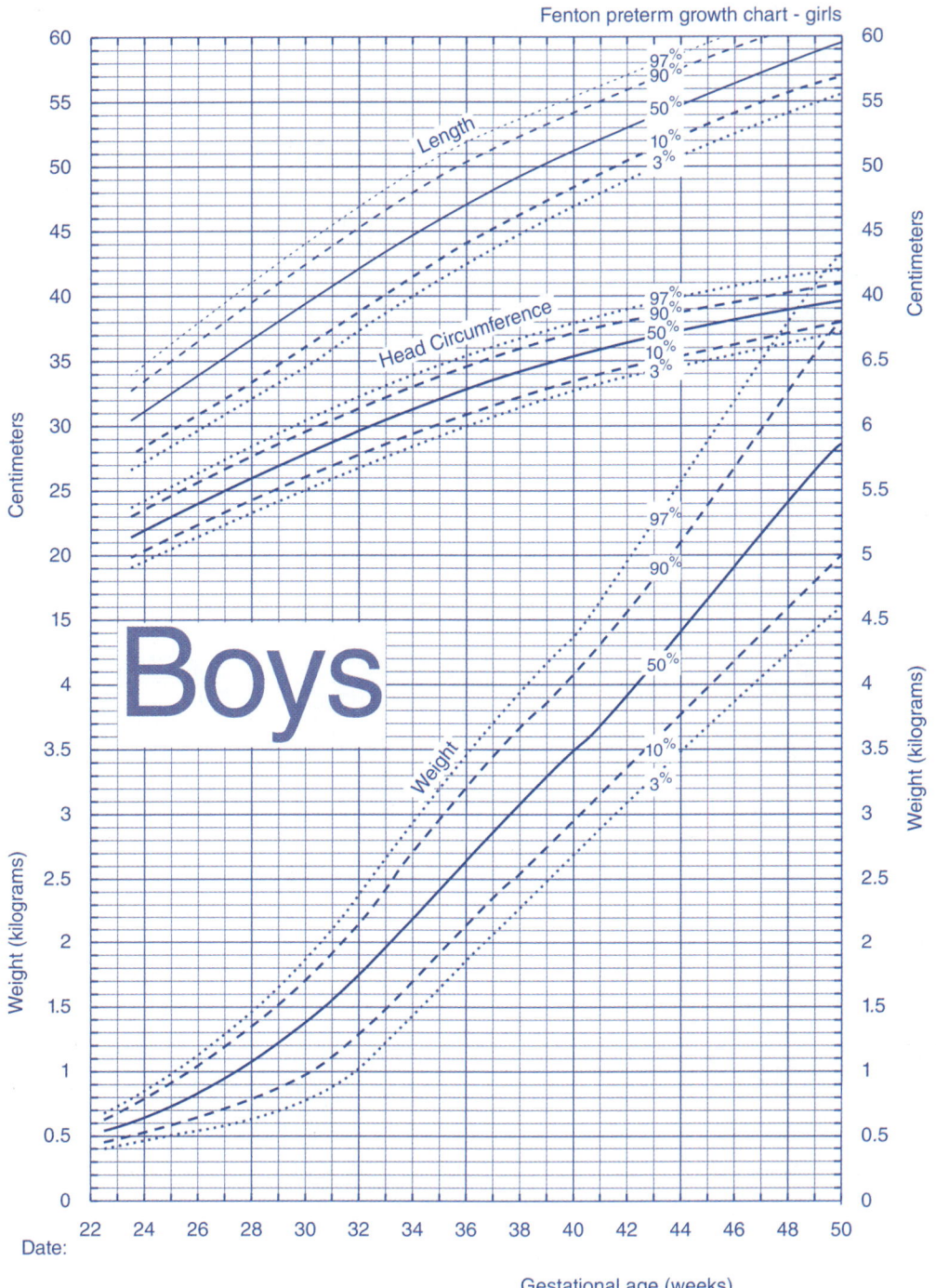

FIGURE 22.7 Fenton Preterm Growth Chart: Boys
Reproduced from Fenton TR, Kim JH. A systematic review and meta-analysis to revise the fenton growth chart for preterm infants. *BMC Pediatr*. 2013;13:59-2431-13-59.

restriction during this time period has been associated with reduced exacerbation of respiratory disease and reduced incidence of bronchopulmonary dysplasia (BPD), a form of chronic lung disease commonly found in premature infants caused by mechanical ventilation and long-term use of oxygen, later in life.[26] Also, hypernatremia may result from increased sodium intake. Therefore, sodium provision should be limited to less than 1 mEq/kg/day until postnatal diuresis is completed.[15] At this point, sodium intake can be advanced to 2 to 4 mEq/kg/day.[10,19] Some VLBW or ELBW infants may require more sodium, up to 10 mEq/kg/day, due to limited renal tubular sodium reabsorption resulting in increased losses through the kidney. To manage this, adjust fluid provision to maintain hydration and then adjust sodium intake by 1 to 2 mEq/kg/day as needed until serum sodium values are within normal limits.

Potassium

ELBW infants are at increased risk to develop nonoliguric hyperkalemia, usually within the first 72 hours of

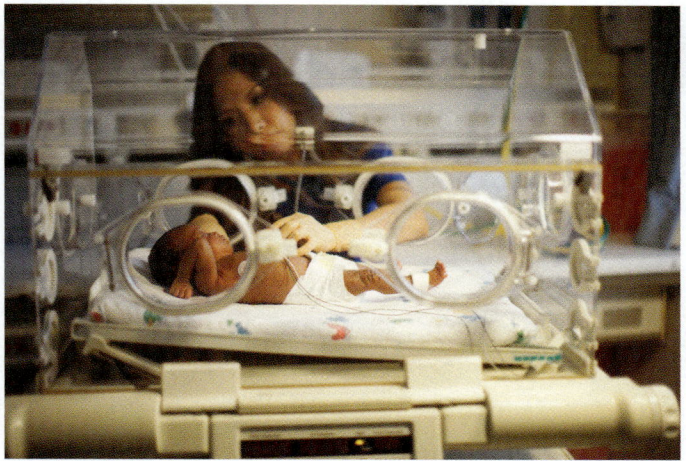

FIGURE 22.8 Preterm Infant in an Incubator
© ERproductions Ltd/Blend Images/Getty Images.

life, especially those who are born extremely premature, have blood group incompatibility with their mother, are catabolic, are bruised, have metabolic acidosis, or receive excessive potassium intake.[25] The incidence of this has decreased with earlier administration of amino acids in initial PN solutions and improved fluid management.[25] Potassium should not be provided until the infant is urinating regularly and serum potassium is normalized. Once this occurs, potassium can be introduced at 0.5 to 1 mEq/kg/day and advanced to 2 to 3 mEq/kg/day.[10,19] Further adjustments may be made as needed based upon changes in renal function or serum levels, especially if diuretic therapy is being used.

Acid–Base Balance

Increased losses of bicarbonate through immature kidneys of premature infants may result in shifts in acid–base balance, most commonly metabolic acidosis, in the first week or two of life. When this occurs, the infant will require alkalotic supplementation in the form of acetate.[25] Because acetate and chloride must be paired with cations in solution, intake of these anions should be restricted until the neonate is able to receive sodium and potassium as previously discussed.[25] Additional chloride supplementation may be required in neonates being treated with diuretic therapy resulting in contraction alkalosis or an increase in blood pH due to fluid losses.

TABLE 22.2 MACRONUTRIENT REQUIREMENTS IN PREMATURITY

Macronutrient	Premature Infant Requirements
Carbohydrate	10-14 g/kg/day
Protein	3.5-4.5 g/kg/day
Fat	5-7 g/kg/day

Calcium and Phosphorus

Approximately 80% of bone mineral stores are laid down during the last trimester of intrauterine development.[27] Calcium is readily transferred across the placenta during the third trimester of gestation, providing the fetus with optimal bone growth and calcium stores.[19] Low phosphate intake will cause the kidneys to retain phosphate, eliminating phosphate excretion in the urine and resulting in hypercalcemia and hypercalciuria.[14] Phosphate deficiency results in bone demineralization, further exacerbating osteopenia of prematurity.[14] Optimal provision of supplemental calcium and phosphorus are of extreme importance to optimize bone retention and growth.

A growing premature infant will require 3 to 4 mEq calcium/kg/day (60-90 mg/kg/day) and 1.3 to 2.25 mMol phosphorus/kg/day (40-70 mg/kg/day) via PN.[14] The ideal calcium-to-phosphorus ratio to promote optimal mineral retention and bone growth is 1.3 to 1.7 mg elemental calcium : 1 mg phosphorus weight ratio (2.2 to 2.6 mEq Ca : 1 mMol P).[25] VLBW infants on PN for longer than 2 weeks should receive increased monitoring for developing osteopenia. Increased losses of urinary calcium may result from certain medications, such as diuretics and steroids, especially with long-term use. This can lead to **nephrocalcinosis**, (deposition of calcium in the kidney parenchyma) and increased risk for metabolic bone disease. SGA infants may have increased phosphorus requirements to prevent refeeding syndrome resulting from rapid growth and increases in lean tissue mass. Calcium and phosphorus provision may be limited in PN solutions due to limitations in solution stability and solubility. In order to optimize solubility, higher concentrations of amino acids and dextrose can be added, lipids should be given separately, and cysteine should be added to the PN solution. In addition, neonatal amino acid solutions are more acidic than standard solutions, which increases calcium and phosphorus solubility.

Relatively high amounts of calcium and phosphorus are also required for preterm neonates being enterally fed. Bovine or human milk–based multinutrient fortifiers that may be added to breast milk are called **human milk fortifiers**. Human milk fortifiers are meant for preterm infants and contain high amounts of calcium and phosphorus to meet the increased demand and support bone turnover and development. Commercial preterm infant formulas also contain more calcium and phosphorus than any other infant formulas to meet the needs of this population.

> **CORE CONCEPT 6**
>
> Neonates born prior to completing their third trimester are born relatively calcium deficient and osteopenic.

Magnesium

The magnesium requirement for infants on PN is 0.2 to 0.5 mEq/kg/day.[14] Magnesium may be omitted from initial or transitional PN solution if the mother received significant amounts of magnesium sulfate prenatally to prevent premature

CASE STUDY REVISITED

Quinn is now 24 hours old, DOL1. The neonatology team has asked you to provide recommendations for starting and advancing PN for Quinn. Her current labs are:

Biochemical Data:
Sodium 143 (127-143 mEq/L)
Potassium 5.1 (3.5-5.0 mEq/L)
Chloride 113 (98-110 mEq/L)
Carbon dioxide 18 (20-30 mEq/L)
Blood urea nitrogen 25 (5-17 mg/dL)
Creatinine 0.55 (0.4-1.3 mg/dL)
Glucose 70 (70-139 mg/dL)

Clinical Data:
Urine output: 4 mL/kg/hour

Questions

1. What are Quinn's estimated energy needs?
2. What GIR would you provide and how much protein and fat (in g/kg/day) would you put in her initial PN?
3. At what rate would you advance each of these macronutrients?
4. What glucose, protein, and fat amounts (in g/kg/day) would recommend for Quinn's final goal PN?
5. Considering Quinn's GA, labs, and urine output as a reflection of her postnatal diuresis, what are Quinn's fluid requirements?
6. How would you recommend her fluid intake from PN be advanced?
7. How would you describe her electrolytes?
8. Which electrolytes would you monitor closely?

---

labor or to treat preeclampsia. High amounts of circulating magnesium in a newborn may result in symptoms of increased tiredness or fatigue, sluggish GI motility, and constipation. Magnesium supplementation may be provided once the infant is passing stool normally. **Table 22.3** summarizes maintenance electrolyte requirements in premature infants.

TABLE 22.3 MAINTENANCE ELECTROLYTE REQUIREMENTS IN PREMATURITY

Electrolyte	Premature Infant Requirements
Sodium	2-4 mEq/kg/day
Potassium	2-3 mEq/kg/day
Calcium	3-4 mEq/kg/day (60-90 mg/kg/day)
Phosphorus	1.3-2.25 mMol/kg/day (40-70 mg/kg/day)
Magnesium	0.2-0.5 mEq/kg/day

Methods of Feeding

Parenteral Nutrition (PN)

Due to the extreme prematurity of the GI tract of VLBW neonates, meeting their high calorie demand enterally may be challenging, if not impossible, in the first days or weeks of life. The small stomach capacity, immaturity of the GI tract, and critical illness make advancing to full enteral feeds a slow and cautious process. PN has been a life-saving intervention not only for premature infants, but also surgical infants who may have prolonged periods when they are unable to receive any nutrition via their GI tract. Providing PN is most critical for VLBW and ELBW infants. PN is used as a vehicle to maintain fluid requirements and deliver electrolytes the same way it would be done with intravenous fluids. Being able to meet the macronutrient and micronutrient needs of premature infants is what make PN necessary for these patients to thrive.

CORE CONCEPT 7

Parenteral nutrition is a critical element of neonatal care in terms of the survival, development, and prevention of extrauterine growth restriction of premature infants.

Vascular Access

PN can be given whether a patient has central or peripheral access. Peripheral PN (PPN) is most useful in conjunction with enteral nutrition to meet the nutrition needs of the patient. Because of the restrictions in osmolarity and dextrose concentration, PPN is not able to meet the nutrition needs of preterm infants alone. Current American Society of Parenteral and Enteral Nutrition recommendations state that the maximum osmolality of a safe PPN is 900 mOsm/L and that dextrose concentration must not exceed 12.5%.[27] PPN is good for short-term use to supplement calorie and micronutrient needs, but is not optimal for achieving nutrition needs for growth. PPN also carries the risks of intravenous infiltrates due to the hyperosmotic solution running through small vessels and the caustic nature of some of the PN additives, such as calcium. Running high volumes or high rates of fluid may also lessen the viability of a peripherally placed intravenous line.

Central PN (CPN) is the recommended delivery of PN in patients who will require PN for more than a few days. The larger vessels can tolerate a higher osmotic solution and higher dextrose concentrations. Complete nutrition and fluid needs can be met with CPN run through centrally placed intravenous catheters. Central catheters will always carry the risk of sepsis; therefore, diligent line care is necessary to maintain safe access for long-term PN delivery.

Energy Requirements

Energy needs of parenterally fed preterm infants are 15% to 20% less than those of enterally fed infants because calorie expenditure of digestion and absorption loss does not occur when the nutritional provision bypasses the GI tract. Energy needs are based on body size, need for nutrient accretion, and losses to assure that postnatal growth will approximate the in utero growth of a normal healthy fetus of the same postconception age. ELBW infants have the lowest estimated resting energy expenditure (REE), while larger infants have a higher REE. Calorie requirement for ELBW on PN are estimated at approximately 90 to 95 kcal/kg/day.[16,17] VLBW infants are estimated to require 100 to 110 kcal/kg/day, while LBW infants require 110 to 115 kcal/kg/day while on PN.[16,17] It is generally accepted that estimated requirements for infants of these respective sizes are based on the above recommendations regardless of whether the infant was born extremely premature or SGA. This is because it is believed that infants born SGA did not acquire the necessary nutrient stores or develop to their full potential and, therefore, have catch-up growth needs. However, the necessity of catch-up growth for neonates, as well as the expectation that preterm infants will grow at the same velocity of their in utero counterparts, continues to be controversial.

Glucose

Glucose tolerance is limited in VLBW and smaller infants due to insufficient insulin production, relative insulin resistance, and the continued hepatic release of glucose from the starvation response triggered when placental transfer of nutrients is terminated. Glucose provision must be fairly low when initially administered and advanced slowly to prevent the reactive hyperglycemia caused by the physiologic glucose intolerance. Hyperglycemic response will be lessened when dextrose is administered with amino acids, as amino acids stimulate insulin production and release. It is important to prevent hyperglycemia because glucose overload will be spilled into the kidneys, causing an osmotic diuresis potentially leading to dehydration. It is equally important to prevent hypoglycemia because glucose is the primary fuel to maintain brain function, growth, and development. IUGR infants are at increased risk of developing hyperglycemia due to delayed insulin production and response and increased risk of developing hypoglycemia due to increased metabolic demand of catch-up growth. In order to maintain blood glucose in a normal range, the glucose infusion rate must be closely monitored and controlled. **Glucose infusion rate (GIR)** is a function of the concentration of dextrose and the rate at which the dextrose is administered and is typically measured in milligrams of dextrose per kilogram per minute (mg/kg/min).

> **PRACTICE POINT**
>
> Initial glucose infusion rate for premature infants must be between 4 and 6 mg/kg/min to maintain adequate glucose provision for the brain.

The demand for low GIR along with relatively high fluid requirements of ELBW infants may require the use of fluids with low dextrose concentration. The minimum dextrose concentration of fluids delivered should be 5% so that a hypotonic solution is not administered.

> **PRACTICE POINT**
>
> Dextrose can be advanced maintaining blood glucose levels above 50 mg/dL and below 120 mg/dL, by 1 to 2 mg/kg/min daily.

It is common practice in the neonate population to aim for a maximum GIR administration at 14 to 16 mg/kg/min. Excessive glucose intake may induce lipogenesis.[14,20] It may also negatively affect respiratory gas exchange by increasing carbon dioxide production, which the preterm infant has a harder time expelling, exacerbating respiratory distress.[14,20]

> **CORE CONCEPT 8**
>
> Carbohydrate in the form of dextrose, providing 3.4 kcal/gram, is the major energy source in parenteral nutrition.

Amino Acids

While it has always been common to start premature neonates on dextrose-containing intravenous fluids soon after birth, the early administration of intravenous amino acids has only become common practice in the past decade.[20] Prior to this practice, amino acids were not given until several days after birth. It is now understood that protein provision promotes anabolism and weight gain. The type of amino acid solution used for infants contains high amounts of essential amino acids and emulates the serum amino acid profile of a breastfeeding infant.[25,28] Intravenous protein requirements are based on fetal requirements, amino acid delivery across the placenta throughout gestation, and the extrauterine environment after birth. In a fetal environment, 50% of the amino acids passed across the placenta are utilized for energy, while the other half are used for protein synthesis.[20] Preterm infants have higher requirements than their fetal counterparts because of postnatal nitrogen excretion.

For preterm infants who were neither IUGR nor born SGA, 2.5 g protein/kg daily, in conjunction with receiving 50 nonprotein kcal/kg/day, is the minimum dose needed to maintain positive nitrogen balance.[21] In order to achieve protein accretion and growth rates to match those of *in utero* growth rates, the premature infant needs 2.7 to 3.5 g protein/kg/day and 70 nonprotein kcal/kg/day.[21] Because parenteral amino acids are converted to protein in the body at about 75% efficiency, amino acid requirements are as high as 3.7 to 4 g/kg/day. Early administration of amino acids can safely be initiated between 1.5 and 3 g/kg/day within the first few hours after birth to prevent catabolism and promote positive nitrogen balance. Most NICUs have a starter PN solution available that contains dextrose, amino acids, and sometimes calcium to initiate within hours of birth. Amino acids can be incrementally increased to 4 g/kg/day within the first few days of life.

> **PRACTICE POINT**
>
> Providing up to 4 g/kg/day of amino acids is now common clinical practice and has been shown to be safe without clinically significant increases in azotemia, metabolic acidosis, or hyperaminoacidemia.

Monitoring for tolerance of amino acids is not typically necessary unless renal dysfunction is present. Blood urea nitrogen (BUN) is not an effective monitoring tool of protein tolerance because amino acids are used for protein synthesis or oxidized for energy, which reflects metabolism. In the first few days to weeks of life, BUN is more reflective of hydration status rather than protein metabolism or tolerance. BUN levels as high as 40 mg/dL have been observed in neonates in the first week of life whether or not they were receiving parenteral amino acids.

> **CORE CONCEPT 9**
>
> Provision of amino acids within the first hours of life prevents postnatal growth failure, reduces complications and morbidities, and promotes neurodevelopment even at low calorie intake.

Lipids

> **PRACTICE POINT**
>
> Provision of intravenous lipids is an essential component of neonatal PN.

Long chain fatty acids are necessary for newborn brain development. Essential fatty acid deficiency (EFAD) can develop in VLBW infants within the first week of life because of minimal fat tissue stores and high demand for rapid growth.[20] VLBW infants have very minimal tissue stores of essential fatty acids, primarily linoleic acid; *in utero*, a fetus relies entirely on essential fatty acid transfer from the placenta.[15] Lipid injectable emulsion (ILE), which contains linoleic acid, can prevent essential fatty acid deficiency if provided at least at approximately 0.5 g/kg/day.[20,25] Lipids are also an important source of energy and are calorically dense. When given in greater volumes, lipids

Clinical Roundtable

Topic: Determining adequacy of protein in the preterm population

Background: It is known that premature infants have high protein needs for adequate weight gain and growth. There are several references for estimating protein requirements for premature infants, but there is no established standard of practice for measuring adequacy of protein provided. Serum albumin and prealbumin, while measures of circulating proteins, can also be altered by severity of illness and fluid shifts. Some NICU clinicians have begun looking at BUN levels, a measure of protein turnover, to determine the adequacy of protein provided in their patients.

Roundtable Discussion

Consider the available ways to assess protein adequacy in the preterm populations.

1. Do you think BUN could be a more accurate marker of protein adequacy compared to albumin or prealbumin in this population?
2. When might you use each?
3. How would you suggest manipulating the protein provided based on BUN levels?

Reference

1. Arslanoglu S, Moro GE, Zieler EE. Adjustable fortification of human milk fed preterm infants: does it make a difference? *J Perinat.* 2006;26:614-621.

can balance the calorie breakdown of the macronutrient components of PN, lessening the demand to give an excessive amount of calories as carbohydrate.[15] This concentrated source of nonprotein calories promotes nitrogen retention.

Standard 20% lipid emulsions contain a lower phospholipid emulsifier to triglyceride ratio, which leads to more rapid lipid clearance than standard 10% lipid emulsions and therefore are preferable for use in the neonatal population.[15,25] Lipids can be safely initiated in the first 24 to 48 hours of life to aid in nitrogen balance and prevent EFAD. The initial dose recommendation is 0.5 to 1 g/kg/day.[20]

> **PRACTICE POINT**
>
> Lipids should be advanced slowly each day, by 0.5 to 1 g/kg/day, and maximum dose should not exceed 3 g/kg/day to prevent ketosis.

For neonates, lipids should be administered over 20 to 24 hours for optimal clearance, although it is recommended that infusion of lipid emulsion alone hang for no more than 12 hours at a time.[25,29] Some institutions choose to change the lipid source and tubing every 12 hours in this population to accommodate a longer infusion time, while others opt to allow a 20- to 24-hour hang time in order to minimize additional manipulation of the lipid line to reduce potential contamination. Triglyceride levels should be monitored after advancing lipids to 2 g/kg/day and 3 g/kg/day to ensure normal serum levels. If serum triglyceride levels exceed 200 mg/dL, ILE should be reduced by 0.5 to 1 g/kg/day until serum triglyceride levels return to normal.[19]

In recent years there has been some concern regarding the high polyunsaturated fatty acid content of the ILE as linoleic acid (omega-6) from soybean oil used in the United States. It is thought that linoleic acids increase the production of inflammatory mediators, leading to the synthesis of prostaglandins, leukotrienes, and thromboxanes when converted to arachidonic acid.[15] These inflammatory agents have been identified in exacerbating pulmonary hypertension and increasing the risk of developing PN-associated liver disease (PNALD).[20] A fat emulsion has been developed from fish oil that contains the omega-3 fatty acids eicosapentaenoic acid and docosahexaenoic acid, which are anti-inflammatory.[30] This fat emulsion is currently used in Europe and is under investigation in the United States. It is available through the Food & Drug Administration for compassionate use and for studies to examine their utility for preventing and reversing PNALD. Another fat emulsion developed contains a mixture of soybean oil, MCT oil, olive oil, and fish oil.[31] This fat blend has a more physiologic mix of omega-3 and omega-6 fatty acids, balancing the pro-inflammatory and anti-inflammatory effects, and is now available for use in adult patients in the United States. Until there are more data supporting the use of these fat emulsions in the premature population, it is recommended to reduce ILE provision to 1 g/kg/day for infants who have PNALD, defined as having a conjugated bilirubin level >2 mg/dL.[31]

Plasma carnitine levels are low in premature infants and decrease further in the first 2 weeks of life if the infants are exclusively on PN. **Carnitine** is an amino acid derivative that aids in the oxidation of fatty acids. Studies have shown little, if any, clinical benefit to supplementing carnitine in PN as a means of improving fatty acid oxidation. However, it is commonly recommended to add carnitine to neonatal PN for patients who are receiving exclusively PN for longer than 2 weeks or if carnitine deficiency is determined.[15]

Electrolytes

Electrolytes are withheld or restricted in the first few days of life prior to the neonate diuresis of initial fluid and to prevent exacerbation of pulmonary disease and later development of BPD. Once postnatal diuresis has occurred, sodium and potassium can be added to PN in limited amounts (1-2 mEq/kg/day) and advanced incrementally to meet physiologic needs. Neonatal needs during the first weeks of life will vary depending on renal function, hydration status, and the use of systemic diuretics. While metabolic acidosis may be common during the first few weeks of life, requiring increased acetate provision in the PN, once the diuresis period is over, chloride can be added back into the PN to maintain optimal acid–base balance.

Minerals

Calcium and phosphorus supplementation are an important part of PN therapy. Premature neonates are at elevated risk of developing osteopenia of prematurity. Receiving PN with little or no calcium or phosphorus increases this risk further. Providing required amounts of calcium and phosphorus can be difficult due to solubility limitations and the high risk of precipitation. A severe fluid restriction will significantly decrease the ability to add appropriate amounts of calcium and phosphorus to the PN solution due to limitations related to solution concentration. Calcium and phosphorus will also need to be limited in PPN due to their high osmolalities and the risk of calcium causing intravenous infiltrates or extravasation. Neonatal amino acid solutions are more acidic compared to standard amino acid solutions. This increases the solubility of calcium and phosphorus, which may allow more to be added to the PN solution. The addition of cysteine hydrochloride and higher concentrations of amino acids and dextrose, and providing lipids as a separate infusion, helps to prevent the precipitation of calcium and phosphorus. Preterm infants, particularly LBW infants, receiving prolonged PN are likely to experience poor bone mineralization and should be monitored regularly. Serum calcium and phosphorus levels along with alkaline phosphatase, an enzyme that correlates with bone growth, should be checked every 1 to 2 weeks for patients requiring long-term PN. Although normal alkaline phosphatase levels are higher in preterm neonates (upwards of 600 IU/L) due to their rapid bone growth, levels above 800 IU/L require additional workup, including skeletal radiographs to look for bone demineralization and rickets.

Vitamins

All newborn infants are born with a relatively sterile GI tract. Without the colonization of appropriate bacteria, they are unable to synthesize their own vitamin K. Prenatal stores of vitamin K and initial dietary intakes are limited. Therefore, neonates are at increased risk of having hemorrhagic disease of the newborn from vitamin K deficiency. To prevent this, all neonates born in a U.S. hospital receive an intramuscular injection of vitamin K soon after birth.

Pediatric solutions of multivitamins are available and recommended for use in PN solution. Use of an adult multivitamin PN solution would put a neonate at increased risk of vitamin toxicities. All water- and fat-soluble vitamins are contained in the pediatric vitamin solution. Vitamins are photosensitive, putting them at risk of oxidation and degradation with light exposure on a PN bag. Protecting the PN bag and tubing with an opaque bag may aid in the preservation of these vitamins. There is also a relative risk of vitamins adhering to the plastic PN bag and tubing. Higher infusion rates and using the shortest IV tubing possible will help reduce this risk. Because VLBW infants have limited stores of vitamins, not receiving the full, expected dose of vitamins due to these issues should be considered.

Vitamin A has been of particular interest for premature neonates in relation to the reduction of BPD. Premature neonates are born with low stores of vitamin A. Vitamin A has a role in tissue repair and cell differentiation and turnover. Supplemental vitamin A may be provided intravenously in addition to the multivitamin solution in the PN or by providing a high-dose intramuscular injection. While benefits have been shown in reducing risk of BPD development with vitamin A supplementation in multiple studies, individual neonatal intensive care units may choose to use or not use additional supplemental A depending on the BPD rates in their unit.

Trace Elements

Trace elements are required for all premature infants because adequate passage of trace elements across the placenta and storage do not occur without completion of gestation to term. Premature neonates also have increased demand due to rapid growth rates. These factors put them at increased risk of trace element deficiencies. Neonatal and pediatric multitrace solutions are available for addition to PN solution. Some trace elements may also be added individually.

For infants with cholestatic jaundice, manganese can be reduced or removed in PN to prevent toxicity. However, zinc and selenium should always be provided. Inadequate selenium has been associated with increased risk of developing BPD and retinopathy of prematurity.[15] Zinc is required for energy metabolism, tissue accretion, and wound healing. VLBW infants have high requirements due to their rapid growth rates, so it is recommended that additional zinc sulfate be provided to PN solutions beyond what is provided in the multitrace solution.[15] This practice should also be considered for infants with increased losses from diarrhea, stomal losses, or severe skin disease.

While iron is not recommended for routine addition to PN, it may be added in limited amounts to PN solutions without lipids if a neonate is receiving the majority of their nutrition from PN for 2 months or longer. It may also be required if a neonate develops iron deficiency anemia while receiving PN. Recent red blood cell transfusions, which are also sources of iron, should be taken into account when considering the addition of iron to a PN solution.

Enteral Nutrition

Enterally feeding infants, including preterm infants, is the preferred method of providing nutrition. Feeding the premature GI tract provides luminal nutrients to help the tissue mature, develop, and colonize appropriately. When the GI tract is not fed, it begins to atrophy, making it more susceptible to infections. Necrotizing enterocolitis (NEC),

CASE STUDY REVISITED

The neonatology team has stated that given the IUGR status of Quinn, they are feeling cautious about starting enteral feeds and are considering waiting until she is 3 days old before feeding her.

Questions:
1. What recommendations would you provide to them about early enteral feeding?
2. When would you start MEN feeds for Quinn?
3. After 5 days of MEN feeding, at what rate would you advance her enteral feeds?

a condition characterized by inflammation and cell death within the intestinal wall, can occur. However, feeding premature infants too quickly and with large volumes have also been associated with increased risk of developing NEC.

> **PRACTICE POINT**
>
> Enteral nutrition should be started as soon after birth as possible, optimally in the first 48 hours of life, but started carefully and in small volumes.

Early enteral feedings provide several benefits to the premature infant. For all ELBW infants and some VLBW infants, providing minimal enteral nutrition (MEN), or trophic feedings, will provide luminal nutrients and promote the secretion of gastric hormones and enzymes to prime the gut for larger volumes of enteral feeding. Stimulating the GI tract with MEN decreases PN-related problems, such as the development of PNALD, and helps improve weight gain. MEN is defined as a subnutritional volume of enteral feeding, 10 to 20 mL/kg/day, provided at that volume for a predetermined length of time, typically 3 to 7 days.[27] Once the trophic feeding period is completed, it has been shown that feeding advancements of 10 to 30 mL/kg/day are safe and do not increase the incidence of developing NEC.[28,29] Advancing enteral feeds at this rate allows for the relatively quick achievement of full feeding volume and more rapid weight gain.[28,29] Many institutions have developed standardized methods of starting and advancing enteral feeds. Evidence has shown that developing and following a standardized feeding regimen can decrease the incidence of NEC in an institution.[30] Conditions that may delay the initiation and advancement of enteral feedings include hemodynamic instability, hypotension, indomethacin treatment, abnormal GI exam or GI dysfunction, severe metabolic acidosis, severe respiratory instability, hypoxia, or hypoxemia.[33]

> **PRACTICE POINT**
>
> Premature infants may lack the ability to feed orally on their own because of the inability to suck, swallow, and breathe simultaneously, which develops around 33-36 weeks gestational age.

Infants who lack the ability to suck, swallow, and breathe simultaneously need to be fed via a nasogastric or orogastric tube (**Figure 22.9**). Frequent intermittent or bolus feeding is the most physiologic way to feed premature infants. This method allows for the natural rise and fall of gastric hormones and enzymes, aids in the development of hunger cues, and teaches the infants to wake at appropriate times to feed. Feeding small volumes more frequently (every 2 hours) has been shown to improve feeding tolerance compared to feeding larger volumes less frequently (every 4 hours). Bolus feeds delivered via gravity or over an electronic pump infusion decreases the nutrient loss seen with

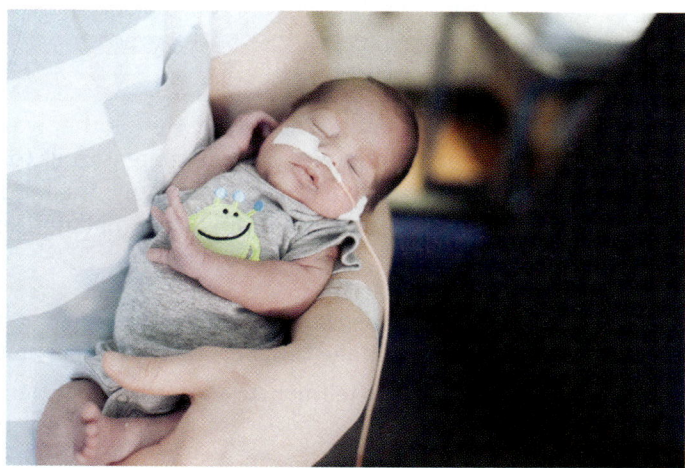

FIGURE 22.9 Preterm Infant with Nasogastric Tube
©Jill Lehmann Photography/ Moment/Getty Images.

continuous feeding related to the adherence of fats, minerals, and vitamins by extended dwell time of the milk or formula in the plastic tubing.[19] For this reason, bolus or intermittent feeding promotes better delivery of nutrients and may lead to improved weight gain for premature infants with intact, functional GI tracts compared to continuous feeding.[34] Once an infant reaches 33 to 34 weeks PMA, small oral feedings may be trialed. Transition to oral feeding should be initiated based on the infant's readiness cues, including waking or fussiness around the time of feeding, rooting, and putting hands near or around mouth.[36-38]

Continuous feedings may be advantageous for infants with severe lung disease, gastroesophageal reflux (GER), malabsorption, poor motility, GI surgery, or severe or multiple episodes of feeding intolerance.[25,39,40] Continuous feeds may promote better absorption of nutrients and increased weight gain in infants with malabsorption as a result of short-bowel syndrome or intestinal failure, or during recovery from NEC.[25,39] When feeding continuously, intragastric feeds are preferred to transpyloric or postpyloric feeding.[41] Transpyloric feeding has been associated with such complications as intestinal perforation and mortality. Transpyloric feedings should only be used as a last resort for infants who are at risk of aspiration, extremely severe GER, or severe respiratory compromise.[42]

Common issues that complicate enteral feeding are GER, emesis, and gastric residuals. All three occur commonly in premature infants and often lead to concerns of feeding intolerance. The premature GI tracts of preterm infants have an underdeveloped lower esophageal sphincter and gastro-esophageal junction. Therefore, GER and mild emesis is very common in premature infants and tend to resolve over time because these organ connections are not tight at birth and develop and tighten throughout infancy.[40] Most GER and emesis should not be concerning or indicate feeding intolerance.[40] GER becomes problematic when reflux is bilious or causes respiratory instability or aspiration. Emesis is concerning when the amount of emesis is 50% or more of the volume fed, if the amount of

> **CASE STUDY REVISITED**
>
> Quinn is now nearly 36 hours old. Her mother was very sick from the preeclampsia after delivery. Despite her intentions of providing breast milk for her baby, she has not been pumping as often as needed to establish an adequate supply. The medical team would like you to speak with the mother to establish a feeding plan with her so that feeds can be started for Quinn.
>
> **Questions**
> 1. How would you educate Quinn's mother about breastfeeding, pumping breast milk, and the role of mother's milk and donor milk in feeding her preterm daughter?
> 2. What might you tell mom to encourage her to pump more regularly in order to be able to provide breast milk?

emesis is inhibiting weight gain, or if the emesis contains bile or blood.[15] Gastric residuals are also fairly common in infants and more common in preterm infants. Gastric residuals are more commonly seen in the setting of continuous feeds compared to bolus feedings, and do not likely indicate feeding intolerance if the abdominal exam is normal. Similarly to emesis, gastric residuals that are 50% or more of the volume fed or residuals that contain bile or blood may be concerning indicating lack of effective gastric motility or feeding intolerance.[43]

> **CORE CONCEPT 10**
>
> Feeding the gastrointestinal (GI) tract early has been shown to promote endocrine adaptation and to accelerate early motility patterns. Premature infants also have better tolerance of feeds, achieve full feeding volume sooner, and have a reduced risk of feeding aversion when fed early; all of which may lead to decreased length of hospital stay.

Feeding Selection

Breast Milk, Breastfeeding, and Donor Milk

For the premature infant, human milk is ideally used for enteral feeds. The options for human milk are mother's own milk or pasteurized donor human milk. Mother's own milk is the optimal choice compared to donor milk. Mothers can express their milk using a breast pump so that the milk can be fed to the premature infants in controlled volumes, at specific times, and via a feeding tube (**Figure 22.10**). During the first month of a premature infant's life, the composition of the mother's breast milk is slightly different than that of the milk of the mother of a term infant.[19] Preterm breast milk contains higher amounts of protein and sodium compared to term breast milk. After the first month of lactation, the breast milk produced by the mother of the preterm infant will transition to a composition more similar to term human milk.

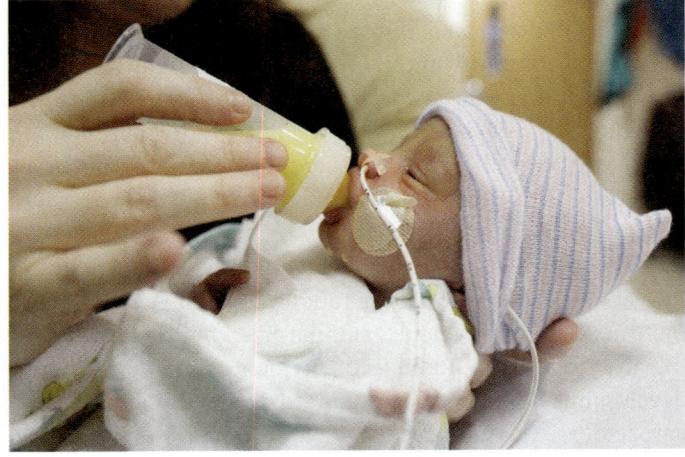

FIGURE 22.10 Preterm Infant with Nasogastric Feeding Tube in Place Being Bottle Fed with Breast Milk
©Tbd/E+/Getty Images.

There are several reasons why human milk is the preferred food for premature infants. Human milk contains many nonnutritive components that have been shown to be protective or beneficial to the GI tract of premature infants. There are anti-infectious compounds including lactoferrin, nucleotides, cytokines, and oligosaccharides, as well as immune cells such as neutrophils, macrophages, and T-lymphocytes.[20] Feeding the premature infant with human milk has been shown to decrease the incidence of NEC and sepsis, likely due to these components.[19] These immune-protective components have anti-inflammatory, antibacterial, antiviral, and prebiotic effects that help the GI tract develop a healthy microbiome.[20] Multiple types of growth factors and enzymes are found in human milk and likely contribute to the fact that preterm infants fed human milk tolerate their feeds better, are able to advance their feedings more rapidly, and achieve full enteral feeds earlier. This may lead to an earlier discharge from the hospital. Human milk also contains many different hormones that may contribute to better neurodevelopment. It has been suggested that these beneficial and protective effects of human milk are likely dose-dependent, with the most benefits seen in infants that receive exclusively human milk.[34,44-46]

> **PRACTICE POINT**
>
> The concentrations of macro- and micronutrients are lower in human milk when compared to infant formulas; however, the nutrients are more readily absorbed from human milk. This is especially true for zinc and iron, as well as fat due to the presence of lipases in breast milk.

> **PRACTICE POINT**
>
> Even with optimal absorption, the nutrient concentrations of human milk are insufficient to meet the high calorie demands and calcium and phosphorus needs of preterm infants to maintain rapid growth and bone mineralization rates.

Human milk fortifiers are often added to human milk to increase macro- and micronutrient concentrations. Human milk fortifiers are available as bovine-based powders, bovine-based concentrated liquids, and human milk–based liquids. They all contain macro- and micronutrients, but in varying amounts. Depending on which fortifier is used, additional supplementation of sodium, chloride, protein, iron, or vitamins may be necessary. These fortifiers are not available for retail purchase. If growth is still inadequate after the addition of these fortifiers, modular products may be added such as liquid hydrolyzed protein, MCT oil, emulsified lipids, vegetable oils, or glucose polymers. It is important to try to use these modulars in appropriate ratios so the natural distribution of calories from carbohydrate, protein, and fat is not altered and the protein–energy ratio used to preserve optimal growth of lean body mass is maintained. Providing too much fat from an oil modular may put the infant at risk of developing ketosis, providing too much carbohydrate from glucose polymers may promote lipogenesis, and providing too much protein fortifier may unnecessarily strain the premature kidneys. Infant formula powders or concentrates can also be used instead of modular products, although sterile liquids are preferred to nonsterile powders for premature infants.

Breastfeeding and providing expressed breast milk can be emotionally rewarding for the mothers of premature infants during a frightening and stressful time when the infants are in the hospital. Providing this type of nutrition promotes involvement in the infant's care and direct interaction with the infant at a time when the typical development of the mother–infant dyad is inhibited due to the complex care needs of the premature infant. Mothers who are interested in breastfeeding are encouraged to do so as soon as possible for premature infants. After a mother expresses her breast milk, a premature infant may be put to the breast for nonnutritive suckling. This practice helps develop the oral skills of the infant, enhances mother's milk production, and encourages mother–infant bonding. Once the premature infant reaches 33 weeks PMA and is showing cues for oral feeding readiness, actual breastfeeding prior to breast milk pumping may be started.[37,38] Because of the high metabolic demands of premature infants, supplemental high-calorie, fortified breast milk or formula feeds are typically needed in conjunction with direct breastfeeding.

There are some instances in which a mother may wish to provide breast milk for her infant, but is unable. For these infants, especially the ones at highest risk of developing NEC, sepsis, or feeding intolerance, pasteurized donor human milk is available. Donor milk is generally term milk from later in lactation; however, some milk banks collect and are able to supply preterm donor milk. The risks and benefits of donor milk are still being investigated. Some evidence has suggested that it may decrease the risk of

⚠ Clinical Controversy

There have been many studies published documenting the decreased risk of developing necrotizing enterocolitis on an exclusively human milk diet compared to bovine milk–based products. Work such as that of Sullivan et al. has led to the widespread use of pasteurized donor human milk when maternal milk is not available. However, Chowning et al. report poor weight gain in premature infants being fed pasteurized donor human milk.

Questions

1. Based upon this research, discuss how you would balance the well-established benefits of a human milk diet for premature infants and the need for adequate growth and weight gain.
2. How would you decide which neonates would most benefit from the protective effects of an exclusive human milk diet?

References:

1. Sullivan S, Schanler RJ, Kim JH, et al. An exclusively human milk-based diet is associated with a lower rate of necrotizing enterocolitis than a diet of human milk and bovine milk-based products. *J Pediatr*. 2010; 156:562-7
2. Chowning R, Radmacher P, Lewis S, Serke L, Pettit N, Adamkin DH. A retrospective analysis of the effect of human milk on prevention of necrotizing enterocolitis and postnatal growth. *J Perinatol*. 2016;36:221-224

developing NEC.[47-50] Growth and development rates of infants receiving donor milk tend to be slower. Donor milk typically has lower concentrations of protein, sodium, and chloride, which may be caused by the pasteurization, handling, and storage of donor breast milk.[51,52] The lower amounts of these nutrients may be why growth and development rates are lower in infants receiving donor milk.

> **CORE CONCEPT 11**
>
> Human milk is the ideal choice for enterally feeding premature infants.

Preterm and Transitional Formulas

Because the nutritional needs and capabilities of the GI tract of premature infants are so different from that of term infants, commercial formula companies have developed infant formulas to meet the specific needs of this population. The protein provided is whey predominant and the fat contained in the formula is 50% MCT oil for improved absorption and easier digestion.[53] The formulas are only available as ready-to-feed liquid and are made in concentrations of 20, 24, and 30 kcal/fl oz.[53] These different calorie forms can be mixed with one another to create various calorie concentrations between 22 and 28 kcal/fl oz. The 30 kcal/fl oz concentrated preterm formula can also be used as a liquid fortifier for human milk. All premature infants born before 34 weeks gestation and born at a weight less than 1,800 g who are not receiving breast milk or who need supplemental feeds with formula should receive preterm formula. These formulas are not available for retail purchase.

> **PRACTICE POINT**
>
> Preterm formulas contain higher amounts of protein, calcium, phosphorus, and vitamins to meet the high needs of preterm infants.

Specialty formulas have also been developed for infants who are born closer to term or for preterm infants once they reach at least 34 weeks PMA and weigh at least 2,000 g. These transitional formulas come in a standard formulation of 22 kcal/fl oz. They contain higher concentrations of nutrients than term infant formulas, but less than preterm formulas. This is specifically true for protein, calcium, phosphorus, and vitamins.[53] These formulas contain 25% to 30% MCT oil for improved digestion.[53] It is recommended that infants stay on this formula for the first 9 to 12 months of life or until the infant's weight-for-length is maintained above the 25th percentile. These formulas are available as powder or ready-to-feed. The powder form can be concentrated to make a formula of greater calorie density than 22 kcal/fl oz if higher calories are needed to promote weight gain. The powder can also be added to the breast milk of late premature infants to increase the calorie density of the breast milk as the infant is getting ready to transition to home. Transitional formulas are available for retail purchase and, therefore, can be used outside of the hospital.

Preparing for Discharge

It is common that premature infants will need increased calorie feedings upon discharge to continue to support their rapid growth rates and high metabolic demand. The method of how a premature infant feeds will impact discharge planning. In rare cases, an infant may be discharged with a feeding tube or may need to be woken up for feedings at least every 4 hours. It is important for all parents of premature infants to receive discharge teaching and education about the special needs and risks of bringing home a baby born prematurely.

> **PRACTICE POINT**
>
> In order to be ready to go home, a premature infant must be able to take all of their feedings by mouth via a bottle, breastfeeding, or a combination of both; be demonstrating adequate weight gain; wake for feedings every 2 and 4 hours; and maintain their body temperature without the use of an incubator.

The premature infant is still likely to be smaller than they would have been if born at term. These infants should be monitored closely once discharged. Many hospitals with NICUs also have a NICU graduates or follow-up outpatient clinic for continuity of care. These clinics target premature infants who are at highest risk for growth failure or developmental delay and follow up with them at least every 6 months for growth measurements, weight checks, and developmental testing. Home services are also available for high-risk infants that can provide physical and occupational therapy, speech therapy, and feeding therapy once per week or more. Premature infants are at risk of physical and cognitive developmental delays, and the risks are higher the more prematurely an infant is born. Intensive support, follow-up, and intervention may prevent or lessen delays in this population as they reach childhood and adulthood.

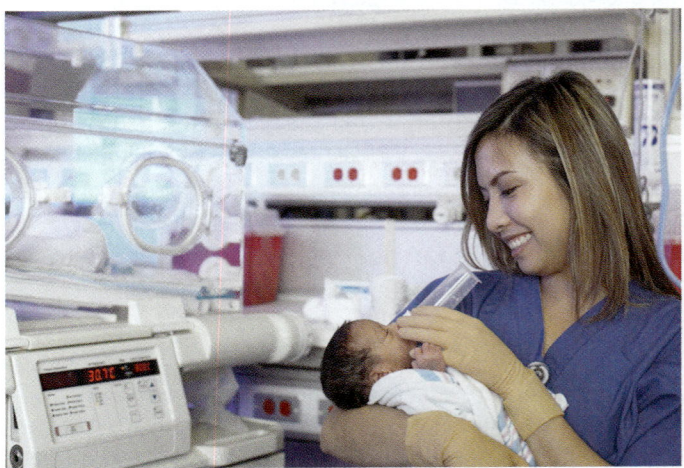

FIGURE 22.11 Neonatal Nurse Feeding Preterm Infant
©Blend Images - ERproductions Ltd/ Brand X Pictures/Getty Images.

CASE STUDY

Quinn is now 35 weeks PMA (about 1 month old). Her mom is noticing that her breast milk supply is starting to slow down. She would like to directly breastfeed Quinn as much as possible in order to stimulate her breast milk supply.

Questions

1. Is Quinn developmentally ready to start feeding by mouth?
2. If the mother's supply is still inadequate, what would you suggest as a backup option?
3. Quinn's mother is also asking when Quinn will be ready to come home. What goals will Quinn have to achieve to be discharged home from the hospital?

⚠ Clinical Controversy

The standard of weight gain and growth expectations in premature infants have always been to match the *in utero* weight gain potential of a growing fetus of the same gestation. This continues to be the recommendation of the American Academy of Pediatrics. However, long-term follow-up of former premature infants has started to suggest that rapid weight gain of growth-restricted neonates may predispose them to the development of metabolic syndrome as adults, as first published by epidemiologist David Barker and later became known as the Barker Hypothesis.

Questions

1. Based upon this research, discuss how you would balance the need for catch-up growth early in life versus the increased risk of early weight gain and risk of metabolic syndrome later in life.
2. How would you determine energy needs and weight gain goals?

References:

1. Kleinman RE, Greer FR. American Academy of Pediatric Nutrition Committee on Nutrition. *Pediatric Nutrition*. American Academy of Pediatrics: Elk Grove, IL; 2013
2. Barker DJ. The fetal and infant origins of adult disease. *BMJ*. 1990; 301 (6761): 1111

Chapter Summary

Nutritional management of the preterm population presents many challenges, including, but not limited to, increased nutrient needs and immature organ function. Appropriate utilization and timing of provisions of parenteral, enteral, and/or oral nutrition are necessary for successful growth. The achievement of extrauterine growth through specialized nutrition support is vital for the health and development of the premature neonate.

Key Terms

oligohydramnios, low birth weight (LBW), very low birth weight (VLBW), extremely low birth weight (ELBW), small-for-gestational-age (SGA), appropriate-for-gestational-age (AGA), large-for-gestational-age (LGA), intrauterine growth restriction (IUGR), growth discordance, postnatal diuresis, patent ductus arteriosus (PDA), nephrocalcinosis, human milk fortifiers, glucose infusion rate (GIR), carnitine

References

1. 2016 Premature Birth Report Card. March of Dimes Website. http://www.marchofdimes.org/mission/prematurity-reportcard.aspx. Accessed July 15, 2017.
2. The American College of Obstetricians and Gynecologists Committee on Obstetric Practice Society for Maternal-Fetal Medicine Committee Opinion No.579: Definition of term pregnancy. *Obstet Gynecol*. 2013;122(5):1139-1140.
3. American Academy of Pediatrics Committee on Fetus and Newborn: Age terminology during the perinatal period. *Pediatrics*. 2004;114(5):1362-1364.
4. ACOG Committee on Obstetric Practice. Guidelines for perinatal care. *AAP Books*. 2012.
5. Fenton TR. A new growth chart for preterm babies: Babson and Benda's chart updated with recent data and a new format. *BMC Pediatrics*. 2003;3(1):13.

6. Fenton TR, Kim JH. A systematic review and meta-analysis to revise the Fenton growth chart for preterm infants. *BMC Pediatrics*. 2013;13:59.
7. Lubchenco LO, Hansman C, Boyd E. Intrauterine growth in length and head circumference as estimated from live births at gestational ages from 26 to 42 weeks. *Pediatrics*. 1966;37(3):403-408.
8. Lubchenco LO, Hansman C, Dressler M, Boyd E. Intrauterine growth as estimated from liveborn birth-weight data at 24 to 42 weeks of gestation. *Pediatrics*. 1963;32:793-800.
9. Olsen IE, Groveman SA, Lawson ML, Clark RH, Zemel BS. New intrauterine growth curves based on United States data. *Pediatrics*. 2010;125(2):e214-e224.
10. Cloherty J, Stark A. Identifying the high-risk newborn and evaluating gestational age. *Manual of Neonatal Care*. Philadelphia, PA: Lippincott Williams Wilkins; 2010:41-58.
11. Cetin I, Alvino G. Intrauterine growth restriction: implications for placental metabolism and transport. *Placenta*. 2009;30:77-82.
12. Cetin I, Foidart J, Miozzo M, et al. Fetal growth restriction: a workshop report. *Placenta*. 2004;25(8):753-757.
13. Hendrix N, Berghella V. Non-placental causes of intrauterine growth restriction. *Semin Perinatol*. 2008;32(3):161-165.
14. Martin JA, Hamilton BE, Osterman MJ, Driscoll AK, Matthews TJ. Births: Final data for 2015. *Natl Vital Stat Rep*. 2017 Jan 5;66(1):1-70.
15. Adamkin DH. *Nutritional strategies for the very low birthweight infant*. New York, NY: Cambridge University Press; 2009.
16. Rigo J, Senterre J. Nutritional needs of premature infants: current issues. *J Pediatr*. 2006;149(5):S80-S88.
17. Ziegler EE. Nutrient requirements of premature infants. *Nestle Nutr Workshop Ser Pediatr Program*. 2007;59:161-172; discussion 172-176.
18. Babson SG, Benda GI. Growth graphs for the clinical assessment of infants of varying gestational age. *J Pediatr*. 1976;89(5):814-820.
19. Kleinman RE, American Academy of Pediatrics. *Pediatric Nutrition Handbook*. 6th ed. Elk Grove Village, IL: American Academy of Pediatrics; 2009:1470.
20. Koletzko B, Poindexter B, Uauy R, eds. *Nutritional care of preterm infants: Scientific basis and practical guidelines*. Karger Medical and Scientific Publishers; Basel, CH, 2014.
21. Ziegler EE. Protein requirements of very low birth weight infants. *J Pediatr Gastroenterol Nutr*. 2007;45 Suppl 3:S170-S174.
22. Kien CL. Digestion, absorption, and fermentation of carbohydrates in the newborn. *Clin Perinatol*. 1996;23(2):211-228.
23. Tsang RC, Uauy R, Koletzko B, Zlotkin S. *Nutrition of the Preterm Infant: Scientific Basis and Practical Guidelines*. Digital Educational Publishing, Inc., Cincinnati, Ohio, USA. 2005.
24. Wirth Jr F, Numerof B, Pleban P, Neylan M. Effect of lactose on mineral absorption in preterm infants. *J Pediatr*. 1990;117(2):283-287.
25. Groh-Wargo S, Thompson M, Cox JH. *ADA Pocket Guide to Neonatal Nutrition* Academy of Nutrition and Dietetics, Chicago Illinois, USA. 2016.
26. Baumgart S, Costarino AT. Water and electrolyte metabolism of the micropremie. *Clin Perinatol*. 2000;27(1):131-146.
27. Nehra D, Carlson SJ, Fallon EM, et al. A.S.P.E.N. clinical guidelines: nutrition support of neonatal patients at risk for metabolic bone disease. *J Parenter Enteral Nutr*. 2013;37(5):570-598.
28. Helms RA, Christensen ML, Mauer EC, Storm MC. Comparison of a pediatric versus standard amino acid formulation in preterm neonates requiring parenteral nutrition. *J Pediatr*. 1987;110(3):466-470.
29. Erratum for Guidelines for preventing catheter-related infections. *Morb Mortal Wkly Rep*. 2002;August 16:711.
30. Gura KM, Duggan CP, Collier SB, et al. Reversal of parenteral nutrition-associated liver disease in two infants with short bowel syndrome using parenteral fish oil: Implications for future management. *Pediatrics*. 2006;118(1):e197-201.
31. Wales PW, Allen N, Worthington P, George D, and Compher C. ASPEN clinical guidelines: support of pediatric patients with intestinal failure at risk of parenteral nutrition–associated liver iesase. *J Parenter Enteral Nutr*. 2014;38:538-557.
32. Tomsits E, Pataki M, Tolgyesi A, Fekete G, Rischak K, Szollar L. Safety and efficacy of a lipid emulsion containing a mixture of soybean oil, medium-chain triglycerides, olive oil, and fish oil: a randomised, double-blind clinical trial in premature infants requiring parenteral nutrition. *J Pediatr Gastroenterol Nutr*. 2010;51(4):514-521.
33. Duggan C, Watkins JB, Walker WA. *Nutrition in pediatrics: Basic science, clinical applications*. Shelton, Connecticut People's Medical Publishing House-USA; 2007.
34. Schanler RJ, Shulman RJ, Lau C, Smith EO, Heitkemper MM. Feeding strategies for premature infants: randomized trial of gastrointestinal priming and tube-feeding method. *Pediatrics*. 1999;103(2):434-439.
35. Jesse N, Neu J. Necrotizing enterocolitis relationship to innate immunity, clinical features, and strategies for prevention. *NeoReviews*. 2006;7(3):e143-e150.
36. Kirk A, Alder S, King J. Cue-based oral feeding clinical pathway results in earlier attainment of full oral feeding in premature infants. *J Perinatol*. 2007;27(9):572-578.
37. Puckett B, Grover VK, Holt T, Sankaran K. Cue-based feeding for preterm infants: a prospective trial. *Am J Perinatol*. 2008;25(10):623-628.
38. McCain GC. An evidence-based guideline for introducing oral feeding to healthy preterm infants. *Neonatal Netw*. 2003;22(5):45-50.
39. Hwang ST, Shulman RJ. Update on management and treatment of short gut. *Clin Perinatol*. 2002;29(1):181-194.
40. Poets CF. Gastroesophageal reflux: a critical review of its role in preterm infants. *Pediatrics*. 2004;113(2):e128-e132.
41. Macdonald PD, Skeoch CH, Carse H, et al. Randomised trial of continuous nasogastric, bolus nasogastric, and transpyloric feeding in infants of birth weight under 1400 g. *Arch Dis Child*. 1992;67(4 Spec No):429-431.
42. Pereira GR. Nutritional care of the extremely premature infant. *Clin Perinatol*. 1995;22(1):61-75.
43. Mihatsch WA, von Schoenaich P, Fahnenstich H, et al. The significance of gastric residuals in the early enteral feeding advancement of extremely low birth weight infants. *Pediatrics*. 2002;109(3):457-459.
44. Meinzen-Derr J, Poindexter B, Wrage L, Morrow A, Stoll B, Donovan E. Role of human milk in extremely low birth weight infants' risk of necrotizing enterocolitis or death. *J Perinatol*. 2009;29(1):57-62.
45. Schanler R, Shulman R, Lau C. Feeding strategies for premature infants: beneficial outcomes of feeding fortified human milk versus preterm formula. *Pediatrics*. 1999;103:1150-1157.
46. Sisk P, Lovelady C, Dillard R, Gruber K, O'Shea T. Early human milk feeding is associated with a lower risk of necrotizing enterocolitis in very low birth weight infants. *J Perinatol*. 2007;27(7):428-433.
47. Arslanoglu S, Ziegler EE, Moro GE, WAPM Working Group on Nutrition. Donor human milk in preterm infant feeding: evidence and recommendations. *J Perinat Med*. 2010;38(4):347-351.
48. Boyd CA, Quigley MA, Brocklehurst P. Donor breast milk versus infant formula for preterm infants: systematic review and meta-analysis. *Arch Dis Child Fetal Neonatal Ed*. 2007;92(3):F169-75.
49. Henderson G, Anthony MY, McGuire W. Formula milk versus maternal breast milk for feeding preterm or low birth weight infants. *The Cochrane Library*. 2007.
50. Section on Breastfeeding. Breastfeeding and the use of human milk. *Pediatrics*. 2012;129(3):e827-e841.

51. Ewaschuk J, Unger S, O'Connor D, et al. Effect of pasteurization on selected immune components of donated human breast milk. *J Perinatol.* 2011;31(9):593-598.
52. Moro GE, Arslanoglu S. Heat treatment of human milk. *J Pediatr Gastroenterol Nutr.* 2012;54(2):165-166.
53. Klein CJ. Nutrient requirements for preterm infant formulas. *J Nutr.* 2002;132(6 Suppl 1):1395S-577S.
54. Rayyis SF, Ambalavanan N, Wright L, Carlo WA. Randomized trial of "slow" versus "fast" feed advancements on the incidence of necrotizing enterocolitis in very low birth weight infants. *J Pediatr.* 1999;134(3):293-297.
55. Patole SK, de Klerk N. Impact of standardised feeding regimens on incidence of neonatal necrotising enterocolitis: a systematic review and meta-analysis of observational studies. *Arch Dis Child Fetal Neonatal Ed.* 2005;90(2):F147-F151.
56. Kleinman RE, Greer FR. American Academy of Pediatric Nutrition Committee on Nutrition. *Pediatric Nutrition*. American Academy of Pediatrics: Elk Grove, IL; 2013.
57. Barker DJ. The fetal and infant origins of adult disease. *BMJ.* 1990;301(6761):1111.
58. Sullivan S, Schanler RJ, Kim JH, et al. An exclusively human milk-based diet is associated with a lower rate of necrotizing enterocolitis than a diet of human milk and bovine milk-based products. *J Pediatr.* 2010;156:562-567.
59. Chowning R, Radmacher P, Lewis S, Serke L, Pettit N, Adamkin DH. A retrospective analysis of the effect of human milk on prevention of necrotizing enterocolitis and postnatal growth. *J Perinatol.* 2016;36:221-224.
60. Arslanoglu S, Moro GE, Zieler, EE. Adjustable fortification of human milk fed preterm infants: does it make a difference? *J Perinat.* 2006;26:614-621.

Chapter 23

Nutrition in Pediatrics

Angela Goscilo
Kathy Prelack

Chapter Outline

Core Concepts
Introduction
Growth and Development
Nutrition Screening and Assessment
Assessing Patterns of Growth and Etiology
Normal Pediatric Nutrition

Pediatric Malnutrition
Calculating Energy Needs for Catch-Up Growth
Nutrition Support During Times of Illness or Chronic Disease
Immunonutrition in Nutrition Support of Children

CORE CONCEPTS

1. Growth velocity and rates of gain in weight and length are well described, with the most rapid rates of gain the first few months of life.

2. Body composition changes throughout childhood. Nutritional risk is greater in children 0 to 2 years of age due to a greater fat versus fat-free mass content and lower percentage of body protein.

3. Underweight is defined as low weight-for-age. Failure to gain weight may indicate acute or short-term deficits, history of insult, or long-term illness.

4. Stunting, or low height-for-age, may be indicative of long-term ongoing illness, genetic or endocrine abnormalities, or a history of insult.

5. Wasting refers to low weight-for-height or BMI-for-age and is an indication of recent and severe state of undernutrition. Wasting may be the result of disease and is responsive to nutrition intervention.

6. Growth charts are used to evaluate growth from birth to age 20 years. Serial measures of weight and height and their patterns can be used to determine nutritional status, as well as growth abnormalities and their potential etiology.

7. Energy and protein needs, per kilogram of body weight, are the highest at birth and plateau through early childhood, as a consequence of changes in growth.

8. Vitamins and minerals, especially calcium, iron, and vitamin D, provide essential nutrients for growth and development. Without adequate micronutrient status, children may have impaired growth.

9. At each stage, children should consume a well-balanced diet. Eating environment, parental modeling, and nutrition knowledge can all influence eating practices.

10. Failure to thrive must be addressed using an interprofessional approach, including feeding based on

catch-up energy and nutrient requirements to prevent developmental delays and child mortality.

11. Nutrition support may be indicated in pediatric patients when oral feeding does not provide enough energy or nutrients. Timely initiation, particularly in children younger than 2 years of age, prevents rapid deterioration of nutritional status.

Learning Objectives

1. Compare and contrast body composition in different stages of growth and the implications for nutrition therapy.
2. Assess growth utilizing standardized growth charts, as appropriate for age.
3. Differentiate among patterns of growth abnormalities, including failure to gain weight, failure to grow, and stunting, and identify causal factors and etiology for each.
4. Assess malnutrition in children using anthropometric indices and standardized z-scores.
5. Relate introduction and progression of food with developmental cues in children.
6. Describe how pediatric macronutrient and micronutrient requirements change throughout childhood.
7. Identify common feeding problems among children and determine appropriate interventions.
8. Assess nutritional status using anthropometric, biochemical, clinical, dietary, and physical examination information.
9. Define failure to thrive and its contributing factors.
10. Determine catch-up growth needs.
11. Develop an enteral nutrition care plan for the pediatric patient.
12. Describe parenteral nutrition needs of the pediatric patient.

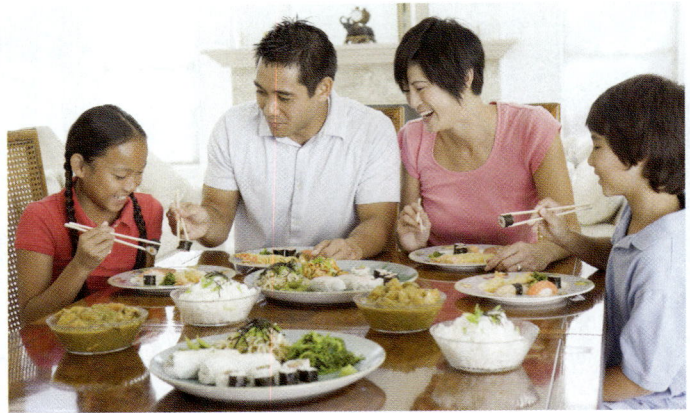
© Monkey Business Images/Shutterstock.

Introduction

Childhood is a period of rapid growth and development. From birth to age 20 years, a child undergoes many physical, social, and developmental changes. Nutrition plays a vital role in this process. Assuring adequate nutritional status requires a multifaceted approach at each stage of development, with attention given to the role of increasing independence, peer influence, and environmental factors. When faced with disease and critical illness, children are vulnerable to altered growth and malnutrition. A comprehensive nutritional assessment and prompt initiation of nutrition intervention, including nutritional support, may be necessary to prevent complications such as dehydration and weight loss, as well as long-term consequences in growth.

This chapter will explore the foundations of pediatric nutrition. Child-specific nutrition assessment and normal nutrient requirements from birth to young adulthood will be discussed. The case study will prompt evaluation of growth trends and abnormalities, identification of common nutrition problems, and development of appropriate nutrition intervention strategies, including nutrition support therapy.

Growth and Development

Physical Growth and Its Characteristics

Growth is defined as an increase in physical size or mass of body tissues that occurs from infancy to adulthood. Growth is a defining process of childhood. It indicates more than just nutritional status because it can be a predictor of overall health and disease risk later in life. Growth is measured throughout childhood, beginning immediately after birth. Head circumference, recumbent length, and weight are key indices of growth among infants. As children grow older, the appropriate measures of growth become height and weight.

Children typically grow in **growth channels**, which are trajectories of growth. Although some deviations are expected, larger variations in growth can be a cause for concern. Growth occurs at the greatest rate in the first few months of life and then plateaus through early to mid-childhood. It is expected that birth weight will double in 4 to 5 months and triple by 1 year. Similarly, length is expected to increase by 50% during the first year of life. By age 4, it can be expected that a child will have doubled his or her birth length.[1] Although there are general rules of thumb for growth in the healthy infant, each individual should be evaluated according to other factors such as ethnicity, parental size, and a child's natural growth disposition.

For pediatric inpatients, weight is assessed frequently. In newborns throughout infancy, weight gain is measured daily and recorded in grams per day. Changes in length are not evident on a daily basis and are evaluated over a longer time span. On average, babies are born at approximately

CASE STUDY INTRODUCTION

Peter is a 4-month-old baby boy with two older siblings: a brother, age 5 years, and a sister, age 3 years. At his routine visit, his parents express to the nurse practitioner their concern that he is not gaining enough weight. His mother reports that her first two children had hearty appetites and rapidly gained weight throughout the first few months of life. You are consulted to assess Peter's growth and meet with him and the family after the pediatrician examines Peter. As you screen for the medical record, you obtain the following information.

Anthropometric Data:

Age	Birth	3 months	4 months
Weight (kg)	3.3 (6.6 lbs)	5.2 (11.4 lbs)	5.4 (11.9 lbs)
Length (cm)	50 (20")	58 (23")	62 (24")

Biochemical Data: None

Clinical Data:
Past Medical History: Peter was the product of a healthy, term pregnancy delivered via an uncomplicated vaginal delivery.
Medications: He is not currently on any medications. He has had no previous ailments and is up to date with his vaccinations.
Vital Signs: Normal

Questions

1. Using the correct growth chart, chart Peter's anthropometric data at birth, 3 months, and 4 months. What are your concerns? How might you classify Peter's pattern of growth?
2. What is the expected rate of gain in weight and length for Peter?
3. What other data might you want to obtain from the medical record? What information could this provide?
4. What additional questions might you ask Peter's parents when you meet?

---

50 cm and grow to around 75 cm by their first birthday. **Table 23.1** contains the expected weight and length gains for an infant in the first 12 months.

Growth velocity is the rate at which a child grows.[2] Growth velocity is greatest in the first year. Infants grow at approximately 6.5 kg per year and gain 25 cm/year. The rate of growth then declines from age 1 to the onset of puberty. Once a child enters puberty, they again experience greater rates of growth. **Table 23.2** shows the approximate length/height and weight growth rates for children from infancy to adolescence. As indicated in the table, during childhood, males and females grow at similar rates, with growth velocities diverging at the onset of puberty.

> **CORE CONCEPT 1**
>
> Growth velocity and rates of gain in weight and length are well described, with the most rapid rates of gain the first few months of life.

Body Composition During Growth

Body composition of children greatly differs from that of adults. In this respect, children are not just small adults. Generally, younger children have less lean body mass (LBM) as well as less fat mass, but have far greater energy needs per kilogram of body weight than adults. In addition, in the early stages of life, LBM tends to be comprised of less protein and more water, making it of poorer quality. When injured or facing metabolic stress, these alterations in body

TABLE 23.1 EXPECTED GAINS IN WEIGHT AND LENGTH DURING THE FIRST 12 MONTHS OF LIFE

Expected Rate of Growth in First Year of Life		
Age (months)	Weight (g/day)	Length (cm/month)
0–3	24–28	3.3–3.6
3–6	19–21	2.0
6–9	14–15	1.5–1.6
9–12	11	1.1–1.3

TABLE 23.2 LENGTH/HEIGHT AND WEIGHT GROWTH VELOCITY FROM BIRTH TO ADOLESCENCE

Age Group	Growth Velocity	
	Height (cm/year)	Weight (kg/year)
0-1 year	25	6.5
1-2 years	12	2.5
2-5 years	7.5	2.5
6-12 years	6	2.5

CORE CONCEPT 2

Body composition changes throughout childhood. Nutritional risk is greater in children 0 to 2 years of age due to a greater fat versus fat-free mass content and lower percentage of body protein.

composition and metabolism can put particularly infants and young children at greater nutritional risk.

Body composition varies based on stage of development (**Figure 23.1**). At birth, the body composition of children is primarily composed of water (70%), with diminished lean body protein and fat masses. Preterm infants are at an even greater risk because they have marginal fat stores and LBM of poorer quality (meaning more water and less protein content). As they grow, infants gain proportionally more fat than LBM. Furthermore, the quality of their LBM with respect to protein content remains low, at approximately 13% throughout the first year of life.[3-5] Because infants preferentially rely on glucose versus fat as an energy source, they are at high risk for LBM depletion. In situations of stress that result in accelerated gluconeogenesis, LBM reserves are quickly exhausted. This can sometimes be masked by their abundant fat stores. Lastly, given their larger proportion of viscera skin to overall body mass, infants are at greater risk for heat and evaporative water losses, making them prone to dehydration and electrolyte imbalance.[4]

After age 2 years, there is a gradual increase in the quantity and quality of LBM. Increases in both protein and bone mineral content take place. By age 10 years, a child's protein content is approximately 17% and bone mineral content is 4%. Combined with this is a diminished reliance on glucose as a primary energy source, making older children at lower risk for LBM depletion than infants.[4] Fat content as a proportion of body weight is less than that of infancy and young age. However, prolonged calorie deficits in prepubertal children are still harmful, because they result in an increased rate of fat mass depletion.

Adolescence is the next stage of development, which begins around age 10 years and continues until age 17 to 18 years in females and age 20 years in males. This is a time of increased growth velocity. Increases in fat mass once again occur, a phenomenon referred to as the **adiposity rebound**.[6-8] Sexual dimorphism begins at age 13 years, which marks the onset of puberty. Up until then, males and females have a similar body composition. After this point, females experience a greater rate of increase in fat in preparation for puberty than males.[4] This is also a time when girls become more aware of their bodies and have increased body sensitivity. Due to their changing body composition, iron and calcium become key nutrients of concern.[6-8]

In contrast, males have a leaner and taller growth spurt. It is estimated that the pubertal growth spurt in males accounts for 17% to 18% of their final height.[7] Calcium is also a nutrient of concern for boys, as 90% of bone growth occurs by age 19 years. The timing of the adiposity rebound can be an indicator of adult body composition. Research has indicated that those who experience an early adiposity rebound are at a greater risk for adult obesity.[6] The fat-free mass plateaus around age 17 years for females and age 20 years

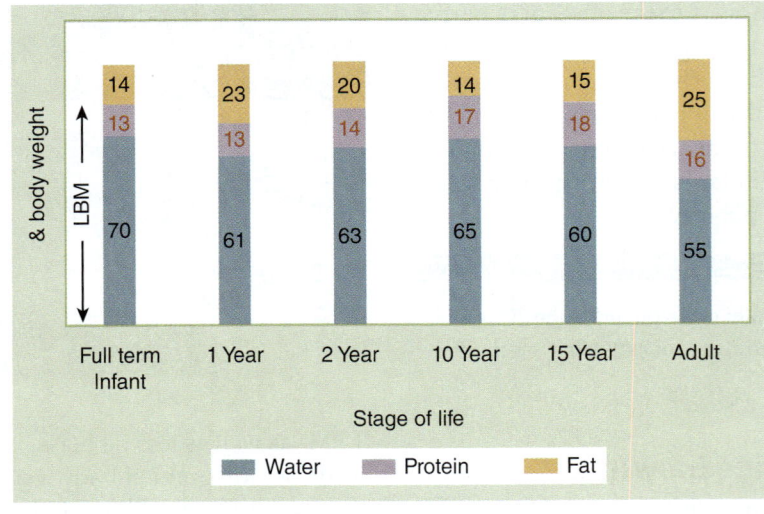

FIGURE 23.1 Changes in Body Composition During Growth

for males. When faced with metabolic stress or illness, older adolescents are at a lower risk than younger children because they have greater energy reserves compared to their metabolic rate.[4]

Nutrition Screening and Assessment

Nutrition assessment is a process of evaluating several different components to determine nutritional risk and status, diagnose malnutrition if it exists, identify problems that need intervention, and establish a plan of care. Information is drawn from anthropometrics, biochemical data, medical history, nutrition-focused physical exam, diet history, and discussion with other healthcare team members. In children, obtaining laboratory values is less routine than in adults. Similarly, children typically have a brief medical history, if any. Therefore, anthropometrics, along with a detailed diet history and nutrition-focused physical exam, serve as the cornerstones of a nutritional assessment.

Anthropometric Measures

Anthropometrics are the measurement of physical characteristics of the human body. Anthropometric measurements include height, weight, head circumference, body mass index (BMI), skin fold thickness, and arm circumference. These measures are used to evaluate the growth of a child and can also provide indicators of overall well-being and nutritional status. Anthropometrics are evaluated using growth charts, which will be discussed in the subsequent section. Accurate measurement of growth in children is critical for nutrition evaluations. Measures of weight and length or height should be taken at every hospital or physician office visit. Anthropometric data are most useful when **serial measures** are taken because they demonstrate patterns of growth and enable the clinician to determine etiology and hence the appropriate intervention.[1]

> **PRACTICE POINT**
>
> Measures of weight and length or height should be taken at every hospital or clinic visit.

Stature: Length or Height

In infants, recumbent length is used instead of height. Recumbent length is measured using a fixed headboard with a moveable footboard. The child lies flat on the length board with their head positioned against the headboard and eyes looking straight up. Length is measured from the vortex to the soles of their feet. It is best to have two individuals taking this measurement because it can be difficult to have a child maintain a straight position while they are measured (**Figure 23.2**). Recumbent length is typically greater than height by about 0.5 cm. This is the most difficult measurement to accurately obtain in young children.

Once children are older and can stand up straight, their height is measured using a stadiometer, as shown in

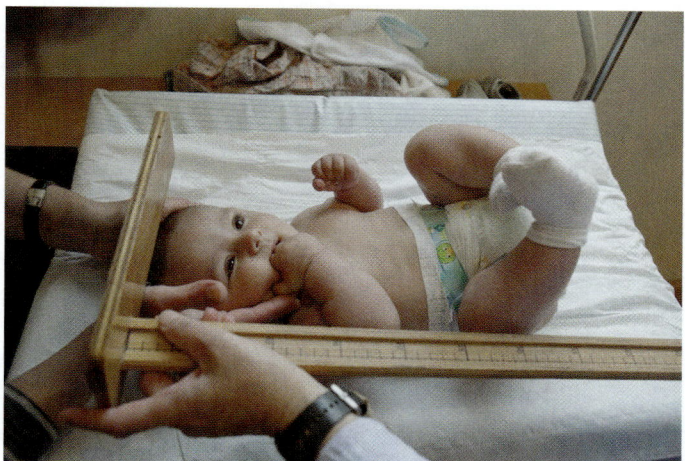

FIGURE 23.2 Two-person Method of Measuring Length in an Infant Child
© B. BOISSONNET / BSIP/BSIP SA / Alamy Stock Photo.

Figure 23.3. The height of a child when they are standing up can be referred to as their stature. The child should stand in bare feet with their occipital part of the cranium, shoulder blades, and buttocks against the wall.

Another reference point of height is the **mid-parental height** of the child. This can provide an indication of how the child is expected to grow. It is important to note that if parents are unusually tall or short, the resulting mid-parental height can be a poor indicator of child stature.[9] The target height, when estimated by mid-parental, is the parent's height ± two standard deviations, which is about 10 cm.

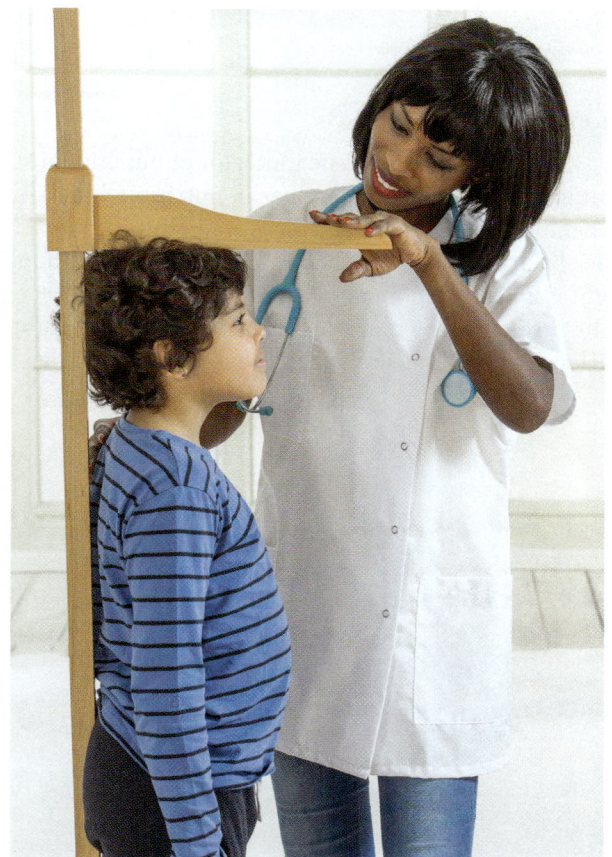

FIGURE 23.3 Measurement of Height in Older Child by Stadiometer
©JPC-PROD/Shutterstock.

For Girls

$$\text{Mid-parental Height} = \frac{(\text{Maternal Height (cm)} + \text{Paternal Height (cm)} - 13)}{2}$$

For Boys

$$\text{Mid-parental Height} = \frac{(\text{Maternal Height (cm)} + \text{Paternal Height (cm)} + 13)}{2}$$

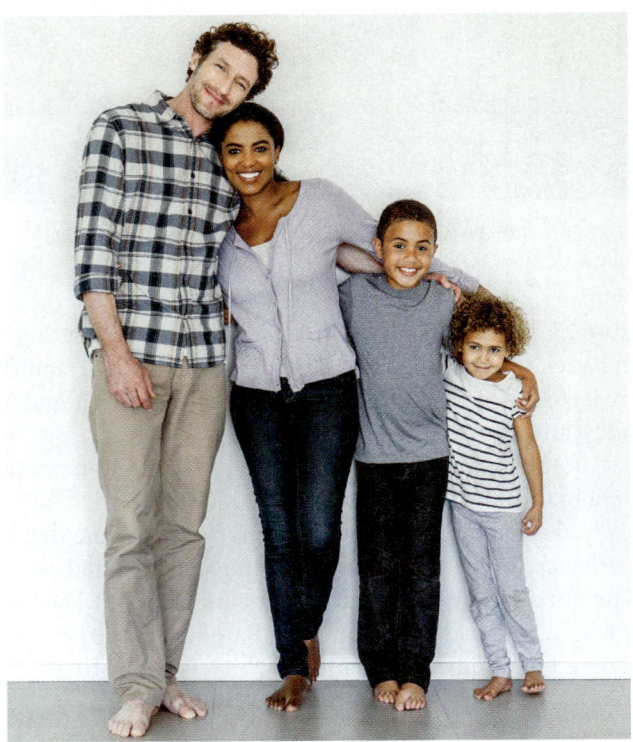

Weight

Body weight is used as a basic indicator of nutritional status. It is most sensitive to changes in nutritional intake and health. Infants should be measured nude (**Figure 23.4**), while children can be weighed in light clothing. Although weight is a key component to assessment measures, it can be influenced by many factors. For example, weight is influenced by fluid status, fed or fasting state, scale accuracy, and inter-observer error. It is best to control for some of these factors by taking serial measures using the same scale and the same trained observers.

Infants can also be measured using the tare method. Using this method, the parent first steps on the scale, which is then tared. Next, the parent holds the child and together they are weighed, and the weight recorded on the scale is that of the infant.

Head Circumference

Head circumference (HC) is taken by wrapping a tape measure around the most prominent area on the back of the head, immediately above the supraorbital ridge, to just above the patient's eyebrows. This will provide the greatest circumference (**Figure 23.5**). This measure is only performed up to 36 months of age. HC that is ± 2 standard deviations below the mean or below the 2nd percentile may indicate microcephaly. Microcephaly at birth can be due to a variety of genetic disorders. Normal HC at birth followed by a decline in HC is known as acquired **microcephaly**. Acquired microcephaly can be the result of an infectious process such as meningitis and may indicate poor brain growth or development. **Macrocephaly** is when HC is more than ± 2 standard deviations larger than the mean.[10] HC is the least sensitive to undernutrition, and changes in height and weight will occur before those in HC. Like height and weight, HC can be analyzed using a growth chart.

Body Mass Index

In younger children, weight-for-height can be used to determine BMI. BMI is a key indicator used in a nutrition assessment. It represents weight in kilograms divided by stature in meters squared. In essence, BMI is an index

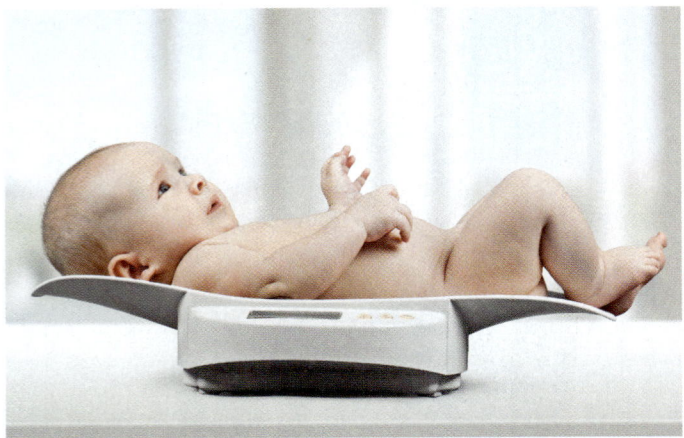

FIGURE 23.4 Measurement of Weight in Infant Child

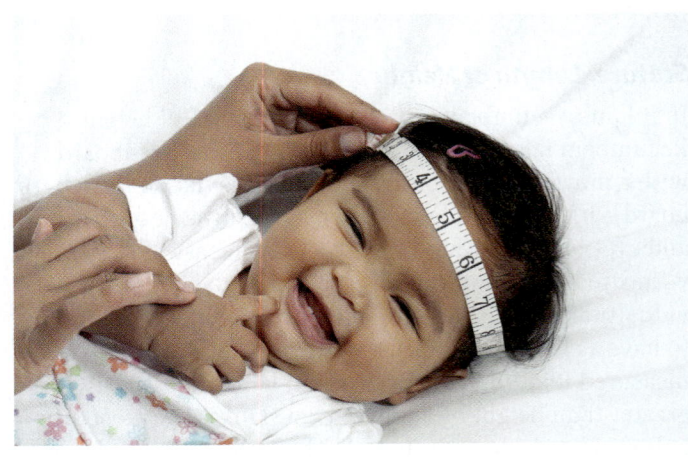

FIGURE 23.5 Measurement of Head Circumference in Infant Child

of weight relative to height. BMI is calculated beginning at age 2 years (prior to age 2 years, weight-for-length is used) and is interpreted using BMI percentiles (BMI-for-age). BMI-for-age is useful in determining overweight and obesity, as well as wasting.[11] Children with a BMI-for-age greater than the 95th percentile are considered obese. Those within the 85th to 94th percentile are considered overweight.[11–13]

$$BMI = \frac{Weight\ (kg)}{Stature\ (m)^2}$$

Skinfold Thickness and Arm Circumference Measurements

Skinfold thickness is a measure of body composition. Skinfold thickness is measured using a skinfold caliper at the midpoint of the arm between the acromion and olecranon.[14] Measurements should be taken from the same arm each time, with the arm relaxed. A skinfold caliper is used to pull the layer of skin along with the subcutaneous fat tissue away from the muscle. Measurements are then recorded to 0.5 mm. Using predictive equations, the percentage of body fat, and therefore fat-free mass, can be determined. Research suggests that caution should be used when predicting body fat mass from skinfold measurements in children. Use of the predictive equations should match the population being measured.[15] In addition, these measurements should be taken carefully and repeated for accuracy. Effort should be made to ensure that the muscle layer is not included in the measurement.

Arm circumference is another anthropometric measurement that can be used to determine body composition in children. Similar to skinfold thickness, the circumference is taken from the midpoint of the arm between the acromion and olecranon.[14] Equations are then used to determine the body composition of the child. Arm circumference is a quick method of determining body composition.

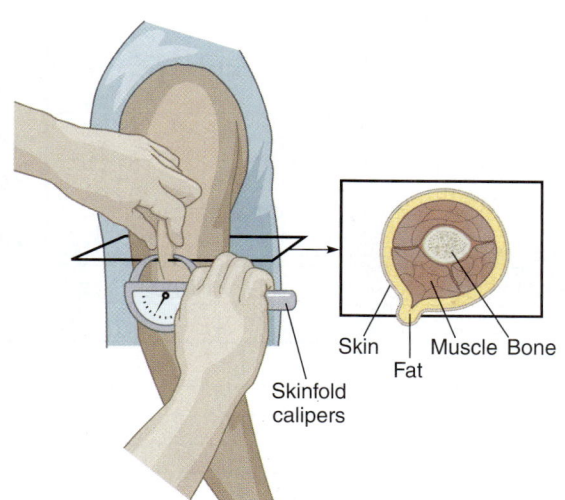

Skinfold Thickness

Evaluating Growth Using Standardized Growth Charts

Anthropometric measures are interpreted using growth charts. Use of growth charts dates back to the late 1800s.[2] **Growth charts** describe the normal or expected amount of growth based on well-child data. They depict the growth channels and velocity that correlate to patterns of growth in healthy children. There are two sets of charts, the **World Health Organization (WHO) growth charts** and the **Centers for Disease Control and Prevention (CDC) growth charts**.

WHO Growth Charts

The WHO charts were updated in April 2006 using data from the WHO Multicentre Growth Reference study, which included six different countries: Brazil, Ghana, India, Oman, Norway, and the United States.[2,16,17] The WHO charts begin at birth and describe growth of infants who were exclusively breastfed for the first 4 to 6 months (**Figure 23.6**). Infants in this sample then had complimentary foods introduced at 6 months, in addition to breast milk.

The WHO growth charts are considered **growth standards**. They represent optimal growth or how normal children should grow when breastfed, which serves as the gold standard for feeding.[2,11,17] Compared to other growth data, the WHO data set is superior, compiled from more frequent serial measures from a significantly larger sample size, beginning at birth.[16] The WHO growth chart is the first to describe optimal growth for children.[2]

The WHO charts should be used from birth to age 2 years, according to the CDC and American Academy of Pediatrics (AAP).[17] There are several parameters that can be evaluated on these charts, including **weight-for-age**, **height-for-age**, **head-circumference-for-age**, and **weight-for-height**. Growth curves range from the 2nd to the 98th percentile.

CDC Growth Charts

The CDC charts were updated in May 2000 using NHANES II and NHANES III data.[18,19] The CDC charts also include data from Vital Statistics because the NHANES data do not include infants younger than 3 months. As a result, these charts fail to accurately capture the rapid weight gain that occurs during the first 6 months of life.[16] In contrast to the WHO data, relatively few infants in this data set were exclusively breastfed for more than a few months. In addition, the data are more cross-sectional in design.

The CDC growth charts are a **growth reference**. These charts describe growth in a specific time or place (**Figure 23.7**).[17] The CDC and AAP recommend that CDC charts are used to evaluate growth in children older than 2 years of age.[17] Like the WHO charts, they are gender specific. There are several curves that can be used to evaluate a child's growth status, using percentiles or z-scores.[18,19] These include weight-for-age, height-for-age, and BMI-for-age. BMI-for-age curves were recently developed when the CDC charts were updated in 2000.[18,19]

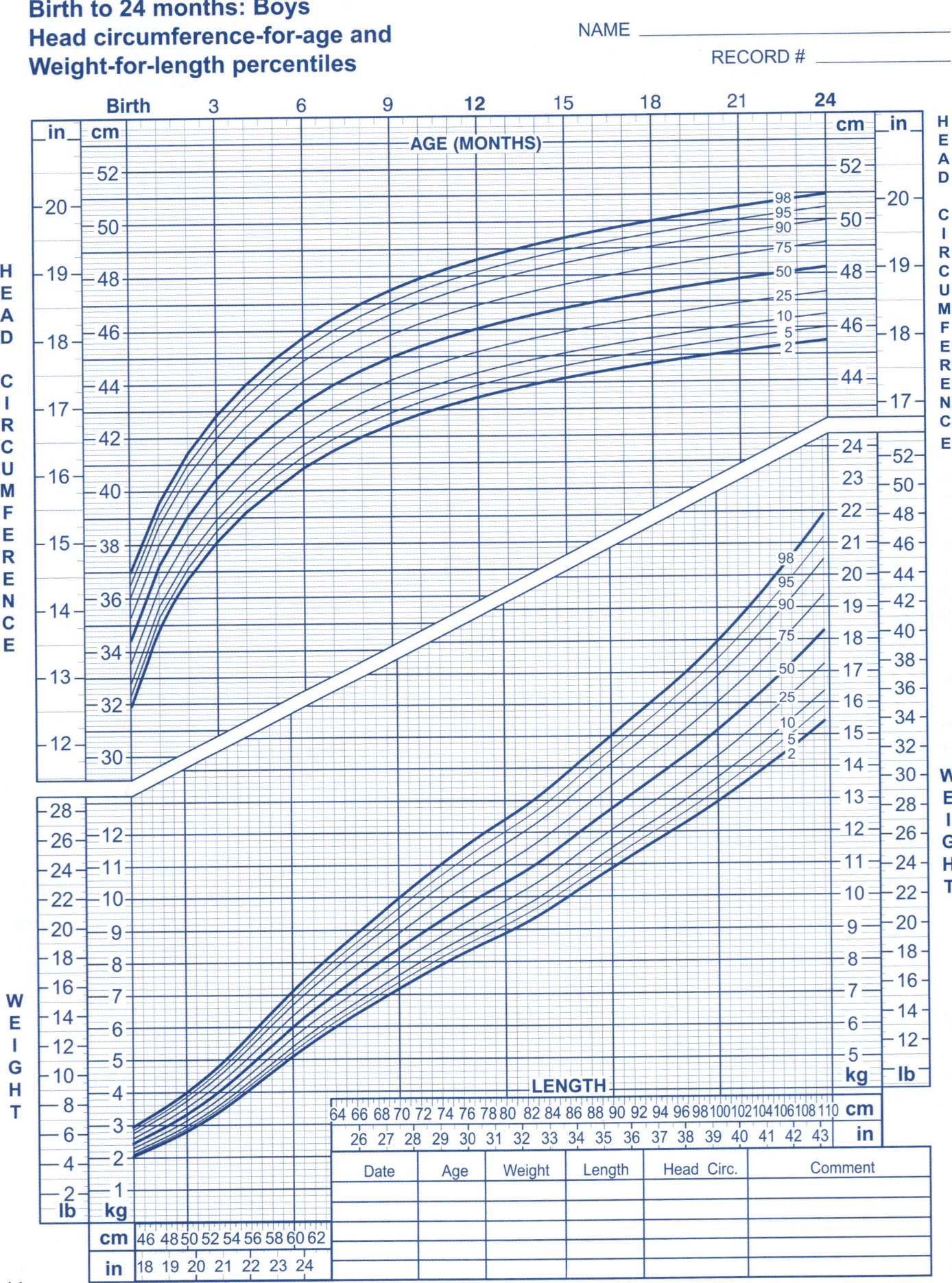

FIGURE 23.6 WHO Growth Charts for Weight for Age and Length for Age (*continued*)

Chapter 23 Nutrition in Pediatrics 645

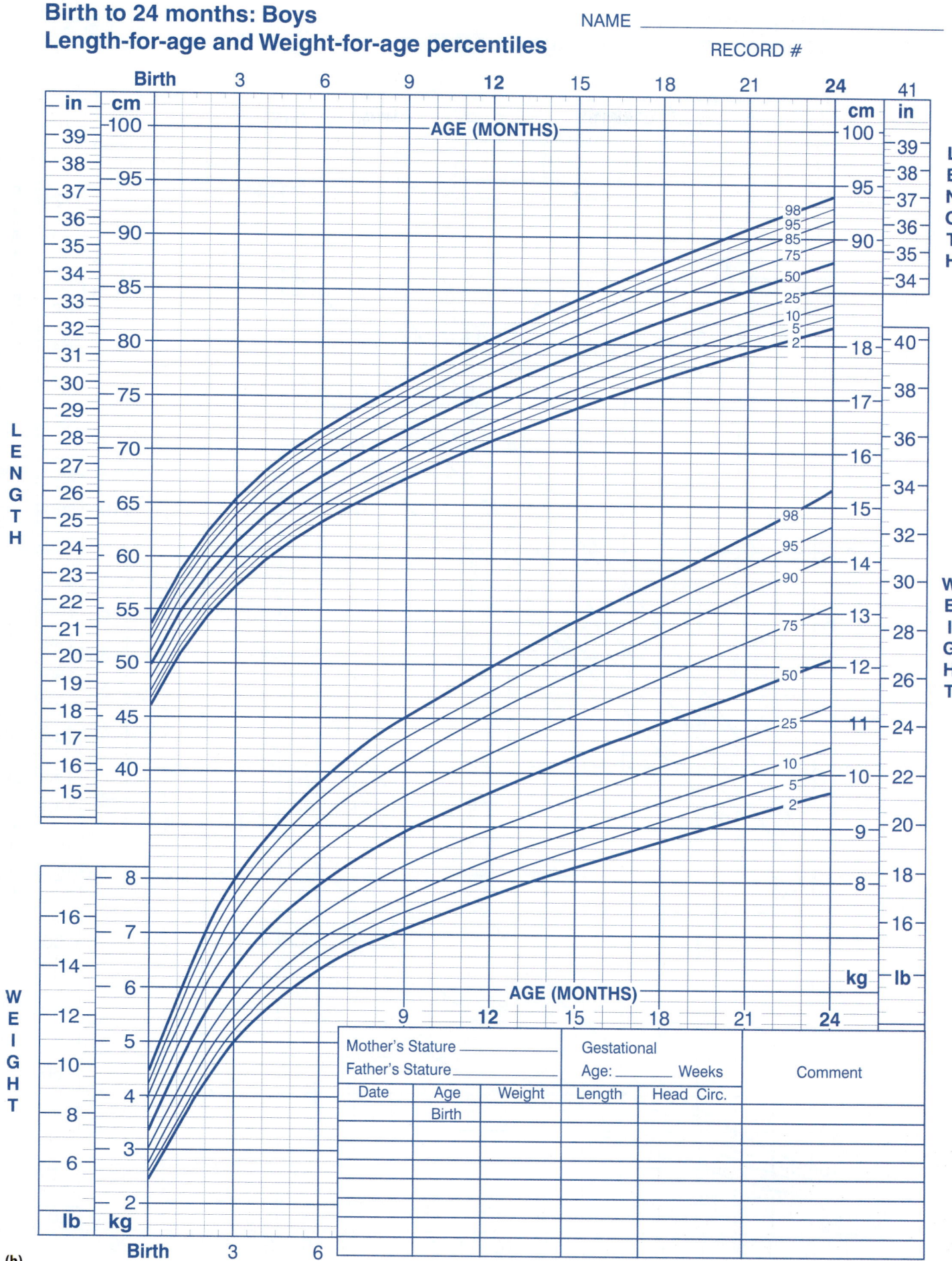

Birth to 24 months: Boys
Length-for-age and Weight-for-age percentiles

FIGURE 23.6 (continued)
Courtesy of the Centers of Disease Control and Prevention, November 1, 2009.

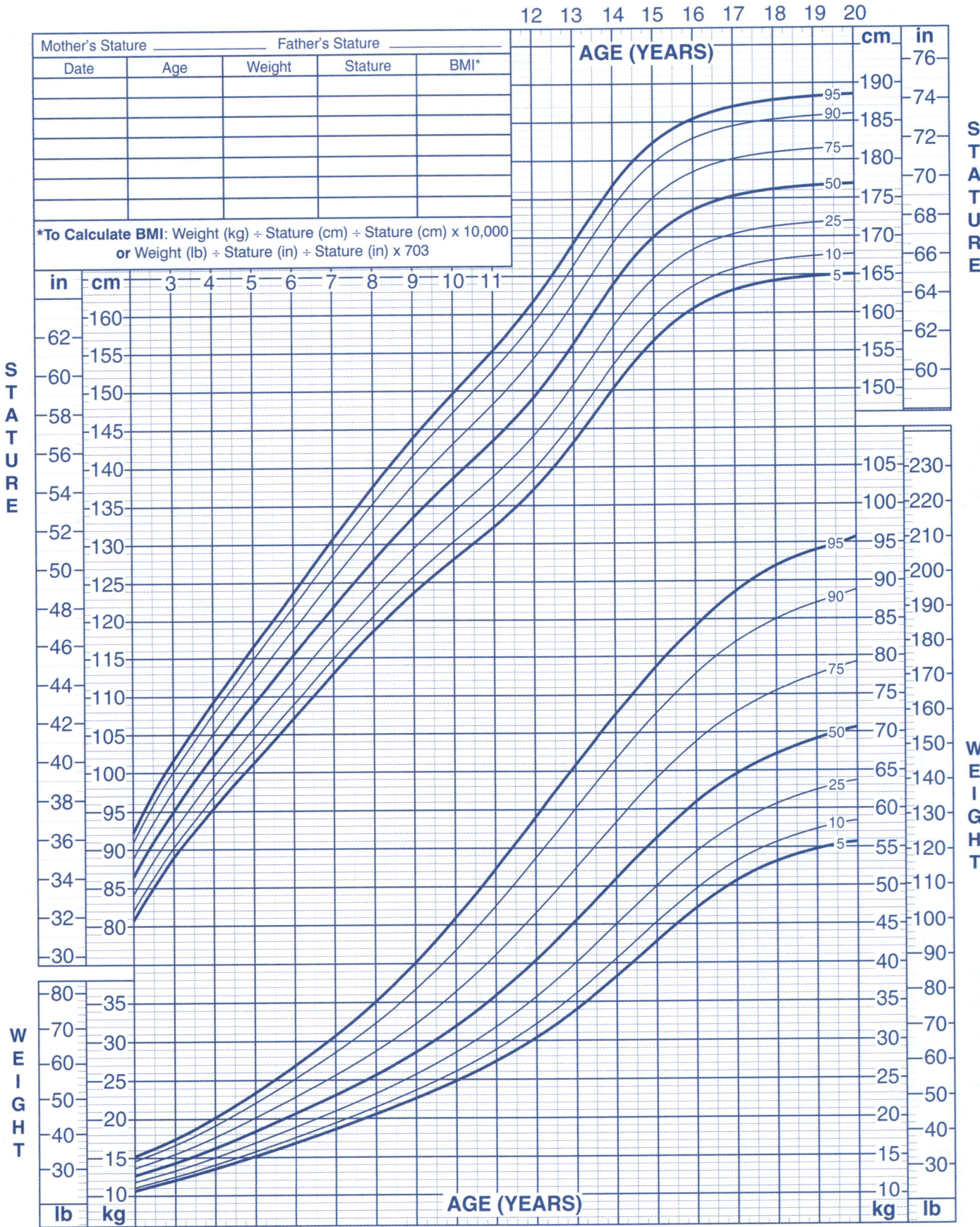

FIGURE 23.7 CDC Growth Charts for Weight for Age and Height for Age (*continued*)
Centers for Disease Control and Prevention (CDC). Developed by the National Center for Health Statistics in collaboration with the National Center for Chronic Disease Prevention and Health Promotion.(2000) http://www.cdc.gov/growthcharts.

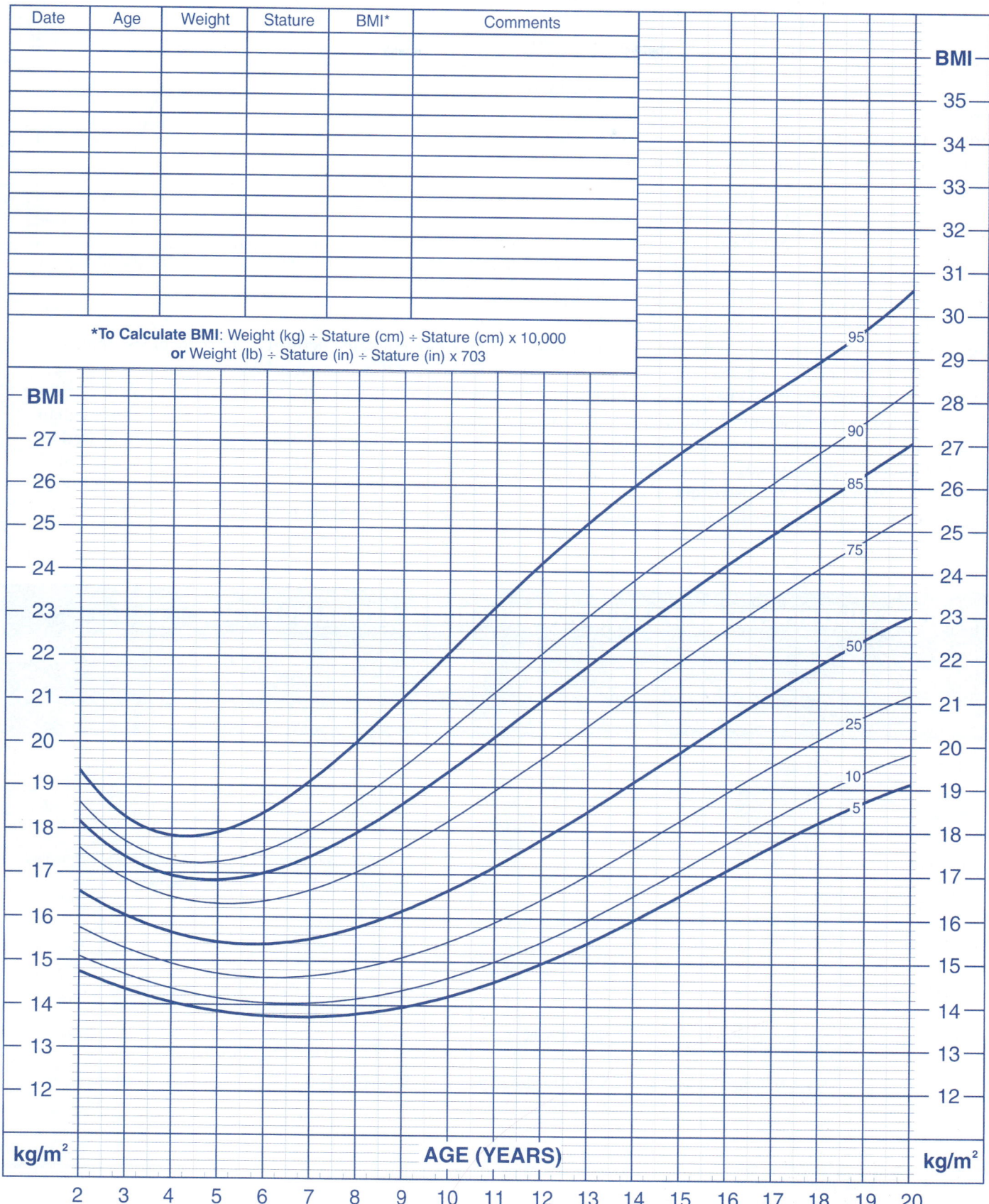

FIGURE 23.7 (continued)

Application of Z-Score Growth Charts to Evaluate Growth and Malnutrition

WHO routinely applies **z-scores** to assess growth and nutritional status in children.[11] A z-score can provide more specific information than the percentiles given by growth charts for weight-for-age, height-for-age, BMI–for-age, and weight-for-height evaluations. Z-scores also enable a more precise assessment of change within an individual child's growth pattern or nutritional status. A z-score is a representation of the individual difference from the median.[20]

$$\text{Z-score} = \frac{\text{(Individual Anthropometric} - \text{Median Anthropometric)}}{\text{Standard Deviation}}$$

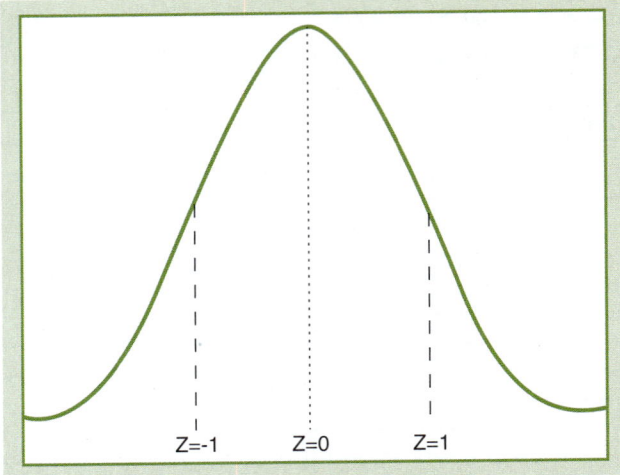

A z-score of 0 is considered normal, because it represents the median or the 50th percentile. Z-scores can range three standard deviations above or below the median. Positive z-scores indicate height, weight, or BMI that are above the median, whereas negative z-scores indicate height, weight, or BMI below the median.[21] It is recommended by the Academy of Nutrition and Dietetics and A.S.P.E.N. that z-scores be used to classify children who are underweight, stunted, or wasted based on WHO standards (**Table 23.3**).[11,22] **Underweight** is defined as a low weight-for-age, with a z-score less than –2, with severe underweight being defined as a z score of less than –3. Stunting, defined as a low height-for-age, and wasting, defined as a low weight-for-height or low BMI-for-age, are similarly classified based on z-scores below the median. Z-scores can be calculated and are increasingly used to evaluate growth, often being included in the medical record (**Figure 23.8**).[11] Most healthy children will "track" along a certain z-score percentile. Patterns of concern

TABLE 23.3 INTERPRETATION OF Z SCORES DURING GROWTH AND MALNUTRITION[11]

	Growth indicators			
Z-score	Length/height-for-age	Weight-for-age	Weight-for-length/height	BMI-for-age
Above 3	See note 1	See note 2	Obese	Obese
Above 2			Overweight	Overweight
Above 1			Possible risk of overweight (see note 3)	Possible risk of overweight (see note 3)
0 (median)				
Below –1				
Below –2	Stunted (see note 4)	Underweight	Wasted	Wasted
Below –3	Severely stunted (see note 4)	Severely underweight (see note 5)	Severely wasted	Severely wasted

Notes:
1. A child in this range is very tall. Tallness is rarely a problem, unless it is so excessive that it may indicate an endocrine disorder such as a growth-hormone-producing tumor. Refer a child in this range for assessment if you suspect an endocrine disorder (e.g., if parents of normal height have a child who is excessively tall for his or her age).
2. A child whose weight-for-age falls in this range may have a growth problem, but this is better assessed from weight-for-length/height or BMI-for-age.
3. A plotted point about 1 shows possible risk. A trend towards the 2 z-score shows definite risk.
4. It is possible for a stunted or severely stunted child to become overweight.
5. This is referred to as very low weight in IMCI training modules. (Integrated Management of Childhood Illness, In-service training. WHO, Geneva, 1997).

Reproduced from World Health Organization. Training Course on Child Growth Assessment. Geneva, WHO, 2008.

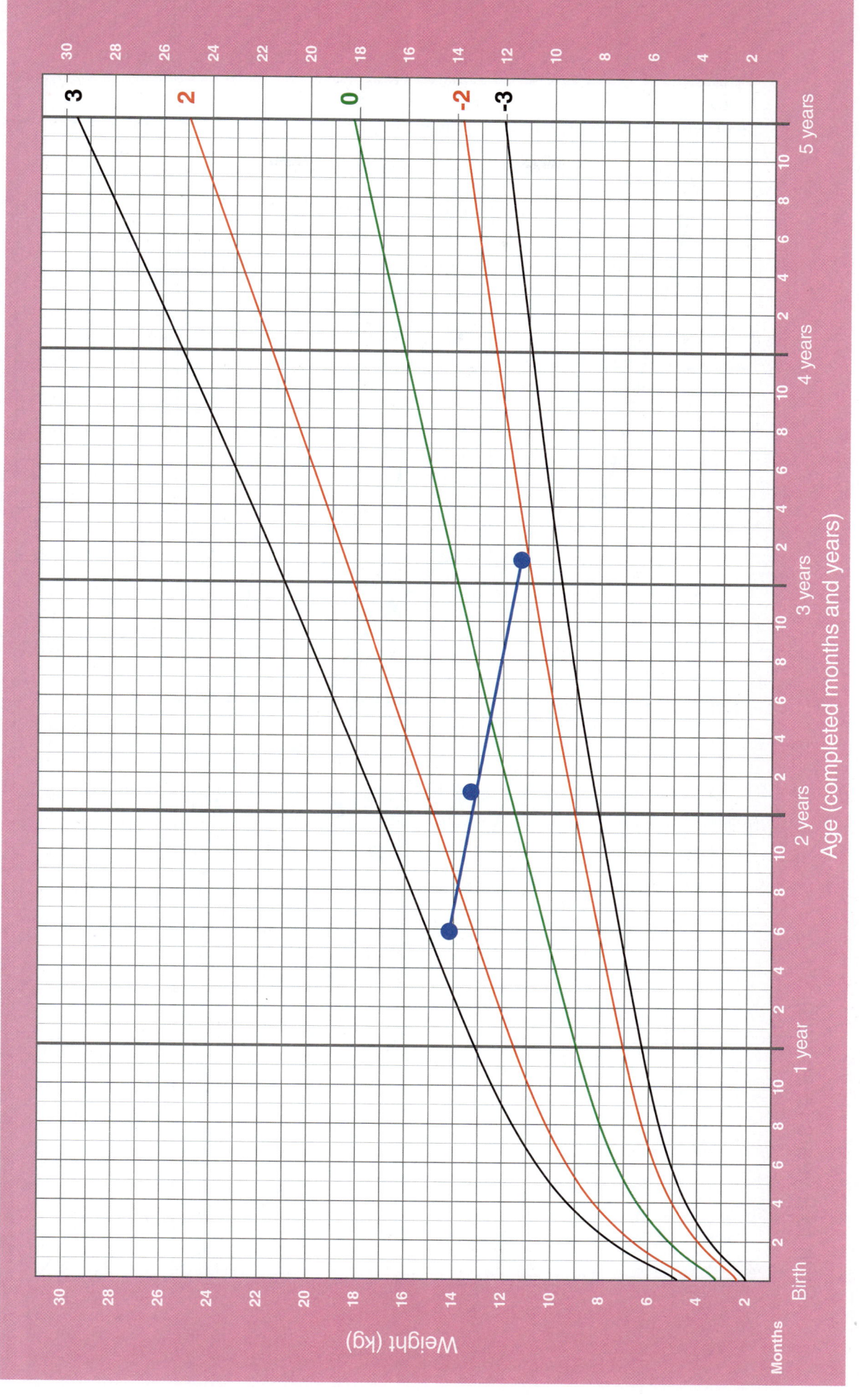

FIGURE 23.8 Using Trends in Z-Scores to Evaluate Growth *(continued)*

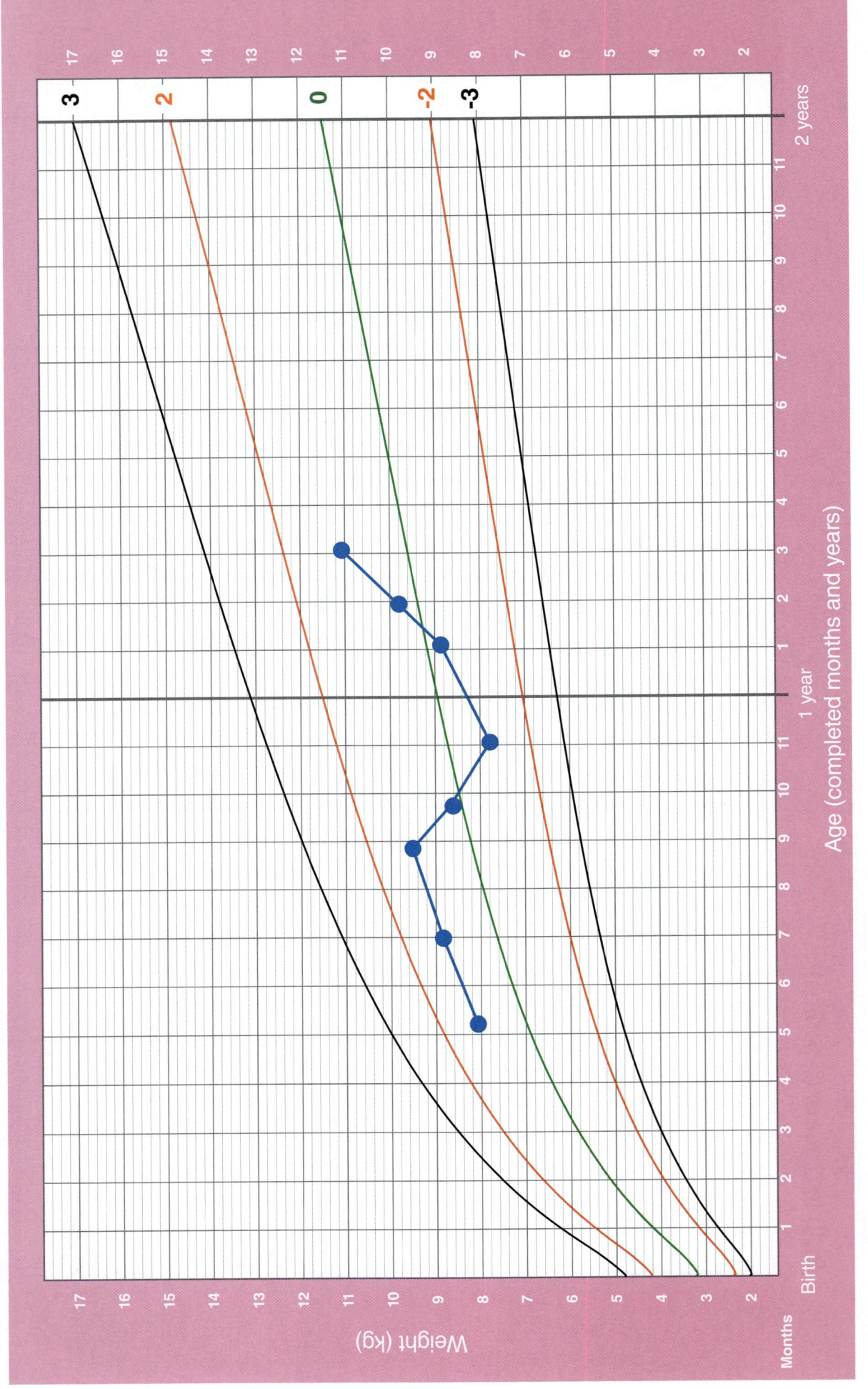

FIGURE 23.8 (continued)

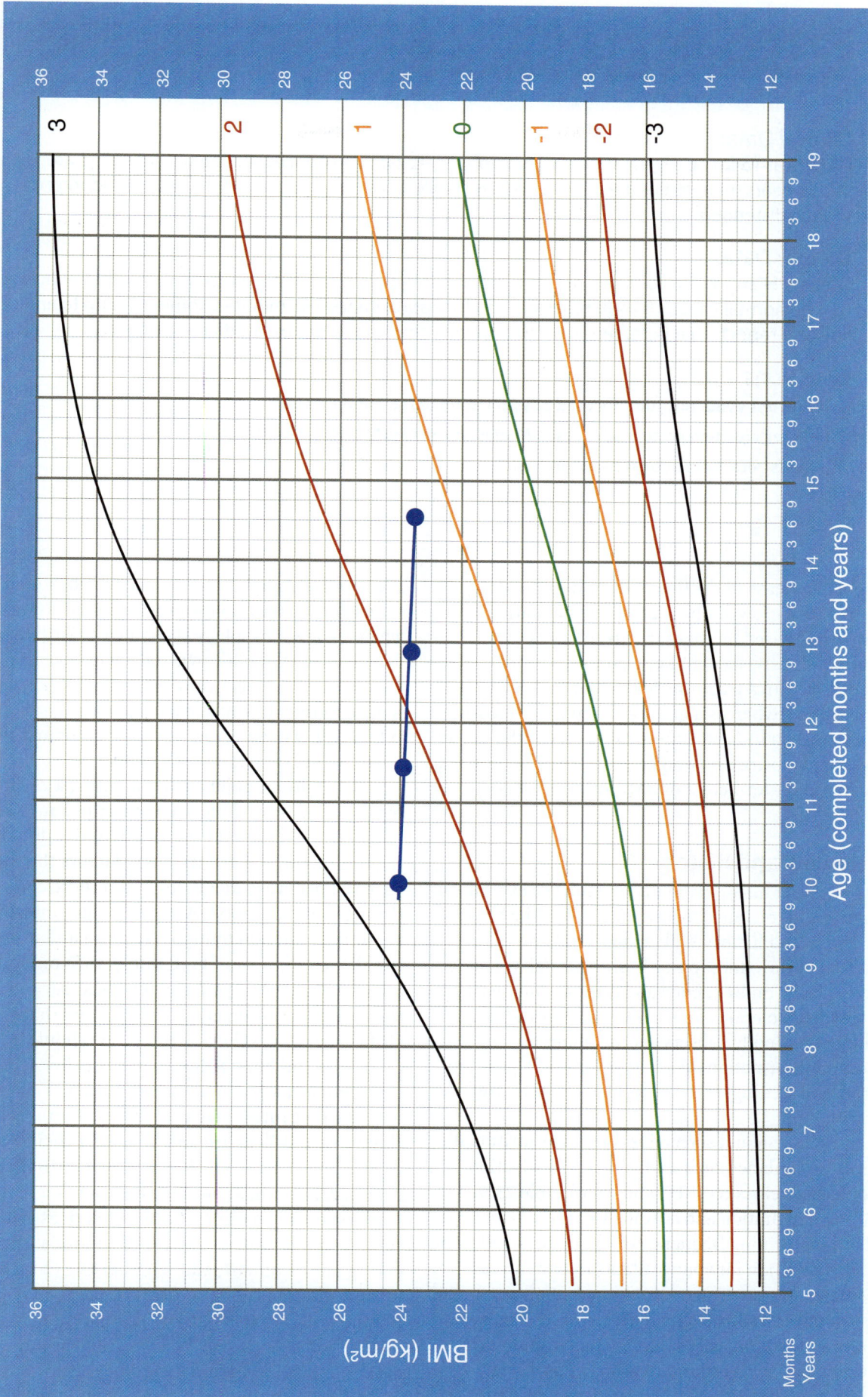

FIGURE 23.8 (continued)

> ## CASE STUDY REVISITED
>
> Later that day, you meet with the patient and gather additional information to complete your assessment.
>
> ### Clinical Data:
> **Nutrition-focused Physical Exam:** Upon physical exam you notice that Peter is difficult to arouse and appears thin. His lips are dry and slightly swollen. His eyes appear sunken and his abdomen is slightly distended.
>
> ### Dietary Data:
> **Dietary History:** For the past 4 months, Peter has been exclusively breastfed. His mother indicates that he normally feeds 8 to 10 times per day for approximately 45 minutes, sometimes up to an hour. She also reports that Peter tends to "spit-up" after most feedings in significant amounts.
>
> ### Questions
> 1. What does your nutrition-focused physical exam tell you about Peter?
> 2. Is Peter's feeding pattern adequate? What is concerning?
> 3. Assess Peter's nutritional status and risk.

include sharp increase or decline in trendline, crossing a z-score line, or a growth line that is flat (stagnation). Interpreting risk based on these trends requires consideration of many factors. For example, a rapid transient decrease in a trendline for weight may occur with short-term illness, whereas a gradual decline or a crossing of a z-score line can indicate chronic illness. On the other hand, children who are overweight may show a downward trendline in weight-for-height or BMI-for-age that is desirable.

Diet Interview and History

The goal of the diet history is to understand the overall pattern of eating and tolerance to food in a child. The focus of a diet interview and history will change based on the age and condition of the child. In newborns through infancy, emphasis is placed on frequency and duration of breast or formula feedings, tolerance to feedings, and introduction of complimentary foods. Observing the infant feeding can provide useful information on adequacy of suck, positioning, tolerance to feeding, and comfort level of the caregiver (**Table 23.4**).

Diet interview should screen for common nutritional problems during infancy such as diarrhea, constipation, gastroesophageal reflux (GERD), and colic (**Table 23.5**). Information on hydration and adequacy of intake can be assessed by determining frequency of wet diapers and stool patterns. It is common for young infants to have up to 8 to 10 wet diapers or stools per day. Normal stools can be liquid or soft in the earlier stages of life. Breastfed babies tend to have softer, more yellow stools than formula-fed infants. Constipation is a common problem useful to screen for during the interview. When identified, a proactive bowel regimen along with fiber and fluid intake can alleviate constipation. GERD occurs when food from the stomach refluxes into the esophagus. GERD often occurs when the lower esophageal sphincter is still immature. It usually resolves on its own and is rarely serious. However, anorexia, poor weight gain, and malnutrition can occur in some children, in which case medication is often then used. When GERD is refractory to medications and the baby is not growing, surgery may be indicated.

For children older than 6 months, a 24-hour diet recall or 3-day food record, similar to adults, can be taken. However, food type and quantity do not describe the full picture. There are many factors that influence the pediatric diet history and these can change throughout childhood. As a child ages, information about introduction to foods, vitamin and mineral supplementation, and food intolerance or food allergies are important. At every age, it is necessary to understand the cultural and socioeconomic factors that influence a child's nutrition. The diet interview should address parental beliefs and knowledge, dietary customs, eating behaviors, and developmental cues to eating.

The diet interview in toddlers should recognize that most toddlers are able to eat on their own. Their eating practices are influenced by familial choices; therefore, asking about familial diet is useful.[23–25] Understanding a child's eating practices—how well they respond to newly introduced foods; their typical eating environment; and whether the child eats at the table with the family, in front of the television, or while playing—facilitates patient and parent education. A 3-day food record may be necessary because a child's eating habits vary from day to day. Information should be gathered about snack time, grazing between meals, and beverage consumption.[14]

TABLE 23.4 DIETARY ASSESSMENT OF BREAST FEEDING AND FORMULA INTAKE IN INFANTS

Feeding Method	Questions to Ask	General Guidelines
Breastfed	Frequency and duration Complementary feedings/foods Is the mother expressing her breast milk? Vitamin/mineral or other supplements?	On-demand feeding suggested Feed every 2 to 3 hours, or 8 to 12 feedings in 24 hours. *If feeds are shorter than 10 minutes* Possible insufficient breast milk *If feeds are longer than 50 minutes* Possible ineffective sucking, an anatomic cause, or low milk production
Formula fed	Formula intake and preparation Nipple used Complementary foods Vitamin/mineral supplementation	Approximately 3 to 4 oz (90 to 120 mL) per feeding for the first month (6 to 8 times per day) Individual variation; look for hunger and satiety cues Volume increases and frequency decreases By 2 to 4 months, baby consumes enough formula to sleep through the night

In children aged 3 to 10 years, diet interview should focus on food eaten outside of the home, such as school lunch.[14] Nutrition knowledge, beliefs, and food intolerances or avoidances should be explored.[23,24] This concept extends to adolescence, where eating behavior is highly influenced by body image, peer-pressure, home life, and eating environment.

Conferring with other clinicians can provide additional information on developmental milestones and social and environmental factors that arise in their individual assessments. An interprofessional approach to pediatric assessment lends itself to a better rounded, more comprehensive model of care and is considered best practice.

TABLE 23.5 COMMON NUTRITION-RELATED PROBLEMS IN INFANTS

Problem	Evaluation	Signs and Symptoms	Recommended Treatment
Stool patterns	Normal *Breastfed:* 4 to 6/day; loose, soft to runny, seedy, yellow *Formula fed:* Thick, pasty consistency; green, tan, or yellow	Diarrhea Difficult to define stool frequency can be high in first 1 month Decreases over 1 year Look for change in pattern to more frequent and watery Constipation Dry, hard, infrequent stools	Diarrhea Treat dehydration-normal diet if hydrated Fat restriction Lactose free Constipation Fluid Fiber
Colic	Babies usually cry if hungry or wet. Rule of Threes: Cries more than 3 hours per day, 3 days per week, for 3 weeks or more	Excessive crying or distress when otherwise healthy; predictable time of day or episodes; posture changes, such as clenched fists and abdominal tension	Short-lived, usually resolves over 3 to 6 months; mother may omit common allergens, hydrolyzed formula may help (avoid switching formula too much)
Gastroesophageal reflux (GERD)	Small amount of reflux several times per day is common in healthy babies	Symptoms include regurgitation, coughing, weight loss, anorexia, arching of the back when feeding	Position changes: Hold baby upright for 20 to 30 minutes after feeding; interrupt feeding to burp baby Dietary changes: Switch formula, thicken formula with rice cereal, use a different-sized nipple Medications: omeprazole or ranitidine

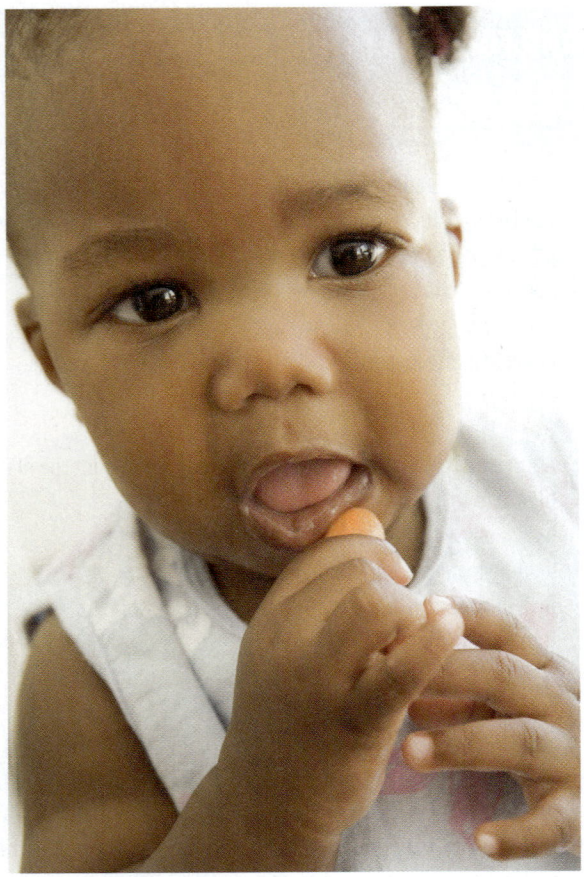
© Monkey Business Images/Shutterstock.

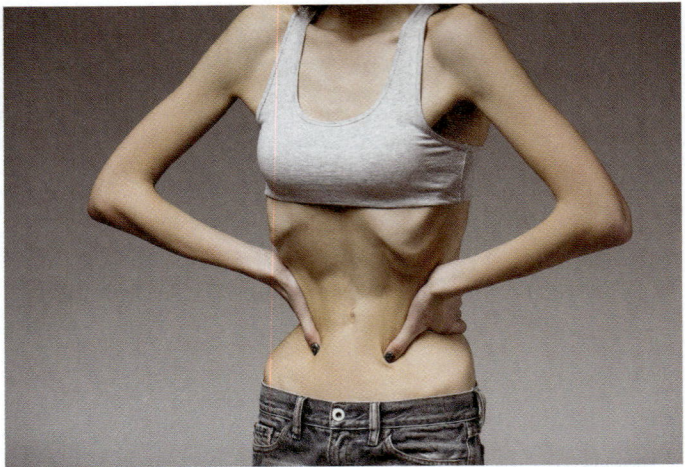
© VGstockstudio/Shutterstock.

Nutrition-focused Physical Exam

The physical exam is another vital piece of information for nutrition assessment. The physical exam should be done in collaboration with the medical team. During the exam, the accuracy of anthropometric measures can be confirmed and signs of malnutrition can be detected.[10] The exam also provides the opportunity to developmentally assess the child. Development delays, such as an inability to hold the head up or hold utensils, may impact nutritional status and the child's ability to advance their diet. The nutrition-focused physical exam is critical in children because they are at the greatest risk for change in nutritional status and malnutrition.[10,26] Malnutrition can result in delays in growth and development if left undetected.

Physical examination of a pediatric patient uses similar techniques to those used in adults. Inspection is the visual examination of the patient, with particular emphasis on body color, symmetry, and shape. Palpation, or the touching and feeling of the patient, is another technique used to evaluate temperature, moisture, and tenderness. Percussion is a technique used on the abdomen to determine the presence of solids and air. The final technique used is auscultation, or listening to the sounds of the bowel using a stethoscope.

General Inspection

The first step of the exam is to inspect the patient. General inspection can confirm the patient's height and weight status, giving information beyond the actual anthropometric measure, particularly with respect to body composition and musculature. Overall appearance is important to assess, noting whether the child is restless, engaged, or lethargic. Look for signs of labored breathing or a fruity odor to the breath. During this first step, it is important to monitor for signs of subcutaneous fat loss, muscle wasting, and edema.[10,26]

> **PRACTICE POINT**
>
> Assessing overall appearance provides useful information about the patient's overall health and disposition.

Head and Face

The next area to examine is the head and face. Inspect the head and face, looking specifically for symmetry; temporal wasting, an indication of malnutrition; or puffiness of the eyes/eyelids, suggesting edema.[10,26] The patient's hair quality should be examined for fullness, texture, and symmetry. Hair quality may deteriorate with essential fatty acid, zinc, or biotin deficiency, as well as during insufficient protein or calorie intake. The examiner should also palpate the top of the head. Lack of closure in the anterior fontanelle by 18 months of age suggests that the infant may have a vitamin D deficiency.[26] A child's eyes should be inspected as part of the physical exam. Healthy eyes will appear shiny, bright, and clear with moist membranes. Abnormalities of the eyes can be related to vitamin A deficiency.

Oral Cavity

It is important to examine the oral cavity, which includes the lips, tongue, teeth, and gums, because many nutritional deficiencies can present in the mouth.[27] Many B-vitamin deficiencies manifest in the oral cavity. Lips may appear dry and swollen.[27,28] A magenta coloration on the tongue is an indication of folate, riboflavin, niacin, vitamin B_{12}, or iron deficiency.[26] Lesions discovered in the mouth should be noted, because they may indicate iron or vitamin C

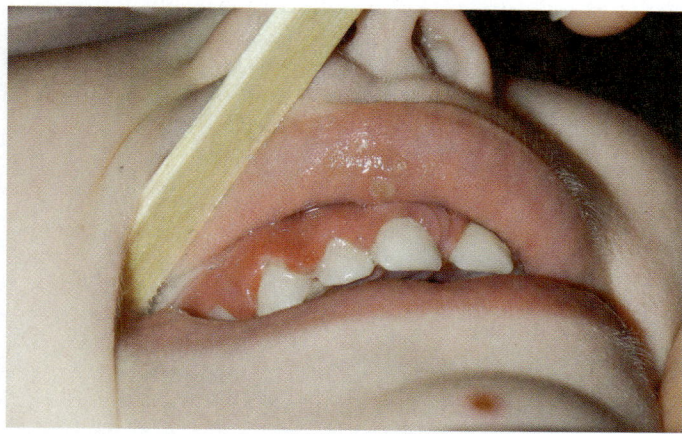

deficiency. Vitamin C deficiency may also be indicated by bleeding gums. In addition to revealing micronutrient deficiencies, oral lesions may impair food intake. Children with stomatitis or soreness in the mouth may refuse to eat. Conditions such as GERD, bulimia, or celiac disease may result in the erosion of tooth enamel.[27,28]

Skin and Nails

Skin integrity is clinically meaningful. Pallor, dry skin, or moist, clammy skin can be indicative of poor health or nutrition-related problems. Many micronutrient deficiencies first appear on the skin. The skin should

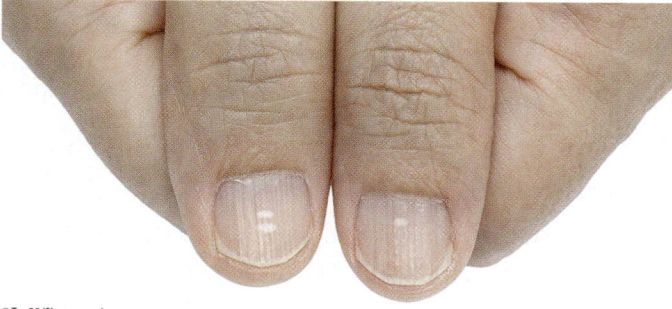

be thoroughly examined for color, symmetry, marks or rashes, bruises, lacerations (cuts, scrapes, or tears), turgor, and flaking.[26] Skin abnormalities may be associated with iron, folate, vitamin B_{12}, essential fatty acid, or zinc deficiency. Nails are easy to inspect and signal potential deficiencies of iron, protein, or vitamins A or C. Nails that are dull appearing, spoon shaped, or ridged, or that contain white spots, can be a sign of iron, protein, or other nutrient deficiencies.

Abdominal Examination

The examination of the abdomen should begin with the practitioner standing over the child. The symmetries and delineation of the region should be examined. Next, observe the abdomen from the horizontal view in order to note the shape. A flat abdomen is considered to be normal and healthy. A scaphoid shape (sunken abdomen) indicates decreased subcutaneous fat stores, likely as a result of poor intake, whereas a protuberant abdomen is a sign of obesity.[26] Next, palpitation of the area, feeling for texture, distention, and tenderness, is performed. The abdomen may feel firm or distended as a result of gas, fluid, or bowel obstruction.[26] Using the nondominant hand, gently tap over each quadrant of the abdomen and note the resulting sounds. A dull sound will result when the area above organs, fluid, or fecal matter is tapped. The last component to the nutrition-focused abdominal examination is auscultation of the bowel sounds. Using a stethoscope, gently press into the right lower quadrant of the abdomen. Bowel sounds can be defined in three categories: normal or high pitched gurgling that occurs 5 to 35 times per minute, hypoactive or softer than normal, with decreased frequency, or hyperactive or loud rustling.[26] It should be noted if no bowel sounds are heard.

Biochemical Data

Biochemical markers are highly disease dependent. As such, laboratory data can be quite useful for identifying nutritional deficiency, diet inadequacy, and disease. There are many different markers that can be analyzed to gain a better understanding of a patient's nutritional status. However, minimal lab work is done in pediatric patients unless history, signs and symptoms indicate it necessary. For growing children, vitamin D, calcium, and iron are nutrients of concern. In children who are vegan, it is critical to ensure adequate vitamin B_{12} consumption through lab work. Also, overweight and obese children should have a lipid profile. If additional lab work is available, it should be compared to pediatric standards.

Electrolytes

Electrolytes such as sodium, potassium, chloride, glucose, calcium, magnesium, and phosphorous should be evaluated in children who are not eating or feeling well. Electrolytes can be an indication of hydration status, renal function, and hemodynamics. For critically ill patients, analysis of electrolytes may indicate how well they are tolerating treatments and feeding.

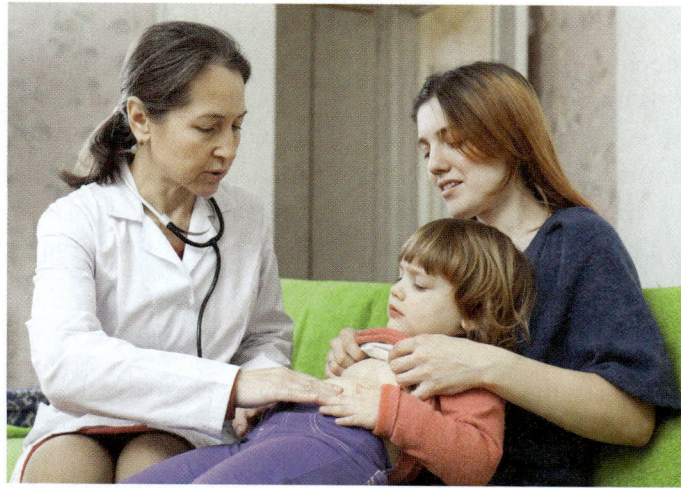

CASE STUDY REVISITED

You next see Peter 5 months later at his 9-month visit. His anthropometric and diet history are as follows.

Anthropometric Data:

Age (months)	Birth	3	4	6	9
Weight (kg)	3	5.2	5.4	5.6	5.8
Length (cm)	50	58	62	63	64

Dietary History:
Dietary History: Peter's mother has gone back to work and transitioned him to bottle feeds using a standard baby formula. He continues to spit up frequently and seems "colicky." On average, he feeds 5 to 6 times per day and drinks 4 to 6 oz per feed (although spits up frequently).

Questions

1. How would you assess Peter's growth since you last saw him at 4 months? How would you describe his pattern of growth? What has changed?
2. What might you look for in a nutrition-focused physical exam?
3. What labs might you obtain?
4. What is your assessment of his dietary intake? Is it sufficient?
5. What might a dietary intervention be for Peter?

Iron Status Indicators

Iron status should be checked in preschool- and school-aged children, as well as adolescents. Preterm or low birth weight infants, as well as infants who are fed non-iron-fortified formulas or who are not consuming enough iron-rich foods, are considered at risk and should be screened at 9 to 12 months of age.[29] Hemoglobin, hematocrit, iron, total iron binding capacity, and mean corpuscular volume should be analyzed in the pediatric patient. Iron-deficiency anemia and other types of anemia, such as macrocytic anemia, can be detected through these markers. **Table 23.6** lists the normal hemoglobin and hematocrit levels for children ages 2 to 18 years.[30,] Monitoring of iron status is especially important for children who follow vegetarian diets.

Bone Health Markers

Vitamin D, calcium, and parathyroid hormone are three critical values to assess in pediatric patients. All three of these markers work together in bone mineralization. Sufficient amounts of vitamin D and calcium are necessary for growth. Unfortunately, many older children do not consume the recommended amount of calcium and vitamin D.

> **PRACTICE POINT**
>
> There are no routine lab values monitored for pediatric patients, unless warranted by signs and symptoms.

Medical and Social History

Medical and social history help the healthcare team to better understand the patient. These data provide a more comprehensive picture of the patient.

Medical History

In the hospital setting, a patient's medical history will be a part of their medical record. This may include information about chronic illness, trauma, surgery, or infection. In addition, a child's birth history, any current illness or diagnosis, and medications will be listed. History of nausea, vomiting, and diarrhea; any problems with reflux; and stool patterns should be noted. It is important to review this information, because it can provide greater detail about the child's current state and guide further evaluation and discussion. In an outpatient setting, some of the medical history may be provided if the patient was referred by a physician. However, it may be necessary to consult the parent to get a complete history.

Social History

The social history is an essential component to a child's nutrition assessment. The social history will provide information about the child's family's education, values, and beliefs; family stressors; or other personal details.

TABLE 23.6 NORMAL HEMOGLOBIN AND HEMATOCRIT LEVELS IN PEDIATRIC PATIENTS, BY GENDER AND AGE GROUP[31]

Hemoglobin and Hematocrit Levels by Age Group		
Age Range (Sex)	Hemoglobin (g/dL)	Hematocrit (%)
2 to 6 years (Both)	12.5	37
6 to 12 years (Both)	13.5	40
12 to 15 years (Female)	11.8	35.7
12 to 15 years (Male)	12.5	37.3
15 to 18 years (Female)	12	35.9
15 to 18 years (Male)	13.3	39.7

Modified from 3Academy of Nutrition and Dietetics. Pediatric Nutrition Care Manual. https://www.nutritioncaremanual.org/topic.cfm?ncm_category_id=12&lv1=144610&ncm_toc_id=144610&ncm_heading=&.Accessed 8/19/17.

TABLE 23.7 DIAGNOSTIC INTERPRETATIONS OF GROWTH CHART ANALYSIS

	Growth Chart Interpretations		
Diagnosis	Underweight (low weight-for-age)	Stunted (low height-for-age)	Wasted (low weight-for-height)
Acute, short-term deficit	X		
Normal for ethnicity History of insult	X	X	
Long-term, ongoing illness	X	X	X
Genetic Endocrine		X	

Assessing Patterns of Growth and Etiology

Plotting growth on percentile growth curves is the most common method of tracking growth in a hospital or clinical setting. Measures are more valuable when there are several data points to interpret. One data point is not as meaningful because it does not indicate a pattern of development. When analyzing growth data, it is important to consider the interval between measurements. Also, growth can occur in bursts and is not necessarily linear. If a value seems irregular, a repeat measurement should be requested. As discussed earlier, there are several different growth indices that can be interpreted by charting growth (**Table 23.7**).

Interpreting Changes in Weight-for-Age

Weight-for-age is a reflection of body mass for age. It represents how a child's weight compares to other children of the same age. Along with nutritional intake, weight-for-age is influenced by both ethnicity and genetics and is related to height and BMI. As stated previously, changes in weight are most sensitive to short-term alternations in nutritional status. Low weight-for-age or underweight may indicate acute or short-term deficits, history of insult, or long-term illness. For some ethnicities, low weight-for-age may be considered normal. Generally speaking, children who are low weight-for-age are defined as being underweight. However, an index of weight-for-age alone is difficult to interpret because it does not distinguish between overall size and weight status. A child who is small but of adequate proportional weight will have the same weight-for-age as a child who is tall, but extremely thin. Likewise, the duration and identification of any pattern of decline provides more meaningful information and insight on cause and treatment. Children who have a low weight-for-age, but track along that same percentile, are likely not to be at risk, as opposed to children who demonstrate a drop in their weight-for-age percentile channel. Minor changes in weight that are transient may represent a brief lapse in nutritional intake or overall health. Changes in weight-for-age are significant when they cross percentiles and continue over time. This is a cue to thoroughly assess diet history, because weight is strongly linked to caloric intake or an energy deficit due to increased energy expenditure or malabsorption. Monitoring changes in stature that accompany alterations provide valuable insight. A decline in weight-for-age without a drop in length or height can be defined as failure to gain weight (**Figure 23.9**). Weight-for-length in this instance will begin to fall.[32] Failure to grow describes a drop in length or height without a drop in weight (**Figure 23.10**).

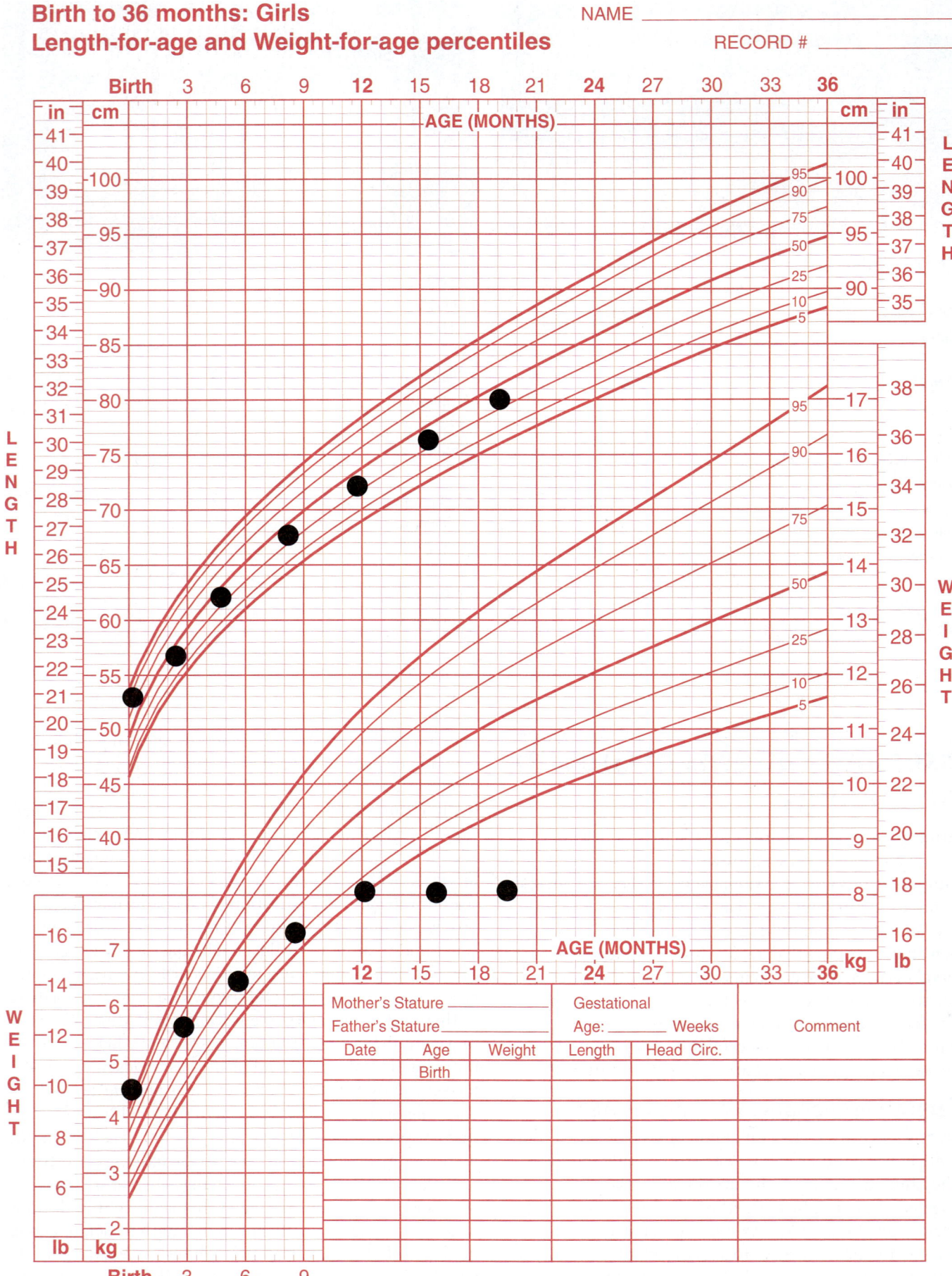

FIGURE 23.9 Failure to Gain Weight
Centers for Disease Control and Prevention (CDC). Features of the CDC Growth Charts. (2015, April 30). Retrieved from https://www.cdc.gov/nccdphp/dnpao/growthcharts/training/overview/page3.html.

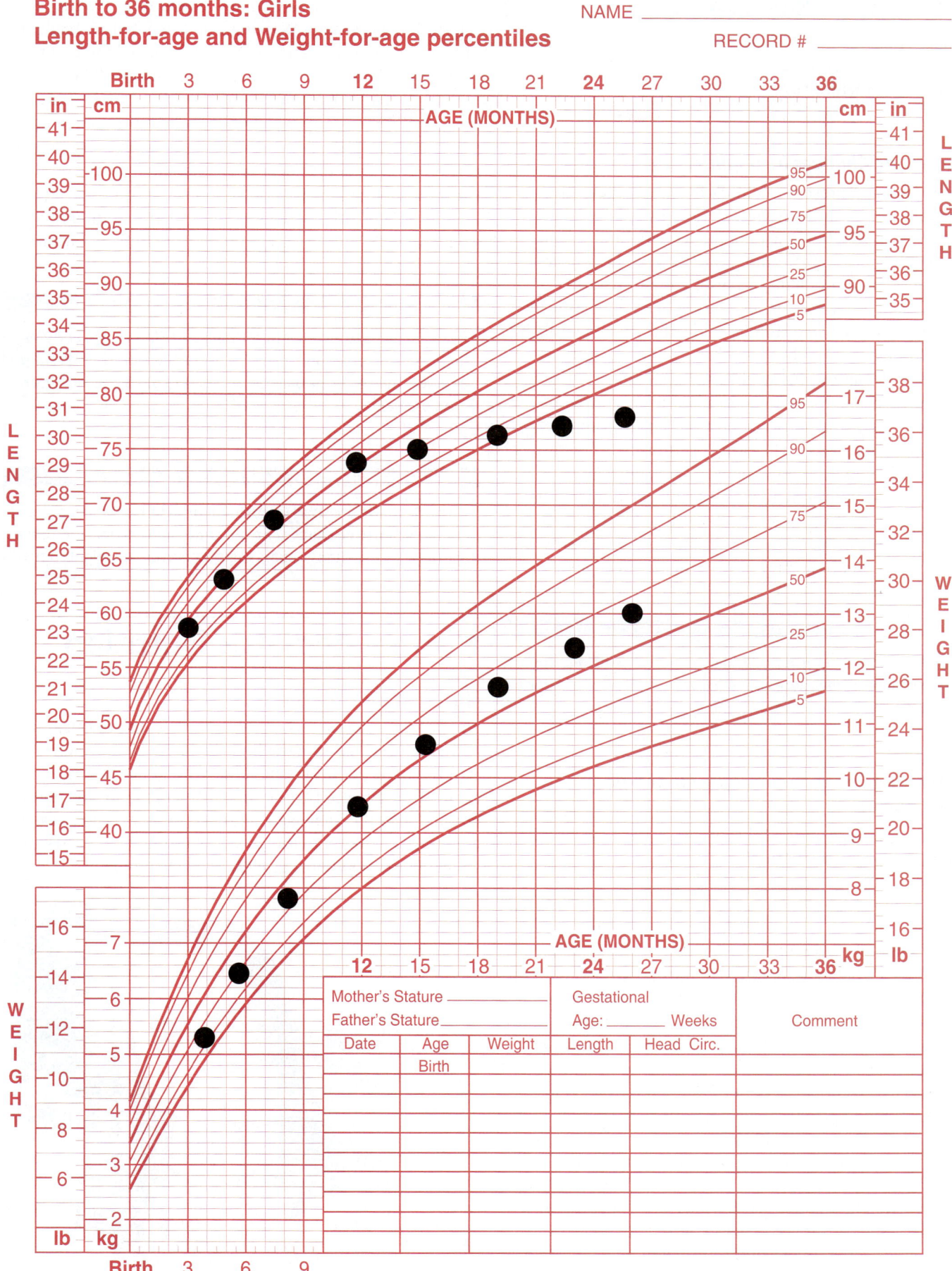

FIGURE 23.10 Failure to Grow is Represented by a Decline in Stature Without a Decline in Weight. The Etiology May Relate to Non-nutritional Factors. In Patients Where Stunting is not Accompanied by a Decline in Weight-for-age, Overweight or Obesity can Occur

Kuczmarski RJ, Ogden CL, Guo SS, et al. 2000 CDC growth charts for the United States: Methods and development. National Center for Health Statistics. Vital Health Stat 11(246). 2002.

> **CORE CONCEPT 3**
>
> Underweight is defined as low weight-for-age. Failure to gain weight may indicate acute or short-term deficits, history of insult, or long-term illness.

Interpreting Changes in Height-for-Age

Height-for-age represents a child's height compared to other children of the same age. Height is a less-sensitive indictor than weight in cases of inadequate intake. Thus, a drop in height-for-age is more indicative of long-term nutrition-related problems or chronic malnutrition.

Low height-for-age can also be a reflection of **stunting**. Stunting occurs when a child is below the 5th percentile in height-for-age or when he or she has a z-score less than 2 standard deviations below the median. Failure to reach linear growth suggests long-term insufficient nutrient intake or suboptimal health conditions, such as an infection or chronic disease. The cause of stunting is not always known and often prompts a medical work up. Certain disease states, environmental causes, repeated infections, or micronutrient deficiencies can all result in low height-for-age. Depending on the etiology for impaired linear growth, nutrition interventions may or may not be effective in reversing stunting.

> **CORE CONCEPT 4**
>
> Stunting, or low height-for-age, may be indicative of long-term on-going illness, genetic or endocrine abnormalities or a history of insult.

Interpreting Changes in Weight-for-Length or BMI-for-Age

Like height-for-age and weight-for-age, weight-for-length or BMI-for-age are analyzed based on percentiles in pediatric patients. BMI-for-age is similar to weight-for-height or length, the latter being the equivalent indicator in children younger than age 2 years. BMI-for-age and weight-for-length, when plotted on the CDC growth charts, help identify children who are underweight, normal, overweight, or obese. Z-scores can also be used to classify BMI-for-age or weight-for-length. Children who have a z-score of one standard deviation above the median, which is the equivalent to 25 kg/m² at 19 years of age, are considered overweight. Those with a z-score greater than two standard deviations are considered to be obese.[6] Pediatric obesity is often a predictor of adult obesity. BMI-for-age is one of the easiest methods to screen for overweight and obesity in children. High BMI-for-age may be an indicator of increased adiposity or overweight and obesity. BMI-age does not account for the differences between fat and fat-free masses.[4] However, in some cases, high weight-for-height may not be an indication of obesity but a result of lean body mass. This occurs in very active children.

Low BMI-for-age or weight-for-height (or length) is referred to as **wasting**. Wasting is defined by the Academy of Nutrition and Dietetics as a weight-for-height lower than 2 standard deviations below the median.[22] Wasting is not influenced by genetics or ethnicity. It is a strong predictor of mortality among children younger than age 5 years. Low BMI-for-age or weight-for-height (or length) results from an acute short-term change in intake or the onset of disease. Those who present with wasting are likely to positively respond to nutritional intervention. Table 23.7 provides a guide for the interpretation of growth charts.

> **CORE CONCEPT 5**
>
> Wasting refers to low weight-for-height or BMI-for-age and is an indication of recent and severe state of undernutrition. Wasting may be the result of disease and is responsive to nutrition intervention.

> **CORE CONCEPT 6**
>
> Growth charts are used to evaluate growth from birth to age 20 years. Serial measures of weight and height and their patterns can be used to define wasting, stunting, and underweight status.

Normal Pediatric Nutrition

Nutrient Requirements

Nutritional needs are assessed in relation to growth and activity. Children have the highest energy and protein requirements per kilogram of body weight of any age group. Energy needs are significantly higher in this population due to the increased synthesis of new tissue, as well as storage of energy in the tissue. Micronutrient needs are also greatest to support growth and development.

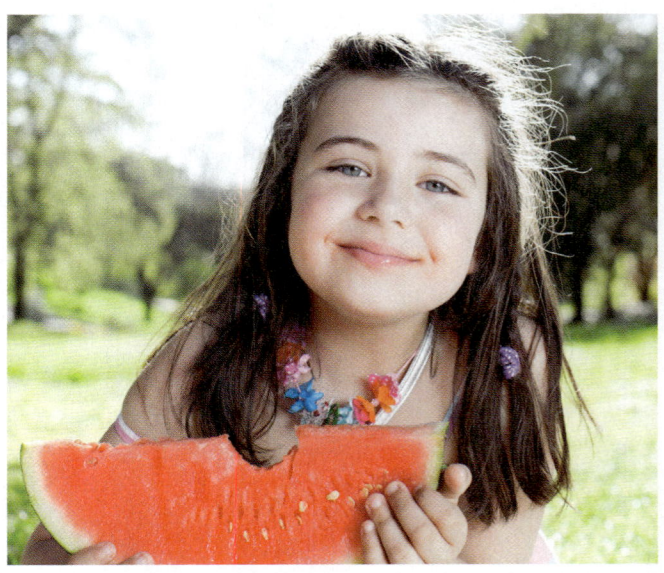

©JW LTD/DigitalVision/Getty Images.

Recommendations for a Healthy Eating Pattern

After the age of 2 years, toddlers transition to eating more like adults than infants. The U.S. Department of Agriculture's MyPlate focuses on a healthy eating pattern for all ages and suggests portion sizes for fruits, vegetables, grains, protein, dairy, and oil for each age range and gender. These guidelines are written for the general public to promote healthy eating. **Table 23.8** summarizes these recommendations for children ages 2 to 18 years.[33] It is the role of the dietitian to promote healthy eating in all settings.

In addition to MyPlate, the 2015 Dietary Guidelines provide recommendations for healthy eating patterns at all ages. The Guidelines suggest that Americans consume a diet composed of a variety of fruits and vegetables, whole grains, lean protein, oils, and low-fat or fat-free dairy.[34] In addition, it is recommended that Americans limit added sugars and saturated fat to 10% of their total calories and reduce sodium intake to 2,300 mg. The 2015 Dietary Guidelines emphasize the importance of healthy eating patterns, particularly the Healthy Mediterranean Style Eating Pattern and a Healthy Vegetarian Eating Pattern.[33] These patterns are intended for individuals of all ages to promote a healthy lifestyle and prevent chronic diseases such as obesity, type 2 diabetes, and cardiovascular disease.

Despite these recommendations, many children do not get adequate amounts of fiber and key vitamins and minerals such as vitamin D, calcium, and potassium. In addition, children often have a positive energy balance; excessive intakes of fat, saturated fat, sugar, and sodium; and inadequate intakes of fruits, vegetables, whole grains, dairy, and seafood.[34]

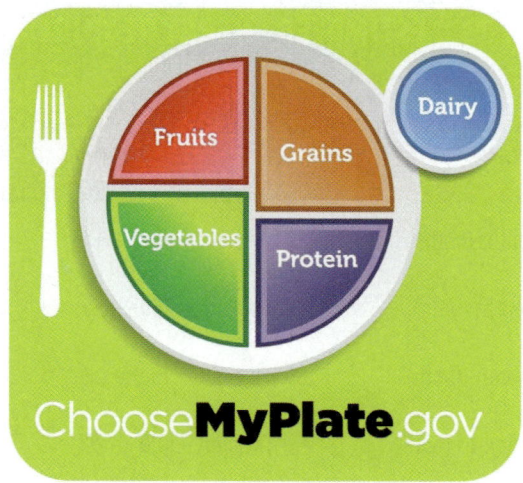

Reproduced from U.S. Department of Agriculture. ChooseMyPlate.gov.

Energy Requirements

Estimated energy requirements (EER) in the healthy child include the energy required for growth and tissue deposition. Energy needs can be predicted for healthy children using the Dietary Reference Intakes (DRIs). These requirements are based on studies of energy metabolism in healthy populations and incorporate additional needs for growth and physical activity. The DRI equations are meant to include all children with weight- and height-for-age from the 3rd to the 95th percentile (**Table 23.9**).[35] The DRIs are not appropriate to use in children with an altered clinical status. Instead, standardized equations must be used that account for stress and activity factors.

TABLE 23.8 MYPLATE FRUIT, VEGETABLE, GRAINS, PROTEIN, DAIRY, AND OIL RECOMMENDATIONS

Age (Sex)	Food Group Requirements					
	Fruit (cups per day)	Vegetables (cups per day)	Grains (ounce equivalents per day)	Protein (ounce equivalents per day)	Dairy (cups per day)	Oil (teaspoons per day)
2 to 3 years (Both)	1	1	3	2	2	3
4 to 8 years (Both)	1 to 1½	1 to 1½	5	4	2½	4
9 to 13 years (Female)	1½	2	5	5	3	5
9 to 13 years (Male)	1½	2½	6	5	3	5
14 to 18 years (Female)	1½	2½	6	5	3	5
14 to 18 years (Male)	2	3	8	6½	3	6

Modified from ChooseMyPlate.gov.

TABLE 23.9 ESTIMATED ENERGY REQUIREMENTS

Estimating Energy Expenditure

Age Range (Sex)	Energy Expenditure Equation (kcal) Weight in kg, Height in m, Age in years
0-3 months (both)	$(89 \times \text{weight} - 100) + 175$
4-6 months (both)	$(89 \times \text{weight} - 100) + 56$
7-12 months (both)	$(89 \times \text{weight} - 100) + 22$
13-36 months (both)	$(89 \times \text{weight} - 100) + 20$
3-8 years (Males)	$88.5 - (61.9 \times \text{age}) + \text{Physical Activity Factor}^{**} \times (26.7 \times \text{weight}) + (903 \times \text{height}) + 20$
3-8 years (Females)	$135.3 - (30.8 \times \text{age}) + \text{Physical Activity Factor} \times (10 \times \text{weight}) + (934 \times \text{height}) + 20$
9-18 years (Males)	$88.5 - (61.9 \times \text{age}) + \text{Physical Activity Factor} \times (26.7 \times \text{weight}) + (903 \times \text{height}) + 25$
9-18 years (Females)	$135.3 - (30.8 \times \text{age}) + \text{Physical Activity Factor} \times (10 \times \text{weight}) + (934 \times \text{height}) + 25$

**Physical Activity (PA) Factors for EER Equations

	Male	Female	Physical Activity
Sedentary	1.0	1.0	Typical daily living activities
Low active	1.13	1.16	Plus 30-60 minutes moderate activity
Active	1.26	1.31	Plus ≥ 60 minutes moderate activity
Very active	1.42	1.56	Plus ≥ 60 minutes moderate activity and 60 minutes vigorous or 12 minutes moderate activity

Modified from the DRI Report, National Academy of Sciences.

TABLE 23.10 RDA ENERGY REQUIREMENTS

RDA for Calories

Age (Sex)	Calories Per kg Body Weight	Calories Per Day
0-6 months (Both)	108	650
6-12 months (Both)	98	850
1-3 years (Both)	102	1,300
4-6 years (Both)	90	1,800
7-10 years (Both)	70	2,000
11-14 years (Males)	55	2,500
15-18 years (Males)	45	3,000
11-14 years (Females)	47	2,200
15-18 years (Females)	40	2,200

Modified from National Academies Press, National Research Council. Recommended Dietary Allowances. 10th ed. Chapter 3: Energy.

In addition to the EER equations, the Recommended Daily Allowance (RDA) can be used to determine energy needs.[36] Similar to the DRI equations, the RDA is based upon a healthy population. However, it uses the median height and weight to determine the caloric needs per kilogram of body weight or per day. From birth to age 10 years, the energy requirements for males and females are the same; they diverge once children reach adolescence. **Table 23.10** contains a summary of the RDA for energy needs from birth to age 18 years. It is important to note how the changes in energy needs correlate to the changes to growth velocity. During periods of rapid growth, such as the first year of life and early adolescence, energy requirements are increased.

Protein

Protein is a critical nutrient for growth. In the first year of life, LBM of a child increases by approximately 11% to 15%.[36] In addition, recall that body weight doubles within the first year. These increases require more protein per kilogram of body weight than in later stages of development. **Table 23.11** contains the RDA for protein, based on age range and gender. Like energy requirements, males and females have identical requirements through middle childhood, which then differ at the time of adolescence. The differences in protein requirements occur as a result of the sex-specific changes in body composition. These standards account for tissue maintenance, tissue growth, variation in growth, and efficiency of utilization.

TABLE 23.11 RDA FOR PROTEIN BASED ON AGE RANGE AND GENDER

Age (Gender)	RDA for Protein	
	Grams of Protein/kg Body Weight	Grams of Protein/Day
0-6 months (Both)	2.2	13
6-12 months (Both)	1.6	14
1-3 years (Both)	1.2	16
4-6 years (Both)	1.1	24
7-10 years (Both)	1.0	28
11-14 years (Males)	1.0	45
15-18 years (Males)	0.9	59
11-14 years (Females)	1.0	46
15-18 years (Females)	0.8	44

Modified from National Academies Press, National Research Council. Recommended Dietary Allowances. 10th ed. Chapter 6: Protein and Amino Acids.

CORE CONCEPT 7

Energy and protein needs, per kilogram of body weight, are the highest at birth and steadily decline through early childhood until the adolescent growth spurt.

Micronutrients: Vitamins and Minerals

As children grow, they require vitamins and minerals for adequate development and cellular processes. A summary of the key nutrients required for children is provided in **Table 23.12** and an overview of nutrients of concern and supplementation recommendations is provided in **Table 23.13**. It should be noted that for vegetarian or vegan children, calcium, vitamin D, vitamin B_{12}, and iron are particular nutrients of concern because the major dietary sources of these nutrients are from animal products.

CORE CONCEPT 8

Vitamins and minerals, especially calcium, iron, and vitamin D, provide essential nutrients for growth and development. Without adequate micronutrient status, children may have impaired growth.

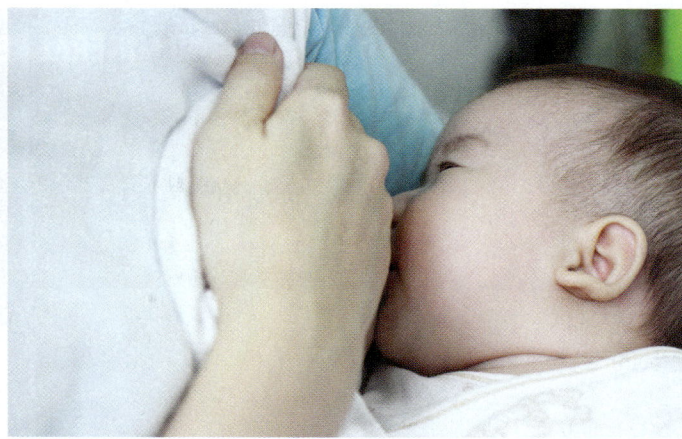

©kdshutterman/Shutterstock.

Full-term Infants

From birth through the first 4 to 6 months of life, infants are fed exclusively breast milk or commercial baby formula. The AAP recommends that breast milk be the sole source of infant nutrition from birth to approximately 6 months, because it provides specific energy and nutrients necessary for the developing infant.[39] It is recommended that breastfeeding be continued through 12 months, along with the addition of complimentary foods.

Breast Milk Breast milk provides complete nutrition for the infant in their first months of life. Breast milk is composed of fat, carbohydrates, and protein and contains approximately 20 kcal per ounce. Fat makes up 40% to 55% of the total energy of the milk. The majority of the fat is composed of triglycerides, of which approximately 17% are fatty acids.[40] Carbohydrates are in the breast milk as lactose and oligosaccharides. Lactose is the primary carbohydrate in the milk and fuels the high energy demands of the brain. Oligosaccharides also comprise a large portion of the carbohydrates but are not able to be digested by the infant. Instead, they feed the gut microbiota, functioning as prebiotics.[40,41] Lastly, protein is present in three different classes: whey, casein, and mucins. Protein in the milk has an antimicrobial and immune-modulating effect, as well as a nutrient role. The concentration of these macronutrients changes throughout lactation.

Human milk is classified into three groups—**colostrum**, transitional milk, and mature milk—based on the changes in composition that occur throughout lactation. In the early stages, colostrum is produced, which has a very high concentration of whey protein. Colostrum is also highly bioactive, providing immunoglobulins to promote the development of the immune system in the infant.[40] In addition, colostrum contains growth factors, which promote development in the newborn. From the 2nd to 7th months of lactation, the protein concentration decreases and ultimately levels off. In contrast, the fat concentration gradually increases. Carbohydrate content in breast milk is at its greatest concentration between 4 and 7 months. Mature human milk is approximately 55% whey and 44% casein. The composition of milk is thought to be unique to each infant because it is

TABLE 23.12 SELECTED VITAMIN AND MINERAL RECOMMENDED DAILY ALLOWANCE, BIRTH TO 18 YEARS

Age (Sex)	Vitamin A (ug/d)	Vitamin C (mg/d)	Vitamin D (ug/d)	Vitamin E (mg/d)	Vitamin K (ug/d)	Thiamin (mg/d)	Riboflavin (mg/d)	Niacin (mg/d)	Vitamin B_6 (mg/d)	Folate (ug/d)	Iron (mg/d)	Zinc (mg/d)
0-6 months (Both)	400	40	10	4	2.0	0.2	0.3	2	0.1	65	0.27	2
6-12 months (Both)	500	50	10	5	2.5	0.3	0.4	4	4	80	11	3
1-3 years (Both)	300	15	15	6	30	0.5	0.5	6	0.5	150	7	3
4-8 years (Both)	400	25	15	7	55	0.6	0.6	8	0.6	200	10	5
9-13 years (Female)	600	45	15	11	60	0.9	0.9	12	1.0	300	8	8
9-13 years (Male)	600	45	15	11	60	0.9	0.9	12	1.0	300	8	8
14-18 years (Female)	700	65	15	15	75	1.0	1.0	12	1.2	400	15	9
14-18 years (Male)	900	75	15	11	60	0.9	0.9	16	1.3	400	11	11

Modified from Dietary Reference Intakes for energy, carbohydrate, fiber, fat, fatty acids, cholesterol, protein and amino acids (2002/2005) and Dietary reference intakes for water, potassium, sodium, chloride and sulfate (2005).

associated with maternal characteristics such as age and diet, as well as the birth weight of the infant.[40]

In addition to its nutritional benefits, breast milk contains many biologically active components that serve other roles. The immunoglobulins present in milk help to protect the newborn from illness while their immune system is still developing. Separately, breast milk also functions to develop the infant's intestinal microbiota. Research indicates that breastfed infants have a more stable and less diverse microbiota, with double the amount of bacterial cells.[42]

PRACTICE POINT

Exclusive breastfeeding is recommended by the AAP to approximately 6 months, because it provides complete nutrition and changes in nutrient composition based on the infant's needs.

Infant Formula Infant formulas are designed to provide infants with adequate nutrition through the first 6 months of life. They are formulated to mimic the effect that breast milk has on the infant's growth and development, immunity, and microbiota.[43] There are many different formulas on the market, available as ready to use, liquid concentrate, and powder. They are composed of similar protein and carbohydrates as breast milk. Formulas are available in different varieties as well, including iron-fortified formulas, cow's milk–based formulas, and soy formulas, among others. Infant formulas typically provide 20 kcal per ounce, when mixed at standard concentrations.

Cow's milk formulas provide 1.45 to 1.6 g/dL of protein, which is higher than the protein content in breast milk. The protein sources in these formulas are casein and whey. Like breast milk, lactose is the main source of carbohydrates. Fat provides 40% to 50% of total calories. Vegetable oil, in a blend of palm, soy, coconut, safflower, and sunflower oils, is used as the fat source to provide essential fatty acids and improve digestibility.[43] Docosahexaenoic acid and arachidonic acid, as well as antioxidants, are often added to infant formulas. These are used to enhance the immune system

TABLE 23.13 NUTRIENTS OF CONCERN IN THE PEDIATRIC POPULATION

	Nutrients of Concern	
Age Range	Nutrients of Concern	Recommendations for Potential Need for Supplementation
Full-term infants	Vitamin D Iron Fluoride (after 6 months)	Vitamin D, *within the first few days after birth* Iron, *after 4 to 6 months for breastfeeding infant; for formula-fed infants, the AAP recommends use of an iron-fortified formula*
Preschool-aged children	Vitamin A Calcium Iron Zinc, *especially in vegetarians*	If nutrient intake is low or varied, a vitamin supplement may be necessary.
School-aged Children	Calcium Vitamin D It is important to ensure that children in this age range consume a variety of calcium-rich foods.	If nutrient intake is low or varied, a vitamin supplement may be necessary.
Adolescence	Vitamin A Vitamin D Vitamin E Folate Iron Zinc Magnesium Calcium	If nutrient intake is low or varied, a vitamin supplement may be necessary.

Data from What We Eat in America: NHANES Survey.

and potentially aide in the development of the infant's vision and neurological development.[43]

Iron-fortified formulas contain 40% to 55% of total calories from carbohydrates, 5% to 6% of total calories from protein, and 50% of calories from fat. These can also be concentrated to provide 24 kcal or higher per ounce for infants with suboptimal growth. Iron-fortified formulas are indicated for preterm infants, as they help to replenish iron stores. The AAP recommends the use of iron-supplemented formulas in infants who are formula fed.[1] The use of these formulas can have a positive effect on the long-term iron stores of the infant.[44] Despite this recommendation, some argue against iron fortification in formula because it far exceeds the concentration in breast milk. Opponents of iron fortification suggest that the decreased iron concentration in breast milk is an evolutionary adaptation.[45]

Infant formulas continue to evolve in other ways to better imitate breast milk. Additives such as prebiotics and probiotics are being used to enhance infant formulas with varying success as far as growth and clinical benefit.[46–50] Prebiotics have been shown to reduce respiratory infections in infants through the first 6 months of life.[49] However, formulas supplemented with prebiotics have not improved growth rates beyond that of non-prebiotic-fortified supplements.[50] While probiotics are proven to be safe, they do not offer any clinical advantage over non-probiotic formula in full-term infants. Probiotics may reduce necrotizing enterocolitis in preterm infants and are thought to also be beneficial for infants with GI distress, because they alter the gut microbiota.[46] Thus overall, despite their proposed benefits, research has not substantiated the clinical value in prebiotic and probiotic supplementation of infant formula.

PRACTICE POINT

Iron is a nutrient of concern in newborns, especially those receiving formula. An iron-fortified formula is recommended.

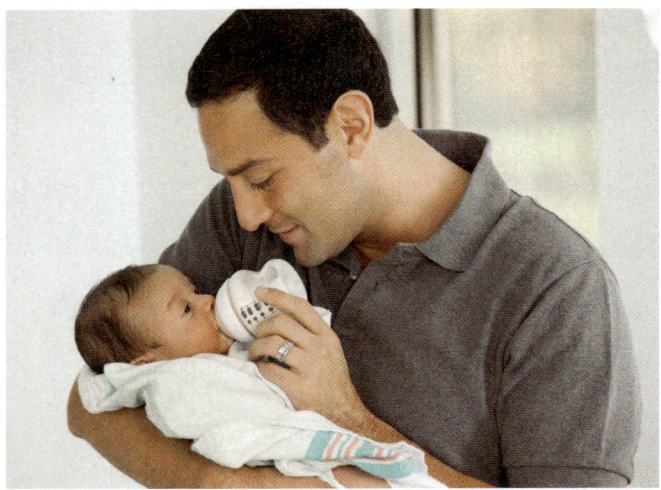

©Ariel Skelley/DigitalVision/Getty Images.

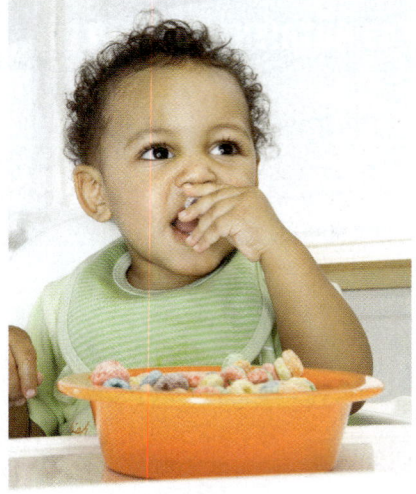

© James Woodson/Digital Vision/Thinkstock.

Introduction of Food and Developmental Cues

After 4 to 6 months of breastfeeding or formula feeding, it is necessary to begin to introduce the baby to solid foods. Breastfeeding is no longer sufficient to sustain the nutritional requirements of the infant. The AAP recommends introducing complimentary foods at 6 months of age; however, the exact time when exclusive breastfeeding no longer provides adequate energy and nutrients is unknown.[50] Introducing new foods is guided by the development of the child. Grains and fruits are typically the first to be introduced because they are the least allergenic. Table 23.14 summarizes the introduction of foods and corresponding developmental cues. Development is the key determining factor in whether a child can eat new foods; feeding a child solid foods before they are developmentally ready can delay additional feeding milestones.

As solid foods are introduced, it is necessary to postpone exposure to foods that may pose a risk to the infant. In the first year, both cow's milk and honey should be avoided. The AAP recommends that cow's milk be introduced only after 12 months.[51] Early introduction of cow's milk can diminish the iron status of the infant.[53] Consumption of honey in infants can result in botulism. Botulism results from ingestion of spores, which may be present in honey, that release a nerve-damaging toxin.[52] Foods that pose a choking hazard for infants, such as hot dogs, popcorn, grapes, nuts, and raisins, should also be avoided until the child has further developed their oral motor skills.

Toddlers

Nutrition at this stage is important for continuation of growth and development and maintenance of life-long health. Toddlers are still continuing to develop oral motor skills. By 18 months, a toddler is able to handle a cup, self-feed, and self-regulate. They begin to consume more textured foods, but are cautious to accept new foods. It may take several attempts at introducing new foods before a toddler will try them. Parents should allow them to explore the look, smell, and taste of new foods.

Toddlers, because they have increased energy requirements but cannot eat large portions, require smaller, frequent meals. This can be in the form of three meals and two to three snacks or or six smaller meals per day in order to meet their nutritional needs. It is important that children be allowed to learn to feed themselves and decide how much to eat in a comfortable yet structured atmosphere. However, like infants, toddlers are at risk for choking, because they are still developing their oral motor muscles. Most toddlers fail to eat the recommended amount of fruits and vegetables. Early introduction of fruits and vegetables are associated with greater consumption of fruits and vegetables later in life.[54–57]

> **PRACTICE POINT**
>
> Toddlers may need to be exposed to certain foods on numerous occasions to create familiarity before trialing it. Early introduction of healthy foods promotes life-long positive eating habits.

Preschool-aged Children

Preschool-aged children, like toddlers, require multiple smaller meals each day to meet their energy requirements. It is recommended that they consume nutrient-dense foods and avoid consumption of excess sugar-sweetened beverages.

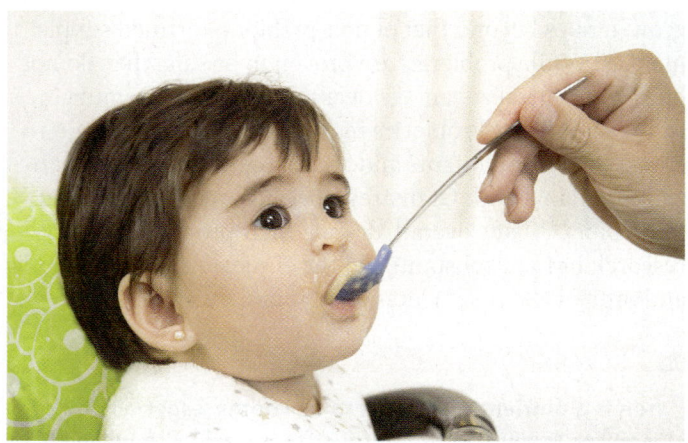

© Marcos Mesa Sam Wordley/Shutterstock.

TABLE 23.14 INTRODUCTION TO FOODS

Introduction to Foods

Age Range	Nutrition-related Developmental Cues	Food Type Consumed	Feeding Behavior
0 to 4 months	Sucking and tongue thrusting	Breast milk Infant formula	Newborn: feed every 1.5 to 2 hours 1 to 4 months: feed every 2 to 3 hours
4 to 6 months	Mature sucking Munching pattern Steady head control Briefly sits independently	Continue to breast feed or bottle feed Baby cereal introduced Strained fruit/vegetables	Feed every 3 to 4 hours Messy spoon feeding, suckling motion on spoon
7 to 9 months	Normal gag reflex Sits alone for 3 to 5 minutes Holds bottle Steady head control (no bobbing)	Continue to breast feed or bottle feed Stage 1 baby food introduced Stage 2 introduced at 8 months Soft mashed table food at 9 months	Feed every 3.5 to 4 hours Hand-to-mouth play
10 to 12 months	Finger feeds Reaches for spoon Learning mature chewing; by 12 months, chewing skills advance	Continue to breast feed or bottle feed Table foods Foods that dissolve introduced at 10 months Foods that are easily chewed introduced at 11 months	Feed every 4 to 6 hours Use food as toy, mouth play

Modified from A.S.P.E.N. Pediatric Nutrition Support Curriculum. 2nd ed. 2015.

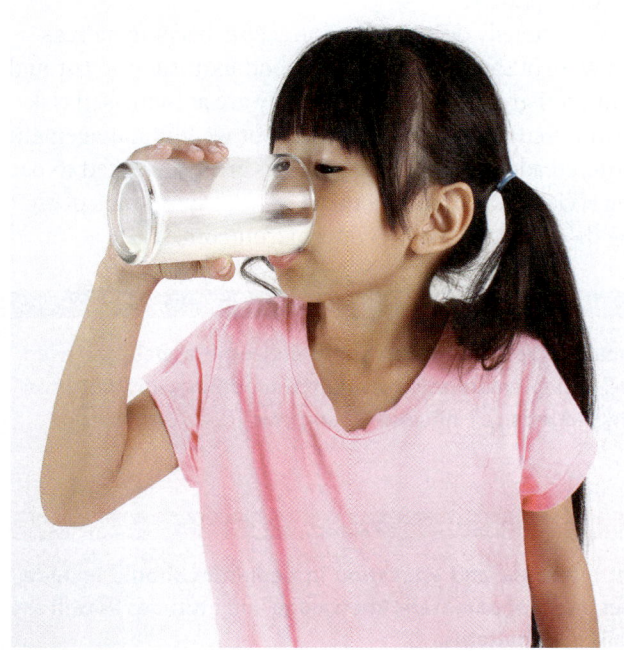

©paulaphoto/Shutterstock.

Also, preschool-aged children can begin to switch to lower-fat foods. At this age, children continue to learn how to self-regulate. Parents should practice division of responsibility as their child is able to feed him- or herself. Research has indicated that when children fill their own plates, they consume less food and begin to recognize their own satiety cues. Forceful or restrictive environments can have a negative impact on children. In these atmospheres, children are prone to overeating and later weight gain, because they are not able to exercise control. The diet of preschool-aged children is largely reflective of their parents' diet.

School-aged Children

School-aged children begin to better understand and describe food. They are able to categorize food by their likes and dislikes, as well as if they are healthy. At the same time, school-aged children have the potential to consume more sugar-sweetened beverages and high-fat foods and less wholesome foods like low-fat dairy, fruits, vegetables, and whole grains. School-aged children who eat meals with their family are less likely to drink sugar-sweetened

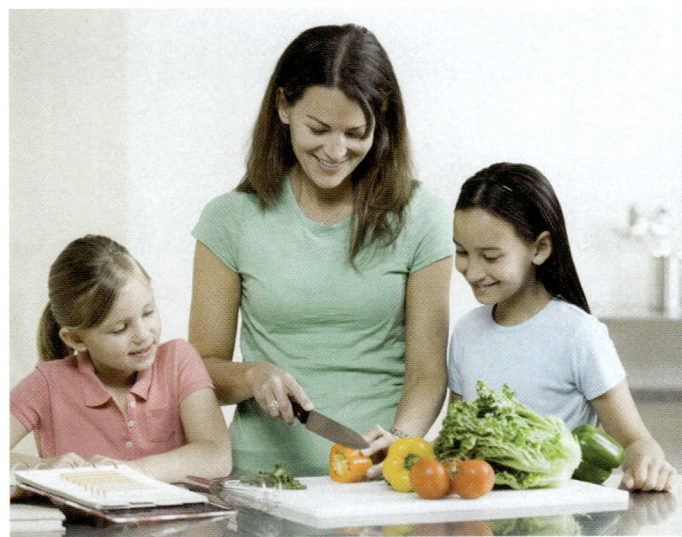

© Artemis Gordon/ShutterStock, Inc.

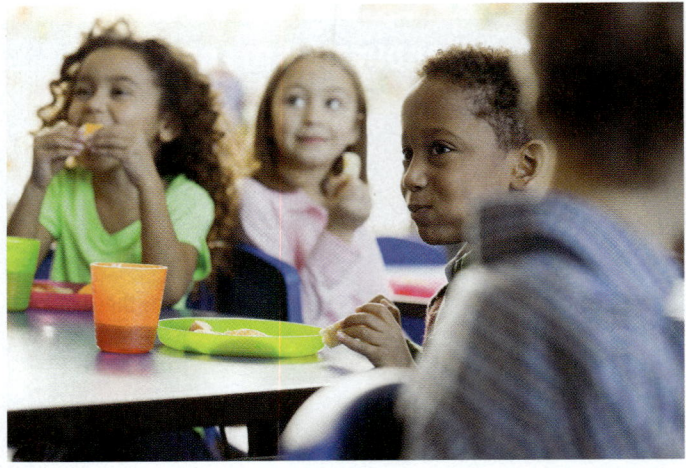

©Hero Images/Getty Images.

beverages.[56] Unlike toddlers and preschoolers, school-aged children consume a wider variety of foods. School-aged children also have lower energy needs, thus balance between energy intake and activity becomes increasingly important. It is recommended by the AAP that school-aged children exercise for a minimum of 60 minutes per day. This should be a combination of aerobic exercise and muscle- and bone-strengthening activities. However, fewer than half of American children meet this requirement.

There are many factors that influence a child's eating behavior, including his or her eating environment. As a dietitian, it is important to provide education about how the environment promotes the development of healthy eating practices. Children's early eating practices are highly affected by their parents. Family feeding practices can influence a child's perception on meal size and satiety.[54] As children grow and develop, their tastes develop as well. The eating environment is especially important as children try new foods. Enthusiastic modeling and repeated exposures can help a child to try new foods. A healthy home environment is most closely associated with healthy eating habits, such as increased fruit and vegetable consumption and decreased soda and snack food consumption.[56]

Adolescents

Adolescents have increased energy and nutrient needs compared to preschool and school-aged children due to an increase in growth velocity. Older children's eating habits are largely influenced by their friends, often resulting in decreased consumption of nutrient-dense foods and increased intake of sugar-sweetened beverages and high-fat, nutrient-poor foods. Despite increased intake of calories, lack of certain nutrients such as calcium and iron are problematic for this age group. Adolescents are at increased risk for osteoporosis later in life due to suboptimal bone mineralization. Iron-deficiency anemia, poor weight management, and chronic diseases such as type 2 diabetes and heart disease may also result from poor dietary habits.[14] While older children should be encouraged to make their own healthy food choices, it is important to continue family meals. Assuring a good breakfast is associated with more healthful eating behaviors as well as better diet quality.[56–60]

As previously described, adolescents become increasingly aware of the changes in their bodies as they go through the pubertal growth spurt. Thus, they are at increased risk for disordered eating patterns and poor weight management. Disordered adolescent eating patterns are also related to parenting styles.[61] Recognizing the signs and symptoms of an eating disorder may help to improve outcomes.

> **CORE CONCEPT 9**
>
> At each stage, children should consume a well-balanced diet. Eating environment, parental modeling, and nutrition knowledge can all influence eating practices.

> **PRACTICE POINT**
>
> Diet interview and education in pediatrics should include assessment of parenteral knowledge and attitudes as well as family meal patterns.

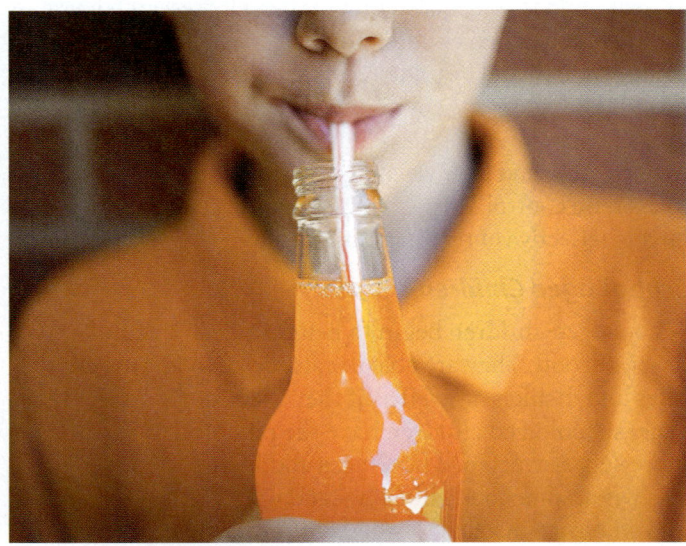

©Melissa Lomax Speelman/Moment/Getty Images.

> ## CASE STUDY REVISITED
>
> At Peter's 1-year visit, it is determined that he has failure to thrive. His information is below.
>
> **Anthropometric Data:**
>
> | Age (months) | Birth | 3 | 4 | 6 | 9 | 12 |
> |---|---|---|---|---|---|---|
> | Weight (kg) | 3 | 5.2 | 5.4 | 5.6 | 5.8 | 6.2 |
> | Length (cm) | 50 | 58 | 62 | 63 | 64 | 65 |
>
> **Biochemical Data:**
> Iron 49 (60-170 mcg/dL)
> Transferrin 395 (170 to 370 mg/dL)
> Transferrin saturation 10.7% (20%–50%)
> Total Iron Binding Capacity 455 (240–450 mcg/dL)
>
> **Clinical Data:**
> **Past Medical History:** Failure to gain weight, persistent GERD
> **Medications:** omeprazole
> **Vitals Signs:** Normal
> **Nutrition-focused Physical Exam:** Appears thin, slightly pale, lethargic
>
> **Dietary Data:**
> **Diet Recall:**
> Breakfast: 4 ounces low-fat milk, ¼ pancake with syrup, 2 apple slices
> Mid-morning snack: 10-15 Cheerios, 4 oz water
> Lunch: 2 slices of turkey, 1 slice of cheese, juice box
> Afternoon snack: Refuses food, 4 oz chocolate milk (2%)
> Dinner: Chicken or fish (1 oz), mashed potato or rice (2-3 tablespoons), corn or peas (1/3 cup)
> **Diet Prescription:** Age appropriate
>
> ### Questions
>
> 1. Assess Peter's current nutritional status. Using www.peditools.org, determine Peter's weight-for-age, length-for-age and weight-for-length z-scores.
> 2. What are Peter's current nutritional problems?
> 3. Assess Peter's energy requirement for normal growth. Is Peter's dietary intake sufficient?
> 4. Determine Peter's needs for catch-up growth.
> 5. Provide recommendations to Peter's typical diet to help meet his needs for catch up growth.

Pediatric Malnutrition

Pediatric malnutrition affects many children worldwide. A.S.P.E.N. defines pediatric malnutrition as "an imbalance between nutrient requirement and intake resulting in cumulative deficits of energy, protein or micronutrients that may negatively affect growth, development and other relevant outcomes."[62] In the United States, pediatric malnutrition is often secondary to disease, chronic illness, trauma. or surgery.[62] Although hospitalized pediatric patients are at the greatest nutritional risk, children should be screened at their routine physical exams.[21] Lack of standard definitions and screening criteria allows malnutrition to go undetected. Pediatric malnutrition can be defined through five domains: anthropometrics, growth charts, chronicity, etiology, and functional status.[21,62] Chronicity refers to the time span in which malnutrition was documented; it can be defined as acute (less than 3 months in duration) or chronic (ongoing for more than 3 months).

Failure to Thrive

Failure to thrive (FTT) is a condition of pediatric malnutrition, often identified within the first 3 years of a child's life. It is estimated that 5 out 100 children suffer from FTT.[63] The term FTT is used less frequently with the development of malnutrition criteria based on z-scores. Malnutrition defined by z-scores describes infants and children who lost weight or deviated from their age- and gender-specific growth patterns as indicated by the standardized growth charts. It is solely defined by anthropometrics.[21] However, FTT describes the cause and etiology behind malnutrition and remains clinically useful. There are two types of FTT: **organic FTT** and **nonorganic FTT**. Over 90% of FTT cases are not disease related. Children with FTT are more vulnerable to infection and behavioral problems.[64]

Criteria for Diagnosis

Children with FTT will present with inadequate physical growth and an inability to maintain expected growth over a period of time. There is no clear consensus on diagnosis for FTT. Generally, FTT is characterized by delayed growth: less than 3rd percentile weight-for-age, less than 10th percentile weight-for-height, and weight less than 80% of ideal weight-for-height. In addition, these children have decreased growth velocity, which is traditionally defined as weight decreasing more than two major percentiles or standard deviations over a 3- to 6-month time frame. As mentioned, z-scores, as opposed to percentiles, are increasingly used in describing malnutrition, including FTT, as 3% of normal children fall below the 3rd percentile for weight and height. A z-score that falls below two standard deviations is a clear indication of FTT.

In addition to the anthropometric indicators of FTT, an accurate summary of a child's eating habits, caloric intake, and parent–child interaction is necessary to better determine the cause of FTT.[63] For infants, it is important to ask the parent how much milk or formula the child consumes and how long it takes them to feed. In toddlers, FTT may be caused by picky eating or insufficient caloric intake. If possible, observing the child eating and stress level of the parent at mealtime is useful. Understanding the cause of FTT can help to design more appropriate nutrition interventions.

Etiology and Pathophysiology

Organic FTT defines a child with poor growth related to an underlying medical condition. Nonorganic FTT, or psychosocial FTT, refers to a child younger than age 5 years with poor growth and no underlying medical condition. Because most children have FTT with mixed etiologies, it is best to classify them based on cause. Inadequate caloric intake or absorption, excess metabolic demand, and defective utilization are all possible causes of FTT. There are also some non-disease-related causes of FTT, such as nutritional information deficit, consumption of a mostly liquid diet, family stressors, maternal depression, and food shortage.[64] FTT is not only a medical condition, but one with social and environmental roots. Dietitians can further educate parents on appropriate diets for children or help the family to utilize support programs.

Management of FTT

Successful management of FTT requires a multidisciplinary approach. Because the disease is multifactorial, the treatment must be as well. The healthcare team should include a psychologist and social worker, especially if inadequate access to resources is the cause of FTT. In order to manage FTT, the child's energy needs for **catch up growth** must be assessed. First, determine the ideal body weight for the child based on age or height. The ideal body weight can be based on the 50th percentile on the growth charts, when stunting has occurred. If the child being evaluated falls below the 3rd percentile, the 5th to 25th percentile can be used as the goal weight. In nonstunted children, the ideal weight-for-length can be used as well. Once the ideal body weight has been determined, the nutritional requirements, for catch-up growth, should be set for the child. The nutrient requirements may be affected by the underlying medical conditions.

> **PRACTICE POINT**
>
> If a child falls below the 3rd percentile, setting the ideal body weight at the 5th percentile is slightly conservative. The ideal body weight can be set up to the 25th percentile.

Calculating Energy Needs for Catch-Up Growth

$$\frac{\text{RDA for age} \times \text{Ideal Weight-for-height}}{\text{Actual Weight}}$$

Or

$$\frac{\text{RDA for age} \times \text{Ideal Weight-for-age}}{\text{Actual Weight}}$$

Because there are many causes and contributing factors to FTT, there are many steps that can be taken to facilitate further growth. First, adequate nutrition should be provided. This can be accomplished by supplying concentrated infant formulas or using high-calorie and high-protein solid foods, in addition to a supplement. In cases of severe undernutrition, calories should be added back slowly to prevent refeeding syndrome. For children suffering from nonorganic FTT, in addition to providing a nutrient-dense diet, lifestyle changes may be necessary to provide an appropriate eating environment. These changes involve the parents as well as the child. Determining a meal and snack schedule and including a personalized meal plan for the child may be necessary. Furthermore, parents and caregivers should receive education about setting limits on meal times, reinforcing good eating behavior, and limiting grazing and distractions.

> **PRACTICE POINT**
>
> Mealtimes in FTT patients should be limited to approximately 20 to 30 minutes. Parents should be educated on reinforcing good eating behavior and limiting grazing and distractions.

> **CORE CONCEPT 10**
>
> Failure to thrive must be addressed using an interprofessional approach, including feeding based on catch-up energy and nutrient requirements to prevent developmental delays and child mortality.

CASE STUDY REVISITED

At 13 months, Peter returns for a follow-up. His height and weight are the same. His mother reports that he continues to have significant reflux and often refuses to eat. It is determined that he will need surgery to repair his GERD. Given his history of FTT, the team asks you for a recommendation for nutrition support for 2 weeks prior to surgery and 1 week after until Peter can resume eating.

Questions

1. What is the most appropriate form of nutrition support for Peter?
2. Provide your recommendation for nutrition therapy, including type of nutrition, route of administration, nutrition formulation, and volume needed for catch up growth.
3. How will you monitor Peter's nutritional adequacy?

Nutrition Support During Times of Illness or Chronic Disease

Because children have lower LBM, they are especially vulnerable to malnutrition during illness. Critically ill pediatric patients are at the greatest risk for malnutrition. Research estimates that 40% to 50% of hospitalized patients are at risk for malnutrition.[63–65] Failure to provide optimal nutrition combined with the metabolic response to critical illness contributes to these rates of malnutrition in hospitalized pediatric patients. All children admitted into a pediatric intensive care unit (PICU) should have measures of height and weight done with z-scores.[66]

Nutrition support is a strategy used to minimize the risk for and treat malnutrition. Enteral nutrition (EN) and parenteral nutrition (PN) are the two forms of nutrition therapy that are used. The goal of nutrition therapy is to provide adequate nutrition to minimize LBM losses and minimize the long-term consequences of critical illness.

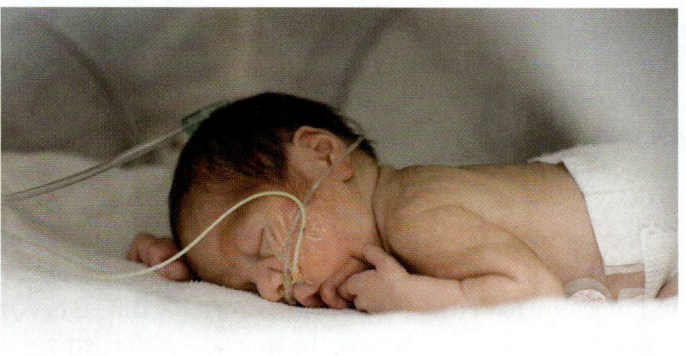
©Annedehaas/E+/Getty Images.

Providing sufficient nutrients can improve the patient's immune response, prevent reduced gut function, and decrease length of hospital stay.[66]

> **PRACTICE POINT**
>
> Enteral nutrition is the preferred mode of nutrient delivery in children.

Enteral and parenteral nutrition are both considered in the critically ill pediatric patient. The enteral route is beneficial in maintaining mucosal immunity and is associated with improved mortality in critically ill children.[66] However, PN should be used when EN is not tolerated, particularly in children at nutritional risk or if the gut is dysfunctional. The current A.S.P.E.N. guidelines on the provision of nutrition support state that while EN is the preferred modality, delaying PN for 7 days, as is common in adults, should not be broadly applied in the pediatric population. Timing and use of supplemental PN should be individually determined based on the status of the patient. PICU patients who cannot receive EN during the first week of admission may receive supplemental PN. Malnourished patients or those at risk for rapid deterioration, such as in metabolic stress, should also receive PN if EN cannot be advanced beyond a low volume. **Table 23.15** presents the indications and contraindications for enteral and parenteral nutrition in the pediatric patient.[67]

> **CORE CONCEPT 11**
>
> Nutrition support may be indicated in pediatric patients when oral feeding does not provide enough energy or nutrients. Timely initiation, particularly in children younger than 2 years of age, prevents rapid deterioration of nutritional status.

Enteral Nutrition

EN initiated within the first 24 to 48 hours following admission, and at rates up to two-thirds of goal, is associated with improved clinical outcomes in children.[66] In a

TABLE 23.15 INDICATIONS AND CONTRAINDICATIONS FOR ENTERAL AND PARENTERAL NUTRITION

Enteral versus Parental Nutrition

	Indications	Contraindications
Enteral Nutrition	**Inadequate oral intake** *Causes:* developmental, behavioral, or anatomical complications **Increased nutritional needs** *Causes:* chronic disease, malabsorption, metabolic disorders, inadequate intestinal function, increased energy expenditure, critical illness	**GI tract cannot be safely accessed** *Causes:* facial or esophageal injury **Gut is not functional** *Causes:* feedings cannot be advanced, excessive diarrhea, ileus, obstruction, fistulas **Hemodynamic instability** *Causes:* critical illness, as evidenced by vasopressor or extracorporeal membrane oxygenation utilization
Parenteral Nutrition	GI tract is not functional or it cannot be accessed Nutrient needs exceed what can be provided by enteral nutrition and oral intake Premature infants: GI tract is not fully developed Certain disease states: congenital heart disease, congenital abnormalities, necrotizing enterocolitis, short bowel syndrome Critical illness Failure to thrive with diarrhea	Oral and enteral nutrition provides enough energy and nutrients Poor central line access Low nutritional risk

Modified from: A.S.P.E.N. Pediatric Nutrition Support Core Curriculum. 2nd ed. Corkins, 2015.[67]

critical care setting, there are many barriers to EN progression, such as use of vasoactive drugs, prolonged periods of holding feeds for procedures, and gastrointestinal intolerance. Use of step-wise algorithms to guide initiation and progression of EN are advised for safe and timely EN support (**Figure 23.11**).[66] Evaluation of nutritional risk based on malnutrition or the severity of disease and accompanying metabolic stress should be incorporated into this decision-making process. Given their decreased LBM, children 0 to 2 years of age should be presumed high risk.

> **PRACTICE POINT**
>
> Standard feeding algorithms should be used to guide nutrition support therapy, including parameters for bedside monitoring of feeding tolerance.

Enteral Access

Enteral nutrition can be given through gastric feeds or postpyloric feeds. Gastric feeds are more physiologic and mimic normal nutrition, particularly when given as a bolus feed. Gastric feeding is preferred in pediatric patients, as larger volumes of formula can be administered at once. However, in children where gastric feedings are not tolerated, or those with neurologic dysfunction, anatomical abnormalities, gastroparesis, or high risk for aspiration, postpyloric feedings should be used.[66]

There are several different enteral access points. Feeding tubes such as nasogastric, nasojejunal, gastrostomy, percutaneous endoscopic gastrostomy (PEG), jejunostomy, and percutaneous endoscopic jejunostomy (PEJ) are all options for feeding the pediatric patient. Nasoenteric tubes can be used in the short term, for a maximum of 8 weeks, as they can cause nasal erosion and oral feeding aversion in children.[68]

Gastrostomy and PEG tubes are also commonly used in the pediatric patient when they require long-term EN or if they cannot have a nasoenteric feeding tube.[68] Gastrostomies are indicated when a patient will be fed through a tube for longer than 6 to 12 weeks. Gastrostomies feed directly into the stomach, but differ in the techniques used to insert the tubes. PEG tubes are associated with greater complications in children, because there is potential to damage the bowel or create an obstruction; however, they are presumed safe in infants as small as 6 kg. Gastrostomy tubes are generally preferred by families because they maintain quality of life and are more aesthetically pleasing.[68] Jejunostomy and PEJ tubes are placed similarly to a gastrostomy tube. They can either be advanced or have the stoma created postpylorically. Because patients with jejunostomy tubes will be less tolerant to higher volumes or unable to receive bolus feedings, a schedule that works for the child and family will need to be established.

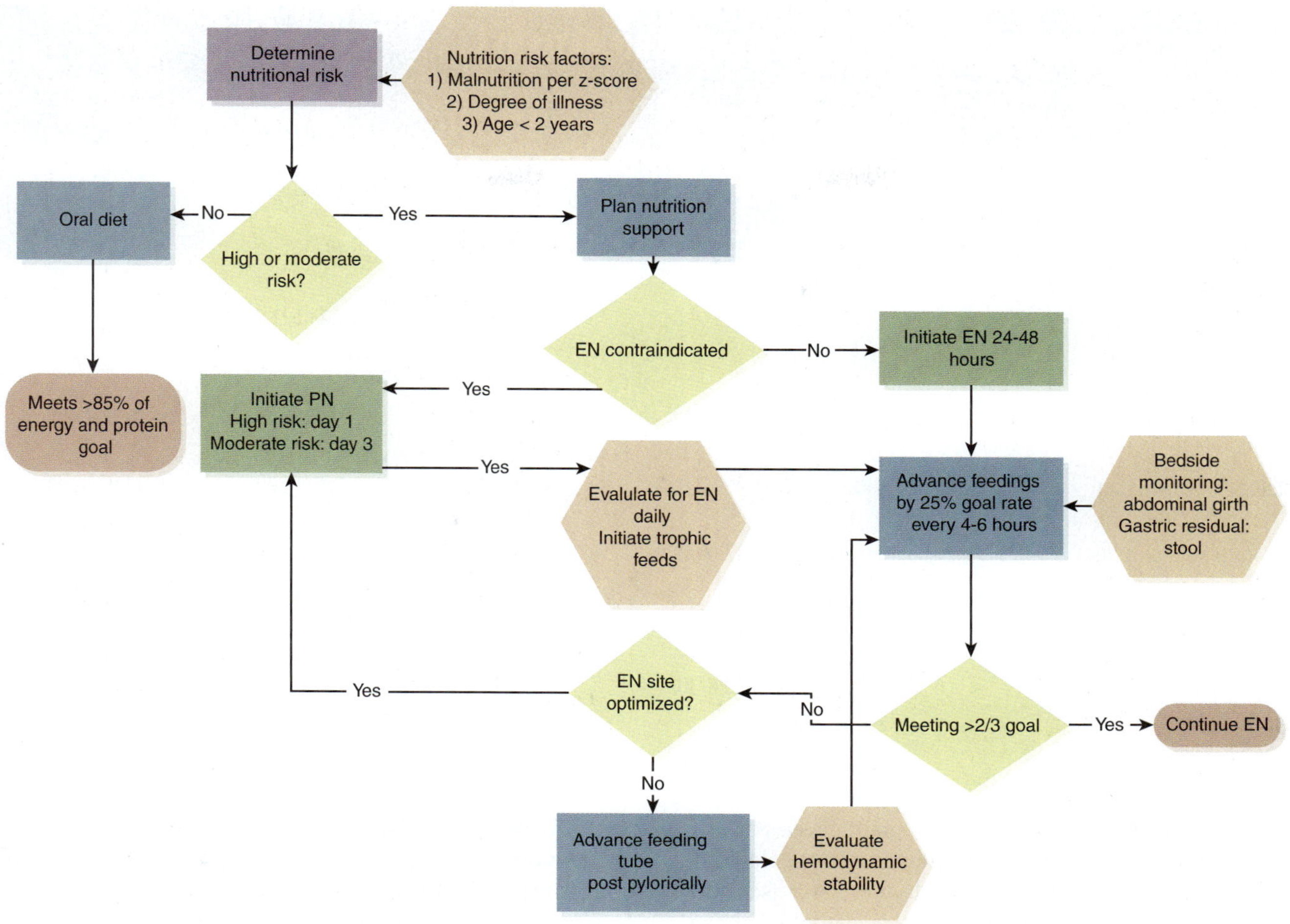

FIGURE 23.11 Example of an Algorithm for Nutrition Support Therapy in Children

> **PRACTICE POINT**
>
> If enteral nutrition is expected to be used for longer than 6 to 12 weeks, a semi-permanent tube, such as a PEG, PEJ, gastrostomy, or jejunostomy, should be inserted instead of a nasoenteric tube.

Enteral Formulas

There are many factors, including growth and diet history, biochemical data, level of GI function, and current feeding regimen, that should be considered when choosing an enteral formula for a pediatric patient (**Table 23.16**). Age of the patient is also a consideration. For infants, concentrated infant formulas and fortified breast milk are often necessary. Pediatric formulas are designed for patients aged 1 to 13 years. Adult formulations may be indicated for the adolescent population and are also well suited for younger patients with burns or trauma, as they are higher in protein and micronutrients that support wound healing.

The osmotic load of most adult formulas is likely acceptable for older children. In general, children require a lower renal solute load. Children younger than age 4 years should receive formulas less than 400 mOsm/kg. Older children can tolerate slightly more concentrated formulas, but should not exceed 600 mOsm/kg. Presence of abdominal distension, delayed gastric emptying, vomiting, and diarrhea may indicate that the osmotic load is too great for the patient.

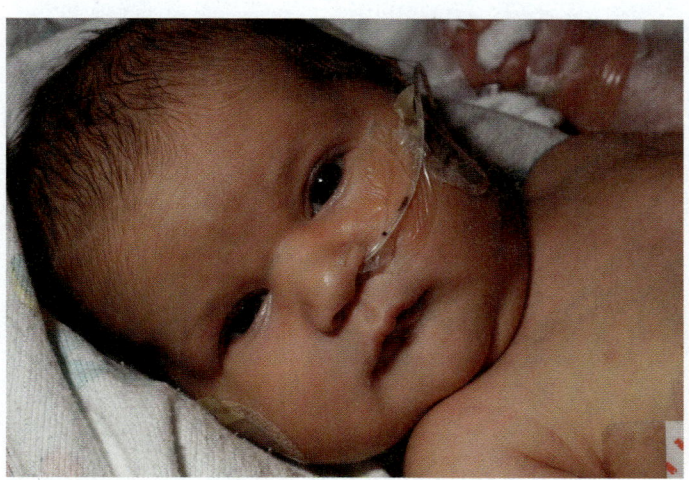

> **PRACTICE POINT**
>
> Pediatric enteral formulas are appropriate to feed children during early childhood. After age 10 years, adult formulas should be considered because they can better meet the needs for the patient.

TABLE 23.16 ENTERAL FORMULAS USED IN PEDIATRIC PATIENTS

Formula Name	Pediasure	Nutren Jr	Jevity	Peptamen	Promote
Concentration (kcal/mL)	1.0	1.0	1.06	1.0	1.0
Protein g/1000 mL (% kcal)	30 (12)	30 (12)	41.8 (16.7)	40 (16)	62.5 (25)
Carbohydrate g/1000 mL (% kcal)	143 (54)	110 (40)	146 (54.3)	128 (51)	130 (32)
Fat g/1000 mlL (% kcal)	38 (34)	50 (44)	32.8 (29)	33 (39.2)	26 (23)
Sodium/potassium (mg)	380/1,310	460/1,320	878/1,482	560/1,500	1,000/1,980
Calcium/phosphorus (mg)	1,055/84	1,000/800	859/717	800/700	1,200/1,200
Vitamin D (IU)	675	560	288	528	400
Zinc (mg) /selenium (mcg)/ copper (mg)	6.3/30/0.8	10.8/30/1	18/54/1.6	24/50/2	24/70/2

Types of Formulas There are three main classes of enteral formulas: polymeric, semi-elemental, and elemental. Pediatric formularies differ from adult ones, because there are not as many disease-specific formulas available for the pediatric popluation. In these situations, adult formulations may be necessary to provide a better nutrient composition or to promote recovery. For infants younger than 1 year, concentrating infant formula to 24 to 30 calories per ounce is common practice. In addition, modular protein and fat in the form of vegetable oil can be added. Breast milk can be given through a feeding tube as well. This is ideal, because it can promote continuation of breastfeeding once the child recovers. Breast milk can be fortified to meet the increased needs of a child during illness.

Polymeric formulas can be used when the entire digestive tract is normally functioning. Polymeric formulas are characterized by the presence of intact proteins. These formulas provide 30 kcal per ounce, 12% to 15% of which are from protein, 44% to 53% from carbohydrates, and the remaining 35% to 45% from fat. Vitamins and minerals are also provided to reach 100% of the RDA when 1 L is given. Polymeric formulas are available as standard, calorie dense, and fiber enriched. The variations in the formulations help individualize nutrition therapy based on patient needs and for different disease states. Fiber-enriched formulas typically contain 5 to 8 g/L of fiber. For example, a child who presents with diarrhea may benefit from the use of a polymeric fiber-enriched formula. Calorie-dense pediatric

Clinical Roundtable

Topic: Micronutrient Supplementation in Children Receiving Enteral Nutrition

Background: Children receiving nutritional support are often metabolically stressed, resulting in increased micronutrient losses and/or requirements. Despite a lack of evidence defining micronutrient needs in conditions of stress and illness, certain antioxidant nutrients such as selenium, vitamins C and E, and wound-healing trace elements zinc and copper can often be supplemented in high amounts. Some clinicians advocate that use of adult formulas, particularly in amounts needed to meet increased energy and protein requirements of critically ill children, will provide sufficient amounts of these micronutrients.

Roundtable Discussion

1. What are the risks associated with single-nutrient supplementation in high doses?
2. What are the advantages and disadvantages in using adult formulas to meet requirements in children younger than age 10 years?
3. Given the lack of evidence, how might you determine best practice for meeting micronutrient requirements in children receiving nutrition support?

formulas are designed for children younger than age 10 years and are concentrated to 1.5 kcal/mL.

Semi-elemental formulas are specially designed to enhance nutrient absorption when the GI tract has been compromised. These formulas are indicated when children present with GI conditions due to malabsorption or maldigestion. Semi-elemental formulas contain proteins that have been broken down into peptides and amino acids. The macronutrient composition of these formulas is similar to that of the polymeric formulas. Calorically dense semi-elemental formulas can also be used when children do not tolerate large volumes of formula.

Elemental formulas are also indicated in several situations, such as a compromised GI tract, short-bowel syndrome, malabsorption, and multiple protein allergies. These formulas contain only free amino acids. The macronutrient composition of elemental formulas varies greatly. Carbohydrates provide approximately 46% to 63% of total calories, fat contributes 25% to 45% of total calories, and protein adds the remaining 10% to 15% of calories. Elemental formulas are provided in powdered form, which allows the osmotic load to be changed based on the energy concentration of the order. Elemental formulas typically have a greater osmolality than semi-elemental or polymeric options.

Monitoring of Enteral Tolerance

Patients receiving enteral nutrition should be closely monitored. There are several complications that may result from enteral feeds; they can be related to tube function or gastrointestinal intolerance. Signs of intolerance include large gastric residuals, presence of GI symptoms (abdominal distention, constipation, diarrhea, nausea, vomiting), which may lead to an inability to receive sufficient volume to obtain necessary nutrients from enteral nutrition.[69] While commonly practiced, use of gastric residual monitoring is not directly associated with feeding tolerance and gastric emptying.[70] Furthermore, in patients with soft, pliable enteroflex feeding tubes, aspiration of gastric contents is difficult. Therefore, clinicians must use clinical judgment and signs of intolerance as described above to determine advancement schedule or when to hold feeds. Measurement of abdominal girth prior to starting enteral feedings and at every nursing shift is a useful way to anticipate the onset of tube feeding intolerance through monitoring of abdominal distention.

It is also important to evaluate all potential causes of intolerance to enteral feedings. Children may also have adverse reactions to some of the medications they are receiving. In addition, enteral supplementation of electrolytes such as sodium, potassium, or phosphorus via feeding tube can result in a high osmolality, contributing to signs of dumping syndrome. Patients on prolonged antibiotics may develop altered gut flora, resulting in diarrhea. It is useful to evaluate these other factors first before switching the formula.

Feeding tubes should be monitored for placement by marking the tube. Feeding tubes can migrate or be improperly placed, which can lead to aspiration and poor tolerance. The use of a nasal bridle to secure a nasoenteric feeding tube is often used in children to prevent migration and dislodgement (**Figure 23.12**). Feeding tubes may also become clogged and should be checked for signs of occlusion. Fine bore tubes that are placed nasoenterically are more comfortable for the patient but pose a greater risk for occlusion.

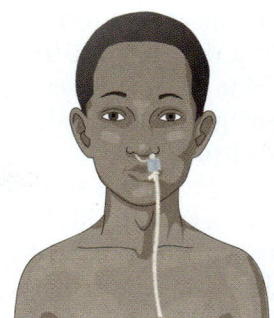

FIGURE 23.12 Nasal Bridle Used to Secure Nasoenteric Feeding Tube

Patients who begin nutrition support after a period of decreased intake are at risk for refeeding syndrome. These patients are prone to hypophosphatemia, hypokalemia, and hypomagnesemia. Physiologic alterations include tachycardia and fluid retention. Feedings are advanced slowly in the setting of refeeding syndrome. Initiating feeds at one-third of calorie goal and slowly advancing by one-third each day with monitoring of electrolytes is necessary in this setting.

Parenteral Nutrition

Parenteral nutrition may be indicated in pediatric patients who are unable to feed orally and do not tolerate enteral feedings. Indications for PN include short-bowel syndrome, pseudo-intestinal obstruction, and intestinal failure.[67] PN is also indicated in premature infants as their GI tract is underdeveloped. Critically ill children, children on extracorporeal membrane oxygenation, or those at nutritional risk may also require parenteral nutrition.[66]

Parenteral Access

Parenteral nutrition can be administered through a central or a peripheral line. A **central venous catheter** is placed with the catheter tip into the superior vena cava. Access through a main, central vein is often preferred as more concentrated solutions can be provided. Peripheral parenteral nutrition (PPN) is delivered via a smaller vein and is limited to 10% to 12% dextrose solutions. PPN cannot meet the nutritional needs of premature infants.

Energy Targets in Parenterally Fed Patients

For critically ill pediatric patients, the goal is set for maintenance, not growth. As such, pediatric patients can sometimes appear to have lower energy needs than when in health because they are not laying down new tissue or being physically active. Newborns who require PN need, at minimum, 75 kcal/kg/day for homeostasis. Infants in a thermoneutral environment require 50 kcal/kg/day for maintenance. Generally, the energy distribution in these patients should be 15% to 25% of total energy from protein, 30% to 40% of total energy from fat, and 50% to 60% of total energy from carbohydrates.

Commonly, predictive equations are used to determine the energy requirements of critically ill children. However, as in adults, these equations do not accurately estimate energy needs, given that many disease states produce variable metabolic responses. This can be particularly concerning in parenterally fed patients, where overfeeding and underfeeding lead to serious respiratory and hepatic complications.[66,70–72] Thus, use of indirect calorimetry is considered by A.S.P.E.N. to be the gold standard in determining the patient's energy expenditure.[66,74] Indirect calorimetry can estimate what substrates are being metabolized, as well as the resting energy expenditure of the individual.[75] A.S.P.E.N. states that patients who do not meet their calorie goals, fail to wean off respiratory support, require increased respiratory support, need muscle relaxants for 7 days, are hypermetabolic, or have an expected length of stay longer than 4 weeks in the intensive care unit are candidates for indirect calorimetry. In this context, patient populations who would benefit from indirect calorimetry include critically ill, ventilator-dependent, burn-injured patients; patients who are underweight or overweight; oncology patients; and those with neurological trauma.[76] If indirect calorimetry is not available, empiric formulas may be used.[66,77]

Carbohydrate Glucose should be the primary carbohydrate source for patients receiving PN. It is a preferred fuel source for the brain, red and white blood cells, and wounded tissue. Provision of intravenous dextrose blunts gluconeogenesis, thereby minimizing erosion of lean body mass. In children aged 0 to 2 years, who are highly reliant on glucose as their primary fuel source, intravenous dextrose should comprise a majority of calories. Intakes of at least 50% to 60% of total energy requirement are suggested. Likewise, intake can be based on the glucose infusion rate (GIR), which represents the amount of glucose that is oxidized. This varies according to age and weight of the child. The GIR is highest in young children, gradually declining to rates similar to adults by ages 2 to 5 years. The GIR must be about 2 mg/kg/min in order to prevent ketosis, but below 15 mg/kg/min to prevent hepatic steatosis and lipogenesis. **Table 23.17** summarizes the pediatric guidelines for glucose infusion. Notably, glucose oxidation can be altered due to malnutrition, stress, and overall composition of diet.[67,78]

Fat Intravenous lipid injectable emulsions (ILEs) offer the advantage of being energy dense and low in osmolality. Compared to dextrose as an energy source, they stimulate less carbon dioxide production. Lipid turnover and fatty acid oxidation are increased during critical illness in children, indicating that fat is a good source of energy in this setting. ILEs also provide essential fatty acids, even

TABLE 23.17 PEDIATRIC GIR (MG/KG/MIN) BY BODY WEIGHT[67,78]

Weight (kg)	Maximum Glucose Infusion Rate GIR (mg/kg/min)
<3	8.3
3 to 10	13
10 to 15	8.5
15 to 20	7
20 to 30	<9
<30	<7

in small amounts (5% of energy requirement from linoleic and linolenic fatty acids). For pediatric patients receiving PN, fat in general accounts for approximately 30% to 40% of energy intake. Infants can receive as little as 25% of their total calories from fat, or 2.5 to 3 g/kg/day. Older children with decreased fat needs may receive a higher percentage approximating 1.5 to 2.5 g/kg/day of fat. Energy intake from fat that exceeds 60% is associated with a risk of pulmonary complications, alteration in neutrophil function, aggregation of platelets, and mitochondrial defects.[77] Most ILE are soy based and thus higher in linoleic (omega-6) fatty acid. Because omega-6 fatty acids stimulate the production of inflammatory mediators, soy-based lipid emulsions are somewhat undesirable.[77]

Protein Protein is provided as amino acids in PN solutions. In infants, pediatric-specific formulations contain amino acid compositions that simulate the amino acid composition of human milk and can stimulate growth in non–critically ill patients. PN provision in neonates has added cysteine, which is conditionally essential in this population. A dose of 30 mg/day is recommended. Supplemental cysteine has been shown to have no added benefit in older children.

Protein needs vary based on age as well as disease state. During critical illness, amino acids are redistributed from the skeletal muscle to the liver and other organs for wound healing, immunity, and overall recovery. Typically, during critical illness and the stress response, the rates of protein breakdown exceed synthesis, placing children at high risk for prolonged negative nitrogen balance and catabolism. When protein losses are profound and occur in critical organs such as the heart and lungs, clinical manifestations take place that can hinder breathing and weaning from the mechanical ventilator. The recommended minimum amount of protein in critically ill children is 1.5 g/kg per day.[66] However, protein needs can be much higher, particularly in severe trauma or burn injury, rising to greater than 3 to 4 g/kg per day. Ultimately, protein targets should promote positive nitrogen balance. In neonates, 1.5 to 3 g/kg of protein are required. From ages 1 to 3 years, 2 to 3 g/kg of protein are necessary as a minimum, while older children require 1 to 2.5 g/kg of protein in PN solutions. Amino acid solutions should not exceed 4 g/kg to prevent azotemia.[79]

Fluid and Electrolytes In PN solutions, fluid and electrolytes are provided based on the clinical condition of the patient. Often, requirements are determined based on the biochemical indices, hydration, and clinical condition. Electrolyte management is best managed in IV fluids outside of the PN solution to avoid wasting solution once abnormalities are corrected. Table 23.18 summarizes the general electrolyte requirements in children.

Additives There are many micronutrients and medications that can be administered through a PN solution. Vitamin and trace element solutions are added to formulas. In patients younger than 11 years, pediatric vitamin mixes are provided based on the weight of the child. Similar to normal pediatric patients, calcium and phosphorus are both nutrients of concern because they are required for bone mineralization; however, their amounts are limited due to risk of precipitation. Deficiencies in zinc, selenium, and copper are common in patients receiving PN. Adequate levels of these minerals are necessary for development, as well as wound healing and immunity. Carnitine, an amino acid derivative, is required for lipid oxidation in patients receiving PN for more than 4 weeks. It can also benefit patients who have high triglycerides. Carnitine should be provided at a rate of 2 to 5 mg/kg/day.

TABLE 23.18 ELECTROLYTE REQUIREMENTS IN PEDIATRIC PATIENTS

Electrolyte	Infants and Children	Adolescents >50 kg
Sodium	2-5 mEq/kg	1-2 mEq/kg
Potassium	2-4 mEq/kg	1-2 mEq/kg
Calcium	0.5-4 mEq/kg 500-600 mg/L	10-20 mEq/day 200-400 mg/L
Phosphorus	0.5-2 mmol/kg 400-450 mg/L	10-40 mmol/day 150-300 mg/L
Magnesium	0.3-0.5 mEq/kg 50-70 mg/L	10-30 mEq/d 20-40 mg/L

Administration of Parenteral Nutrition

Parenteral nutrition can be administered continuously or cyclically. There are benefits and risks associated with both methods of administration. Continuous infusion of parenteral nutrition results in a continuous supply of glucose to the child, which causes constant release of insulin. It also allows for a lower osmotic load to be delivered to the patient. There are additional risks associated with continuous glucose infusion, however, such as the development of liver dysfunction, hepatomegaly, and parenteral nutrition–associated liver disease (PNALD).

Parenteral Nutrition–associated Liver Disease

PNALD is a difficult condition that affects from 30% to 70% of infants on PN, which is far higher than its prevalence in adults.[80] PNALD presents most commonly as cholestasis in children. Factors such as prematurity and low birth weight, short-bowel syndrome, bacterial overgrowth, decreased enterohepatic circulation, and lack of certain amino acids may be to blame. Length of time on PN is directly related to incidence of PNALD.[81,82] Currently in the forefront of understanding the etiology and treatment of PNALD is the lipid source used in parenteral solutions. Traditional ILE is soybean oil (SO) based, which is high in omega-6 fatty acids. Use of fish oil (FO)–based ILE is proven to decrease incidence of cholestasis and PNALD. The mechanism appears to be a reduction in cytokines and inflammatory mediators, due to a higher omega-3 fatty acid content. Use of FO-based ILE is also associated with reduced morbidity and mortality or need for liver transplant in children requiring longer term PN.[83–85]

> **PRACTICE POINT**
>
> Pediatric patients on parenteral nutrition support are at an increased risk for PNALD, so it is important to monitor children for signs of this condition.

Monitoring

Parenteral feeding needs to be closely monitored. In the critically ill pediatric patient, overfeeding and underfeeding can both be problematic. Overfeeding is sometimes difficult to observe given the ease at which PN can be provided with little signs of intolerance that would otherwise be seen with EN feedings. However, overfeeding of PN can negatively impact the liver, potentially resulting in hepatic steatosis. In addition, overfeeding results in increased carbon dioxide production, making it difficult to wean off of the ventilator. Exacerbation of hyperglycemia, a common problem during metabolic stress, is another risk of overfeeding with PN. Underfeeding is equally problematic because patients present with a negative nitrogen balance, malnutrition, and impaired immunity. In addition, increased catabolism, accelerated

> ## ⚠ Clinical Controversy
>
> ### IV Lipid Emulsions in Intestinal Failure–associated Liver Disease
>
> PN is required in children with intestinal failure (IF). IF can be caused by short bowel syndrome or dysfunctional bowel due to necrotizing enterocolitis and a number of congenital diseases of the gastrointestinal system. The incidence of IF in children is 3 to 5 per 100,000 cases. PN is necessary in supporting these children during bowel adaptation until enteral nutrition can be tolerated. Unfortunately, the process of bowel adaptation is lengthy and may take months to years to occur. During this time, IF-associated liver disease (IFALD) is a common complication. The primary consequence of IFALD is cholestasis, which in some patients leads to end-stage liver disease and the need for liver transplant. Research shows that replacement of soybean oil (SO) with fish oil (FO) reduces the effects of IFALD. Several studies describe the potential benefits of FO ILE as decreased inflammation, improvement in the lipid panel, decreased bilirubin levels, and reversal of PNALD.[84–86] Calkins et al.[87] report that 75% of infants receiving FO versus 6% receiving SO have resolution of cholestasis. However, intravenous FO therapy is not yet approved by the FDA. Lacking this therapeutic option, researchers have looked at the efficacy of reducing the administration of SO ILE to less than 1 g/kg/d. Calkins et al.[88] demonstrated that giving low-dose SO at 1 g/kg/day versus conventional SO at 3 g/kg/day was also associated with decreased levels of conjugated bilirubin without impacting growth parameters. This raises the question of whether lower doses of SO ILE could be sufficient in treatment and prevention of ILALD. Given the cost and lack of FDA approval, this could be valuable therapeutic option to FO ILE.
>
> The recent introduction of composite lipid emulsions that contain less soybean oil (30%) and inclusion of medium chain triglycerides (30%), olive oil (25%), and fish oil (15%) has brought yet another alternative for treating and preventing ILALD. Diamond et al.[89] demonstrate a reduction in IFALD in patients receiving composite lipid versus conventional SO ILE. This is contrary to a case report by Lee et al.[90] where ILALD only improved when using solely FO. Controversy therefore remains as to whether the best treatment and prevention of IFALD lies in monotherapy with FO as the sole lipid source, reduction in SO lipid, or a combined approach where SO is reduced and FO is given.
>
> ### Question
>
> 1. Evaluate the type and strength of the studies described above. What is your opinion on the ideal approach to treating and preventing ILALD in children with intestinal failure?
>
> ### References
>
> 1. Calkins KL, Dunn JC, Shew SB, Reyen L, Farmer D, Devaskar SU, Venick RS. Pediatric intestinal failure associated liver disease is reversed in 6 months with intravenous fish oil. *J Parenter Enteral Nutr.* 2014; 38(6):682–692.
> 2. Calkins KL, Havraneck T, Kelley-Quon LI, Cerny L, Flores M, Grogan T, Shew SB. Low-dose parenteral soybean oil for the prevention of parenteral associated liver disease in neonate with gastrointestinal disorders: A multicenter randomized controlled pilot study. *J Parenter Enteral Nutr.* 2017; 41(3):404–411.
> 3. Diamond IR, Grant RC, Pencharz PB, et al. Preventing the progression of intestinal failure-associated liver disease in infants using a composite lipid emulsion: a pilot randomized controlled trial of SMOFlipid. *J Parenter Enteral Nutr.* 2017;41(5):866–877.
> 4. Lee S, Park HJ, Yoon J, et al. Reversal of intestinal failure-associated liver disease by switching from a combination lipid emulsion containing fish oil to fish oil monotherapy. *J Parenter Enteral Nutr.* 2016;40(3):437–440.

loss of LBM, and respiratory muscle mass loss all result from underfeeding.[76,77,91] Clinicians wishing to avoid the negative consequences of overfeeding PN may be overly judicious in providing adequate calories. Likewise, given the risk of ILE as described above, lipids are sometimes omitted. Routine assessment of nutritional parameters such as weight, nitrogen balance, and healing is useful to assure patients are being fed adequately.

Monitoring of electrolytes and other biochemical parameters are important in PN-fed children. **Table 23.19** shows a recommended schedule in PN-fed patients. Often, because these patients are critically ill, many of these parameters are monitored as part of acute care management. It is therefore important not to duplicate lab monitoring to avoid excess blood loss with multiple blood draws.

Immunonutrition in Nutrition Support of Children

Given the paucity of data and potential harm of immune-modulating nutrients as evidenced in adults, A.S.P.E.N. currently does not recommend use of immune-enhancing nutrients in children.[66] The most common nutrients studied, either alone or in combination, are glutamine,

TABLE 23.19 BIOCHEMICAL MONITORING OF CHILDREN RECEIVING PN

Biochemical Indices	Monitoring Schedule
Electrolytes Calcium (ionized), phosphorus, magnesium	Prior to PN; every 6 hours after the initiation of PN; then daily
Glucose	Prior to PN; every 6 hours after the initiation of PN; then daily *Requires more frequent monitoring with insulin therapy*
Liver function tests	Weekly
Triglycerides	Prior to initiating IVLE; then weekly
Urinary urea nitrogen	Weekly
Blood urea nitrogen, creatinine	Daily
Amylase, lipase	Weekly

arginine, omega-3 fatty acids, and antioxidants such as selenium. An overview of the rationale for use and current findings is provided below.

Glutamine

Glutamine is involved in immune response, metabolic function, and tissue production; however, it is a conditionally essential amino acid during the inflammatory response. It is thought that glutamine may improve outcomes when administered during critical illness.[92,93] However, in a meta-analysis, glutamine supplementation was not proven to have a benefit on pediatric patients with severe gastrointestinal disease.[94] Similarly, in a randomized control trial of children receiving PN for greater than 5 days, no significant reduction in inflammatory markers was found.[95] There is limited research to support the use of glutamine supplementation in nutritional support of the pediatric population.

Arginine

Like glutamine, arginine plays a critical role in the body. Arginine is a precursor to growth hormone–promoting anabolism. It is also a precursor to nitric oxide, which in proper doses can be effective for bronchial dilation and respiratory mechanics. However, there is limited research to support the supplementation of arginine in critically ill children.[96] Knowledge, for the most part, is extrapolated from research in critically ill adults. Because arginine has the potential to do harm in hemodynamically unstable patients, there may be negative consequences to supplementation, so it is not recommended for the pediatric population.[97]

Omega-3 Fatty Acids

Omega-3 fatty acids are hypothesized to have immune benefits for critically ill patients. Apart from research described above in PNALD, where omega-3 fatty acids in ILE decrease release of pro-inflammatory cytokines, their clinical benefit is lacking. Omega-3 fatty acids provided in combination with antioxidants and other immune-enhancing nutrients to children with respiratory failure, to date, do not show improved clinical outcome.[66]

Overall, the use of immunonutrition in pediatric nutrition support formulations is not consistently recommended.[47,64,93] Research indicates that immune-enhanced formulas may provide better nutritional markers, but do not have an impact on key endpoints such as length of hospital stay or mortality. Further research needs to be done to better understand the impact of these factors in hard clinical outcomes.

Chapter Summary

Childhood is a time of growth and development that requires adequate nutritional status. Nutrition assessment in the pediatric patient revolves around assessment of growth patterns and their etiology. Diet history and a nutrition-focused physical exam are key components of a nutritional assessment as well. Evaluating social factors, including parental education, nutrition beliefs, and socioeconomic status can guide nutrition interventions. As children grow and develop, nutritional risk factors and concerns vary. Nutrient concerns will change. Focus on calcium, iron, and vitamin D is often needed.

As a result of the changes in body composition experienced during childhood, children are at the greatest risk for malnutrition. Nutrition support therapies such as enteral and parenteral nutrition can prevent and reverse signs of malnutrition in this population. However, instances of malnutrition still remain. Failure to thrive is problematic in the first 3 years of life, and must be treated using an interprofessional approach.

Key Terms

growth, growth channels, growth velocity, adiposity rebound, serial measures, mid-parental height, head circumference, microcephaly, macrocephaly, growth charts, WHO growth charts, CDC growth charts, growth standards, growth reference, z-scores, underweight, weight-for-age, height-for-age, stunting, wasting, weight-for-height, colostrum, pediatric malnutrition, failure to thrive, organic FTT, nonorganic FTT, catch-up growth

References

1. Marcdante KJ, Kliegman R, Nelson WE. *Nelson essentials of pediatrics*. 7th ed. Philadelphia, PA: Elsevier/Saunders; 2015.
2. Cole TJ. The development of growth references and growth charts. *Ann Hum Biol*. 2012;39(5):382-394.
3. Fomon SJ, Haschke F, Ziegler EE, Nelson SE. Body composition of reference children from birth to age 10 years. *Am J Clin Nutr*. 1982;35(suppl):1169-1175.
4. Forbes GE. Human body composition. *Growth, aging, nutrition, and activity*. 12th ed. Boston, MA: Springer-Valeg; 2012.
5. Tori-Romos T, Paley C, Pi-Sunyer FX, Gallager D. Body composition during fetal development and infancy through the age of 5 years. *Nutrition*. 2015;69:1279-1289. doi:10.1038/ejcn.2015.117.
6. Whitaker RC, Pepe MS, Wright JA, Seidel KD, Dietz WH. Early adiposity rebound and the risk of adult obesity. *Pediatrics*. 1998;101(3):E5.
7. Abbassi V. Growth and normal puberty. *Pediatrics*. 1998;102(2 Pt 3):507-511.
8. Williams SM, Goulding A. Patterns of growth associated with the timing of adiposity rebound. *Obesity* (Silver Spring). 2009;17(2):335-341.
9. Wright CM, Cheetham TD. The strengths and limitations of parental heights as a predictor of attained height. *Arch Dis Child*. 1999;81(3):257-260.
10. Sniderman A. Abnormal head growth. *Pediatr Rev*. 2010;31(9):382:384.
11. World Health Organization. Training Course on Child Growth Assessment. Geneva, WHO, 2008.
12. Ogden CL, Flegal KM. Changes in terminology for childhood overweight and obesity. *Natl Health Stat Report*. 2010;(25):1-5.
13. Division of Nutrition, Physical Activity and Obesity, National Center for Chronic Disease Prevention and Health Promotion. Defining childhood obesity. Centers for Disease Control and Prevention Web site. http://www.cdc.gov/obesity/childhood/defining.html. Updated 2015. Accessed April 4, 2016.
14. Secker DJ, Jeejeebhoy KN. How to perform subjective global nutritional assessment in children. *J Acad Nutr Diet*. 2012;112(3):424-431.e6.
15. Sonneville K, Duggan C, eds. *Manual of pediatric nutrition*. 5th ed. Shelton, CT: People's Medical Publishing House; 2014.
16. de Onis M, Garza C, Onyango AW, Borghi E. Comparison of the WHO child growth standards and the CDC 2000 growth charts. *J Nutr*. 2007;137(1):144-148.
17. Grummer-Strawn LM, Reinold C, Krebs NF, Centers for Disease Control and Prevention (CDC). Use of World Health Organization and CDC growth charts for children aged 0–59 months in the United States. *MMWR Rec Rep*. 2010;59(RR–9):1-15.
18. Ogden CL, Kuczmarski RJ, Flegal KM, et al. Centers for Disease Control and Prevention 2000 growth charts for the United States: Improvements to the 1977 National Center for Health Statistics Version. *Pediatrics*. 2002;109(1):45-60.
19. Kuczmarski RJ, Ogden CL, Guo SS, et al. 2000 CDC growth charts for the United States: Methods and development. *Vital Health Stat 11*. 2002;(246)(246):1-190.
20. Dibley MJ, Staehling N, Nieburg P, Trowbridge FL. Interpretation of Z-score anthropometric indicators derived from the international growth reference. *Am J Clin Nutr*. 1987;46(5):749-762.
21. Becker PJ, Nieman Carney L, Corkins MR, et al. Consensus statement of the Academy of Nutrition and Dietetics/American Society for Parenteral and Enteral nutrition: Indicators recommended for the identification and documentation of pediatric malnutrition (undernutrition). *J Acad Nutr Diet*. 2014;114(12):1988-2000.
22. Holt KA. *Bright futures: Nutrition*. 3rd ed. Elk Grove Village: American Academy of Pediatrics; 2011:278.
23. Cooke LJ, Wardle J, Gibson EL, Sapochnik M, Sheiham A, Lawson M. Demographic, familial and trait predictors of fruit and vegetable consumption by pre-school children. *Public Health Nutr*. 2004;7(2):295-302.
24. Briefel RR, Reidy K, Karwe V, Devaney B. Feeding infants and toddlers study: Improvements needed in meeting infant feeding recommendations. *J Am Diet Assoc*. 2004;104(1 Suppl 1):s31-7.
25. Loth KA, MacLehose RF, Fulkerson JA, Crow S, Neumark-Sztainer D. Are food restriction and pressure-to-eat parenting practices associated with adolescent disordered eating behaviors? *Int J Eat Disord*. 2014;47(3):310-314.
26. Green Corkins K. Nutrition-focused physical examination in pediatric patients. *Nutr Clin Pract*. 2015;30(2):203-209.
27. Radler DR, Lister T. Nutrient deficiencies associated with nutrition-focused physical findings of the oral cavity. *Nutr Clin Pract*. 2013;28(6):710-721.
28. Touger-Decker R, Mobley C, Academy of Nutrition and Dietetics. Position of the Academy of Nutrition and Dietetics: Oral health and nutrition. *J Acad Nutr Diet*. 2013;113(5):693-701.
29. Baker R, Greer FR. Diagnosis and prevention of iron deficiency and iron-deficiency anemia in infants and young children (0-3 years of age). *Pediatrics*. 2010;126(5).
30. Gibson RS, Heath AL, Szymlek-Gay EA. Is iron and zinc nutrition a concern for vegetarian infants and young children in industrialized countries? *Am J Clin Nutr*. 2014;100 Suppl 1:459S–68S.
31. Academy of Nutrition and Dietetics. Pediatric Nutrition Care Manual. Full Term Infants.https://www.nutritioncaremanual.org/topic.cfm?ncm_category_id=12&lv1=144610&ncm_toc_id=144610&ncm_heading=&. Accessed August 19, 2017.
32. Nofal AA, Schwenk WF. Growth failure in children. A symptom or disease? *Nutr Clin Prac*. 2013;28(6):651-658.
33. US Department of Health and Human Services, US Department of Agriculture. 2015-2020 Dietary Guidelines for Americans. 2015.
34. Ogata BN, Hayes D. Position of the Academy of Nutrition and Dietetics: Nutrition guidance for healthy children ages 2 to 11 years. *J Acad Nutr Diet*. 2014;114(8):1257-1276.
35. A Report of the Panel on Macronutrients, Subcommittees on Upper Reference Levels of Nutrients and Interpretation and Uses of Dietary Reference Intakes, Standing Committee on the Scientific Evaluation of Dietary Reference Intakes, Food and Nutrition Board, Institute of Medicine. Chapter 3: Energy. In: *Dietary reference intakes for energy, carbohydrate, fiber, fat, fatty acids, cholesterol, protein, and amino acids (macronutrients)*. 2005:53.
36. National Research Council (US) Subcommittee on the Tenth Edition of the Recommended Dietary Allowances. 3, Energy. In: *Recommended dietary allowances*. 10th ed. Washington, DC: National Academies Press; 1989.
37. National Research Council (US) Subcommittee on the Tenth Edition of the Recommended Dietary Allowances. Chapter 6, Protein and Amino Acids. In: *Recommended Dietary Allowances*. 10th ed. Washington, DC: National Academies Press; 1989.
38. US Department of Agriculture, Agricultural Research Service. Nutrient intakes from food and beverages: Mean amounts consumed per individual, by gender and age. What we eat in America: NHANES 2013-2014. 2016.

39. American Academy of Pediatrics. Breastfeeding and the use of human milk. *Pediatrics*. 2012; 129(3): e827–e841. Accessed November 19, 2017 from http://pediatrics.aappublications.org/content/129/3/e827.full.pdf+html
40. Andreas NJ, Kampmann B, Mehring Le-Doare K. Human breast milk: A review on its composition and bioactivity. *Early Hum Dev*. 2015;91(11):629-635.
41. Vandenplas Y, Zakharova I, Dmitrieva Y. Oligosaccharides in infant formula: More evidence to validate the role of prebiotics. *Br J Nutr*. 2015;113(9):1339-1344.
42. Lonnerdal B. Infant formula and infant nutrition: Bioactive proteins of human milk and implications for composition of infant formulas. *Am J Clin Nutr*. 2014;99(3):712S–7S.
43. Joeckel RJ, Phillips SK. Overview of infant and pediatric formulas. *Nutr Clin Pract*. 2009;24(3):356-362.
44. Committee on Nutrition. Iron fortification of infant formulas. *Pediatrics*. 1999;104(1):February 20, 2016-119-123.
45. Quinn EA. Too much of a good thing: Evolutionary perspectives on infant formula fortification in the United States and its effects on infant health. *Am J Hum Biol*. 2014;26(1):10-17.
46. Mugambi MN, Musekiwa A, Lombard M, Young T, Blaauw R. Probiotics, prebiotics infant formula use in preterm or low birth weight infants: A systematic review. *Nutr J*. 2012;11:58-2891-11-58.
47. Vandenplas Y, De Greef E, Veereman G. Prebiotics in infant formula. *Gut Microbes*. 2014;5(6):681-687.
48. Arslanoglu S, Moro GE, Boehm G. Early supplementation of prebiotic oligosaccharides protects formula-fed infants against infections during the first 6 months of life. *J Nutr*. 2007;137(11):2420-2424.
49. Ashley C, Johnston WH, Harris CL, Stolz SI, Wampler JL, Berseth CL. Growth and tolerance of infants fed formula supplemented with polydextrose (PDX) and/or galactooligosaccharides (GOS): Double-blind, randomized, controlled trial. *Nutr J*. 2012;11:38.
50. Committee on Nutrition of the American Academy of Pediatrics. Complementary feeding. In: Kleinman RE, ed. *Pediatric nutrition handbook*. 6th ed. Elk Grove Village, IL: AAP; 2009:113.
51. American Academy of Pediatrics Committee on Nutrition: The use of whole cow's milk in infancy. *Pediatrics*. 1992;89(6 Pt 1):1105-1109.
52. Cox N, Hinkle R. Infant botulism. *Am Fam Physician*. 2002;65(7):1388-1392.
53. Corkins M, ed. *A.S.P.E.N. Pediatric Nutrition Support Core Curriculum*. 2nd ed. Silver Springs, MD: A.S.P.E.N; 2015.
54. Frankel LA, Hughes SO, O'Connor TM, Power TG, Fisher JO, Hazen NL. Parental influences on children's self-regulation of energy intake: Insights from developmental literature on emotion regulation. *J Obes*. 2012;2012:327259.
55. Fink SK, Racine EF, Mueffelmann RE, Dean MN, Herman-Smith R. Family meals and diet quality among children and adolescents in North Carolina. *J Nutr Educ Behav*. 2014;46(5):418-422.
56. Loth KA, MacLehose RF, Larson N, Berge JM, Neumark-Sztainer D. Food availability, modeling and restriction: How are these different aspects of the family eating environment related to adolescent dietary intake? *Appetite*. 2016;96:80-86.
57. Larson N, MacLehose R, Fulkerson JA, Berge JM, Story M, Neumark-Sztainer D. Eating breakfast and dinner together as a family: Associations with sociodemographic characteristics and implications for diet quality and weight status. *J Acad Nutr Diet*. 2013;113(12):1601-1609.
58. Neumark-Sztainer D, Wall M, Fulkerson JA, Larson N. Changes in the frequency of family meals from 1999 to 2010 in the homes of adolescents: Trends by sociodemographic characteristics. *J Adolesc Health*. 2013;52(2):201-206.
59. Woodruff SJ, Campbell K, Campbell T, Cole M. The associations of meals and snacks on family meals among a sample of grade 7 students from southwestern Ontario. *Appetite*. 2014;82:61-66.
60. Neumark-Sztainer D, Hannan PJ, Story M, Croll J, Perry C. Family meal patterns: Associations with sociodemographic characteristics and improved dietary intake among adolescents. *J Am Diet Assoc*. 2003;103(3):317-322.
61. Zubatsky M, Berge J, Neumark-Sztainer D. Longitudinal associations between parenting style and adolescent disordered eating behaviors. *Eat Weight Disord*. 2015;20(2):187-194.
62. Mehta NM, Corkins MR, Lyman B, et al. Defining pediatric malnutrition: A paradigm shift toward etiology-related definitions. *J Parenter Enteral Nutr*. 2013;37(4):460-481.
63. Atalay A, McCord M. Characteristics of failure to thrive in a referral population: Implications for treatment. *Clin Pediatr*. 2012;51(3):219.
64. Cole SZ, Lanham JS. Failure to thrive: An update. *Am Fam Physician*. 2011;83(7):829-834.
65. Prieto MB, Cid JL. Malnutrition in the critically ill child: The importance of enteral nutrition. *Int J Environ Res Public Health*. 2011;8(11):4353-4366.
66. Mehta NM, Skillman HE, Irving SY, Cass-Bu J, Vermilyea S, Farringorn EA, Mckeever L, Hall AM, Goday PS, Braunschweig C. Guidelines for the provision and assessment of nutrition support therapy in pediatric critically ill patient: Society of Critical Care Medicine and American Society for Parenteral and Enteral Nutrition. *J Parenter Enteral Nutr*. 2017;4(5):706-742.
67. A.S.P.E.N. Pediatric Nutrition Support Core Curriculum. 2nd ed. Corkins. Silver Spring, MD;2015.
68. Vermilyea S, Goh VL. Enteral feedings in children: Sorting out tubes, buttons, and formulas. *Nutr Clin Pract*. 2016;31(1):59-67.
69. Martinez EE, Pereira LM, Gura K, Stenquist N, Ariagno K, Nurko S, Mehta NM. Gastric emptying in critically ill children. *J Parenter and Enteral Nutr*. 2017; 41(7):1100-1109.
70. Blaser AR, Starkopf J, Kirsimagi U, Deane AM. Definition, prevalence, and outcome of feeding intolerance in intensive care: A systematic review and meta-analysis. *Acta Anaesthesiol Scand*. 2014;58(8):914-922.
71. Hardy CM, Dwyer J, Snelling LK, Dallal GE, Adelson JW. Pitfalls in predicting resting energy requirements in critically ill children: A comparison of predictive methods to indirect calorimetry. *Nutr Clin Pract*. 2002;17(3):182-189.
72. Sion-Sarid R, Cohen J, Houri Z, Singer P. Indirect calorimetry: A guide for optimizing nutritional support in the critically ill child. *Nutrition*. 2013;29(9):1094-1099.
73. Coss-Bu JA, Jefferson LS, Walding D, David Y, Smith EO, Klish WJ. Resting energy expenditure in children in a pediatric intensive care unit: Comparison of Harris Benedict and Talbot predictions with indirect calorimetry values. *Am J Clin Nutr*. 1998;67(1):74-80.
74. Dokken M, Rustoen T, Stubhaug A. Indirect calorimetry reveals that better monitoring of nutrition therapy in pediatric intensive care is needed. *J Parenter Enteral Nutr*. 2015;39(3):344-352.
75. McClave SA, Lowen CC, Kleber MJ, McConnell JW, Jung LY, Goldsmith LJ. Clinical use of the respiratory quotient obtained from indirect calorimetry. *J Parenter Enteral Nutr*. 2003;27(1):21-26.
76. Mehta NM, Bechard LJ, Leavitt K, Duggan C. Cumulative energy imbalance in the pediatric intensive care unit: Role of targeted indirect calorimetry. *J Parenter Enteral Nutr*. 2009;33(3):336-344.

77. Kyle UG, Arriaza A, Esposito M, Coss-Bu JA. Is indirect calorimetry a necessity or a luxury in the pediatric intensive care unit? *J Parenter Enteral Nutr.* 2012;36(2):177-182.

78. Guidelines on pediatric parenteral nutrition. *J Pediatr Gastroenterology Nutr.* 2005;41:S28–S32.

79. Mehta NM, Compher C, A.S.P.E.N. Board of Directors. A.S.P.E.N. Clinical Guidelines: Nutrition support of the critically ill child. *J Parenter Enteral Nutr.* 2009;33(3):260-276.

80. Kumpf VJ. Parenteral nutrition-associated liver disease in adult and pediatric patients. *Nutr Clin Pract.* 2006;21(3):279-290.

81. Lauriti G, Zani A, Aufieri R, et al. Incidence, prevention, and treatment of parenteral nutrition-associated cholestasis and intestinal failure-associated liver disease in infants and children: A systematic review. *J Parenter Enteral Nutr.* 2014;38(1):70-85.

82. Koseesirikul P, Chotinaruemol S, Ukarapol N. Incidence and risk factors of parenteral nutrition-associated liver disease in newborn infants. *Pediatr Int.* 2012;54(3):434-436.

83. Nandivada P, Fell GL, Gura KM, Puder M. Lipid emulsions in the treatment and prevention of parenteral nutrition-associated liver disease in infants and children. *Am J Clin Nutr.* 2016;103(2):629S–634S.

84. Calkins KL, DeBarber A, Steiner RD, et al. Intravenous fish oil and pediatric intestinal failure–associated liver disease: changes in plasma phytosterols, cytokines, and bile acids and erythrocyte fatty acids. *J Parenter Enteral Nutr.* 2017. [Epub ahead of print] doi: /10.1177/0148607117709196

85. Nandivada P, Fell GL, Mitchell PD, et al. Long-term fish oil lipid emulsion use in children with intestinal failure–associated liver disease. *J Parenter Enteral Nutr.* 2017;41(6):930-937. http://dx.doi.org/10.1177%2F0148607116633796

86. Lee SI, Valim C, Johnston P, et al. Impact of fish oil-based lipid emulsion on serum triglyceride, bilirubin, and albumin levels in children with parenteral nutrition-associated liver disease. *Pediatr Res.* 2009;66(6):698-703.

87. Calkins KL, Dunn JC, Shew SB, Reyen L, Farmer D, Devaskar SU, Venick RS. Pediatric intestinal failure associated liver disease is reversed in 6 months with intravenous fish oil. *J Parenter Enteral Nutr.* 2014; 38(6):682-692.

88. Calkins KL, Havraneck T, Kelley-Quon LI, Cerny L, Flores M, Grogan T, Shew SB. Low-dose parenteral soybean oil for the prevention of parenteral associated liver disease in neonate with gastrointestinal disorders: A multicenter randomized controlled pilot study. *J Parenter Enteral Nutr.* 2017; 41(3):404-411.

89. Diamond IR, Grant RC, Pencharz PB, et al. Preventing the progression of intestinal failure-associated liver disease in infants using a composite lipid emulsion: a pilot randomized controlled trial of SMOFlipid. *J Parenter Enteral Nutr.* 2017;41(5):866-877. doi: 10.1177/0148607115626921.

90. Lee S, Park HJ, Yoon J, et al. Reversal of intestinal failure-associated liver disease by switching from a combination lipid emulsion containing fish oil to fish oil monotherapy. *J Parenter Enteral Nutr.* 2016;40(3):437-440. doi: 10.1177/0148607114567200. Epub 2015 Jan 5.

91. Mehta NM, Bechard LJ, Dolan M, Ariagno K, Jiang H, Duggan C. Energy imbalance and the risk of overfeeding in critically ill children. *Pediatr Crit Care Med.* 2011;12(4):398-405.

92. Mok E, Hankard R. Glutamine supplementation in sick children: Is it beneficial? *J Nutr Metab.* 2011;2011:617597.

93. Zhou YP, Jiang ZM, Sun YH, Wang XR, Ma EL, Wilmore D. The effect of supplemental enteral glutamine on plasma levels, gut function, and outcome in severe burns: A randomized, double-blind, controlled clinical trial. *J Parenter Enteral Nutr.* 2003;27(4):241-245.

94. Brown JV, Moe-Byrne T, McGuire W. Glutamine supplementation for young infants with severe gastrointestinal disease. *Cochrane Database Syst Rev.* 2014;12:CD005947.

95. Jordan I, Balaguer M, Esteban ME, et al. Glutamine effects on heat shock protein 70 and interleukines 6 and 10: Randomized trial of glutamine supplementation versus standard parenteral nutrition in critically ill children. *Clin Nutr.* 2016;35(1):34-40.

96. Argaman Z, Young VR, Noviski N, et al. Arginine and nitric oxide metabolism in critically ill septic pediatric patients. *Crit Care Med.* 2003;31(2):591-597.

97. Zhou M, Martindale RG. Arginine in the critical care setting. *J Nutr.* 2007;137(6 Suppl 2):1687S–1692S.

Chapter 24

Nutritional Management of Childhood Obesity

Adi Goldberg
Ashley Abbott
Kathy Prelack

Chapter Outline

Core Concepts
Introduction
Prevalence
Defining Childhood Obesity
Childhood Obesity and Medical Comorbidities
Other Comorbidities: Orthopedic, Dental, and Nonalcoholic Fatty Liver

Psychological Effects of Childhood Obesity
Factors Associated with Childhood Obesity
Assessment, Management, and Intervention
Intervention Approaches
Surgical Intervention

CORE CONCEPTS

1. The medical and psychosocial comorbidities associated with childhood obesity present unique challenges to the healthcare provider in the prevention, diagnosis, and treatment of this disease.

2. Childhood obesity is associated with many of the risk factors for cardiovascular disease, including high blood pressure, high cholesterol and poor glycemic control that could eventually lead to diabetes.

3. Overweight and obese children are at an increased risk for multiple risk factors associated with cardiac dysfunction, increasing the likelihood of CVD progression with age.

4. Type 2 diabetes in children and adolescents is associated with early onset of micro- and macrovascular complications and increased risk of mortality in middle age, making prevention of this disease extremely important.

5. Obese children and adolescents who seek medical treatment for obesity have demonstrated elevated rates of depression, anxiety, social anxiety, loneliness, and preference for isolative activities.

6. The etiology of childhood obesity is multifactorial; individual factors, social factors, and environmental factors all play a role in a child's health status.

7. For successful weight loss, it is recommended to introduce children to healthy eating and behavioral patterns instead of placing them on calorie-restricted diets, which may set them up for failure and future weight gain.
8. Behavioral change in children can be achieved by employing motivational interviewing during counseling, providing positive reinforcement from the child's support system, and identifying cues that lead to unhealthy behaviors.
9. Three procedures that are recommended for weight loss in adolescents include the adjustable gastric binding procedure, the Roux en Y gastric bypass, and the sleeve gastrectomy.

Learning Objectives

1. Define childhood obesity and list the available indicators used by health practitioners to assess obesity, along with the pros and cons to each of them.
2. Learn the pathophysiology of childhood obesity and related medical comorbidities.
3. Recognize the potential psychological effects that obesity and weight gain can have on children.
4. Understand the etiology of childhood obesity and the interplay of multifactorial aspects, particularly with the growing field of nutrigenomics.
5. Explore the different models of nutritional care and intervention used for childhood obesity.
6. Learn about the different techniques used for behavioral intervention with obese children and the correlation between BMI and the development of mental health conditions.
7. Discuss the significance of childhood obesity prevention and the most recent Centers for Disease Control and Prevention (CDC) guidelines.
8. Identify the different types of weight loss surgical procedures that are safe and available for children.

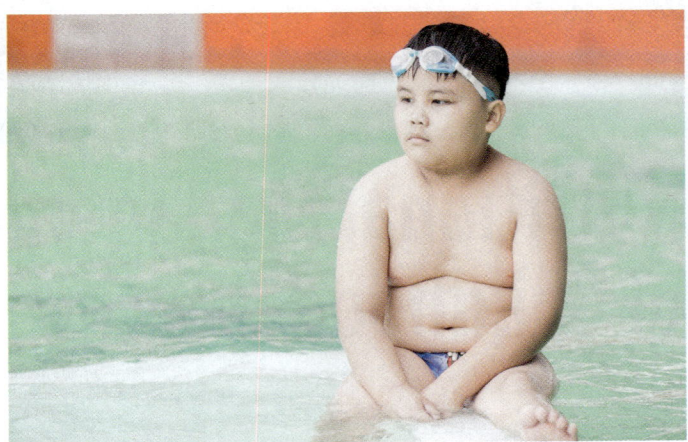
©kwanchai.c/Shutterstock.

Introduction

Childhood obesity is a significant health problem in the United States and a major focus of many public health efforts. The medical and psychosocial comorbidities associated with childhood obesity present unique challenges to the healthcare provider in the prevention, diagnosis, and treatment of this disease. The etiology of childhood obesity varies among individuals; however, numerous genetic and environmental factors have been identified as key risk factors for this disease. Medical nutrition therapy is indicated in the prevention, treatment, and management of childhood obesity.

CORE CONCEPT 1

The medical and psychosocial comorbidities associated with childhood obesity present unique challenges to the healthcare provider in the prevention, diagnosis, and treatment of this disease.

Prevalence

Childhood obesity is an extremely common childhood disease, affecting 12.7 million children and adolescents. Although its prevalence has remained fairly stable, at 17%, over the past decade, and has even declined in children aged 2 to 5 years, it continues to be a problem for older children and particular subgroups of our population.[1,2] According to the 2013 Heart Disease and Stroke Statistics Update, 23.9 million (31.8%) children aged 2 to 19 years are overweight.[3] **Figure 24.1** shows the obesity prevalence in children and adolescents from 1999/2000-2013/2014. The U.S. Preventative Services Task Force recommends that clinicians screen for obesity in children 6 years or older with intensive behavioral interventions to promote weight regulation when indicated.[4]

Defining Childhood Obesity

A unique challenge presented in the pediatric population when considering obesity is how to identify and define it. The determination of obesity for children in the United States is typically made using the 2000 CDC body mass index (BMI) sex- and age-specific charts. These BMI charts illustrate the distribution of BMI in U.S. children aged 2 to 20 years using percentile curves, allowing healthcare providers to track an individual's height and weight over time. These charts are useful when considering increasing or decreasing trends in a patient's weight.[5]

CASE STUDY INTRODUCTION

Nora is a 14-year-old female referred to you for medical nutrition therapy by her primary care provider (PCP). Nora has gained over 20 pounds this past year. Her PCP is concerned that with continuous weight gain and high low-density lipoprotein (LDL)/triglyceride levels, Nora will develop type 2 diabetes and chronic cardiac disease. Nora came to her initial appointment with her mother, who is morbidly obese. At the initial meeting, Nora explained that her favorite foods include fast-food options and processed desserts such as Yodels and cinnamon buns. Nora does very little physical activity during the week and claims that she does not find any enjoyment from exercise.

Anthropometric Data:
Height: 165 cm (64")
Weight: 85 kg (187 lb)
BMI: 31 kg/m2
Waist circumference: 101.6 cm (40")

Biochemical Data:
Total cholesterol 275 mg/dL (Desirable: <200 mg/dL)
Low-density lipoprotein cholesterol (LDL-C) 145 mg/dL (Desirable: <100 mg/dL)
High-density lipoprotein cholesterol (HDL-C) 22 mg/dL (Desirable: ≥40 mg/dL)
Triglycerides 220 mg/dL (Desirable: <150 mg/dL)
Glycated hemoglobin A1C 6.0% (4.3-5.8%)
Fasting blood sugar 115 mg/dL (70-99 mg/dL)

Clinical Data:
Past Medical History: Asthma, prehypertension, prediabetes
Medications: Sertraline (anxiety), corticosteroids (asthma)
Vital Signs: Blood pressure 140/90 mm Hg; Temperature 97.5°F; Heart rate 80 beats/min
Nutrition-focused Physical Exam: Appears well nourished. Adiposity consistent with android body type. Oral exam, hair, and nails appear normal. Skin is warm and intact. No evidence of acanthosis nigricans. Abdominal exam unremarkable. No evidence of lower or upper extremity edema.

Dietary Data:
24-hour Diet Recall:
Breakfast (7 am): 2 bowls of Cocoa Puffs, whole milk, 1 cup of orange juice, 1 Pop-Tart
Snack (10 am): 1 bag of Chex Mix, 8 to 10 mini Oreos, 8 oz of chocolate milk
Lunch (12:30 pm): 1 hamburger with bun with ketchup and mayonnaise, French fries, steamed peas and carrots, 1 bag of potato chips, 1 medium soda (Nora receives school lunch)
Snack (4 pm): 2 Eggo chocolate chip waffles, 1 mini bag of Cheez-it crackers
Dinner: 2 bowls of boxed macaroni and cheese, 1 Italian roll, steamed green beans, 1 can of Dr. Pepper, 1 brownie for dessert
Pre-bedtime snack: 1 bowl of vanilla ice cream with whipped cream and Hershey's chocolate chips

Questions

1. Plot Nora's data on the Centers for Disease Control and Prevention (CDC) growth chart. In what percentile is her weight-for-age? Height-for-age? BMI-for age? sex?
2. Does this information classify Nora as underweight, normal weight, overweight, or obese?
3. What risk factors does Nora have for diabetes and cardiovascular disease (CVD)?
4. Access Nora's diet recall. What recommendations can be made to improve her diet?
5. Identify a nutrition intervention to help improve Nora's lipid panels.
6. Would you recommend scheduling a follow-up with Nora? What are the benefits of a follow-up session?

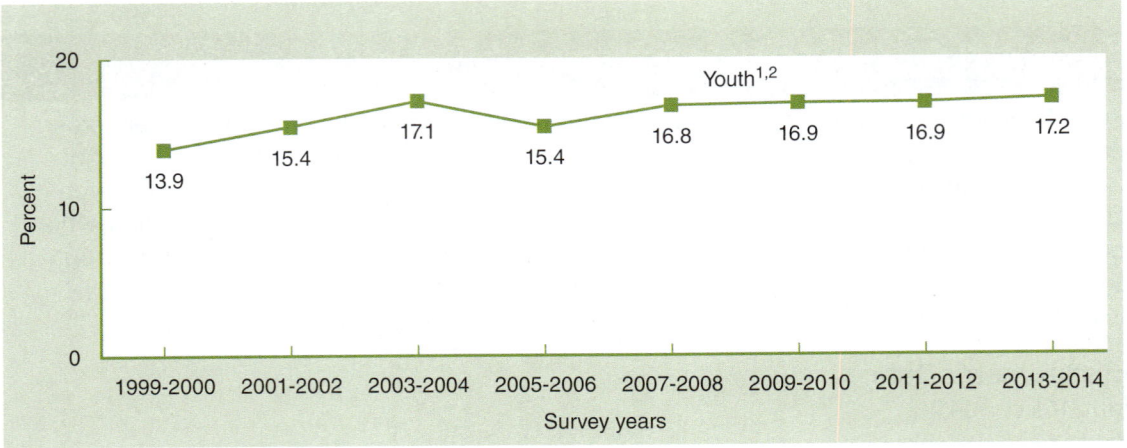

[1] Significant increasing linear trend from 1999–2000 through 2013–2014.
[2] Test for linear trend for 2003–2004 through 2013–2014 not significant ($p > 0.05$).

FIGURE 24.1 Trends in Obesity Prevalence among Children and Adolescents Aged 2 to 19 Years: United States, 1999/2000 through 2013/2014

Reproduced from CDC/NCHS, National Health and Nutrition Examination Survey.

When BMI is calculated, it is plotted on one of the sex-specific CDC BMI-for-age growth charts. Age- and sex-specific percentiles are used in children and adolescents because body fat percentage changes with age and differs between sexes. Weight classifications are as follows: 5th to 85th percentile considered normal weight, 85th to 95th percentile considered overweight, and greater than 95th percentile considered obese.[6] Children's height and weight should be measured at least annually to assess any upward or downward trends in growth.

It has been determined that measuring BMI may not always be the best indicator of total body adiposity in adults, and this same finding has been demonstrated in the pediatric population. The reason for this is because BMI does not take into account body composition and the difference between lean body mass, including bone, and fat mass. In addition to the CDC recommendations for measuring obesity in children and adolescents, there are several other organizations that identify different cutoff points for assessing when a patient is considered overweight or obese. Standardizing BMI would permit tracking global trends of increasing weight.[3]

BMI is the assessment tool that is most often used to identify overweight or obese individuals; however, other tools may also be used. Waist circumference, skinfold thickness, hip circumference, waist/hip ratio and waist/height ratio are alternative measurements used to assess body fat.[4] Measurements of skinfold thickness have proven to be more accurate predictors of adiposity in children than BMI. However, measuring height and weight in children is a much simpler process than measuring skinfold thickness, which often can be inaccurate due to human error. Thus, BMI continues to be the preferred measurement when identifying overweight or obese children.[7]

Measuring waist circumference is an inexpensive method that has been highly effective in measuring body fat and predicting the development of obesity-related chronic disease in adults. The CDC provides guidelines for

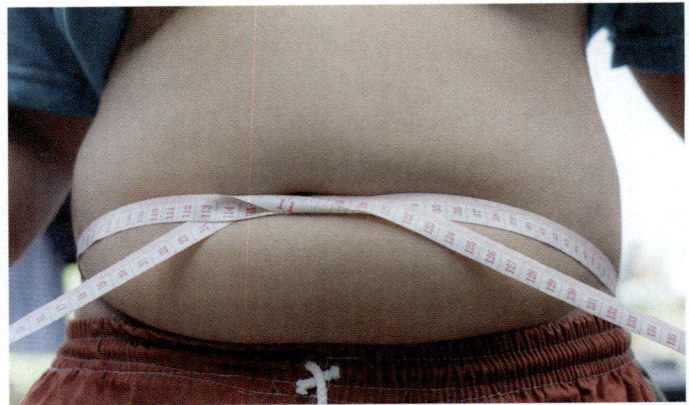

©chanchai plongern/Shutterstock.

healthcare professionals to use when measuring waist circumference to access childhood obesity (**Table 24.1**).[5] Waist circumference measurements are used less often in the pediatric population, although it is an important assessment method that may predict future adverse health complications. Emerging evidence suggests that central obesity is increasing at an even faster rate than BMI.[8] An upward trend in waist circumference is seen even when BMI is stabilized, which is alarming as substantial evidence suggests that measurements of central adiposity may be a better predictor of adverse health outcomes than overall adiposity.

In order to implement appropriate interventions, it is necessary to assess and classify the weight status of an individual. Establishing a consistent and effective way to do this in the pediatric population is highly important. Currently, use of BMI age- and sex-specific growth charts is the method most often used in the United States. Measurement of waist circumference should be considered due to its effectiveness in predicting the likelihood of health complications in the future. Childhood obesity is associated with many of the risk factors for cardiovascular disease (CVD), including high blood pressure, high

Childhood Obesity and Medical Comorbidities

Given the current prevalence of childhood obesity, there is concern that these overweight and obese children will become overweight and obese adults at high risk for CVD. It has been predicted that the number of additional cardiovascular events related to obesity in adolescence will be more than 100,000 by 2035. As unsettling as these predictions are, perhaps most unsettling are the reports of cardiovascular abnormalities in obese children, suggesting cardiovascular dysfunction may not only be a concern in the future for these children, but a concern to be dealt with at present.[3,9]

Left Ventricular Hypertrophy, Hypertension, and Epicardial Fat

Obesity is associated with increased metabolic demand due to greater adipose tissue and lean mass, increased blood volume, and increasing preload to the heart. **Left ventricular hypertrophy (LVH)** is a disease in which the muscle of the left ventricle becomes thickened and enlarged (**Figure 24.2**). LVH is caused by the increase in workload the heart experiences as a response to hypertension. It has been well documented as a risk factor for the development of CVD morbidity and mortality in adults and has been shown that, on average, obese children and adolescents have greater left ventricular mass than their healthy counterparts of the same sex and age. This increase in LVH is of particular concern for children and adolescents with hypertension, because this combination of CVD risk factors has demonstrated an increased risk of cardiovascular events.[9,10]

The clustering of risk factors that have been identified in pediatric metabolic syndrome may also be significant for the acceleration of atherosclerosis in adolescents. Observations from autopsy studies by the Bogalusa Heart Study, a long-term epidemiologic study of cardiovascular risk factors from birth through age 38 years, demonstrated a strong relationship between coronary atherosclerosis and cardiovascular risk factors in young people. Elevated BMI was reported to have been significantly related to the extent of atherosclerotic lesions in adolescents, along with other identified risk factors including increase systolic blood pressure, high serum LDL cholesterol, serum triglyceride concentration, and smoking. Although the development of atherosclerosis is not often documented as clinically significant before adulthood is reached, the development of fatty streaks and thickening of the arterial media begin in the obese pediatric population.[11]

In addition to the clustering of risk factors for CVD mentioned above, obese children have been observed to have greater **epicardial fat** deposition as compared to their peers with a healthy BMI. Epicardial fat is a fat deposit that surrounds that heart and is enclosed by the viscera pericardium. Epicardial fat has multiple important

TABLE 24.1 CDC WAIST CIRCUMFERENCE MEASUREMENTS FOR ASSESSING CHILDHOOD OBESITY

Waist Circumference Measurements in Centimeters

Age	Male Percentiles			Female Percentiles		
	85th	90th	95th	85th	90th	95th
2 years	51.2	52.0	53.4	51.6	52.9	54.7
3 years	53.3	54.6	56.9	54.3	55.0	57.3
4 years	56.7	57.5	62.7	56.2	58.3	60.2
5 years	58.3	60.8	66.0	60.4	63.3	†
6 years	65.3	69.6	78.7	63.5	64.3	67.9
7 years	68.1	71.3	74.6	67.3	72.9	78.1
8 years	73.0	78.1	81.0	75.2	78.7	82.7
9 years	79.5	85.0	91.2	79.6	83.0	88.1
10 years	81.1	85.6	89.9	82.0	84.1	88.8
11 years	87.2	90.4	97.0	87.2	93.6	103.0
12 years	91.6	93.7	98.5	87.3	95.1	98.8

Data from CDC/NCHS, National Health and Nutrition Examination Survey. 2008.
†Standard error not calculated by SUDAAN.

cholesterol, along with poor glycemic control that could eventually lead to diabetes. As the rates of childhood obesity continue to be high, so too are the medical comorbidities that accompany this disease.[9]

CORE CONCEPT 2

Childhood obesity is associated with many of the risk factors for cardiovascular disease, including high blood pressure, high cholesterol, and poor glycemic control that could eventually lead to diabetes.

PRACTICE POINT

Use BMI as the general screening tool when identifying childhood obesity. Further measurements that may be beneficial to include in the assessment are measuring waist circumference, skinfold thickness, hip circumference, waist/height ratio, and waist/hip ratio.

> ## CASE STUDY REVISITED
>
> Nora reports feeling "exhausted" no matter what time she falls asleep. Nora's mother says she is a loud snorer, and the doctor notices Nora is having increased work of breathing just sitting in the doctor's office.
>
> **Biochemical Data:**
> Triglycerides 220 mg/dL (Desirable: <150 mg/dL)
> Total Cholesterol (TC) 275 (Desirable: <200 mg/dL)
> Low Density Lipoprotein Cholesterol (LDL-C) 145 (Desirable: <100 mg/dL)
> High Density Lipoprotein Cholesterol (HDL-C) 22 (Desirable: ≥40 mg/dL)
>
> **Clinical Data:**
> **Vital Signs:** Blood pressure 140/90 mm Hg
>
> ### Questions
> 1. What comorbidities associated with obesity might Nora be experiencing?
> 2. Based on these labs, what would you say Nora is at risk for?

functions, such as acting as an endocrine and paracrine gland and providing an energy reservoir for cardiomyocytes. Although epicardial fat is necessary for numerous metabolic and bodily functions, increased epicardial fat deposition has been associated with insulin resistance, coronary artery disease, carotid intima-media thickness, and arterial stiffness.[12]

Overweight and obese children are at an increased risk for multiple risk factors associated with cardiac dysfunction, increasing the likelihood of CVD progression with age. Establishing standardized values to evaluate measures of cardiovascular risk in the pediatric population will be an important consideration, because this population would benefit from early intervention to slow or stop the progression of cardiovascular disease into adulthood.

> ### CORE CONCEPT 3
> Overweight and obese children are at an increased risk for multiple risk factors associated with cardiac dysfunction, increasing the likelihood of CVD progression with age.

Metabolic Syndrome

Metabolic syndrome in adults is identified when an individual has three or more of the following metabolic risk factors: increased waist circumference, high systolic or diastolic blood pressure, elevated fasting glucose and triglyceride levels, and low HDL-C (**Figure 24.3**). Threshold values determining high and low risk levels for these components were established in the ATP III guidelines. Meeting the criteria for metabolic syndrome indicates increased

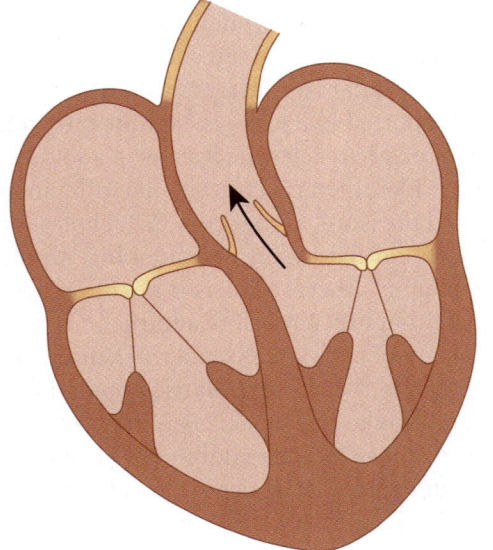
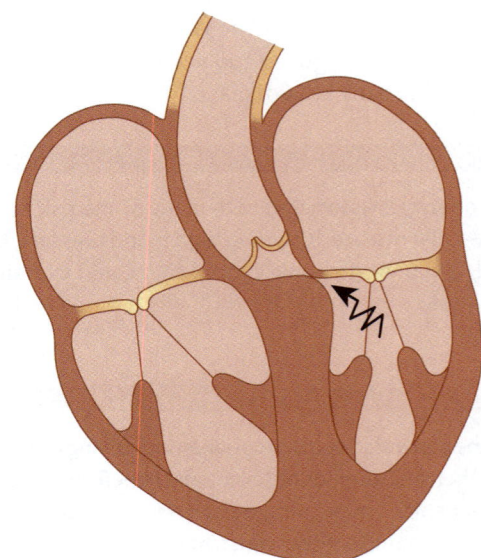

FIGURE 24.2 Left Ventricular Hypertrophy. Hypertrophy of the Left Ventricle Leads to Obstructed Blood Flow

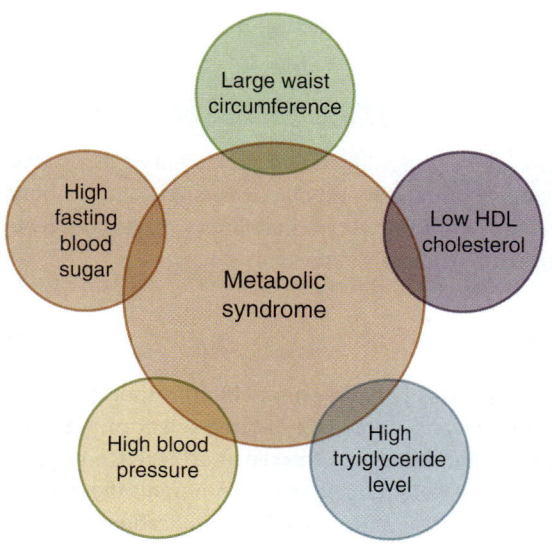

FIGURE 24.3 Factors Contributing to Metabolic Syndrome

risk for cardiovascular disease and type 2 diabetes, fatty liver, gallstones, asthma, and sleep disturbances.[13]

In the past decade, there has been a greater focus on defining metabolic syndrome as it relates to the pediatric population. Pediatric metabolic syndrome has been defined in over 27 different pediatric studies and over 40 varying definitions have been established.[14] There is currently no clear definition of metabolic syndrome in the pediatric population, but a similar clustering of risk factors has been shown in children as compared with adults. Additionally, studies of populations have found the prevalence of metabolic syndrome in obese children and adolescents may be as high as 30% and note increases in BMI to correlate with increased risk for metabolic syndrome in children.[9] Furthermore, studies have also shown that measuring waist circumference is a better predictor than BMI when identifying the presence of metabolic syndrome and cardiovascular disease in children.[15] A large waist circumference is reflective of the total body fatness and the excess visceral abdominal fat, which increases the risks of developing cardiovascular disease and diabetes.[16]

Insulin Resistance and Type 2 Diabetes

Insulin resistance occurs when peripheral tissues are insensitive to insulin action, resulting in increased insulin production by the pancreatic beta cells. When the beta cells are no longer able to compensate for the lack of insulin sensitivity in the tissues, high levels of glucose remain in the blood and hyperglycemia results. This increased demand on the pancreatic beta cells to hypersecrete insulin influences the progressive beta cell failure that is characteristic of type 2 diabetes (**Figure 24.4**).[17]

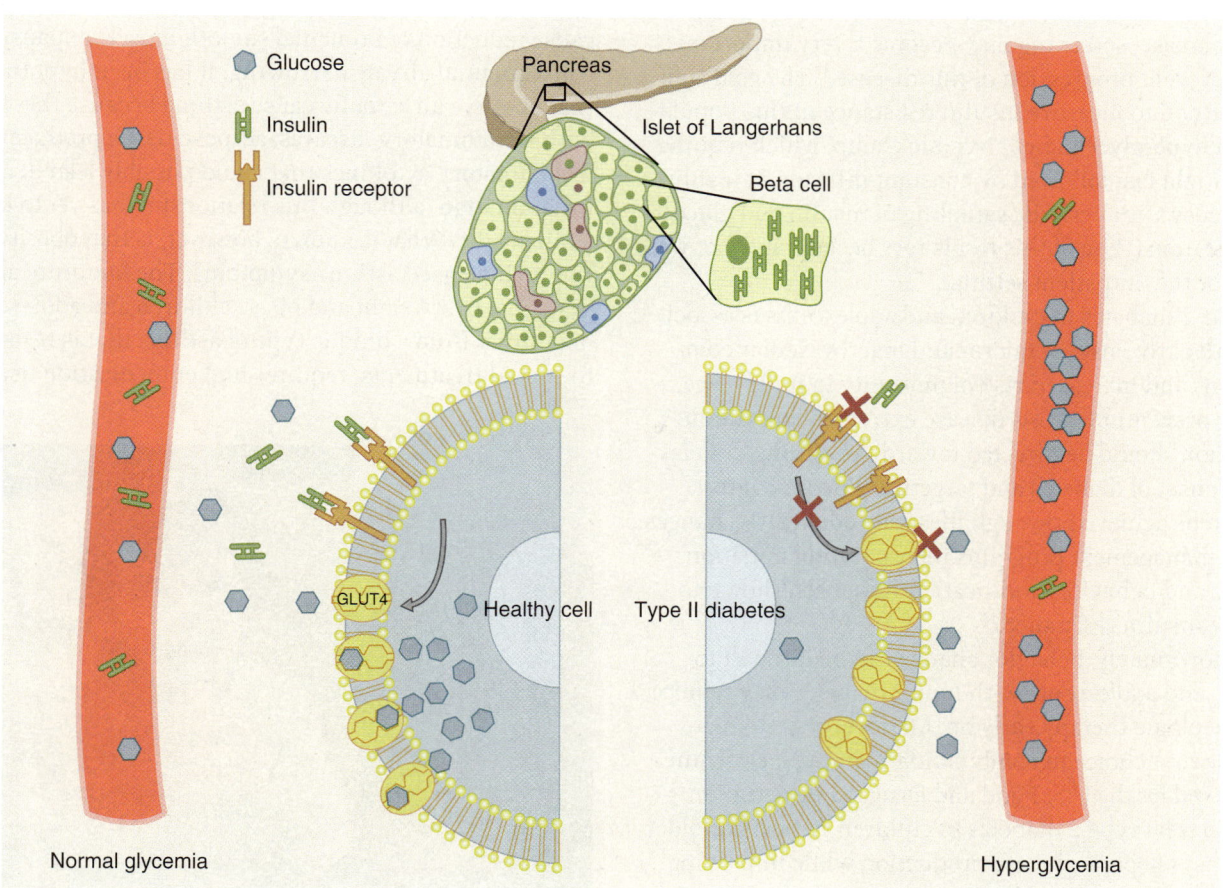

FIGURE 24.4 Insulin Resistance in Type 2 Diabetes

Type 2 diabetes was rarely diagnosed in children before the 1990s, which is why it was often referred to as "adult-onset" diabetes, whereas type 1 diabetes was referred to as "juvenile onset" diabetes.[17] "Adult-onset" is no longer an accurate depiction of type 2 diabetes, because it now accounts for 45% of new-onset diabetes in adolescents, with the highest rates observed among minority populations aged 15 to 19 years.[18]

Inflammation in the setting of obesity has been associated with insulin resistance. Increased **intramyocellular lipid deposition** has been linked to decreased uptake of glucose; adolescents with impaired glucose tolerance (IGT) often present with increased intramyocellular lipid content and increased visceral fat deposition. Impaired glucose tolerance may then lead to prediabetes and eventually diabetes in adolescence, making early intervention essential in this population.[18]

Prediabetes in adults is characterized by impaired glucose tolerance and/or impaired fasting glucose. Increased prevalence of prediabetes among adolescents and children characterized by IGT has been documented.[16] IGT in adolescence has been reported in obese children and adolescents, indicating prevalence of prediabetes in this population.[15]

If insulin resistance and IGT are detected early, it is possible to stop the progression of and even reverse type 2 diabetes. Screening is not universally performed, however, and there are relatively few reports on the epidemiology and history of complications in adolescents with type 2 diabetes. As the rates of obesity and type 2 diabetes in this population increase, screening may become a very important tool to prevent progression of this disease.[17] The gold standard method to measure insulin resistance in this population is a hyperglycemic-euglycemic clamp, which requires an overnight fast followed by constant infusion of insulin and glucose with periodic sampling of insulin and glucose concentrations. Use of this test is rare because it is not well suited for the outpatient setting.

Type 2 diabetes in children and adolescents is associated with early onset of micro- and macrovascular complications and increased risk of mortality in middle age, making prevention of this disease extremely important.[19] Prevention should be directed toward preventing or delaying the onset of diabetes and targeting glucose control. This can be achieved through lifestyle and dietary changes. Weight management programs incorporating nutrition, exercise and behavior modification have been shown to improve insulin resistance.[17]

Unfortunately, behavior change can be difficult to achieve, and adolescents with type 2 diabetes may require pharmacologic therapy early on. Metformin with insulin is the first choice in combination therapy; metformin is approved by the U.S. Food and Drug Administration (FDA) to treat type 2 diabetes in children 10 years or older. It decreases hepatic glucose production while improving insulin resistance. Combination treatments of metformin, insulin therapy, and lifestyle intervention have proven to be most effective in the treatment of type 2 diabetes in the pediatric population.[17]

> ### CORE CONCEPT 4
> Type 2 diabetes in children and adolescents is associated with early onset of micro- and macrovascular complications and increased risk of mortality in middle age, making prevention of this disease extremely important.

> ### PRACTICE POINT
> Type 2 diabetes prevention for children should be directed toward preventing or delaying the onset of diabetes and targeting glucose control. This can be achieved through dietary changes and weight management programs that incorporate nutrition, exercise, and behavioral modifications.

Asthma

As the rate of childhood obesity has risen over the years, so too have the rates of asthma, making overweight/obesity and asthma two of the most significant health problems worldwide. Asthma affects about 9.1% of children in the United States. Prevalence has been attributed to air pollution, tobacco smoke, and dietary or lifestyle choices, and now a link between obesity and asthma is being suggested.[20]

Excess body fat affects the free movement of air and compresses the lungs. In addition, lack of deep breathing resulting from restricted lung movements and obesity can cause reduction of bronchial smooth muscle expansion and consequential airway narrowing. It has been hypothesized that obesity can actually cause asthma because these are both inflammatory diseases; adipose tissue produces pro-inflammatory cytokines that could possibly lead to airway inflammation, although this relationship has yet to be confirmed.[21] What is known, however, is that obesity can lead to increased asthma symptoms. The literature also suggests that overweight and obese children and adolescents may suffer from a unique type of asthma that is resistant to steroid treatments, requires higher medication use, and

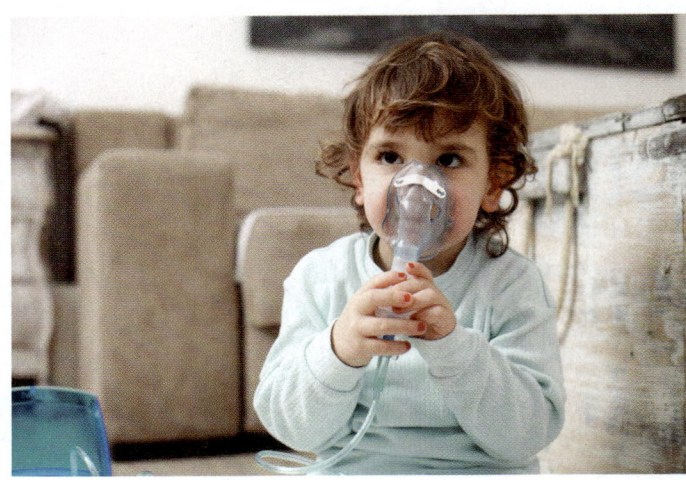
©Nikodash/Shutterstock.

results in more hospitalizations as compared to the asthma in children within the healthy BMI range.[22] Weight loss has demonstrated improvement in pulmonary function and research suggests possible benefits of an anti-inflammatory diet connected to relief of asthma symptoms.[21,22]

Sleep Apnea

Studies show that about 33% of severely overweight children have symptoms of **obstructive sleep apnea**, while about 5% have severe obstructive sleep apnea. As defined by the American Thoracic Society, obstructive sleep apnea is "a disorder of breathing during sleep characterized by prolonged partial upper airway obstruction and/or intermittent complete obstruction that disrupts normal ventilation during sleep and normal sleep patterns."[23] Evidence supports adult obesity as a risk factor for sleep apnea; a link between childhood obesity and sleep apnea has also been established. Fatty infiltration of upper airway structures, subcutaneous fat deposits in the anterior neck region promoting pharyngeal collapse, and increased respiratory load secondary to increased adipose tissue in the abdominal wall and cavity may result in decreased lung volumes and increased work of breathing during sleep.[24] Obstructive sleep apnea is associated with cardiovascular complications and can lead to systemic hypertension, increased ventricular mass, and diastolic dysfunction, further adding to the health complications already associated with childhood obesity.

Improvement in obstructive sleep apnea has been demonstrated with weight loss, making lifestyle intervention an important part of prevention and treatment of this disorder. Weight loss may be particularly challenging for this population because increased daytime sleepiness and changes in appetite and eating patterns are often a result of obstructive sleep apnea and can promote weight gain and severity of obesity.[9]

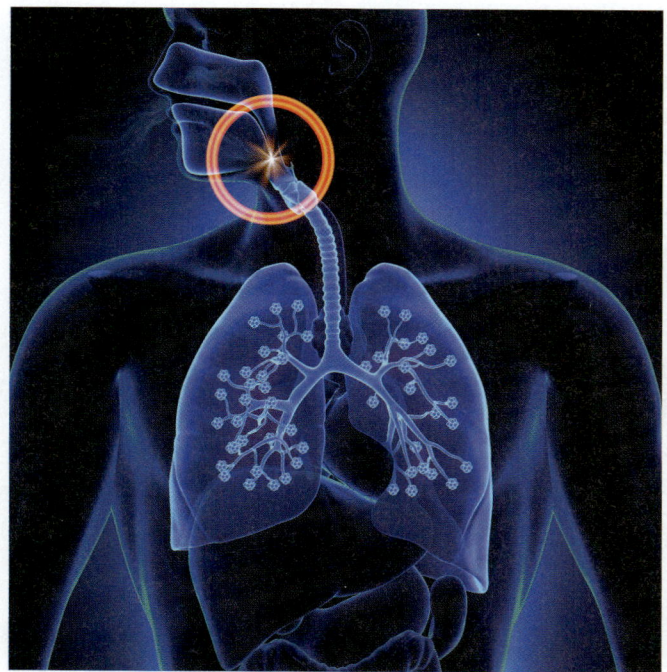
©decade3d - anatomy online/Shutterstock.

Other Comorbidities: Orthopedic, Dental, and Nonalcoholic Fatty Liver

The medical comorbidities associated with childhood obesity are vast. In addition to those mentioned, obese children and adolescents are at risk for orthopedic problems as a result of excess weight and stress on the musculoskeletal system, nonalcoholic fatty liver disease, and dental caries.[17,25]

Nonalcoholic fatty liver disease (NAFLD) has been found to be the number one cause of chronic liver disease in children and adolescents in the United States.[26] NAFLD is a condition where macrovesicular fat accumulates in hepatocytes, resulting in the enlargement of the liver. Along with liver fat accumulation, NAFLD causes the liver cells to become damaged and inflamed (**Figures 24.5A and 5B**).[27] The development of NAFLD in children can lead to cirrhosis, a disease that can eventually lead to liver failure. NAFLD is caused by an array of conditions, such as metabolic syndrome, obesity, high levels of cholesterol and LDL, and insulin resistance.[20] NAFLD is more prevalent in boys than girls due to the absence of estrogen, which has been found to reduce lipid peroxidation in lipoproteins.[27] Specific ethnicities, ages, and genetic factors can also have an impact on the development of NAFLD in children. The most common treatment recommended for children with NAFLD is healthy eating and weight loss, as weight loss can reduce fibrosis and fat in the liver. There are currently no approved medications for childhood NAFLD, and thus living a healthy lifestyle is the only solution for this disease.

Psychological Effects of Childhood Obesity

Along with the medical comorbidities that accompany childhood obesity, there are also many psychological comorbidities to consider. Children who are overweight or

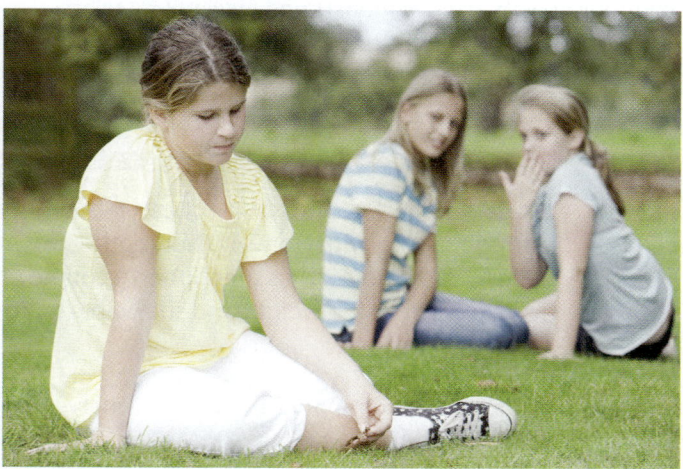
©Monkey Business Images/Shutterstock.

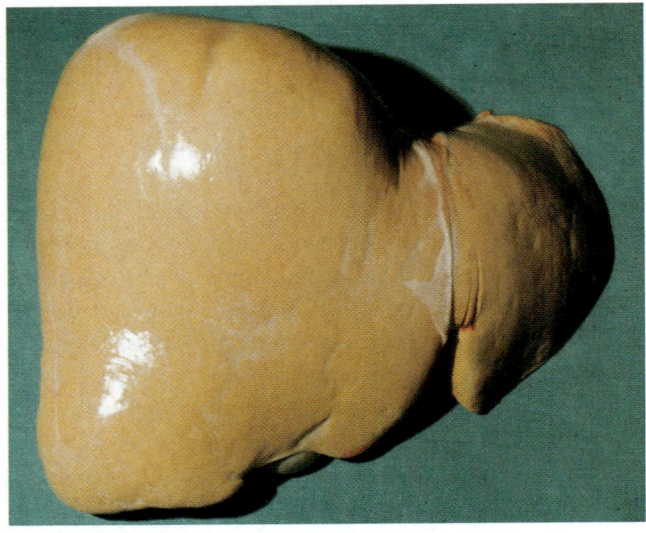
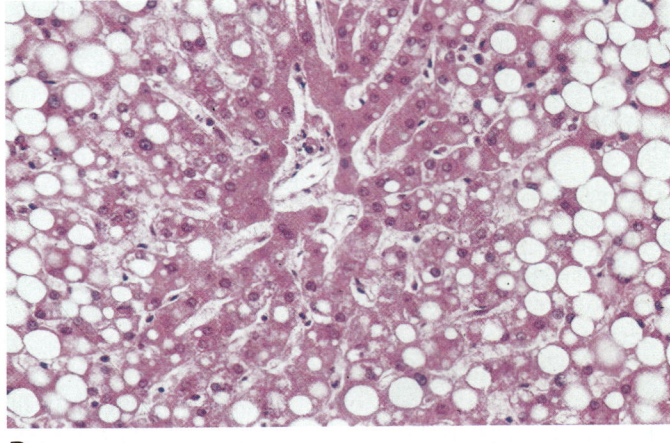
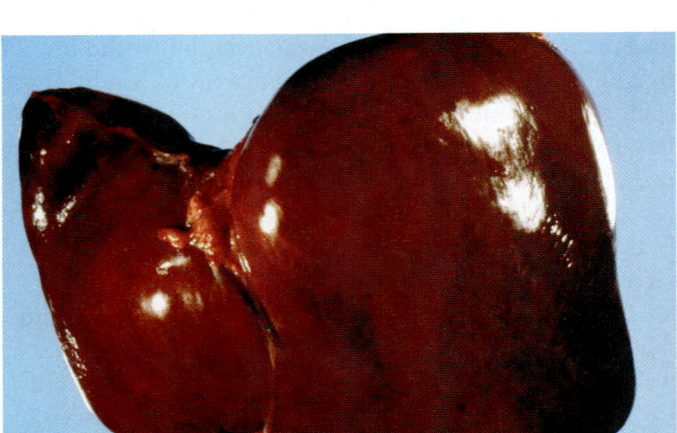
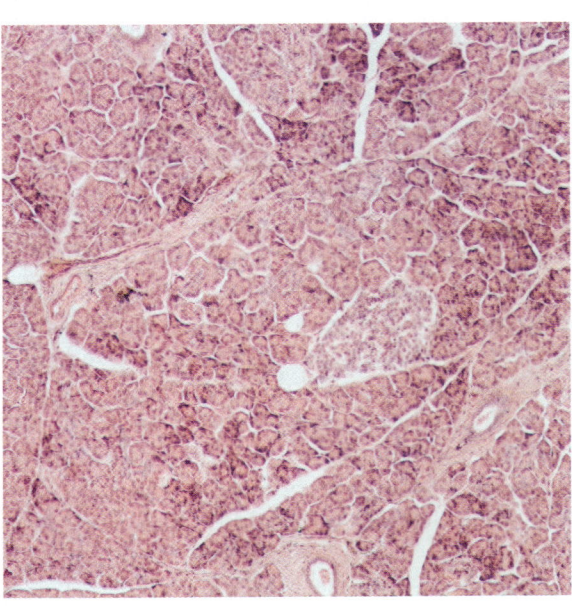

FIGURE 24.5 Fatty Liver in Nonalcoholic Steatohepatitis
(a) and (b) Courtesy of Leonard V. Crowley, MD, Century College; (c) ©Southern Illinois University/Science Source/Getty Images; (d) ©Pan Xunbin/Shutterstock.

obese often face stigma and prejudice from their peers that can lead to serious psychological damage.[29]

Depression and Obesity Stigma

Obese children and adolescents who seek medical treatment for obesity have demonstrated elevated rates of depression. Rates of children who meet depression criteria in those seeking obesity treatments through bariatric surgery have been reported as high as 45%.[28] These rates greatly exceed that of the general pediatric population. Studies have found a correlation between high BMI and greater risk for depression in the pediatric population.[29]

Psychological complications may result from teasing and obesity stigma. These overweight and obese children often face negative stereotypes from their peers, educators, and parents.[30] Obesity stigma has been associated with

CASE STUDY REVISITED

Through talking with Nora and her mother, you notice a strained relationship between the two. Nora seems depressed and has mentioned a couple of times the bullying she experiences in school. She wants to start losing weight and she wants to do it fast!

Question

1. How would you approach behavioral interventions with Nora?

adverse effects on self-esteem and body image. In addition, obesity stigma may contribute to weight gain because it can lead to decreased desire to participate in physical activity, lower academic achievement, and perpetuation of adverse eating habits such as binge eating.[28]

Peer Relationships

Bullying by peers of overweight and obese youth has been associated with self-reported depression, anxiety, social anxiety, loneliness, and preference for isolative activities.[15] Peer relationships during childhood and adolescence have proven to be essential; healthy social and cognitive development depends on interactions with peers. Literature has shown that obese adolescents may have poor social functioning and have a more difficult time making friends with peers.[28]

Family Relationships

Parents are very important role models for children, and their participation in childhood obesity intervention and prevention is essential for success. A support system provided by parents and siblings is key as a child transforms to a healthier lifestyle. It can be difficult for parents to realize when their child is overweight or obese. Often parents of overweight and obese children deny that their child's weight is a problem; it is the role of the health professional to help the parent realize the adverse health consequences of their child's future and recommend healthy modifications to make at home.

Cognitive Impairment

Early onset of obesity is associated with cognitive impairments. Children with early-onset morbid obesity displayed lower levels of cognitive functioning than their nonobese siblings. Research suggests that obesity and/or a high fat diet leads to local inflammation within the hypothalamus that alters synaptic plasticity, contributes to neurodegeneration, and even initiates brain atrophy.[31] Obese youth have also been found to have significantly more negative behaviors and poor adaptive functioning.[9] Interventions to treat obesity and central inflammation have proven effective in improvement of some aspects of cognitive function.[29]

> **CORE CONCEPT 5**
>
> Obese children and adolescents who seek medical treatment for obesity have demonstrated elevated rates of depression, anxiety, social anxiety, loneliness, and preference for isolative activities.

> **PRACTICE POINT**
>
> To gain a better understanding of the psychological factors impacting the patient, it is recommended to determine the peer and parental relationships present in the patient's life.

Health-Related Quality of Life

The Pediatric Quality of Life Inventory is a tool designed to measure health-related quality of life for children and adolescents; using this tool to assess measures of fatigue in pediatric patients revealed those with obesity to experience fatigue comparable with pediatric patients receiving cancer treatments.[32] Overweight and obese patients often experience difficulty completing daily tasks or engaging in physical activity. When impairment of everyday functioning occurs, the child's quality of life may suffer greatly; the likelihood of quality of life impairment in obese individuals was found to be 5.5 times greater than that of a healthy-weight child.[28] When tasks of daily living become difficult for the child, it is often at that time that parents and adolescents seek weight management therapy.[28]

Factors Associated with Childhood Obesity

The etiology of childhood obesity is multifactorial; individual factors, social factors, genetic factors, and environmental factors all play a role in a child's health status. Understanding the main reason or reasons that a child is overweight/obese is extremely important in effective treatment and management.

Low Socioeconomic Status

There is an association between low family income and a higher percentage of overweight or obese youth. Children living in communities with lower mean annual income are more likely to have decreased physical activity, increased time watching television, and steady consumption of school lunches that are frequently energy dense.[33] Poorer communities often have less access to supermarkets with fresh produce and poor access to recreational parks and afterschool exercise programs. Low-income communities also have significantly more street food vendors and convenience stores than higher-income neighborhoods, which tend to have supermarkets that provide more healthful food options.[33] Additionally, fast food restaurants tend to populate low-income neighborhoods, leading to greater consumption of inexpensive, higher-calorie foods.[34]

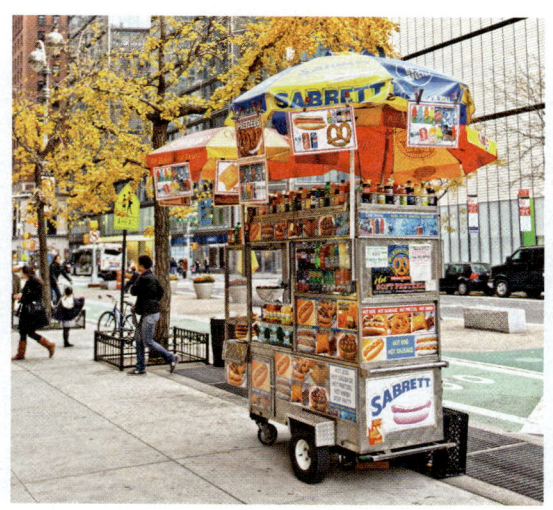

©Stuart Monk/Shutterstock.

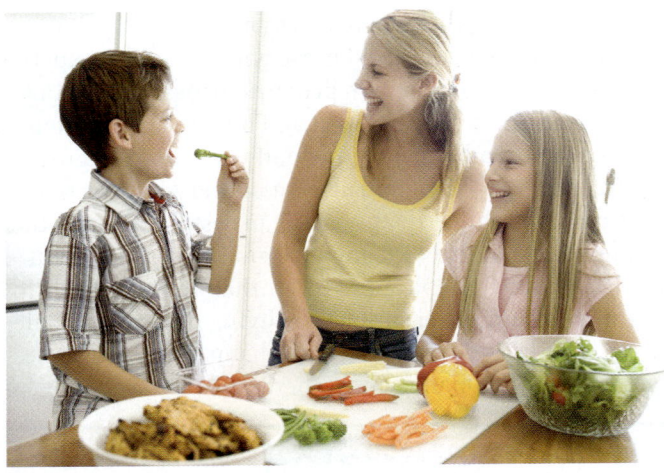

Family Patterns

The family environment is an important factor in a child's development and lifestyle habits. Children often mirror their parent's lifestyle choices, and they are affected by exposure to certain foods, portion sizes provided, and family routines. Children who grow up in sedentary households are less likely to engage in physical activity. Part of the parent's role is to provide young children with nutrient-dense foods and encourage physical activity. As children grow up, they will be able to make their own decisions regarding dietary and exercise habits, although they are still likely to mirror their parents' actions. Thus, it is the responsibility of the parents to act as role models.[17]

Parenting style can have an effect on a child's eating patterns.[17] Authoritative feeding style, which is characterized by parental sensitivity and high expectations for child self-control, has shown to be effective in promotion of healthy eating behaviors and increased consumption of fruits and vegetables.[35] Evidence shows that encouragement to try fruits and vegetables is effective, whereas pressure to do so is often ineffective. In similar fashion, restriction of some unhealthy food items to promote a healthy diet is often beneficial, while extreme restriction has actually proven to facilitate unhealthy eating behaviors and relationships with food.[35]

Genetic Factors

Genetic Factors and Nutrigenomics

Genetic factors play a strong role in the development of childhood obesity. Parental obesity has a large impact on the trajectory of their child's BMI and future health status. When both parents are overweight, their children have an 80% chance of becoming obese, whereas obesity prevalence reduces by 14% when both parents have a normal BMI.[36]

In fact, the interaction between genes and the environment is a rapidly progressing field of research. It is estimated that genetic factors account for greater than 40% of population variation in BMI.[37] With the discovery of leptin, a hormone that stimulates appetite derived in the adipose tissue, the proposed number of obesity-susceptible genes is growing. Mutations in the genes that code for leptin and leptin receptors have been linked to human obesity, and leptin administration has proven effective in treating obesity.[38] In children, increased sleep duration resulted in lower leptin levels, decreased appetite, and decreased weight. Conversely, ghrelin levels were not effected,[39] Both leptin and ghrelin, the hunger hormone, are hereditary and also increase the probability of childhood obesity.[40] The regulation of leptin and ghrelin is outlined in **Figure 24.6**.

Nutrigenomics, the study of how genes and nutrients interact, is another factor that contributes to childhood obesity. Numerous studies have demonstrated that consumption of specific macronutrients and micronutrients control gene expression in various ways. The research of nutrigenomics focuses on the association between single-nucleotide polymorphisms (SNPs), a specific genetic code that varies among people, and how they are altered by the consumption of specific nutrients.[41] These SNPs act as biological markers in research to help determine which genes are associated with specific diseases. An association was discovered between fat mass and SNPs in obesity-associated FTO gene regions with BMI. Children who inherit the FTO gene are more likely to struggle with obesity and the onset of type 2 diabetes.[42]

CORE CONCEPT 6

The etiology of childhood obesity is multifactorial; individual factors, social factors, and environmental factors all play a role in a child's health status.

PRACTICE POINT

When children are frustrated with the hardships that come with losing weight, it is important to teach them about the genetic and environmental factors that can contribute to weight gain. This conversation can help childhood patients recognize the areas where they have the ability to improve their health (i.e., physical activity, dietary changes) as opposed to certain genetic factors that are beyond their control.

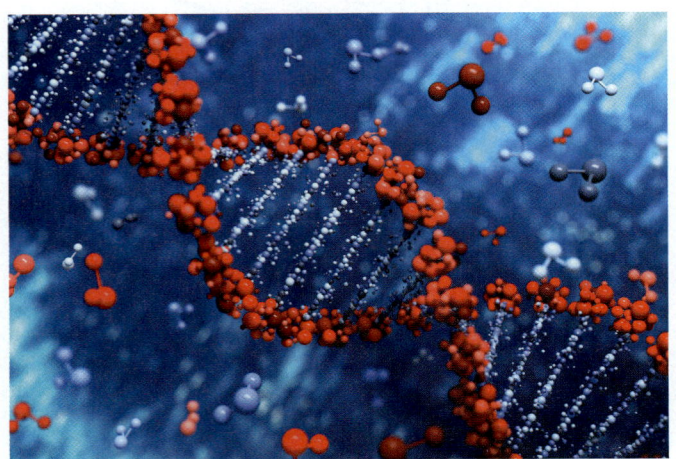

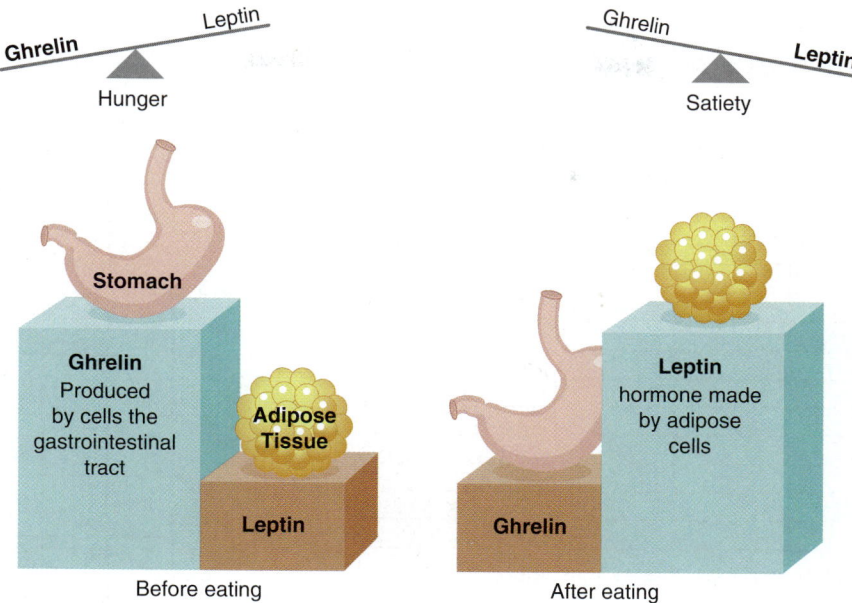

FIGURE 24.6 Regulation of Appetite by Hormones Leptin and Ghrelin

Assessment, Management, and Intervention

Nutrition Assessment of Childhood Obesity

The American Medical Association Expert Committee has established guidelines for assessing childhood obesity. At every doctor visit, the pediatric patient's height and weight should be measured and their BMI should be plotted on the CDC BMI sex- and age-specific charts (**Figure 24.7**). From there, the child's medical risk (i.e., child history and exam, parental obesity, and family history), behavior risk (i.e., sedentary time, dietary habits, and physical activity), and attitudes (i.e., family and patient motivation) should be assessed. For those children with a BMI in the 85th to 94th percentiles, classified as overweight, laboratory values should be assessed as needed. For the patient charting greater than or equal to the 95th percentile, classified as obese, laboratory values should be collected and assessed.[43] Refer to Figure 24.7 for the BMI-for-age percentile growth charts for girls and boys.

> **PRACTICE POINT**
>
> For children with a BMI classified as overweight or obese, collect and monitor laboratory values to assess early signs of hypertension, diabetes, and cardiovascular disease.

Primary and Secondary Prevention: Approaches to Weight Loss

As seen in adult populations, primary strategies for weight maintenance or weight loss for children focus on energy balance; energy intake should be equal to energy expended. In their position paper on interventions for prevention and treatment of pediatric obesity, the Academy for Nutrition and Dietetics identifies key areas for primary prevention, which include integrating education with supportive environment change in school and child care settings, including physical activity and parent engagement. As for secondary prevention, for children already overweight and obese, a staged approach based on BMI percentiles is recommended. Each stage increases in intensity based on obesity risk. Stages 1 to 3 focus primarily on behavioral changes, while Stage 4 is a tertiary-based intervention that can include a combination of dietary, behavioral, pharmacological, and surgical interventions.[44]

For children considered overweight or obese, intervention goals can include slowing the rate of weight gain, stopping weight gain, or losing weight. For successful weight loss, it is recommended to introduce children to healthy eating and behavioral patterns instead of placing them on calorie-restricted diet, which may set them up for failure and future weight gain.[45] While restrictive dieting is not recommended for children, success in weight loss has been seen in children who were introduced to the concepts of calories and portion control. The National Institutes of Health (NIH) provides calorie guidelines for children and parents that are based on age, sex, and the child's level of physical activity (**Table 24.2**).[46] Other governmental organizations also offer various suggestions and tools regarding weight loss and living a healthy lifestyle for children (**Figure 24.8**).

Children and adolescents experience periods of rapid growth, and as height continues to increase, interventions related to portion control and healthy eating should result in a decrease in BMI. For many children who are overweight, it is recommended that the child maintain their weight and allow for growth in height to normalize their BMI. Children experience an adiposity rebound period

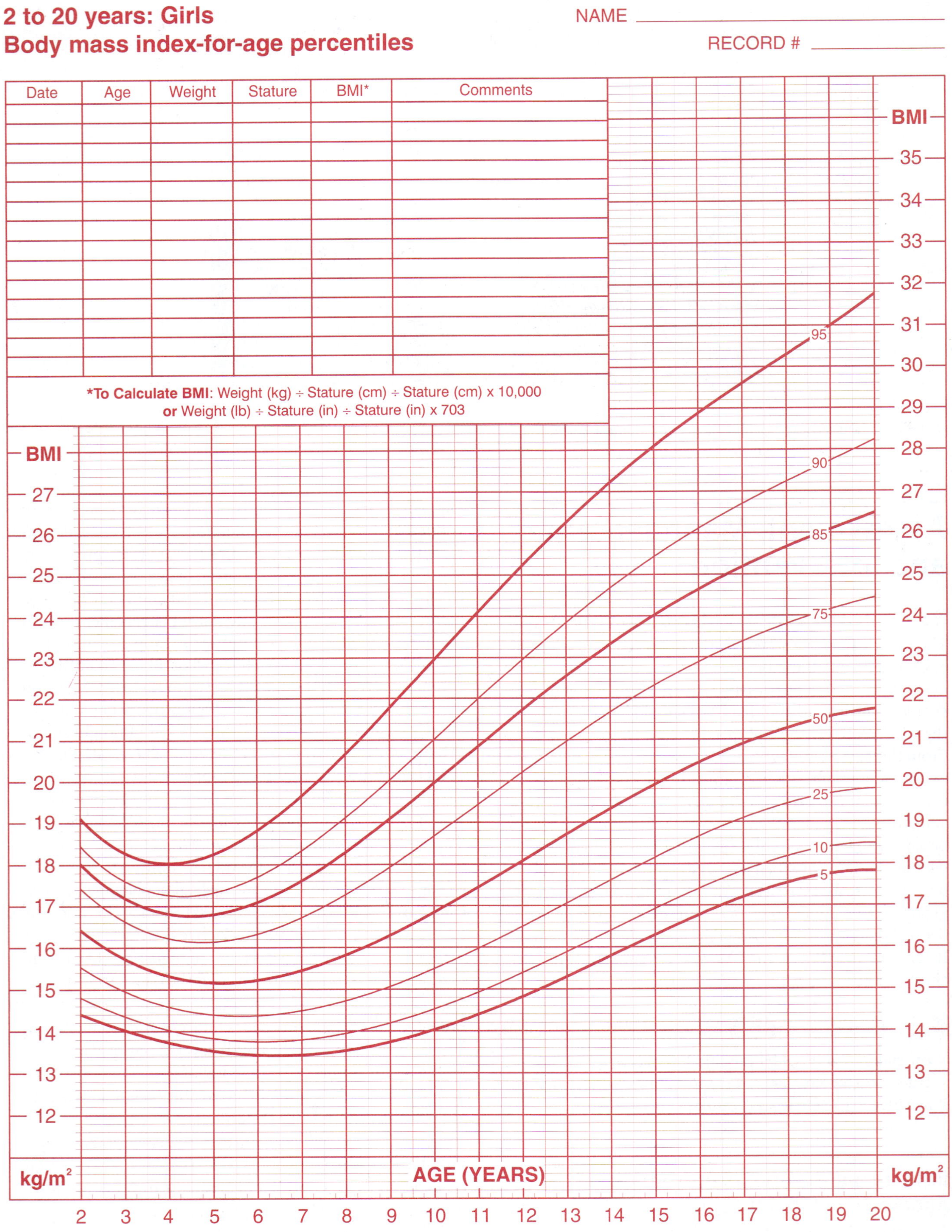

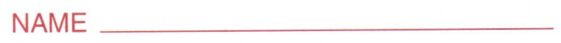

FIGURE 24.7 Body Mass Index-for-Age Percentiles: (A) Girls and (B) Boys Ages 2 to 20 Years[5]

Reproduced from Natioanl Center for Health Stastics in Collaboration with National Center for Chronic Disease and Health Promotion, 2000. www.cdc.gov/growthCharts.

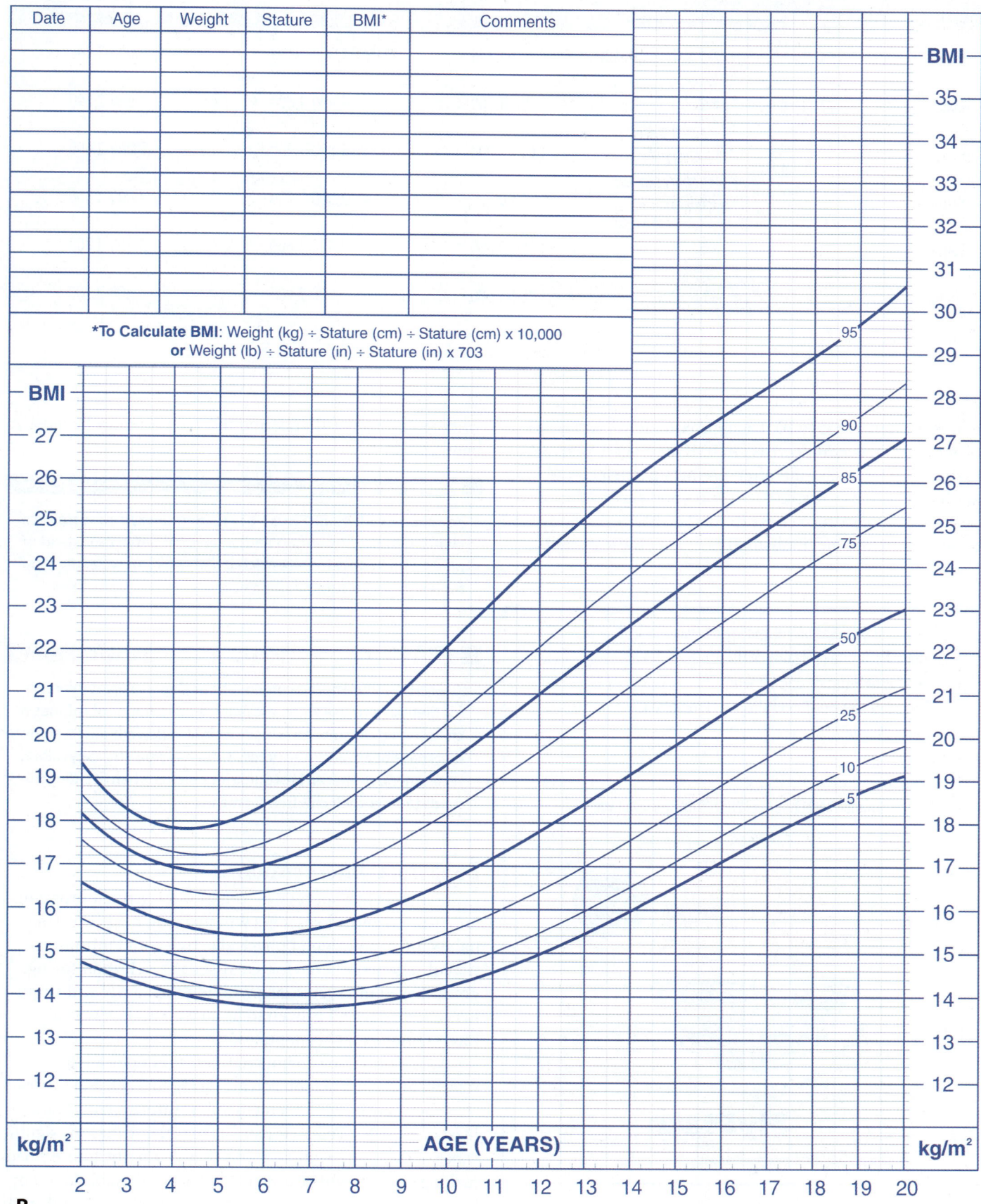

FIGURE 24.7 Body Mass Index-for-Age Percentiles: (A) Girls and (B) Boys Ages 2 to 20 Years[5]

Reproduced from National Center for Health Statistics in Collaboration with National Center for Chronic Disease and Health Promotion, 2000. www.cdc.gov/growthCharts.

TABLE 24.2 NIH DAILY ENERGY RECOMMENDATIONS (IN CALORIES)

Gender	Age (Years)	Not Active	Somewhat Active	Very Active
Male	2-3	1,000-1,200	1,000-1,400	1,000-1,400
Male	4-8	1,200-1,400	1,400-1,600	1,600-2,000
Male	9-13	1,600-2,000	1,800-2,200	2,000-2,600
Female	2-3	1,000	1,000-1,200	1,000-1,400
Female	4-8	1,200-1,400	1,400-1,600	1,400-1,800
Female	9-13	1,400-1,600	1,600-2,000	1,800-2,200

Data from HHS/USDA Dietary Guidelines for Americans, 2010

which is an increase in BMI at approximately 5 to 7 years of age after an initial decrease in BMI after age 1 year. An earlier adiposity rebound often predicts persistent and adulthood obesity. Similarly, the pre- and early pubertal periods of adolescence cause dramatic changes in body composition and metabolism. It is during these periods where weight surveillance and intervention may be most beneficial.[43]

CORE CONCEPT 7

For successful weight loss, it is recommended to introduce children to healthy eating and behavioral patterns instead of placing them on calorie-restricted diet, which may set them up for failure and future weight gain.

PRACTICE POINT

The NIH daily caloric recommendations chart is a great reference for dietitians to use when estimating the amount of calories a child should consume to achieve weight loss. While strict calorie diets have been found unsuccessful for children, the daily caloric recommendations can be a guide for parents when deciding the foods to offer their children for meals.

- Centers for Disease Control and Prevention (CDC)
- National Institute of Health (NIH)
- Academy of Nutrition and Dietetics
- USDA Center for Nutrition Policy and Promotion
- Healthy People 2020
- Nutrition.gov
- Let's Move!
- Women, Infants, and Children (WIC) Nutrition Program

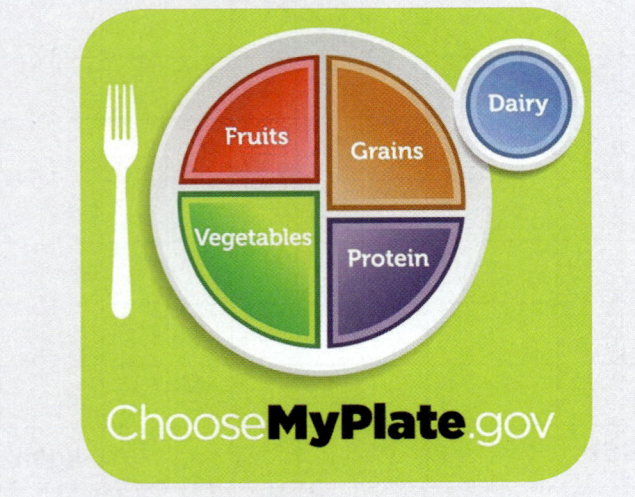

FIGURE 24.8 Government Organizations and Programs that Offer Information and Tools for Parents and Children Regarding Living a Healthy Lifestyle

Reproduced from U.S. Department of Agriculture. ChooseMyPlate.gov.

Behavioral Intervention

Components of a successful weight management program for children and adolescents will focus on healthy eating habits, incorporation of physical activity, and minimization of sedentary behavior. Goal-setting, self-monitoring, group-based interventions involving the family and stimulus control have all proven to be successful behavioral interventions for this population.[17]

When providing an intervention, it is important to remember the population you are trying to reach and the reasons they may find it difficult to follow through with healthy lifestyle changes. Pediatric patients may not realize the significance of the health complications they face in the future when making changes will be difficult and uncomfortable for them in the present. Cardiovascular risks are invisible to youth and their parents; symptoms are often not felt and thus even presentation of elevated laboratory values may not be effective.

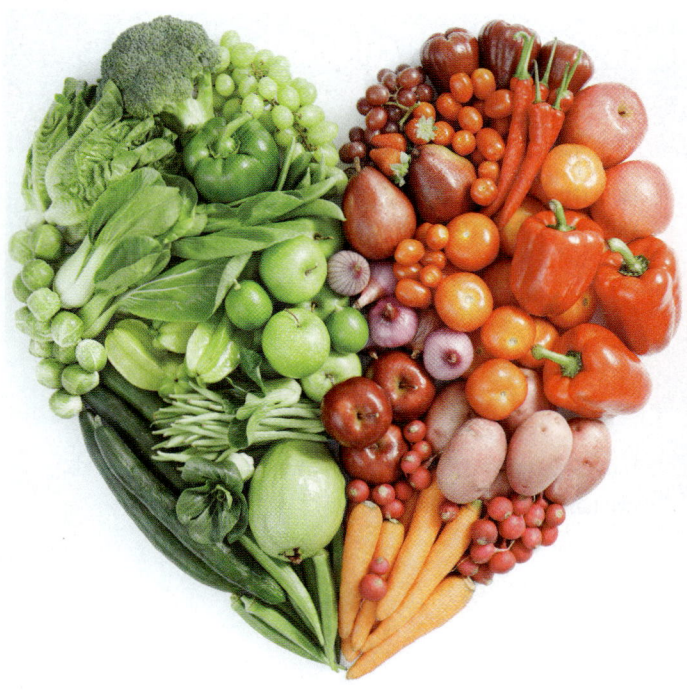
©ifong/Shutterstock.

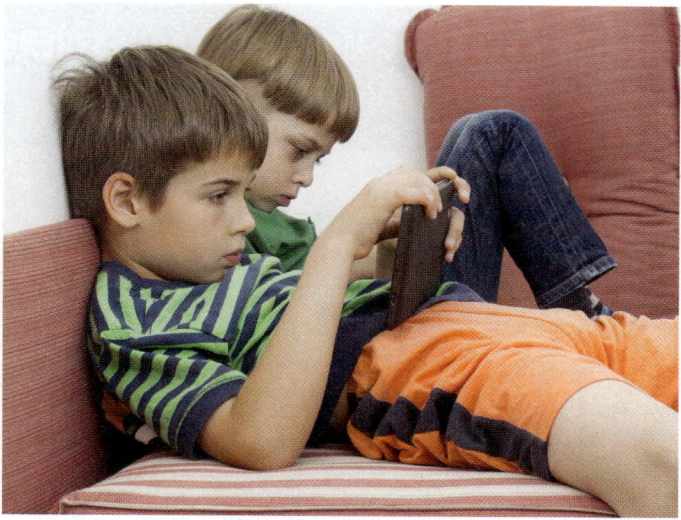
©vesna cvorovic/Shutterstock.

Dietary Intervention

The dietary approach to pediatric obesity that is recommended by most healthcare providers is a moderate energy restriction. The goal is to encourage healthy relationships with food; overrestriction may lead to sneaking behaviors and subsequent weight gain. The goals of intervention should focus on developing nutritionally balanced and portion controlled eating that is age appropriate. To assess the best dietary approaches for weight management in children, the Academy of Nutrition and Dietetics systematically reviewed the efficacy of the Stop Light Diet for Children, the Low Carbohydrate diet and the Reduced Glycemic Load diet. The impact on outcome were inconsistent, leading the Academy of Nutrition and Dietetics Expert Committee to conclude that a variety of dietary approaches may be useful. Of note, studies indicate that emphasis on increasing intake of healthy foods is more effective in reducing weight and preventing rebound as is reducing intake of high-energy foods. This finding correlates with less parental restriction on eating behaviors and less focus on a child's weight.[44]

> **PRACTICE POINT**
>
> A number of dietary approaches may be effective in promoting a healthy weight in children. A focus on eating healthy food, as opposed to energy restriction, may be more effective.

Physical Activity

Sedentary behaviors, such as watching TV, playing video games, or using the computer, should be limited. These sedentary activities may take the place of physical activity in a child's routine and, most importantly, can lead to excess calorie intake. Media has a big role in the childhood obesity epidemic, as children are bombarded with ads promoting high-energy, high-sugar foods that can act as triggers to consume these food items. The American Academy of Pediatrics recommends limiting all screen time to a maximum of 2 hours per day; additionally, special care should be taken to eat meals away from the TV, to limit distractions.

Increasing physical activity level is an important part of a weight management program. Studies have shown that structured or programmed aerobic exercises are actually less effective than simply increasing the activity of everyday living. Recent guidelines for physical activity recommend at least 60 minutes of activity on most days of the week. Children should be encouraged to make small changes that incorporate more activity throughout the day (Table 24.3). Physical activity has been shown to improve lipid and glucose metabolic profiles, insulin resistance, and respiratory function, and reduce adiposity.[47]

Intervention Approaches

Group Based

Family-based behavioral intervention that focuses on dietary and physical activity changes has been shown to be effective for long-term weight management. Parental influence on children and adolescents as role models is often overlooked, but these relationships are extremely important for weight management.[17]

Motivational Interviewing

This counseling style is patient centered and elicits behavior change by having the patient identify a behavior change they would like to make and come up with their own solutions on how to go about doing so. Motivational interviewing can be very successful in the pediatric population because it allows the patient to be in charge of their own

TABLE 24.3 AEROBIC, MUSCLE AND BONE STRENGTHENING EXERCISES IN CHILDREN

Exercise	Examples
Moderate to Vigorous Aerobic 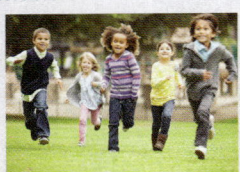 ©Monkey Business Images/Shutterstock.	Moderate intensity: hiking, biking, walking, rollerblading Vigorous intensity: running, jump roping, swimming, tennis
Muscle-Strengthening Activities 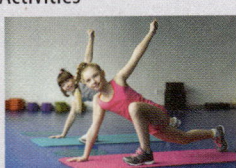 ©Dreams Come True/Shutterstock.	Yoga, resistance exercises using body weight or resistance bands, gymnastics, modified push-ups
Bone-Strengthening Activities 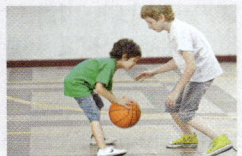 ©Robert Kneschke/Shutterstock.	Jumping, hopping, skipping, and running Sports such as basketball, tennis, and volleyball

Data from CDC Youth Physical Activity Guidelines, 2017. Retrieved from: https://www.cdc.gov/physicalactivity/basics/children/what_counts.htm

---

Box 24.1
CDC Youth Physical Activity Guidelines

Children and adolescents should have 60 minutes (1 hour) or more of physical activity daily.

- **Aerobic:** Most of the 60 or more minutes a day should be either moderate- or vigorous-intensity aerobic physical activity and should include vigorous-intensity physical activity at least 3 days a week.
- **Muscle-strengthening:** As part of their 60 or more minutes of daily physical activity, children and adolescents should include muscle-strengthening physical activity on at least 3 days of the week.
- **Bone-strengthening:** As part of their 60 or more minutes of daily physical activity, children and adolescents should include bone-strengthening physical activity on at least 3 days of the week.

Reproduced from CDC. 2008 Physical Activity Guidelines for Americans. Retrieved from: https://health.gov/paguidelines/guidelines/summary.aspx

---

behavior changes. Key concepts of motivational interviewing include the following[17]:

- **Express empathy:** It is important for the healthcare provider to show the patient and family understanding about where they are coming from; this helps them to feel comfortable and be more willing to listen to suggestions made by the healthcare provider.
- **Develop discrepancy:** Listening for inconsistencies between future goals and current behavior can help the patient make connections as to how their current behavior is hindering their future progress towards achieving their goal.
- **Roll with resistance:** Using different ways to confront resistance from the patient about making a behavior change that do not include arguing with the patient. These approaches might include shifting focus away from the area of contention, establishing patient control over choices, or restating the patient's concern from a new perspective.
- **Support self-efficacy:** Building the patient's confidence in their ability to make the behavior change.

Positive Reinforcement

Positive reinforcement, such as praise and acknowledgement, is demonstrated to be effective in promoting behavior

Clinical Roundtable

Topic: The Use of Media in Nutrition Intervention for Obese Children

Background: The influence media has on children is one of the main factors that promotes sedentary behaviors and the development of childhood obesity. Due to constant technological advancements, children are spending more hours sitting in front of electronic devices than engaging in physical activity. According to a study on the role media has with childhood obesity, children today spend an average of 5.5 hours daily using electronic devices. Not only does media consumption foster sedentary behaviors, but it also encourages unhealthy eating patterns through constant food commercials for fast-food restaurants and unhealthy snacks. Multiple studies have found a direct link between weight gain in children and media consumption. Thus, it is worthwhile to develop nutrition interventions that utilize media to promote physical activity and healthy lifestyle choices.

Roundtable Discussion: Consider the use of media when developing nutrition interventions for obese children.

1. What are some examples of ways to incorporate social media and electronic devices with nutrition interventions for obese children?
2. What are challenges that can come with this development?
3. How might you overcome these challenges?

References

1. Chou S-Y, Rashad I, Grossman M. Fast-Food restaurant advertising on television and its influence on childhood obesity. *J Law Econ*. November 2008. doi:10.3386/w11879.
2. Henry J. Kaiser Family Foundation. The role of media in childhood obesity. Issue brief #7030, 2004.

changes. Rewards unrelated to food are also effective. Rewards that encourage extra physical activity, such as a trip to the park or a new piece of sports equipment, can be used.[17]

Stimulus Control

The focus of this behavioral intervention is to minimize the cues for undesirable behavior and promote the cues for desirable behavior. This approach recommends the removal of certain foods from the home so that the temptation to eat unhealthy foods is no longer there. Similarly, having healthy foods readily available and in clear view can trigger healthful eating.[17]

Goal Setting

Patients who set clear and achievable goals have been proven to have more success following through with a behavior change than those who did not set goals or who set goals that were too broad. Small, specific goals encourage slow and steady changes that are likely to be more sustainable as well as increase self-efficacy in the child. An example of a small, specific goal would be to recommending for the child to "walk the dog for 30 minutes, 5 times per week," as opposed to the broader goal of "get more exercise."[17]

> **CORE CONCEPT 8**
>
> Behavioral change in children can be achieved by employing motivational interviewing during counseling, providing positive reinforcement from the child's support system, and identifying cues that lead to unhealthy behaviors.

CASE STUDY REVISITED

Nora returns in 2 years for a check-up. Her BMI is now 35 and she is charting at the 99th percentile for her sex and age. Nora is now 17 years old and has been seeing a dietitian for the past year, but she has not been able to lose more than 20 pounds before quickly putting it back on. Her lab values have not improved. Nora is inquiring about the possibility of bariatric surgery.

Questions

1. Is Nora now a candidate for surgery?
2. Which bariatric procedure(s) would be appropriate for Nora?
3. What nutrition parameters would you monitor in Nora after surgery?

Surgical Intervention

For some individuals, behavioral interventions are not effective, and thus surgical interventions may be considered. A clinical controversy that exits today is the long-term effectiveness and degree of risk weight loss surgery has on children.

Indications for Surgical Intervention

Guidelines for surgical intervention in the pediatric population vary in medical literature. The Betsy Lehman Center of Patient Safety and Medical Error Reduction provides selection criteria for childhood bariatric surgery by patients aged 12 to 18 years, BMI >35 kg/m^2 with serious comorbidities, and BMI >40 with other comorbidities. Serious comorbidities are defined as type 2 diabetes, moderate to severe obstructive sleep apnea, nonalcoholic fatty liver disease, or pseudotumor cerebri, or idiopathic intracranial pressure. Other comorbidities include mild sleep apnea, mild nonalcoholic fatty liver disease, hypertension, dyslipidemia, and significantly impaired quality of life.[48] In addition to the above-mentioned criteria, patients must have reached 95% of skeletal growth if planning a divisional or malabsorptive surgery. The patient must demonstrate that they understand the significant lifestyle changes they will have to make regarding diet and physical activity after the surgery. Often, an interprofessional team approach is used to guide these patients through a multistep process and evaluate their readiness for this life-changing operation.

> **PRACTICE POINT**
>
> Prior to the weight loss procedure, it is important for the patient to understand the health risks and benefits of the surgery. Along with the parents and the interprofessional team, determine whether the patient is mature enough to have surgical procedure done and has the proper support system.

Weight Loss Procedures

All bariatric procedures promote weight loss, but they differ in the way negative energy balance is achieved. Weight loss may be achieved through restricted intake or malabsorption.[48]

Malabsorptive Procedures

Biliopancreatic diversion with or without duodenal switch is a malabsorptive procedure that prevents absorption by allowing ingested nutrients to mix with bile and pancreatic secretions and be absorbed in a very small segment of the distal small intestine. This often results in significant macro- and micronutrient malabsorption, diarrhea, gas, and nutrient deficiencies. Malabsorptive procedures are often not used in the pediatric population due to severity of symptoms and tendency for deficiencies to develop.

Roux en Y gastric bypass is the most commonly performed bariatric surgery and is considered the gold

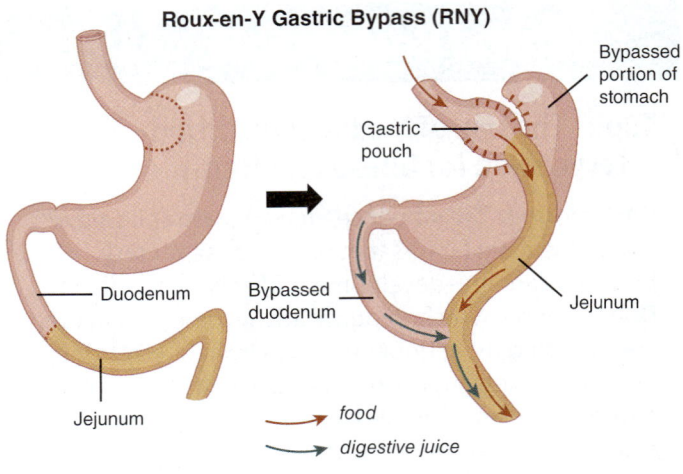

standard for effectiveness.[41] It has been used in adolescents since the 1980s.[33] This surgery results in the creation of a 15- to 30-mL gastric pouch that severely restricts intake and bypasses the distal stomach, duodenum, and part of the jejunum, resulting in malabsorption.[49,50] This surgery results in appetite reduction and an average weight loss of one-third initial body weight is demonstrated. Data from the adolescent population show significant decreases in body fat after gastric bypass. Studies have found that individuals who underwent the Roux en Y gastric bypass procedure have lower levels of ghrelin, reducing their appetite and leading to greater weight loss.[25] As with any surgery, complications should be considered. Major complications include intestinal leakage, pulmonary embolism, and bleeding.[49] Intestinal leakage occurs when there is a hole all the way through the stomach, gallbladder, small intestine, or large intestine. As the hole progresses, bacteria, bile, stomach acid, partially digested food, and stool can leak into the abdominal cavity and cause peritonitis, an inflammation to the abdominal peritoneum. Symptoms of intestinal leakage include severe stomach pain, diarrhea, fever, nausea, vomiting, and a tender abdomen. Children who develop intestinal leakage should seek immediate medical care to treat this condition and determine whether surgical procedures are necessary.[51]

Restricted Intake Procedures

Vertical Banded Gastroplasty The vertical banded gastroplatsy procedure involves the creation of a small gastric pouch, which empties into the distal stomach. This procedure uses a band and staples to create the pouch. The goal of this procedure is to slow the passage of food into the stomach, which will ultimately limit the amount of food the individual can eat and lead to weight loss. This procedure is no longer as popular as it once was and is now rarely used in adolescents due to lack of sustained weight loss.

Adjustable Gastric Banding Adjustable gastric banding was approved for use in the United States in 2001. It involves the placement of a prosthetic band with an

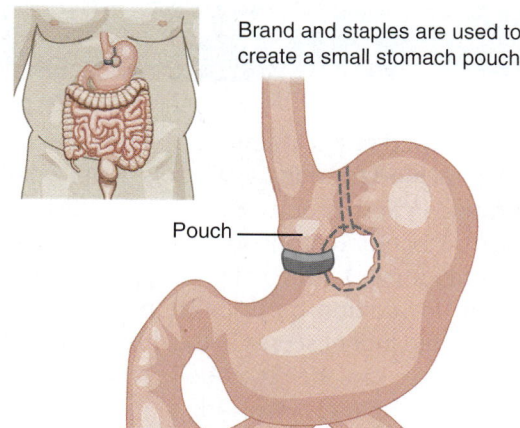

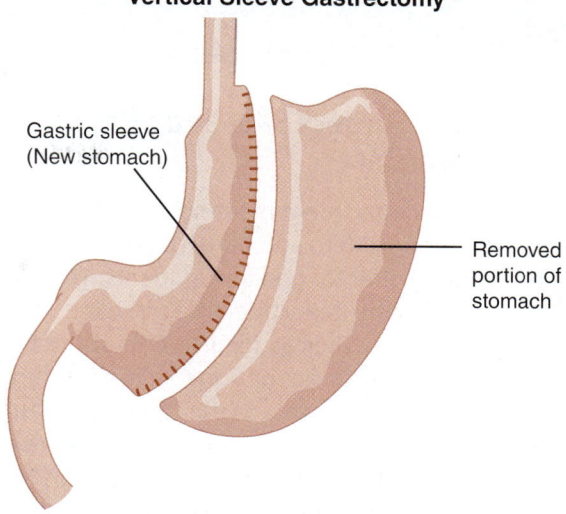

adjustable inner diameter around the proximal stomach to restrict food entry, filling the gastric pouch instead. This procedure is the least invasive and is reversible. Weight loss occurs more slowly; maximal weight loss is usually achieved over 2 to 3 years. Results indicate adjustable gastric banding is comparable in efficacy to gastric bypass.[49] The safety of the lap band procedure, along with the absence of associated nutritional deficiencies, makes the procedure attractive for the pediatric population.

Sleeve Gastrectomy The **sleeve gastrectomy (SG)** involves a left partial gastrectomy that removes the majority of the stomach including the fundus and greater curvature. The SG has been found to be effective and well tolerated in the adolescents with severe obesity.[52] Although the SG is mainly restrictive, it is thought that decreased appetite is influenced by the removal of the portion of the stomach that produces ghrelin.[53] The SG has some advantages compared to other bariatric procedures including the fact that the upper GI tract remains intact leading to a decreased risk of **dumping syndrome** and there is a reduced risk of obstruction. Although the SG has grown in popularity in adult bariatric surgical options, few data are currently available comparing outcomes of different bariatric surgery techniques in adolescents.

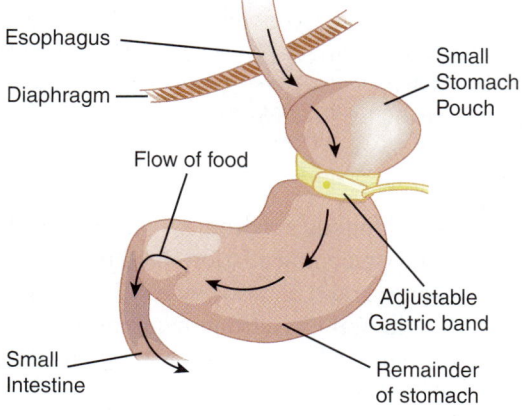

CORE CONCEPT 9

Three procedures that are recommended for weight loss in adolescents include the adjustable gastric binding procedure, the Roux en Y gastric bypass, and the sleeve gastrectomy.

PRACTICE POINT

The following criteria indicate when weight loss surgery is appropriate and recommended for pediatric patients: patient age is 12 to 18 years, BMI >35 kg/m^2 with serious comorbidities, and BMI >40 with other comorbidities.

Nutritional Considerations

Daily supplementation is needed after bariatric surgery due to dietary vitamin and mineral intake restriction and possible malabsorption. In the Roux en Y procedure, levels of vitamin B$_{12}$, calcium, vitamin D, iron, and thiamine may be insufficient and should be monitored.[50] Consistent use of nutritional supplementation is essential and should be stressed to the adolescent. Due to the reduction of the gastric reservoir size, dumping syndrome is a common condition that often develops after bariatric surgery. Dumping syndrome is a condition where large particles of food rapidly travel from the stomach to the small intestine, making it difficult for the small intestine to digest and absorb nutrients. Early dumping syndrome occurs 30 to 60 minutes after consumption and is caused by rapid food movement from the stomach, followed by a surplus of fluid from the bloodstream into the small intestine. Symptoms of early dumping syndrome include abdominal cramping, severe diarrhea, nausea or vomiting, and a rapid heartbeat. Late dumping syndrome occurs 1 to 3 hours after ingestion and is caused by rapid movement of sugar into the small intestine, raising the body's blood glucose levels and increasing the release of insulin from the pancreas. The rapid release of insulin levels causes blood glucose levels to drop, resulting in hypoglycemia. Symptoms of the late dumping syndrome include fatigue, sweating, dizziness, shakiness, fainting, and rapid heartbeat.[54] Medical nutritional therapy is the first step in treating early and late phases of the

⚠ Clinical Controversy

Is Bariatric Surgery Safe and Effective for Children?

At a hospital department meeting, the hospital administrator is proposing to add bariatric surgery as a new service line to offer for pediatric patients. There is much debate among the department heads in medicine, surgery, and ancillary clinical departments about the safety of this surgical treatment option for children and adolescents. They are asking you, as the Director of Nutrition, to weigh in on this initiative. You agree to review the literature and return with your formal opinion.

As childhood obesity rates continue to rise nationwide, there is a growing need to determine the appropriate forms of intervention available for chronic diseases associated with obesity. Bariatric surgery is a controversial solution that has been found to help weight loss and decrease long-term risks associated with extreme obesity. While some studies have proven the effectiveness in bariatric surgery for children, others have stated that these procedures can leave children with long-term medical and psychological complications and thus bariatric surgery is not recommended.[49] Dr. Joan C. Han, the director of Pediatric Obesity Program at the National Institutes of Health, discusses in her article that the risks of bariatric surgery for children and long-term efficacy is an area where more research needs to be developed and thus should be only recommended to children with extreme caution.[50] You find two studies that seem to match your population, described below.

A prospective study completed in Australia compared the weight loss adolescents experienced after a lifestyle intervention program (reduced energy intake, behavioral intervention, and increased physical activity) with bariatric surgery.[55] Fifty participants aged 14 to 18 years, with a BMI ≥35 and existing medical complications of hypertension, asthma, or metabolic syndrome, were randomized to participate in either the gastric banding program or the lifestyle program. The participants in the gastric banding program underwent the lap band adjustable gastric surgery and were given detailed dietary recommendations by dietitians and advised to be physically active for 30 minutes each day after recovery. The participants in the lifestyle program were given individualized diet plans (800-2000 kcal/day), recommended physical activity schedules, and behavioral modifications. While successful weight loss was found in both groups, 84% of the participants in the gastric banding group lost more than 50% of their excess weight versus 12% of participants in the lifestyle program. In addition, participants in the gastric banding program had higher scores in the quality of life assessment and also saw their metabolic syndrome and insulin resistance completely resolved.[56]

The Medical University of Vienna conducted a follow-up study regarding the lives of 10 adolescents who participated in an original study on adolescent obesity and bariatric surgery. The 10 participants in this study were ages 14 to 20 years, had a BMI of ≥49, and were unsuccessful in previous forms of weight loss interventions. Although weight loss was found 24 months after the procedure, 6 out of the 10 patients regained the weight 3 years later. Participants also felt exhausted and weak and experienced stomach pains 44 months after the procedure. In addition, 40% of the participants suffered from rheumatic pains and 60% experienced daily drowsiness, palpitations, and chest pains.[57] Participants turned to food when coping with emotional stress, experienced a negative body image, and received high scores on the depression screening tools.

Based on this research, describe what the conflicting issues are and how they may affect your hospital's decision? What are the strengths and weaknesses of the studies? What factors might need to be implemented for a successful outcome? What recommendation might you make for initiation of a bariatric surgery program at your institution?

References

1. O'Brien PE, Sawyer SM, Laurie C, etal. Laparoscopic adjustable gastric banding in severely obese adolescents. A randomized trial. *JAMA*. 2010;303(6):519-526. doi:10.1001/jama.2010.81.

2. Han JC, Lawlor DA, Kimm SYS. Childhood Obesity—2010: Progress and Challenges. *Lancet*. 2010;375(9727):1737-1748. doi:10.1016/S0140-6736(10)60171-7.

3. Dietrich S, Widhalm K, Prager G, Silberhummer G, Orth D. Bariatric surgery in morbidly obese adolescents: a 4 years follow-up of ten patients. *Aktuelle Ernährungsmedizin*. 2008;33(03). doi:10.1055/s-2008-1079394.

---

dumping syndrome. The dietary measures recommended for patients with dumping syndrome include delaying the intake of any liquids until 30 minutes after the meal, consuming six small meals per day, and eliminating rapidly absorbed carbohydrates from the diet. Patients are also advised to lie down for 30 minutes after the meal to delay gastric emptying and symptoms of dumping syndrome.[54] The patient should follow these dietary recommendations for 3 to 4 weeks, and weekly monitoring should be made by a PCP or registered dietitian (RD). If dumping syndrome symptoms do not improve, various surgical procedures or alternate forms of therapy should be considered.

Follow-up with an RD is important to help the patient make positive dietary changes and improve or maintain nutritional status following surgery. RDs can work with the patient to understand the micronutrient deficiencies they are at risk for, as well as help develop a plan for dietary intervention. Patients may experience symptoms such as nausea, vomiting, or diarrhea, which an RD can help link to certain foods in a patient's diet.

Postoperative Care

Postoperatively, patients should follow an interprofessional program that encourages follow-up with different members of the medical team.[50] The team should include a pediatrician, psychologist, dietitian, bariatric surgeon, and program coordinator. A strong postoperative program that offers ample support for these patients is important for long-term success and maintenance of weight loss.[48]

Chapter Summary

Rates of childhood obesity are following a concerning upward trend, and as rates of obesity in children and adolescents increase, so too do the related comorbidities. Children are now facing serious health complications, such as type 2 diabetes, metabolic syndrome, hypertension, obstructive sleep apnea, and cardiac dysfunction that had previously only been seen in adulthood.

A standardized method to assess and evaluate these overweight and obese individuals should be established. Currently, BMI and age- and sex-specific growth charts are the most common ways to assess overweight and obesity. Individuals considered overweight or obese should be evaluated for comorbidities, and interventions should be implemented as early as possible so that the patient does not carry adverse health complications into adulthood. Behavioral interventions can be used to address dietary and physical activity lifestyle changes. In some individuals, behavioral changes may not be effective and surgical intervention can then be considered.

Childhood obesity carries with it much medical and psychological comorbidity that can affect almost all aspects of the child's life. Health professionals should attempt to identify trends of overweight and obesity early so as to implement an intervention plan as soon as possible, because it has been demonstrated that early intervention is associated with reduced health complications and progression on obesity into adulthood.

Key Terms

childhood obesity, left ventricular hypertrophy, epicardial fat, metabolic syndrome, insulin resistance, intramyocellular lipid deposition, obstructive sleep apnea, nonalcoholic fatty liver disease, nutrigenomics, biliopancreatic diversion, Roux en Y gastric surgery, adjustable gastric binding, sleeve gastrectromy, dumping syndrome

References

1. Ogden, CL, Carroll, MD, Fryar, CD, Flegal, KM. Prevalence of obesity among adults and youth: United States, 2011–2014. NCHS data brief, no. 219; Hyattsville, MD: National Center for Health Statistics, 2015.
2. Ogden CL, Carroll MD, Fryar CD, Kit BK, Flegal KM. Prevalence of adult and childhood obesity in the United States, 2011-2014. *JAMA*. 2016;315(21):2292-9.
3. Balakrishnan PL. Identification of obesity and cardiovascular risk factors in childhood and adolescence. *Pediatr Clin North Am*. 2014;61(1):153-171.
4. US Preventative Service Task Force, Grossman DC, Bibbins-Domingo K, et al. Screening for obesity in children and adolescents: US Preventive Services Task Force Recommendation Statement. *JAMA*. 2017 Jun 20;317(23):2417-2426. doi: 10.1001/jama.2017.6803.
5. Centers for Disease Control and Prevention, National Center for Health Statistics. http://www.cdc.gov/nchs. Last updated September 2010. Accessed December 2, 2017.
6. Division of Nutrition, Physical Activity and Obesity, National Center for Chronic Disease Prevention and Health Promotion. Defining childhood obesity. Centers for Disease Control and Prevention Web site. http://www.cdc.gov/obesity/childhood/defining.html. Published 2015. Updated October 20, 2016. Accessed December 2, 2017.
7. Freedman DS, Wang J, Ogden CL, et al. The prediction of body fatness by BMI and skinfold thicknesses among children and adolescents. *Ann Hum Biol*. 2007;34(2):183-194. doi: 10.1080/03014460601116860.
8. Griffiths C, Gately P, Marchant PR, Cooke CB. A five year longitudinal study investigating the prevalence of childhood obesity: Comparison of BMI and waist circumference. *Public Health*. 2013;127(12):1090-1096.
9. Daniels SR. Complications of obesity in children and adolescents. International Journal of *Obesity*. 2009;33:S60. doi: doi:10.1038/ijo.2009.20.
10. Berenson GS, Srinivasan SR, Bao W, Newman WP, Tracy RE, Wattigney WA. Association between multiple cardiovascular risk factors and atherosclerosis in children and young adults. *N Engl J Med*. 1998;338(23):1650-1656. doi: 10.1056/NEJM199806043382302.
11. DeBoer MD. Obesity, systemic inflammation, and increased risk for cardiovascular disease and diabetes among adolescents: A need for screening tools to target interventions. *Nutrition*. 2013;29(2):379-386.
12. Salazar J, Luzardo E, Mejías JC, et al. Epicardial fat: physiological, pathological, and therapeutic implications. *Cardiol Res Prac*. 2016;2016;1291537. doi:10.1155/2016/1291537.
13. Grundy SM, Brewer HB, Cleeman JI, Smith SC, Lenfant C, for the Conference Participants. Definition of metabolic syndrome: Report of the National Heart, Lung, and Blood Institute/American Heart Association conference on scientific issues related to definition. *Circulation*. 2004;109(3):433-438. doi: 10.1161/01.CIR.0000111245.75752.C6.
14. Schubert CM, Sun SS, Burns TL, Morrison JA, Huang TT. Predictive ability of childhood metabolic components for adult metabolic syndrome and type 2 diabetes. *J Pediatr*. 2009;155(3):S6.e1-S6.e7.
15. Sarría A, Moreno LA, Garcí-Llop LA, Fleta J, Morellón MP, Bueno M. Body mass index, triceps skinfold and waist circumference in screening for adiposity in male children and adolescents. *Acta Paediatrica*. http://onlinelibrary.wiley.com/doi/10.1111/j.1651-2227.2001.tb00437.x/full. Published January 2, 2007. Accessed July 10, 2017.
16. Després J-P. Cardiovascular disease under the influence of excess visceral fat. *Crit Pathways Cardiol*. 2007; 6(2):51-59. doi:10.1097/hpc.0b013e318057d4c9.
17. Kim G, Caprio S. Diabetes and insulin resistance in pediatric obesity. *Pediatr Clin North Am*. 2011;58(6):1355-1361.

18. D'adamo E, Caprio S. Type 2 diabetes in youth: Epidemiology and pathophysiology. *Diabetes Care*. 2011;34:S161. doi: 10.2337/dc11-s212.
19. Craig ME, Huang C. Type-2 diabetes in childhood: Incidence and prognosis. *Pediatr Child Health*. 2009;19(7):321-326. doi: 10.1016/j.paed.2009.03.011.
20. Pulgarón ER. Childhood obesity: A review of increased risk for physical and psychological comorbidities. *Clin Ther*. 2013;35(1):A18-A32. doi: 10.1016/j.clinthera.2012.12.014.
21. Rance K, O'Laughlen M. Obesity and asthma: A dangerous link in children: An integrative review of the literature. *J Nurse Pract*. 2011;7(4):287-292. doi: 10.1016/j.nurpra.2010.06.011.
22. Papoutsakis C, Priftis KN, Drakouli M, et al. Childhood overweight/obesity and asthma: Is there a link? A systematic review of recent epidemiologic evidence. *J Am Nutr Dietet*. 2013;113(1):77-105. doi: http://dx.doi.org/10.1016/j.jand.2012.08.025.
23. Lumeng J, Chervin R. Epidemiology of pediatric obstructive sleep apnea. *Proc Am Thorac Soc*. 2008;5:242. doi: 10.1513/pats.200708-135MG.
24. Tauman R, Gozal D. Obesity and obstructive sleep apnea in children. *Paediatr Respir Rev*. 2006;7(4):247-259. doi: 10.1016/j.prrv.2006.08.003.
25. Cummings DE, Shannon MH. Roles for ghrelin in the regulation of appetite and body weight. *Arch Surg*. 2003;138(4):389-396. doi:10.1001/archsurg.138.4.389.
26. Shneider BL, González-Peralta R, Roberts EA. Controversies in the management of pediatric liver disease: Hepatitis B, C and NAFLD: Summary of a single topic conference. *Hepatology*. 2006;44(5):1344-1354. doi:10.1002/hep.21373.
27. Spengler EK, Loomba R. Recommendations for diagnosis, referral for liver biopsy, and treatment of NAFLD and NASH. *Mayo Clinic Proc*. 2015;90(9):1233-1246. doi:10.1016/j.mayocp.2015.06.013.
28. Dreyer ML, Egan AM. Psychosocial functioning and its impact on implementing behavioral interventions for childhood obesity. *Prog Pediatr Cardiol*. 2008;25(2):159-166. doi: http://dx.doi.org/10.1016/j.ppedcard.2008.05.007.
29. Dockray S, Susman EJ, Dorn LD. Depression, cortisol reactivity, and obesity in childhood and adolescence. *J Adolesc Health*. 2009;45(4):344-350. doi: 10.1016/j.jadohealth.2009.06.014.
30. Vander Wal JS, Mitchell ER. Psychological complications of pediatric obesity. *Pediatr Clin North Am*. 2011;58(6):1393-401.
31. Miller AA, Spencer SJ. Obesity and neuroinflammation: A pathway to cognitive impairment. *Brain Behav Immun*. 2014;42:10-21. 10.1016/j.bbi.2014.04.001.
32. Maloney AE. Pediatric obesity: A review for the child psychiatrist. *Child Adolesc Psychiatr Clin N Am*. 2010;19(2):353-370. doi: 10.1016/j.chc.2010.01.005.
33. Hilmers A, Hilmers DC, Dave J. Neighborhood disparities in access to healthy goods and their effects on environmental justice. *Am J Public Health*. 2012;102(9):1644-1654. doi:10.2105/AJPH.2012.300865.
34. Eagle TF, Sheetz A, Gurm R, et al. Understanding childhood obesity in America: Linkages between household income, community resources, and children's behaviors. *Am Heart J*. 2012;163(5):836-843. doi: 10.1016/j.ahj.2012.02.025.
35. Blissett J. Relationships between parenting style, feeding style and feeding practices and fruit and vegetable consumption in early childhood. *Appetite*. 2011;57(3):826-831. doi: j.appet.2011.05.318.
36. Lifshitz F. Obesity in children. *J Clin Res Pediatr Endocrinol*. 2008;1(2):53-60. doi:10.4008/jcrpe.v1i2.
37. Hjelmborg JVB, Fagnani C, Silventoinen K, et al. Genetic influences on growth traits of BMI: a longitudinal study of adult twins. *Obesity*. 2008;16(4):847–852.
38. Cheung WW, Peizhong M. Recent advances in obesity: genetics and beyond. *ISRN Endocrinol*. 2012; 2012: 536905.
39. Hart CN, Carskadon MA, Considine RV, et al. Changes in children's sleep duration on food intake, weight, and leptin. *Pediatrics*. 2013;6(2):1-10.
40. Aznar LM, Pigeot I, Ahrens W. *Epidemiology of obesity in children and adolescents: prevalence and etiology*. New York, NY: Springer; 2011.
41. Mead MN. Nutrigenomics: The Genome–Food Interface. Environmental Health Perspectives. *Environ Health Perspect*. 2007;115(12):A582-A589.
42. Frayling TM, Timpson NJ, Weedon MN, et al. A common variant in the FTO gene is associated with body mass index and predisposes to childhood and adult obesity. *Science*. 2007;316(5826):889-894.
43. Barlow SE, for the Expert Committee. Expert committee recommendations regarding the prevention, assessment, and treatment of child and adolescent overweight and obesity: summary report. *Pediatrics*. 2007;120(suppl 4):S164-S192.
44. Hoelscher, DM, Kirk S, Ritchie, L, Cunningham-Sabo, L for the Academy Positions Committee. Position of the Academy of Nutrition and Dietetics: Interventions for the prevention and treatment of pediatric overweight and obesity. *J Acad Nutr Diet*. 2013;113:1375-1394.
45. Tanofsky-Kraff M, Faden D, Yanovski SZ, Wilfley DE, Yanovski JA. The perceived onset of dieting and loss of control eating behaviors in overweight children. *Int J Eating Disord*. 2005;38(2):112-122. doi:10.1002/eat.20158.
46. U.S. Department of Health and Human Services/USDA Dietary Guidelines for Americans, 2010. https://health.gov/dietaryguidelines/dga2010/dietaryguidelines2010.pdf. Published December 2010. Accessed December 2, 2017.
47. Centers for Disease Control and Prevention. Aerobic, Muscle- and Bone-Strengthening: What counts? https://www.cdc.gov/physicalactivity/basics/children/what_counts.htm. Accessed December 2, 2017.
48. Lenders CM, Gorman K, Lim-Miller A, Puklin S, Pratt J. Practical approaches to the treatment of severe pediatric obesity. *Pediatr Clin North Am*. 2011;58(6):1425-1438. doi: 10.1016/j.pcl.2011.09.013.
49. Inge TH, Zeller MH, Lawson ML, Daniels SR. A critical appraisal of evidence supporting a bariatric surgical approach to weight management for adolescents. *J Pediatr*. 2005;147(1):10-19. doi: 10.1016/j.jpeds.2005.03.021.
50. Brei MN, Mudd S. Current guidelines for weight loss surgery in adolescents: A review of the literature. *J Pediatr Health Care*. 2014;28(4):288-94. 10.1016/j.pedhc.2013.04.005.
51. Henne-Bruns D, Kramer K. Incidence of, risk factors for, and prevention of intestinal leakage. *Zentralblatt Fur Chirurgie* [serial online]. n.d.;138(3):301-306.
52. Al-Sabah SK, Almazeedi SM, Dashti SA, Al-Mulla AY, Ali DA, Jumaa TH. The efficacy of laparoscopic sleeve gastrectomy in treating adolescent obesity. *Obes Surg*. 2015;25(1):50–4. doi:10.1007/s11695-014-1340-9.
53. Frezza EE, Chiriva-Internati M, Wachtel MS. Analysis of the results of sleeve gastrectomy for morbid obesity and the role of ghrelin. *Surg Today*. 2008;38(6):481-483.
54. Tack J, Arts J, Caenepeel P, De D, Bisschops R. Pathophysiology, diagnosis and management of postoperative dumping syndrome. *Nat Rev Gastroenterol Hepatol*. 2009 6(10):583-90.
55. O'Brien PE, Sawyer SM, Laurie C, et al. Laparoscopic adjustable gastric banding in severely obese adolescents. A randomized trial. *JAMA*. 2010;303(6):519-526. doi:10.1001/jama.2010.81.
56. Han JC, Lawlor DA, Kimm SYS. Childhood Obesity—2010: Progress and Challenges. *Lancet*. 2010;375(9727):1737-1748. doi:10.1016/S0140-6736(10)60171-7.
57. Dietrich S, Widhalm K, Prager G, Silberhummer G, Orth D. Bariatric surgery in morbidly obese adolescents: a 4 years follow-up of ten patients. *Aktuelle Ernährungsmedizin*. 2008;33(03). doi:10.1055/s-2008-1079394.

Chapter 25

Nutrition in Eating Disorders

Natalie Faella

Chapter Outline

Core Concepts
Introduction
Background and Etiology
Prognosis
Psychological Treatment

Pharmacotherapy
Nutrition Assessment
Medical Nutrition Therapy
Counseling
Patient Monitoring and Evaluation

CORE CONCEPTS

1. The etiologies of eating disorders generally comprise a complex interaction of genetic, biological, behavioral, psychological, and social factors, requiring that diagnosis and treatment incorporate a interprofessional team of psychiatric, medical, and nutrition professionals.

2. Eating disorders are spectral disorders because they exist on a continuum of severity and often become more severe the longer they are present.

3. Research has shown when cessation of disturbed eating behaviors and physical restoration occurs early in the treatment process, the result is better response to psychotherapy and improved overall prognosis.

4. In the eating disorder community, laboratory values within normal limits do not reflect nutrition stability; conservation mechanisms, like the body's adaptive ability to maintain visceral protein metabolism in chronic starvation mode, can initially hide nutrient deficiencies.

5. Individuals with eating disorders can present with fluid and electrolyte abnormalities secondary to purging methods, fluid restriction or overload, metabolic changes, or a combination of these.

6. Medical nutrition therapy guidelines for eating disorders are largely based on clinical experience.

7. Changes in resting energy expenditure must be considered during the refeeding process because the reintroduction of food causes a dramatic increase in diet-induced thermogenesis, or the thermic effect of food.

8. Indirect calorimetry is the best method to determine whether an eating disorder patient is hypometabolic or hypermetabolic.

9. Refeeding syndrome is a serious and potentially fatal condition that can occur in severely malnourished patients if aggressive oral, enteral, or parenteral nutrition intake is introduced within the first week of treatment

Learning Objectives

1. Describe the interprofessional approach needed to diagnose and treat individuals with eating disorders and the role of the registered dietitian (RD) in detection and treatment.
2. Specify the signs and clinical complications of anorexia nervosa and bulimia nervosa and their subtypes.
3. Define binge eating disorder and explain its treatment.
4. Recognize the signs and three major complications of the female athlete triad.
5. Define refeeding syndrome, specify those at risk, and state the serum shifts that are characteristic of the syndrome.
6. Identify the treatment goals for each eating disorder.
7. Describe obstacles that clinicians may encounter in treating patients with eating disorders.

Introduction

An **eating disorder (ED)** is a psychiatric illness characterized by chronic disturbances of eating habits and weight control behaviors that debilitate both physical health and psychological functioning. EDs are different from disordered eating, such as frequent dieting, refusing to eat certain macronutrients, and skipping meals, in that disordered eating typically does not negatively impact health as significantly as an ED. Anorexia nervosa (AN), bulimia nervosa (BN), and binge eating disorder (BED) are of the most widely known EDs. In addition to AN, BN, and BED, other categories of EDs defined by the fifth edition of the *Diagnostic and Statistical Manual of Mental Disorders (DSM-V)* include pica; rumination disorder; avoidant restrictive food intake disorder (ARFID); and two additional categories of EDs, "other specified feeding or eating disorder" and "unspecified feeding or eating disorder."[1]

Eating disorders are relatively rare, with a lifetime prevalence estimates ranging from 0.3% to 1.6%.[2] AN is associated with the lowest prevalence, followed by BN, and then BED.[2] In the United States, 20 million women and 10 million men suffer from an ED at some point in their life.[3] Eating disorders represent a large public health issue due to their life-threatening nature and potentially long-lasting impacts on health. The etiologies of EDs are multifactorial, comprising a complex interaction of genetic, biological, behavioral, psychological, and social factors. Thus, diagnosis and treatment must incorporate a interprofessional team of psychiatric, medical, and nutrition professionals. Due to the complex nature of EDs, it is imperative for team members to work together and coordinate care plans to provide consistent and efficacious care in the treatment of ED.

> **CORE CONCEPT 1**
>
> The etiologies of eating disorders generally comprise a complex interaction of genetic, biological, behavioral, psychological, and social factors, requiring that diagnosis and treatment incorporate a interprofessional team of psychiatric, medical, and nutrition professionals.

Background and Etiology

Anorexia Nervosa

Anorexia nervosa (AN) is characterized by an intense fear of weight gain that leads to overrestriction of dietary intake, significantly low body weight, and a distorted self-perception of body weight or shape. The lifetime prevalence of AN in the U.S. adult population is 0.6%.[4] This illness predominately manifests in females, with a female-to-male ratio of 10:1.[1] Incidences of AN are commonly seen in postindustrialized, high-income countries such as the United States, New Zealand, Australia, Japan, and many European countries, with a steady increase documented among 15 to 19 year olds worldwide since the 1930s.[5] Of those affected, only 33.8% are receiving treatment.[4]

AN develops as one of two subtypes: the restrictive type or the binge-purge type. Individuals with the restrictive type achieve a low body weight through extreme dietary restraint. Excessive exercise is often characteristic of this subtype. Exercise is considered excessive when it occurs at inappropriate times or settings, continues despite injury, or when it significantly interferes with important activities. Individuals with the binge-purge type have recurrent episodes of binge eating followed by compensatory behaviors that may include self-induced vomiting; misuse of laxatives, enemas, or diuretics; or a combination of these. Both subtypes share an intense fear of gaining weight and a disturbed perception of body shape (**Figure 25.1**). Crossover between the two subtypes is common, because patients may start with the restrictive type and adopt the binge-purge type over time.[5,6]

Patients with AN are often described as having a weight deficit, or being of "significantly low body weight." The World Health Organization classifies adult thinness from mild to severe as body mass index (BMI) values between 17 and 18.5 to less than 16, respectively.[1] An individual's weight history, body frame, and experienced physiological disturbances should be taken into account and may

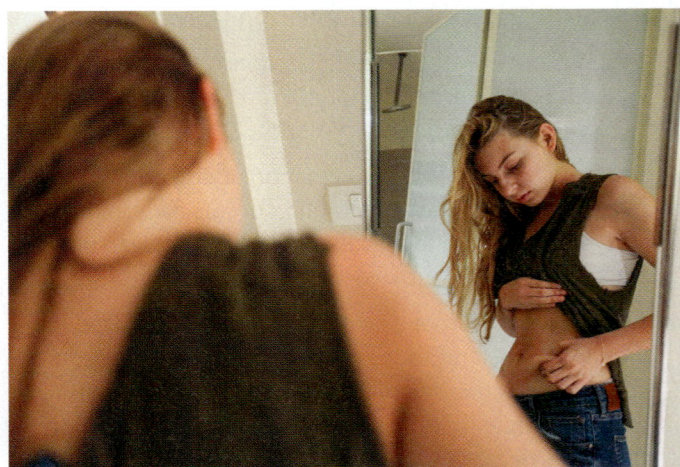

FIGURE 25.1 Individuals with Eating Disorders often Have a Distorted Self-perception of Body Weight or Shape
© PhotoStock-Israel/Cultura/Getty Images.

CASE STUDY INTRODUCTION

Emma is a 22-year-old woman with anorexia nervosa. Her disordered eating habits started at age 20 years, during her second year of college. Her senior year of college brought on more stress as she finished up difficult classes, searched for jobs, and ended a relationship with her long-term significant other. For the last few months, Emma reported eating fewer than 600 calories per day and performing cardiovascular exercise for 1 to 2 hours daily. She states that she has not experienced a menstrual period for the past 6 months. Emma presents to the emergency department for suspected dehydration after fainting in class.

Anthropometric Data:
Height: 167.7 cm (66")
Weight: 40 kg (88 lbs)
BMI: 14.2 kg/m^2
Weight history
52 kg (115 lbs) 2 years ago
45 kg (99 lbs) 6 months ago
Lowest adult weight: current weight of 40 kg (88 lbs)

Biochemical Data:
Sodium 150 (135-145 mEq/L)
Potassium 2.9 (3.6-5.0 mEq/L)
Chloride 94 (98-110 mEq/L)
Carbon dioxide 32 (20-30 mEq/L)
Blood urea nitrogen 33 (6-24 mg/dL)
Creatinine 0.8 (0.4-1.3 mg/dL)

Phosphorus 2.8 (2.7-4.5 mg/dL)
Magnesium 1.4 (1.3-2.1 mEq/L)
Glucose 70 (70-99 mg/dL)
Total cholesterol 202 mg/dL (Desirable<200 mg/dL)
Albumin 3.5 (3.5-5.0 g/dL)
Vitamin B$_{12}$ 150 (160-950 pg/mL)

Clinical Data:
Past Medical History: None
Medications: None
Vital Signs: Blood pressure 93/55 mm Hg (sitting), 70/50 mm Hg (standing); Temperature 95.7°F; Heart rate 50 beats/min
Nutrition-focused Physical Exam: Appears pale with dry skin and lanugo on extremities. Clavicular muscle wasting and thin extremities noted. Hair appears thin, dry, easily plucked. Nails are thin and brittle. Oral exam notable for dry oral mucosa, cracked and reddened areas at corners of mouth, atrophic tongue. Mild abdominal distention noted.

Dietary Data:
Dietary History: Follows a vegetarian, low-fat diet. Limits dairy intake, although eats yogurt. Drinks water and coffee daily.

Questions
1. What is Emma's nutritional status?
2. What are her nutritional risk factors?
3. What are your nutrition priorities for Emma during her inpatient hospitalization?
4. What additional information would you like to obtain?

---

better indicate a weight deficit than a BMI value. Postmenarcheal women with AN may develop **amenorrhea**, which is the absence of three consecutive menstrual cycles. Prepubescent males and females can experience sexual maturation arrest, in which males may develop a testosterone deficiency and females may experience primary amenorrhea or delayed menarche, which is not achieving first menses by age 14 years.

Many risk factors are thought to play a role in the development of AN. Drug or alcohol abuse and psychiatric disorders such as anxiety disorders, panic disorder, and obsessive-compulsive disorder are some of the psychosocial factors associated with AN.[1] Influential social factors include cultural settings where thinness is valued. Professions that encourage a lean physique, such as modeling or elite athleticism, can also be instrumental in the development of an ED. Personality traits such as rigid and inflexible thinking, lack of spontaneity, feelings of perfectionism, low self-esteem, and need for control are characteristic to AN as well.

The genetic component of the disorder is unclear; however, it has been seen that the likelihood of developing an ED is significantly increased in first-degree biological relatives of individuals with EDs. There is also a higher concordance rate of AN in monozygotic twins versus dizygotic twins. Alterations in brain serotonin levels, neuropeptide systems, and brain neurocircuitry are also thought to be components of etiology.[5,6]

Bulimia Nervosa

Bulimia nervosa (BN) is an ED characterized by recurrent episodes of binge eating followed by one or more compensatory behaviors to avoid weight gain. A binge is defined as the consumption of an unusually large amount of food within a discrete period of time, generally within 2 hours.[1] Feelings of loss of control over binging and purging behaviors and an intense sense of body dissatisfaction are central to diagnosis.[7] Patients generally maintain a body weight at or above minimally normal, differentiating this disorder from the binge-purge type of AN. The lifetime prevalence of BN is 0.9% in the U.S. population, and only 43.2% of those are receiving treatment.[2,4] BN is primarily seen in Caucasian women, and like AN, the highest occurrences are in postindustrialized countries.[1]

The compensatory behaviors employed in BN categorize individuals into one of two subtypes: purging type and nonpurging type. Purging behaviors include self-induced vomiting (**Figure 25.2**) and laxative, enema, and/or diuretic misuse. Nonpurging behaviors include excessive exercise and fasting. Type 1 diabetics with BN may reduce or omit insulin doses as a compensatory behavior in attempt to decrease

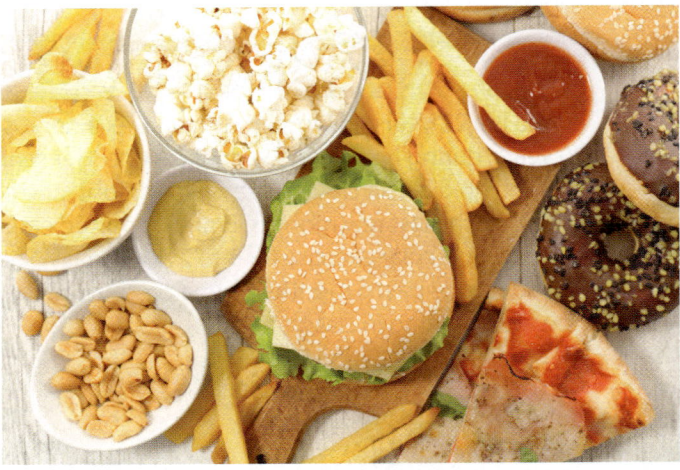

FIGURE 25.3 Foods that Are Consumed During a Binge Typically Include Energy-Dense Snacks and Desserts that Individuals would Normally Avoid
© margouillat photo/Shutterstock.

the uptake and utilization of carbohydrates consumed during a binge.[1] Binging is central to the diagnosis of BN. Episodes of binge eating usually take place in secrecy and are accompanied by feelings of guilt and shame. Foods that are consumed during a binge vary on an individual basis, but typically include energy-dense snacks and desserts the individual would normally avoid (**Figure 25.3**). Certain "triggers" may stimulate binge eating episodes, such as interpersonal stressors; dietary restraint; boredom; and negative feelings related to body shape, weight, and food.[8]

Like AN, there are many potential contributing factors to the development and course of BN. Psychosocial factors such as feelings of low self-esteem and anxiety; parental obesity and substance abuse; and childhood experiences such as sexual or physical abuse, early pubertal maturation, and obesity are associated with BN. Individuals with BN tend to have a strong desire to lose weight and have attempted to diet many times in the past. They may also experience adverse emotional states like anxiety, frustration, and labile mood, and have psychiatric issues such as depression, personality disorders, and social anxiety disorders.[1]

> **PRACTICE POINT**
>
> Patients with BN generally maintain a body weight at or above minimally normal, which differentiates this disorder from the binge-purge type of anorexia nervosa.

Binge Eating Disorder

Binge eating disorder (BED) is characterized by recurrent binge eating episodes that are not followed by compensatory purging or nonpurging behaviors. The lifetime prevalence of adults in the United States with BED is 1.6%.[2] The gender ratio for BED is far less skewed than other EDs with the U.S. lifetime prevalence being 3.5% for females and 2.0% for males.[4] BED is similarly prevalent among different racial and ethnic groups. Children and adolescents are

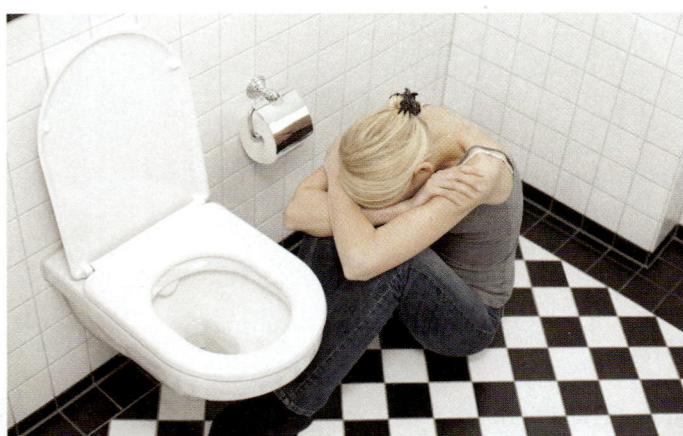

FIGURE 25.2 Individuals with Bulimia Nervosa Use Compensatory Behaviors, such as Self-Induced Vomiting, Misuse of Laxatives/Diuretics, Fasting, and/or Excessive Exercise
© Westend61/Getty Images.

less likely than adults to meet the criteria for the disorder; however, they may still experience some of the symptoms such as loss of control over eating.[9] Individuals with BED are generally overweight or obese. The highest incidence of BED is found in individuals seeking weight loss treatment, particularly those interested in bariatric surgery.

Binge eating episodes are typically characterized by rapid eating and eating when not physically hungry, and are followed by feelings of guilt, disgust, and embarrassment. Comparable to BN, individuals with BED tend to feel powerless over their eating behaviors and unhappy with their weight or body shape. BED also seems to occur in families, which may reflect a possible influence of genetic addictive traits.[5]

> **PRACTICE POINT**
>
> The highest incidence of binge eating disorder is found in individuals seeking weight loss treatment, particularly those interested in bariatric surgery.

Other Specified Feeding or Eating Disorder

The DSM-V defines Other Specified Feeding or Eating Disorders as "presentations of characteristics of feeding and eating disorders that cause clinically significant distress or impairment in social, occupational, or other areas of functioning," but do not meet the full criteria for any other disorder in the feeding and ED diagnostic class.[1] There is very limited knowledge of the prevalence and clinical manifestations of this class of disorders due to the lack of empirical attention.[10]

Night eating syndrome (NES) falls under this category of EDs and is a disordered eating pattern characterized by morning anorexia, evening hyperphagia, and insomnia.[11] NES is comparable to BED in that both disorders are characterized by episodes of hyperphagia or binging and occur in individuals with body shape, weight, and eating concerns. NES is also associated with psychiatric issues such as anxiety and depression.[11] Individuals with NES differ in that they experience nocturnal anxiety, which is not symptomatic of BED. Crossover between the two disorders often occurs and approximately 9% of individuals with BED have NES as well.[12]

Unspecified Feeding or Eating Disorder

The diagnosis of Unspecified Feeding or Eating Disorder is used when a clinician chooses not to specify the reasons an individual does not meet the full criteria for a specific ED. This could be used in situations when the clinician lacks sufficient information to make a more specific diagnosis. For instance, if the patient is in an emergency room setting, or unwilling to provide information, the clinician may be unable to formulate an accurate diagnosis.[1]

Avoidant Restrictive Food Intake Disorder and Orthorexia

Avoidant restrictive food intake disorder (ARFID) is included in the DSM-V feeding and eating disorder class and is characterized as a persistent disturbance in eating that leads to significant clinical consequences, such as weight loss, inadequate growth, significant nutrient deficiencies, and/or impaired psychosocial functioning (such as an inability to eat with others). ARFID differs from AN in that the preoccupation with body weight and shape is not the driving force of restrictive behaviors.[1]

Orthorexia is a more recently coined term that describes an excessive preoccupation with healthy eating. It may begin as an attempt at healthy eating and turn into an obsession of food-related topics, the quality of food in the diet, and rigid beliefs about food. Orthorexia differs from AN and BN by the lack of associated fear of weight gain and preoccupation with weight loss. This pathological fixation on health-conscious eating behaviors is not recognized in the DSM-V as a clinical diagnosis.[13]

Prognosis

EDs are associated with significant medical complications, physical and psychological morbidities, relapse, and mortality. They are considered spectral disorders because they exist on a continuum of severity and often become more severe the longer they are present. Even with psychiatric treatment and nutritional rehabilitation, relapse is common in EDs, with rates ranging from 25% to 51% in both AN and BN.[14]

> **CORE CONCEPT 2**
>
> Eating disorders are spectral disorders because they exist on a continuum of severity and often become more severe the longer they are present.

Anorexia Nervosa

The course and outcome of AN are extremely variable. The average age of onset is 19 years and is generally associated with a stressful life event, such as leaving home for college.[1] Many individuals adopt a new eating behavior, such vegetarianism, prior to developing the disorder.[15] Such changed behaviors may serve as a red flag for clinicians to intervene.[2] During the course of the disorder, crossover between the AN subtypes often occurs. For instance, individuals with the restricting type may begin to engage in binge eating and purging behaviors. Crossover between subtypes post-ED treatment is even more likely to occur.[14]

> **PRACTICE POINT**
>
> Many individuals develop a new eating behavior, such as vegetarianism, prior to developing anorexia nervosa.

Clinical Complications

Many physiological changes can occur during the course of AN. These may include development of brittle hair and nails; **lanugo** or soft, downy hair growth on the face and body; ketotic breath caused by ketosis; cyanosis of the

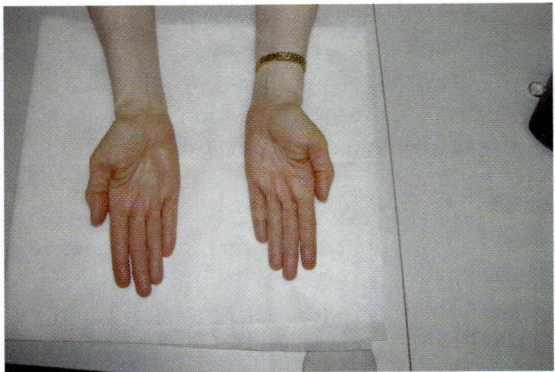

FIGURE 25.4 Individuals Who Consume a Diet Excessively High in Carotenoid Containing Foods May Develop Orange Pigment in the Skin
Reproduced with permission from Atlas Dermatológico. Accessed at, http://www.atlasdermatologico.com.br/disease.jsf?diseaseId=69

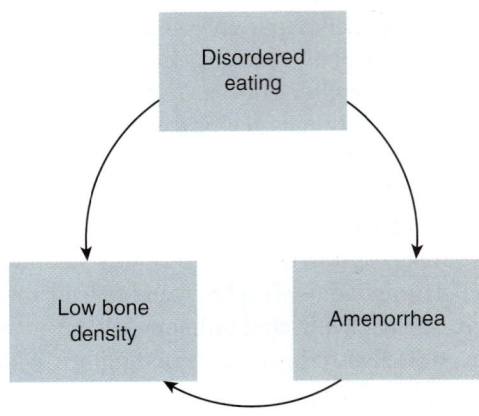

FIGURE 25.5 The Female Athlete Triad

extremities; hypercarotenemia, or the presence of orange pigment in the skin typically related to overconsumption of carotenoid-containing foods (**Figure 25.4**); hypothermia; and/or cold intolerance. Protein-energy malnutrition often results from inadequate intake causing a loss of adipose tissue and somatic protein stores. Resultant cachetic and prepubescent-appearing bodies are distinct features of AN.[7] Serious cardiac complications such as bradycardia, arrhythmias, and orthostatic or postural hypotension, which is a drop in blood pressure that occurs upon standing from a sitting or lying down position, are often seen in AN, but are largely reversible with restoration and correction of dietary deficiencies.[8] Gastrointestinal (GI) issues that can result include delayed gastric emptying, severe constipation, and decreased small-bowel motility. Peripheral edema can also occur from cessation of diuretics that may have been used in the binge–purge type.[15]

A decrease in resting energy expenditure (REE) will occur secondary to weight loss, decreased lean body mass, energy restriction, and decreased leptin levels. As patients refeed and restore weight, REE increases and often results in hypermetabolism.[16] Physical activity can account for up to 50% of total energy expenditure in patients with AN due to decreased REE.[17]

Bone mineral density significantly decreases early in the course of illness and may not be fully reversed by recovery. In a state of starvation, bone metabolism will favor resorption, which impedes bone formation.[18] In an 8-year follow up of patients with AN, it was found that low body weight was associated with low bone mineral density in the spine, and 2 or more years of amenorrhea was associated with reduced bone mineral density in the hip and spine.[19] Hormonal alterations may also occur in individuals with AN. Low leptin levels are a key feature of AN and reflect a low body fat mass, as adipocytes secrete this hormone in proportion with the body's adipose stores. Leptin helps regulate the oscillating levels of lutenizing hormone and estradiol, thus low levels of estradiol are characteristic to AN as well.[6] A decrease in the thyroid hormone triiodinethyroxine (T3), known as T3 syndrome, can also occur and may alter metabolic functioning.

Bone mineral loss and hormonal alterations are two key features of a syndrome known as **female athlete triad**, which consists of disordered eating habits, osteoporosis, and menstrual disorders (**Figure 25.5**). These females typically utilize at least one unhealthy weight control method and exhibit characteristics of perfectionism, competitiveness, and high self-motivation. Female athletes may have classifiable eating disorders, but not all meet the criteria for AN. The term "anorexia athletica," is often used to distinguish the disrupted eating behaviors associated with training and sports performance from pathological AN.[20]

The three areas of this triad are interrelated through physiological and psychological mechanisms. Psychological pressures for elite performance are often perceived as requiring low body mass, which may lead to high-volume training and low energy intake. Chronic low energy intake can temporarily pause the menstrual cycle to conserve energy; low body weight, excessive exercise, and stress can halt the cycle as well. Resultant amenorrhea causes a decrease in the production of estrogen, a major hormone required for maintaining bone mineral density. Hypoestrogenic states are associated with low bone mineral density and high osteoporosis risk.[20]

Psychosocial symptoms of AN may include social withdrawal, irritability, insomnia, and depressed mood. Patients also may exhibit obsessive-compulsive features, both related and unrelated to food. Preoccupation with food and weight-related thoughts might manifest as a desire to cook for others, collect recipes, or hoard food. The Minnesota Starvation Experiment, a well-known study conducted by Ancel Keys during World War II, suggested a link between these obsessive and compulsive behaviors and undernutrition.[21,22]

Relapse and Mortality

Disordered cognitions about food and eating behaviors can be difficult to overcome, making relapse in AN very common. Predictors of AN relapse include age, psychosocial functioning, preoccupation with and misperception of body weight or shape, and individual psychotherapy.[14]

CASE STUDY REVISITED

Emma is admitted to the hospital and the medical team immediately provides intravenous fluids to treat her dehydration as they devise a plan for nutrition therapy.

Questions

1. What physiological complications of AN does Emma exhibit?
2. How would you interpret Emma's labs?
3. How might you expect her labs to change after she receives intravenous fluids?
4. Is her REE expected to be high or low at this time, and why?
5. How would you expect it to change during the refeeding process?

Sometimes relapse may involve a brief return of ED behaviors that self-resolve; other times relapse may be more severe, requiring the patient to seek medical treatment again. Hospital readmissions for AN have been significantly associated with three major factors: prior admission to the hospital, length of initial hospital stay, and rapid regain of weight.[23]

The crude mortality rate for AN is approximately 5% per decade.[14] Mortality rates and risk of suicide are higher for individuals with AN compared to other EDs.[24] Risk of mortality is higher in individuals with poor psychosocial functioning, low body weight, abuse of substances, and a longer duration of illness.[25]

Bulimia Nervosa

The average age of onset for BN is 20 years, and it is typically initiated during or after an attempt at dieting for weight loss or multiple stressful events.[4] Disordered eating patterns associated with BN generally occur for several years and exhibit either a chronic or intermittent course. Crossover from BN to AN occurs in 10% to 15% of cases and usually results in return of BN behaviors. Other individuals may continue to binge eat, but no longer engage in compensatory behaviors at a certain point.[1]

Clinical Complications

Individuals with BN are usually of normal weight and keep their ED behaviors secretive, making clinical detection difficult. When vomiting is the compensatory mechanism utilized, certain signs and symptoms can help identify the disorder, such as eroded dental enamel, increased incidence of dental caries, gingivitis, enlarged parotid glands, and **Russell's sign** (the scarring by teeth of the lower dorsum of the hand used to stimulate the gag reflex). Chronic vomiting can result in dehydration, alkalosis, and hypokalemia, and can manifest as a sore throat, esophagitis, subjunctival hemorrhage, and mild hematemesis. More serious complications include **Mallory-Weiss tears**, or tears in the mucosa at the stomach–esophagus junction; esophageal rupture; and acute gastric dilation. Laxative misuse may result in dehydration, elevated serum aldosterone and vasopressin levels, rectal bleeding, abdominal cramps, and intestinal atony. Individuals with BN may experience rectal prolapse or become dependent on laxatives to stimulate bowel movements.[6,7]

Compensatory behaviors put individuals with BN at increased risk for serious electrolyte abnormalities. Hypokalemia, one of the most common abnormalities seen with self-induced vomiting, can lead to atrial and ventricular arrhythmias. It has been found that generally 40% of individuals who purge twice or more a day are hypokalemic.[8] Individuals who utilize ipecac syrup, an emetic agent typically used to induce vomiting after ingestion of poison, as a compensatory behavior are at risk for cardiomyopathy due to emetine, a cardiac toxin found in ipecac. Death from ventricular arrhythmias or congestive heart failure can occur when excessive amounts are taken.[8] **Figure 25.6** outlines the clinical complications seen in both AN and BN.

The effect of compensatory behaviors on REE is not entirely clear. Some studies have shown that purging decreases metabolic rate, while other studies have shown its effects are insignificant.[26,27] Dietary restriction, seen in both AN and BN, is thought to decrease REE by putting the body into semi-starvation mode, while binge eating behaviors may partially compensate this reduction.[28]

Relapse and Mortality

Patients who experience full remission for 1 year after treatment have better long-term outcomes than those that relapse within the first year. Some predictors of relapse have been identified as level of psychosocial functioning; anxiety about weight or body shape; lower scoring on the Global Assessment Functioning Scale, a numeric scale used by mental health clinicians to subjectively rate an individual's social, occupational, and psychological functioning; and higher mania scoring on the Psychiatric Status

Clinical Roundtable

Topic: The Minnesota Starvation Experiment

Background: During World War II, Ancel Keys and his colleagues conducted a study to gain insight to the physical and psychological effects of semi-starvation and the obstacles involved in refeeding in order to better understand how to refeed civilians who had been starved during the war. The findings of this study have been helpful in understanding the implications of food deprivation on both physiological and cognitive functioning in individuals with AN and BN.

At a Minnesota lab in 1944, 36 male volunteers, many of whom were conscientious objectors who wanted to contribute to the war effort, were observed at baseline for 3 months, during a semi-starvation phase for 6 months, and in a nutrition rehabilitation phase for 3 months. The research protocol was designed to have volunteers lose 25% of their normal body weight by following a hypocaloric meal plan. Additionally, participants expended energy walking 22 miles/week and tending to various duties like housekeeping, laboratory work, and participating in university classes and activities. Measurements of physical strength, body weight, and endurance were taken in addition to clinical monitoring that included laboratory measures and electrocardiograms.

Some of the side effects reported during the semi-starvation state were physical symptoms such as decreased stamina and libido, intolerance to cold temperatures, hair loss, and dizziness. Participants also reported experiencing fatigue, apathy, introversion, irritability, and decreased ability to concentrate. Some participants began reading and collecting cookbooks; hoarding or hiding food instead of eating it; and savoring food by eating slowly, taking very small bites, or adding water to meals to increase volume. Some participants would "cheat" from their diet; for instance, on a trip into town, one participant demonstrated binge-like behaviors where he consumed excessive amounts of milkshakes and ice cream sundaes instead of following the hypocaloric meal plan. Excessive gum chewing and caffeine intake also emerged for some during this malnourished stage, with reports of intake up to 40 packs of gum per day and 15 cups of coffee per day between meals. Participants also experienced distorted body image, not seeing themselves as excessively thin despite appearing cachetic.

In the 3-month rehabilitation phase, calorie increases were distributed among four subgroups: initially an additional 400, 800, 1,200, and 1,600 kcal/day each. It was found that vitamin and protein supplements were ineffective for weight gain at this stage and only abundant calories aided restoration. Keys found a positive effect when 800 kcal/day were added to each group, and concluded that around 4,000 kcal/day for some months was necessary for rehabilitation.

Almost 60 years after the experiment, 18 of the participants were interviewed about their experience in the Minnesota study. They all felt it took longer than 3 months of rehabilitation to feel back to normal, and that there were some lingering aftereffects of the study. They all spoke passionately about what made them volunteer for the study and that even after going through the grueling experience, they would make the sacrifice again.

Roundtable Discussion

The Minnesota Experiment participants and Keys may not have known the insight this experiment would provide in the treatment and understanding of EDs.

1. How might the physical side effects experienced by the participants be similar to symptoms seen in AN?
2. One of the surprising findings of the study was the psychological impact of the hypocaloric diet. How do the psychological side effects described by the Minnesota Experiment correlate with EDs in general and AN in particular?
3. Describe how Keys's findings of the refeeding process help us to understand hypermetabolism in the refeeding process and caloric requirements necessary to restore weight.

References

1. Franko DL, Keshaviah A, Eddy KT, et al. A longitudinal investigation of mortality in anorexia nervosa and bulimia nervosa. *Am J Psychiatry*. 2013;170(8):917-925.
2. Kalm FL, Semba RD. They starved so that others be better fed: remembering Ancel Keys and the Minnesota Experiment. *J Nutrition*. 2005;135(6):1347-1352.

Rating Scale, a rating scale used by mental health clinicians to evaluate degree of mental illness.[14] Like AN, the suicide risk is also elevated for individuals with BN. The crude mortality rate is 2% per decade and individuals with BN are considered to have a significantly elevated risk for mortality.[1]

Binge Eating Disorder

Little is known about the development and course of BED, as it has more recently begun to gain empirical attention. The average age of onset is 25 years; however, onset later in adulthood has been documented as well.[4] Unlike BN, attempts at dieting often follow the development of the

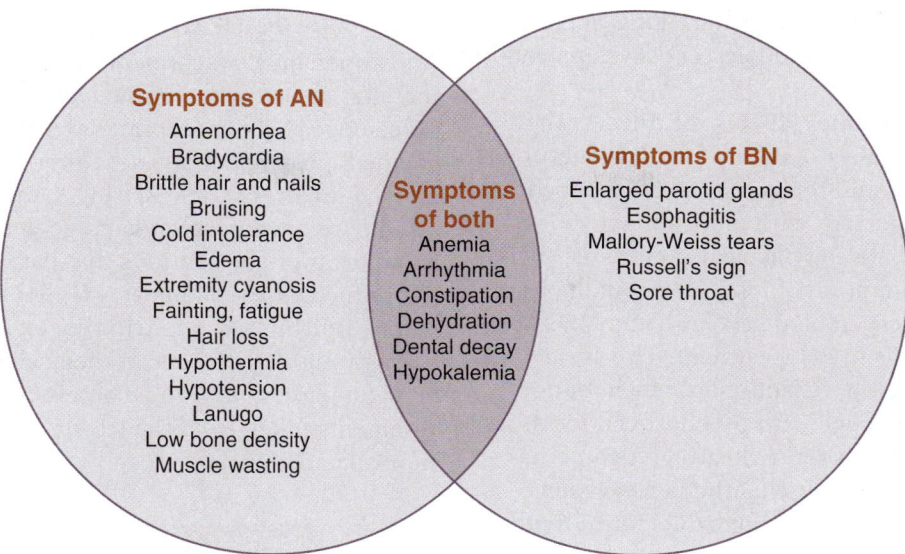

FIGURE 25.6 Comparison of Clinical Complications of AN and BN

disorder. BED is a relatively persistent disorder and its course is generally comparable to BN in terms of severity and duration.[1]

Clinical Complications

BED is associated with increased risk for weight gain and development of obesity. Obesity, and obesity in BED, are two distinct conditions in that most obese individuals do not engage in binge eating behaviors and on average consume fewer calories than obese individuals with BED.[1] This puts individuals with BED at a significantly higher risk for developing type 2 diabetes and cardiovascular diseases.[9] Compared to obese, BMI-matched controls, individuals with BED experience greater functional impairment, lower quality of life, and increased healthcare utilization. They also experience a higher lifetime prevalence of substance abuse problems and psychological comorbidities like major depression disorder and personality disorders.[1]

Relapse and Mortality

Those who seek treatment for BED tend to be older than those seeking treatment for other EDs, and their rate of relapse tends to be higher. Many times, weight that was lost during treatment is regained within the first year. Like AN and BN, BED increases the risk for medical morbidities and mortality.

Psychological Treatment

EDs are complex psychiatric illnesses that require ongoing psychological treatment. Nutrition education and physical restoration alone do not constitute recovery; cognitive and emotional restoration must be achieved in treatment as well. Research has shown when cessation of disturbed eating behaviors and physical restoration occur early in the treatment process, better responses to psychotherapy and overall prognosis result.[6] Family-based treatment, cognitive behavioral therapy (CBT), interpersonal psychotherapy, and dialectical behavioral therapy (DBT) are forms of psychotherapeutic treatment that have been shown effective in the treatment of EDs.

> **CORE CONCEPT 3**
>
> Research has shown when cessation of disturbed eating behaviors and physical restoration occur early in the treatment process, the result is be tter responses to psychotherapy and improved overall prognosis.

The **Maudsley approach** or Maudsley method, also known as family-based treatment, has been shown to be an effective treatment for adolescents with AN.[29] This approach empowers parents to take on the responsibility of weight restoring their child, transforming their relationship to involve issues other than food, and helping their child resume normal adolescent behavior without having an ED.[30] Involving family members in treatment may also provide a more reliable recollection of a patient's history of weight loss, dietary intake prior to ED onset, and other features of the illness, as ED patients generally deny or lack insight to their disorder.[1]

The Maudsley approach consists of three phases: weight restoration, returning control over eating to the adolescent, and establishing a healthy adolescent identity.[31,32] The first phase focuses on empowering parents to disrupt the ED and support their adolescent. It seeks to separate the adolescent's behaviors from the adolescent and encourages parental action. The second phase of treatment begins once disordered eating has ceased and parents begin to transition control over eating back to the adolescent. The third phase occurs when weight is able to be maintained and focuses on the ways the family can help to address the effects of the ED on adolescent developmental processes.[31,32]

Cognitive behavior therapy (CBT) is regarded as the first-line treatment for BN.[24] CBT is a highly structured therapy that identifies and replaces maladaptive behaviors and cognitive processes with more suitable ones (i.e., discrimination between physical symptoms, such as bloating, with resumption of food intake and body weight changes).[6] Interpersonal psychotherapy has also been shown efficacious in BN treatment. This form of therapy may reduce the risk of relapse by helping patients recognize and cope with psychosocial stressors that contribute to their disordered eating. A combination of these psychotherapeutic methods have been effective in decreasing binge eating habits for individuals with BED as well.[14]

Dialectical behavior therapy (DBT) is designed to help individuals change unhelpful patterns of behavior by identifying triggers and applying new coping skills. When used in ED treatment, it involves teaching new coping skills, replacing ED behaviors with more constructive ones, and enhancing self-respect. This method holds potential for decreasing episodes of binge eating, which may be influenced by emotional dysregulation and used as a maladaptive coping skill.[6]

Pharmacotherapy

Pharmacotherapy for treatment of EDs is an area of ongoing research. Recent trials have shown that olanzapine, an atypical neuroleptic agent, improved both weight and dysfunctional thinking in patients with AN.[33] Medications such as **selective serotonin reuptake inhibitors (SSRIs)** may also be prescribed to patients with AN to alleviate mood symptoms or reduce anxiety; however, they have demonstrated low efficacy in treatment of AN. It is important to note SSRIs may not be effective in the severely malnourished.[33] Fluoxetine, a type of SSRI, is currently the only U.S. Food and Drug Administration–approved drug to treat BN.[6] Antidepressants have been found to alleviate some symptoms of BN and BED.[34] Certain anti-epileptic medications have been efficacious in suppression of binge eating episodes and reduction of body weight.[34]

Nutrition Assessment

The nutrition assessment will depend on the stage of illness and treatment setting, but will generally include measuring anthropometrics, evaluating dietary and fluid intake, assessing eating behaviors and attitudes, interpreting biochemical data, and applying a nutrition diagnosis to create a treatment plan for nutritional rehabilitation.

Anthropometric Assessment

Anthropometric assessment in the ED population includes measurement of body weight and body fat percentage. A daily preprandial weight should be taken gowned, post-void, and first thing in the morning for patients in an inpatient setting. Outpatients should also be weighed post-void and gowned once a week. It is important to be cautious that patients may attempt to produce false weights by withholding bowel movements, waiting to void, drinking excessive fluids, or hiding weighted objects on themselves. Estimation of body fat percentage can be obtained from skinfold measurements taken from the tricep, bicep, subscapular, and suprailiac regions.[7]

> **PRACTICE POINT**
>
> Eating disorder patients may try to produce false weights by withholding bowel movements, waiting to void, drinking excessive fluids, or hiding weighted objects on themselves.

Dietary Assessment

In obtaining diet history, the RD should assess the patient's overall energy intake, macronutrient distribution, and fluid consumption.[6] Patients with AN tend to overestimate their caloric intake and fail to recognize that their eating habits are extremely restrictive. The distributions of macronutrients consumed are affected as a result. Aversion of high-fat foods and adoption of a vegetarian diet are common; reasons for following a vegetarian diet should be evaluated by the RD to determine whether they are genuine or being used as a guise to limit intake.[7]

Micronutrient intake generally parallels macronutrient intake: fat-restricted diets may result in deficiencies of fat-soluble vitamins and essential fatty acids (EFA). Avoidance of fats puts individuals at greater risk for EFA deficiencies. Vegetarian diets are commonly low in protein, vitamin B_{12}, iron, and zinc, while vegan diets may additionally be low in calcium and vitamin D. B vitamin deficiencies, particularly riboflavin, vitamin B_6, thiamin, folic acid, and vitamin B_{12}, are commonly reported in EDs, especially in lower-weight patients with AN. Both insufficient intake of meats and carbohydrates and alcohol abuse can cause or intensify these deficiencies.[35] A deficiency in vitamin B_6 can exacerbate EDs due to its effects on serotonin and appetite.

Fluid intake should also be assessed to identify whether the patient is restricting intake to avoid feeling full, or drinking excessively to ward off hunger. Water loading, or excessive water intake, may be utilized as a weight manipulation method prior to weigh-ins to produce a falsely elevated weight. A urine-specific gravity level below 1.010 may indicate water loading.[6]

A 24-hour dietary recall may not provide an accurate representation of a BN patient's diet, because they are known for chaotic eating patterns ranging from restrictive, to adequate, to binge eating. Assessing their intake over a week and averaging the total caloric intake over 7 days would provide a more accurate depiction of their diet. Despite reports of feeling "empty" after compensatory behaviors like self-induced vomiting and laxative abuse, the majority of calories consumed prior are retained, making these behaviors ineffective for weight loss. Evidence has shown that up to 1,200 calories are retained after a binge, whether that binge was 1,500 or 3,500 calories.[36] Laxative abuse also has minimal effects in removal of calories, because it has been shown to reduce calorie absorption by only up to 12%.[37]

RDs can begin to assess the patient's eating habits, behaviors, and attitudes while obtaining the diet history. Eating habits include the pattern of intake (i.e., number of meals per day, time and duration of meals, eating environment, etc.), avoidance of specific food groups, amount of variation in the diet, and fluid intake. A common intake pattern among EDs is to be restrictive in the morning, saving the majority of caloric intake for later in the day. Patients with EDs may also have an eating cut-off time where they are fearful to take in calories past a certain hour. Duration of meals varies among EDs, in that patients with BN tend to eat very quickly, demonstrating their difficulty with satiety cues, while those with AN may eat very slowly to avoid eating too much. The amount of variation in the diet is typically low in EDs and patients tend to consume the same foods in the same-sized portions every day.[6,7] It is not uncommon for the amount of accepted or "safe" foods and portion sizes to continually decrease over time.

> **PRACTICE POINT**
>
> The amount of variation in the diet is typically low in eating disorder patients and they tend to consume the same foods in the same-sized portions every day.

Many ritualistic, atypical behaviors are exhibited in EDs. Ritualistic behaviors include cutting food into very small pieces, eating foods in a certain order, not allowing different food items to touch, and moving food around the plate to avoid consumption. Patients may also use atypical seasonings like lemon juice and spices to avoid salt, and may use excessive amounts of nonnutritive sweeteners knowing they do not have caloric value. Unusual combinations of food and unusual use of utensils or fingers to eat are also characteristic to EDs.[6]

Attitudes about food include dichotomous thinking about foods that trigger binges as well as distorted ideas about portion sizes. Patients with EDs tend to view certain foods as being "good" or "bad," or foods that feel safe versus unsafe to eat. Foods that are higher in fat, sugar, or starch are often regarded as "bad," while fruits, vegetables, and lean proteins are regarded as "good." Patients with AN tend to avoid "bad" foods similarly to how individuals with BN may try to avoid foods that trigger binge eating episodes. For some, overrestriction of "bad" foods can lead to intense cravings for them, causing them to trigger episodes of binging when encountered. Portion sizes of foods also tend to be inaccurately estimated in patients with EDs. Individuals with BN, for example, have been shown to overestimate the portion size of foods by greater than 125% to 700%.[38]

⚠ Clinical Controversy

Vegetarianism and Eating Disorders

While many individuals adopt a vegetarian lifestyle due to environmental awareness, health concerns, and/or animal rights, some may use the diet as a tactic for weight loss or masking of an ED. Bardone-Cone et al. found that women with EDs are four times more likely to be vegetarian than women without EDs. It also found that more than 52% of women with a history of EDs had been vegetarians at one point in their lives, of which 42% were motivated by weight-related reasons and 68% perceived their vegetarianism to be related to their ED. Timko et al. sought to identify whether various types of vegetarian diets (vegan, vegetarian, and semi-vegetarian) were related to the development of an ED. This study found that semi-vegetarians, but not full vegetarians or vegans, were most likely to engage in disordered eating behaviors. It was found that vegans and vegetarians appeared to have the healthiest attitudes toward food.

1. Given the contradictory findings, how might clinicians interpret vegetarianism and eating pathology?
2. Should individuals at high risk of eating disorders be discouraged from following a vegetarian diet?
3. How might the adoption of a various forms of vegetarianism guide a clinician in assessing dietary intent?
4. How would you determine whether it is appropriate to allow ED clients to continue their vegetarian lifestyle?

References

1. Bardone-Cone AM, Fitzsimmons-Craft EE, Harney MB, et al. The inter-relationships between vegetarianism and eating disorders among females. *J Acad Nutr Diet.* 2012;112(8):1247-1252.
2. Timko Ca, Hormes JM, Chubski J. Will the real vegetarian please stand up? An investigation of dietary restraint and eating disorder symptoms in vegetarians versus non-vegetarians. *Appetite.* 2012;58(3):982-990.

Biochemical Assessment

It is generally accepted in the ED treatment community that laboratory values within normal limits do not reflect nutrition stability. The etiology behind this phenomenon relates to the metabolic changes that occur during starvation. During periods of low energy intake, there is a greater reliance on fatty acids and ketones as a source of energy to decrease use of protein for gluconeogenesis in order to spare lean body mass. If dietary protein is also lacking, amino acid recycling is increased, with reprioritization toward visceral protein synthesis. This conservation mechanism, which supports the body's adaptive ability to maintain visceral protein metabolism in chronic starvation mode, can initially hide nutrient deficiencies.[39] In addition, dehydration may mask serum albumin levels, making them appear normal. It may not be until the refeeding process begins, when metabolic activity improves and tissue repair and cell turnover start utilizing already low nutrient stores, that true deficiencies will be revealed.[35]

> **CORE CONCEPT 4**
>
> In the eating disorder community, laboratory values within normal limits do not reflect nutrition stability; conservation mechanisms, like the body's adaptive ability to maintain visceral protein metabolism in chronic starvation mode, can initially hide nutrient deficiencies.

Despite generally low fat intake, abnormal lipid values are a common feature of EDs. Malnutrition may affect the functionality of the liver, resulting in high serum cholesterol levels. A low intake of EFAs may also be related to elevated cholesterol levels. Postprandial hypoglycemia is another clinical feature of AN due to depleted hepatic glycogen reserves. Without these reserves, the liver is unable to normalize blood glucose levels following the elevated release of insulin that occurs in response to increased food intake.[15] Low thyroid-stimulating hormone and low T3 levels may also result as an adaptation to fasting, starving, and protein-energy malnutrition.

> **PRACTICE POINT**
>
> Abnormal lipid levels are a common feature in EDs. Malnourished patients with AN can present with elevated cholesterol levels secondary to impaired liver functioning.

Low zinc and vitamin B_{12} levels are common in EDs and can result from insufficient energy intake, avoidance of red meat, or adoption of a vegetarian diet.[6] Zinc deficiency may also exacerbate EDs due to its effects on the sense of taste and symptoms of depression.[35] Low vitamin D levels are often reported for patients with EDs related to decreased dairy intake. Inadequate calcium intake is also common; however, it is unlikely to be reflected in serum calcium levels. A food frequency

CASE STUDY

On hospital day (HD) 2, you meet with Emma to get additional information about her diet prior to admission.

Dietary Data:
Usual diet recall for 2 months prior to admission:
Breakfast (7 am): 24 oz black coffee with artificial sweetener
Lunch (12 pm): 1 apple, 1 veggie burger (no roll), 12 baby carrots, 12 oz water
Snack (3 pm): 6 oz fat-free plain Greek yogurt
Dinner (6 pm): salad with 2 cups romaine lettuce, 1 cup baby spinach, 1 tomato, 1 green pepper, ½ cup shredded carrots, ¼ chopped onion, ½ cup black beans, 3 tbsp balsamic vinegar, 12 oz water

In collecting Emma's diet history, she reveals that she became vegetarian as an attempt to lose weight 2 years ago. Additionally, she reports finding it difficult to consume her goal calories while hospitalized because she continues to almost exclusively choose low-calorie, high-volume foods like vegetables. Emma's mother requests that her daughter take an iron supplement given her meat avoidance for the past 2 years.

Questions
1. How would you address Emma's vegetarianism and her mother's request?
2. How could incorporating more animal proteins potentially help with food volume?
3. Considering her diet history and the nutrition-focused physical exam findings during her admission assessment, in addition to iron, what other micronutrients may Emma be lacking?

questionnaire or dietary recall would more accurately reveal low calcium intake. Iron-deficiency anemia is common in women of childbearing age, with or without EDs. Vegetarian or vegan patients are also at increased risk for deficiency, as well as excessive exercisers due to red blood cell hemolysis.[35]

Fluid and electrolyte abnormalities secondary to purging methods, fluid restriction or overload, metabolic changes, or a combination normally present in EDs. Elevated blood levels of sodium, potassium, blood urea nitrogen, and creatinine may reflect dehydration, while overhydration or water loading may be reflected by low sodium and low chloride levels. GI losses from purging most commonly cause hypokalemia, but purging may also be revealed by decreased chloride and elevated bicarbonate and amylase levels. Laxative abuse may be reflected by elevated bicarbonate and decreased chloride levels as well.[6,35]

> **CORE CONCEPT 5**
>
> Individuals with eating disorders can present with fluid and electrolyte abnormalities secondary to purging methods, fluid restriction or overload, metabolic changes, or a combination of these.

Medical Nutrition Therapy

There is no professional consensus on restoring health and weight in AN, stopping binge-purge behaviors in BN, or modifying the disturbed thoughts and attitudes about food and body weight central to all EDs. Medical nutrition therapy guidelines for EDs are largely based on clinical experience. RDs provide medical nutrition therapy for the normalization of nutritional status and play an essential role in the treatment team.[4] Communication among the interprofessional team members is imperative to ensure coordination of care, consistency of and adherence to treatment plans, and avoidance of drug–nutrient interactions. RDs may also act as a resource of nutrition education for other healthcare professionals and family members of patients.

> **CORE CONCEPT 6**
>
> Medical nutrition therapy guidelines for eating disorders are largely based on clinical experience.

Treatment for EDs may begin at one of five levels of care: inpatient hospitalization, residential treatment centers, partial hospitalization/full-day treatment, intensive outpatient, and outpatient.[38] The level of care required may depend on several factors, including severity of malnutrition and ED behaviors, degree of medical and psychiatric instability, weight percentage of ideal body weight (IBW), amount of structure needed for eating or restoring weight, and geographic availability. Patients with EDs may require treatment at multiple levels of care. Whether a patient begins at an outpatient level of care and eventually requires inpatient stabilization, or gradually moves from higher to lower levels of care, it is not uncommon for ED patients to require more than one level of care throughout their course of treatment.

Goals and Guidelines

Anorexia Nervosa

Nutrition rehabilitation goals for AN are to restore body weight and normalize eating patterns. Weight restoration is essential for recovery and will generally require supervision in a residential ED treatment program or specialized hospital unit for those who are severely malnourished. Treatment plans generally include a targeted weight gain of 2 to 3 lbs per week in an inpatient setting, and 0.5 to 1 lb per week in an outpatient setting.[40] It is important to note common weight fluctuations in AN. Body water loss can occur simultaneously with the depletion of glycogen stores and loss of lean tissue, while edema can occur secondary to constipation, malnutrition, and refeeding. Even in the most cautious approaches to refeeding, fluid retention will occur at first.[15]

Goal weights, or IBWs, may be established as a range instead of a specific number of pounds and should be determined on an individual level. Ranges should be individualized based on age, height, pubertal stage, premorbid weight, and previous growth trajectories. Return of menses provides an objective measure of health in postmenarcheal females.[33] Goals may include being within 10% of IBW or achieving a weight where menses is restored for amenorrheic females.[15]

Growth charts containing multiple points of references provide crucial information for expected growth trajectories and can be used to set a more accurate, individualized IBW for patients up to 20 years old. For example, setting IBW at the population average BMI-for-age (50th percentile) would not be a realistic expectation for an adolescent who previously trended between the 10th to 25th percentile, or the 75th to 90th percentile, BMI-for-age. Research has shown that when IBW was set with growth charts to estimate BMI-for-age versus the standard 50th percentile BMI-for-age, it more closely estimated the weight at which menses returned in adolescents.[41] Growth charts also paint a picture of weight history prior to ED onset. Input from the treatment team and parents is crucial in setting IBW for preadolescents and adolescents, because an IBW set too low may perpetuate EDs. For children, energy needs and weight goals must be readjusted every 3 to 6 months to account for growth.[6,33]

Adult IBW ranges are more of a state of health that the treatment team can assess based on endocrine status, laboratory values, cognitive improvements, and overall nutrition status.[6] There is limited research on setting IBW for adult patients. The Hamwi method, which includes height, weight, and gender factors, may be used as a guide and adjusted on individual basis. For example, if a patient has historically settled at a weight higher or lower than estimated while not using ED behaviors and demonstrating medical stability, this may be a more appropriate weight goal.

> **PRACTICE POINT**
>
> Goal weights, or ideal body weights (IBWs), may be established as a range instead of a specific number of pounds and should be determined on an individual level. Ranges should be individualized based on age, height, pubertal stage, premorbid weight, and previous growth trajectories.

Changes in REE must be considered during the refeeding process. The reintroduction of food causes a dramatic increase in diet-induced thermogenesis (DIT), or the thermic effect of food. In healthy individuals, DIT can account for 14% to 16% of REE and up to 30% of energy expenditure in AN patients during the refeeding process.[42] During refeeding, REE begins to increase and patients become hypermetabolic, causing them to lose weight easily and require increasing amounts of energy to gain weight. REE eventually normalizes as food intake becomes adequate and weight and lean body mass are restored, although individuals may remain hypermetabolic for 3 to 6 months after weight restoration.[6,42] Additionally, energy intake may convert to heat before it can be used to build tissue, which can manifest as night sweats. These effects are obstacles to weight gain, and ongoing adjustments in caloric intake should be made to account for them. Cessation of physical activity will likely be necessary in the initial phases of treatment to promote weight gain, maintain or improve cardiac health, or normalize laboratory values.

> **CORE CONCEPT 7**
>
> Changes in resting energy expenditure must be considered during the refeeding process because the reintroduction of food causes a dramatic increase in diet-induced thermogenesis, or the thermic effect of food.

Prescribed daily caloric intakes should be individualized and involve vigilant clinical and laboratory monitoring to promote weight gain and prevent refeeding syndrome. Indirect calorimetry is the best method to determine whether the patient is hypometabolic or hypermetabolic; however, this is not always available for use. Instead, REE equations such as the Mifflin–St. Jeor and Dietary Reference Intake for age are often used. These equations may overestimate calorie needs in the initial stages of restoration and underestimate needs in the later stages of restoration, because increasingly more energy is needed to maintain the same rate of weight gain.[43] For instance, compared to women without eating disorders, patients with AN require higher caloric intake to maintain and restore weight. In order to maintain weight, 30 kcal/kg body weight/day, on average, is required for healthy women, while patients with AN, over time, may require between 60 and 100 kcal/kg body weight/day to restore weight.[42] The American Psychological Association treatment guidelines for AN recommend an initial calorie prescription of 30 to 40 kcal/kg body weight/day, or 1,000 to 1,600 kcal/day.[40] Adjustments may need to be made often to promote continued weight gain; an incremental increase of 200 to 300 kcal/day can ensure weight restoration continues.[44] For some patients, caloric prescription may progress up to 70 to 100 kcal/kg body weight/day.[40,42] Males and females generally peak at 4,000 and 3,500 kcal/day, respectively.[15]

It is important to observe and address eating behaviors during times of high energy intake to confirm patients are not discarding or hiding food, or engaging in compensatory behaviors like vomiting or being excessively active. Behaviors such as excessive standing, pacing, or weight manipulation may increase as patients are required to consume higher calorie meal plans.

> **CORE CONCEPT 8**
>
> Indirect calorimetry is the best method to determine whether an eating disorder patient is hypometabolic or hypermetabolic.

The amount of empirical data regarding optimum food choices to support weight gain is limited. Increased dietary variety has been associated with better weight restoration and increases probability of meeting macro- and micronutrient needs.[6,42] Currently, there are no specific recommendations for macronutrient distribution for ED patients. RDs can promote nutritional adequacy by creating meal plans that incorporate appropriate balance of macronutrients. The Institute of Medicine provides the daily macronutrient intake recommendations for weight maintenance in adolescents and adults of 110 to 140 g of carbohydrate/day, 1g protein/kg body weight/day, and 15 to 20 g of EFAs/day.[45]

Fat intake is crucial during refeeding to replenish depleted lipids and correct lipid alterations. Lipids play a major role in neuronal wiring between brain regions. EFAs are present in high concentrations in the brain and appear to play a role in memory, brain performance, and mental well-being. Deficiency in omega-3 fatty acids has been linked to psychiatric disorders like depression and psychological traits such as hostility.[1,46] Due to their high fat content, fatty fish and oils like canola and flaxseed, which are rich sources of omega-3 fatty acids, are likely to be avoided by AN patients.

Vegetarian and vegan diets may need to be discouraged during the initial phases of refeeding to promote adequate EFA intake and high biological value (HBV) sources of protein.[6] Adequate protein intake from a mix of HBV sources and vegetable sources can increase restoration rate of nutrient status.[42] It may be helpful to initially incorporate "safer" HBV sources like fish or chicken when reintroducing animal proteins, because individuals with AN may be uncomfortable consuming red meat. Patients may find HBV sources more appealing because it takes a larger volume of a vegetable protein to provide the same amount of protein provided from an animal source. Intake of HBV sources of protein, such as red meat, will also increase zinc intake. Zinc needs are higher in children and adolescents for proper growth, making this a particular micronutrient of concern in young vegetarians.

Promoting adequate fluid intake is also important to correct electrolyte imbalances and further assist any problems with constipation. Fiber intake may promote early satiety and increase GI discomfort.[8] High fiber foods should be introduced slowly with appropriate water intake to prevent GI discomfort. Nonstimulant laxatives, such as polyethylene glycol, may be more appropriate treatments for constipation for this population. Supplementation with a 100% Recommended Daily Allowance multivitamin—with the exception of iron, as iron can exacerbate constipation as well—is recommended for AN patients in the initial weight restoration phase.[6]

Oral feeding is the first choice of treatment because it provides a safer, less invasive, and more therapeutic form of refeeding. Refractory cases may require nutritional support during treatment. Multiple failed attempts at oral feeding, life-threatening weight loss of more than 40% below IBW, and a worsening or severe psychological or physical state are indicators for nutritional support. Enteral feeds supplying 1 to 1.5 kcal/mL of polymeric formula via nasogastric tube are typically the first choice for nutrition support in such situations.[15] Nocturnal enteral feeds may be beneficial in assisting weight gain in patients who have plateaued or continued to restore at a slow rate. Parenteral nutrition (PN) is prescribed for severe and refractory cases only. PN increases risk for catheter-related infections, and could result in an air embolism if an agitated patient refusing nutrition support attempted removal of the intravenous line. Medical teams must use utmost discretion around PN use in AN patients.[15]

Refeeding syndrome is a serious and potentially fatal condition that can occur in severely malnourished patients if aggressive oral, enteral, or parenteral nutrition intake is introduced within the first week of treatment. The metabolic shift that occurs from starvation to refeeding causes increased cellular uptake of glucose, potassium, phosphate, and magnesium, causing resultant low serum concentrations.[47,48] The etiology of refeeding syndrome begins when starvation or malnutrition leads to a catabolic condition in the body where glycogenolysis, gluconeogenesis, and lean body mass catabolism occur. When a concentrated carbohydrate source is introduced, the production of insulin, an anabolic hormone, leads to a shift from catabolism to anabolism. This results in an increase in thiamine utilization and the cellular uptake of glucose, potassium, phosphorus, and magnesium, as well as an increased demand for phosphorus to phosphorylate ADP to ATP.[49] These serum shifts, particularly hypophosphatemia, are hallmarks of refeeding syndrome. Left untreated, this electrolyte imbalance can progress into acute fluid overload due to sodium and water retention, respiratory compromise due to hypophosphatemia, cardiac involvement due to hypokalemia and hypomagnesemia, and/or neurologic complications due to thiamine deficiency.[49] Providing supplemental potassium, phosphorus, magnesium, and thiamine prior to the introduction of feeds and throughout the refeeding process can correct any imbalances and prevent potential complications.[47,48]

> **CORE CONCEPT 9**
>
> Refeeding syndrome is a serious and potentially fatal condition that can occur in severely malnourished patients if aggressive oral, enteral, or parenteral nutrition intake introduced within the first week of treatment.

CASE STUDY REVISITED

It is HD 7 and Emma has been better tolerating the volume of meals since reintroducing chicken and fish. She has been following the meal plan consistently for 1 week and has restored some weight. Emma also reports constipation, with her last bowel movement being 4 days ago. She privately discloses that she engaged in purging behaviors (self-induced vomiting) one to two times per day prior to admission.

Anthropometric Data:
Weight: 40.5 kg (89.2 lbs) increased from admission weight of 40 kg (88 lbs)
BMI: 14.4 kg/m^2

Questions
1. Could other factors in addition to true restoration be contributing to this weight increase?
2. Is this an appropriate rate of weight restoration in the inpatient setting?
3. If not, what adjustments would you make to her meal plan?
4. How can Emma's constipation be addressed?

Prevention and treatment of refeeding syndrome advises hypocaloric nutritional treatment and electrolyte supplementation for those identified as being at risk. The National Institute of Health and Clinical Excellence criteria for identifying those at risk are as follows[47]:

- Individuals with one or more of the following: BMI <16; unintentional weight loss of >15% of body weight in the last 3 to 6 months; very little or no nutritional intake for more than 10 days; low serum potassium, phosphate, or magnesium levels prior to feeding
- Individuals with two or more of the following: BMI <18.5; unintentional weight loss of >10% of body weight in the past 3 to 6 months; very little or no nutritional intake for more than 5 days; history of chronic drug use (insulin, diuretics, antacids); alcohol or drug abuse

> **PRACTICE POINT**
>
> Prevention and treatment of refeeding syndrome advises hypocaloric nutritional treatment and electrolyte supplementation for those identified as being at risk.

The feeding prescription for at-risk patients should contain conservative carbohydrate content. The general feeding regimen prescribed is 10 kcal/kg body weight on day 1 of treatment; increase by 5 kcal/kg body weight/day on days 2 to 4; increase by 20 to 30 kcal/kg body weight/day on days 5 to 7; then remain at 30 kcal/kg body weight/day or increase if necessary for weight restoration.[6] While weight is restoring, serum concentration of phosphorus, magnesium, potassium, sodium, and glucose should initially be monitored daily or every other day, and eventually decreased to biweekly monitoring once indicated stable.[15]

Bulimia Nervosa

Goals for nutrition rehabilitation in BN typically include weight maintenance, cessation of binge–purge cycle, restoration of normal eating behavior, correction of nutrient deficiencies, balance of electrolyte levels, and recognition of hunger and satiety cues. Although weight loss may be the intention of the patient's purging behaviors, and may be a reasonable long-term goal for some individuals, it should not be the initial goal of intervention and should not be explored until after treatment. RDs can provide appropriate calorie prescriptions, information related to correcting electrolyte abnormalities, and nutrition education while assisting the establishment of a normal eating pattern. Additional guidelines for medical nutrition therapy include meal planning to provide adequate macro- and micronutrient intake and establishing a meal pattern to promote dietary structure.[2]

Like AN, changes in REE must be considered when calculating calorie prescriptions in BN. Generally, patients with BN will require lower calorie intake to restore or maintain weight than patients with AN.[42] Clinical signs of hypometabolism, such as cold intolerance or low T3 levels, are also useful assessments of metabolic efficiency. Body weight should be monitored and caloric adjustments made accordingly to support weight maintenance or restoration goals. Weight fluctuations due to purging are common because weight loss may initially result from dehydration, followed by weight gain from rebound fluid retention. Individuals who abruptly stop abusing laxatives or diuretics may experience significant fluid retention for several weeks.[40] Edema, fluid retention, and swollen salivary glands that can result from purging behaviors may be mistaken as true weight gain. It is important to educate patients on this side effect to potentially prevent an increase in compensatory behaviors triggered by this presumed weight gain.

Patients may be resistant to meal plans, or structured food plans, at first; they typically fast for the first half of the day to avoid contributing to caloric intake consumed during binges later. Restricting intake below energy needs can trigger binge eating episodes. A structured meal plan that avoids long periods of fasting by providing three meals and snacks daily along with a balanced intake of macronutrients can decrease cravings and promote satiety and nutritional adequacy. Menu planning and self-monitoring have been shown effective in decreasing binge–purge behaviors. Additionally, meal and snack consistency and cessation of binge–purge behaviors together can help to strengthen hunger and satiety cues in these patients.[6]

During treatment for BN, patients will require a great deal of encouragement to follow a structured dietary plan and cease purging and nonpurging compensatory behaviors. As excessive exercisers begin to decrease frequency and/or duration of physical activity, a focus of treatment would likely be to avoid increasing restrictive eating habits as a means of making up for this difference in physical activity. They should be reminded that overrestriction increases the likelihood of binge eating, a behavior that was unhelpful for weight loss in the past.[6] Patience and support are crucial for facilitating positive changes in eating habits of BN patients.

Binge Eating Disorder

The goals of BED treatment include interrupting binge eating behaviors, improving body image and nutrition status, increasing physical activity, and promoting self-acceptance. A combination of dietary counseling and psychotherapy are generally used to treat BED and lead to the most desirable outcomes.[50] An RD's role includes helping identify patients with the disorder, evaluating their nutrition requirements, and educating them on normal eating habits to prevent future binges. Like BN, weight loss may be appropriate long-term goal, but the initial emphasis of treatment should be on reduction of binge eating episodes.

CASE STUDY REVISITED

It is now HD 12. The team plans to continually increase Emma's caloric prescription in small increments over time. The team decides to review Emma's biochemical data since her admission to the hospital. The nutrition therapy goals for Emma are to prevent further weight loss, correct nutrient deficiencies, and work toward a restoration goal of being within 10% of her ideal body weight.

Current Anthropometric Data:
Weight: 41 kg (90.7 lbs) increased from 40.5 kg (89.2 lbs)
BMI: 14.6 kg/m^2

Biochemical Data:

	Normal Range	HD 1	HD 3	HD 5	HD 7	HD 9	HD 11
Sodium	135-145 mEq/L	150	147	145	144	143	143
Potassium	3.6-5 mEq/L	2.9	3.8	3.3	3.2	3.4	3.6
Chloride	98-110 mEq/L	94	96	100	100	99	99
CO_2	20-30 mEq/L	32	31	29	28	29	28
BUN	6-24 mg/dL	33	29	25	24	24	22
Phosphorus	2.7-4.5 mg/dL	2.8	2.3	2.1	2.8	3	3.1
Magnesium	1.3-2.1 mEq/L	1.4	1.2	1.1	1.4	1.5	1.5
Albumin	3.5-5 g/dL	3.5	----	----	----	----	2.9

Questions

1. Did Emma meet the National Institute of Health and Clinical Excellence criteria for those at risk for refeeding syndrome? Why or why not?
2. How might you describe Emma's biochemical data trends?
3. Did she demonstrate signs of refeeding syndrome? Why or why not?
4. What other factors might have played a role in her labs increasing or decreasing?
5. What is Emma's ideal body weight? What is her goal weight?
6. Why is it necessary to refeed in this slow, nonaggressive approach?
7. On HD 12, approximately how many calories should Emma be consuming in her meal plan?
8. What other factors should be considered in determining her calorie goals?
9. What questions can you ask Emma to assess her attitude and approach to food and eating as she progresses through the refeeding process?

Counseling

Not all individuals with EDs will be ready to change or willing to participate in treatment because they may not be ready to let go of their ED or want recovery. For example, individuals with AN may interpret their disorder as an identity that is more meaningful to them than the disorder's detrimental health effects, potentially including death.[44] Providing nutrition recommendations and counseling for this patient population can be quite difficult. Clinicians should always provide support and positive reinforcement when counseling patients with EDs (**Figure 25.7**). Training in motivational interviewing can be beneficial for the treatment process as this client-centered counseling method can help clinicians determine individuals' motivation or readiness for making health behavior changes. It also allows for a collaborative approach to treatment, which enhances individuals' intrinsic motivation to change.[6]

Weight restoration and fluctuations during treatment can be extremely difficult, both physiologically and psychologically. Symptoms of delayed gastric emptying, constipation, fluid retention, and edema are uncomfortable and can impair the ability to meet nutritional needs, especially in AN patients who may be consuming large amounts of food to restore weight. For some patients, weight may initially restore in the abdominal region.[44] While the weight will redistribute over time, the abdominal region tends to be a particularly sensitive area for AN patients, making this change incredibly difficult. As they begin to notice changes in their body weight or shape, they may experience increased symptoms of anxiety, depression, irritability, and, for some, suicidal thoughts. With sustained weight gain and maintenance, these mood symptoms improve.[40] In AN, weight restoration is associated with improved cognitive and physical symptoms and is essential for psychotherapy. It is important to be thoughtful of these changes during the refeeding process and offer education and support around them during nutrition counseling with ED patients.

RDs and other members of the treatment team should be aware of the various pro-anorexia ("pro-ana") and pro-bulimia ("pro-mia") websites that glorify EDs. These sites view EDs in a positive light, as something that takes great strength, determination, and self-control. Thinness is depicted as an ideology, with pictures of extremely thin models and encouraging messages to continue working towards this valued goal. They also provide tips for achieving this goal such as very low calorie diet plans, ways to ward off hunger without eating, and secretive purging methods. It is important for RDs to view the content of these sites because they can provide insight to strategies used by their patients to continue ED habits during treatment.[6]

Nutrition Education

Nutrition education is an essential part of treatment and is most helpful after malnutrition is corrected, when the ability to process new information is no longer impaired. Some ED patients may already spend significant amounts of time learning about nutrition-related topics, but their ED or unsound resources cause them to misinterpret the information. Topics to consider during treatment include guidelines for balanced eating; the impact of malnutrition on growth, development, behavior, and mood; set-point theory; hunger and satiety cues; the effects of restrictive diets on metabolism; the ineffectiveness of compensatory behaviors and their physiological effects; and exercise and energy balance. An RD may need to consult with the clinical team before providing certain education topics. Topics like sports nutrition and healthy eating while dining out may not be appropriate until the patient is in remission.[6,7]

> **PRACTICE POINT**
>
> Nutrition education is an essential part of treatment and is most helpful after malnutrition is corrected, when the ability to process new information is no longer impaired.

Patient Monitoring and Evaluation

Monitoring methods for ED treatment include measurements of height and weight, anthropometric measures, resting and postprandial energy expenditure, diet records, eating behaviors and attitudes, and laboratory data, if indicated. Daily weights should be taken for patients in the hospital and weekly weights should be taken for those receiving outpatient treatment. A baseline height should be obtained in adults, while monthly or bi-monthly measures should be taken for children. Anthropometric skinfold tests should be monitored as medically indicated for both inpatients and outpatients. Food records for outpatients with AN or BN should include fluid intake, artificial sweetener use, physical activity, and eating behaviors. BN patients should also include feelings experienced while eating, types of foods consumed during binges, and the time and method of compensatory behaviors.[6]

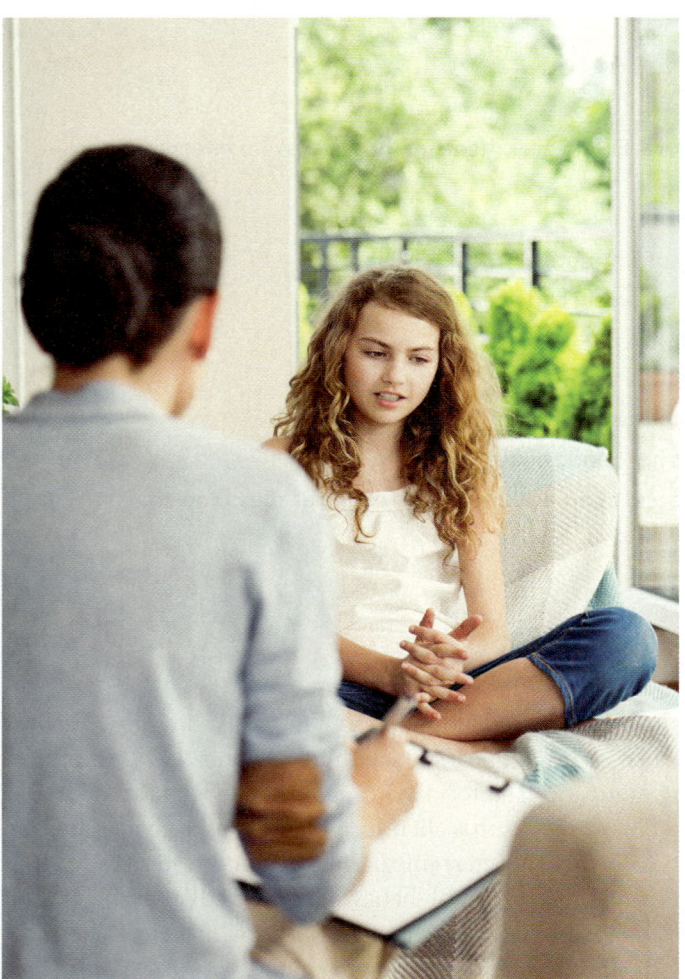

FIGURE 25.7 Providing Support and Positive Reinforcement when Counseling Patients with EDs is Critical
© Izusek/E+/Getty Images.

Screening tools may be helpful for identifying patients with suspected EDs. The SCOFF (Sick, Control, One stone [equal to 14 lbs], Fat, Fear) questionnaire is a validated, simple screening tool that can be used in adjunct with physical examination and laboratory studies.[8] The Eating Disorder Examination Questionnaire (EDE-Q) is widely used to assess the change in ED symptoms over the course of treatment, and found to be reliable in assessing ED attitudes.[51] RDs working with bariatric surgery candidates should be mindful that individuals with BED often seek weight loss surgery. Screening for this major contraindication of surgery and educating BED patients on the role it plays in nutrition and lifestyle, both pre- and postsurgery, can be used to address this disordered eating behavior.[6]

Early detection and prevention of EDs is one of the best treatment practices and can be achieved through patient monitoring. Being cautious of red flags (e.g., an adolescent recently adopting a vegetarian diet or a type 1 diabetic skipping insulin doses with the intention of weight control) during counseling sessions can help the RD to address disordered eating habits before they develop into a serious ED. The main focus of nutrition counseling sessions with all individuals should support health-centered behaviors rather than weight-centered behaviors to decrease risk of ED development.

PRACTICE POINT

Early detection of eating disorders is one of the best treatment practices and can be achieved through patient monitoring. Be cautious of red flags in counseling sessions such as recent adoption of a vegetarian diet or a type 1 diabetic skipping insulin doses with the intention of weight control.

Chapter Summary

EDs are multifactorial conditions associated with significant physical and psychological morbidities that require management through an interprofessional approach. Disordered thoughts and behaviors related to food and eating can be extremely difficult to overcome and relapse is common. Medical nutrition therapy is essential for nutritional rehabilitation. The refeeding process can lead to significant physiologic changes and a gradual reintroduction of the provision of energy can reduce the risk of refeeding syndrome as well as corresponding fluid and electrolyte abnormalities. Treatment of EDs may include various types of inpatient and/or outpatient care. The restoration of body weight and the normalization of eating patterns are essential for successful outcomes and prognosis.

Key Terms

eating disorder (ED), anorexia nervosa (AN), amenorrhea, bulimia nervosa (BN), binge eating disorder (BED), night eating syndrome (NES), avoidant restrictive food intake disorder (ARFID), orthorexia, lanugo, female athlete triad, Russell's sign, Mallory-Weiss tears, Maudsley approach, cognitive behavioral therapy (CBT), dialectical behavioral therapy (DBT), selective serotonin reuptake inhibitor (SSRI), refeeding syndrome

References

1. American Psychiatric Association. *Diagnostic and statistical manual of mental disorders: DSM-5*. 5th ed. Arlington, VA: American Psychiatric Association; 2013.
2. Swanson SA, Crow SJ, Le Grange D, Swendsen J, Merikangas KR. Prevalence and correlates of eating disorders in adolescents: results from the national comorbidity survey replication adolescent supplement. *Arch Gen Psychiatry*. 2011;68(7):714-723. doi: 10.1001/archgenpsychiatry.2011.22.
3. Wade Td, Keski-Rahkonen A, Judson J. Epidemiology of eating disorders. In: Tsuang M, Tohen M, eds. *Textbook in Psychiatric Epidemiology*. 3rd ed. New York, NY: Wiley; 2011:343-360.
4. Hudson J, Hiripi E, Pope H, Kessler R. The prevalence and correlates of eating disorders in the national comorbidity survey replication. *Biol Psychiatry*. 2007;61:348.
5. Keski-Rahkonen A, Hoek HW, Susser ES, et al. Epidemiology and course of anorexia nervosa in the community. *Am J Psychiatry*.2007;164(8):1259-1265.
6. Ozier AD, Henry BW. Position of the American Dietetic Association: nutrition interventions in the treatment of eating disorders. *J Am Diet Assoc*. 2011;111(8):1236-1241.
7. Luder E, Schebendach J. Nutrition management of eating disorders. *Top Clin Nutr*. 1993;8(3):48-63.
8. Trent SA, Moreira ME, Colwell CB, Mehler PS. ED management of patients with eating disorders. *Am J Emerg Med*. 2013;31(5):859-865.
9. Iacovino JM, Gredysa DM, Altman M, Wilfley DE. Psychological treatments for binge eating disorder. *Curr Psychiatry Rep*. 2012;14(4): 432-446. doi: 10.1007/s11920-012-0277-8.
10. Le Grange D, Swanson SA, Crow SJ, Merikangas KR. Eating disorder not otherwise specified presentation in the US population. *Int J Eat Disord*. 2012;45(5):711-718. doi: 10.1002/eat.22006.
11. Fischer S, Meyer AH, Hermann E, Tuch A, Munsch S. Night eating syndrome in young adults: delineation from other eating disorders and clinical significance. *Psychiatry Res*. 2012;200(2-3):494-501.
12. Berner LA, Allison KC. Behavioral management of night eating disorders. *Psychol Res Behav Manag*. 2013;6:1-8.
13. Gramaglia C, Brytek-Matera A, Rogoza R, et al. Orthorexia and anorexia nervosa: two distinct phenomena? A cross-cultural comparison of orthorexic behaviours in clinical and non-clinical samples. *BMC Psychiatry*. 2017;17:75. doi: 10.1186/s12888-017-1241-2.
14. Keel PK, Dorer DJ, Franko DL, Jackson SC, Herzog DB. Postremission predictors of relapse in women with eating disorders. *Am J Psychiatry*. 2005;162(12):2263-2268.
15. Mehler P, Winkelman A, Andersen D, Gaudiani J. Nutritional rehabilitation: practical guidelines for refeeding the anorectic patient. *J Nutr Metab*. 2010;2010. doi: 10.1155/2010/625782.
16. Forman-Hoffman VL, Ruffin T, Schultz SK. Basal metabolic rate in anorexia nervosa patients: using appropriate predictive equations during the refeeding process. *Ann Clin Psychiatry*. 2006;18(2):123-7.
17. Melchior J. From Malnutrition to refeeding during anorexia nervosa. *Curr Opin Clin Nutr Metab Care*. 1998;1(6):481-485.
18. Swenne I, Stridsberg M. Bone metabolism markers in adolescent girls with eating disorders and weight loss: effects of growth, weight trend,

18. developmental and menstrual status. *Arch Osteoporos*. 2012;7(1-2):125-133. doi: 10.1007/s11657-012-0090-3.

19. Halvorsen I, Platou D, Hoiseth A. Bone mass eight years after treatment for adolescent-onset anorexia nervosa. *Eur Eat Disorders Rev*. 2012;20(5):386-392. doi: 10.1002/erv.2179

20. Birch K. Female athlete triad. *BMJ*. 2005;330(7485):244-246.

21. Kalm LM, Semba RD. They starved so that others be better fed: remembering Ancel Keys and the Minnesota Experiment. *J Nutr*. 2005;135(6):1347-1352.

22. Tucker T. *The Great Starvation Experiment: Ancel Keys and the Men Who Starved for Science*. Minneapolis, MN: University of Minnesota Press; 2007.

23. Willer MG, Thuras P, Crow SJ. Implications of the changing use of hospitalization to treat anorexia nervosa. *Am J Psychiatry*. 2005;162(12):2374-2376.

24. Touyz S, Le Grange D, Lacey H, et al. Treatment for severe and enduring anorexia nervosa: a review. *Aust N Z J Psychiatry*. 2012;46(12):1136-1144. doi: 10.1017/S0033291713000949.

25. Franko DL, Keshaviah A, Eddy KT, et al. A longitudinal investigation of mortality in anorexia nervosa and bulimia nervosa. *Am J Psychiatry*. 2013;170(8):917-925.

26. Kotler LA, Devlin MJ, Matthews DE, et al. Total energy expenditure as measured by doubly-labeled water in outpatients with bulimia nervosa. *Int J Eat Disord*. 2001;29(4):470-476. doi: 10.1002/eat.1044.

27. Obarzanek E, Lesem MD, Goldstein DS, et al. Reduced resting metabolic rate in patients with bulimia nervosa. *Arch Gen Psychiatry*. 1991;48(5)456-462.

28. Castellini G, Castellani W, Lelli L, et al. Association between resting energy expenditure, psychopathology and HPA-axis in eating disorders. *World J Clin Cases*. 2014;2(7):257-264. doi: 10.12998/wjcc.v2.i7.257.

29. Hay P. A systematic review of evidence for psychological treatments in eating disorders: 2005-2012. *Int J Eat Disord*. 2013;46(5):462-469. doi: 10.1002/eat.22103.

30. Attia E, Walsh BT. Anorexia nervosa. *Am J Psychiatry*. 2007;164(12):1805-1810.

31. Lock J, Le Grange D, Agras WS, Dare C. *Treatment Manual for Anorexia Nervosa: A Family-Based Approach*. New York, NY: Guilford Press; 2001.

32. Le Grange D, Lock J. *Treating Adolescent Bulimia: A Family-Based Approach*. New York, NY: Guilford Press; 2007.

33. Rosen DS and the Committee on Adolescence. Clinical report identification and management of eating disorders in children and adolescents. *Pediatrics*. 2010;126(6):1240-1253. doi: 10.1542/peds.2010-2821

34. Mitchell JE, Roerig J, Steffen K. Biological therapies for eating disorders. *Int J Eat Disord*. 2013;46(5):470-477. doi: 10.1002/eat.22104.

35. Setnick J. Micronutrient deficiencies and supplementation in anorexia and bulimia nervosa: a review of literature. *Nutr Clin Pract*. 2010;25(2):137-142. doi: 10.1177/0884533610361478

36. Kaye WH, Weltzin TE, Hsu LK, et al. Amount of calories retained after binge eating and vomiting. *Am J Psychiatry*. 1993;150(6):969-971. doi: 10.1176/ajp.150.6.969.

37. Bo-Linn GW, Santa Ana CA, Morawski SG, et al. Purging and calorie absorption in bulimic patients and normal women. *Ann Intern Med*. 1983;99(1):14-17.

38. Stang JS, R.D., Story M, Zollman M. Food risk ratings and food portion size estimations among women with bulimia nervosa. *Top Clin Nutr*. 1997;12(4):50-57.

39. Jensen GL, Bistrian B, Roubenoff R, Heimburger DC. Malnutrition syndromes: a conundrum vs continuum. *JPEN J Parenter Enteral Nutr*. 2009;33(6):710-716.

40. American Psychiatric Association. Treatment of patients with eating disorders, third edition. *Am J Psychiatry*. 2006;163:15.

41. Harrison ME, Obeid N, Fu MCY. Growth curves in short supply: a descriptive study of the availability and utility of growth curve data in adolescents with eating disorders. *BMC Family Practice*. 2013;14:134.

42. Marzola E, Nasser JA, Hashim SA. Nutritional rehabilitation in anorexia nervosa: review of the literature and implications for treatment. *BMC Psychiatry*. 2013;13:290.

43. Scalfi L, Marra M, DeFilippo E, et al. The prediction of basal metabolic rate in female patients with anorexia nervosa. *Int J Obes*. 2001;25:359-364. DOI:10.1038/sj.ijo.0801547.

44. Cockfield A, Philpot U. Symposium 8: Feeding size 0: the challenges of anorexia nervosa managing anorexia from a dietitian's perspective. *Proc Nutr Soc*. 2009; 68:281-288. doi: 10.1017/S0029665109001281.

45. Otten J, Hellwig J, Meyers L. *DRI: Dietary Reference Intakes: The Essential Guide to Nutrient Requirements*. Washington DC: National Academies Press; 2006.

46. Iribarren C, Markovitz JH, Jacobs Jr DR, et al. Dietary intake of n-3, n-6 fatty acids and fish: relationship with hostility in young adults—the CARDIA study. *Eur J Clin Nutr*. 2004;58(1):24-31.

47. National Institute for Health and Clinical Excellence. *Nutrition support in adults*. National Collaborating Center for Acute Care. London, The Royal Surgeons of England; 2006.

48. Rio A, Whelan K, Goff L, et al. Occurrence of refeeding syndrome in adults started on artificial nutrition support: prospective cohort study. *BMJ Open*. 2013;3. doi: 10.1136/bmjopen-2012-002173

49. Solomon SM, Kirby DF. The refeeding syndrome: a review. *JPEN J Parenter Enteral Nutr*. 1990;14:90-97.

50. Wonderlich SA, de Zwaan M, Mitchell JE, Peterson C, Crow S. Psychological and dietary treatments of binge eating disorder: conceptual implications. *Int J Eat Disord*. 2003;34. doi: 10.1002/eat.10206.

51. Rose JS, Vaewsorn A, Rosselli-Navarra F, et al. Test-retest reliability of the eating disorder examination-questionnaire (EDE-Q) in a college sample. *J Eat Disord*. 2013;1:42.

52. Bardone-Cone AM, Fitzsimmons-Craft EE, Harney MB, et al. The inter-relationships between vegetarianism and eating disorders among females. *J Acad Nutr Diet*. 2012;112(8):1247-1252. doi: 10.1016/j.jand.2012.05.007.

53. Timko CA, Hormes JM, Chubski J. Will the real vegetarian please stand up? An investigation of dietary restraint and eating disorder symptoms in vegetarians versus non-vegetarians. *Appetite*. 2012;58(3):982-990. doi: 10.1016/j.appet.2012.02.005

Chapter 26

Nutrition in Developmental Disabilities

Jennifer Hall

Chapter Outline

Core Concepts
Introduction
Background on Developmental Disabilities
Prader Willi
Spina Bifida
Cerebral Palsy
Down Syndrome
Autism Spectrum Disorders

CORE CONCEPTS

1. Developmental disabilities are life-long conditions that can present along a wide spectrum within the same condition.

2. Developmental disabilities are associated with a variety of medical and nutritional complications, of which the potential for obesity is present for all and can further complicate care.

3. Prader Willi is a genetic condition that occurs due to a chromosomal microdeletion.

4. The hallmark characteristic of Prader Willi is hyperphagia, which persists despite many attempts at intervention.

5. Weight management is one of the biggest challenges in caring for a Prader Willi patient.

6. Spina bifida is a neural tube defect that can be prevented, in part, through folate supplementation.

7. Myelomeningocele is the most common form of spina bifida and is characterized by incomplete fusion of the spine, often resulting in swallowing, bowel, and bladder dysfunction.

8. Cerebral palsy patients are classified based upon type of movement and limbs affected, with the main distinctions being between spastic and nonspastic.

9. Muscle tone and ambulatory status can vary within cerebral palsy patients and greatly impact energy assessment.

10. Down syndrome is a disability that can occur as a result of chromosomal alterations.

11. Patients with Down syndrome have a higher prevalence of celiac disease compared to their peers without Down syndrome.

12. Autism spectrum disorder (ASD) is a group of disorders that impact behavior, communication, and development.

13. Food selectivity can be one of the biggest challenges in caring for a patient with autism.

SECTION 3 NUTRITION IN THE LIFECYCLE

> **Learning Objectives**
>
> 1. Discuss the similarities and differences among each of the presented developmental disabilities.
> 2. Describe potential nutritional issues secondary to a patient's developmental disability.
> 3. Identify how a nutritional assessment differs in a patient with each of these developmental disabilities.
> 4. Assess and develop nutritional care plans unique to each disability.
> 5. Formulate education plans and strategies for dietary management in each of the developmental disabilities.

Introduction

This chapter and its case studies present basic nutritional concepts from which to understand each of these unique conditions. Basic nutritional parameters, as well as medical nutrition therapy needed for specific complications found within each condition, are described.

A **developmental disability** is a condition that becomes evident at birth or early childhood and has varying impacts on the individual throughout the life cycle. The developmental disabilities covered in this chapter are common and have the most frequent secondary medical and nutritional issues within the category of developmental disabilities. The Centers for Disease Control and Prevention (CDC) estimates that 1 in 6 children in the United States ages 3 to 17 years have one or more developmental disabilities.[1] While each condition faces its own unique challenges, the common nutritional themes of developmental disabilities are feeding difficulties, weight challenges, and the need for consistent long-term follow up throughout the life cycle.

> **CORE CONCEPT 1**
>
> Developmental disabilities are life-long conditions that can present along a wide spectrum within the same condition.

The developmental disabilities that will be covered in this chapter include Prader Willi syndrome, spina bifida, cerebral palsy, Down syndrome, and autism. Prader Willi syndrome is a genetic condition whose main symptom is hyperphagia leading to obesity, which necessitates the need for nutritional counseling and interventions.[2] Spina bifida is a neural tube defect that occurs as a result of the failure of spinal closure in the first month of fetal life, and can result in a variety of specific defects, each with unique medical and nutritional challenges.[3] Cerebral palsy is a neurological disorder that affects muscle tone, movement, and coordination; it presents on a wide spectrum from mild to severe.[4] Down syndrome and autism each present with unique nutritional needs, the management of which can be complicated by cognitive and behavioral challenges.

The tools of nutritional assessment are important to revisit, because they play a large part in the care of this patient population. In cases of patients with developmental disabilities, it is important to look for and assess potential medical and nutritional complications unique to each condition, and to continue to re-assess over time for changes. Practitioners should note the variations within each condition and assess each patient as an individual, while keeping in mind what to look for. It may also be necessary to additionally interview parents or caretakers to ensure accuracy when collecting patient information.

Common topics to assess and discuss in this population include any recent weight changes or history of unplanned weight loss/gain, previous or current feeding issues, any supplemental enteral needs past or present, and any previous work with a feeding team. In addition, bowel management is a topic that may need further questioning in order to adequately assess potential issues. Another important point to consider is whether the client has previously worked with a registered dietitian (RD), in order to assess what their learning needs are and what they may have been taught by another provider.

An important comorbidity that can impact patients with any type of developmental disability is obesity. Rates of obesity have been climbing in the United States, with recent estimates that 1 out of 3 U.S. adults are obese (roughly 72 million people).[5] Developmentally disabled patients can be at greater risk of obesity due to physical limitations, dietary habits, medications, and lack of resources. Overweight and obesity rates are higher for children with special health care needs: 36% of children 10 through 17 years of age who have special health care needs are overweight or obese compared with 30% of children of the same ages without special health care needs.[6] As obesity rates continue to climb in the general population, this will likely translate to higher obesity rates seen in the developmentally disabled, making this an important population for nutrition counseling and education. In addition, many of the secondary health conditions that these patients will face, such as chronic pain, will likely become worse with any excess weight challenges.[7]

> **CORE CONCEPT 2**
>
> Developmental disabilities are associated with a variety of medical and nutritional complications, of which the potential for obesity is present for all and can further complicate care.

In general, it is important to ask the standard nutrition and nutrition-related questions when assessing a patient with a developmental disability. Client history is an essential part of a full nutritional assessment and can encompass a variety of topics. Client history can set the framework for determining previous and current nutritional issues, as well as methods that have led to success in the past. Obtain

CASE STUDY INTRODUCTION

Logan is an 8-year-old male coming for outpatient nutrition counseling after diagnosis with Prader Willi syndrome and referral from his pediatrician. Logan was referred due to recent dramatic increase in weight over the past 3 months, now above the 99th percentile on the CDC growth charts. His parents report that Logan is constantly asking for food and snacking throughout the day, and he has started sneaking food into his room at night.

Anthropometric Data:

Visit	Weight kg (lb)	Weight/Age Percentile (%)	Height cm (in)	Height/age Percentile (%)	Body Mass Index (BMI)	BMI/Age Percentile (%)
3 months ago	30 (66)	76	120 (47")	4	20.8	96
Today	40 (88)	97	120 (47")	3	27.8	99

Biochemical Data:
HbA1c 6.5 (4.3%-5.8%)

Clinical Data:
Past Medical History: None
Medications: Somatotropin
Vital Signs: Blood pressure: 130/68 mm Hg
Nutrition-focused Physical Exam: Patient appears obese consistent with android body type. Hair and nails appear normal. Skin is pale, warm, and intact. Exam is limited due to patient's irritability.

Dietary Data:
24-hour Diet Recall:
Breakfast: Bacon, eggs, pancakes, orange juice
Snack: Granola bar, milk, fruit
Lunch: Sandwich (turkey/cheese), chips, pickles, crackers, cookie, milk
Snack: Cheese, crackers, juice
Dinner: Mac and cheese, peas, bread and butter, chicken, milk, water
Snack: Ice cream, candy

Questions
1. How would you describe Logan's nutritional status?
2. What are his calorie goals?
3. What education might you provide for Logan?
4. Identify an intervention to adress Logan's nutritional issues.

---

information about birth and early history, including any feeding issues, growth issues, and any failure to thrive, as well as trends along growth charts, such as changes in percentiles. Additionally, learning about any previous feeding practices, any previous work with a registered dietitian (RD), food allergies, medications, and dietary supplements taken are all points to highlight in a patient interview. It may also be important to have input from parents/guardians in addition to patient report in order to ensure accuracy. Having background knowledge about the common issues seen in each condition will help to determine which questions may need further exploration and probing.

Prader Willi

Prader Willi syndrome (PWS) is a genetic condition first described in 1956 by Prader, Labhart, and Willi, and was determined in 1981 to be a condition that occurs as a result of a genomic imprinting, which means that the gene expression is altered based upon which parent the genes came from.[8] The majority of PWS patients, roughly 70%, have PWS due to the deletion on the 15q11-q13 area in chromosome 15 from the paternal region.[9] PWS is a prime example of genomic imprinting because, were this deletion to occur on the maternal side, it would result in Angelman Syndrome and not PWS.[9] Most of the remaining cases of PWS are found to be caused by maternal uniparental disomy, which is when two copies of the maternal side are included.[9] Very rarely (fewer than 5% of cases) is the cause due to other imprinting center defects such as a deletion or epimutations.[10]

> **CORE CONCEPT 3**
>
> Prader Willi is a genetic condition that occurs due to a chromosomal microdeletion.

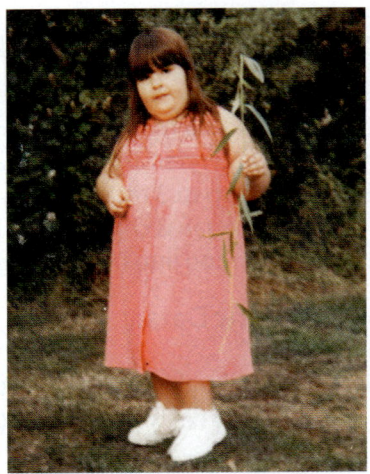

FIGURE 26.1 21-Year-Old Woman with Prader Willi Syndrome.
© Barcroft / Contributor/Getty Images.

PWS occurs in 1 in 10,000 to 20,000 live births,[11] although the prevalence is thought to be underestimated due to potential late diagnosis. A clinical indicator that would lead to testing for PWS in an infant is central hypotonia. Typical presentation of a baby with PWS and central hypotonia will include lethargy, poor sucking ability, weak cry, and decreased movement, with the potential to develop failure to thrive as a result of these symptoms.[8] Other facial characteristics that can be seen are almond-shaped eyes, thin upper lip, and hypopigmentation of hair and skin compared to other family members.[8] If PWS is suspected, testing will involve methylation analysis, which, if positive, will prompt FISH (florescence in situ hybridization) testing in order to determine the cause of the deletion.[8]

> **PRACTICE POINT**
>
> Presenting symptoms of PWS in infancy can include lethargy, decreased movement, weak suckling ability, and faint cry.

Additionally, as PWS patients grow, they are also characterized by short stature, small hands and feet, low IQ, and behavioral problems.[11] **Figure 26.1** demonstrates the short stature associated with Prader Willi in a young adult.

Common nutritional issues that can present include early failure to thrive until about age 2 years, followed by increasing weight gain related to hyperphagia, often leading to eventual overweight and obese status if left uncontrolled.[8] **Hyperphagia** (insatiable hunger) is a hallmark symptom of PWS, thought to occur as a result of a hypothalamic abnormality.[8] Prader Willi is the most common syndromic cause of life-threatening obesity. Many of the complications associated with obesity, such as diabetes mellitus, can also be seen over time with increasing weight gain in these patients. Additionally, these patients can present with bowel issues, typically constipation, which may be due to a combination of dietary choices, inactivity, or medications, and will require consistent management. Typical medical nutrition therapy strategies should be used, with education on the importance of a high fiber and fluid diet, as well as encouraging increased activity. This may be difficult for patients to follow, so the use of medications (stimulants, laxatives) may be needed. Patients with PWS may experience issues with osteopenia and osteoporosis. While there are a multitude of nutritional and medical issues that require attention, a large piece of this condition is behavioral and psychological, stemming from the hyperphagia and mental deficiency. Common behavioral issues that arise are obsessive compulsive disorder, food-seeking behavior, temper tantrums, and skin picking.[11] Persistent hyperphagia can lead patients with PWS to seek out and eat nonfood items such as garbage or pet food, or to go as far as to steal food or money in order to try and obtain food.

> **CORE CONCEPT 4**
>
> The hallmark characteristic of Prader Willi is hyperphagia, which persists despite many attempts at intervention.

Anthropometrics

As previously mentioned, patients with PWS typically have initial feeding problems that can impact growth and, if not addressed, can suffer from failure to thrive, which is then followed by eventual obesity. All of this makes the collection and monitoring of anthropometric data essential in order to adequately monitor the patient. For PWS patients, short stature is commonly seen, which is important to keep in mind when taking anthropometrics and assessing growth charts.[11] Proposed growth charts are shown in **Figure 26.2**. According to Chen, short stature is almost always present by the mid-20s, and the average adult heights to be expected in PWS are for 155 cm (61 in) for males and 148 cm (58 in) for females.[8] Chen also noted these patients have slow growth of hands and feet, resulting in hands that are usually small and narrow and feet that tend to be short and broad, with an average shoe size of 5 for men and 3 for women.[8] The lack of growth seen in these patients is due to a deficiency of growth hormone (GH), with 50%

of infants and children with PWS diagnosed as GH deficient.[12]

Due to the growth issues seen in PWS, GH treatment has been used to help make up for lack of normal growth. In 2000, the U.S. Food and Drug Administration (FDA) approved growth hormone for use in PWS patients.[8] An article from the *Journal of Clinical Endocrinology and Metabolism* states that, from their general consensus, GH can be an appropriate part of the treatment plan for PWS when combined with other therapies such as dietary and lifestyle changes.[12] Trials have shown significant benefit from using GH, including increased rate of growth, adolescent growth spurt and some normalization of height, and decreased fat mass by approximately 10%.[8] Patients have also shown improvements in motor development in infancy and body composition in adulthood.[8] In addition, GH therapy decreases fat mass and increases muscle mass, potentially having a beneficial effect on appetite and weight gain.[13] Possible side effects include sleep apnea, joint pain, and peripheral edema, but the reported rate of these side effects is low.[12]

> **PRACTICE POINT**
>
> Growth hormone can be used in the PWS population as part of a treatment plan.

When assessing PWS children's growth, it is recommended to use the typical World Health Organization (WHO)/CDC growth charts, but to also keep in mind the growth expectations or potential use of GH and how this may affect the growth charts.[14] There are no standardized growth charts available; however, there are some growth charts that have been developed specifically for children with PWS who are not taking GH. These growth charts may better estimate a PWS child's growth than the traditional WHO growth charts,[11] but the major limitation is that they were created based on a small sample size. Further research is needed in this area, and for now it is recommended to use the traditional growth charts, with the PWS-specific ones potentially as a supplement.[14]

Biochemical and Clinical

Proper diagnosis of PWS will require genetic testing for confirmation and to determine the cause of microdeletion, as previously mentioned. As patients age, should there be suspicion of osteopenia or osteoporosis, patients may receive a bone mineral density scan as well as measurements of vitamin D and calcium to determine course of action.[9]

Medical nutrition therapy for age-appropriate weight maintenance and weight loss should be used in helping to curb weight gain that can often occur due to the hyperphagia experienced by these patients. A healthy diet full of

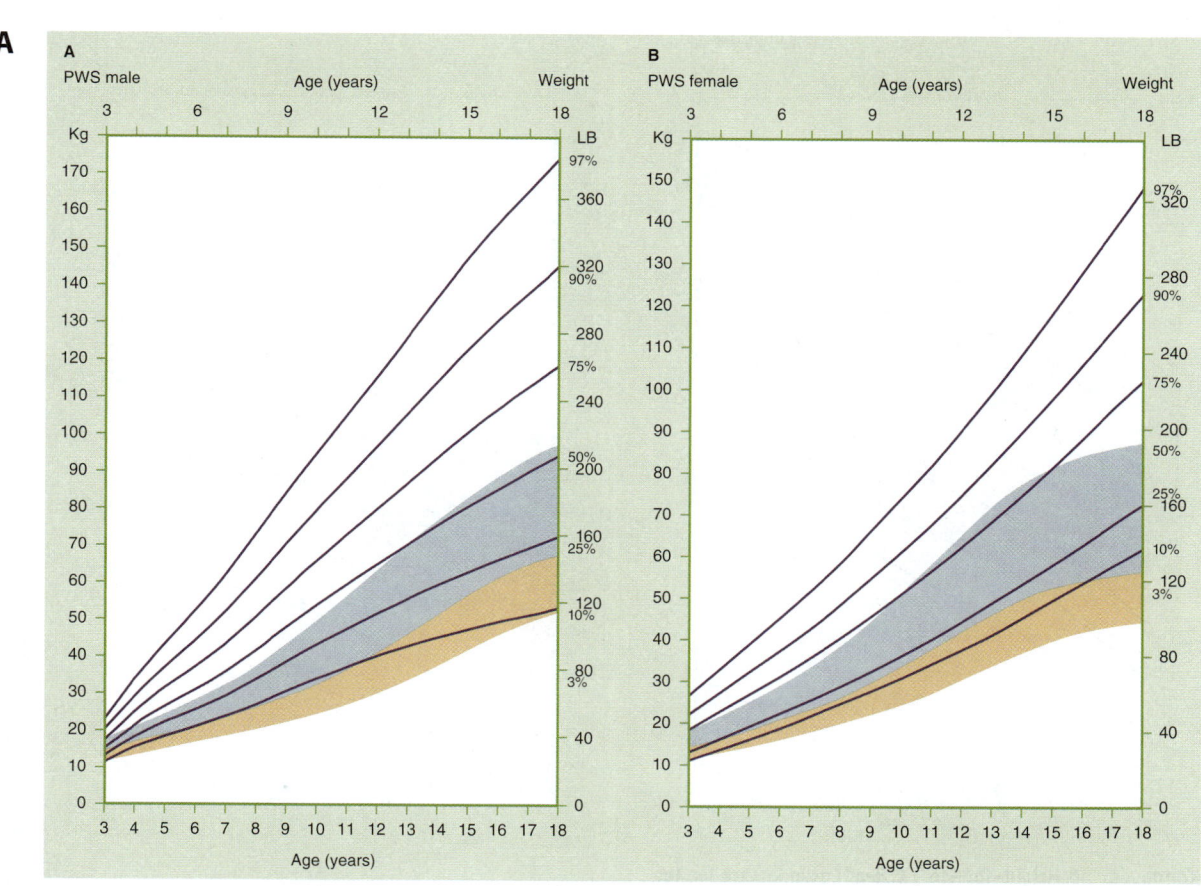

FIGURE 26.2 Proposed Growth Charts for Prader Willi Syndrome. A. Weight-for-Age *(continues)*

Reproduced from Butler et al. Growth Charts for Non-Hormone Treater Prader-Willi Syndrome. *Pediatrics*. 2015;135(1).

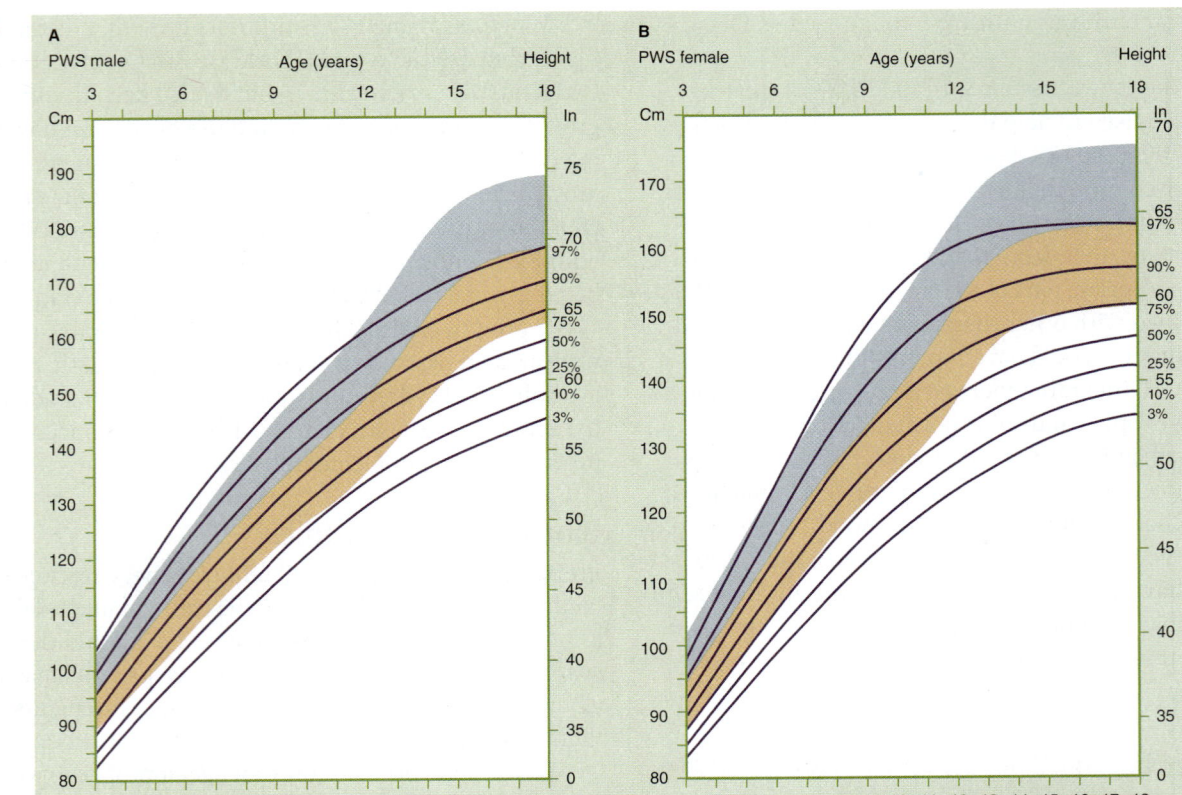
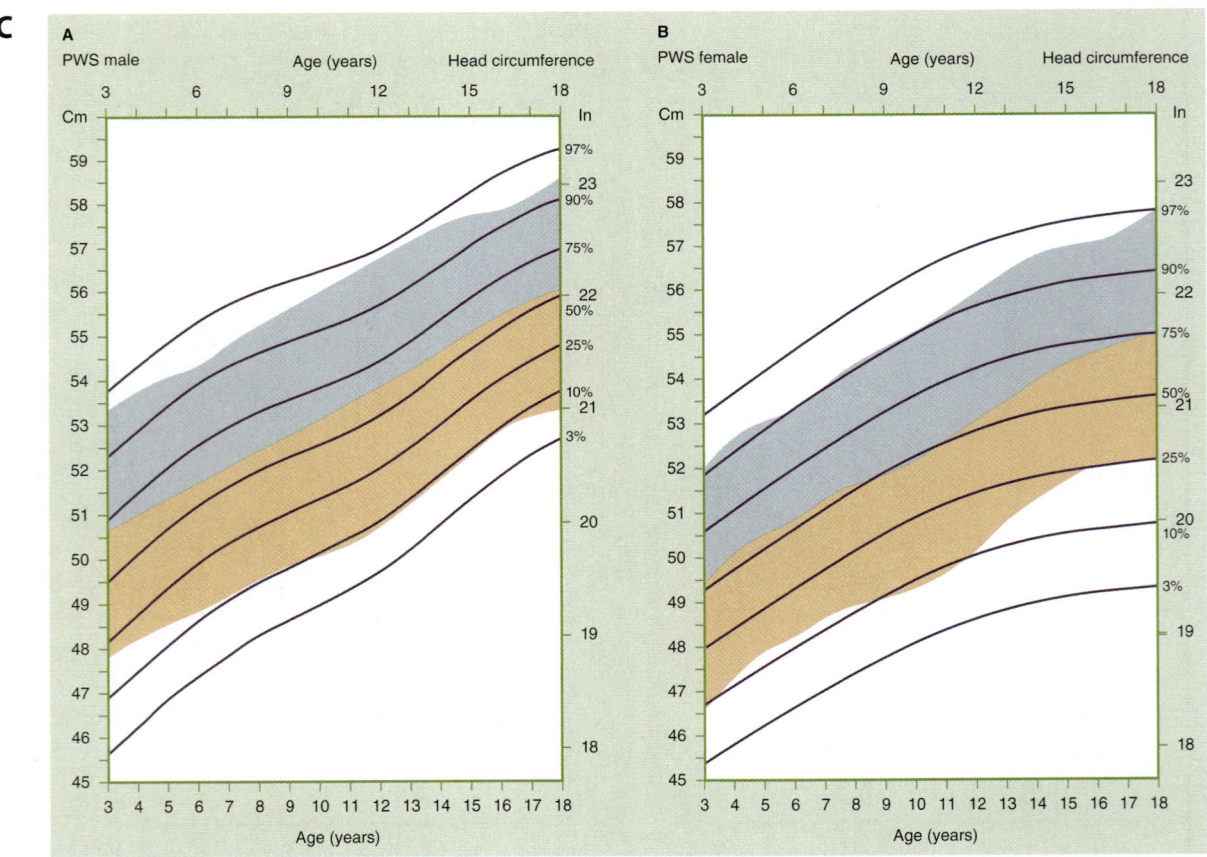

FIGURE 26.2 (Continued)   **B. Height–for-Age**   **C. Head Circumference-for-Age**

Reproduced from Butler et al. Growth Charts for Non-Hormone Treater Prader-Willi Syndrome. *Pediatrics*. 2015;135(1).

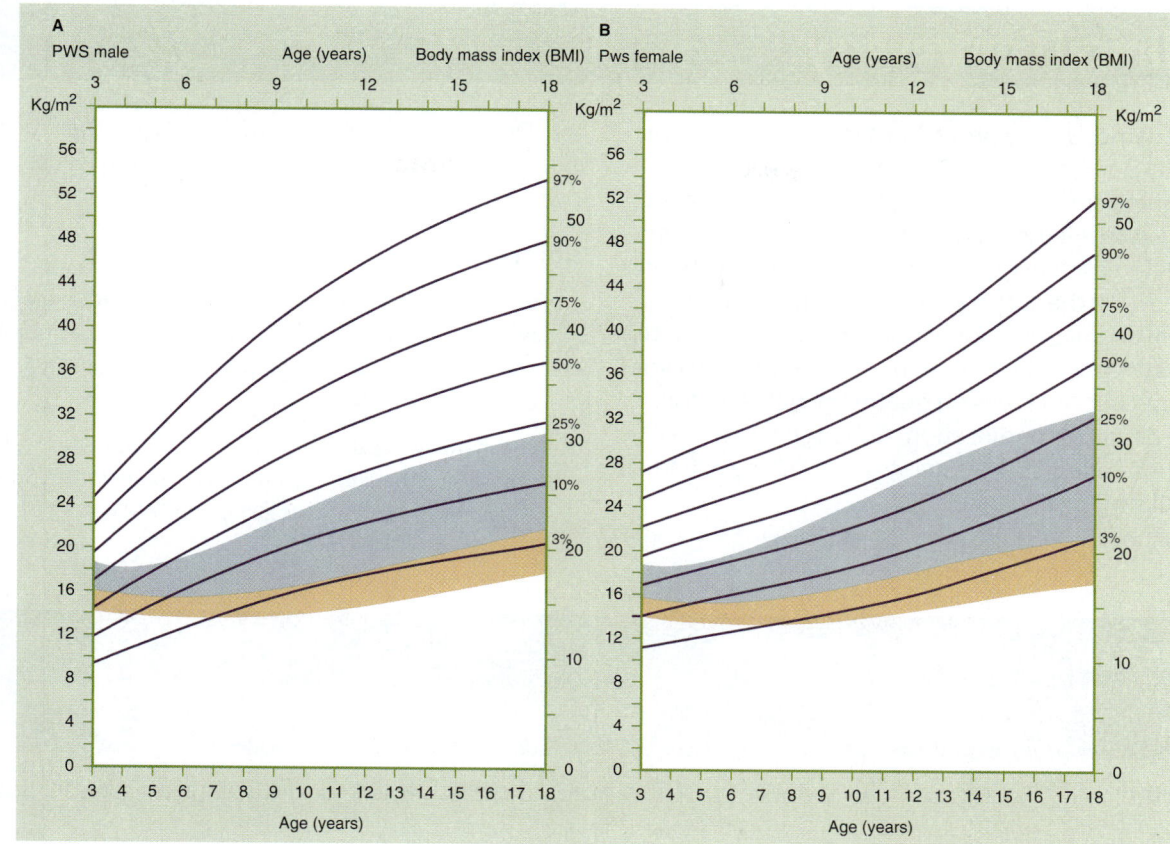

FIGURE 26.2 D. BMI–for-Age
Reproduced from Butler et al. Growth Charts for Non-Hormone Treater Prader-Willi Syndrome. *Pediatrics*. 2015;135(1).

fruits, vegetables, lean proteins, and whole grains should be encouraged. Lower calorie options for foods and drinks should be explored.[15] Use of My Plate for meal planning is a common tool used for education on healthful diets. Physical activity should be encouraged as tolerated in order to help combat weight gain. A plan for monitoring weight trends should be instituted to determine when food changes and activity are no longer enough to prevent excessive weight gain.

Weight-loss surgery has been increasing in popularity as a treatment option for obesity in patients who fit specific criteria based on BMI and comorbidities. With obesity being the hallmark problem in patients with Prader Willi, the question is then whether weight-loss surgery is a viable option in treatment of PWS patients. There are limited data on this subject, but there are case reports and small reviews present in the literature. In general, there has been some short-term success, but overall long-term results are not in favor of this practice.[16] Risk of complications associated with the surgery, such as gut perforation, nutritional anemia, osteopenia, and even death, as well as limited weight reduction seen, are all reasons to avoid weight-loss surgery and instead focus on treatment with exercise, diet, and behavior modification.[16] While some patients with PWS have had successful surgeries, the general recommendations at this time are that further research is needed about the long-term effects in this population, so recommendations for surgical interventions cannot be made at this time.[12]

Another clinical topic of interest is the potential use of weight-loss medications in the PWS population. Various medications have been trialed in order to enhance weight loss and energy expenditure, but have been shown to be unsuccessful in short-term trials.[12] Antiepileptics, specifically topiramate, have been used in attempts to affect food-seeking behavior, but no clinical trials have been done and there is a potential for many adverse side effects.[12] Additionally, anorexigenic agents have shown no benefit in treating hyperphagia, but research is limited.[2] Limited study data and lack of efficacy seen in prior research necessitate the need for further research to evaluate pharmacotherapy's role in the treatment plans for Prader Willi patients. Pharmacotherapy, which has been used in an attempt to improve appetite/hunger, may be ineffective for appetite as well as behavior management.[12] A list of PWS options for medications are listed in **Table 26.1**.

> **CORE CONCEPT 5**
>
> Weight management is one of the biggest challenges in caring for a Prader Willi patient.

⚠ Clinical Controversy

Use of bariatric surgery procedures to manage obesity in the PWS population continues to be a topic for debate. Some small studies, such as that by Fong et al., have shown that it is effective for weight loss. However, questions over safety remain. The risk of complications associated with the surgery, such as gut perforation, nutritional anemia, osteopenia, and even death, as well as limited weight reduction seen, are all reasons to avoid surgery and instead focus on treatment with exercise, diet, and behavior modification. Although more research is needed, some patients with PWS have had successful surgeries.

Discuss the use of bariatric surgery in the Prader Willi population. What are the pros and cons to its use? What is your position?

References

1. Fong AK, Wong SK, Lam CC, Ng EK. Ghrelin level and weight loss after laparoscopic sleeve gastrectomy and gastric mini-bypass for Prader–Willi syndrome in Chinese. *Obesity Surg.* 2012;22(11): 1742-1745.

2. Scheimann AO, Butler MG, Gourash L, Cuffari C, Klish W. Critical analysis of bariatric procedures in Prader-Willi syndrome. *J Pediatr Gastroenterol Nutr.* 2008;46(1):80-83.

TABLE 26.1 PWS MEDICATION OPTIONS

Medication	Proposed Use	Implications/Evidence for Use
Antiepileptics (topiramate)	• Alter food seeking behavior	• Numerous potential negative side effects such as confusion, dizziness, fatigue • No published clinical trials related to use in PWS
Anorexigens (phentermine)	• Appetite control	• No benefit seen to appetite control or weight status for PWS patients
Somatostatin	• Suppress ghrelin • Reduce hyperphagia	• No benefit seen to appetite or weight status for PWS patients
Lipase Inhibitors (orlistat)	• Inhibit pancreatic lipase (prevent some fat absorption)	• Known gastrointestinal side effects • Evidence of some weight loss

Data from Deal CL, Tony M, Höybye C, et al. Growth hormone research society workshop summary: Consensus guidelines for recombinant human growth hormone therapy in prader-willi syndrome. The Journal of Clinical Endocrinology & Metabolism. 2013;98(6; Scheimann AO, Butler MG, Gourash L, Cuffari C, Klish W. Critical analysis of bariatric procedures in prader-willi syndrome. J Pediatr Gastroenterol Nutr. 2008;46(1):80-83.

Assessment of Energy Needs

Energy needs of patients with PWS will change with age. As an infant, patients should be prescribed standard age-appropriate recommendations unless there is a diagnosis of failure to thrive, in which case the infant will need to be placed on a higher-calorie formula or breast milk to promote weight gain. As patients age, there are specific guidelines on energy-needs assessment for the PWS population. For weight maintenance, it is recommended to prescribe 10 to 11 calories/cm of height. For a patient who needs weight reduction, 8 to 9 calories/cm are recommended.[17] Both recommendations are listed in **Table 26.2**. These recommendations are lower than the standards used for the average population in order to account for hyperphagia, shorter stature, and obesity seen in these patients. It is also important to note that because recommendations are for fewer calories than average patients, vitamin and mineral intake should be monitored to ensure patients are still achieving recommended daily allowances despite overall recommended lower intake.[12]

As previously mentioned, patients in this population often struggle with feeding difficulties and weight

TABLE 26.2 PRADER WILLI SYNDROME CALORIE GOALS

Weight maintenance	10-11 calories/cm height
Weight reduction	8-9 calories/cm height

Data from Holland M, Murray M. Diet and nutrition. In: Lucas BL, Feucht SA, Grieger LE, eds. *Children with Special Health Care Needs: nutrition care handbook.* Pediatric Nutrition Practice Group and Dietetics in Developmental and Psychiatric Disorders, American Dietetic Association; 2004.

> **CASE STUDY REVISITED**
>
> Logan is seen 1 month after his initial visit, and he continues to gain weight. His parents report that Logan continues to frequently request food throughout the day, and he has escalated his habit of sneaking and hiding food.
>
> **Questions**
> 1. What strategies would you use to help Logan and his family?
> 2. What other practitioners would you want to get involved, and why?

challenges. It is often very difficult for patients to maintain weight or prevent weight gain due to hyperphagia. Consistent follow up and routines are needed for patients and families to stay on track.

> **PRACTICE POINT**
>
> Many patients will resort to eating nonfood items because of their hyperphagia, which necessitates the need for interventions from various disciplines to help manage behaviors.

Long-term Monitoring and Evaluation

There is no cure for PWS, so patients within this population will require life-long education and support in order to manage associated problems. Practitioners will need to follow weight trends over time to assess adequacy of nutritional management and make any needed changes. Behavioral management is another large piece of a PWS patient's long-term management that will require consistent work, reassessment, and follow up. Managing a patient's hyperphagia and weight will likely be the biggest challenges for the medical team in the long-term care of a patient with PWS.

Spina Bifida

Both genetic and environmental factors play a role in spina bifida (SB), a primarily neurological condition that can often result in orthopedic complications. The prevalence of SB has been declining in North America due to improved prenatal diagnosis and the dietary fortification of many foods with folate. In 1998, the FDA began requiring manufacturers to fortify grain products with folic acid in order to help increase intake.[18] This was done because of the association between low folate intake and increased risk of children being born with neural tube defects, although the exact mechanism for this is still unknown.[18]

> **CORE CONCEPT 6**
>
> Spina bifida is a neural tube defect that can be prevented, in part, through folate supplementation.

There are four classifications of SB: myelomeningocele (the most common form, at 80%-90% of all births), meningocele, closed neural tube defects, and occulta.[19] The differences among these are based on the impact to the spine and are listed in **Table 26.3**. Myelomeningocele (myelo) is the most common form of SB and is an incompletely fused spine from which there is a protrusion of the spinal cord, including nerves. Meningocele also results in an incomplete fusion but does not include any nerves—only spinal fluid—which makes this a less-severe form of SB.[20] Closed neural tube defects are a result of bone, meninges, or fat malformations.[20] **Figure 26.3** shows a comparison of the three classifications. An example of a closed defect

TABLE 26.3 CLASSIFICATION OF SPINA BIFIDA

Myelomeningocele	• Most common • Most severe • Spinal cord and nerves extend through part of the spine • Possible nerve damage, hydrocephalus, and other disabilities
Meningocele	• Exposed meninges and spinal fluid • Fewer disabilities and overall lower severity due to lack of nerve exposure
Occulta	• Least severe form • Malformation of one or more vertebrae • Typically minimal to no symptoms
Closed neural tube defects	• Malformations of bone, fat, or meninges • Wide range of symptoms and severity • Example: Lipomeningocele (fatty tissue deposit)

Data from http://www.ninds.nih.gov/disorders/spina_bifida/detail_spina_bifida.htm http://www.spinabifidaassociation.org/site/c.evKRI7OXIoJ8H/b.8277225/k.5A79/What_is_Spina_Bifida.htm

CASE STUDY INTRODUCTION

Sadie is a 6-year-old female with spina bifida who comes to the outpatient nutrition clinic after a referral from her pediatrician. Sadie is wheelchair-bound and her parents are interested in a nutrition appointment because Sadie is overweight and has decreased interest in activities, which has decreased her mobility.

Anthropometric Data: N/A

Biochemical Data: None

Clinical Data:
Past Medical History: Spina bifida, constipation
Vital signs: Normal
Medications: Multivitamin (gummy), Colace, senna

Dietary Data:
24-hour Diet Recall:
Breakfast: 1 bowl of cereal, whole milk (6 oz)
Snack: 6 peanut butter crackers
Lunch: Sandwich (tuna), 1 small bag of chips, whole milk (6 oz)
Snack: 2 oatmeal cookies, whole milk (4 oz)
Dinner: 1 bowl pasta with 2 meatballs, water
Snack: 1 cup ice cream

Questions
1. How would you obtain anthropometrics? Describe the pros and cons of various alternative methods.
2. How would you educate parents about energy balance and adjustments in Sadie's diet?

---

is **lipomeningocele**, which is the deposition of fatty tissue tumors. Lastly, occulta, which tends to be an asymptomatic form of SB, is often not detected until a patient presents with specific back or urologic problems.[19]

The most commonly encountered nutrition-related issues with patients who have SB include bowel problems such as constipation and incontinence and under- or overweight status. Swallowing difficulties can also occur as a result of Chiari II malformation, which is present in 80% to 90% of patients with myelomeningocele SB.[19] This malformation can lead to feeding problems as a result of the swallowing difficulties, requiring further work with nutrition, medical, and occupational therapy teams.

CORE CONCEPT 7
Myelomeningocele is the most common form of spina bifida and is characterized by incomplete fusion of the spine, often resulting in swallowing, bowel, and bladder dysfunction.

Anthropometrics

Anthropometrics can be difficult to obtain due to potential physical limitations of patients, in which case a variety of alternative methods may have to be used. For weight measurements, the first option is to use the standard digital or balance beam scale. However, if patients are unable to stand on the scale, there are a few alternatives. Patients who are small enough can be held by their parent on the scale, with parent's weight then subtracted. Additionally, a pan/bucket scale, bed scale, or platform scale in which a wheelchair can be placed are all viable options.[21] A bed scale is shown in **Figure 26.4**. It is also important to note the mode of weight measurement on the growth chart for consistency. For children who are unable to stand to obtain a traditional height measurement, alternatives include use of a lengthboard, sitting height measurement, and arm span measurements.[21] Selecting a mode of height measurement should be done based upon specific needs of the child as well as the competency of the clinician in obtaining height through alternative methods. As with weight, it is important to note the method used to obtain height in order to maintain consistent and accurate measurements. Also of note, the standard CDC growth charts should be used to plot and track anthropometrics, because there are no available standardized growth charts for this population.

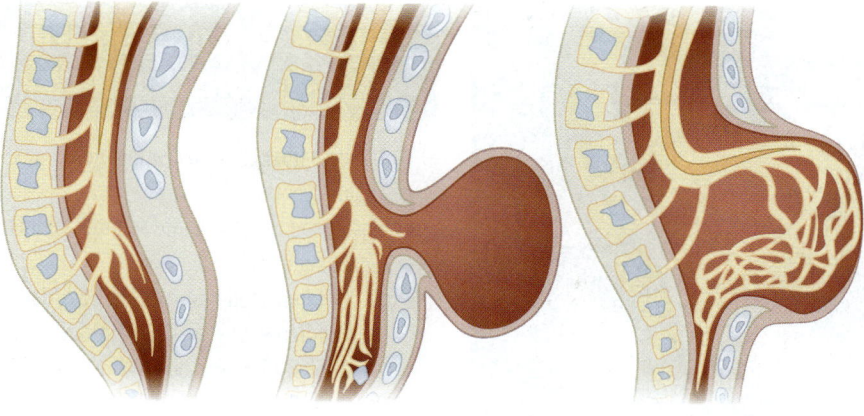
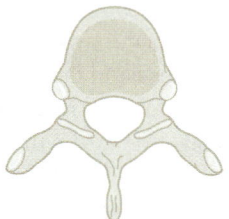
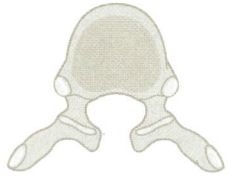

FIGURE 26.3 Comparison of Occulta, Meningocele, and Myelomeningocele

> **PRACTICE POINT**
>
> Accurate and consistent measurement of weight is important, preferably taken using the same measurement techniques over time. Large aberrations in weight should be verified by rechecking.

Biochemical and Clinical

Specific biochemical measurements obtained and medical procedures performed will depend on the patient, their age, any secondary conditions or issues, and their unique needs. The necessity of surgical intervention is dependent upon the type of SB, with early surgery needed only for patients with open defects. The typical clinical path has been for surgery to be done in the first few days of life to close the defect, and to then provide life-long care for associated disabilities. Recently the option of in-utero surgery has been developing as a viable option. The MOMS (Management of Myelomeningocele Study) Trial, a prospective clinical trial funded by the National Institutes of Health, has yielded promising results. This study has shown that in-utero surgery at 19 to 25 weeks' gestation may reduce occurrence of Chiari malformation and need for **ventriculoperitoneal (VP) shunting**, as well as improved overall neuromotor function. In-utero surgery for spina bifida repair is not without potential risks of membrane rupture and preterm delivery, and further research is still needed.[22]

CASE STUDY REVISITED

Sadie presents for follow up after parental concern for her dramatic weight increase per her recent pediatrician appointment. She does not have any physical signs of a weight increase. Her parents report using the nutrition strategies previously discussed.

Questions

1. What could be happening? What would be the course of action?
2. What strategies might be used to assure accurate and consistent weight?

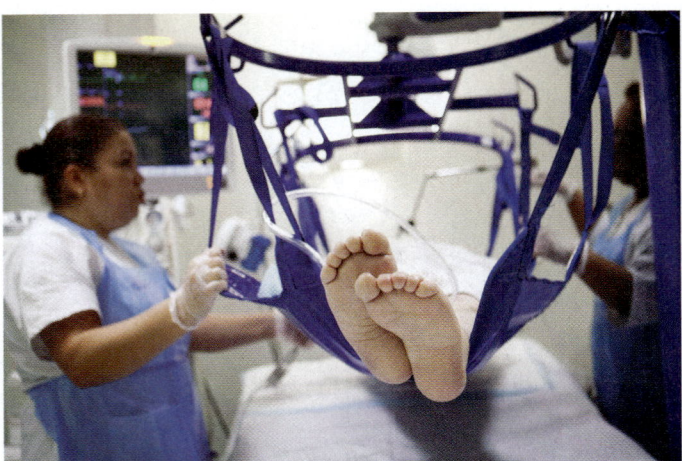

FIGURE 26.4 Digital Bed Scale
©BSIP/UIG via Getty Images.

TABLE 26.4 RECOMMENDATIONS FOR CONSTIPATION PREVENTION

- Increase fiber intake by eating more fruits, vegetables, and whole grains
- Encourage use of MyPlate as a tool for increasing fiber intake
- Goal fiber intake:
  - Children aged 1-8 years: 19-28 g/day
  - Children 9-13 years: 26-31 g/day
  - Adults: 25-35 g/day
- Increase fluid intake in addition to fiber, to avoid worsening constipation

Patients may additionally need surgical management of potential complications such as hydrocephalus. Signs of this can be seen in the neonatal period, including enlarged head circumference and bulging anterior fontanel.[23] Hydrocephalus can be managed through VP shunting, which drains excess cerebrospinal fluid into a peritoneal space to alleviate pressure and prevent progression of hydrocephalus.[23]

In addition to the typical surgical interventions seen in SB patients, there is also the potential for many other associated conditions, each with their own unique challenges that need to be managed in addition to SB. Approximately 15% to 20% of SB patients will experience seizures, occurring more often in patients with shunts.[23] Management for this will likely require antiepileptic medication. SB patients may also face challenges with orthopedic issues such as club foot, which has been seen in 50% of myelo patients.[23] Club foot management requires physical and occupational therapy, potential casting, releases, and/or splinting, with the possibility of further surgical management around age 1 to 2 years. An infant with club foot is shown in **Figure 26.5**. Additionally, rates of scoliosis are approximately 15% to 20% of patients with SB.[23] Two conditions that tend to be common and challenging for this population are neurogenic bladder and bowel. **Neurogenic bladder**, often seen in myelo patients, occurs when patients are unable to perceive bladder fullness and lack coordination between contraction and relaxation.[23] **Neurogenic bowel** is found in most patients with SB and results in decreased bowel motility leading to constipation. The decreased motility, in turn, necessitates the need for the establishment of a bowel regimen. Methods for management can include stimulation, suppositories, enemas, or work with an RD for medical nutrition therapy for constipation, highlighting the importance of adequate fiber and fluids. Specific recommendations are listed in **Table 26.4**.

Assessment of Energy Needs

Patients with SB may have significantly lower energy needs than children without SB due to lower measured resting energy expenditure as well as low lean body mass levels as a result of increased adiposity.[24] Additionally, any motor paralysis can lead to decreased caloric expenditure and presents the potential for obesity.[23] Obesity can be prevalent in this population, not due to the spina bifida diagnosis itself, but as a result of comorbidities.[24] For these reasons, alternative methods to estimate the energy needs of patients with SB are available and based on height. Recommendations are for 9 to 11 kcal/cm for weight maintenance, or 7 kcal/cm for weight loss.[25] These recommendations, listed in **Table 26.5**, are lower than what a child of the same age without SB would receive using the traditional energy needs assessment with the Schofield method or other resources.[26]

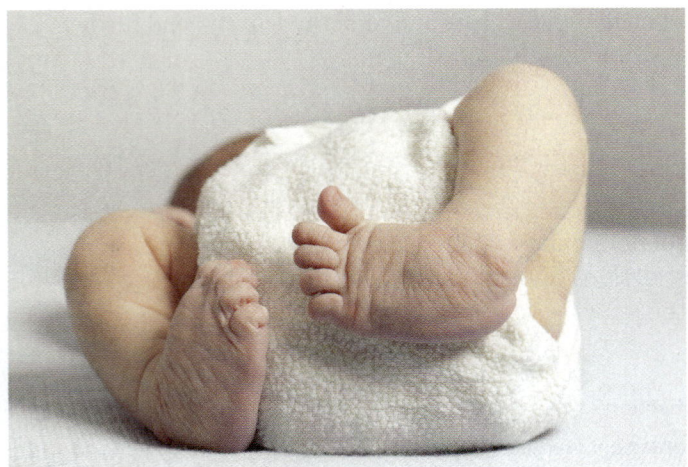

FIGURE 26.5 Infant with Club Foot
©Alis Leonte/Shutterstock.

TABLE 26.5 ENERGY NEEDS OF SPINA BIFIDA PATIENTS

Low energy needs	7-9 kcal/cm
Moderate energy needs	9-11 kcal/cm
High energy needs	12-15 kcal/cm

> **PRACTICE POINT**
>
> Spina bifida patients have lower energy needs than peers their age.

Feeding Difficulties

Patients with SB, as with other developmental disabilities, have the potential to experience feeding difficulties. Specific to SB are feeding problems due to a Chiari II malformation, which can cause swallowing problems. **Chiari II malformation**, also known as Arnold-Chiari malformation (**Figure 26.6**) is more often seen in myelomeningocele-type SB patients than other types of SB.[27] This malformation is an extension of the cerebellar and brain stem tissue into the foramen magnum with the cerebellar vermis (connects the two halves of the cerebellum) appearing as incomplete or damaged.[27] These malformations result in a change in pressure to the brain stem, potentially leading to blockages of cerebrospinal fluid and altering functions controlled by these areas, such as swallowing. Potential causes for this malformation can include genetic mutations, structural defects, or vitamin/mineral deficiencies (e.g., folic acid).[27] Patients can be asymptomatic or can appear with a variety of symptoms such as neck pain, balance issues, poor feeding, headaches, and drooling. Roughly 5% of myelomeningocele patients have a severe malformation and initially present with symptoms such as apnea, failure to thrive and **cyanosis** (bluish coloring of the skin).[23]

Treatment of the Chairi II is based upon presentation of clinical symptoms, with the potential for surgical interventions for patients who present symptomatically or appear as if their symptoms will worsen.[28] Type of surgical intervention will depend upon symptoms present, severity of symptoms, and surgeon preference, and there is no clear consensus on the ideal surgical intervention for Chiari II malformation.[29] However, common surgical procedures include occipital craniectomy and laminectomy or cervical laminectomy, all of which are procedures to provide decompression in hopes of improving craniospinal pressure and/or potentially altered cerebrospinal fluid circulation.[28]

> **PRACTICE POINT**
>
> Chiari II malformation can be found in myelo patients, with the potential for severe symptoms such as apnea, cyanosis, and failure to thrive.

Weight Challenges

Studies have shown that patients with developmental disabilities tend to be overweight and obese, including patients who have SB.[30] Some estimates show that up to 18% of children and adolescents with SB classify as obese.[30] Overweight and obesity can result due to typical factors such as diet and exercise, but with the diagnosis of SB presenting unique challenges on top of the usual patient experience. These patients may be less active than reference populations; inactivity increases risk of obesity, which, in turn, will negatively impact whatever mobility the patient does have and serve as a risk factor for other comorbidities.[23] RDs will need to employ typical practices of medical nutrition therapy with changes made to counseling style or goal setting as needed to fit individual patients and accommodate for any challenges as a result of SB.

Long-term Monitoring and Evaluation

Long-term monitoring will include evaluation of growth, any feeding issues, potential need for a consistent bowel management program, and potential for overweight and obesity. Additionally, dealing with any secondary health issues that come with normal aging, while taking into account the SB diagnosis and its unique challenges, will be important.

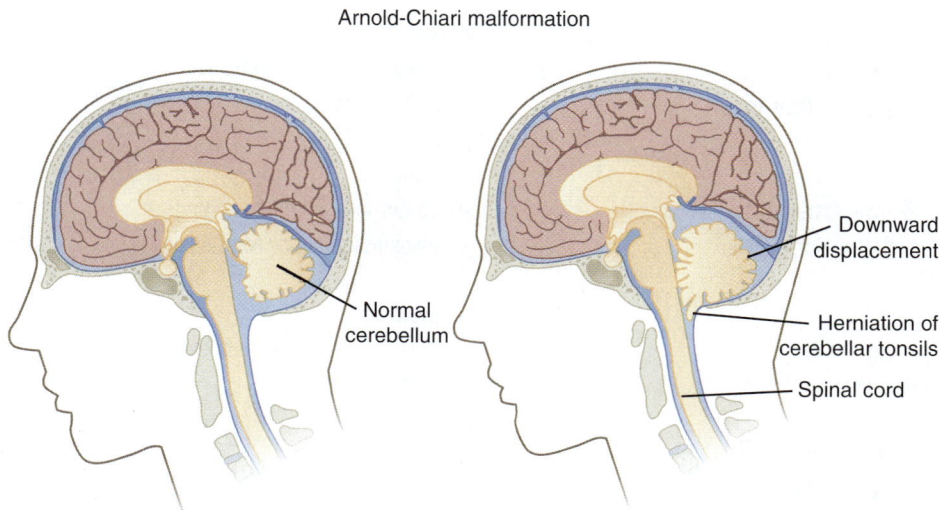

FIGURE 26.6 Arnold-Chiari Malformation

Cerebral Palsy

Cerebral palsy is one of the most common disabilities, presenting in 1 of every 500 live births.[31] A cerebral palsy (CP) diagnosis encompasses a variety of manifestations as well as many secondary issues. Potential causes of CP include prematurity, brain malformations, in utero stroke, hypoxic ischemic encephalopathy, meningitis, anoxic insult, and accidental head trauma.[4]

The different CP classifications listed in **Table 26.6** are made based on the type of movement and limbs affected. CP can be **spastic** (increased muscle tone), which can present as hemiplegia (unilateral involvement), diplegia (disproportionate lower extremity movement), and quadriplegia (whole body involvement).[4] Nonspastic CP is a lack of ability to control movement, which can present in a variety of ways, such as hypotonia (low postural tone) or ataxia (unbalanced walking).[32] Mixed CP is a combination of characteristics of both spastic and nonspastic types of CP.

> **CORE CONCEPT 8**
>
> Cerebral palsy patients are classified based upon type of movement and limbs affected, with the main distinctions being between spastic and nonspastic.

Patients in the CP population can face a variety of medical issues secondary to their diagnosis, such as seizures, which occur in approximately 30% of patients.[4] Other issues may include deficits in learning and cognition and respiratory, vision, hearing, and orthopedic issues. According to the CDC, in 2008, 58.2% of children with CP were able to walk independently, 11.3% walked with a handheld mobility device, and 30.6% had limited or no walking ability.[33] A walking frame for assistance with movement is shown in **Figure 26.7**. Nutrition concerns in a patient with CP are swallowing problems, underweight status, gastrointestinal problems, osteopenia, and constipation.

Anthropometrics

As with other developmentally disabled patients, CP patients can also present challenges when trying to collect and assess anthropometrics. In addition to the challenges in obtaining anthropometrics is the fact that CP patients often have issues with poor growth that can negatively affect overall health and well-being, which makes data collection and monitoring so essential in providing the best care.[34]

In general, it is recommended that CDC sex-specific growth charts be used in assessing growth of children with CP.[34] Of note, there are multiple specialized growth charts available that are categorized depending upon type of CP, with various distinctions that can be used to assess growth.[35] However, these growth charts are more for a descriptive purpose and should be used with caution.[34]

In addition to using specialized growth charts, patients will likely need alternative methods to measure weight and height based on the extent of the disability. Patients with more severe disability will require more assistance and alternatives in collecting these data. Obtaining an accurate weight can be challenging, so alternative methods should be considered. Alternative methods can include a bed scale, weight with a parent and subtracting parent weight, platform scale, chair scale (if patient can sit alone), or another adaptive device for assistance.[36] An accurate height/length can also be difficult to obtain due to potential contractures and/or inability to stand. In these cases, alternatives include crown to rump length, sitting height, arm span, and tibia length or knee length.[36] It is also important to note the type of alternative measuring method used in order to continue

TABLE 26.6 CEREBRAL PALSY CLASSIFICATIONS

Pyramidal (Spastic): Increased Muscle Tone	Extrapyramidal (Nonspastic): Decreased Ability to Control Movement
Diplegia • Bilateral extremity involvement • Usually presents in legs rather than arms	**Ataxia** • Uncoordinated movement • Unbalanced walking
Hemiplegia • Unilateral upper and lower extremity involvement • Usually arm and leg of same side affected	**Dystonia** • Contortions of limbs, twisting • Involuntary muscle contractions
Triplegia • Involvement of three extremities • Usually both legs and one arm affected	**Athetosi** • Slow, involuntary movements • Writhing
Quadriplegia • Involvement of all four extremities • Usually legs more affected than arms	**Chorea** • Repetitive, irregular movements • Can be brief and somewhat rapid

Data from Dodge NN. Cerebral palsy: Medical aspects. *Pediatr Clin North Am.* 2008;55(5):1189-1207

CASE STUDY INTRODUCTION

Millie, a 4-year-old female, is new to this clinic and is admitted for your evaluation. Her parents report she has been losing weight and her status overall has been declining. They also report they were previously told that their daughter will likely need enteral nutrition support through tube feeding.

Anthropometric Data:
Weight: 12 kg (26.4 lb), <3 percentile weight/age (CDC growth chart)
Height: 95 cm (37"), 10 percentile height/age (CDC growth chart)
Weight/height: <3% (CDC growth chart)
BMI: 13.6 kg/m^2, <3 percentile BMI/age (CDC growth chart)

Biochemical Data:
Hemoglobin 8 (12.0-15.5g/dL)

Clinical Data:
Past Medical History: Cerebral palsy, non-spastic
Nutrition-focused physical exam: Appears pale and thin. Skin noted to be dry with poor skin turgor. No wounds noted. Oral exam notable for a dry tongue and mucosa. Hypotonic muscle tone observed.

Dietary Data:
24-hour Diet Recall:
Breakfast: 2 oz whole milk (to thickened consistency), 1 silver dollar pancake, 3 tbsp vanilla yogurt
Lunch: ½ grilled cheese sandwich, apple juice (to thickened consistency)
Dinner: 1 small bowl of pasta with tomato sauce, 1 turkey meatball, 3 oz whole milk (to thickened consistency)
Snack: Chocolate pudding
Diet Prescription: high calorie/protein diet; enteral supplementation

Questions

1. What criteria are used in the decision about the necessity of a gastric feeding tube?
2. What would you say to family and Millie about the plan moving forward?

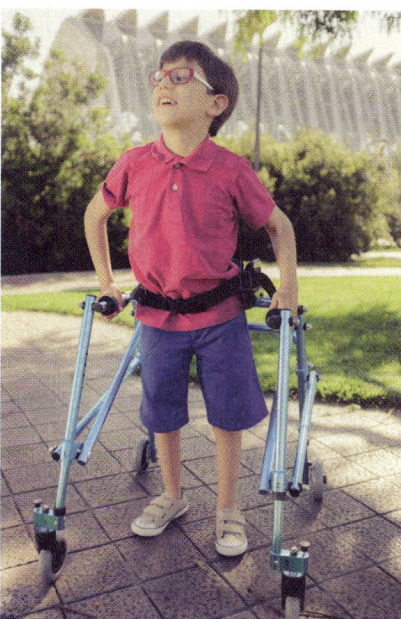

FIGURE 26.7 Walking Frame for Assistance with Movement

using the same method, which will provide further accuracy in assessing growth and show more meaningful trends in growth charts.[34] Additionally, use of triceps skinfold thickness can be useful for assessing fat stores in patients with CP, as BMI/age will most likely not be a useful measure due to alterations in growth with CP.[34]

> **PRACTICE POINT**
>
> Alternative methods for obtaining anthropometrics are necessary for accurate assessment of a CP patient, and noting which method was used is important for follow-up measurements.

Biochemical and Clinical

Specific biochemical measurements obtained will depend on the patient, their age, any secondary conditions or issues, and their unique needs. One major issue that many CP patients face is spasticity, which inhibits normal functioning due to increased muscle tone and tightness.

Management of spasticity is important for overall quality of life for the patient, and there are various methods, including medications.[37] One class of medications used is benzodiazepines, which serve as antispasticity medications to reduce spasms by affecting gamma-aminobutyric acid (GABA) receptors.[37] Note that potential side effects include increased secretions and/or salivation, as well as constipation and urinary retention.[37]

Baclofen, which also acts by affecting GABA receptors, can be used as an oral medication or by insertion of a pump to deliver this medication.[37] Baclofen has been seen to act as a muscle relaxant to help with spasticity and reduce muscle tone, which supports its use in this population. The potential benefits of choosing provision through a pump mechanism rather than orally are potential improved salivation, communication, and speech in addition to the improvements in spasticity.[37] Another medication that can be used to combat spasticity in CP patients is botulinum toxin, which has been used in this population since 1988.[37] Studies show this medication can help improve comfort and ease of care of patient who has spastic CP while also increasing fine motor function and improving upper limb spasticity.[37]

> **PRACTICE POINT**
>
> Medications can be helpful in the management of spasticity, and the ones most often used for this population at this time include baclofen, botulinum toxin, or benzodiazepines.

Other secondary medical issues often seen in patients with CP include seizures, which are present in up to 30% of patients; typical treatment will include use of antiepileptics.[4] An important consideration in using antiepileptics in children is that use of these drugs can negatively impact bone mineral density, making children more susceptible to fractures.[38] Supplementation of calcium and vitamin D to prevent depletion would be warranted. Additionally, patients taking antiepileptic medications are also at risk for decreased levels of folic acid and other essential B vitamins.[39] Clinicians should ensure patients are achieving adequate intake from dietary or supplemental sources. Hearing and vision abnormalities can also occur, likely as a result of the prematurity that is often connected with CP.[4] Potential orthopedic issues that can arise as secondary complications to CP include scoliosis, contractures, and joint dislocations.[4] Additionally, bone health is of concern in this population due to medication use, immobility, and potential poor nutritional intake of necessary nutrients including calcium and vitamin D.[40] Studies have shown low bone mineral density for age in children with CP, which suggests the need for early identification and intervention to promote good bone health and prevent consequences such as fractures.[40]

Gastrointestinal (GI) problems, specifically with gastric motility, often present as a result of the nature of CP and its effect on muscles, leading to issues with reflux and constipation.[4] As mentioned, constipation occurs in up to 80% of CP patients as a result of GI issues, lack of fiber and/or fluids, and inactivity.[4] Recommended management will include medical nutrition therapy for constipation (fiber and fluids) as well as the possible use of bowel medications such as laxatives. Recommendations for assistance in reflux prevention are detailed in **Table 26.7**.

TABLE 26.7 COMMON TIPS FOR REFLUX PREVENTION

- Avoid spicy or acidic foods
- Avoid heavy, fatty meals
- Avoid coffee
- Remain upright after meals (do not lie down immediately after eating)
- Avoid eating right before bed time

Assessment of Energy Needs

There are several equations available in use to estimate the energy needs of a patient with CP, each with a different point of focus. One energy estimation equation by Holland recommends basing energy needs for children on height, with different ranges based on low to high energy needs.[25] Similarly, another equation uses height plus the presence or absence of motor dysfunction to determine a similar range of calorie needs. Krick recommended a different approach, estimating energy needs in children by taking into account multiple factors such as muscle tone, activity, and growth.[41] The starting equation used for an estimate with this method is as follows:

$$\text{Resting energy expenditure} \times \text{muscle tone} \times \text{activity} + \text{growth factors} = \text{kcal/day}$$

Note that although this equation is broader in scope than some others, it runs the risk of inaccuracies due to potential errors in estimating each factor. Clinical judgment should be used in deciding which equation to use, and any adjustments needed based upon each individual patient and their unique needs. **Table 26.8**, **Table 26.9**, and **Table 26.10** provide further considerations of muscle tone and ambulatory status when estimating energy needs in this population.

> **CORE CONCEPT 9**
>
> Muscle tone and ambulatory status can vary within cerebral palsy patients and greatly impact energy assessment.

Feeding Difficulties

There are a variety of potential feeding difficulties that could arise in a CP patient. Most commonly, CP patients present with oromotor problems, which can lead to risk of aspiration, prolonged feeding times, and malnutrition. One study showed that 58% of patients with moderate to severe CP experienced feeding difficulties: 60% of those experienced mild to moderate problems and 40% of those

TABLE 26.8 ENERGY NEEDS ADJUSTMENT BY MUSCLE TONE AND AMBULATORY STATUS[41]

Low muscle tone	Subtract 10%
Normal muscle tone	No adjustment
High muscle tone	Add 10%
Bedridden	Add 15%
Wheelchair-bound	Add 20%
Ambulatory	Add 30%
Growth	Add 5 kcal/kg for expected/desired growth or catchup growth

Data from Krick J, Miller P. Nutritional implications in children with cerebral palsy. *Nutrition Focus*. 2003;18(3).

TABLE 26.9 ENERGY NEEDS IN CP[25]

Low energy needs	7-9 kcal/cm
Moderate energy needs	9-11 kcal/cm
High energy needs	12-15 kcal/cm

Data from Holland M, Murray M. Diet and nutrition. In: Lucas BL, Feucht SA, Grieger LE, eds. *Children with Special Health Care Needs: nutrition care handbook*. Pediatric Nutrition Practice Group and Dietetics in Developmental and Psychiatric Disorders, American Dietetic Association; 2004.

TABLE 26.10 ENERGY NEEDS BY AMBULATORY STATUS[33]

Nonambulatory CP	11 kcal/cm
Ambulatory with motor dysfunction CP	14 kcal/cm
Non–motor dysfunction CP	15 kcal/cm

Developed from Centers for disease control, disability and health: Disability and obesity. http://www.cdc.gov/ncbddd/disabilityandhealth/obesity.html#ref. Accessed October, 21, 2013.

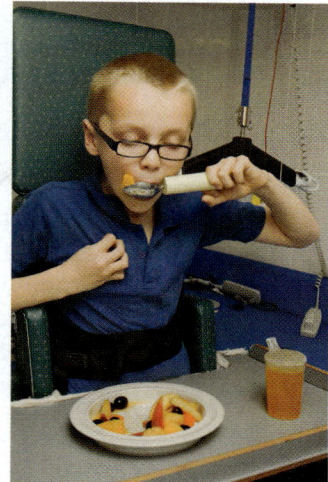

FIGURE 26.8 Adaptive Feeding Devices Help Meet the Individual Needs of the Patient
© BRIAN MITCHELL/Getty Images.

experienced severe problems.[42] Pharyngeal phase abnormalities can include swallow delay, food residue after swallowing, pharyngeal dysmotility, and aspiration (usually related to specific food textures).[42] There is increased risk of dysphagia in this population, with the potential to present with silent aspiration, which is why proper assessment of feeding safety is important.[4] Gastroesophageal reflux disease (GERD) is also common in this population, often presenting with symptoms such as food refusal, failure to thrive, small-volume feeds, and vomiting. Patients will need to work with appropriate resources in order to address these feeding problems, which may include involving speech-language pathologists and occupational therapists to assess swallowing function and to ensure feeding is safer and easier. Tools such as adaptive feeding devices can be instituted by occupational therapists to improve feeding ability. This can include specialized utensils, cups, and bowls; hand cuffs for holding special tools; and seating devices. Adaptive feeding devices (**Figure 26.8**) are patient specific and tailored to their individual needs and abilities.

> **PRACTICE POINT**
>
> An interprofessional team approach, consisting of an RD, speech-language pathologist, occupational therapist, physician, and other healthcare professionals is necessary in order to fully treat a patient and their unique feeding problems.

If patients continue to struggle with meeting their nutritional needs orally, or if it is deemed unsafe to do so, consideration of nutritional support is appropriate. Gastric tube placement for feeding support is appropriate for severe cases in which patients are unable to safely feed (determined by failed speech/swallow evaluation), prolonged feeding times, and/or inadequate intake to maintain nutritional status.[43] Evidence shows that patients are able to gain weight after feeding-tube placement, but there are no clear data on improvements in growth.[43]

Weight Challenges

Most CP patients historically have been underweight and at risk of malnutrition. This generally remains true within the moderate-to-severe cohorts of CP patients because children with CP often present with feeding difficulties, which, if unaddressed, can lead to growth failure, underweight status and malnutrition.[34] However, CP patients can also

Clinical Roundtable

Topic: Calculating Growth and Energy Needs for CP Patients

Background: Use of traditional formulas for estimating energy requirements in pediatric patients is imprecise in CP patients. Differences in body composition, mainly decreased muscle mass, and activity render these formulas inaccurate. Multiple equations have been developed for the calculation of growth and energy requirements in CP patients. However, patients will differ, particularly based on muscle spasticity and ambulatory status.

Roundtable Discussion

1. Consider the differences in the tables shown. How would you choose which to use in your assessment?
2. How would you determine whether you are using the proper calculation?

have weight challenges regarding overweight status. Studies have shown that overweight status tends to be increasingly seen in ambulatory patients, while nonambulatory and more severe patients are on the lower side of the weight spectrum.[44] Recent studies have shown that patients with less-severe CP have fewer feeding issues, are more mobile, and can be at risk for overweight just like peers within the same age group.[45]

Recommendations for nutritional management of these patients will include individualized nutritional care plans to meet unique needs. For underweight patients, strategies could include but are not limited to high-calorie diets; small, frequent meals; nutritional supplements; or supplemental tube feeding. For patients working on overweight status, use of behavior modification techniques, portion control, and general healthy eating tips should be considered. For patients on both sides of the spectrum, nutritional education and goal setting, as well as monitoring of weight trends to assess progress, will be vital.

Long-term Monitoring and Evaluation

CP is a life-long condition and there is no cure, so patients within this population will require continued education and support in order to manage this condition as well as associated problems. Practitioners will need to follow weight trends over time to assess the adequacy of nutritional management and make any needed changes. Patients with more severe forms of CP will require long-term follow up for nutritional support management as well as management of bowel regimens. Long-term work with other practitioners, especially physical and occupational therapy for management, will be important to best meet a goal of function and mobility.

Down Syndrome

Down syndrome (DS), also known as trisomy 21, is a developmental/intellectual disability that occurs in 1 out of 700 babies born in the United States.[46] There are three types of DS that can occur: trisomy 21, translocation DS, and mosaic. The majority of DS cases (95%) present as trisomy 21, in which there is an extra copy of chromosome 21, making for a total of three rather than the typical two chromosomes. Translocation DS represents 3% of cases and occurs as a result of the translocation of extra chromosome 21 material onto another chromosome, rather than remaining independent as seen in classic trisomy 21.

CASE STUDY REVISITED

Millie returns 2 months later with further weight loss. The decision is made to start supplemental tube feeding.

Anthropometric Data:
Weight: 11.5 kg (25.3 lb), <3 percentile weight/age (CDC growth chart)
Height: 95 cm (37"), 5 percentile height/age (CDC growth chart)
BMI: 12.7 kg/m^2 <3 percentile BMI/age (CDC growth chart)

Questions

1. What would you recommend as a nutrition regimen?
2. What goals for oral intake would you recommend for the patient?
3. What parameters might you monitor?

CASE STUDY INTRODUCTION

Nolan is a 5-year-old male with Down syndrome who has been referred by his pediatrician to see an RD due to a recent diagnosis of celiac disease. Nolan presents as slightly underweight and his parents report issues with constipation.

Anthropometric Data:
Weight: 15 kg (33 lb), 5% weight/age (CDC growth chart)
Height: 109 cm (43"), 50% height/age (CDC growth chart)
Weight/height: <3% (CDC growth chart)
BMI: 12.6 kg/m^2, <3% BMI/age (CDC growth chart)

Biochemical Data:
tTG-IgA result Positive for celiac disease

Clinical Data:
Nutrition-focused Physical Exam: Thin appearing, but otherwise normal for age; healthy-looking hair and skin. Abdominal exam notable for mild distention. No edema noted.
Medications: Miralax PRN, multivitamin

Dietary Data:
Dietary History: Previously eating a regular diet for age, but with reported GI symptoms when eating various carbohydrates (pasta, bread).

Questions
1. What nutritional risk factors does Nolan have?
2. What type of education is necessary for this family?
3. How would you adapt education based upon his diagnosis of Down syndrome?

Lastly, mosaic makes up approximately 2% of cases and occurs when there is a mixture of typically formed pairs of chromosome 21 as well as trios.[46]

Although there are variations, DS patients typically present with a certain grouping of physical characteristics. These can include almond-shaped eyes, short neck, flattened face, small hands and feet, short stature, and small ears (**Figure 26.9**).[46] Additionally, people with DS often have lower IQs compared to their peers.[46] Associated health problems for people with DS can include congenital heart disease (40%-50%), hearing and vision problems (60%-75%), obstructive sleep apnea (50%-75%), celiac disease (5%), autism (1%), and Hirschsprung disease (<1%).[47]

Risk of DS increases as the mother's age during pregnancy increases, with higher prevalence seen in mothers older than age 35 years.[46] Diagnosis of DS can be done either during pregnancy or after birth. During pregnancy, the first step is to conduct standard screening tests, which can include an ultrasound and blood work, to be used for an initial assessment for DS. If there are findings consistent with DS, the next step would be to perform a diagnostic test, which could include amniocentesis, percutaneous umbilical cord testing, or chorionic villus sampling,[46] which all look for changes in chromosomes consistent with DS. Diagnosis after birth can be made through physical examination in combination with blood testing for alterations in chromosomal patterns.[46]

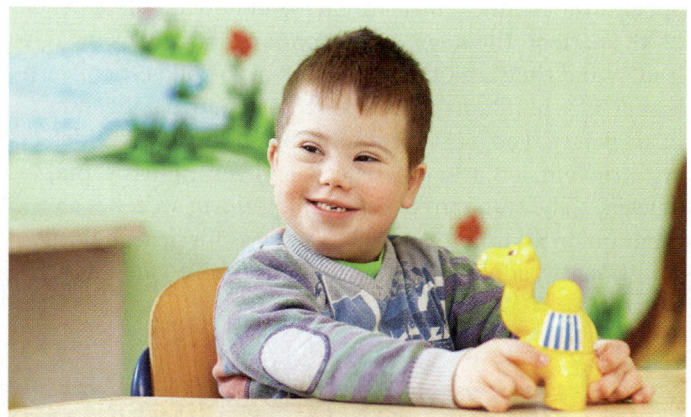

FIGURE 26.9 Child with Down Syndrome
©Olesia Bilkei/Shutterstock.

> **CORE CONCEPT 10**
>
> Down syndrome is a disability that can occur as a result of chromosomal alterations.

Anthropometrics

In general, people with DS tend to be of shorter stature and grow slower than their peers.[48] DS growth charts were created in 1988 after a study done by Cronk et al. showed that these differences in growth were true to this population, with growth rates in infancy almost 20% lower for children with DS.[49] Growth can be altered based on present comorbidities such as cardiac or gastrointestinal issues, which may lead to initial issues with poor feeding and weight gain.[48] However, with medical advances and increased life expectancy, these charts are no longer widely used and current recommendations are instead to monitor growth via standard CDC and WHO growth charts based on sex.[50]

However, a research study has compiled a data set of over 600 children with DS to try and create a disease-specific growth chart.[50] It was found that children in the more recent study were seen to have better initial weight gain from birth to age 3 years, and increases in height for both males and females.[50] Current recommendations are to continue using the CDC/WHO growth charts but with the potential to use these new charts in the future, in the hopes of one day having established growth charts for DS to better monitor and track growth trends in this population.

> **PRACTICE POINT**
>
> Down syndrome–specific growth charts are available, but current recommendations are to use CDC/WHO growth charts to monitor growth.

Biochemical and Clinical

Specific biochemical measurements obtained will depend on the patient, their age, any secondary conditions or issues, and their unique needs. One of the biggest concerns is that 50% of infants with DS are born with a congenital heart defect. The most commonly occurring cardiac defects are atrioventricular septal defects and ventricular septal defects.[51] The standard of care is to perform an echocardiogram on all infants with DS to assess for heart defects. Additionally, adolescents and adults with DS can develop cardiac issues such as mitral valve prolapse, even without any preexisting problems.[51] Another medical complication that is associated with DS is Hirschsprung disease. **Hirschsprung disease** is a blockage of the large intestine that is a result of missing nerves in the bowel that function to move material through. This is treated through surgical repair, but studies have found that many DS patients will still suffer from residual bowel problems even after repair.[52] This can include incontinence, soiling, constipation, and even enterocolitis, all of which have the potential for long-term management needs.[52]

Obesity can become a problem for people with DS, because they have reduced resting metabolic rates compared to their peers, likely due to the composition of fat-free mass or a cellular metabolism abnormality.[53] The combination of lower metabolic rates and slower growth rates contribute to development of obesity. Studies have shown that people with DS are more likely to be overweight or obese than nondisabled peers, and additionally have a higher prevalence of secondary health problems compared to healthy-weight peers.[54] Close monitoring of growth charts and trends is important in combination with a healthy diet, regular physical activity, and limiting sedentary activities to help prevent obesity.[51]

An increased prevalence of celiac disease has been seen in patients with DS compared to the general population.[55] Some studies estimate that roughly 4% to 7% of people with DS will develop celiac disease, often with delayed diagnosis.[51] Current recommendations from the American Academy of Pediatrics suggest a discussion of celiac disease and its symptoms and presentation at child's well visits to assess the potential for celiac disease.[47] If patients are exhibiting known signs of celiac such as abdominal pain/bloating, constipation, diarrhea, or growth changes, then testing should be done to confirm a diagnosis.[47] There is currently no consensus on whether or not testing should be done in nonsymptomatic DS patients, even with the increased prevalence.[47] Positive diagnosis of celiac disease will mean following a gluten-free diet (avoidance of wheat, barley, and rye) in order to help alleviate and manage symptoms. **Table 26.11** provides an overview of common foods that contain gluten. The current market has numerous gluten-free

CASE STUDY REVISITED

Nolan has overall been following the dietary instructions provided at the last appointment on gluten-free eating quite well. His family reports improved symptoms and intake. Anthropometrics today show a 1 kg weight gain, placing him at roughly the 10th percentile for weight.

Questions

1. What would be your educational focus for this appointment?
2. What goals would you set, keeping in mind the potential for growth slowing and future obesity in this population?

TABLE 26.11 COMMON FOODS THAT CONTAIN GLUTEN	
Pastas	Wheat-based noodles (spaghetti, ravioli), dumplings, ramen noodles, couscous
Breads	Wheat and white bread, croissants, bagels, flatbread, donuts, rolls, muffins, pita, naan
Baked Goods	Cake, cookies, pies, brownies
Cereals/Breakfast foods	Wheat-based cereals, corn flakes and rice puffs that contain malt, pancakes, waffles, French toast

options that can help ease the transition, which, combined with nutrition education and a focus on fruits, vegetables, and lean proteins, should lead to improvements.

CORE CONCEPT 11

Patients with Down syndrome have a higher prevalence of celiac disease compared to their peers without Down syndrome.

Assessment of Needs

As previously mentioned, patients with DS have lower resting energy expenditure and growth rates relative to their peers. As a result, energy estimates and caloric needs for DS can be lower than average. Patients can have increased energy needs, especially in infancy, as a result of cardiac issues, poor growth, or decreased feeding abilities.[56] Estimates for energy needs can be made using equations specifically for this population; for children with DS, aged 5 to 11 years, starting estimates are 16.1 kcal/cm (males) and 14.3 kcal/cm (females).[56] More research is needed to help determine guidelines for this patient population, especially for other age groups.

PRACTICE POINT

Calorie estimates based on height can be used to estimate energy needs of some Down syndrome patients.

Long-term Monitoring/Evaluation

Long-term monitoring for the DS population will include the potential cardiac issues in the future, even without issues in childhood; obesity; potential for celiac disease; vision/hearing problems; and the typical problems or comorbidities that can be seen with aging such as diabetes, high blood pressure, or high cholesterol. Also important to note is that advances in medicine have greatly impacted the life expectancy for patients with DS. Life expectancy has increased dramatically from 25 years of age in 1983 to 60 years of age in 2015.[57]

Autism Spectrum Disorders

Autism spectrum disorder (ASD) is a group of disorders that impact behavior, communication, and development. ASD prevalence has been increasing over the past 15 years and affects 1 in 68 children in the United States, occurring roughly 5 times more often in boys.[58] The American Psychiatric Association's Diagnostic and Statistical Manual, (DSM) 4th edition classified ASD into the following subcategories: autism disorder, Asperger's, or pervasive developmental disorders not otherwise specified. However, the current DSM, 5th edition has changed the criteria in that each of these subcategories is now diagnosed as Autism Spectrum Disorder.[59] Typical features of ASD include challenges with behaviors, such as preforming repetitive behaviors; difficulty with change; and limited communication and social interactions.[60] ASD can sometimes occur due to genetics, but more often than not the cause is unknown. ASD is challenging to diagnose as there are no specific medical tests; instead, diagnosis is based upon looking for specific "red flags" (Table 26.12) combined with assessment of behavior and development. Treatment includes behavioral/education interventions and sometimes medications to manage corresponding diagnoses such as depression, anxiety, or obsessive compulsive disorder, but there are no specific medications to treat or manage ASD itself.[60] Figure 26.10 shows a child with autism.

CORE CONCEPT 12

Autism spectrum disorder (ASD) is a group of disorders that impact behavior, communication, and development.

Health problems commonly found in this population include GI issues, seizures, and sleep difficulties.[61] GI issues can include chronic diarrhea and constipation, with some studies reporting a prevalence of 46% to 85% in children with ASD, although the association is still unknown.[61] Seizures can be associated with ASD (11%-39%), but are more commonly found in ASD patients who have an additional neurological impairment (roughly 42%). Sleep difficulties can be common in patients with ASD and can be the result of medical problems such as sleep apnea, but more often manifest as a result of behavioral issues or stressors. Further research is needed to determine the best approach for managing sleep difficulties in this population, but some preliminary studies have shown melatonin to be effective in improving sleep.[61]

Anthropometrics

There are no specialized growth charts for monitoring the growth of children with ASD, as this does not typically impact normal growth. Monitoring of growth in this population will include using standard CDC growth charts on a routine basis and use of BMI/age to assess weight status.[62] Identified issues of under- or overweight status can be

TABLE 26.12 RED FLAGS FOR ASD

Neurological	Signs/Symptoms	Medical	Signs/Symptoms
Speech/Language	Delay in first words beyond 12-18 months	Seizures	Mild-eye gaze, auras, decreased muscle tone
Eye Contact	Lack of joint attention and shared gazes, does not look when called upon	Gastrointestinal	GERD, constipation, irritable bowel syndrome, gastritis
Sensory Processing	Refusal to touch various textures	Food Allergies	Diarrhea, pain with eating, fussiness, arching of the back
Sleep Patterns	Poor sleeper	Ear Infections	Irritability, pain, sleeplessness
Maladaptive Behaviors	Tantrums, aggression	Eczema	Itching, discomfort, eczema patches

treated with the appropriate medical nutrition therapy. Of note, research has shown that children with ASD were found more likely to be overweight or obese than children without this diagnosis.[63] Specifically, older children with autism had higher likelihood of obesity than younger children with autism, and the odds of overweight or obesity in children who also had a sleep condition were higher still.[63] The reason for increased likelihood of overweight and obesity in this population is likely multifactorial and due to potential issues with food selectivity/preferences, limited physical activity, and possible use of medications with side effects of weight gain.[63]

Biochemical and Clinical

Because there is no definitive form of treatment for ASD, parents will often seek complementary alternative medicine options such as following restrictive diets, taking nutritional supplements, or using alternative treatments such as yoga or chiropractors. Use of restrictive diets to try and improve behavioral symptoms includes gluten/casein-free, ketogenic, food additive avoidance, and other elimination diets.[64]

Gluten-free or casein-free diets are often used in this population with the thought that eliminating these proteins from the diet will improve ASD symptoms.[65] Some small studies have suggested minor improvements, but more research is needed, and nutrition education is necessary for patients who will be following these diets to ensure good nutritional status when eliminating foods with these nutrients. Patients eliminating these foods can risk calcium, vitamin D, and vitamin B deficiencies.[66]

The ketogenic diet is most recognized for its use in patients with epilepsy, but interest has grown in use of this diet for patients with ASD, specifically for those with ASD who experience seizures. The ketogenic diet involves high fat consumption (ranging from 60%-89% of caloric needs), moderate protein, and low carbohydrates, so that the body will burn fat for fuel.[67] At this time, only limited research is available; small studies have shown improved behavior and seizure activity, but further research on a larger scale is needed to determine the true effects.

Elimination of food additives can also be used in an attempt to improve behavioral symptoms and concurrent medical problems, with the idea that food additives have the potential to contribute to hyperactivity, GI problems, and behavior changes.[66] This type of **elimination diet** can encompass a variety of potential items to eliminate such as artificial sweeteners and flavorings, high fructose corn syrup, and food colorings.[66] Working with an RD is important in order to ensure that good overall nutrition is maintained.

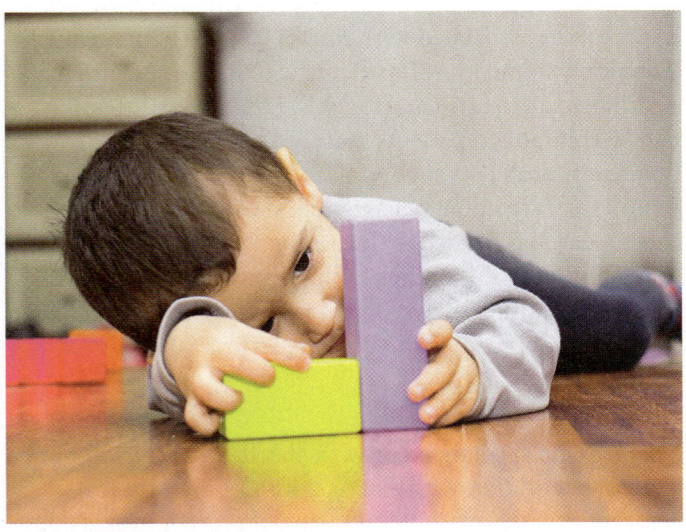

FIGURE 26.10 Child with Autism
©Nazarova Mariia/Shutterstock.

CASE STUDY INTRODUCTION

Billy is a 4-year-old male, diagnosed with Autism 1 year prior, who has been referred to the RD from his pediatrician due to "picky eating" and continued weight gain that now classifies him as obese. Billy is also on medication for anxiety, which is likely contributing to his weight gain.

Anthropometric Data:
Weight: 20 kg (44 lb), 95% weight/age (CDC growth chart)
Height: 99 cm (3' 3"), 25% height/age (CDC growth chart)
Weight/height: >95% (CDC growth chart)
BMI: 20.4 kg/m^2, >95% BMI/age (CDC growth chart)

Biochemical Data:
Labs within normal limits, including vitamin D level of 35 ng/mL

Clinical Data:
Medications: Gummy multivitamin daily
Nutrition-focused Physical Exam: Obese but well appearing. Oral exam, hair, and nails appear normal. Skin is warm and intact. Abdominal exam unremarkable.

Dietary Data:
24-hour Diet Recall:
Breakfast: Strawberry milk (8 oz), 2 medium pancakes with syrup, 1 strawberry yogurt
Lunch: Strawberry milk (8 oz), turkey sandwich (turkey, cheese, mayo), small bag potato chips
Snack: 4 vanilla wafer cookies, strawberry yogurt
Dinner: Strawberry milk (8 oz), 1 large bowl macaroni and cheese, 2 breadsticks

Questions

1. What are Billy's nutritional risk factors?
2. How would you assess Billy's energy needs?
3. Should Billy be on a special diet for autism?

> **PRACTICE POINT**
>
> There is currently no scientific evidence to support use of restrictive or elimination diets for patients with autism.

Selectivity with foods can lead to potential alterations in micronutrient intake. Some research has shown an increased risk of inadequate intake of calcium, vitamin D, zinc, and vitamin B$_{12}$ in patients with autism who are selective eaters.[68] Potential for deficiencies will be dictated by which foods are included on a routine basis and which are avoided, either by following a particular diet or through selectivity choices. Additionally, it is important to take into consideration the potential impact ASD may have on oral health. There is a potential for increased risk of caries and dental issues due to patient specific sensory issues and how this would impede performing necessary oral hygiene.

Feeding Difficulties

Children with ASD tend to have more feeding challenges than their peers, which can include aversions, hypersensitivities, and sensory issues.[69] These challenges can translate into avoiding foods of a certain texture, color, taste, smell, or other various determining factors. The overarching term that can be used to describe this phenomenon is food selectivity. Issues with food selectivity have the potential to lead to nutrient inadequacies, depending on the foods consumed by the child.[70] It is important to assess the diet for nutritional adequacy and determine any macro- and micronutrient deficiencies. Treatment in hopes of overcoming food selectivity will likely involve multiple disciplines, including therapists, RDs, and occupational therapists. Depending on the child and their unique needs, adaptations can be made such as different settings for meal times; modified utensils and food textures; or employing strategies to help prepare and guide patients through trials of new and different foods.[70]

> **CORE CONCEPT 13**
>
> Food selectivity can be one of the biggest challenges in caring for a patient with autism.

> ### CASE STUDY REVISITED
>
> Billy and his family have returned for a follow-up appointment and his weight has continued to increase. His diet recall remains mostly the same, and his parents report that Billy is still resistant to trying fruits and vegetables.
>
> #### Questions
> 1. What other healthcare providers might you consult?
> 2. What types of modifications could be helpful?

Assessment of Needs

Estimation of energy and protein needs should be calculated by using standard pediatric growth charts and energy estimation equations. No condition-specific caloric estimates are established for this population. Goals should be based on weight status or other medical issues that impact energy needs. It is important to also take into account the potential impact of selectivity or specificity in food changes and how this might translate into over- or undernutrition in regards to certain macro- and micronutrients.

> **PRACTICE POINT**
>
> There are currently no autism-specific growth charts, as it has not been shown to greatly impact normal growth expectations.

Long-term Monitoring and Evaluation

Long-term monitoring will include evaluation of growth, potential need for a bowel management program, and the potential for overweight and obesity. Additionally, dealing with any secondary health issues that come with normal aging while taking into account an autism diagnosis and its unique challenges will be important.

Chapter Summary

Developmental disabilities are a group of conditions that are both diverse in nature but share similarities in secondary complications and necessary management. Each patient should be treated as a unique individual, using an interprofessional approach to help with management of care across the life span. As there is the potential for a variety of secondary complications with each developmental disability, it is important to know the hallmarks of each condition and work with a team approach to ensure all aspects of care are addressed.

Key Terms

developmental disability, hyperphagia, myelomeningocele, lipomeningocele, ventriculoperitoneal shunting, neurogenic bladder, neurogenic bowel, Chiari II malformation spastic, cyanosis, Hirschpsrung disease, autism spectrum disorder, elimination diet

References

1. Boyle CA, Boulet S, Schieve LA, et al. Trends in the prevalence of developmental disabilities in US children, 1997-2008. *Pediatrics*. 2011;127(6):1034-1042.
2. Goldstone A, Holland A, Hauffa B, Hokken-Koelega A, Tauber M. Recommendations for the diagnosis and management of Prader-Willi syndrome. *J Clin Endrocinol Metabol*. 2008;93(11):4183-4197.
3. Spina bifida: Basics. Centers for Disease Control and Prevention website. http://www.cdc.gov/ncbddd/spinabifida/facts.html. Reviewed September 11, 2017. Accessed December 3, 2017.
4. Dodge NN. Cerebral palsy: Medical aspects. *Pediatr Clin North Am*. 2008;55(5):1189-1207.
5. Ogden C, Carroll M, Kit B, Flegal K. Prevalence of obesity among adults: United States, 2011–2012. NCHS data brief, no 131. https://www.cdc.gov/nchs/data/databriefs/db131.pdf. Accessed December 3, 2017.
6. Disparities Snapshot: Children with Special Health Care Needs. National Survey of Children's Health (NSCH) 2007. Child and Adolescent Health Measurement Initiative, Data Resource Center for Child and Adolescent Health website. http://childhealthdata.org/browse/data-snapshots/nsch-profiles/special-health-care-needs?geo=1&ind=465. Accessed December 3, 2017.
7. Rimmer JH, Yamaki K, Davis BM, Wang E, Vogel LC. Obesity and overweight prevalence among adolescents with disabilities. *Prev Chronic Dis*. 2011;8(2):A41.
8. Chen C, Visootsak J, Dills S, Graham JM Jr. Prader-Willi syndrome: An update and review for the primary pediatrician. *Clin Pediatr (Phila)*. 2007;46(7):580-591.
9. Butler MG. Prader-Willi syndrome: Obesity due to genomic imprinting. *Curr Genomics*. 2011;12(3):204-215.
10. McCandless SE. Committee on Genetics. Clinical report-health supervision for children with Prader-Willi syndrome. *Pediatrics*. 2011;127(1):195-204.
11. Butler MG, Sturich J, Lee J, et al. Growth standards of infants with Prader-Willi syndrome. *Pediatrics*. 2011;127(4):687-695.
12. Deal CL, Tony M, Höybye C, et al. Growth hormone research society workshop summary: Consensus guidelines for recombinant human growth hormone therapy in Prader-Willi syndrome. *J Clin Endrocinol Metabol*. 2013;98(6);E1072-E1087.
13. Miller JL, Lynn CH, Driscoll DC, et al. Nutritional phases in Prader–Willi syndrome. *Am J Med Genet A*. 2011;155(5):1040-1049.
14. Academy of Nutrition and Dietetics. Pediatric Nutrition Care Manual. Prader Willi syndrome: Anthropometrics. https://www.nutritioncare

15. Academy of Nutrition and Dietetics. Pediatric Nutrition Care Manual. Prader Willi Syndrome: Nutrition Intervention. https://www.nutritioncaremanual.org/topic.cfm?ncm_category_id=13&lv1=144620&lv2=144745&lv3=2977&ncm_toc_id=269977&ncm_heading=Nutrition%20Care%20home%20page. Accessed December 3, 2017.

16. Scheimann AO, Butler MG, Gourash L, Cuffari C, Klish W. Critical analysis of bariatric procedures in Prader-Willi syndrome. *J Pediatr Gastroenterol Nutr*. 2008;46(1):80-83.

17. Academy of Nutrition and Dietetics. Pediatric Nutrition Care Manual. Prader Willi: Comparative standards. https://www.nutritioncaremanual.org/topic.cfm?ncm_category_id=13&lv1=144620&lv2=144745&lv3=269974&ncm_toc_id=269974&ncm_heading=Nutrition%20Care%20home%20page. Accessed December 3, 2017.

18. Williams LJ, Rasmussen SA, Flores A, Kirby RS, Edmonds LD. Decline in the prevalence of spina bifida and anencephaly by race/ethnicity: 1995-2002. *Pediatrics*. 2005;116(3):580-586.

19. Fletcher JM, Brei TJ. Introduction: Spina bifida—A multidisciplinary perspective. *Dev Disabil Res Rev*. 2010;16(1):1-5.

20. Spina bifida information page. National Institute of Neurological Disorders and Stroke website. http://www.ninds.nih.gov/disorders/spina_bifida/detail_spina_bifida.htm. Accessed December 3, 2017.

21. Academy of Nutrition and Dietetics. Pediatric Nutrition Care Manual. Spina Bifida: Anthropometrics. https://www.nutritioncaremanual.org/topic.cfm?ncm_category_id=13&lv1=144620&lv2=144744&lv3=269958&ncm_toc_id=269958&ncm_heading=Nutrition%20Care%20home%20page. Accessed December 3, 2017.

22. Adzick NS. Fetal surgery for spina bifida: Past, present, future. *Semin Pediatr Surg*. 2013;22(1):10-17.

23. Sandler AD. Children with spina bifida: Key clinical issues. *Pediatr Clin North Am*. 2010;57(4):879-892.

24. Liusuwan RA, Widman LM, Abresch RT, Styne DM, McDonald CM. Body composition and resting energy expenditure in patients aged 11 to 21 years with spinal cord dysfunction compared to controls: Comparisons and relationships among the groups. *J Spinal Cord Med*. 2007;30(suppl 1):S105-111.

25. Holland M, Murray M. Diet and nutrition. In: Lucas BL, Feucht SA, Grieger LE, eds. *Children with special health care needs: Nutrition care handbook*. Pediatric Nutrition Practice Group and Dietetics in Developmental and Psychiatric Disorders. Chicago, IL: American Dietetic Association; 2004.

26. Bunting K, Mills J, Philips S, Ramsey E, et al. Alternative methods to determine energy needs, energy requirements in children with developmental disabilities. In: *Pediatric Nutrition Reference guide*. 9th ed. Houston, TX: Texas Children's Hospital; 2010:21-22.

27. Chiari malformation fact sheet. National Institute of Neurological Disorders and Stroke website. http://www.ninds.nih.gov/disorders/chiari/detail_chiari.htm. Accessed December 3, 2017.

28. Tubbs RS, Oakes WJ. Treatment and management of the Chiari II malformation: An evidence-based review of the literature. *Child's Nervous System*. 2004;20(6):375-381.

29. Akbari SHA, Limbrick DD Jr, Kim DH, et al. Surgical management of symptomatic chiari II malformation in infants and children. *Child's Nervous System*. 2013;29(7):1143-1154.

30. Reinehr T, Dobe M, Winkel K, Schaefer A, Hoffmann D. Obesity in disabled children and adolescents: An overlooked group of patients. *Dtsch Arztebl Int*. 2010;107(15):268-275.

31. Schoendorfer NC, Vitetta L, Sharp N, et al. Micronutrient, antioxidant, and oxidative stress status in children with severe cerebral palsy. *JPEN J Parenter Enteral Nutr*. 2013;37(1):97-101.

32. Academy of Nutrition and Dietetics. Pediatric Nutrition Care Canual: Cerebral palsy: Disease process. https://www.nutritioncaremanual.org/topic.cfm?ncm_category_id=13&lv1=144620&lv2=144742&lv3=269920&ncm_toc_id=269920&ncm_heading=Nutrition%20Care%20home%20page. Accessed December 3, 2017.

33. Data and Statistics for Cerebral Palsy. Center for Disease Control and Prevention Website. https://www.cdc.gov/ncbddd/cp/data.html. Accessed December 3, 2017.

34. Andrew MJ, Parr JR, Sullivan PB. Feeding difficulties in children with cerebral palsy. *Arch Dis Child Educ Pract Ed*. 2012;97(6):222-229.

35. Academy of Nutrition and Dietetics. Pediatric Nutrition Care Manual. Cerebral palsy: Anthropometrics. https://www.nutritioncaremanual.org/topic.cfm?ncm_category_id=13&lv1=144620&lv2=144742&lv3=269925&ncm_toc_id=269925&ncm_heading=Nutrition%20Care%20home%20page. Accessed December 3, 2017.

36. Baer M, Harris A, Trahms C, Ogata B. Pacific west MCH distance learning network: Nutrition for children with special health care needs. http://depts.washington.edu/pwdlearn/web/intro.php. Accessed December 3, 2017.

37. Verrotti A, Greco R, Spalice A, Chiarelli F, Iannetti P. Pharmacotherapy of spasticity in children with cerebral palsy. *Pediatr Neurol*. 2006;34(1):1-6.

38. Sheth RD, Binkley N, Hermann BP. Progressive bone deficit in epilepsy. *Neurology*. 2008;70(3):170-176.

39. Sener U, Zorlu Y, Karaguzel O, Ozdamar O, Coker I, Topbas M. Effects of common anti-epileptic drug monotherapy on serum levels of homocysteine, vitamin B12, folic acid and vitamin B6. *Seizure*. 2006;15(2):79-85.

40. Finbråten A, Syversen U, Skranes J, Andersen G, Stevenson R, Vik T. Bone mineral density and vitamin D status in ambulatory and non-ambulatory children with cerebral palsy. *Osteoporosis Int*. 2014:1-10.

41. Krick J. A proposed formula for calculating energy needs of children with cerebral palsy. *Dev Med Child Neurol*. 1992;34:481-487.

42. Rogers B. Feeding method and health outcomes of children with cerebral palsy. *J Pediatr*. 2004;145(2):S28-S32.

43. Ferluga ED, Archer KR, Sathe NA, et al. Interventions for Feeding and Nutrition in Cerebral Palsy. Comparative Effectiveness Review No. 94. (Prepared by the Vanderbilt Evidence-based Practice Center under Contract No. 290-2007-10065-I) AHRQ Publication No. 13-EHC015-EF. Rockville, MD: Agency for Healthcare Research and Quality. March 2013. https://effectivehealthcare.ahrq.gov/topics/cerebral-palsy-feeding/research. Accessed December 3, 2017.

44. Hurvitz EA, Green LB, Hornyak JE, Khurana SR, Koch LG. Body mass index measures in children with cerebral palsy related to gross motor function classification: A clinic-based study. *Am J Phys Med Rehabil*. 2008;87(5):395-403.

45. Rogozinski BM, Davids JR, Davis RB, et al. Prevalence of obesity in ambulatory children with cerebral palsy. *J Bone Joint Surg*. 2007;89(11):2421-2426.

46. Birth Defects: Facts About Down Syndrome. Center for Disease Control and Prevention. http://www.cdc.gov/ncbddd/birthdefects/downsyndrome.html. Reviewed July 27, 2017. Accessed December 3, 2017.

47. Bull MJ, Committee on Genetics. Health supervision for children with Down syndrome. *Pediatrics*. 2011;128(2):393-406.

48. Academy of Nutrition and Dietetics. Pediatric Nutrition Care Manual. Down Syndrome: Anthropometrics. https://www.nutritioncaremanual.org/topic.cfm?ncm_category_id=13&lv1=144620&lv2=144743

&lv3=269940&ncm_toc_id=269940&ncm_heading=Nutrition%20Care%20home%20page. Accessed December 3, 2017.

49. Cronk C, Crocker AC, Pueschel SM, et al. Growth charts for children with Down syndrome: 1 month to 18 years of age. *Pediatrics*. 1988;81(1):102-110.

50. Zemel BS, Pipan M, Stallings VA, et al. Growth charts for children with down syndrome in the United States. *Pediatrics*. 2015;136(5):e1204-11.

51. Roizen NJ, Patterson D. Down's syndrome. *Lancet*. 2003;361(9365):1281-1289.

52. Friedmacher F, Puri P. Classification and diagnostic criteria of variants of Hirschsprung's disease. *Pediatr Surg Int*. 2013;29(9):855-872.

53. Murray J, Ryan-Krause P. Obesity in children with Down syndrome: background and recommendations for management. *Pediatr Nurs*. 2010;36(6):314.

54. Rimmer JH, Yamaki K, Davis BM, Wang E, Vogel LC. Obesity and overweight prevalence among adolescents with disabilities. *Prev Chronic Dis*. 2011;8(2):A41.

55. Zachor DA, Mroczek-Musulman E, Brown P. Prevalence of celiac disease in Down syndrome in the United States. *J Pediatr Gastroenterol Nutr*. 2000;31(3):275-279.

56. Academy of Nutrition and Dietetics. Pediatric Nutrition Care Manual. Down Syndrome: Nutrition Therapy Efficacy. https://www.nutritioncaremanual.org/topic.cfm?ncm_category_id=13&lv1=144620&lv2=144743&lv3=269943&ncm_toc_id=269943&ncm_heading=Nutrition%20Care%20home%20page. Accessed December 3, 2017.

57. Down Syndrome Facts. National Down Syndrome Society website. http://www.ndss.org/Down-Syndrome/Down-Syndrome-Facts/. Accessed December 3, 2017.

58. Autism Spectrum Disorder (ASD): Data and Statistics. Center for Disease Control and Prevention website. http://www.cdc.gov/ncbddd/autism/data.html. Reviewed March 10, 2017. Accessed December 3, 2017.

59. Autism Spectrum Disorder: Diagnostic Criteria. Center for Disease Control and Prevention website. https://www.cdc.gov/ncbddd/autism/hcp-dsm.html. Accessed Updated April 18, 2016. December 3, 2017.

60. Anagnostou E, Zwaigenbaum L, Szatmari P, et al. Autism spectrum disorder: advances in evidence-based practice. *CMAJ*. 2014;186(7):509-519.

61. Myers SM, Johnson CP. American Academy of Pediatrics Council on Children with Disabilities. Management of children with autism spectrum disorders. *Pediatrics*. 2007;120(5):1162-1182.

62. Academy of Nutrition and Dietetics. Pediatric Nutrition Care Manual. Autism Spectrum Disorders: Anthropometrics.https://www.nutritioncaremanual.org/topic.cfm?ncm_category_id=13&lv1=144620&lv2=145108&lv3=269987&ncm_toc_id=269987&ncm_heading=Nutrition%20Care%20home%20page. Accessed December 3, 2017.

63. Broder-Fingert S, Brazauskas K, Lindgren K, Iannuzzi D, Van Cleave J. Prevalence of overweight and obesity in a large clinical sample of children with autism. *Acad Pediatr*. 2014;14(4):408-414.

64. Berry RC, Novak P, Withrow N, et al. Nutrition management of gastrointestinal symptoms in children with autism spectrum disorder: Guideline from an expert panel. *J Acad Nutr Dietet*. 2015;115(12):1919-1927.

65. Levy SE, Hyman SL. Complementary and alternative medicine treatments for children with autism spectrum disorders. *Child Adolesc Psychiatr Clin N Am*. 2008;17(4):803-820.

66. Privett D. Autism spectrum disorder—Research suggests good nutrition may manage symptoms. *Today's Dietitian*. 2013;15(1):46.

67. Napoli E, Duenas N, Giulivi C. Potential therapeutic use of the ketogenic diet in autism spectrum disorders. *Front Pediatr*. 2014;2:69.

68. Graf-Myles J, Farmer C, Thurm A, et al. Dietary adequacy of children with autism compared with controls and the impact of restricted diet. *J Dev Behav Pediatr*. 2013;34(7):449-459.

69. Academy of Nutrition and Dietetics. Pediatric Nutrition Care Manual. Autism Spectrum Disorders: Feeding Skills. https://www.nutritioncaremanual.org/topic.cfm?ncm_category_id=13&lv1=144620&lv2=145108&lv3=269988&ncm_toc_id=269988&ncm_heading=Nutrition%20Care%20home%20page. Accessed December 3, 2017.

70. Cermak SA, Curtin C, Bandini LG. Food selectivity and sensory sensitivity in children with autism spectrum disorders. *J Am Diet Assoc*. 2010;110(2):238-246.

Chapter 27

Nutrition in Geriatrics

Jennifer Cho
Andrea Hurwitz

Chapter Outline

Core Concepts
Introduction
Background and Etiology
Changes in Body Composition in the Geriatric Population
Malnutrition Risk in Geriatrics

Physiologic Factors
Nutrition Screening and Assessment in Geriatrics
Nutrient Needs
Physiologic Alterations Effecting Micronutrient Metabolism
Nutrition Management

CORE CONCEPTS

1. Among other factors, reduced energy requirement is largely due to decreases in lean body mass and physical activity in the older population.
2. Unlike body water and lean body mass, fat mass increases with age; adipose tissue does not have significant metabolic activity compared to muscle.
3. Sarcopenia is not a treatable condition; however, measures can be taken to slow progression.
4. Sarcopenia and obesity can coexist in an individual; the presence of both sarcopenia and obesity has been shown to put older adults at a higher risk for adverse outcomes and functional impairment than sarcopenia or obesity alone.
5. Individuals with dysphagia may limit food and liquid intake or avoid certain types of food, potentially leading to malnutrition.
6. With aging, social support becomes a valuable tool in optimizing the quality and quantity of the food consumed.
7. If etiologies are identified and if appropriate interventions are made, progression of malnutrition can be slowed or reversed and quality of life and function can be improved.
8. Differences in nutrient needs from younger adults can be seen in energy, fluid, protein requirements as a result of changes associated with aging.

Learning Objectives

1. Describe how the age structure of the American population has changed over the years.
2. Explain how age affects body composition and nutritional needs.
3. Determine which screening tool to use to identify older adults at nutritional risk.
4. Differentiate between sarcopenia and cachexia.
5. State the contributing factors to geriatric malnutrition.
6. Discuss the implications of sarcopenia and geriatric malnutrition.
7. Determine which particular micronutrient deficiencies to monitor in the geriatric population.
8. Formulate appropriate nutrition recommendations/intervention that is in line with goals of care for older adults.

Introduction

The age structure of the overall American population has changed dramatically since World War II. Much of this change has been driven by the aging baby boomers. Significant growth in the population after World War II, coupled with improvements in health care, allowed for an increase in life expectancy and has contributed to the change in composition of the American population.

Older Americans are currently defined as those who are age 65 years and older.[1] They constitute a large proportion of our population, and there is a growing focus on health care of elderly people. Geriatrics, the study of the chronic diseases often associated with aging, including diagnoses, treatment, and/or management of these conditions, was created to address the shift in age structure of the American population and its impact on the healthcare system and management.

Changes associated with normal aging, chronic diseases, and social and environmental factors increase nutritional risk for older adults. Data from studies of acute hospitalization in older patients suggest that up to 71% are at nutritional risk or are malnourished.[2] This increase in nutritional risk can further exacerbate existing health problems in older populations. Therefore, nutrition status of older adults should be carefully monitored. **Geriatric nutrition**, or the medical nutrition therapy for older adults, helps to screen, assess, and intervene when appropriate. This chapter will focus on nutritional concerns in older persons and recommend options to help improve or manage these issues using a case study as a guide throughout the chapter.

Background and Etiology

In the United States, the proportion of the older population has increased and is expected to continue to grow over the next 40 years. By 2060, the number of Americans aged 65 years and older is projected to be 98 million, more than double its population of 47.8 million in 2015[1] (**Figure 27.1**). The number of people aged 85 years and older is also expected to more than double from 6.3 million in 2015 to 14.6 million in 2040. In 2040, those aged 65 years and older are predicted to account for 21.7% of the population.[3]

Not only has the U.S. population grown, but it is living longer. The life expectancy of humans has progressively increased since 1900 due to advancements in research, science, and technology, as well as improvement in healthcare provision. The life expectancy at birth for females and males in the United States is 81.2 and 76.4 years, respectively, and has remained stable since 2012. Moreover, the age-adjusted mortality rate declined 1% to a record low in 2014.[4] Age-specific death rates also decreased significantly in 2014 for all age groups 65 years and older. Thus, older

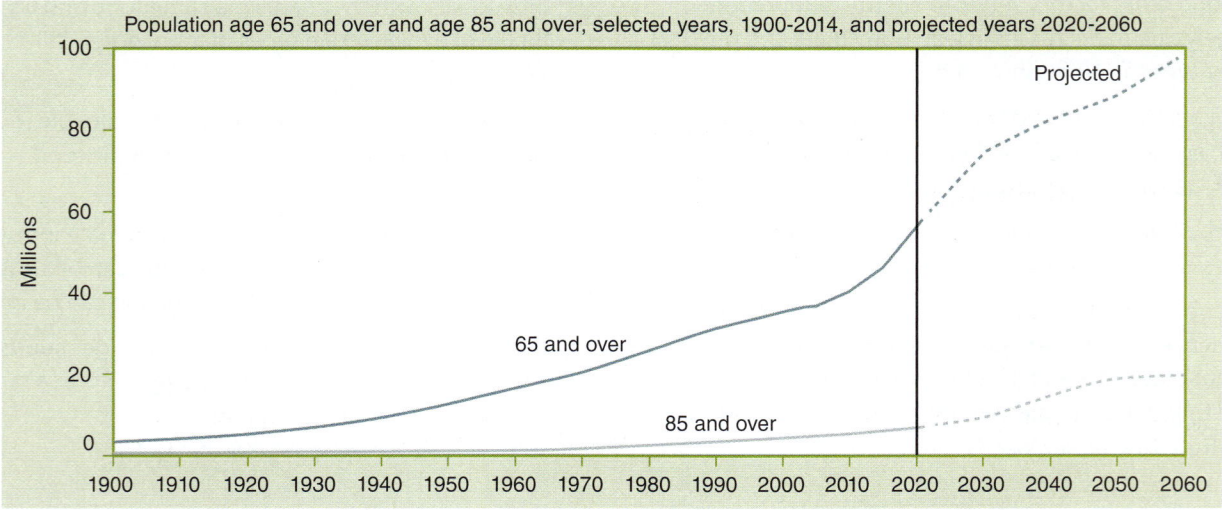

FIGURE 27.1 Population 65 Years and Older and 85 Years and Older: Selected Years and Projected Years

Reproduced from Federal Interagency Forum on Aging-Related Statistics. Older Americans 2016: Key Indicators of Well-Being. Washington, DC: U.S. Government Printing Office. August 2016. https://agingstats.gov/docs/LatestReport/Older-Americans-2016-Key-Indicators-of-WellBeing.pdf.

CASE STUDY INTRODUCTION

Esther is an 84-year-old female who lives in an in-law apartment attached to her daughter's home. Her family reports that she appears to have lost weight. She is usually able to perform activities of daily living, but presents with altered mental status, decreased oral intake of foods and fluid, and increased lethargy for 2 weeks.

Anthropometric Data:
Height: 152.4 cm (60")
Weight: 40.9 kg (90 lbs)
BMI 17.6 kg/m^2
Weight history
Usual body weight: 45 kg (100 lbs) 2 months ago

Biochemical Data:

Sodium 150 (135-145 mEq/L)
Potassium 3.1 (3.6-5.0 mEq/L)
Chloride 107 (98-110 mEq/L)
Carbon dioxide 22 (20-30 mEq/L)
Blood urea nitrogen 45 (6-24 mg/dL)
Creatinine 2.4 (0.4-1.3 mg/dL)

Glucose 100 (70-139 mg/dL)
HbA1c 4.5% (4.3-5.8%)
Hematocrit 36 (35 to 47%)
Hemoglobin 13 (12.0 to 15.5 gm/dL)
Albumin 3.9 (3.5 to 5.0 g/dL)
Mean corpuscular volume 110 (80-99 fL)

Clinical Data:
Past Medical History: Hypertension (HTN), gastroesophageal reflux disease (GERD), osteoporosis, arthritis
Medications: Atenolol, protonix, seroquel, Os-Cal, Vitamin B$_{12}$, nonsteroidal anti-inflammatory drugs (NSAIDs)
Vital Signs: Blood pressure: 89/60 mm Hg
Nutrition-focused Physical Exam: Patient is tired and lethargic. She has dark circles under both eyes and mild temporal muscle depression. Her oral exam is notable for edentulism, dry, sticky mouth, dry tongue, and chapped lips. Her skin is cool and dry with poor skin turgor. No wounds observed. She has evident clavicular muscle wasting. No upper or lower extremity edema noted. Nails reveal slow capillary refill.

Dietary Data:
Dietary History:
Breakfast: Instant oatmeal and black coffee
Lunch: 1 cup of canned tomato soup (mixed with water)
Dinner: Baked chicken with steamed vegetables, 1 cup of rice, 8 oz of low-fat milk
Diet prescription: 2 g sodium

Questions

1. Describe Esther's nutritional status and nutritional risk.
2. What are the priorities in treating Esther? Is her diet order appropriate?
3. What additional information/labs would you like to obtain?
4. Evaluate Esther's diet. Would she benefit from a multivitamin?

Americans are living longer and contributing to the changes in age composition of the U.S. population.

However, the aging of the population has wide-ranging implications for the country. According to data from the Centers for Disease Control and Prevention, those who are 65 years and older have the highest rates of emergency room visits, hospitalization, and prescription drug use.[4] In addition, there has been a major shift in the leading causes of death for all age groups, from infectious and acute illnesses to chronic and degenerative diseases. Currently, more than one-fourth of all Americans and two of every three older Americans have multiple chronic conditions, their treatment accounting for 66% of the country's healthcare budget.[5]

The aging population is largely responsible for the major shift in the leading causes of death. Aging leads to a gradual and progressive decline in cell or tissue structure and function, resulting in loss of organ system reserves and weakened homeostatic controls. This physiological change associated with aging is influenced by both genetic and environmental factors. However, despite advances in molecular biology and genetics, the reason as to how aging occurs remains unanswered.

Several theories have been proposed to help explain the process of aging. The theories of aging fall into two main categories: preprogrammed theories and damage or error theories.[6] The preprogrammed view is that genes are preprogrammed to control the course of a cell's life and death, and the regulation of these genes would depend on the body's maintenance, repair, and defense systems. An example of the preprogrammed theory would be a family of anti-aging genes known as the sirtuins that may control pathways in the cell cycle that increase life span and influence aging.[7] The damaged or error theories emphasize exogenous factors that lead to the accumulation of reactive or toxic free radicals, which can induce cumulative damage at various levels (i.e., DNA, mitochondria or telomeres, RNA, and protein synthesis). This damage leads to genetic abnormalities, loss of hormonal function, and immunosenescence. **Immunosenescence** is the gradual deterioration of the immune system that occurs with aging, which irreversibly causes decreased function, morbidity, and eventual death.

Health, physiologic, and functional changes associated with the aging process increase nutritional risk for older adults.[8] In the United States, five of the eight most common causes of death for adults aged 65 years or older have a known nutritional influence (**Figure 27.2**).[4] Most older adults consume foods that are high in fat and added sugars ("empty calories") instead of more nutrient-dense foods; greater than 80% of Americans older than 71 years old consumed more than the recommended amount of discretionary calories.[9] Moreover, the mean Healthy Eating Index 2005 score for persons aged older than 65 years who participated in the Chicago Health and Aging Project was 61.2 out of 100, revealing that their diets needed improvement.[10] Having a poor-quality diet over a lifetime can adversely affect health as individuals age. Older persons who follow a diet consisting of high-fat and sugary foods have a higher risk of mortality than those with a healthy dietary pattern.[11] On the other hand, those who followed a diet consistent with current dietary guidelines (increased amounts of vegetables, fruits, whole grains, poultry, fish, and low-fat dairy products) had health outcomes associated with better nutritional status, more years of healthy life, and survival.

Changes in Body Composition in the Geriatric Population

Health, physiologic, and functional changes that occur with aging affect nutrient metabolism and energy needs. These changes in metabolism affect body composition and, ultimately, weight. In Western society, weight typically increases until around 50 years of age in men and 60 years of age in women and thereafter declines.[12] Among other factors, it can be attributed in a large part to decreases in physical activity, which subsequently reduce energy expenditure. Despite weight gain, however, lean body mass tends to decline in the older adult population even with a good diet. The loss of lean body mass, also known as **sarcopenia**, further decreases the basal metabolic rate and, together with reduced expenditure, lowers energy requirements.

CORE CONCEPT 1

Among other factors, reduced energy requirement is largely due to decreases in lean body mass and physical activity in older population.

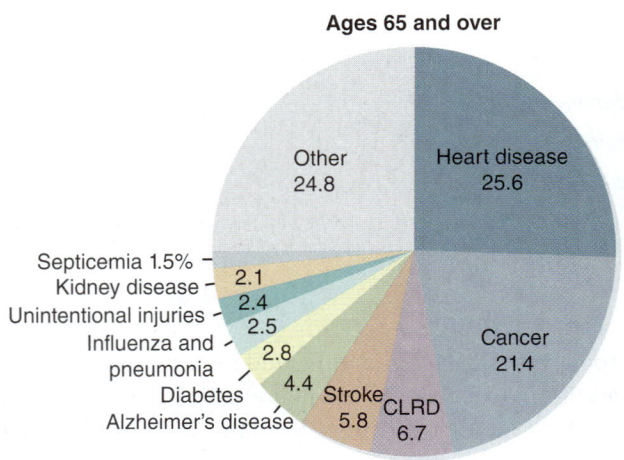
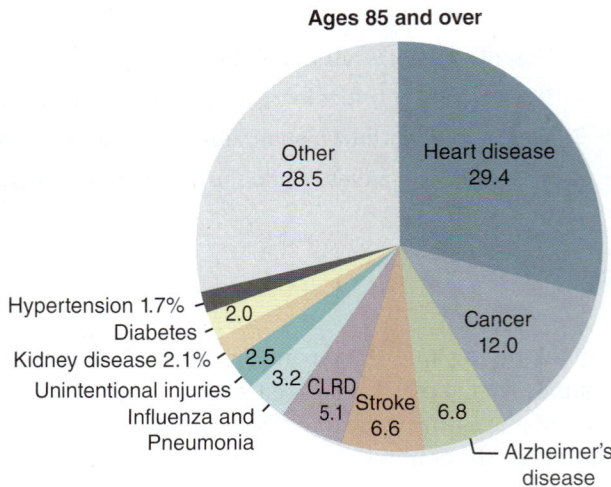

FIGURE 27.2 Leading Causes of Death Ages 65 and Older and 85 and Older

Physiological changes and age of onset of changes in body composition are variable. Gender, physical activity, and hormones additionally influence when body changes occur. First, a decline in body water occurs with age. Body water makes up about 60% of body weight in young and middle-aged adults and close to 50% in older adults.[13] Additionally, **insensible water loss**, the loss of water through the skin and respiration, increases with age. As a consequence, older adults have a higher risk for dehydration than young adults.

Another significant change occurs with lean body mass. Lean body mass consists of muscle, bone, and non-fatty tissue; it is the body weight minus fat. Unfortunately, it may decline by as much as 40% between the third and eighth decade of life.[14] As a consequence, the decline in muscle strength amounts to 1.5% per year between ages of 50 and 60 years and 3% per year thereafter. However, through appropriate nutrition and resistance training, the rate of decline in muscle mass can be slowed.[15]

Unlike body water and lean body mass, fat mass increases with age. Typically, an adult male's body contains 6% to 24% fat, while a female's body contains 14% to 31% fat.[14] By the seventh decade, however, fat comprises about 30% of the body of males, with higher proportions in females. In particular, visceral fat, especially of the central abdomen, and intramuscular fat tend to increase, while subcutaneous fat in other regions of the body declines.[16,17] Consequently, abdominal obesity increases with age. Unfortunately, adipose tissue has no significant metabolic activity and the basal metabolic rate decreases by about 2% per decade.

> **CORE CONCEPT 2**
>
> Unlike body water and lean body mass, fat mass increases with age; adipose tissue does not have significant metabolic activity compared to muscle.

Aging is also associated with changes in bone remodeling: Bone remodeling takes longer to complete and the rate of mineralization also declines. Consequently, bone mass declines after age 30 years by about 1% in women and 0.7% in men.[18] In women, the loss accelerates to 3% to 5% in the postmenopausal period due to estrogen loss. This change is important, because decline in bone mass increases the risk of osteoporosis in older adults. Therefore, vitamin D and calcium requirements change with age due to their crucial role in the prevention and delay of the progression of osteoporosis.

The changes in body water content, lean body mass, fat composition, and bone mass that accompany aging ultimately impact metabolism, weight, and health. For instance, a decline in body water increases the serum concentration of water-soluble drugs (such as digoxin, diuretics, warfarin, etc.), which enhances their pharmacodynamic effects.[14] Fluid administration requires awareness of differences in water distribution across various cellular compartments (intracellular, extracellular, and interstitial). Fat-soluble drugs are kept in the body longer due to increased fat stores, increasing the risk of adverse effects on mind, gait, and balance. These changes in composition also contribute to insulin resistance, putting older adults at a higher risk for diabetes. Overall, changes in body composition associated with aging lead to decreased metabolic rate and muscle mass, which makes the older adult more susceptible to falls and chronic illnesses.

Sarcopenia

Sarcopenia is characterized by the loss of muscle mass, strength, and performance in the aging population.[19,20] It has a complex, multifactorial etiology, which includes disuse of muscle, changing endocrine function, chronic diseases, inflammation, insulin resistance, and suboptimal protein intake (**Figure 27.3**). In addition, there is an increased fat infiltration in

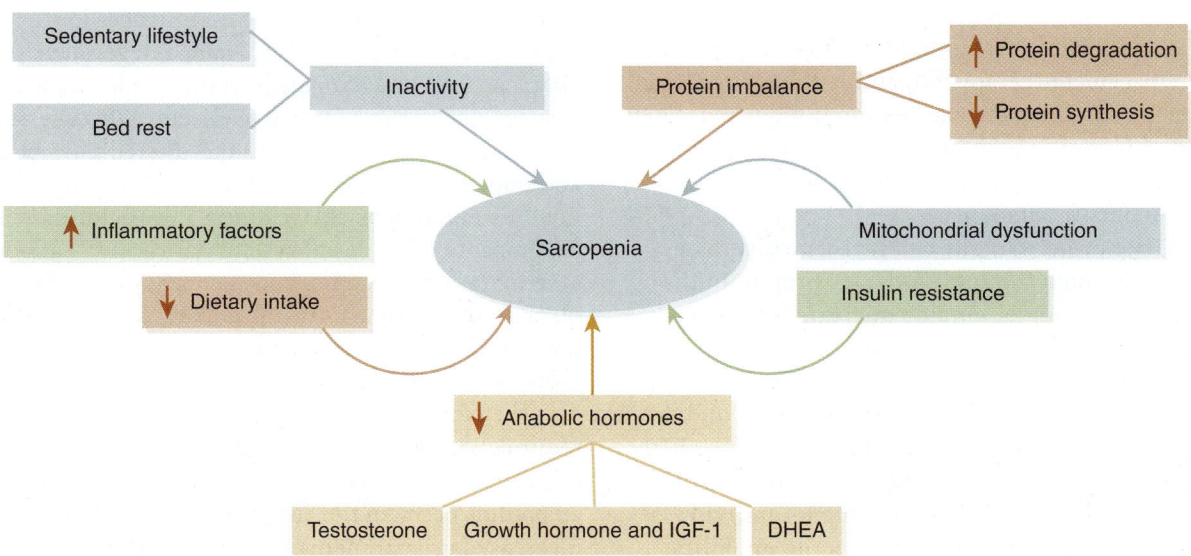

FIGURE 27.3 Contributing Factors to Sarcopenia

Reprinted from Farshidfara F, Shulginaa V, Myrie SB. Nutritional supplementations and administration considerations for sarcopenia in older adults. Nutrition, Health, and Aging, Volume 3. 2015;3:147-170. Copyright with permission from IOS Press. The publication is available at IOS Press through http://dx.doi.org/10.3233/NUA-150057

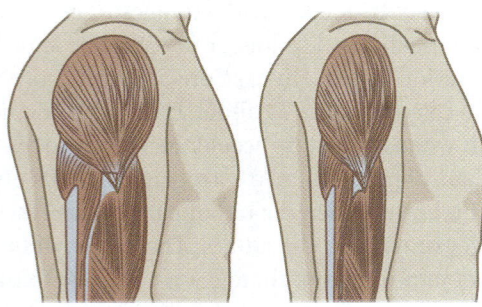

FIGURE 27.4 Normal Muscle versus Muscle Wasting

muscle, which leads to decreased muscle quality and strength (**Figure 27.4**).

This term should not be confused with cachexia.[21] **Cachexia** is a general wasting and malnutrition usually associated with chronic disease. Whereas most people with cachexia are sarcopenic, most sarcopenic individuals are not considered cachectic. Also unlike cachexia, sarcopenia does not require the presence of an underlying illness.

The decline in muscle use is attributable to the decline in physical activity as individuals age. In the United States, 28% to 34% of adults ages 65 to 74 years and 35% to 44% of adults ages 75 years or older are inactive. This not only exacerbates the ongoing muscle loss but also increases fat mass, which does not have a significant metabolic activity. Sarcopenia is not only a key precursor to the development of frailty, but also a powerful predictor of late-life disability.[22]

Changes with endocrine function also accompany aging. Testosterone and estrogen production in the body declines in older adults, which appears to accelerate the development of sarcopenia.[23] Various studies suggest that relative deficiencies of estrogen and testosterone contribute to muscle catabolism. Some studies have shown an increase in muscle mass with testosterone replacement.[24,25] However, studies have not demonstrated similar improvement with estrogen replacement therapy.[26] Insulin also plays a role in the progression of sarcopenia, as insulin inhibits muscle breakdown.[27] Unfortunately, insulin resistance increases with age, and the reduction of insulin action on muscle may contribute to muscle catabolism.

Inadequate protein intake can further exacerbate sarcopenia. Although the role of dietary protein in the prevention of sarcopenia remains unclear,[28] some evidence suggests that protein intake moderately greater than the Recommended Daily Allowance (RDA) may be beneficial to promote muscle protein anabolism and deter progressive loss of muscle mass with age.[29] Current RDA of protein is 0.8 g/kg for older adults. However, adequate protein consumption can be challenging for individuals with limited resources, reduced appetite, mobility issues, and environmental limitations.[30] National Health and Nutrition Examination Survey data indicate that the average protein intake of Americans meets or exceeds the RDA; however, a significant proportion of older adults (approximately 10%-25%) consume less protein than the RDA.[31] Subsequently, protein undernutrition can contribute to sarcopenia.

Sarcopenia has a wide range of health-related implications for older adults and can significantly affect their quality of life. It is estimated to affect 8% to 40% of adults aged 60 years or older and approximately 50% of those aged 75 years or older.[32,33] Sarcopenia is estimated to cost an estimated $18.5 billion in healthcare dollars, as it is associated with increased rates of functional impairment, disability, falls, and mortality. Therefore, slowing the progression of muscle loss with aging can help improve the overall health status of the older population.

Sarcopenia is not a treatable condition. However, measures can be taken to slow its progression. Lack of activity is an important contributor to loss of muscle mass and strength at any age.[34-36] Thus, the primary intervention for sarcopenia currently is resistance training. Recent studies suggest that muscle strength, as opposed to muscle mass, is independently associated with lower extremity performance, which is a factor for disability among older persons.[37] Moreover, even with aging, muscle fibers are still prone to plasticity in response to different functional demands (i.e., physical activity).[38] Therefore, regular exercise that includes resistance and aerobic training, coupled with adequate intake of high-quality protein, can enhance muscle mass and function in older adults and decelerate the progression of sarcopenia.[39]

> **CORE CONCEPT 3**
>
> Sarcopenia is not a treatable condition; however, measures can be taken to slow progression. The current, most effective intervention for sarcopenia is resistance training.

Frailty

Sarcopenia has considerable consequences for the development of frailty and disability. **Frailty** is a geriatric syndrome characterized by age-related declines in multiple organ systems due to the cumulative effects of disease, inactivity, stress, poor nutritional intake, altered physiology, and impaired homeostatic reserve.[40] Thus, frailty does not only entail physical weakness due to muscle loss, but encompasses the central system (i.e., brain), endocrine system, immune system, and skeletal system. As a result, older adults become vulnerable to adverse health outcomes including falls, hospitalization, institutionalization, and mortality.

The most widely used criteria for diagnosis for frailty requires at least three of the following characteristics to be present in an individual: unintended weight loss of 10 pounds or 5% in the last year, exhaustion, weakness (decreased grip strength), decreased walking speed, and low physical activity.[41] Older persons who meet at least three of the criteria are at a higher risk of adverse health outcomes

Decrease in the prevalence or severity of frailty likely will have benefits for individuals, their families, and society. Across various studies, exercise has been shown to improve functional ability. Although the effect of exercise on frailty may be small to moderate,[42-44] a Cochrane review that incorporated 67 randomized controlled trials of exercise interventions for long-term care residents concluded that strength and balance training interventions can help increase muscle strength and functional abilities.[45] The most effective exercise intervention (type, duration, and frequency) is uncertain, but even a small gain in strength of older individuals might translate into important functional gains. The effectiveness of nutrition interventions on impaired nutrition and weight loss of frailty has also been studied. Unfortunately, evidence is scarce and nutrition interventions have not yielded positive outcomes for frailty. A systematic review of clinical trials that included community-dwelling frail older individuals found no evidence of nutrition interventions' effectiveness on disability measures.[46]

Nutrition (dietary quality) appears to play a role in the development of frailty. According to a cross-sectional analysis of 802 persons aged 65 years or older in Europe, low daily energy intake (≤21 kcal/kg) was significantly associated with frailty.[47] The study also found that independent of energy intake, a low intake of protein; vitamins D, E, and C; and folate were all significantly associated with frailty in this older population. Analysis of the data from the Third National Health and Nutrition Examination Survey (NHANES III) indicated that low serum 25-hydroxyvitamin D levels (less than 15 ng/mL) were associated with increased risk of frailty in older adults.[48] Given well-established associations between 25-hydroxyvitamin D deficiency and numerous chronic diseases (i.e., diabetes and hypertension),[49-51] in addition to potential correlation between 25-hydroxyvitamin D status and muscle weakness,[52-54] vitamin D supplementation is being investigated as a treatment option for frailty.

Pressure Injury

Pressure injuries are another major consequence of sarcopenia. **Pressure injury** is defined as a localized injury of the skin and/or underlying tissue as a result of pressure, or pressure in combination with friction (usually over a bony prominence).[55] Pressure injuries develop when blood flow to the skin and the underlying tissue is impeded by constant pressure. The most common sites are the sacrum, coccyx, heels, or the hips, but other sites can be affected as well.

Pressure injuries affect an estimated 3 million adults in the United States.[56] Of the 3 million, 70% occur in persons older than 65 years.[57] Pressure injury is now a prominent national healthcare issue with aging population. In a review article published by the National Pressure Ulcer Advisory Panel in 2001, the prevalence of pressure injuries in the United States between 1990 and 2000 estimated to range from 10% to 18% in general acute care and up to 29% in home care.[58] Pressure injuries not only have a huge financial burden on the healthcare system, but increased mortality rates have been observed in older patients who develop pressure ulcers.[59]

Various intrinsic (i.e., limited mobility, poor nutrition, comorbidities, aging skin, etc.) and extrinsic (i.e., pressure, friction, shear, moisture, etc.) factors contribute to the formation of pressure ulcers in older adults.[60] However, it occurs most commonly in persons experiencing prolonged immobility, humidity (i.e., urinary incontinence), friction, and shear force.[61] When a person is not able to move for a long time, constant pressure is applied to the area that sits on a surface; this pressure decreases blood flow to the tissue in the area and causes ischemia and hypoxia. Gradual accumulation of tissue damage leads to the development of pressure ulcers.

Pressure injuries can be characterized into four progressive stages, which indicate the severity of the pressure injury.[55] In addition to the four stages, there is an unstageable stage and a deep tissue injury stage. Depending on the stage of the pressure injury, nutritional intervention varies. Unfortunately, insufficient evidence exists to support the employment of nutritional support for the prevention and/or management of pressure ulcers. According to a systematic review on pressure ulcer treatment strategies, most studies that utilized protein supplementation found greater reduction in ulcer size than without, but not more complete wound healing.[56] Because of the small number of trials, evidence about micronutrient supplementation (vitamin C and zinc) is insufficient to draw conclusion.

Sarcopenic Obesity

The decline in lean body mass accompanied by an increase in adipose tissue is the most relevant change leading to a reduction of the basal metabolic rate in older adults. In addition, older adults are generally less physically active and acquire health conditions that put them at risk for prolonged immobility (i.e., arthritis), further contributing to the decrease in total energy requirements. Although energy needs decline with age, individuals often do not make a comparable reduction in energy intake, and this results in weight gain.[62] Additionally, older adults tend to have lower protein intake in their diet, and this may impair protein muscle turnover. These two phenomena combined can lead to a geriatric condition called sarcopenic obesity.

Sarcopenic obesity is the coexistence of age-related loss of skeletal mass and strength and excess body fat.[63] It has been found to increase in prevalence with advancing age.[64] The presence of both sarcopenia and obesity has shown to put older adults at a higher risk for adverse outcomes and functional impairment than sarcopenia or obesity alone.[63] Moreover, sarcopenic obesity has been modestly associated with increased cardiovascular disease in older adults.[65]

Multiple etiologies have been implicated in the pathophysiology of sarcopenic obesity, including excess energy intake, physical inactivity, low-grade inflammation, insulin resistance, and changes in hormonal environment.[66] As is widely established, a sedentary lifestyle is a risk factor for obesity.[67] Also, obese persons tend to be less physically active, which may contribute to decreased muscle strength.[68] Thus, both factors—physical inactivity and obesity—can contribute to sarcopenic obesity.

A pro-inflammatory state may also contribute to sarcopenic obesity. The adipocytes in the adipose tissue and/or infiltrating macrophages produce pro-inflammatory cytokines such as interleukin (IL-6) and tumor necrosis factor-α. These pro-inflammatory cytokines have been positively associated with fat mass and negatively with muscle mass.[69] Furthermore, Schrager et al.,[70] in the InCHIANTI study, found that obese, community-dwelling older adults with low muscle strength had elevated C-reactive protein and IL-6 levels than those with normal strength. Therefore, a pro-inflammatory state may be one of the contributing factors to decreased muscle strength among obese persons.

Currently, geriatric nutritional assessment is based on weight, weight history, and body mass index (BMI). Unfortunately, BMI cannot detect sarcopenic obesity; an individual may be categorized as overweight or obese according to BMI but may not have enough lean body mass to maintain normal physical function. Therefore, the effect of sarcopenic obesity on morbidity and mortality may be underestimated.[66] It is imperative that better methods be developed to help screen those with sarcopenic obesity.

> **CORE CONCEPT 4**
>
> Sarcopenia and obesity can coexist in an individual; the presence of both sarcopenia and obesity has shown to put older adults at a higher risk for adverse outcomes and functional impairment than sarcopenia or obesity alone.

Malnutrition Risk in Geriatrics

Undernutrition in older individuals is more common and has a greater impact on healthcare outcomes (i.e., physical function, healthcare utilization, and length of stay for hospitalizations) than in younger adults.[71-73] In community-dwelling older individuals, a BMI less than 22 has been associated with higher risk of 1-year mortality as well as impaired functional status.[74] Older persons with a BMI less than 20 are more likely to die while in the hospital, and those who are discharged are more likely to die in the following year.[75] These relationships hold true even after adjusting for illness severity and functional status.[76] Thus, routine screening should be performed in this vulnerable population to prevent or treat malnutrition.

The prevalence of malnutrition in older persons also depends on the population studied; it tends to vary depending on the geography, age distribution, and living situation of the population. In a multinational study (the United States, Europe, South Africa) using the Mini Nutritional Assessment to estimate the frequency of undernutrition in older adults, the prevalence of malnutrition among 4,507 older persons was 22.8%.[77] The highest rates were observed in the rehabilitation setting (50.5%) and lowest rates were seen in community dwellers (5.8%). Moreover, more than one-third of hospitalized older adults (38.7%) were considered malnourished by the study criteria.

Physiological changes associated with normal aging increase nutritional risk for older adults. Additionally, other factors affect nutritional needs of an older individual: presence or absence of a disease and related organ system compromise; the ability to access, prepare, ingest, and digest food; and personal food preferences (**Figure 27.5**). These factors combined prevent older individuals from consuming an adequate amount of nutrient-dense foods and can adversely affect the nutritional status of an older individual. Identifying and treating contributing factors can improve quality of life and function in older adults. However, interventions' benefits and risks should be weighed and should be in line with patient's goal of care.

> **PRACTICE POINT**
>
> In the older adult population, benefits and risks of nutrition interventions should be weighed prior to implementation and should be in line with the patient's goals of care.

Physiologic Factors

A number of age-related physiologic factors can affect nutritional status of older individuals, such as decrease in taste and smell sensitivity, delayed gastric emptying, early satiety, and dysregulation of food intake.

With aging, there is an increased threshold for detecting odor and a decrease in perceived odor intensity.[78] Additionally, although the number of taste buds remains constant, the threshold for recognition of salt and other specific tastes increases. Consequently, changes in odor and taste perception likely alter the **cephalic phase of digestion**, adversely affecting learned associations between the taste and smell of foods with cues involved in meal initiation, volume of food intake, and meal termination. The cephalic phase of digestion is the first of three phases of digestion; it begins with the sight,

CASE STUDY REVISITED

Once Esther's dehydration was corrected and her oral intake improved, she was discharged home under the care of her family. Unfortunately, her mental status continued to decline. Esther now needs assistance with activities of daily living (primarily cooking food and climbing stairs). After 3 weeks, Esther was readmitted with failure to thrive and dehydration; she had lost an additional 5 pounds within a month. She appears very weak, at times incoherent, and is not responding appropriately to your questions.

Anthropometric Data:
Height: 152.4 cm (60")
Weight: 38.5 kg (85 lbs)
BMI: 16.6 kg/m^2

Biochemical Data:

Sodium 152 (135-145 mEq/L)
Potassium 3.0 (3.6-5.0 mEq/L)
Chloride 111 (98-110 mEq/L)
Carbon dioxide 24 (20-30 mEq/L)
Blood urea nitrogen 40 (6-24 mg/dL)
Creatinine 2.8 (0.4-1.3 mg/dL)

Glucose 88 (70-139 mg/dL)
Hematocrit 33 (35% to 47%)
Hemoglobin 12 (12.0-15.5 gm/dL)
Albumin 3.4 (3.5-5.0 g/dL)
Mean corpuscular volume 118 (80-99 fL)

Clinical Data:
Vital signs: Blood pressure: 95/72 mm Hg
Medications: Atenolol, Protonix, Seroquel, Os-Cal, vitamin B_{12}, NSAID

Dietary Data:
Dietary History: Family states that Esther continues to have a poor appetite. She reports some difficulty swallowing and frequently coughs after drinking fluids. Once a week they take her out to eat at her favorite restaurant where she eats 100% of her meal of fish, mashed potatoes, and carrots.

Questions

1. What is Esther's current nutritional status? How has it changed?
2. Assess her biochemical indices. What are your concerns?
3. How does her medical history and overall health impact her nutritional risk?
4. Would you recommend adding or deleting anything to her medication regimen?
5. What should be considered when developing nutrition interventions for Esther?

---

smell, or taste of food and ends once the first bite is swallowed. It is the point at which the brain sends a signal through the vagus nerve to the stomach, triggering the production of gastric juices.

Earlier satiety can also occur from a combination of factors, including decreased rate of gastric emptying, increased sensitivity to gastric distention, and hormonal changes. Decreases in gastric emptying rates in older adults may result in prolonged distention of the antral stomach, reducing hunger and increasing satiety.[79] The production of several digestive hormones thought to be involved in satiety (such as GLP-1, CCK, and leptin) may be affected by aging[80]; moreover, aging may decrease the central nervous system's sensitivity to these hormones.

Studies have also suggested that older persons may have impaired ability to regulate food intake and are less able to adapt to underfeeding. Roberts et al.[81] found that after a period of underfeeding, older adults experienced less-frequent hunger than younger adults and did not regain the weight they had lost when they were allowed to freely consume food for 6 months, while, on average, younger adults regained all their lost weight. This decrease in ability to compensate for periods of reduced food intake due to illness or other issues can result in

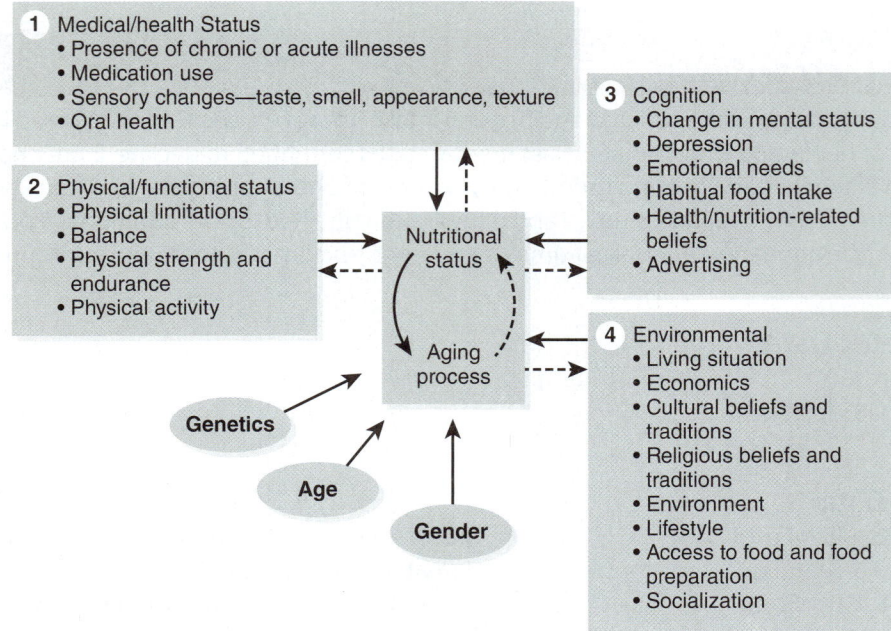

FIGURE 27.5 Factors that Influence Nutritional Status
Modified from American Dietetic Association. Position paper of the American Dietetic Association: Nutrition across the spectrum of aging. J Am Diet Assoc. 2005; 105(4): 616–633.

continual weight loss, especially when combined with social and psychological factors.

Overall Health Status

Acute and chronic diseases affect people of all ages. However, older persons are more likely to have acquired one or more illnesses such as stroke, dementia, cancer, arthritis, osteoporosis, rheumatoid arthritis, and chronic kidney disease due to bodily damages accumulated through the years. According to a study by Drewnowski and Shultz,[82] it is estimated that 85% of all older Americans have at least one chronic disease that affects nutrient intake. As a consequence, older adults often unintentionally alter their food intake because of pain, restricted mobility, anorexia, nausea, loss of dexterity and coordination, and fatigue.[83] They may also need to restrict their diet due to changes in nutrient absorption, metabolism, and excretion associated with certain chronic illnesses like diabetes and cardiovascular disease.

Unfortunately, medications used to manage and/or treat chronic illnesses can also interfere with nutrient absorption, metabolism, and excretion, and thus may contribute to nutrient deficiencies and malnutrition. Due to the high prevalence of older adults experiencing a number of pathologic conditions, polypharmacy is frequent. Certain drugs that are commonly used in this population are well known to adversely affect food intake and nutrient absorption.[84] For example, digoxin, which is used to treat heart failure; ACE inhibitors, which are used for hypertension; metformin, an oral antidiabetic agent; and antidepressants can cause nausea, anorexia, or dysgeusia. Proton pump inhibitors can impair nutrient absorption through effects on gastric pH, and laxatives promote rapid intestinal transit, thereby reducing nutrient absorption times.

Physiologic changes, presence of chronic diseases, and polypharmacy adversely affect the oral cavity. Oral health is an important but often neglected branch of medicine. As with other organs, the oral cavity also deteriorates with aging, and poor oral health directly limits food intake by older persons.[85] Decreased salivary flow due to various medical conditions, medications, and inadequate fluid intake can affect taste or alter the oral antimicrobial environment, increasing the risk of dental caries and oral candidiasis.[86] Painful dental caries, loss of teeth, edentulous states combined with ill-fitting dentures, and gingivitis can affect the older person's ability to chew and/or swallow.[85] Subsequently, older people may resort to the use of texture-modified diets or avoidance of foods.

Psychological/Neurocognitive Status

Progressive aging has been associated with a rise in the prevalence of depression and other psychological problems, including loss of interest and forgetfulness.[87] The anorexia, lethargy, confusion, and disorientation associated with various cognitive and mood disturbances can contribute to poor nutritional adequacy.[88]

Depression is a common phenomenon among older adults, but remains underrecognized and undertreated. In various studies, depression was identified as the most frequent identifiable cause of weight loss and undernutrition.[89,90] Depression increases the release of hypothalamic corticotrophin-releasing factor, a powerful anorectic agent.[84] Additionally, depression often diminishes an individual's motivation to obtain, prepare, and consume foods. Therefore, older adults with continued weight loss should be screened for depression.

Dementia

Dementia is a common geriatric condition that has an important implication for the nutritional status of older adults. It is characterized by a progressive, irreversible deterioration of cognition that can eventually cause an individual to be dysphagic, immobile, and unable to carry out **activities of daily living (ADLs)**. Additionally, the individual may no longer recognize friends and family members, have decreased ability to communicate, be totally dependent for care, and be incontinent.

Dementia has many etiologies, including neurodegenerative diseases, endocrine disorders, vascular disease, and even nutritional deficiencies. Alzheimer's disease, which is one of the most common neurodegenerative diseases, primarily affects the geriatric population.[91] The cause for most cases is still unknown, except that Alzheimer's disease is caused, at least in part, by genetics. Vascular dementia, which is the second most common form of dementia, can occur due to inadequate blood flow to the brain, resulting in brain damage. Vitamin B deficiencies (such as thiamin, vitamin B_6, and vitamin B_{12}) can also present with dementia-like symptoms, but may be reversible with appropriate supplementation.

Those with dementia typically experience a progressive decline in memory and increased confusion; as memory declines and confusion increases, things such as grocery shopping, cooking, and self-feeding become disorganized and impaired.[84] Subsequently, the frequency of eating nutritionally inadequate meals increases and may lead to a decrease in oral food intake altogether, ultimately resulting in malnutrition.

Functional Status

As discussed earlier, sarcopenia and sarcopenic obesity adversely affect functional capabilities in older persons. Ongoing muscle loss that occurs with sarcopenia is not only a key precursor to the development of frailty, but also a powerful predictor of late-life disability.[22] Similarly, sarcopenic obesity has been independently associated with the onset of **instrumental activities of daily living (IADLs)** disability in community-dwelling elderly.[92] Excess weight in persons with low muscle mass can further decrease the ability to perform physical activity and contribute to muscle disuse, especially in individuals with joint problems, as the excess weight is a burden on the muscle, joints, and bones. This continual cycle of low muscle mass and decreased activity can eventually lead to loss of functional capacity.

In addition to the physiological changes, older individuals often experience limitations in physical function due to illness, chronic disease, injury, or a combination of these factors. As a consequence, the ability of an older person to independently perform ADLs and/or IADLs diminishes. For example, 20% of stroke survivors, 11% of older adults with diabetes, and 10% of older adults with ischemic heart disease need help executing ADLs.[93] In 2009, approximately 41% of people older than 65 years of age reported a functional limitation (ADL and/or IADL), with a higher percentage reported in women and those who are poor.[94]

Dysphagia

The physiological changes and illnesses associated with aging can also impair the swallowing mechanism, leading to dysphagia. **Dysphagia** is a condition categorized by difficulty swallowing. **Oropharyngeal dysphagia** (OD), defined as the difficulty in forming or moving an alimentary bolus safely from the oral cavity to the esophagus, is one of the most common types of dysphagia in older patients.[95] Among common diseases or conditions affecting the geriatric population, stroke and dementia are the primary causes of dysphagia in older adults. OD is reported in 20% to 30% of dementia patients and identified through testing in 57% to 84% of Alzheimer's patients. Approximately 64% to 78% of acute stroke patients demonstrate OD by instrumental measure, while 40% to 80% of chronic stroke patients continue to have signs of OD. Other individuals at risk include those undergoing radiation therapy for head and neck cancer and patients with neurodegenerative diseases such as Parkinson's disease, amyotrophic lateral sclerosis, and multiple sclerosis.[95]

One of the primary concerns with dysphagia is aspiration. **Aspiration** is the entry of material into the airway below the vocal cords. Silent aspiration is when a bolus of food, liquid, or saliva enters the airway without eliciting a response. This is different from overt aspiration, which leads to symptoms of coughing and clearing of one's throat. Both can cause pneumonitis or pneumonia. As people age, they may experience predysphagia, which is an impairment in swallowing that does not result in significant dysfunction. Predysphagia may be due to decreased lingual (tongue) strength and pressure, xerostomia (dry mouth), cognitive decline, and medications.[96]

Screening for dysphagia is critical. Diagnosis can be made by a fiberoptic endoscopic examination of swallowing or radiographically through a videofluoroscopic swallowing exam, also known as a modified barium swallow. In this evaluation, a food in three forms (liquid, paste, and solid) is mixed with barium paste, allowing the movement of food to be evaluated as it passes through the oral, pharyngeal, and esophageal phases of swallowing. The Dysphagia Outcome and Severity Scale classifies severity of dysphagia from Severe (Level 1) to Normal (Level 7), with each stage defining oral intake restrictions, including nothing by mouth when severe; the degree of assistance needed when eating; and dietary modifications that

TABLE 27.1 DIETARY MODIFICATIONS BASED ON SEVERITY OF DYSPHAGIA[96,97]

Dysphagia Outcome and Severity Scale Score	Functional Impairment	Level of Assistance Needed with Oral Intake	Dietary Restrictions	Diet Modifications
Level 1: Severe	Severe pharyngeal bolus retention; unable to clear foods, silent aspiration	Maximum assistance needed	No oral intake	Enteral tube feeding
Level 2: Moderate to Severe Dysphagia	Aspiration without cough or weak cough	Maximum assistance needed	Partial oral intake allowed based on consistency tolerated. No thin liquids.	Pureed diet: Pureed or pudding-like foods. Examples: Pureed meats, fruits, and vegetables; puddings; hummus; partial enteral tube feedings
Levels 3 and 4: Mild to Moderate Dysphagia	Moderate retention in the pharynx and oral cavity that can be cleared with cue; aspiration with at least one consistency	Total or intermittent supervision, cueing, strategies	Avoid hard fruits and vegetables, corn skins, nuts, seeds, coarse cereals, and thin liquids	Mechanical soft diet: Cohesive, soft, and moist textured foods Examples: Pancakes with syrup, scrambled eggs, ground or bite-sized meats, soft cooked vegetables
Levels 5 and 6	Retention in pharynx cleared when cued, reduced mastication, aspiration of thin liquids only	Intermittent or distant supervision	Avoid hard, sticky, crunchy foods	Soft diet, thickened liquids. Examples: Most foods allowed. Encourage soft, moist foods.
Level 7	Normal function	None	Regular	All foods

Data from Ney DM, Weiss JM, Kind AJ, Robbins J. Senescent swallowing: Impact, strategies, and interentions. *Nutr Clin Pract*. 2009;24:395. O'Neil KO, Purdy M, Falk J, Gallo L. The dysphagia outcome and severity scale. *Dysphagia*. 1999;14:139-145.

should be prescribed based on the degree of impairment (**Table 27.1**).

Many individuals with dysphagia may need to limit food and liquid intake or avoid certain types of food. As a consequence, the frequency of eating nutritionally and calorically inadequate meals increases, leading to malnutrition. Additionally, modified texture diets, such as puree or mechanically softened, that are used to reduce the risk of aspiration can decrease the palatability of food, another cause of decreased meal intake and subsequent malnutrition.

CORE CONCEPT 5

Individuals with dysphagia may limit food and liquid intake or avoid certain types of food potentially leading to malnutrition.

Disability brought on by a combination of the abovementioned factors has implications for the nutrition status of the older Americans. Those who are frail and functionally impaired often need to rely on others for transportation to and from the grocery store, meal preparation, feeding, and cleaning up.[98] Unfortunately, older persons may not be able to receive the assistance they need for adequate intake, and this may contribute to nutritional deficiencies. Therefore, social support is critical, especially in this population, in preventing malnutrition (**Figure 27.6**).

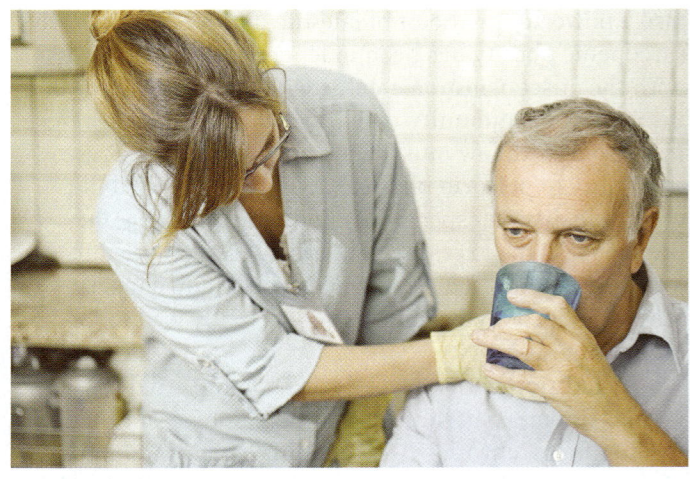

FIGURE 27.6 Swallow Evaluation by a Speech-Language Pathologist
© jeangill/E+/Getty Images.

Clinical Roundtable

Topic: Calcium Supplementation for Osteoporosis

Background: It is well established that adequate calcium intake can help prevent and/or delay osteoporosis, particularly in postmenopausal women. As a consequence, calcium supplements have been widely used to combat osteoporosis, especially in those with a diet deficient in calcium. However, excess calcium consumption has been associated with increased risk of cardiovascular disease and death. Recent meta-analysis data suggest that high calcium intake may increase the risk of myocardial infarction (MI).[102] Although it is uncertain as to how calcium supplements can increase the risk of MI, calcium supplements have been shown to increase vascular calcification and mortality in patients with renal failure.[103]

Roundtable Discussion

Is calcium supplementation necessary in older population? If so, is it safe? Would you recommend it?

Social Factors

Various environmental factors such as living situation, access to food and food preparation, and socialization can impact the quality and quantity of the food eaten by an older individual. A significant proportion of older adults live near the poverty line and may need to use money on medications and other necessities. In 2010, an estimated 3.5 million older persons were below the poverty level, and another 2.1 million were considered near poor (<125% of the poverty level)[94]; almost 16% of persons aged 65 years and older attributed their financial difficulty to medical expenses. This food insecurity adversely affects adequate food intake and financial support may be needed to acquire food.

Additionally, as people age, there is an increased frequency of isolation at mealtimes. Various studies have shown that eating alone can profoundly affect nutritional practices; for instance, surveys of people living alone indicate that independently living people eat less and are at a higher risk of malnutrition than those living and/or eating with others.[87,99] Moreover, several studies have demonstrated that older adults who eat with others consume more than those who eat alone.[100,101] Therefore, it is important to recognize that with aging, social support becomes a valuable tool in optimizing the quality and quantity of the food consumed (**Figure 27.7**).

> **CORE CONCEPT 6**
>
> With aging, social support becomes a valuable tool in optimizing the quality and quantity of the food consumed.

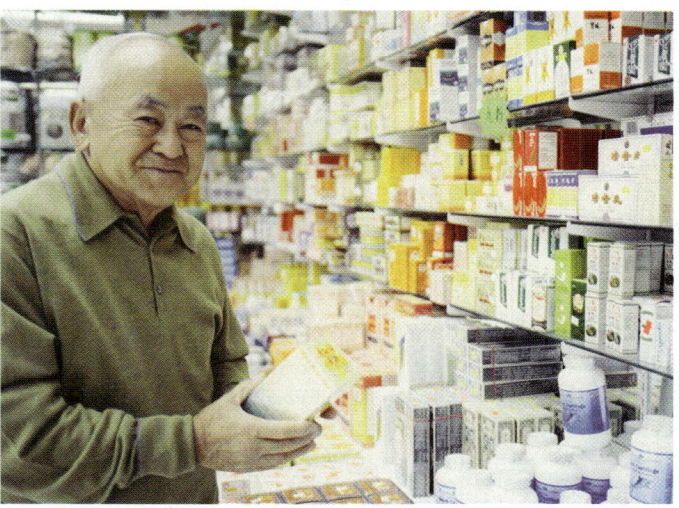
© Paul Edmondson/Corbis.

FIGURE 27.7 Social Interaction is a Key Part in Maintaining Nutritional Status in Older Adults
© Tetra Images/Getty Images.

Nutrition Screening and Assessment in Geriatrics

Overall, physiological changes associated with normal aging increase nutritional risk for older adults. Decreased metabolic rate and muscle mass make the older adult more susceptible to falls and chronic illnesses. Therefore, it is imperative that routine nutritional screening be performed for the geriatric population to prevent malnutrition, or to recognize it at an early stage and address it before it progresses and adversely affects health and quality of life.

Studies of acute hospitalization in older patients have suggested that up to 71% are at nutritional risk or are malnourished.[2] Malnutrition is associated with increased morbidity and mortality, functional disability, decreased quality of life, and increased frequency and length of hospital stay.[104-107] However, if the contributing factors are identified and if appropriate interventions are made, progression of malnutrition can be slowed or reversed and quality of life and function can be improved.

> **CORE CONCEPT 7**
>
> If etiologies are identified and appropriate interventions are made, progression of malnutrition can be slowed or reversed and quality of life and function can be improved.

A number of screening tools have been developed for identifying older persons at risk for undernutrition. Of the various tools, the **Mini Nutritional Assessment (MNA)** and Malnutrition Screening Tool (MST) are recommended for use in assessing nutritional status in the geriatric population due to their high sensitivity (>83%) and specificity (>90%).[108] The MST was developed for use in acutely hospitalized patients and has been validated for use in cancer patients.[109] However, the average age for which it was validated was 57 to 60 years, and thus not applicable for the geriatric population.

The MNA has been more frequently used than the MST because evidence suggests that the MNA is the most valid assessment tool for malnutrition and is predictive of poor outcomes in ambulatory older adults and those residing in long-term care facilities.[110] The MNA consists of a global assessment and subjective view of health in addition to questions specific to diet and a series of anthropomorphic measurements[111]; it consists of 6 questions (**Figure 27.8**) and has shown good sensitivity compared to the full version.[112,113] The full MNA is often used for complete nutrition assessment.

The Academy of Nutrition and Dietetics (AND) and the American Society for Parenteral and Enteral Nutrition (A.S.P.E.N.) published a consensus statement regarding the criteria for the diagnosis of malnutrition. According to their statement, having two or more of the six characteristics (insufficient energy intake, weight loss, loss of muscle mass, loss of subcutaneous fat, localized or generalized fluid accumulation that may sometimes mask weight loss, and diminished functional status as measured by hand-grip strength) is recommended for diagnosis.[114]

Although collecting periodic body weights can be challenging, it is the simplest screening method for detecting changes in nutritional status and the risk of mortality. Among community-dwelling older persons, loss of as little as 5% of weight over a 3-year period has been associated with increased mortality.[115] According to the Minimum Data Set, a standard clinical assessment tool used in Medicare- and Medicaid-certified long-term care facilities, weight loss is considered clinically significant when an individual experiences a loss of 5% of usual body weight in 1 month, or 10% in 6 months.[116] It is important to determine whether there is a true significant weight loss from a loss of muscle or adipose tissue, or whether it is water loss caused by a medication, such as a diuretic used for treatment of a chronic condition such as congestive heart failure.

> **PRACTICE POINT**
>
> Although collecting periodic body weights can be challenging, it is the simplest screening method for detecting changes in nutritional status and the risk of mortality.

> **PRACTICE POINT**
>
> Older adults often do not check their weight. In the absence of a measured or stated weight, a clinician can ask how clothes are fitting to assess for weight loss or gain.

Unfortunately, accurate nutrition screening and assessment for undernutrition in older persons can be difficult due to other confounding factors such as inflammation, sarcopenia, frailty, and the presence of chronic diseases and their physiologic and metabolic abnormalities. For instance, underweight adults are not the only population at risk of malnutrition. Weight, height, and BMI can provide misleading information regarding the nutrition status of an individual due to the physiologic changes associated with aging, as can be seen with sarcopenic obesity. In addition to older adults with sarcopenic obesity, well-nourished overweight or obese adults who develop a severe acute illness or experience a major traumatic event are at risk for malnutrition.[117-119] Moreover, because nutrition status in older adults is also affected by their functional capacity, screening for and assessing functional ability and their ability to procure and prepare food is important in this population. For functional assessment, ADLs and IADLs are commonly used. Refer to **Table 27.2** for the components of these two assessment tools.[120]

> **PRACTICE POINT**
>
> Older adults can often be poor historians. Always try to speak to family members, if available, to obtain or verify information that the patient stated.

Nutrient Needs

Physiologic and health changes, as well as functional decline, affect nutrient requirements in older adults. Nutrient needs of the geriatric population are quite similar to the needs in young adults, but differences can be seen in energy, fluid, protein, and a few micronutrient requirements as a result of changes associated with aging (i.e., sarcopenia, chronic disease, physical inactivity, senescence). Unfortunately, although the knowledge of the nutrient requirements of older persons is expanding, there is insufficient evidence to support establishment of standards for some nutrients. Furthermore, even though guidelines (i.e., Dietary Reference Intake [DRI], RDA) have been developed for the older population to use as a reference to maintain or achieve optimal nutrition status, actual nutrient requirements may range widely in this population due to multiple etiologies affecting physiological and functional changes that ultimately affect nutrient metabolism in the body.

Mini Nutritional Assessment
MNA®

Nestlé NutritionInstitute

| Last name: | | First name: | |

| Sex: | | Age: | | Weight, kg: | | Height, cm: | | Date: | |

Complete the screen by filling in the boxes with the appropriate numbers. Total the numbers for the final screening score.

Screening

A Has food intake declined over the past 3 months due to loss of appetite, digestive problems, chewing or swallowing difficulties?
 0 = severe decrease in food intake
 1 = moderate decrease in food intake
 2 = no decrease in food intake

B Weight loss during the last 3 months
 0 = weight loss greater than 3 kg (6.6 lbs)
 1 = does not know
 2 = weight loss between 1 and 3 kg (2.2 and 6.6 lbs)
 3 = no weight loss

C Mobility
 0 = bed or chair bound
 1 = able to get out of bed / chair but does not go out
 2 = goes out

D Has suffered psychological stress or acute disease in the past 3 months?
 0 = yes   2 = no

E Neuropsychological problems
 0 = severe dementia or depression
 1 = mild dementia
 2 = no psychological problems

F1 Body Mass Index (BMI) (weight in kg) / (height in m)^2
 0 = BMI less than 19
 1 = BMI 19 to less than 21
 2 = BMI 21 to less than 23
 3 = BMI 23 or greater

IF BMI IS NOT AVAILABLE, REPLACE QUESTION F1 WITH QUESTION F2.
DO NOT ANSWER QUESTION F2 IF QUESTION F1 IS ALREADY COMPLETED.

F2 Calf circumference (CC) in cm
 0 = CC less than 31
 3 = CC 31 or greater

Screening score
(max. 14 points)

12-14 points: Normal nutritional status
8-11 points: At risk of malnutrition
0-7 points: Malnourished

®Société des Produits Nestlé S.A., Vevey, Switzerland, Trademark Owners.
All of the following references must be included on the MNA® forms: 1. Vellas B, Villars H, Abellan G, et al. Overview of the MNA® - Its History and Challenges. *J Nutr Health Aging*. 2006;10:456-465.
2. Rubenstein LZ, Harker JO, Salva A, Guigoz Y, Vellas B. Screening for Undernutrition in Geriatric Practice: Developing the Short-Form Mini Nutritional Assessment (MNA®-SF). *J Geront*. 2001;56a:M366-377.
3. Guigoz Y. The Mini-Nutritional Assessment (MNA®) Review of the Literature—What does it tell us? *J Nutr Health Aging*. 2006;10:466-487. Page 2
4. Kaiser MJ, Bauer JM, Ramsch C, et al. Validation of the Mini Nutritional Assessment Short-Form (MNA®-SF): A practical tool for identification of nutritional status. *J Nutr Health Aging*. 2009;13:782-788 (Short Form only).

FIGURE 27.8 Mini Nutritional Assessment

Reproduced from www.mna-elderly.com.

TABLE 27.2 ASSESSING THE FUNCTIONAL CAPACITY OF OLDER PERSONS

Activities of Daily Living	Independent	Needs help	Dependent	Cannot do
Feeding				
Grooming				
Toileting				
Ambulating				
Bathing				
Transferring bed/chair				
Instrumental Activities of Daily Living	**Independent**	**Needs help**	**Dependent**	**Cannot do**
Shopping				
Food preparation				
Ability to use the telephone				
Housekeeping				
Doing laundry				
Mode of transportation: driving or using public transportation				
Managing medications				
Managing finances				

Data from Lawton, M.P. The functional assessment of elderly people. *J Am Geriatr Soc.* 1971;19(6):465-481.

CORE CONCEPT 8

Differences in nutrient needs from younger adults can be seen in energy, fluid, and protein requirements as a result of changes associated with aging.

Energy Requirements

Energy requirements decrease progressively with age, due in large part to a decline in physical activity, contributing to further loss of muscle mass in older individuals who are already experiencing loss of lean body mass through the process of senescence. For those older than age 65 years, AND recommends an energy intake of 25 to 35 kcal/kg for females and 30 to 40 kcal/kg for males to maintain weight and prevent unintended weight loss.[121] This recommendation takes into account varying levels of physical activity that older persons may engage in (physical activity factor 1.25 for those who are sedentary to 1.75 for very active individuals). While energy needs decrease, carbohydrate and fat requirements remain similar to those of younger adults.[122] In critically ill adult patients, A.S.P.E.N. recommends, in the absence of indirect calorimetry, that nutritional needs should be determined with published predictive equations or simplistic weight-based equations (25–30 kcal/kg/day).[123]

PRACTICE POINT

For critically ill geriatric patients, follow A.S.P.E.N. guidelines for nutrition support.

As a consequence of physiologic changes, frailty, presence of chronic disease, and overall inadequate intake due to various reasons, older individuals are at risk for unintended weight loss. At the same time, older persons are at risk of unintended weight gain because energy intake is not reduced as requirements decrease. The weight gain can contribute to increased body fat, sarcopenic obesity, and further decline in activity. Therefore, in order to avoid unintended consequences associated with energy imbalance, older individuals should be thoroughly evaluated for their health status, activity level, and physique before assessing their energy needs.

Protein Requirement

Protein intake in older adults should be on the basis of quantity, quality, and timing. Factors related to energy intake, activity level, presence of chronic disease, and overall nutritional status should all be considered in aging adults.

Protein quantity

How much dietary protein older persons need is currently a subject of debate. The DRI for all adults (19 years and older) recommends 0.8 g/kg of protein a day.[123] Unfortunately, achieving adequate protein intake is difficult given multiple physiologic, functional, and environmental challenges that many elderly individuals face, including taste changes, reduced appetite, and mobility issues.[124,125] Evidence from comprehensive short-term nitrogen balance studies suggests that the requirement for protein is not different between healthy younger and older adults and, for most older adults, the DRI of 0.8 g/kg/day is sufficient to meet minimum needs.[126] However, many experts suggest slightly higher protein intake than the amount recommended by the DRI because of protein's role in muscle protein anabolism and its potential to slow the progression of sarcopenia.[29,127] Data from a 3-year prospective study of protein intake and lean body mass loss in community-dwelling older persons indicated that those who had the highest intake (average protein intake of 1.2 g/kg/day) lost the least amount of lean body mass over 3 years.[128] Systematic review and meta-analysis on use of oral nutrition supplements (ONSs) to increase protein intake in aging individuals consistently demonstrate decreased complications related to hip fractures, pressure ulcers, acute illness, infections, and readmission to hospitals.[129] Overall energy intake influences protein efficacy, which can be confounding. When assessing protein intake while controlling for energy intake, there was no impact on lean body mass over a 2-year period in either men or women.[130] Currently, it is suggested that older persons who are sedentary and weight stable consume at least 1 g protein/kg/day, those who are in negative energy balance consume at least 1 to 1.2 g protein/kg/day, and those who preform high-intensity exercises should consume 1.2 to 1.4 g protein/kg/day. For older individuals with chronic disease, protein requirements may be up to 1.5 g/kg/day.[131]

Protein Quality and Timing

The type of protein eaten is also an important factor in building and maintaining muscle mass. Some studies suggest that including foods with the branched chain amino acids, particularly leucine, may increase muscle protein synthesis through a variety of different ways and therefore increase muscle mass.[131] The relationship between plant and animal protein is of interest, but given that plant protein intake is so low, the relationship of protein quality on clinical outcomes is difficult to define. Timing of protein intake should also be considered. Americans tend to eat protein in increasing amounts throughout the day, with dinner being the most protein-heavy meal. By evenly distributing intake of protein during the day, greater muscle growth can be achieved.[132] Additionally, providing protein supplements at breakfast and lunch can increase lean body mass in aging individuals.[133]

Recommendations for Fiber Intake

Adequate dietary fiber intake is also important in the geriatric population due to its widely recognized role in the gastrointestinal (GI) system and its association with nutrient-dense foods. Fiber-rich foods can help curb energy intake without compromising consumption of vitamins, minerals, and antioxidants. Additionally, adequate fiber intake

⚠ Clinical Controversy

Protein Requirements with Aging

Assuring adequate protein intake in aging individuals is difficult given the multiple challenges this population faces with respect to appetite and other barriers to eating, such as poor dentition, immobility, and depression. Current recommendations for protein intake are the same for younger and older adults. However, given their diminished absorption and metabolism of protein, suboptimal anabolic response to protein intake, and increased needs for recovery from disease and inflammatory processes, experts argue that older individuals require higher amounts of protein. The beneficial role that protein may have in maintaining lean body mass, bone mineral density and function in older individuals is under investigation with differing results.[131] Farsijani et al.[130] looked at quartile differences in lean body mass related to energy-adjusted protein at baseline and 2-year follow-up. There was no effect of quantity of protein intake on lean body mass. This is in contrast to the findings of Houston et al.,[128] where energy-adjusted protein intake at the highest quartile resulted in a 40% lower decrease in lean body mass.

Evaluate the research supporting the conflicting results of these two studies. What are factors related to study design might explain the differing results. What is your position?

can help improve gastric motility, glycemic control, and cholesterol levels. Current literature supports dietary fiber intake of 25 to 35 g/day.[134] However, data from national surveys indicate that dietary fiber intake of older adults is lower than recommended levels.[69] Frequent consumption of low-fiber foods can contribute to decreased intakes of vitamins, minerals, and antioxidants, and increased discretionary energy intake, placing older persons at risk for malnutrition and obesity.[8] On the other hand, too much fiber intake is also not recommended in this population, especially frail individuals with poor appetite and anorexia, because a high-fiber diet can lead to satiety and can result in decreased overall food consumption and subsequent weight loss. When recommending fiber intake for older individuals, their fluid intake should also be assessed to prevent uncomfortable side effects associated with increased dietary fiber consumption, such as constipation.

Fluid Requirements

Fluid requirements also decline with age due to decreased lean body mass and daily/physical activity. Current recommendations for daily fluid intake (Table 27.3) have

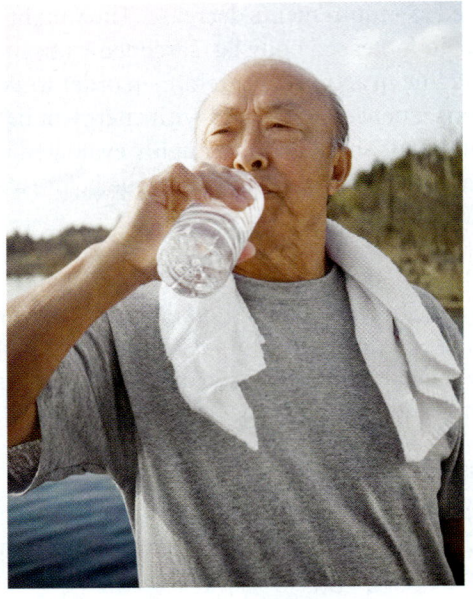

FIGURE 27.9 Hydration Becomes More Important As We Age
© Suprijono Suharjoto/123RF.

been designed to replace normal daily losses and prevent dehydration.[135] Despite the lower requirement, older adults are often at risk of dehydration due to physiological changes and decreased intake. Consequences of dehydration can range from less serious (i.e., constipation and fecal impaction) to detrimental (i.e., cognitive impairment, death). Common risk factors of dehydration in geriatric population include decreased sensitivity to thirst, kidneys' decreased ability to concentrate urine, endocrine changes, alterations in mental status and cognitive abilities, side effects of medications, and limited mobility. Furthermore, fear of incontinence and arthritis pain from taking numerous trips to the bathroom may also decrease older individuals' desire to drink adequate fluid (**Figure 27.9**).

Physiologic Alterations Effecting Micronutrient Metabolism

Aging not only affects macronutrient metabolism, but also micronutrient metabolism. Overall, the body's ability to efficiently utilize micronutrients declines with age, and health, physiologic, and functional status affect adequate oral intake as well. Consequently, older adults are at a higher risk for nutrient deficiencies than young adults, especially of water-soluble vitamins that lack large body stores. Unfortunately, changes in nutritional status often escape recognition until profound physical changes are evident.

Because decreased energy intake associated with aging affects micronutrient intake, the quality of the diet becomes vitally important.[136] Even if the individual is consuming an adequate number of calories, the quality

TABLE 27.3 KEY NUTRITIONAL REQUIREMENTS FOR OLDER ADULTS

Energy	Females: 25–35 kcal/kg Males: 30–40 kcal/kg
Protein	Sedentary and weight-stable older adults: 1 g protein/kg/day With negative energy balance: 1–1.2 g protein/kg/day High-intensity exercise: 1.2–1.4 g protein/kg/day
Fiber	25 to 35 g/day
Fluid[1]	Using Age: Ages 55–65 years: 30 mL/kg/day Ages >65 years: 24 mL/kg/day Using caloric intake: 1 mL/kcal
Vitamin D*	1,000 IU/day
Calcium*	1,200 mg/day
Vitamin B_{12}*	2.4 mcg/day
Iron*	8 mg/day

*Dietary Reference Intake
Modified from Chernoff R. Carbohydrate, fat, and fluid requirements in older adults. In: Chernoff R, ed. *Geriatric Nutrition*. 3rd ed. Sudbury, MA: Jones & Bartlett Publishers; 2006.

of the diet may be poor and may not provide the individual with adequate nutrition for optimal living/function. Moreover, aging brings changes to the GI tract that affects efficiency of digestion, absorption, and metabolism of micronutrients.

A large number of older people are affected by **atrophic gastritis**, or chronic inflammation of the stomach mucosa that characterized by a partial loss of parietal cell mass.[137] Primary causes of atrophic gastritis are autoimmune due to pernicious anemia or chronic *Helicobacter pylori* (*H. pylori*) infection.[138] *H. pylori* causes decreased acid-pepsin digestion in the stomach, decreased secretion of intrinsic factor, bacterial overgrowth of the stomach and proximal small intestine, and elevated pH in the proximal small intestine.[137,139] These factors combined affect nutrient bioavailability of folic acid, vitamin B_{12}, calcium, iron, and beta-carotene because absorption of these nutrients is facilitated by optimal pH and intrinsic factor (vitamin B_{12}).[137,139,140] Atrophic gastritis is difficult to prevent, but one can lower the risk of getting an *H. pylori* infection by practicing good hygiene. Treatment usually focuses on eliminating the *H. pylori* infection with appropriate antibiotics.

In addition to these physiologic changes, chronic illnesses and medications also affect nutrient intake, absorption, metabolism, and excretion. As a result of changes in micronutrient metabolism stemming from multiple etiologies, older adults are at a high risk of developing vitamin and mineral deficiencies. In particular, there is a high prevalence of vitamin B_{12}, vitamin D, and calcium deficiencies among older people.

Vitamin B_{12}

Vitamin B_{12} is a water-soluble vitamin that plays an important role in DNA synthesis and regulation, thereby maintaining the integrity of the nervous system and formation of blood cells. Consequently, vitamin B_{12} deficiency can have detrimental effects on neurologic and hematologic status.

An estimated 6% to 15% of older adults have vitamin B_{12} deficiency, and 20% are estimated to have marginal status.[141] The geriatric population has a high risk of developing low levels of vitamin B_{12} due to malabsorption and poor diet, with malabsorption of vitamin B_{12} being common because of lack of intrinsic factor and atrophic gastritis. Previously, the majority of the vitamin B_{12} deficiencies were believed to result from deficiency in intrinsic factor. However, it is now known that approximately 15% of older persons have poor absorption of protein-bound vitamin B_{12}, which is related to gastric achlorhydria and often associated with atrophic gastritis.[142]

Well-known complications of vitamin B_{12} deficiency include pernicious anemia and neurologic complications affecting sensory and motor function.[143] Other identified effects include osteopenia, neurocognitive impairment, and increased vascular risk associated with elevated homocysteine levels.

Given food-fortification programs with folic acid to reduce the incidence of neural tube defects in the United States, there had been a concern that folate fortification of foods may mask macrocytic anemia in those with vitamin B_{12} deficiency. However, elevated mean corpuscular volume, which is a lab parameter that is often checked for diagnosing anemia, is not a reliable indicator of vitamin B_{12} deficiency, as macrocytosis often has other causes.[144] Additionally, Morris et al., using the NHANES data for older adults in the post-folate fortification years, found that those with vitamin B_{12} deficiency and higher folate levels were more likely to be anemic and to have cognitive impairment than patients with normal folate levels.[145] Given the increase in worldwide food-fortification programs, more research is needed in order to clearly define the relationship between serum folate and vitamin B_{12} levels and their effect on anemia and neurocognition. Some people with low-to-normal serum vitamin B_{12} levels may exhibit changes in mental status that can be overlooked or attributed to symptoms of normal aging. Thus, given the high prevalence of vitamin B_{12} deficiency and the ease and safety of treatment, routine screening should be done in the geriatric population with a serum vitamin B_{12} assay.

DRIs for vitamin B_{12} are not increased for the older population, but given the prevalence of vitamin B_{12} deficiency from age-related changes and prolonged use of certain medications like proton pump inhibitors and metformin,[146] it is recommended that older persons try to increase intake of vitamin B_{12} through food (natural and fortified). However, because there are no identifiable side effects related to excess consumption of vitamin B_{12},[147] supplementation is warranted in persons who cannot achieve optimal intake through food alone. Due to B vitamins' involvement in neuroprotection and prevention of cognitive decline through their role in neutrotransmitter synthesis and participation in the methylation reaction and the homocysteine/methionine metabolic cycle, the effects of vitamin B_{12} supplementation on cognitive function is being investigated.[148] Numerous observational studies have associated low vitamin B_{12} status with more rapid cognitive decline in older adults.[149] However, evidence from randomized trials remains inconclusive.[150]

Vitamin D

Vitamin D has received much attention in the research community and the lay press recently due to its potential implication in reducing the risk of many chronic disorders, including type 2 diabetes, cancer, and heart disease.[151,152] Among its numerous benefits, vitamin D is best known for its role in the prevention and delay of the progression of osteoporosis.

Vitamin D deficiency has been associated with muscle weakness, functional impairment, depression, and increased risk of falls and fractures.[153-155] Additionally, vitamin D insufficiency may lead to hypocalcemia and high serum parathyroid hormone levels, causing secondary hyperparathyroidism. Secondary hyperparathyroidism is the excessive

CASE STUDY REVISITED

After being put on an oral nutrition supplement at her last admission, Esther initially seems to be at baseline but then begins to decline. Esther and her family return for an appointment 2 weeks later due to worsening cognition. They note that she has been eating less than normal and seems to be losing even more weight. Esther is noted to clear her throat multiple times during the visit.

Anthropometric Data:
Height: 152.4 cm (60")
Weight: 38 kg (83 lbs)
BMI: 15.4 kg/m²

Biochemical Data:
Sodium 150 (135-145 mEq/L)   Blood urea nitrogen 74 (6-24 mg/dL)
Potassium 3.6 (3.6-5.0 mEq/L) Creatine 2.8 (0.4-1.3 mg/dL)
Chloride 107 (98-110 mEq/L)
Carbon dioxide 23 (20-30 mEq/L)
Glucose 114 mg/dL (70-139 mg/dL)

Clinical Data:
Medications: Atenolol, Protonix, Seroquel, Os-Cal, vitamin B_{12}, NSAID
Vital signs: Blood pressure: 95/72 mm Hg

Dietary Data:
Dietary History: Family states that Esther does not drink her thickened liquids with meals or throughout the day and, when she does, she drinks them very slowly. They also note that they thought she was drinking her nutrition supplements with thickener but found unused nutrition supplement cans in her room. She states that she tried them for the first week, but she does not like them, so she does not drink them, especially with the thickener.
Diet Recall:
Breakfast: Bowl of oatmeal
Lunch: Mashed potatoes (1 cup) and 1 baked fish stick
Dinner: Elbow macaroni with butter and salt.

Questions

1. What might you recommend for Esther to improve her fluid intake while on thickened liquids?
2. Does Esther need supplemental tube feedings?
3. What should be considered when developing nutrition intervention for Esther?

---

secretion of parathyroid hormone (PTH) in response to hypocalcemia. This increase in PTH level typically occurs when 25-hydroxyvitamin D (25[OH]D) concentrations fall below 30 ng/mL.[156] Consequently, current recommendations for vitamin D deficiency have been developed to prevent 25(OH)D from falling below 30 ng/mL.

In addition to inadequate intake of vitamin D and lack of sun exposure, physiologic changes occur with aging that affect vitamin D status in older adults: There is an impaired skin synthesis of previtamin D and decreased hydroxylation in the kidney.[157] In particular, those who are institutionalized; homebound; and/or have limited sun exposure, obesity, dark skin, osteoporosis, or malabsorption are at a higher risk of vitamin D deficiency.[158] As such, monitoring serum 25(OH)D is recommended for those at high risk, with the goal of achieving levels >30 ng/mL. It is important to note that serum levels do not reflect vitamin D intake status, due to other factors such as sunlight exposure that affect vitamin D production in the body.

Vitamin D deficiency is commonly seen in older people due to reduced intake and skin synthesis. Vitamin D status is typically determined by measuring plasma 25(OH)D levels; however, there is no current consensus on normal 25(OH)D levels. Therefore, the recommended dietary intake is based on maintaining normal PTH levels. The Institute of Medicine proposed that a 25(OH)D level >20 ng/mL (50 nmol/L) is required to maintain normal PTH levels. It is recommended that in addition to sunlight exposure, older persons should consume a higher amount of vitamin D than is recommended for younger adults. Because current research supports a minimum intake of 1,000 IU/day, vitamin D supplementation of that amount is recommended for older adults with poor intake (especially of dairy foods) and/or limited sunlight exposure.

Calcium

Calcium status is also strongly influenced by age. In both sexes, the efficiency of calcium absorption from the GI tract is significantly reduced after age of 60 years. Individuals between the ages of 70 and 90 years absorb about one-third less calcium than younger adults.[159] Therefore, higher calcium intake is recommended for older adults. The current recommendation for those older than 51 years of age is 1,200 mg per day (adequate intake [AI] reference value); however, according to the NHANES 2003-2006 data, women older than 51 years and men older than 70 years of age had intake that fell below the desired value.[160]

In addition to its best-known role in bone health, calcium homeostasis is important for muscle contraction, nerve conduction, hormone regulation, blood coagulation, and other metabolic processes.[161] Serum calcium level depends on dietary intake, diet components, calcium absorption from the GI tract, and renal calcium excretion. Various factors influence calcium absorption in the GI tract. Components in food, such as phytic acid and oxalic acid, bind to calcium and inhibit absorption. Vitamin D concentration in blood directly affects calcium absorption from the GI tract; thus, sufficient vitamin D intake is necessary to maintain optimal serum calcium level without compromising bone homeostasis.

Calcium and vitamin D are intricately related and adequate intakes of both nutrients are important to prevent or manage osteoporosis that is associated with aging. Unfortunately, it can be difficult to have adequate intake of calcium and vitamin D from food alone; thus, it may be necessary to begin supplementation if an individual is at risk of inadequate intake or osteoporosis.

> **PRACTICE POINT**
>
> Inadequate intake of foods as well as changes in the GI tract can affect micronutrient absorption and metabolism.

Aging strongly influences calcium status in the body. The efficiency of calcium absorption from the GI tract decreases significantly after age 60 years in both sexes, which is in part affected by vitamin D status.[147] Calcium balance is also affected by factors that affect renal excretion of calcium, such as high protein and high sodium intake. Furthermore, calcium absorption also depends on the amount of calcium intake; inadequate intake triggers adaptive responses to increase absorption of calcium from the gut, but this compensation mechanism declines with age.

It is generally recommended that the AI level for calcium be met through the diet; however, older persons often cannot consume adequate amount to meet this level and thus supplementation of calcium/vitamin D together is warranted (due to vitamin D's role in absorption of calcium). However, recent literature suggests calcium's potential role in increasing the risk of cardiovascular disease when consumed in excess.[162] As a consequence, supplementation of calcium is not recommended for all persons and caution should be taken to avoid consuming beyond the upper level of 2,500 mg/day.

Nutrition Management

Optimal nutrition care is needed throughout an individual's lifetime and appropriate nutrition intervention should be performed in a timely manner in order to prevent undernutrition and other potential adverse outcomes related to consuming an unhealthy diet. Older persons are at a high risk of malnutrition and the etiology is multifactorial. It is important that healthcare providers, as well as caregivers, identify and treat contributing factors to improve the quality of life and function in older adults. Nutrition intervention for this population can range from eating a healthy and balanced diet to enteral and parenteral nutrition support. Nutrition interventions should be instituted as appropriate and in line with patient's goals of care.

Because most older adults have at least one chronic disease by age 50 years, many are required to follow some type of restrictive diet for their illness(es). Although therapeutic diets are designed to improve health, they can negatively affect the variety and palatability of the food, resulting in decreased desire to eat, reduced intake, unintended weight loss, and undernutrition.[163] For many older adults living in healthcare communities, the benefits of less-restrictive diets outweigh the risks. Therefore, unless absolutely contraindicated, a more liberalized and individualized diet, accounting for individual preferences, should be recommended to improve the quality of life and optimize nutritional status in older adults.

Other nutrition-related interventions include providing assistance for those who are not able to self-feed, modifying food consistency and/or texture, and providing means of socializing during mealtimes. Although feeding assistance typically requires more staff time, it can significantly increase daily caloric intake in an older individual and help them maintain or gain weight.[164] For those who have difficulty with chewing due to oral health problems, providing chopped or ground food can help with mechanical digestion of foods. Socializing during meals can help older persons to consume more than when compared to eating alone.[100,101]

Preventing overnutrition in this vulnerable population is as important as preventing undernutrition. Therefore, the current 2015 Dietary Guidelines for Americans recommend that older adults maintain calorie balance in order to achieve and sustain a healthy weight, as well as eating nutrient-dense foods and beverages.[165] The goal of these recommendations is to prevent unintended weight loss as well as unintended weight gain. To complement this healthy diet for older adults, the Tufts University Jean Mayer U.S. Department of Agriculture Human Nutrition Research Center on Aging developed a plate model (**Figure 27.10**) revised from MyPlate to make it simple and easy for older adults to understand and adopt the 2015 Dietary Guidelines for Americans. Older adults should consume a diet that consists of fruits and vegetables making up half the diet, with vegetables taking up a greater portion of that half. Whole grains and proteins (lean or low-fat meats, fish, legumes, and nuts) should occupy the other half, with grains taking up a greater portion.[163] Dairy products should be low in fat. Unfortunately, data from a recent Older Americans 2010 report reveal that although older individuals are able to meet the standards for fruits, total grains, meat, and beans, intake of vegetables, whole grains, and milk remain below standards.[94]

> **PRACTICE POINT**
>
> Preventing overnutrition in this vulnerable population is as important as preventing undernutrition.

In order to eat a healthy diet, an individual must have access to the food items, as well as the ability to procure, prepare, and consume them. These factors have a profound impact on the nutrition status of older Americans and should be considered when developing a nutrition intervention for an individual. Community-dwelling older persons are at particular risk for food insecurity, and government-funded programs like home-delivered meals have been created to address this problem.[165] However, addressing issues related to food accessibility in the older population remains a challenge.

Nutrition Support

As supported by numerous studies, the following is true: if the gut works, use it. This holds true for any population, including older adults. Currently, the European Society for Parenteral and Enteral Nutrition (ESPEN) provides the

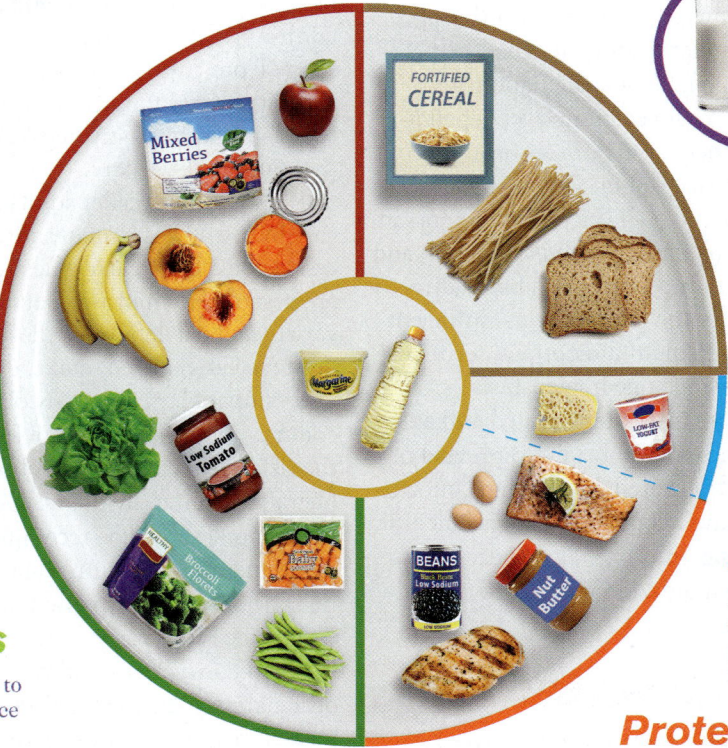

FIGURE 27.10 MyPlate for Older Adults

"MyPlate for Older Adults" Copyright 2016 Tufts University, all rights reserved. "MyPlate for Older Adults" graphic and accompanying website were developed with support from the AARP Foundation. "Tufts University" and "AARP Foundation" are registered trademarks and may not be reproduced apart from their inclusion in the "MyPlate for Older Adults" graphic without express permission from their respective owners.

most comprehensive, evidence-based guidelines on nutrition support provision for the geriatric population.[166,167] According to these guidelines, there are three primary means of providing nutrition support in this population: oral nutritional supplementation (ONS), enteral nutrition (EN) and parenteral nutrition (PN). Nutrition support should be tailored to individual needs after assessing their baseline nutrition status, illnesses, and functional status.

According to ESPEN, ONS is recommended for older persons who are undernourished or at risk of malnutrition, for those with multiple morbidities and/or frailty, and for patients after orthopedic surgery.[166] A meta-analysis that evaluated 55 randomized trials of nutritional supplementation in older patients to prevent malnutrition found that ONS resulted in modest improvement in weight, with a greater increase in patients at home or in long-term care.[168] Overall mortality declined in groups receiving ONS compared to control, but there was no mortality impact for people living at home, and no improvement in functional status. Complication rates were also lower in hospitalized older adults but there was no change in length of stay. Furthermore, some evidence supports the use of ONS, particularly of protein, in postoperative orthopedic patients due to a lower complication rates in the intervention group, but these studies found no reduction in mortality risk.[169]

Unfortunately, older adults who need ONS to maintain and/or improve their nutrition status often have poor compliance due to low palatability of the products, side effects such as nausea and diarrhea, and cost. As such, caregivers and staff should encourage ONS intake and provide a variety of flavors, temperatures, and consistencies, if possible. It is also important that ONS be given between meals as a snack because ONS can increase satiety and contribute to decreased volitional intake during meals. Nutrition interventions using ONS should not only be initiated in persons who are already undernourished, but as soon as there are indications of nutritional risk, irrespective of the underlying illness.[166] Therefore, routine nutritional screening is important in this particular population.

EN may be indicated in those with severe neurologic dysphagia, but it is not recommended in terminal illness, including advanced dementia.[166] In patients who are appropriate to receive EN percutaneous endoscopic gastrostomy (PEG) and nasogastric (NG) tubes are often used for nutrition support for convenience and are associated with less treatment failures and better nutritional status. However, if longer than 4 weeks of tube feeding is anticipated, PEG is the preferred route. Data from various studies reveal that EN delivery via PEG was associated with a greater improvement of nutritional status as compared to EN delivery via NG tube.[170,171] Dysphagia may be reversible in certain types of patients, such as stroke patients; therefore, EN should be accompanied by swallowing therapy until the individual is able to consume sufficient oral intake safely. With severe or advanced disease, including those related to cognitive impairment, there is no evidence that EN affects survival. Conversely, feeding tubes are not recommended for older adults with advanced dementia due to high mortality rates, increased agitation, greater healthcare use, and pressure ulcer development.[172]

Age is not a reason to exclude patients from receiving PN.[167,173] When older patients cannot receive adequate nutrition through EN, PN through a peripheral or central catheter is indicated. PN can be safe and effective when managed correctly and with caution. However, when recommending PN, its contribution to clinical improvement, cost-effectiveness, and potential for developing complications should be considered. Evidence from various studies suggests that PN can improve nutritional status, functional status, and reduce morbidity and mortality. However, because geriatric patients often have insulin resistance as well as impaired cardiac and renal function, they are at a high risk of experiencing metabolic complications (i.e., glucose, electrolyte, and fluid imbalances). Additionally, the restoration of depleted lean body mass is lower in older patients than in younger patients. Therefore, EN should be the first line of intervention and PN should be limited to situations when EN is contraindicated or poorly tolerated.[167]

> **PRACTICE POINT**
>
> In older adults, PN should be limited to situations when EN is contraindicated or poorly tolerated.

Hypodermoclysis, which is the subcutaneous administration of fluid and electrolytes to correct fluid deficit, is indicated in patients with mild to moderate dehydration.[168] It is a relatively safe and easy method of providing hydration, requires less nursing time, is less costly, causes fewer complications, and is more comfortable than IV treatment.

Neither EN nor PN intervention are recommended in patients with terminal illness. Their use should be weighed against a realistic chance of improvement. Comfort is usually the highest priority in these patients, and nutrition support should align with patient's goals of care.

> **PRACTICE POINT**
>
> In older adult population, benefits and risks of nutrition intervention should be weighed prior to implementation and it should be in line with patient's goals of care.

Chapter Summary

Optimal nutrition care is needed throughout an individual's lifetime, and appropriate nutrition intervention should be performed in a timely manner in order to prevent undernutrition, overnutrition, and other potential adverse outcomes related to consuming unhealthy diet. Older persons are at a high risk of malnutrition and the etiology is multifactorial. It is important that healthcare providers as well as caregivers identify and treat contributing factors to improve the quality of life and function in older adults.

Key Terms

geriatric nutrition, immunosenescence, sarcopenia, insensible water loss, cachexia, frailty, pressure injury, sarcopenic obesity, cephalic phase of digestion, dysphagia, oropharyngeal dysphagia, aspiration, activities of daily living (ADL), atrophic gastritis, instrumental activities of daily living (IADL), mini nutritional assessment (MNA)

References

1. Administration for Community Living. Profile of older Americans. https://www.acl.gov/aging-and-disability-in-america/data-and-research/profile-older-americans. Accessed July 13, 2017.
2. de Luis D, Lopez Guzman A. Nutritional status of adult patients admitted to internal medicine departments in public hospitals in Castilla y Leon, Spain—A multi-center study. *Eur J Intern Med* 2006;17(8):556-60.
3. Vincent GA, Velkoff VA. The next four decades: The older population in the United States: 2010 to 2050. 2010: US Department of Commerce, Economics and Statistics Administration, US Census Bureau.
4. Kochanek KD. Murphy S, Xu J, Tejada-Vera B. Deaths: Final data for 2014. *Nat Vital Stat Rep.* 2016;65(4):1.
5. The state of aging and health in America 2013. Atlanta, GA: Centers for Disease Control and Prevention, U.S. Dept of Health and Human Services; 2013.
6. Jin K. Modern biological theories of aging. *Aging Dis.* 2010;1(2):72.
7. Guarente L. Sirtuins, aging, and medicine. *NEJM.* 2011;364(23):2235-2244.
8. Bernstein M, Munoz N. Position of the Academy of Nutrition and Dietetics: Food and nutrition for older adults: promoting health and wellness. *J Acad Nutr Diet.* 2012;112(8):1255-1277.
9. Krebs-Smith SM, Guenther PM, Subar AF, Kirkpatrick SI, Dodd KW. Americans do not meet federal dietary recommendations. *J Nutr.* 2010;140(10):1832-1838.
10. Tangney CC, Kwasny MJ, Li H, Wilson RS, Evans DA, Morris MC. Adherence to a Mediterranean-type dietary pattern and cognitive decline in a community population. *Am J Clin Nutr.* 2011;93(3):601-607.
11. Anderson AL, Harris TB, Tylavsky FA, et al. Dietary patterns and survival of older adults. *J Am Diet Assoc.* 2011;111(1):84-91.
12. Roberts SB, Dallal GE. Energy requirements and aging. *Public Health Nutr.* 2005;8(7a):1028-36.
13. DmitrievaNI Burg MB. Increased insensible water loss contributes to aging related dehydration. *PloS One.* 2011;6(5):e20691.
14. Dharmarajan TS. Geriatric gastroenterology: The geriatrician's perspective. In: Pitchumoni CS, Dharmarajan TS, eds. *Geriatric gastroenterology*. New York, NY: Springer; 2012:3-6.
15. Iannuzzi-Sucich M, Prestwood KM, Kenny AM. Prevalence of sarcopenia and predictors of skeletal muscle mass in healthy, older men and women. *J Gerontol A Biol Sci Med Sci.* 2002;57(12):M772-7.
16. Beaufrere B, Morio B. Fat and protein redistribution with aging: metabolic considerations. *Eur J Clin Nutr.* 2000;54 Suppl 3:S48-53.
17. Enzi G, Gasparo M, Biondetti PR, Fiore D, Semisa M, Zurlo F. Subcutaneous and visceral fat distribution according to sex, age, and overweight, evaluated by computed tomography. *Am J Clin Nutr.* 1986;44(6):739-746.
18. Schulman, RC, Weiss AJ, and Mechanick JI. Nutrition, bone, and aging: an integrative physiology approach. *Curr Osteopor Rep.* 2011;9(4):184-195.
19. Cruz-Jentoft AJ, Baeyens JP, Bauer JM, et al. Sarcopenia: European consensus on definition and diagnosis: Report of the European Working Group on Sarcopenia in Older People. *Age Ageing.* 2010;39(4):412-423.
20. Fielding RA, Vellas B, Evans WJ, et al. Sarcopenia: an undiagnosed condition in older adults. Current consensus definition: prevalence, etiology, and consequences. International working group on sarcopenia. *J Am Med Dir Assoc.* 2011;12(4):249-256.
21. Muscaritoli M. Anker SD, Argilés J, et al. Consensus definition of sarcopenia, cachexia and pre-cachexia: Joint document elaborated by Special Interest Groups (SIG) "cachexia-anorexia in chronic wasting diseases" and "nutrition in geriatrics". *Clin Nutr.* 2010;29(2):154-159.
22. Morley JE, Kim MJ, Haren MT, Kevorkian R, Banks WA. Frailty and the aging male. *Aging Male.* 2005;8(3-4):135-140.
23. Joseph C, Kenny AM, Taxel P, Lorenzo JA, Duque G, Kuchel GA. Role of endocrine-immune dysregulation in osteoporosis, sarcopenia, frailty and fracture risk. *Mol Aspects Med.* 2005;26(3):181-201.
24. Wittert GA, Chapman IM, Haren MT, Mackintosh S, Coates P, Morley JE. Oral testosterone supplementation increases muscle and decreases fat mass in healthy elderly males with low-normal gonadal status. *J Gerontol A Biol Sci Med Sci.* 2003;58(7):618-625.
25. Szulc P, Duboeuf F, Marchand F, Delmas PD. Hormonal and lifestyle determinants of appendicular skeletal muscle mass in men: the MINOS study. *Am J Clin Nutr.* 2004;80(2):496-503.
26. Kenny AM, Dawson L, Kleppinger A, Iannuzzi-Sucich M, Judge JO. Prevalence of sarcopenia and predictors of skeletal muscle mass in nonobese women who are long-term users of estrogen-replacement therapy. *J Gerontol A Biol Sci Med Sci.* 2003;58(5):M436-440.
27. Rasmussen BB, Fujita S, Wolfe RR, et al. Insulin resistance of muscle protein metabolism in aging. *Faseb J.* 2006;20(6):768-769.
28. Millward DJ. Sufficient protein for our elders? *Am J Clin Nutr.* 2008;88(5):1187-1188.
29. Paddon-Jones D, Short K, Campbell W, Eleni E, Wolfe R. Role of dietary protein in the sarcopenia of aging. *Am J Clin Nutr.* 2008;87(5):1562s-1566s.
30. Chernoff R. Protein and older adults. *J Am Coll Nutr.* 2004;23(suppl 6):627s-630s.
31. Fulgoni VL 3rd. Current protein intake in America: analysis of the National Health and Nutrition Examination Survey, 2003-2004. *Am J Clin Nutr.* 2008;87(5):1554s-1557s.
32. Berger MJ, Doherty TJ. Sarcopenia: prevalence, mechanisms, and functional consequences. *Interdiscip Top Gerontol.* 2010;37:94-114. doi: 10.1159/000319997.
33. Kim JS, Wilson JM, Lee SR. Dietary implications on mechanisms of sarcopenia: roles of protein, amino acids and antioxidants. *J Nutr Biochem.* 2010;21(1):1-13.
34. D'Antona G, Pellegrino MA, Carlizzi CN, Bottinelli R. Deterioration of contractile properties of muscle fibres in elderly subjects is modulated by the level of physical activity. *Eur J Appl Physiol.* 2007;100(5):603-611.
35. Degens H, Alway SE. Control of muscle size during disuse, disease, and aging. *Int J Sports Med.* 2006;27(2):94-99.
36. Kortebein P, Ferrando A, Lombeida J, Wolfe R, Evans WJ. Effect of 10 days of bed rest on skeletal muscle in healthy older adults. *JAMA.* 2007;297(16):1772-1774.
37. Visser M, Newman AB, Nevitt MC, Kritchevsky SB, Stamm EB, Goodpaster BH, et al. Reexamining the sarcopenia hypothesis. Muscle mass versus muscle strength. Health, Aging, and Body Composition Study Research Group. *Ann N Y Acad Sci.* 2000;904:456-461.
38. Papa E, Dong X, Hassan M. Resistance training for activity limitations in older adults with skeletal muscle function deficits: a systematic review. *Clin Interven Aging.* 2017;12:955-961.
39. Morley JE, Argiles JM, Evans WJ, et al. Nutritional recommendations for the management of sarcopenia. *J Am Med Dir Assoc.* 2010;11(6):391-396.

40. Ahmed N, Mandel R, Fain MJ. Frailty: an emerging geriatric syndrome. *Am J Med*. 2007;120(9):748-753.
41. Fried LP, Tangen CM, Walston J, et al. Frailty in older adults: evidence for a phenotype. *J Gerontol A Biol Sci Med Sci*. 2001;56(3):M146-156.
42. de Vries NM, van Ravensberg CD, Hobbelen JS, Olde Rikkert MG, Staal JB, Nijhuis-van der Sanden MW. Effects of physical exercise therapy on mobility, physical functioning, physical activity and quality of life in community-dwelling older adults with impaired mobility, physical disability and/or multi-morbidity: a meta-analysis. *Ageing Res Rev*. 2012;11(1):136-149.
43. Theou O, Stathokostas L, Roland KP, Jakobi JM, Patterson C, Vandervoort AA, et al. The effectiveness of exercise interventions for the management of frailty: a systematic review. *J Aging Res*. 2011;2011:569194.
44. Clegg AP, Barber SE, Young JB, Forster A, Iliffe SJ. Do home-based exercise interventions improve outcomes for frail older people? Findings from a systematic review. *Rev Clin Gerontol*. 2012;22(01):68-78.
45. Crocker T, Forster A, Young J, et al. Physical rehabilitation for older people in long-term care. *Cochrane Database Syst Rev*. 2013;2:Cd004294.
46. Daniels R, van Rossum E, de Witte L, Kempen GI, van den Heuvel W. Interventions to prevent disability in frail community-dwelling elderly: a systematic review. *BMC Health Serv Res*. 2008;8:278.
47. Bartali B, Frongillo EA, Bandinelli S, et al. Low nutrient intake is an essential component of frailty in older persons. *J Gerontol A Biol Sci Med Sci*. 2006;61(6):589-593.
48. Wilhelm-Leen ER, Hall YN, Deboer IH, Chertow GM. Vitamin D deficiency and frailty in older Americans. *J Intern Med*. 2010;268(2):171-180.
49. Melamed ML, Michos ED, Post W, Astor B. 25-hydroxyvitamin D levels and the risk of mortality in the general population. *Arch Intern Med*. 2008;168(15):1629-1637.
50. Chonchol M, Scragg R. 25-Hydroxyvitamin D, insulin resistance, and kidney function in the Third National Health and Nutrition Examination Survey. *Kidney Int*. 2007;71(2):134-139.
51. Scragg R, Sowers M, Bell C. Serum 25-hydroxyvitamin D, ethnicity, and blood pressure in the Third National Health and Nutrition Examination Survey. *Am J Hypertens*. 2007;20(7):713-719.
52. Janssen HC, Samson MM, Verhaar HJ. Vitamin D deficiency, muscle function, and falls in elderly people. *Am J Clin Nutr*. 2002;75(4):611-615.
53. Bischoff HA, Borchers M, Gudat F, et al. In situ detection of 1,25-dihydroxyvitamin D3 receptor in human skeletal muscle tissue. *Histochem J*. 2001;33(1):19-24.
54. Endo I, Inoue D, Mitsui T, et al. Deletion of vitamin D receptor gene in mice results in abnormal skeletal muscle development with deregulated expression of myoregulatory transcription factors. *Endocrinology*. 2003;144(12):5138-5144.
55. NUAP Pressure Injury Stages. National Pressure Ulcer Advisory Panel website. http://www.npuap.org/resources/educational-and-clinical-resources/npuap-pressure-injurystages/ Accessed July 18, 2017.
56. SmithME, Totten A, Hickam DH, et al. Pressure ulcer treatment strategies: a systematic comparative effectiveness review. *Ann Intern Med*. 2013;159(1):39-50.
57. Whittington K, Patrick M, Roberts JL. A national study of pressure ulcer prevalence and incidence in acute care hospitals. *J Wound Ostomy Continence Nurs*. 2000;27(4):209-215.
58. Pressure ulcers in America: prevalence, incidence, and implications for the future. An executive summary of the National Pressure Ulcer Advisory Panel monograph. *Adv Skin Wound Care*. 2001;14(4):208-215.
59. Brandeis GH, Morris JN, Nash DJ, et al. The epidemiology and natural history of pressure ulcers in elderly nursing home residents. *JAMA*. 1990;264(22):2905-2909.
60. Bluestein D, Javaheri A. Pressure ulcers: prevention, evaluation, and management. *Am Fam Physician*. 2008;78(10):1186-1194.
61. National Pressure Ulcer Advisory Panel, European Pressure Ulcer Advisory Panel, Pan Pacific Pressure Injury Alliance. Prevention and Treatment of Pressure Ulcers: Quick Reference Guide. 2009 http://www.epuap.org/wp-content/uploads/2016/10/quick-reference-guide-digital-npuap-epuap-pppia-jan2016.pdf. Accessed January 2014.
62. Evans WJ. Exercise and nutritional needs of elderly people: effects on muscle and bone. *Gerodontology*. 1998;15(1):15-24.
63. Zamboni M, Mazzali G, Fantin F, Rossi A, Di Francesco V. Sarcopenic obesity: a new category of obesity in the elderly. *Nutr Metab Cardiovasc Dis*. 2008;18(5):388-395.
64. Houston DK, Nicklas BJ, Zizza CA. Weighty concerns: the growing prevalence of obesity among older adults. *J Am Diet Assoc*. 2009;109(11):1886-1895.
65. Stephen WC, Janssen I. Sarcopenic-obesity and cardiovascular disease risk in the elderly. *J Nutr Health Aging*. 2009;13(5):460-466.
66. Stenholm S, Harris TB, Rantanen T, Visser M, Kritchevsky SB, Ferrucci L. Sarcopenic obesity: definition, cause and consequences. *Curr Opin Clin Nutr Metab Care*. 2008;11(6):693-700.
67. LaMonte MJ, Blair SN. Physical activity, cardiorespiratory fitness, and adiposity: contributions to disease risk. *Curr Opin Clin Nutr Metab Care*. 2006;9(5):540-546.
68. Duvigneaud N, Matton L, Wijndaele K, et al. Relationship of obesity with physical activity, aerobic fitness and muscle strength in Flemish adults. *J Sports Med Phys Fitness*. 2008;48(2):201-210.
69. Cesari M, Kritchevsky SB, Baumgartner RN, et al. Sarcopenia, obesity, and inflammation—results from the Trial of Angiotensin Converting Enzyme Inhibition and Novel Cardiovascular Risk Factors study. *Am J Clin Nutr*. 2005;82(2):428-434.
70. Schrager MA, Metter EJ, Simonsick E, et al. Sarcopenic obesity and inflammation in the InCHIANTI study. *J Appl Physiol*. 2007;102(3):919-925.
71. Shen HC, Chen HF, Peng LN. et al. Impact of nutritional status on long-term functional outcomes of post-acute stroke patients in Taiwan. *Arch Gerontol Geriatr*. 2011;53(2):e149-152.
72. Baumeister SE, Fischer B, Döring A, et al. The Geriatric Nutritional Risk Index predicts increased healthcare costs and hospitalization in a cohort of community-dwelling older adults: results from the MONICA/KORA Augsburg cohort study, 1994-2005. *Nutrition*. 2011;27(5):534-542.
73. Leandro-Merhi VA, de Aquino JL, Sales Chagas JF. Nutrition status and risk factors associated with length of hospital stay for surgical patients. *JPEN J Parenter Enteral Nutr*. 2011;35(2):241-248.
74. Calle EE, Thun MJ, Petrilli JM, Rodriguez C, Heath CW. Body-mass index and mortality in a prospective cohort of U.S. adults. *N Eng J Med*. 1999;341(15):1097-1105.
75. Thomas D, Kamal H, Azharrudin M. The relationship of functional status, severity of illness, and nutritional markers to in-hospital mortality and length of stay. *J Nutr Health Aging*. 2005;9:169-175.
76. Liu L, Bopp M, Roberson P, Sullivan D. Undernutrition and Risk of Mortality in Elderly Patients Within 1 Year of Hospital Discharge. *J Gerontol A Biol Sci Med Sci*. 2002;57(11):M741-M746.
77. Kaiser MJ, Bauer JM, Rämsch C, et al. Frequency of malnutrition in older adults: a multinational perspective using the mini nutritional assessment. *J Am Geriatr Soc*. 2010;58(9):1734-1738.
78. Rolls BJ. Do chemosensory changes influence food intake in the elderly? *Physiol Behav*. 1999;66(2):193-197.

79. Horowitz M, Maddern GJ, Chatterton BE, Collins PJ, Harding PE, Shearman DJ. Changes in gastric emptying rates with age. *Clin Sci (Lond)*. 1984;67(2):213-218.

80. Parker BA, Chapman IM. Food intake and ageing—the role of the gut. *Mech Ageing Dev*. 2004;125(12):859-866.

81. Roberts SB. Regulation of energy intake in relation to metabolic state and nutritional status. *Eur J Clin Nutr*. 2000;54(suppl 3):S64-9.

82. Drewnowski A, Shultz J. Impact of aging on eating behaviors, food choices, nutrition, and health status. *J Nutr Health Aging*. 2001;5(2)75-79.

83. Morley J. Anorexia in Older Persons. *Drugs Aging*. 1996;8(2):134-155.

84. Gammack J. Geriatric assessment and its interaction with nutrition. In: Morley JE, Thomas DR, eds. *Geriatric nutrition*. New York, NY: CRC; 2007:217-234.

85. Garcia N, Miley D. The oral cavity and nutrition. In: Morley JE, Thomas DR, eds. *Geriatric nutrition*. New York, NY: CRC; 2007:249-65.

86. Ritchie CS. Oral health, taste, and olfaction. *Clin Geriatr Med*. 2002;18(4):709-717.

87. Darnton-Hill I. Psychosocial aspects of nutrition and aging. *Nutr Rev*. 1992;50(12):476-479.

88. Brownie S. Why are elderly individuals at risk of nutritional deficiency? *Int J Nurs Prac*. 2006;12(2):110-118.

89. Wilson MM, Vaswani S, Liu D, Morley JE, Miller DK. Prevalence and causes of undernutrition in medical outpatients. *Am J Med*. 1998;104(1):56-63.

90. Thompson MP, Morris LK. Unexplained weight loss in the ambulatory elderly. *J Am Geriatr Soc*. 1991;39(5):497-500.

91. Types of dementia. Alzheimer's Association website. http://www.alz.org/dementia/types-of-dementia.asp. Accessed July 29, 2017.

92. Baumgartner RN, Wayne SJ, Waters DL, Janssen I, Gallagher D, Morley JE. Sarcopenic obesity predicts instrumental activities of daily living disability in the elderly. *Obesity Res*. 2004;12(12):1995-2004.

93. Pfizer Facts. Health status of older adults. Findings from the National Health and Nutrition Examination Survey (NHANES) 1999-2004, the National Health Interview Survey (NHS) 2005, and the Compressed Mortality File (CMF). 2007.

94. Older Americans 2012: Key indicators of well-being 2012. Federal Interagency Forum on Aging-Related Statistics: Washington, DC.

95. Ortega O, Martin A, Clave P. Diagnosis and Treatment of Oropharyngeal Dysphagia in Older Persons: State of the Art. *J Am Med Dir Assoc*. 2017;18(7)576-582.

96. Ney DM, Weiss JM, Kind AJ, Robbins J. Senescent swallowing: Impact, strategies, and interentions. *Nutr Clin Pract*. 2009;24:395.

97. O'Neil KO, Purdy M, Falk J, Gallo L. The dysphagia outcome and severity scale. *Dysphagia*. 1999;14:139-145.

98. Wham CA, Teh RO, Robinson M, Kerse NM. What is associated with nutrition risk in very old age? *J Nutr Health Aging*. 2011;15(4):247-251.

99. Mion L, McDowell J, Heaney L. Nutritional assessment of the elderly in the ambulatory care setting. *Nurse Pract Forum*. 1994;5(1)46-51.

100. de Castro JM, Brewer EM. The amount eaten in meals by humans is a power function of the number of people present. *Physiol Behav*. 1992;51(1):121-125.

101. Locher JL, Robinson CO, Roth DL, Ritchie CS, Burgio KL. The effect of the presence of others on caloric intake in homebound older adults. *J Gerontol A Biol Sci Med Sci*. 2005;60(11):1475-1478.

102. Bolland MJ, Greg A, Gamble G, REid TR. Calcium and vitamin D supplements and health outcomes: a reanalysis of the Women's Health Initiative (WHI) limited-access data set. *Am J Clin Nutr*. 2011;94(4):1144-1149.

103. Russo D, Miranda I, Ruocco C, et al. The progression of coronary artery calcification in predialysis patients on calcium carbonate or sevelamer. *Kidney Int*. 2007;72(10):1255-1261.

104. Jensen GL, Bistrian B, Roubenoff R, Heimburger DC. Malnutrition syndromes: a conundrum vs continuum. *JPEN J Parenter Enteral Nutr*. 2009;33(6):710-716.

105. Jensen GL, Mirtallo J, Compher C, et al. Adult starvation and disease-related malnutrition A proposal for etiology-based diagnosis in the clinical practice setting from the International Consensus Guideline Committee. *JPEN J Parent Ent Nutr*. 2010;34(2):156-159.

106. Obesity at a Glance: Halting the Epidemic by Making Health Easier. National Center for Chronic Disease Control and Prevention and Health Promotion: Atlanta, GA, 2011. https://obesity.procon.org/sourcefiles/CDCobesityatglance2009.pdf. Accessed December 29, 2017.

107. National Alliance for Infusion Therapy and the American Society for Parenteral and Enteral Nutrition Public Policy Committee and Board of Directors. Disease-related malnutrition and enteral nutrition therapy: a significant problem with a cost-effective solution. *Nutr Clin Prac*. 2010;25(5):548-554. doi:10.1177/0884533610378524

108. Skipper A, Ferguson M, Thompson K, Castellanos VH, Porcari J. Nutrition screening tools: an analysis of the evidence. *JPEN J Parenter Enteral Nutr*. 2012;36(3):292-8.

109. Ferguson M, Capra S, Bauer J, Banks M. Development of a valid and reliable malnutrition screening tool for adult acute hospital patients. *Nutrition*. 1999;15(6):458-64.

110. Sieber CC. Nutritional screening tools—How does the MNA compare? Proceedings of the session held in Chicago May 2-3, 2006 (15 Years of Mini Nutritional Assessment). *J Nutr Health Aging*. 2006;10(6):488-492; discussion 492-494.

111. MNA: Mini Nutritional Assessment. http://www.mna-elderly.com. Accessed July 19, 2017.

112. Kaiser MJ, Bauer JM, Ramsch C, et al. Validation of the Mini Nutritional Assessment short-form (MNA-SF): a practical tool for identification of nutritional status. *J Nutr Health Aging*. 2009;13(9):782-8.

113. Dent E, Visvanathan R, Piantadosi C, Chapman I. Use of the Mini Nutritional assessment to detect frailty in hospitalised older people. *J Nutr Health Aging*. 2012;16(9):764-767. doi:10.1007/s12603-012-0405-5

114. White JV, Guenter P, Jensen G, et al. Consensus statement of the Academy of Nutrition and Dietetics/American Society for Parenteral and Enteral Nutrition: characteristics recommended for the identification and documentation of adult malnutrition (undernutrition). *J Am Nutr Diet*. 2012;112(5):730-738.

115. Newman AB, Yanez D, Harris T, et al. Weight change in old age and its association with mortality. *J Am Geriatr Soc*. 2001;49(10):1309-1318.

116. Minimum Data Set (MDS)—Version 2.0 For Nursing Home Resident Assessment and Care Screening. https://www.cms.gov/Medicare/Quality-Initiatives-Patient-Assessment-Instruments/NursingHomeQualityInits/Downloads/MDS-30-RAI-Manual-V113.pdf. Accessed July 19, 2017.

117. Jensen GL, Hsiao PY. Obesity in older adults: relationship to functional limitation. *Curr Opin Clin Nutr Metab Care*. 2010;13(1):46-51.

118. Han T, Tajar A, Lean M. Obesity and weight management in the elderly. *Br Med Bull*. 2011;97(1):169-196.

119. Benton MJ, Whyte MD, Dyal BW. Sarcopenic obesity: strategies for management. *Am J Nurs*. 2011;111(12):38-44.

120. Lawton MP. The functional assessment of elderly people. *J Am Geriatr Soc*. 1971;19(6):465-481.

121. Unintended Weight Loss (UWL) in Older Adults: Energy Needs. Recommendations Summary. http://andevidencelibrary.com/template.cfm?key=2066&auth=1. Accessed December 7, 2017.

122. Dietary Reference Intakes for energy, carbohydrate, fiber, fat, fatty acids, cholesterol, protein, and amino acids. Washington, DC: Institute of Medicine, 2005.

123. McClave SA, Taylor BE, Martindale RG, et al. Guidelines for the provision and assessment of nutrition support therapy in the adult critically ill patient. *JPEN J Parenter Enteral Nutr.* 2016;40(2):159-211.

124. Chernoff R. Protein and older adults. *J Am Coll Nutr.* 2004;23 (suppl 6):627s-630s.

125. Baum JI, Kim IY, Wolfe RD. Protein consumption and the elderly: what is the optimal level of intake? *Nutrients.* 2016;8(6):359. doi:10.3390/nu8060359.

126. Campbell WW, Johnson CA, McCabe GP, Carnell NS. Dietary protein requirements of younger and older adults. *Am J Clin Nutr.* 2008;88(5):1322-1329.

127. Nowson C, O'Connell S. Protein requirements and recommendations for older people: A review. *Nutrients.* 2015;7(8):6874-6899. doi:10.3390/nu7085311. 566s.

128. Houston DK, Nicklas BJ, Ding J, et al. Dietary protein intake is associated with lean mass change in older, community-dwelling adults: the Health, Aging, and Body Composition (Health ABC) Study. *Am J Clin Nutr.* 2008;87(1):150-155.

129. Cawood AL, Elia M, Stratton RJ. Systematic review and meta-analysis of the effects of high protein oral nutritional supplements. *Aging Res Rev.* 2012;11:278-296.

130. Farsijani S, Payette H, Morais JA, Shatenstein B, Gaudreau P, Chevalier S. Even mealtime distribution of protein intake is associated with greater muscle strength, but not with 3-y physical function decline, in free-living older adults: the Quebec longitudinal study on Nutrition as a Determinant of Successful Aging (NuAge study). *Am J Clin Nutr.*, 2017;106(1):113-124. doi:10.3945/ajcn.116.146555

131. Bauer J, Biolo G, Cederholm T, et al. Evidence-based recommendations for optimal dietary protein intake in older people: a Position Paper From the PROT-AGE Study Group. *J Am Med Dir Assoc.* 2013;14:542-559.

132. Paddon-Jones D, Cambell WW, Jacques PF, et al. Protein and healthy aging. *Am J Clin Nutr.* 2015;101:1339S-1345S

133. Norton C, Toomey C, McCormack WG, et al. Protein supplementation at breakfast and lunch for 24 weeks beyond habitual intakes increases whole-body lean tissue mass in healthy older adults. *J Nutr.* 2016;146(1):65-69. doi: 10.3945/jn.115.219022.

134. Chernoff R. Carbohydrate, fat and fluid requirements in older adults. In: Chernoff R, ed. *Geriatric nutrition.* Sudbury, MA: Jones & Bartlett Publishers, 2006.

135. *Dietary Reference Intakes for water, potassium, sodium, chloride, and sulfate.* Washington, DC: Institute of Medicine, 2005.

136. Blumberg J. Nutritional needs of seniors. *J Am Coll Nutr.* 1997;16(6):517-523.

137. Russell RM. Factors in aging that effect the bioavailability of nutrients. *J Nutr.* 2001;131(suppl 4):1359s-1361s.

138. Kapadia CR. Gastric atrophy, metaplasia, and dysplasia: a clinical perspective. *J Clin Gastroenterol.* 2003;36(suppl 5):S29-36; discussion S61-2.

139. Krasinski SD, Russell RM, Samloff IM, et al. Fundic atrophic gastritis in an elderly population. Effect on hemoglobin and several serum nutritional indicators. *J Am Geriatr Soc.* 1986;34(11):800-806

140. Haller J. The vitamin status and its adequacy in the elderly: an international overview. *Int J Vitam Nutr Res.* 1999;69(3):160-8.

141. Allen LH. How common is vitamin B_{12} deficiency? *Am J Clin Nutr.* 2009;89(2):693s-696s.

142. Andrès E, Affenberger S, Vinzio S, et al. Food-cobalamin malabsorption in elderly patients: clinical manifestations and treatment. *Am J Med.* 2005;118(10):1154-1159.

143. Green R. Is it time for vitamin B_{-12} fortification? What are the questions? *Am J Clin Nutr.* 2009;89(2):712S-716S.

144. Carmel R. Mean corpuscular volume and other concerns in the study of vitamin B_{12} deficiency: epidemiology with pathophysiology. *Am J Clin Nutr.* 2008;87(6):1962-1963.

145. Morris MS, Jacques PF, Rosenberg IH, Selhub J. Folate and vitamin B_{12} status in relation to anemia, macrocytosis, and cognitive impairment in older Americans in the age of folic acid fortification. *Am J Clin Nutr.* 2007;85(1):193-200.

146. Langan RC, Zawistoski KJ. Update on Vitamin B_{12} Deficiency. *Am Fam Phys.* 2011;83(12).

147. Bernstein M. Luggen A. *Nutrition for the older adult.* Sudbury, MA: Jones & Bartlett Learning, 2009.

148. Ferry M Roussel AM. Micronutrient status and cognitive decline in ageing. *Eur Geriatr Med.* 2011;2(1):15-21.

149. Clarke R, Birks J, Nexo E, et al. Low vitamin B_{12} status and risk of cognitive decline in older adults. *Am J Clin Nutr.* 2007;86(5):1384-1391.

150. Eussen SJ, de Groot LC, Joosten LW, et al. Effect of oral vitamin B_{12} with or without folic acid on cognitive function in older people with mild vitamin B_{12} deficiency: a randomized, placebo-controlled trial. *Am J Clin Nutr.* 2006;84(2):361-370.

151. Anderson JL, May HT, Horne BD, et al. Relation of vitamin D deficiency to cardiovascular risk factors, disease status, and incident events in a general healthcare population. *Am J Cardiol.* 2010;106(7):963-968.

152. Pludowski P, Holick MF, Pilz S, et al. Vitamin D effects on musculoskeletal health, immunity, autoimmunity, cardiovascular disease, cancer, fertility, pregnancy, dementia and mortality—a review of recent evidence. *Autoimmun Rev.* 2013;12(10):976-989.

153. Milaneschi Y, Shardell M, Corsi AM, et al. Serum 25-hydroxyvitamin D and depressive symptoms in older women and men. *J Clin Endocrinol Metab.* 2010;95(7):3225-3233.

154. Bischoff-Ferrari HA, Dawson-Hughes B, Willett WC, et al. Effect of Vitamin D on falls: a meta-analysis. *JAMA.* 2004;291(16):1999-2006.

155. Gerdhem P, Ringsberg KA, Obrant KJ, Akesson K. Association between 25-hydroxy vitamin D levels, physical activity, muscle strength and fractures in the prospective population-based OPRA Study of Elderly Women. *Osteoporos Int.* 2005;16(11):1425-1431.

156. Steingrimsdottir L, Gunnarsson O, Indridason OS, Franzson L, Sigurdsson G. Relationship between serum parathyroid hormone levels, vitamin d sufficiency, and calcium intake. *JAMA.* 2005;294(18):2336-2341.

157. Holick MF, Matsuoka LY, Wortsman J. Age, vitamin D, and solar ultraviolet. *Lancet.* 1989;2(8671):1104-1105.

158. Rosen CJ. Clinical practice. Vitamin D insufficiency. *N Engl J Med.* 2011;364(3):248-254.

159. Bullamore JR, Wilkinson R, Gallagher JC, Nordin BEC, Marshall CH. Effect of age on calcium absorption. *Lancet.* 1970;296(7672):535-537.

160. Bailey RL, Dodd KW, Goldman JA, et al. Estimation of total usual calcium and vitamin D intakes in the United States. *J Nutr.* 2010;140(4):817-822.

161. Moe, S.M., Disorders involving calcium, phosphorus, and magnesium. *Prim Care.* 2008;35(2):215-237, v-vi.

162. Xiao Q, Murphy RA, Houston DK, Harris TB, Chow WH, Park Y. Dietary and supplemental calcium intake and cardiovascular disease mortality: the National Institutes of Health–AARP Diet and Health Study. *JAMA Intern Med.* 2013;173(8):639-646.

163. Dorner B. Position of the American Dietetic Association: individualized nutrition approaches for older adults in health care communities. *J Am Diet Assoc.* 2010;110(10):1549-1553.

164. Simmons SF, Keeler E, Zhuo X, Hickey KA, Sato HW, Schnelle JF. Prevention of unintentional weight loss in nursing home residents: a controlled trial of feeding assistance. *J Am Geriatr Soc.* 2008;56(8):1466-73.

165. U.S. Department of Health and Human Services and U.S. Department of Agriculture. *2015–2020 Dietary Guidelines for Americans*. 8th ed. http://health.gov/dietaryguidelines/2015/guidelines/. Published December 2015. Accessed December 7, 2017.
166. Volkert D, Berner YN, Berry E, et al. ESPEN guidelines on enteral nutrition: geriatrics. *Clin Nutr*. 2006;25(2):330-360.
167. Sobotka L, Schneider SM, Berner YN, et al. ESPEN guidelines on parenteral nutrition: geriatrics. *Clin Nutr*. 2009;28(4):461-466.
168. Milne AC, Avenell A, Potter J. Meta-analysis: protein and energy supplementation in older people. *Ann Intern Med*. 2006;144(1):37-48.
169. Avenell A, Handoll HG. Nutritional supplementation for hip fracture aftercare in older people. *Cochrane Database Syst Rev*. 2010; CD001880. doi: 10.1002/14651858.CD001880.pub5.
170. BathP, Bath F, Smithard D. Interventions for dysphagia in acute stroke. *Cochrane Database Syst Rev*. 1999;4.
171. Park R, Allison M, Lang J, et al. Randomised comparison of percutaneous endoscopic gastrostomy and nasogastric tube feeding in patients with persisting neurological dysphagia. *BMJ*. 1992;304(6839):1406.
172. American Geriatrics Society Ethics Committee and Clinical Practice and Models of Care Committee. American Geriatrics Society Feeding Tubes in Advanced Dementia Position Statement. *J Am Geriatr Soc*.2014;62:1590-1593.
173. Singh Bajwa SJ, Kulshrestha A. Current clinical aspects of parenteral nutrition in geriatric patients. *J Med Nutr Nutraceuticals*. 2015;4(1): 22-26. doi:10.4103/2278-019X.146157

Glossary

A.S.P.E.N. American Society for Parenteral and Enteral Nutrition

Abscess Occurs when an area of tissue becomes infected, characterized by swollen tissue and accumulation of pus

Absorption The movement of digested food particles from the external environment and into the cells of the gastrointestinal tract, to be utilized by the body

Acetoacetic acid Ketone produced from the metabolism of fat

Acetone Ketone produced from the metabolism of fat

Acidemia Blood pH lower than 7.35

Acidosis The process that raises the hydrogen ion concentration

Acquired immune deficiency syndrome (AIDS) The endpoint of HIV infection, when the T cell lymphocyte CD4 cell count falls below 200 cells/mm^3 and certain AIDS-defining conditions are present

Activities of daily living (ADLs) Routine activities of daily life that are performed independently, including feeding, moving, toileting, and bathing

Activity energy expenditure The energy expenditure associated with physical activity

Actual body weight (ABW) The unadjusted sum of all body compartments without distinction between fat and fat-free mass

Acute decompensated heart failure A rapid onset of heart failure symptoms that requires immediate treatment

Acute hepatitis Liver inflammation lasting up to 6 months

Acute kidney injury (AKI) A rapid decline in kidney function

Acute liver failure Massive hepatic necrosis with the onset of hepatic encephalopathy and coagulopathy within 6 months of known liver disease

Acute pancreatitis Short-term inflammation of the pancreas, most often the result of a biliary tract obstruction or chronic alcoholism

Acute respiratory distress syndrome (ARDS) A type of hypoxemic respiratory failure characterized by acute development of bilateral lung infiltrates that are visible on chest x-ray, an arterial oxygen tension to fraction of inspired oxygen ratio (PaO_2/FiO_2) less than 300 mm Hg, and a systemic inflammatory response

Acute wounds Injuries that heal through a normal sequence of events, usually between 5 and 10 days, or at least within 30 days

Acute-on-chronic hepatitis Acute symptomatic exacerbations in patients with chronic hepatitis

Acute-phase protein Protein that responds to inflammation caused by illness or trauma

Acute-phase reactants plasma proteins whose synthesis and circulating concentrations are regulated in response to inflammation, inflammation and tissue injury

Adaptation changes in small intestinal structure and function in order to adapt to disease or damage

Adaptive hyperfiltration In cases of reduced nephrons, the remaining functional nephrons take on more pressure from the systemic circulation

Adipose Fat tissue

Adiposity rebound Increases in fat mass that occur during adolescence

Adjustable gastric banding A bariatric surgery procedure that involves placement of a prosthetic band with an adjustable inner diameter around the proximal stomach to restrict food entry, filling the gastric pouch instead

Adjusted body weight Algorithm-derived weight used to determine energy expenditure in patients with extremes of body weight

Adjusted edema-free body weight (aBWef) A calculation of body weight in patients undergoing dialysis with edema who are either obese or underweight

Aerophagia Excessive swallowing of air

Air embolism Embolism caused by the introduction of air into a vessel

Alcoholic hepatitis (AH) Steatohepatitis in alcoholic liver disease

Alcoholic liver disease Liver disease caused by excessive consumption of alcohol

Alkalemia Blood pH higher than 7.45

Alkalosis The process that lowers the hydrogen ion concentration

Allogeneic HSCT Stem cell transplant using donor cells

Allograft transplantation Also known as allotransplantation or allogenic transplantation; a graft of tissue transplanted between individuals of the same species, but of disparate genotype

Alveoli tiny sacs within the lungs that allow oxygen and carbon dioxide to exchange between the respiratory space and the bloodstream

Amenorrhea The absence of three consecutive menstrual cycles

AMPK (adenosine monophosphate-activated protein kinase) An enzyme that increases the transport of glucose into the muscles, upregulates fat oxidation, and reduces insulin resistance and serum levels of inflammatory cytokines

Amylorrhea Starch excretion in the feces

Anastomosis The site at which resected sections of intestine are reattached to each other

Anemia A reduction in erythrocytes per unit of blood volume or a decrease in hemoglobin of blood to below level of physiologic needs

Anemia of inflammation and chronic disease (AICD) Anemia caused by chronic inflammatory or infectious disorders

Anencephaly Absence of portions of the brain, skull, and scalp

Angina Chest pain

Angiogenesis The formation of new blood vessels

Ankyloglossia the result of a short, tight, lingual frenulum causing difficulty in speech articulation due to limitation in tongue movement, also called tongue-tie

Anorexia Partial or complete loss of interest in food

Anorexia nervosa (AN) An eating disorder characterized by an intense fear of weight gain that leads to overrestriction of dietary intake, significantly low body weight, and a distorted self-perception of body weight or shape

Anorexigenic Appetite suppressing

Anthropometrics The measurement of physical characteristics of the human body

Anthropometry The assessment of measures and proportions of the human body

Anticariogenic Prevents plaque from recognizing cariogenic foods

Antidiuretic hormone (ADH) The hormone that controls the amount of urine formed

Antiretroviral treatment (ART) The use of pharmacologic agents that have specific inhibitory effects on HIV replication

Antisepsis prevention of infection by inhibiting growth and multiplication of germs

Anuria The absence of urine formation

Apolipoproteins Protein molecules that are a component of the outer layer of lipoproteins

Appliance The plastic pouch that connects to a colostomy to collect stool

Appropriate-for-gestational-age (AGA) Infants born with weights that chart between the 10th and 90th percentiles for their gestational age

Arginine A conditionally essential amino acid required for cell growth, protein synthesis, and collagen deposition

Arterial blood gases (ABGs) Blood gas values used to assess the lungs' ability to oxygenate blood

Ascites Fluid in the abdomen

Asepsis The absence of bacteria, viruses, or other organs

Aspiration The movement of liquid into the patient's lungs

Asthma A chronic disease where the bronchial tubes of the lungs become inflamed and tighten

Asymmetric macrosomia fetal overgrowth, may be associated with maternal diabetes

Atherosclerosis The hardening and narrowing of arteries due to plaque build-up

Atrophic gastritis Chronic inflammation of the stomach mucosa that is characterized by a partial loss of parietal cell mass

Auscultation The assessment of sounds that reflect movement of fluid or air through organs and viscera using a stethoscope

Autism spectrum disorder A group of disorders that impact behavior, communication, and development

Autograft transplantation Also known as autotransplantation; transplantation of a tissue or an organ from one site onto another one or in the body of the same individual

Autologous HSCT Stem cell transplant from the patient's own bone marrow, peripheral blood, or umbilical cord

Avoidant restrictive food intake disorder (ARFID) A persistent disturbance in eating that leads to significant clinical consequences, such as weight loss, inadequate growth, significant nutrient deficiencies, and/or impaired psychosocial functioning such as an inability to eat with others

Azotemia Nitrogenous waste accumulation in the blood

Azotorrhea Excess nitrogen in the urine or feces

Β-hydroxy-β-methylbutyrate (hmb) A metabolite of leucine that may prevent of delay muscle breakdown, increase cell proliferation and protein synthesis, and improve nitrogen balance

Bariatric surgery Weight-loss surgery

Basal metabolic rate Energy expenditure associated with maintaining the metabolic activities of the body's cells and tissues

Basic metabolic panel Blood test that measures glucose, sodium, potassium, carbon dioxide, chloride, blood urea nitrogen, and creatinine

Beta-hydroxybutyric acid Ketone produced from the metabolism of fat

Biliopancreatic diversion A malabsorptive procedure that prevents absorption by allowing ingested nutrients to mix with bile and pancreatic secretions and to be absorbed in a very small segment of the distal small intestine

Bilirubin Yellow pigment that is produced by the destruction of red blood cells

Binge eating disorder (BED) An eating disorder characterized by recurrent binge eating episodes that are not followed by compensatory purging or nonpurging behaviors

Bioelectrical impedance analysis (BIA) A test of the resistance of a high-frequency, low-amplitude electrical current passed through the body; used to make a distinction between fat-free mass and total body water

Biofilm The colonization of bacteria along a surface

Body cell mass All metabolically active tissue

Body mass index (BMI) An anthropometric comparison of body weight to body height independent of frame size; calculated as weight in kilograms divided by the square of height in meters

Bolus a ball of food or single dose of liquid or medication

Bolus feeding A specific volume of feeding is delivered for a specific time interval for a short period of time

Braden Scale for Predicting Pressure Sore Risk A multifactorial scale for predicting the risk of ulcer development; includes sensory perception, moisture, activity, mobility, friction and shear, and nutrition

Brain death Irreversible cessation of all brain activity

Branched chain amino acids (BCAA) Amino acids, including leucine, isoleucine, and valine, that account for 40% of the essential amino acids and are primarily catabolized by skeletal muscle

Bronchi Large air passages that lead from the trachea to the lungs

Bronchioles Small branches in which the bronchus divides

Bronchodilators Oral and inhaled medications used to open up constricted passageways and improve breathing

Brush border Microvilli covered surface of epithelial cells found in certain locations such as the gastrointestinal tract

Bulimia nervosa (BN) An eating disorder characterized by recurrent episodes of binge eating followed by one or more compensatory behaviors to avoid weight gain

Cachexia General wasting and malnutrition usually associated with chronic disease

Cancer cachexia A multifactorial syndrome characterized by an ongoing loss of skeletal muscle mass in cancer patients that cannot be fully reversed by conventional nutritional support

Cardiac cachexia An uncontrollable loss of weight in heart failure patients

Cardiac output A measure of blood pumped per minute that is calculated by multiplying the stroke volume by the heart rate

Cardiogenic shock A severe, life-threatening condition of systemic hypoperfusion

Cardiopulmonary bypass A technique that temporarily takes place of the function of the heart and lungs

Cariogenic Caries promoting

Cariogenicity The caries-promoting properties of a diet or food

Cariostatic Not contributing to decay

Catabolic stress response Significant alterations in physiology, immune function, and metabolism in response to injury, propagated by inflammatory mediators

Catabolism Breakdown of body tissues for energy in response to lack of other energy sources

Catch-up growth Nutritional requirements necessary to achieve ideal body weight

Catecholamines Neurotransmitters that mediate the aberrations seen in cell function and physiology; include epinephrine and norepinephrine

Catheter embolism Embolism caused by a fragment of a broken or damaged catheter

Catheter occlusion The inability to infuse, flush, and/or aspirate on the venous access device

Catheter tip The end of a thin medical tube that is at the site of insertion prone to infection

Catheter-related bloodstream infection (CRBSI) Systemic infection that enters the body via the catheter or insertion site; see central line–associated bloodstream infection (CLABSI)

Catheter-related complications (CRCs) Mechanical (infectious or noninfectious) or metabolic complications of catheter use

Catheter-related venous thrombosis (CRVT) The creation of a thrombus as platelets and fibrin coagulate in a vessel damaged by catheter insertion

CD4 cell count The CD4 T-cell test; a count of the number of T lymphocyte CD4 cells

CDC growth charts Growth charts utilizing data on the growth rates of infants from the United States, starting at age 3 months

Celiac disease An autoimmunue disorder characterized by inflammatory injury to the intestinal mucosa following gluten ingestion

Central line–associated bloodstream infection (CLABSI) Systemic infection that enters the body via the catheter or insertion site; see catheter-related bloodstream infection (CRBSI)

Central parenteral nutrition Nutrition delivered via access to a central vessel, namely the superior or inferior vena cava or the right atrium

Cephalic phase of digestion The first phase of digestion; the point at which the brain sends a signal through the vagus nerve to the stomach, triggering the production of gastric juices

CF transmembrane conductance regulator (CFTR) protein A protein that functions as a channel across the membrane of cells producing mucus, sweat, saliva, tears, and digestive enzymes

CF-related diabetes (CFRD) A type of diabetes found in persons with cystic fibrosis; while it shares similarities with both type 1 and type 2 diabetes, it is its own separate type

Chemotherapy The use of antineoplastic drugs, used as a single agent or in combination with other agents, that disrupt the reproductive cycle of cancer cells

Chiari II malformation An extension of the cerebellar and brain stem tissue into the foramen magnum, with the cerebellar vermis (which connects the two halves of the cerebellum) appearing as incomplete or damaged

Child Pugh classification System used to classify the severity of liver disease and predict patient prognosis

Childhood obesity A condition where a child is significantly overweight for his or her age and height

Cholelithiasis Gallstones

Cholestasis Reduced bile flow

Cholestatic liver disease Liver disease caused by inhibition of bile flow

Chronic hepatitis Liver inflammation lasting greater than 6 months

Chronic inflammation An immune response of the body to ongoing HIV infection

Chronic kidney disease (CKD) A decline in kidney function over time

Chronic obstructive pulmonary disease (COPD) A progressive, systemic disease marked by airflow obstruction; generally encompasses chronic bronchitis, emphysema, and small airways disease

Chronic pancreatitis Long-term, progressive inflammation of the pancreas, leading to loss of exocrine and endocrine function

Chronic wounds Injuries that persist longer than 6 weeks or frequently reoccur and are typically associated with underlying conditions that lead to tissue breakdown, inadequate tissue perfusion, and chronic inflammation

Chylomicrons Spherical vesicles that are part of the class of lipoproteins consisting of a triglyceride core surrounded by apoproteins and cholesterol

Chyme Partially digested food that passes from the stomach to the small intestine

Cilia Hair-like structures within the lungs that normally remove bacteria

Cirrhosis The final stage of liver fibrosis, in which fibrotic tissues form nodules that permanently alter the structure of the liver

Closed tube feeding system A ready-to-use container or bag of formula is connected to the patient's feeding access

Coagulopathy Any condition in which the blood's ability to clot is compromised

Cognitive behavioral therapy (CBT) A highly structured therapy that identifies and replaces maladaptive behaviors and cognitive processes with more suitable ones

Collagen The most abundant protein in the human body; the primary component of the extracellular matrix

Colostomy Removal of the rectum and connecting a portion of the colon as the stoma

Colostrum The first breast milk produced

Complete blood count Blood test that provides a count of the cells in the blood and a description of red blood cells

Comprehensive metabolic panel Blood test that measures all the elements in a basic metabolic panel, plus albumin, total protein, alkaline phophatase, alanine transaminase, aspartate transaminase, and bilirubin

Computed tomography (CT) An imaging modality that utilizes x-ray technology to provide quantitative data on muscle composition and distribution

Continuous ambulatory peritoneal dialysis (CAPD) A form of peritoneal dialysis that requires three to five exchanges daily

Continuous cycling peritoneal dialysis (CCPD) A form of peritoneal dialysis that uses a machine to carry out the exchanges overnight while the patient sleeps

Continuous feeding A slow drip of feedings into the stomach or small intestine on an hourly basis

Continuous infusion Infusion performed for over 24 hours

Continuous renal replacement therapy (CRRT) A type of dialysis utilizing hemofiltration, hemodialysis, or both

Coronary angioplasty See percutaneous coronary intervention (PCI)

Coronary artery bypass graft Surgical procedure in which arterial stenosis is bypassed with the placement of an artificial or saphenous vein graft

Coronary artery disease Atherosclerosis affecting the arteries that supply blood to the heart

Cortisol A glucocorticoid produced by the adrenal cortex, promotes gluconeogenesis and inhibits protein synthesis and inflammation

Counter-regulatory hormones Hormones that oppose the effects of insulin such as glucagon, cortisol, epinephrine, and norepinephrine

Craniorachischisis The most severe type of neural tube defect, in which both the brain and spinal cord remain open

Creatinine height index (CHI) Measurement of creatinine excretion as a percentage

Crohn's disease A form of inflammatory bowel disease characterized by transmural inflammation that can affect any organ of the gastrointestinal tract from mouth to anus

Cross-contamination The passage of pathogens indirectly from one source to another due to the improper use of sterilization procedures, unclean instruments, or recycling of products

Cyanosis Bluish coloring of the skin from a lack of oxygen

Cyclical infusion Infusion performed for 10 to 12 hours per day

Cytokines Cell-signaling molecules that aid in cell-to-cell communication in immune responses and stimulate the movement of cells towards sites of inflammation, infection, and trauma

De ritis ratio The serum AST to ALT ratio

Debridement The removal of dead or damaged tissue

Decompensated cirrhosis See end-stage liver disease (ESLD)

Defined diets Dietary regimens based on an underlying theory or ideology of how food interacts with the body

Delayed gastric emptying A slowing of the movement of food through the gastrointestinal system

Delayed onset lactation Milk production does not begin within 72 hours postpartum

Demineralization The chemical process by which minerals are removed from the teeth

Dental caries Cavities

Dentin The bony tissue forming the bulk of tooth beneath the enamel

Developmental disability A condition that becomes evident at birth or early childhood and has varying impacts on the individual throughout the life cycle

Diabetes distress The intense stress related to the experience of living with diabetes

Diabetic ketoacidosis A condition where excessive ketone bodies cause the blood pH to drop to dangerous levels; can quickly lead to death

Dialectical behavioral therapy (DBT) Therapy that is designed to help individuals change unhelpful patterns of behavior by identifying triggers and applying new coping skills

Diastole Stage of the heartbeat where ventricles are relaxed and blood flows from the atria to refill the ventricles

Diastolic blood pressure The force that pushes against the blood vessels when the heart is at rest

Diet-induced thermogenesis The production of heat associated with the digestion and metabolism of food

Differential count A complete blood count for white blood cells

Digestion The mechanical or enzymatic breakdown of food into its constituents

Digestive enzymes Enzymes that act on the carbohydrates, protein, and lipids contained in food, reducing food into forms the body is capable of utilizing

Digital clubbing Focal enlargement of the terminal ends of the fingers

Direct calorimetry Direct measurement of heat produced or lost

Disaccharide Sugar made up of two monosaccharides

Diverticulosis The accumulation of pouches in the colon

Donation after cardiac death (DCD) Donation of organs after a patient is deceased by means of cardiac death

Doubly labeled water A form of indirect calorimetry based on the assumption of an exponential disappearance of hydrogen and oxygen isotopes from the body

Drug-induced hepatitis Damage to the liver caused by hepatotoxic drugs, chemicals, and supplements

Dry weight An estimated weight in patients with fluid overload (from edema, overhydration, ascites, etc.); determined by subtracting the estimated fluid weight from the actual body weight

Dual energy x-ray absorptiometry (DEXA) A scan used to differentiate bone, lean mass, and bone-free tissues; often used for measuring bone density

Dumping syndrome A range of symptoms that occur when stomach contents are released too quickly and in too large of a volume into the small intestine

Duodenum The proximal portion of the small intestine

Dysgeusia Altered taste perception

Dyslipidemia Alterations in the normal transport of lipids and lipoproteins

Dysphagia Difficulty swallowing

Dyspnea Difficulty breathing

Early childhood carries (ECC) The presence of at least one decayed tooth, a missing tooth, or a tooth surface that has been filled in any primary tooth in a child 6 years or younger

Early enteral nutrition (EEN) The initiation of enteral nutrition within 48 hours of illness or traumatic event

Early-onset preeclampsia Preeclampsia with an onset between 20 and 32 weeks of gestation

Eating disorder (ED) A psychiatric illness characterized by chronic disturbances of eating habits and weight control behaviors that debilitate both physical health and psychological functioning

Eclampsia Severest form of pregnancy induced hypertension, characterized by covulsions, seizure, proteinuria and edema

Edentulism Tooth loss

Ejection fraction The amount of blood being pumped out of the ventricle each time it contracts

Electrocardiogram Diagnostic tool used to measure the heart's electrical activity by placing electrodes on the body surface

Electrolytes Substances that dissolve into ions in solution

Elemental formula A nutritional formula that provides nutrients in predigested forms that are thought to be absorbed within the first few feet of the small intestine

Elimination diet Systematically removing elements of a diet to determine what foods are contributing to symptoms, with the end goal of eliminating offending foods and reintroducing "safe" foods

Embolism A blood clot that breaks free and travels to another area of the body

Enamel The hard mineralized surface of teeth

Enamel hypolpasia An enamel deficiency that increases tooth vulnerability to damage

End-stage liver disease (ESLD) A condition in which the body is unable to make up for the functional deterioration of the liver, resulting in life-threatening complications

End-stage renal disease (ESRD) The most advanced form of chronic kidney disease; also known as Stage 5 kidney disease

Endotoxin Lipopolysaccharide; a toxin produced by gram-negative bacteria

Engorgement Distention of a body part with fluid or other material

Enteral nutrition (EN) The delivery of nutrients into the gastrointestinal tract either by mouth or through a feeding tube

Enterocytes Intestinal absorptive cells

Epicardial fat A fat deposit that surrounds the heart and is enclosed by the viscera pericardium

Epinephrine A hormone produced by the adrenal medulla that aids in the regulation of the sympathetic branch of the autonomic nervous system

Erythropoietin (EPO) The hormone that promotes red blood cell production in bone marrow upon detection of low oxygen levels

Erythropoietin stimulating agent (ESA) Medications that increase production of red blood cells to combat anemia

ESPEN European Society for Parental and Enteral Nutrition

Estimated glomerular filtration rate (eGFR) An estimate of the amount of plasma filtered through the glomeruli within a given period, calculated through the use of various formulas

Euglycemia Normal blood sugar levels in the blood

Exit site The point where the catheter exits the body

Extracellular mass The structural proteins of the body, including skeleton, fascia, cartilage, dermis, and extracellular water

Extravasation Leakage of fluids from an intravenous line into the surrounding tissue

Extremely low birth weight (ELBW) Infants born weighing less than 1,000 grams

Failure to thrive A condition of pediatric malnutrition, often identified within the first 3 years of a child's life

Familial hypercholesterolemia A genetic disorder caused by defective LDL-C receptors that leads to LDL-C levels greater than the 95th percentile for age and gender

Fat lipolysis The hydrolosis (or splitting up) of lipid

Fat oxidation The production of energy from fatty acids

Feeding cues A baby's ability to signal hunger and fullness through signs such as cryting, sucking fingers or fists

Female athlete triad A syndrome comprising disordered eating habits, osteoporosis, and menstrual disorders, often seen in female athletes who utilize at least one unhealthy weight control method

Fetal alcohol syndrome A range of conditions, including irreversible brain damage and growth problems, caused by excessive alcohol consumption during pregnancy

Fetal macrosomia A newborn that is significantly larger than normal

Fibroblast growth factor 23 (FGF23) A hormone produced by bone that acts in the kidney to regulate phosphorus and vitamin D metabolism

Fibrosis A buildup of connective tissue or scar tissue

Fibrostenosis Narrowing of the bowels

Fistula An abnormal tunnel-like connection between the hollow space of an organ and the body

Fluorapatite A crystalline structure that is a naturally occurring form of calcium, phosphorus, and fluoride; it is more resistant than hydroxyapatite

Fluoride A natural element that is important to the integrity of bone and teeth

Fluoroscopic nasoenteric tube placement Using x-ray imaging as a guide when placing the feeding tube from the nose to the stomach or small intestine

Fluorosis Defective tooth mineralization resulting from excessive fluoride ingestion during pre-eruptive tooth mineralization

Foam cells Cells that are laden with fat and macrophages, often the hallmarks of atherosclerotic lesion formation

Food frequency questionnaire (FFQ) A retrospective tool that requires the client to complete a survey about food intake over a specific period of time in an attempt to depict "usual" intake

Food insecurity Anxiety and uncertainty about one's food supply, along with insufficient food intake with or without physical hunger

Food records diary A method of acquiring data on nutritional intake; requires the client to record food intake for a specific time period

Forced expiratory volume (FEV$_1$) The amount of air a person can exhale during forced breathing

Foremilk The first milk released during a feeding

Frailty A geriatric syndrome characterized by age-related declines in multiple organ systems due to the cumulative effects of disease, inactivity, stress, poor nutritional intake, altered physiology, and impaired homeostatic reserve

Fulminant liver failure Liver failure that occurs within 8 weeks of the onset of known liver disease

Functional assay Laboratory test that measures the specific biochemical or physiological functioning of a nutrient, rather than just the quantity of the nutrient

Galactosemia A rare genetically inherited metabolic disorder associated with the inability to metabolize the sugar galactose properly

Gastrectomy Surgical removal of part or all of the stomach

Gastric residual The volume of liquid that remains in the stomach during enteral feeding

Gastric stasis Delayed gastric emptying as a result of the elimination of vagus innervation

Gastroesophageal reflux disease (GERD) A digestive disorder in which the lower esophageal sphincter is relaxed or weakened and remains open, allowing reflux of gastric acid into the esophagus

Gastroparesis Delayed gastric emptying in the absence of a mechanical gastric outlet obstruction

Geophagia Eating dirt

Geriatric nutrition Medical nutrition therapy for older adults

Gestation The time between conception and birth

Gestational diabetes mellitus (GDM) Increased glucose intolerance that is first discovered during the second or third trimester

Gestational hypertension Systolic blood pressure equal to or greater than 140 mm Hg or a diastolic blood pressure equal to or greater than 90 mm Hg that occurs without proteinuria after 20 weeks' gestation

Ghrelin Appetite-inducing gastrointestinal hormone that increases gastrointestinal motility and decreases insulin secretion

Gingiva Gums

Glomerular filtration rate (GFR) The amount of plasma filtered through the glomeruli within a given period

Glomerulus A mass of capillaries that are specifically responsible for producing the ultrafiltrate

Glucagon A hormone produced by the pancreas that works with other hormones to control glucose

Gluconeogenesis Synthesis of glucose from noncarbohydrate sources, usually amino acids

Glucose infusion rate (GIR) A function of the concentration of dextrose and the rate at which the dextrose is administered

Glucose oxidation The aerobic breakdown of glucose for the formation of ATP

Glutamine The most abundant amino acid in the plasma; necessary for protein synthesis, lymphocyte proliferation, and wound healing

Glutamine synthetase The enzyme that removes ammonia from the blood to combine with glutamate to make glutamine

Gluten-free diet A diet that completely avoids dietary gluten

Glycemic index The quantity and rate at which different carbohydrate foods influence blood glucose response

Glycemic load The digestibility rate of foods balanced against the amount of carbohydrate they contain

Glycogenolysis Breakdown of glycogen stores for glucose

Graft Any tissue or organ used for implantation or transplantation

Graft thrombosis Obstruction of blood flow to a graft

Graft versus host disease (GVHD) An immune response designed to eliminate the foreign tissue in the recipient of a allogeneic HSCT, wherein the donor's cells recognize the host's cells are foreign

Granulomas A collection of monocytes and/or macrophages and other inflammatory cells with or without giant cells

Gravida The number of times a female has been pregnant

Growth An increase in physical size or mass of body tissues that occurs from infancy to adulthood

Growth channels Describes growth on or between growth percentiles

Growth charts Data that describe the normal or expected amount of growth based on well-child data

Growth reference Charts that describe growth in a specific time or place

Growth standards Charts that demonstrate optimal growth or how normal children should grow when breastfed

Growth velocity The rate at which a child grows

Gut-liver axis The intricate relationship between the liver and intestines

Half arm span (HAS) The length between the middle of the sternal notch and tip of the middle finger; measured with the patient's arm horizontal and in line with the shoulders; also known as arm length

Handgrip dynamometer A tool used to test handgrip strength

Handgrip strength An assessment of muscle strength used to estimate nutritional status

Hang time The amount of time an enteral formula can safely be at room temperature

Head circumference A measure of head size, taken around the most prominent area on the back of the head, immediately above the supraorbital ridge, to just above the patient's eyebrows

Height Also known as stature; how tall a person is

Height-for-age The plotting of a child's height according to the distribution of height for children of the same age and gender on a growth chart

Helicobacter pylori A bacterial infection that colonizes the stomach by moving through the mucosal lining, attaching to gastric epithelial cells, and sending out cytotoxins to allow for generation of more bacteria

HELLP syndrome A variant of severe preeclampsia characterized by hemolysis, elevated liver enzymes, and low platelet count

Hematemesis The vomiting of blood

Hematopoietic stem cell transplant (HSCT) The infusion of stem cells to treat patients whose bone marrow or immune system is defective or damaged, such as in hematological cancers

Hemochromatosis An autosomal recessive disease characterized by accumulation of iron in the liver, pancreas, heart, adrenals, testes, pituitary, and kidneys

Hemoconcentration Increased red blood cell concentrations and low plasma levels

Hemodialysis (HD) Medical treatment in which blood is removed from the body and processed through a machine containing a dialysis membrane, which acts as an artificial kidney

Hemodilution Decreased red blood cell concentrations and high plasma levels

Hemodynamic instability Inadequate organ and tissue perfusion throughout the body; characterized by hypotension

Hepatic encephalopathy (HE) A neuropsychiatric disorder characterized by personality changes, altered levels of consciousness, and cognitive impairment

Hepatic steatosis The accumulation of fat in the liver

Hepatocellular liver disease Liver disease caused by liver cell injury

Hepatorenal syndrome (HRS) Progressive kidney failure among people with liver disease

High biological value (HBV) Containing all essential amino acids and readily available protein

Hindmilk The last milk released during a feeding

Hirschsprung disease A blockage of the large intestine that is a result of missing nerves in the bowel that function to move material through

HIV wasting syndrome Weight loss of at least 10% of body weight in HIV-positive persons, with symptoms of chronic fever, weakness, or diarrhea in the absence of other related illnesses that could contribute to the weight loss

Home parenteral nutrition (HPN) Parenteral nutrition provided in the home, as opposed to a hospital or other healthcare institution

Host In organ transplantation, the recipient of the organ or tissue

Hydroxyapatite A crystalline structure that is a naturally occurring form of calcium and phosphorus

Hypercalcemia High calcium levels in the blood

Hypercapnia Increased carbon dioxide in the blood

Hyperchloremia High chlorine levels in the blood

Hyperemesis gravidarum (HG) Persistent nausea and vomiting resulting in dehydration, muscle wasting, electrolyte imbalances, ketonuria, nutritional deficiencies, and weight loss of greater than 5% of pre-pregnancy weight

Hyperglycemia High blood sugar levels

Hyperkalemia High potassium levels in the blood

Hypermagnesemia High magnesium levels in the blood

Hypermetabolism The physiological state of increased rate of metabolic activity characterized by an abnormal increase in the body's basal metabolic rate

Hypernatremia High sodium levels in the blood

Hyperphagia Insatiable hunger

Hyperphosphatemia High phosphate levels in the blood

Hypertension Chronic high blood pressure

Hypertonic Having a greater osmolarity than another solution

Hypervolemia Volume overload

Hypocalcemia Low calcium levels in the blood

Hypochloremia Low chlorine levels in the blood

Hypoglycemia Low blood sugar levels

Hypokalemia Low potassium levels in the blood

Hypomagnesemia Low magnesium levels in the blood

Hyponatremia Low sodium levels in the blood

Hypophosphatemia Low phosphate levels in the blood

Hypotonic Having a lower osmolarity than another solution

Hypovolemia Volume depletion

Hypoxemia Low blood oxygen

Ideal body weight (IBW) An adjusted weight-for-height, based on the weights associated with the lowest mortality for a given height

Ileal brake The delay of gastric emptying and slowing of transit time in the proximal portions of the small intestine, allowing extended contact time between nutrients and the mucosa

Ileocecal (IC) valve The valve that separates the ileum of the small intestine from the cecum of the large intestine

Ileostomy Removal of the colon and the rectum and connecting the distal end of the ileum as the stoma

Ileum The distal portion of the small intestine

Immunonutrition The effect of nutrients, including macronutrients, vitamins, minerals, and trace elements, on inflammation, the formation of antibodies, and the resistance to disease

Immunosenescence The gradual deterioration of the immune system that occurs with aging

Immunosuppression Suppression of the immune response by drugs or radiation

Indirect calorimetry Measure of respiratory gas exchange

Inflammation The body's initial response to injury; characterized by redness, warmth, swelling, pain, and loss of function; the first phase of wound healing

Inflammatory bowel disease A group of chronic, relapsing-remitting immune disorders that originate in the gastrointestinal tract

Inflammatory response A complex series of metabolic and physiologic changes that take place following major trauma, disease, sepsis, or surgery

Insensible water loss The loss of water through the skin and respiration

Inspection The visual observation of color, shape, texture, and size

Instrumental activities of daily living (IADLs) Activities that are not required for daily functioning, but are necessary for independent living, such as shopping, food preparation, managing finances, and using the telephone

Insulin resistance The inability of cells to uptake insulin for use in glucose metabolism

Insulin to carbohydrate ratio The amount of carbohydrate processed by one unit of insulin

Intake and output A way of monitoring fluid balance and condition of a patient, includes intake by mouth, feeding tubes, intravenous lines and output primarily through urine, and gastric sections

Intermittent feeding Feeding is delivered over a 20- to 60-minute interval, four to six times per day

Intestinal failure The inability to maintain nutritional autonomy

Intestinal leakage The release of digestive contents into the peritoneum via a hole in the stomach, gallbladder, or small or large intestines

Intra-aortic balloon pump A surgical procedure that provides short-term mechanical support to increase cardiac output via a balloon placed in the aorta via the femoral artery

Intradialytic parenteral nutrition (IDPN) Parenteral nutrition provided via hemodialysis tubing during each hemodialysis treatment

Intramyocellular lipid deposition A condition where macrovescular fat accumulates in hepatocytes, resulting in the enlargement of the liver

Intrauterine growth restriction (IUGR) The condition in which the fetus is unable to grow and develop normally, putting it at high risk of serious consequences after birth

Intravenous Access via a vein, directly to the bloodstream

Intrinsic AKI Kidney injury caused by diseases within the renal parenchyma

Intrinsic factor A glycoprotein produced by the parietal cells of the stomach essential for B_{12} absorption

Involution The final state of mammary gland development, in which the mammnary glands return to their pre-pregnancy state

Iron-deficiency anemia Anemia caused by a lack of iron in the blood

Irritable bowel syndrome A functional gastrointestinal disorder characterized by recurrent abdominal pain and altered bowel habits

Ischemic cardiomyopathy A type of heart failure in which the left ventricle is enlarged because of decreased blood supply to the heart muscle

Ischemic heart disease See coronary artery disease

Isolate Intact, natural form of protein

Isotonic Having the same osmolarity as another solution

Jejunostomy Connecting the distal jejunum as the stoma

Jejunum The middle portion of the small intestine

Kayser-Fleischer ring A brownish or gray-green ring at the rim of the cornea

Kidney Disease Improving Global Outcomes (KDIGO) A group of nephrology experts that provides a source of consolidated, evidence-based clinical practice guidelines to be used in all aspects of kidney disease

Kinetic modeling The method used in hemodialysis to evaluate the effectiveness of dialysis in removing urea from the blood during treatment

Knee-height A measurement taken from the sole of the foot to the anterior surface of the thigh while the lower limb is flexed; used to estimate standing height in nonambulatory patients

Kupffer cells Macrophages dedicated to the liver

Kussmaul's respirations Abnormally deep breathing associated with metabolic acidosis

Kwashiorkor Malnutrition, with or without caloric depletion, that results in depletion of visceral protein

Lactation Secretion of milk from the breasts

Lactogenesis The process of converting inert breast cells to milk-producing cells

Lanugo Soft, downy hair growth on the face and body

Laparoscopic adjustable gastric band (LAGB) Bariatric procedure that physically restricts the stomach by use of an inflatable band that, when filled with saline, squeezes and decreases the size of the stomach

Laparoscopy Using small ports placed on the abdominal wall so that the peritoneal cavity can be accessed

Large-for-gestational-age (LGA) Infants with birth weights that chart above the 90th percentile for their gestational age

Late-onset preeclampsia Preeclampsia with an onset after 34 weeks of gestation

Leaky gut Increased intestinal permeability

Lean body mass The combination of extracellular mass and body cell mass

Left ventricular assist device A surgically implanted mechanical pump that supports heart function by pumping blood from the left ventricle to the aorta to circulate oxygen-rich blood throughout the body

Left ventricular hypertrophy A disease in which the muscle of the left ventricle becomes thickened and enlarged

Leptin A hormone produced by white adipose tissue that inhibits appetite

Let down The release of breast milk

Lipodystrophy A syndrome that includes body fat redistribution and/or metabolic abnormalities

Lipomeningocele A type of closed neural tube defect characterized by deposition of fatty tissue tumors

Lipoproteins Molecules responsible for the transport and delivery of fatty acids

Long-chain triglycerides A chain of fatty acids 14 carbons or more

Low birth weight (LBW) Infants born weighing less than 2,500 grams

Low FODMAP diet A diet low in short-chain carbohydrates (fermentable oligo-, di-, and monosaccharides and polyols)

Macrocytic anemia Large cell anemia; defined as a mean corpuscular volume of greater than 100 fL

Magnetic resonance imaging (MRI) An imaging modality utilizing what is referred to as a free-ionizing radiation technique

Malabsorption The result of defective mucosal uptake or transport of inadequately digested nutrients

Malassimilation The combination of maldigestion and malabsorption

Maldigestion Failure of the enzymatic processes of digestion

Mallory-Weiss tears Tears in the mucosa at the stomach–esophagus junction

Malnutrition A subacute or chronic state of nutrition, in which a combination of varying degrees of overnutrition or undernutrition and inflammatory activity has led to a change in body composition and diminished function

Malnutrition Screening Tool (MST) A nutrition screen tool that was created based on the need for a framework that used routinely available data, was noninvasive and convenient for nondietetics staff, and could be employed across a heterogeneous adult population

Malnutrition Universal Screening Tool (MUST) A nutrition screen tool that utilizes a simple five-step process to arrive at an overall score for risk of malnutrition —either low, medium, or high risk

Marasmus Malnutrition associated with severe caloric depletion, in which the body conserves visceral protein levels

Masticatory function The process of chewing

Mastitis Inflammation of breast tissue

Maternal preeclampsia Preeclampsia in women with a normal placenta, but with low-grade inflammation secondary to obesity, hypertension, or diabetes

Mature milk The final stage of breast milk produced, starting from 2 to 4 weeks postpartum until the end of breastfeeding

Maudsley approach A family-based treatment for eating disorders in adolescents, based on empowering parents to take on the responsibility of restoring weight to their child

Mean arterial pressure The average pressure that pushes blood through the arteries during a cardiac cycle

Medium-chain triglyceride A chain of fatty acids 6-12 carbons long

Melena Dark tarry stools associated with upper gastrointestinal bleeding

Metabolic acidosis A disorder characterized by a low pH, a low HCO_3^- concentration, and a compensatory hyperventilation that contributes to a decreased $PaCO_2$

Metabolic alkalosis A disorder characterized by a high pH, a high bicarbonate concentration, and compensatory hypoventilation that contribute to an increased $PaCO_2$

Metabolic syndrome A syndrome in which an individual has three or more of the following metabolic risk factors: large waist circumference, high systolic or diastolic blood pressure, high fasting glucose and triglyceride levels, and low high-density lipoprotein cholesterol

Metallothionein A protein that binds to copper absorbed into the enterocyte, preventing its absorption

Micelles A combination of digested lipids, phospholipids, and bile acids formed during normal fat absorption

Microalbuminuria The loss of protein in the urine

Microcytic anemia Small cell anemia; defined as a mean corpuscular volume of less than 80 fL

Mid-arm muscle circumference (MAMC) A surrogate measure of lean body mass; cannot be measured directly, but can be estimated using mid-upper arm circumference and triceps skinfold data

Mid-parental height A child's projected adult height based on the height of his or her parents

Mid-upper arm circumference (MUAC) A measure of total arm circumference that provides a measure of both muscle and fat area

Migrating motor complex The source of peristaltic motion in the small intestine

Milk stasis A stoppage in milk flow from the breasts during feeding

Mini Nutritional Assessment (MNA) Screening tool used to assess nutritional status in the geriatric population

Miroablbuminuria Low albumin output; greater than 30 mg but less than 300 mg daily of albumin in the urine

Monosaccharide Simple sugar

Mucolytics Medications that help mobilize mucus and decrease sputum thickness

Myelomeningocele The most common form of spina bifida, in which there is an incompletely fused spine, from which there is a protrusion of the spinal cord, including nerves

Myocardial infarction A blockage in one or more of the arteries that supply blood to the heart; also known as a heart attack

Myocardium Middle layer of the heart

Myocytes Heart cells

Nasoduodenal tube A tube that is placed from the nose, through the stomach, to the duodenum of the small intestine

Nasoenteric See nasogastric

Nasogastric Going through the nose to the stomach

Nasogastric tube A tube that is entered through the nose or mouth and is placed directly to the stomach

Nasojejunal Going through the nose to the jejunum

Nasojejunal tube A tube that is placed from the nose and advanced to the jejunum of the small intestine

Nausea and vomiting of pregnancy (NVP) Nausea and vomiting that is common and typical during the early stages of pregnancy

Nebulizers Medical equipment that utilizes pressurized oxygen to turn liquid medication into a mist for inhalation

Necrotizing enterocolitis A condition in which damaged intestinal tissue causes bloating and diarrhea

Negative acute-phase protein Proteins that decrease during inflammation, such as serum albumin, prealbumin, retinal binding protein, and transferrin

Nephrons The functional units of the kidney

Nephropathy Damage to the kidneys due to diabetes

Nephrotic syndrome A loss of protein through the glomerular membrane

Net secretory response The excretion of more water and sodium than can be ingested

Neural tube A hollow tube that houses the brain, spinal cord, and other neural tissue and eventually differentiates into the respective organs of the central nervous system

Neural tube defect A condition in which the neural tube closes prior to full development, resulting in birth defects

Neurogenic bladder Patients are unable to perceive bladder fullness and lack coordination between contraction and relaxation

Neurogenic bowel Decreased bowel motility leading to constipation

Neuropathy Damage to the nerves

Neutropenia An abnormally low level of neutrophils in the blood

New-onset diabetes after transplant (NODAT) The development of diabetes in a patient who was not diabetic prior to organ transplantation surgery

Night eating syndrome (NES) A disordered eating pattern characterized by morning anorexia and evening hyperphagia and insomnia

Nissen Fundoplication A procedure where the top portion of the stomach is wrapped around the lower esophagus to improve the integrity of the lower esophageal sphincter and reduce reflux

Nitrogen balance Where nitrogen intake (oral, enteral, or parenteral) is equal to nitrogen excretion (urinary, fecal, or wound drainage)

Nitrogenous waste The end products of protein metabolism (urea, creatinine, and ammonia)

Non-celiac gluten sensitivity (NCGS) Gastrointestinal symptoms without inflammation of the gut after consumption of gluten

Nonalcoholic fatty liver disease (NAFLD) Hepatic steatosis from a cause other than alcohol

Nonalcoholic steatohepatitis (NASH) The next stage of liver disease after nonalcoholic fatty liver disease

Nonorganic FTT Failure to thrive not related to an underlying medical condition

Norepinephrine A chemical in the catecholamine family released from the sympathetic nerve fibers and functions as a hormone and neurotransmitter

Normalized PNA (nPNA) PNA normalized to a function of body weight

Normalized protein catabolic rate (nPCR) A clinical tool used to measure the net protein degradation and protein intake in dialysis patients

Normocytic anemia Normal cell anemia; defined as a mean corpuscular volume between 80 and 99 fL

NPO Nil per os; nothing by mouth

Nutrigenomics The study of how genes and nutrients interact

Nutrition assessment The process of evaluating several different components to determine nutritional risk and status, diagnose malnutrition if it exists, identify problems that need intervention, and establish a plan of care

Nutrition Care Process and Model (NCPM) A systematic framework to recognize, diagnose, and intervene upon nutrition-related problems for which a nutrition intervention is the primary treatment

Nutrition Care Process Terminology (NCPT) Standardized terminology used as part of the Nutrition Care Process and Model

Nutrition impact symptoms Nutrition-related side effects of disease

Nutrition screening The process of identifying patients, clients, or groups who may have a nutrition diagnosis and benefit from nutrition assessment intervention by a registered dietitian

Nutrition-focused physical exam (NFPE) A system-based examination of each region of the body that aids in the evaluation of nutrition status by identifying markers of malnutrition and/or nutrient deficiencies

Nutritional Risk Screening (NRS-2002) A nutrition screening tool that measures disease impact in addition to the markers of current or potential malnutrition

Obesity A medical condition in which an individual has excess body fat for a given height

Obesity paradox The protective effect of elevated body mass index in patients with heart failure

Oligosaccharides Carbohydrates made up of monosaccharides (more than two)

Oliguria Low urine volume

Open tube feeding system Formula from a can or package is poured into a separate container that is then attached to the patient's feeding access point

Open tube placement Placement of a gastrostomy tube in which a small incision is made on the abdomen so that the gastrostomy tube can enter

Opportunistic infections Secondary infections that occur in cases of diminished immune system response

Oral rehydration solutions Dilute glucose-water mixtures containing electrolytes

Orexigenic Appetite inducing

Organic FTT Failure to thrive related to an underlying medical condition

Ornithine transcarbamylase (OTC) A key enzyme for ammonia detoxification via the urea cycle

Oroenteric Leading from the mouth to the stomach

Oropharyngeal dysphagia The difficulty in forming or moving a alimentary bolus safely from the oral cavity to the esophagus

Orthorexia An excessive preoccupation with healthy eating

Orthostatic hypotension A fall in blood pressure when a person changes his or her position from recumbent to sitting to standing

Orthotopic Something that occurs in the normal or usual place in the body

Osmotic demyelination syndrome (ODS) Rapid demyelination of the parts of the brain as a result of overly rapid correction of hyponatremia

Osmotic pressure The pressure needed to maintain equilibrium with no net movement of solvent

Osteodystrophy Abnormal development of bone

Ostomy The surgical procedure to create a stoma

Oxalate nephrolithiasis Kidney stones

Pacophagia Eating ice

Palpation The use of touch to assess texture, size, temperature, tenderness, and mobility

Pancreatic enzyme preparations A mixture of the digestive enzymes amylase, lipase, and protease

Pancreatic enzyme replacement therapy Giving of exogenous pancreatic enzymes as treatment for pancreatic exocrine insufficiency

Pancreatic exocrine insufficiency A reduction in pancreatic enzyme activity below the threshold necessary for normal digestion

Pancreatic insufficiency The inability for digestive enzymes to be secreted into the small intestine from the pancreas

Pancreatitis Inflammation of the pancreas

Para/parity The number of times a female has given birth

Paracentesis Aspiration of fluid from peritoneal cavity

Parenteral nutrition A type of nutrition support that relies on the intravenous administration of nutrients to patients who are unable or unwilling to take adequate nutrition orally or enterally

Parenteral nutrition related liver disease (PNALD) A form of NAFLD that occurs with long-term TPN use

Parietal cells Located in the gastric glands within the fundus that secrete hydrochloric acid and intrinsic factor

Pediatric malnutrition Nutritional deficits that may negatively affect growth, development, and other relevant outcomes

Percent ideal body weight (%IBW) The actual body weight divided by the ideal body weight, multiplied by 100; used to compare current and ideal body weights

Percent usual body weight (%UBW) The actual body weight divided by the usual body weight, multiplied by 100; the percentage of the current body weight as related to the normal weight

Percent weight change (%weight change) The amount of weight change divided by the usual body weight, multiplied by 100; the percentage change in body weight between two points in time

Percussion The tapping of fingers against body surfaces for sounds that reflect solids, fluids, or gas

Percussor A hand-held device that helps mobilize bronchial secretions

Percutaneous Through the skin

Percutaneous coronary intervention (PCI) Surgical procedure to correct arterial stenosis by inserting and expanding a balloon-tipped catheter at the site of the narrowing and placing a stent to hold the artery open

Percutaneous endoscopic gastrostomy (PEG) tube A tube that is placed into the stomach via needle puncture into the skin guided by endoscopy

Percutaneous endoscopic jejunostomy (PEJ) A tube that is placed into the jejunum via needle puncture into the skin guided by endoscopy

Perianal disease Often the first signs of Crohn's disease, includes complications of the rectum and anus

Periodontal disease Gum disease

Peripheral artery disease Atherosclerotic narrowing of the arteries that deliver blood to the legs, arms, stomach, or kidneys

Peripheral parenteral nutrition Nutrition delivered via access to a peripheral vessel, such as the vessels of the forearm

Peripherally inserted central catheter (PICC) Access where the catheter is inserted into the subclavian, jugular, femoral, cephalic, or basilic veins, and threaded through the vasculature until the tip reaches the vena cava or right atrium

Peristalsis Contraction of smooth and striated muscles within the gastrointestinal system to allow for the passage of food particles

Pernicious anemia Anemia associated with B_{12} deficiency

Phlebitis Inflammation of the vein

Phlegmon A spreading diffuce inflammatory process associated with formation of pus

Phosphate binders Medications used to reduce the small intestinal absorption of phosphorus from foods

Physicochemical incompatibility Physical or chemical instabilities (such as precipitation) often considered in terms of medications and intravenous infusions

Physiological anemia of pregnancy Anemia in pregnant women caused by the greater increase in plasma compared to red blood cells (hemodilution)

Pica A condition marked by the consumption of nonfood items

PIVKA-II The laboratory test of choice to assess vitamin K status

Placenta A blood-rich structure that develops in the uterus and is responsible for transferring nutrients and gasses from the mother to the fetus via the umbilical vein

Placental barrier A semi-permeable barrier that limits the amount and type of material exchange between the mother and fetus

Placental insufficiency The state in which oxygen, glucose, and amino acid transport through the umbilical vein is hindered

Placental preeclampsia Preeclampsia caused by a poorly developed placenta

Plaque Colonized bacteria on tooth surfaces

Pneumothorax Air accumulation in the pleural space

Polycystic kidney disease (PKD) An inherited disorder causing cysts on the kidneys

Polydipsia Thirst

Polyols Sugar alcohols

Polyphagia Hunger

Polyuria Frequent urination
Porcine-derived pancreatic enzymes Exogenous enzymes taken to treat pancreatic insufficiency
Portal hypertension Pressure greater than 10 mm Hg in the portal vein
Porto-systemic shunting The redirection of blood to veins in the esophagus, stomach, and rectum, which have lower venous pressure
Positive acute-phase protein Proteins that increase during inflammation, such as C-reactive protein, ferritin, and cerulosplasmin
Positive nitrogen balance Taking in more nitrogen than is excreted
Postprandial hyperemic response Increased blood flow to the gastrointestinal tract after enteral feeding
Postrenal AKI Kidney injury caused by urinary tract obstruction
Prebiotics Energy sources for the beneficial bacteria in the colon
Precipitation The settling out of solids in a solution
Preconception health The physical and nutritional health of both men and women in relation to reproduction
Preeclampsia High blood pressure in pregnancy
Prerenal AKI Kidney injury caused by inadequate renal perfusion
Pressure injury A localized injury of the skin and/or underlying tissue as a result of pressure, or pressure in combination with friction
Pressure ulcer Localized injury to the skin and/or underlying tissue caused by external factors, including compression, shear force, friction, moisture, or a combination, primarily occurring on bony prominences; also called pressure injury
Pro-inflammatory cytokines Substances released by the immune cells to regulate the host response to infection, inflammation, and trauma, acting on both the endocrine and organ levels
Probiotics Live microorganisms sold as dietary supplements or as components of foods that are intended to have health benefits through interaction with the body's normal flora
Prokinetics Medications that promote motility by increasing small intestine contractions
Prolamin A major storage protein in some grains; avoidance of the prolamins of wheat, barley, and rye is recommended in celiac disease
Proliferation An increase in the number of cells; the second phase of wound healing
Protein catabolism The release of amino acids for protein synthesis and glucose availability
Protein equivalent of nitrogen appearance (PNA) A method of determining protein needs in hemodialysis patients
Protein-energy malnutrition Malnutrition resulting from an energy deficit concurrent with protein deficit or conditioin of increased protein need
Psuedopolyps Inflammatory polyps
Purkinje fibers Tissues throughout the right and left ventricles that carry the heart's electrical impulse
Pyloroplasty A surgical procedure to enlarge the pyloric sphincter
Radiation therapy The use of high-energy radiation from x-rays, gamma rays, or other sources used to kill cancer cells and shrink tumors
Refeeding syndrome The effects of depletion, repletion, and compartmental shifts in electrolytes, fluids, and other substrates in response to excessive nutritional resuscitation; a serious and potentially fatal condition that can occur in severely malnourished patients
Rejection An immune reaction against grafted tissue that results in failure of the graft to survive
Remineralization The body's natural repair process for noncavitated carious lesions; the rebuilding of enamel on teeth
Remodeling The final phase of wound healing, in which new epithelium and final scar tissue are formed

Renal osteodystrophy A condition that occurs when the kidneys are unable to maintain normal levels of blood calcium and phosphorus
Renal replacement therapy (RRT) A treatment that replaces the normal blood-filtering function of the kidneys used to remove waste and fluid while kidney function is impaired
Respiratory acidosis A disorder characterized by low pH, high $PaCO_2$, and a variable increase in plasma HCO_3^- concentration
Respiratory alkalosis A disorder characterized by a high pH, low $PaCO_2$, and a variable decrease in plasma HCO_3^- concentration
Resting energy expenditure The amount of calories required by the body at rest over a 24-hour period
Retinopathy Damage to the eyes
Root caries Decay on the root surface of the tooth
Roux en Y gastric surgery A bariatric surgery procedure that results in a small gastric pouch that severely restricts intake and bypasses the distal stomach, duodenum, and part of the jejunum, resulting in malabsorption
Russell's sign Tooth-induced scarring on the lower dorsum of the hand used to stimulate the gag reflex
Salvage absorption The normal flora will ferment any unabsorbed carbohydrates that enter the colon to short-chain fatty acids (SCFAs), which are subsequently absorbed and utilized
Sarcopenia The loss of lean body mass
Sarcopenic obesity The coexistence of age-related loss of skeletal mass and strength and excess body fat
Secondary hyperparathyroidism Excessive secretion of parathyroid hormone in response to hypocalcemia
Selective serotonin reuptake inhibitor (SSRI) Antidepressant medications prescribed to patients with anorexia nervosa to alleviate mood symptoms and reduce anxiety
Selective vagotomy Surgery to eliminate innervation from the vagus nerve to the parietal cells of the proximal stomach to decrease secretion of gastric acid and reduce cellular response to gastrin
Self-reported height (SRH) Height information provided by the patient
Sepsis A condition in which the body's normal inflammatory response to infection is amplified
Septic shock Consistent hypotension in patients with sepsis, even with adequate fluid resuscitation
Serial measures Repeated measurements taken over time
Shock liver Acute liver failure as the result of ischemic hepatocellular injury
Short-chain fatty acids Products of soluble fiber fermentation in the colon that promote water and electrolyte absorption
Short bowel syndrome Any malabsorption related to decreased absorptive surface area and/or loss of functional capacity in the small intestine
Short Nutritional Assessment Questionnaire (SNAQ) A nutrition screening tool intended for use during admission to an acute care facility
Sinus tracts A narrow elongated channel in the body that allows the escape of fluid
Skinfold anthropometry Skinfold thickness; measure of one or more anatomical sites using a skinfold caliper device to estimate body fat stores
Sleep apnea A disorder of breathing during sleep characterized by prolonged partial upper airway obstruction and/or intermittent complete obstruction that disrupts normal ventilation during sleep and normal sleep patterns

Sleeve gastrectomy (SG) Bariatric procedure in which portions of the stomach are removed

Small intestinal bacterial overgrowth Where a disproportionate number of bacteria invade the small intestine, competing with the body for ingested nutrients and possibly impairing the individual's nutritional status

Small-for-gestational-age (SGA) Infants born with weights that chart less than the 10th percentile for their gestational age

Somatization Complaint of recurrent medical symptoms of unknown cause

Spastic Increased muscle tone

Spina bifida A birth defect characterized by vertebrae not properly forming around the spine

Spirometry A pulmonary function test that measures how well lungs work by quantifying the amount of air inhaled and exhaled

Spontaneous bacterial peritonitis (SBP) Infection of the ascetic fluid without an apparent source

Stadiometer A piece of equipment designed to measure height constructed of a ruler and sliding horizontal headpiece adjusted to rest on the top of the head

Standard body weight (SBW) The patient's actual body weight expressed as a percentage of a defined normal body weight for Americans of a similar frame size, gender, height, and age

Static assay Laboratory test used to measure the actual level of a nutrient in a specimen

Steatohepatitis Necroinflammation of the liver

Steatorrhea Greasy, foul-smelling diarrhea

Steatosis Accumulation of fat in the liver

Stellate cells Hepatic cells that are responsible for collagen formation and hold 90% of the body's vitamin A stores

Stoma An artificial opening in the skin

Stroke A medical condition in which the blood supply to the brain is interrupted or reduced

Stroke volume The amount of blood pumped per heartbeat

Stunting Low height-for-age

Subjective Global Assessment (SGA) A clinical evaluation of a patient's nutritional status, including the patient's weight history, dietary intake, gastrointestinal symptoms, and functional capacity, as well as a physical exam of subcutaneous fat, muscle wasting, edema, and ascites

Supplemental feedings Artificial feedings meant to augment and support regular oral intake

Sweat test A test to measure the amount of chloride in sweat; at levels about 60 mmol/L, it is diagnostic for cystic fibrosis

Synbiotic A product containing both prebiotic and probiotic strains

Systemic inflammatory response syndrome (SIRS) An inflammatory response that occurs throughout the body in response to infection, inflammation, trauma, and burns

Systole The stage of the heart beat that involves the active pumping of blood out of the heart by the ventricles

Systolic blood pressure The force caused when the heart is actively pumping blood

Tenesmus "Dry heaves" of the rectum

Third spacing The accumulation of fluid in the interstices (edema) or in the potential fluid spaces (effusion) between body cavities

Thromboembolism The blockage of an artery by a thrombus that has detached and traveled to a point elsewhere in the circulatory system

Thrombophlebitis An inflammatory process that causes blood to clot and block one or more veins

Thrombosis A blood clot that interferes with normal blood flow

Thrombotic occlusion Blockage of a blood vessel by a thrombus

Total (truncal) vagotomy A surgical procedure wherein parietal cell innervation is severed and the portion of the vagus nerve that controls gastric emptying is eliminated

Total arm span (TAS) The length between the middle of the sternal notch and tip of either middle finger, doubled; measured with the patient's arm horizontal and in line with the shoulders

Total nutrient admixture A preparation method that allows for extended hang time of parenteral nutrition

Total parenteral nutrition The provision of all nutrients intravenously

Total peripheral resistance Resistance of blood flow in systemic circulation

Toxic megacolon Colonic diameter >6 cm or cecal diameter >9 cm in the presence of systemic toxicity

Transitional milk The second stage of breast milk produced, usually within the 2 weeks between colostrum and mature milk

Transjugular intrahepatic portosystemic shunt (TIPS) A procedure used to reduce portal hypertension and its complications including variceal bleeding

Triceps skinfold (TSF) Skinfold anthropometry measured at the triceps

Tubules The part of the nephron that reabsorbs ultrafiltrate

Tumor necrosis factor A pro-inflammatory cytokine produced by the liver

Ulcerative colitis A form of inflammatory bowel disease characterized by inflammation that is limited to the mucosal layer of the colon

Ultrafiltrate The substance remaining after the kidneys have filtered the waste from the blood

Underfill hypothesis A theory explaining the pathogenesis of ascites related to liver disease, in which peripheral arteriolar vasodilation and splanchnic vasodilation result in fluid accumulation in the peritoneal cavity

Underweight A state of having weight that is less than the median for children of similar age or height

Urea reduction ratio (URR) The reduction in the amount of urea as a result of treatments such as dialysis

Ureters The organs of the genitourinary system that carry urine to the bladder so that it can then be released from the body

Usual body weight (UBW) A patient's normal weight range; usually self-reported

Vagus nerve The longest cranial nerve passing through the neck and thorax to the abdomen

Varices Extremely dilated submucosal veins

Vasopressor Medication that constricts blood vessels, thereby increasing blood pressure

Venipuncture The point where the catheter enters the vasculature

Very low birth weight (VLBW) Infants born weighing less than 1,500 grams

Viral hepatitis A systemic infection that damages the liver

Viral load The amount of virus in the blood

Visceral hypersensitivity Describes the experience of pain within the inner organs often associated with irritable bowel syndrome

Visceral protein An assessment that directly measures protein stores by assessing the proteins made by the viscera, namely, organs (primarily the liver)

VP (ventriculoperitoneal) shunting The draining of excess cerebrospinal fluid into a peritoneal space to alleviate pressure and prevent progression of hydrocephalus

VSL#3 A probiotic consisting of 8 strains of lactic acid bacteria

Vulnerable plaque A thin-cap fibroatheroma that is at risk for rupture

Waist circumference An indicator of fat mass around the waist, used to assess health risk
Waist-hip ratio (WHR) The waist circumference value divided by the hip circumference value
Wasting Low BMI or weight-for-height (or length)
Weight-for-age The plotting of a child's weight according to the distribution of weights for children of similar age and gender on a growth chart
Weight-for-height The plotting of a child's weight relative to his or her height on a growth chart
WHO growth charts Growth charts utilizing data on the growth rates of infants from six countries who were exclusively breastfed for the first 4 to 6 months of life
Wilson's disease An autosomal recessive disorder characterized by excessive deposition of copper in the liver and brain
Wound Damage to the structure and function of tissue
Xanthomas Yellow patches on the skin caused by deposits of excess lipids
Xerostomia Reduced or absent saliva flow
Z-scores Representations of individual differences from the median

Index

A

Abdominal distention, 106
Abdominal pain, 364–365
Absorption, 374–376
    GI malabsorption (*see* Gastrointestinal (GI) malabsorption)
    GI maldigestion (*see* Gastrointestinal (GI) maldigestion)
Academy of Nutrition and Dietetics (AND), 183, 298
Academy of Nutrition and Dietetics Evidence Analysis Library (EAL), 303
ACC/AHA classification, 314
Acetoacetic acid, 254
Acetone, 254
Acid–base physiology
    ABGs, 66–67
    chemical buffers, 66
    disorders, 67–69
    hydrogen ion concentration, 64–66
    kidneys, 66
    lungs, 66
    metabolic and respiratory disorders, 65
Acidemia, 65
Acidosis, 65
Acquired immune deficiency syndrome (AIDS), 546
Activities of daily living (ADLs), 35, 763
Activity energy expenditure (AEE), 155
Actual body weight (ABW), 17–18, 21
Acute decompensated heart failure (ADHF), 314
Acute drug-induced hepatitis, 451–452
Acute hepatitis, 446–447
Acute kidney injury (AKI), 419
    diagnosis, 420, 421
    energy, 421
    etiology, 420
    fluid and sodium, 422
    medical nutrition therapy, 420–421
    medical treatment, 420
    nutrition assessment and intervention, 421
    potassium, 422
    protein, 421
Acute liver disease
    acute liver failure, 452–453
    drug-induced hepatitis, 451–452
    nutrition management, 453
    viral hepatitis, 451
Acute liver failure, 446, 452–453
Acute myelogenous leukemia (AML), 523
Acute pancreatitis (AP), 361–362, 364

Acute Physiology and Chronic Health Evaluation scores (APACHE II), 38
Acute posttransplant phase
    energy, 511
    fluid, 512
    metabolic abnormalities, 512–513
    nutrition support, 513–514
    protein, 511–512
Acute respiratory distress syndrome (ARDS), 477–478
Acute viral hepatitis, 451
Acute wounds, 196
Acute-on-chronic hepatitis, 453
Acute-phase proteins, 71–72, 202
Acute-phase reactants, 176
Adaptive hyperfiltration, 416
Adenosine monophosphate-activated protein kinase (AMPK), 581
Adipocytes, 226
Adipose, 225
Adiposity rebound, 640
Adjustable gastric banding, 702
Adjusted edema-free body weight (aBWef), 425
Adolescence
    nutritional management, 347, 348
    oral health concerns, 347
Adulthood, 348–349
Aerobic, 700
Aerophagia, 476
Age-Related Eye Disease Study (AREDS), 279
Air embolism, 138
AKI. *See* Acute kidney injury
Alanine transaminase (ALT), 76
Albumin, 72
Albumin excretion rate (AER), 277–278
Alcohol, 263
Alcohol consumption, 305
Alcohol intake, 309–310
Alcoholic hepatitis (AH), 453
Alcoholic liver disease (ALD), 453–454
Alkalemia, 65
Alkaline phosphatase (ALP), 76
Alkalosis, 65
Allogeneic HSCT, 536
Allograft transplantation, 504
Alternative medicine, 540
Aluminum-based binders, 428
Alveoli, 488
Amenorrhea, 709
American Burn Association (ABA), 178, 180
American Joint Commission on Cancer (AJCC), 524

American Society for Metabolic and Bariatric Surgery (ASMBS), 241
Amino acids
    parenteral nutrition, 123–125
    wound healing, 208–209
Amylin, 225
Amylorrhea, 365
Anastomosis, 358, 401
Anemia, 78–79, 430–431
Anemia of inflammation and chronic disease (AICD), 84
Anencephaly, 573
Angina, 311
Angiogenesis, 198
Angiotensin receptor blockers (ARBs), 307
Angiotensin-converting enzyme inhibitors (ACEIs), 307
Anorexia, 426
Anorexia nervosa (AN), 708
    clinical complications, 711–712
    female athlete triad, 712
    goals, 719–722
    relapse and mortality, 712–713
Anorexigenic hormones, 225
Anthropometrics, 494, 641
    assessment, 226, 553, 555
    critical illness, acute burn injury, 183–185
    data, 721, 723
Anthropometry
    body composition, 164
    height assessment
        adult height records, 15–16
        knee-height, 16–17
        parameters, 14
        SRH, 16
        stadiometer, 15
        surrogate measures, 15
        total and half arm span, 16–17
    imaging techniques
        BIA, 26–27
        CT, 26
        DXA, 26–27
        MRI, 26
    measurements and proportions, 14
    skinfold anthropometry
        circumference measurements, 23
        hip circumference, 25–26
        MUAC, 23–24
        sites, 22
        TSF, 23
        waist circumference, 24–25

Anthropometry (continued)
  weight
    ABW, 17–18, 21
    BMI, 21–22
    body composition, 22
    body weight modifications, 21
    dry weight, 21
    height-weight tables, 19
    IBW, 19, 20
    predictive equations, 19–20
    UBW, 18–19
    %weight change, 18–19
Anticariogenic foods, 336
Antidiuretic hormone (ADH), 53, 417
Antifluoridation movement, 339
Antioxidants
  heart failure, 321–322
  periodontal disease, 342
  pulmonary diseases, 480
  supplements, 305
Antiretroviral treatment (ART), 548
Apolipoproteins, 299
Appropriate-for-gestational-age (AGA), 614
ARDS. See Acute respiratory distress syndrome
Arginine, 109–111, 208–209
Arterial blood gases (ABGs), 66–67
Arterial puncture, 138
Artificial sweeteners, 263–264
Ascites, 447
Ascorbic acid, 210
ASD. See Autism spectrum disorder
Asepsis, 116
Aspartate transaminase (AST), 75–76
Aspiration, 97, 104, 763
Asthma, 472
  childhood obesity, 690–691
Asymmetric macrosomia, 585
Atherosclerosis, 294, 296
Atrophic gastritis, 771
Auscultation, 28–29
Autism spectrum disorder (ASD)
  anthropometrics, 747–748
  biochemical and clinical data, 748–749
  energy needs, 750
  feeding difficulty, 749–750
  long-term monitoring/evaluation, 750
  red flags, 747–748
  symptoms, 748
Autograft transplantation, 504
Autologous HSCT, 536
Avoidant restrictive food intake disorder (ARFID), 711
Azotemia, 418
Azotorrhea, 365

B

Bacteria-controlled nursing units (BCNU), 182
Bariatric surgery, 234, 704
  inclusion and exclusion criteria, 237, 238
  LAGB, 239
  post-bariatric surgery, 241
  RYGB, 239, 240
  sleeve gastrectomy, 239
  types, 238
Basal energy expenditure (BEE), 154
Basal metabolic rate (BMR), 154
Basic metabolic panel, 48
B-complex vitamins, 321
BED. See Binge eating disorder
Bedside nasoenteral technique, 94–95
Behavior interventions, obesity, 234
Beta-blockers, 307
Beta-hydroxybutyric acid, 254
β-hydroxy-β-methylbutyrate (HMB), 209–210
Bicarbonate, 64
Biliopancreatic diversion, 702
Binge eating disorder (BED), 710–711
  clinical complications, 715
  goals, 722
  relapse and mortality, 715
Biochemical assessment, 45–89, 185–186, 227
  acid–base physiology
    ABGs, 66–67
    chemical buffers, 66
    disorders, 67–69
    hydrogen ion concentration, 64–66
    kidneys, 66
    lungs, 66
    metabolic and respiratory disorders, 65
  anemia
    iron, 83–86
    vitamin B_{12} deficiency, 85–88
  assay types, 48
  endocrine function, 69–70
  enzymes, 75–77
  fluids
    bicarbonate, 64
    calcium, 57–59
    changes in intake, 48
    chloride, 63–64
    distribution, 49–51
    electrolyte disorders, 50–51
    magnesium, 61–63
    phosphorus, 57, 60–61
    potassium, 55–56
    sodium, 51–55
  hematology
    anemia, 78–79
    Hct percentage, 81
    healthy and anemic red blood cells, 79–80
    hemoglobin, 80–81
    MCHC, 82
    MCV, 81–82
    minerals, 80
    primary sites of GI absorption, 80
    RBC count, 81
    RDW, 82–83
    WBC count, 83
  lipid profile, 77–78
  nausea, vomiting, and diarrhea, 47
  ordered groups of tests, 48
  proteins
    cellular growth and metabolism, 70
    somatic protein, 71, 73–75
    total serum, 71
    visceral protein, 71–73
  specimen types, 46
  values, 48
Biochemical markers, 572
Bioelectrical impedance analysis (BIA), 26, 165, 556
Biofilm, 138
Biotherapy, 527
Bi-ventricular assist devices (BIVADs), 315
Blood glucose (BG) management, 320, 321
Blood pressure (BP), 305, 417. See also Hypertension
Blood urea nitrogen (BUN), 75
Blood volume, 417
BMI-for-age, 492, 493
Body cell mass (BCM)
  catabolic disease, 165–166
  differences in body composition, 154
  metabolic support, 167–168
Body composition, 556
  anthropometry, 164
  bioelectrical impedance, 165
  catabolic disease, 165–166
  geriatrics
    frailty, 758–759
    pressure injury, 759
    Sarcopenia, 757–758
    sarcopenic obesity, 759–760
  isotope dilution technique, 165
  models, 163–164
  nutritional status, 163–164
  obesity, 225–226
  prematurity
    carbohydrate requirements, 618–619
    electrolyte requirements, 621–624
    energy requirements, 616–617
    fat requirement, 619
    fluid requirements, 619–621
    protein requirements, 617–618
  two compartment model, 164–165
Body fat, 226
Body mass index (BMI), 21–22, 164, 642–643
  cystic fibrosis, 493
  obesity, 218, 227
Bolus, 356
Bolus feedings, 98, 480
Bone disease
  cystic fibrosis, 500
  IBD, 391
Bone health, 518
Bone-strengthening, 700
Bowel surgery
  bowel resection, 400–401
  colonic involvement, 402

colostomy, 403
Crohn's disease, 400
diet composition, 406, 407
duodenal resection, 401
fluid and electrolyte needs, 406–407
ileal resection, 402
ileocecal valve, 402
ileostomy, 403
intestinal adaptation, 404–405
Jejunal resection, 401–402
jejunostomy, 403
nutritional implications, 403–404
pathophysiology, 404
reconstruction, 402–403
Bowman's capsule, 414
Braden Scale for Predicting Pressure Sore Risk, 204–206
Brain death, 508
Branched chain amino acids (BCAA), 458, 465
Breastfeeding and childhood obesity, 599
Bronchi, 488, 490
Bronchiodilators, 490
Bronchioles, 488, 490
Brush border, 356
Bulimia nervosa (BN), 710
    clinical complications, 713–714
    goals, 722
    relapse and mortality, 713–714

C

Cachexia, 758
Calcitonin, 57
Calcium
    CKD, 427
    corrected serum calcium formula, 58
    electrolytes, 623
    essential functions, 57
    hypercalcemia, 59
    hypocalcemia, 58–59
    recommended adequate intake, 58
Calcium channel blockers (CCBs), 307
Calcium-based binders, 428–429
Caloric sweeteners, 262
Cancer cachexia
    cytokines, 529, 530
    medical management, 530–531
Cancer treatment
    biotherapy, 527
    chemotherapy, 526
    esophageal cancer, 533
    gastric cancer, 533–534
    HNC, 532
    hormone therapy, 527
    intestinal cancers, 534
    lung cancer, 535
    mucositis, 527
    nutrition impact symptoms, 525–526
    oral mucosa, 532
    pancreatic cancer, 534

    radiation therapy, 525
    risk factors, 522
    surgery, 527
Candida, 344
Carbohydrates
    early treatment modality, 259
    enteral nutrition, 100–101
    exercise, 271–272
    glycemic index, 259–260
    glycemic load, 260–261
    liver disease, 457
    metabolism, 570–571
    modification, 259
    organizations, 259
    parenteral nutrition, 123
    requirements, 618–619
Carcinomas, 524
Cardiac cachexia, 317, 319, 322
Cardiac conduction system, 295, 296
Cardiac output, 294
Cardiogenic shock, 322
Cardiopulmonary bypass, 312
Cardiovascular disease (CVD), 262–263, 275–276, 293–325
    added sugar, 305
    alcohol, 305
    antioxidant supplements, 305
    atherosclerosis, 294
    CKD, 430
    clinical course, 298–300
    energy needs, 302
    fiber, 304
    heart failure (*see* Heart failure)
    hypertension (*see* Hypertension)
    medications, 301–302
    monitoring and evaluation, 305
    nutrition assessment, 300–301
    nutrition intervention, 302–303
    nutrition support, 322–324
    nuts, 304
    obesity
        AHA/ACC, 310
        CAD diagnosis and surgical treatment, 311–312
        outcomes, 311
    omega-3 fatty acids, 303–304
    physical activity, 305
    physiology, 294–298
    plant stanols and sterols, 304–305
    saturated/trans fats, replacement, 303, 304
    smoking cessation, 305
Cardiovascular system, obesity, 229–230
Cariogenic foods, 334–335
Cariogenicity, 334
Cariostatic foods, 336
Carnitine, 627
Catabolic stress response, 176
Catabolism, 176
Catch up growth, 670
Catecholamines, 176

Catheter embolism, 138
Catheter occlusion, 138
Catheter-related bloodstream infection (CRBSI), 138–139
Catheter-related complications (CRCs)
    arterial puncture, 138
    embolism, 138
    infectious mechanical complications, 137–139
    noninfectious mechanical complications, 137
    occlusion, 138
    phlebitis, 138
    pneumothorax, 137
    securement, 137
Catheter-related venous thrombosis (CRVT), 138
CD4 cell count, 546
Celiac disease (CD)
    absorption capacity, 375, 377
    clinical manifestations, 376–378
    nutrition interventions, 376–377, 379
    prolamin, 375
Centers for Disease Control and Prevention (CDC), 643, 728
Central line–associated bloodstream infection (CLABSI), 138–139
Central nervous system (CNS), obesity, 223–224
Central parenteral nutrition, 116
    complications, 118
    CVCs, 119–120
    long-term central access, 118–119
    PICC, 118–119
    VADs, 118
Central venous catheters (CVCs), 119–120, 177
Central PN (CPN), 625
Cephalic phase of digestion, 760
Cerebral palsy (CP)
    adaptive feeding devices, 743
    anthropometrics, 740–741
    biochemical and clinical data, 741–742
    classifications, 740
    energy needs, 742–743
    feeding difficulty, 742–743
    long-term monitoring/evaluation, 744
    walking frame, 740–741
    weight challenges, 743–744
CF transmembrane conductance regulator (CFTR) protein, 488
CF-related diabetes (CFRD), 499–500
Chemotherapy, 526
Chiari II malformation, 739
Childhood obesity
    approaches
        goal setting, 701
        group based, 699
        motivational interviewing, 699–700
        positive reinforcement, 700–701
        stimulus control, 701
        weight loss, 695, 698
    asthma, 690–691
    behavioral intervention, 698–699
    CDC waist, 686–687

Childhood obesity (continued)
    definition, 684
    dietary intervention, 699
    epicardial fat, 687
    family patterns, 694
    genetic factors, 694
    IGT, 690
    insulin resistance, type 2 diabetes, 689–690
    low socioeconomic status, 693–694
    LVH, 687–688
    metabolic syndrome, 688–689
    NAFLD, 691
    NIH daily energy, 695, 698
    nutrition assessment, 695–697
    nutritional supplementation, indications, 703–704
    overweight, 684, 686
    physical activity, 699
    psychological effects
        cognitive impairment, 693
        depression, 692–693
        family relationship, 693
        health-related quality of life, 693
        peer relationships, 693
    sleep apnea, 691
    surgical intervention
        indications, 702
        weight loss procedures, 702–703
Child-Pugh classification, 449, 450
Chloride, 63–64
Cholecystokinin (CCK), 225
Cholelithiasis, 141
Cholestasis, 141
Cholestatic liver disease, 446
Cholesterol accumulation, 297
Cholesterol medications, 302
51-chromium-labeled ethylenedaminetetraacetic acid (51-Cr-EDTA), 393
Chronic hepatitis, 446–447
Chronic inflammation, 549
Chronic kidney disease (CKD)
    anemia, 430–431
    calcium, 427
    classification, 422, 423
    definition, 422
    energy, 425
    etiology, 422–424
    fluid and sodium, 426–427
    KDOQI, 422
    lipid disorders, 430
    nutrition intervention, 424–425
    nutritional assessment, 424–425
    nutritional concerns, 424
    phosphorus, 427–429
    potassium, 427
    prevalence, 414
    progression, 417
    protein, 425–426
    PTH, 430
    treatment, 424
    vitamin D deficiency, 429–430

Chronic Kidney Disease Epidemiology (CKD-EPI)
    creatinine equation, 419
    cystatin C equation, 419–420
Chronic liver disease
    ALD, 453–454
    inherited diseases, 456–457
    NAFLD, 455–456
Chronic obstructive pulmonary disease (COPD)
    enteral feeding, 479
    exacerbation, 478
    oxidative stress, 474
    pharmacologic therapies, 474
    REE, 475
    spirometry, 472–473
    TEE, 475
    weight status, 476
Chronic pancreatitis (CP), 360, 364, 365, 367
Chronic posttransplant phase
    bone health and osteoporosis, 518
    cancer, 518
    diabetes, 517
    food–drug interactions and supplement use, 515–516
    hyperlipidemia, 517–518
    hypertension, 517
    long-term metabolic and nutritional consequences, 516
    prevention, 515
    weight gain, 516
Chronic venous ulcers, 199
Chronic wounds, 196
    chronic venous ulcers, 199
    delayed healing, 199
    diabetic ulcers, 199–200
    factors, 198–199
    pathophysiology, 199
    physiological state and metabolism, alterations, 201–203
    pressure ulcers, 200–201
Chyme, 356, 357
Cilia, 488, 489
Cinnamon, 265–266
Cirrhosis
    energy requirements, 461
    enteral nutrition, 463–464
    hepatic encephalopathy, 447, 448
    oral nutrition, 463
    protein requirements, 461
    tissue scarring, 447
    varices, 447
    vitamin D deficiency, 461–462
    Zinc, 462–463
CKD. See Chronic kidney disease
Clinical assessment, obesity, 227
Closed tube feeding system, 97
Coagulopathy, 448–449
Coenzyme Q, 320–321
Cognitive behavior therapy (CBT), 234, 716
Collagen, 198
Colostomy, 403
Colostrum, 596, 663

Combination procedures, bariatric surgery, 238, 239
Combined isotope dilution studies, 166
Complementary medicine, 540
Complete blood count (CBC), 48
Comprehensive lifestyle intervention, 233
Comprehensive metabolic panel, 48
Computed tomography (CT), 26
Constipation, 107
Continuous ambulatory peritoneal dialysis (CAPD), 433
Continuous cycling peritoneal dialysis (CCPD), 433–434
Continuous feeding, 98
Continuous infusion, 135
Continuous renal replacement therapy (CRRT), 421, 434
COPD. See Chronic obstructive pulmonary disease
Coronary angioplasty, 311, 312
Coronary artery bypass graft (CABG), 311
Coronary artery disease (CAD), 311
Corrected bromide space (CBS), 166
Correction factor (CF), 268–270
Craniorachischisis, 573
C-reactive protein (CRP), 72, 230
Creatinine height index (CHI), 74–75
Critical illness, acute burn injury, 175–192
    medical treatment and clinical course, 180–183
    nutritional management
        anthropometrics, 183–185
        biochemical assessment, 185–186
        dietary assessment, 187–188
        energy needs, 188–189
        enteral nutrition support, 190–191
        malnutrition, 183
        NFPE, 186–187
        nutrition screen, 183–185
        parenteral nutrition support, 191–192
        protein needs, 188–189
        vitamins/minerals, 189–190
    pathophysiology
        ABA, 178, 180
        catabolic stress response, 176
        characteristics, 176, 178
        endocrine and metabolic response, 176, 179
        energy expenditure, 176
        energy production, 176–177
        hyperdynamic/flow phase, 176
        hypermetabolism, 176
        macronutrient metabolism, alterations, 176
        morbidity and mortality, 177, 179
        proteolysis, 177
        sepsis, 178–180
        shock (ebb) phase, 176
Crohn's disease, 383
CVD. See Cardiovascular disease
Cyanosis, 739
Cyclical infusion, 135

Cystic fibrosis (CF), 487–500
    CFRD, 499–500
    CF-related bone disease, 500
    CFTR, 488
    clinical manifestations, 488
    diagnosis, 488
    gastrointestinal complications, 499
    infants, 497
    lungs, 488–491
    macronutrients, 497
    micronutrients, 498
    nutrition assessment
        anthropometrics, 494
        biochemical assessment, 494
        clinical manifestations, 492
        diet assessment, 494
        energy and protein needs, 493–494
    nutrition support, 498–499
    nutritional status, 491
    pancreatic insufficiency
        fecal elastase test, 494
        nonenteric-coated enzyme, 496–497
        PERT, 494–496
        porcine-derived pancreatic enzymes, 495
        PPIs, 495
        stool pattern, 497
    sodium chloride, 498
Cytokines, 176, 529, 530

D

Daniel's Crohn's disease, 400
De ritis ratio, 454
Debridement, 203
Decompensated cirrhosis, 448
Defined diets, 393, 394
Delayed gastric emptying (DGE), 368
Delayed onset lactation, 596
Dementia, 763
Demineralization, dental caries, 333
Dental caries
    cariostatic foods, 336
    etiologic factors, 334
    fluoride, 338–340
    fluorosis, 340–341
    food amount, 335
    food combinations, 336–337
    food composition, 334–335
    form and consistency, 335
    frequency and duration of exposure, 335
    host/agent/environment diet, 337
    microorganisms, 334
    pathophysiology, 333
    plaque control, 337
    prevalence and severity, 333
    substrate–dietary factors, 334
    sugar intake, 336
    susceptible tooth, 334
    systemic vs. topical fluoride, 338
    treatment and prevention, 337

Dental disease, 279
Dentures
    pathophysiology, 343
    treatment and prevention, 343–344
Develop discrepancy, 700
Developmental disability, 728
Dextrose infusion, 123
Diabetes
    chronic posttransplant phase, 517
    CKD, 423
    enteral nutrition, 104
    pregnancy, 584–585
Diabetes distress, 275
Diabetes mellitus
    acute complications
        hyperglycemia, 273–274
        hypoglycemia, 274–275
    caring, 252
    chronic complications
        macrovascular, 275–276
        microvascular, 276–280
        psychological, 275
    diagnosis, 258
    exercise
        carbohydrate, 271–272
        type 1 diabetes, 270–271
        type 2 diabetes, 271
    hospital setting
        adverse outcomes, 285–286
        enteral nutrition, 286–287
        noncritical patients, 286
        parenteral nutrition, 287
        rates of mortality, 286
    medical treatment
        American Association of Clinical Endocrinologists, 280
        insulin, 280, 283–285
        oral and injectable noninsulin medications, 280–283
    MNT
        American Diabetes Association, 266
        carbohydrate counting, 267–268
        exchange method, 267–268
        ICR, 268–270
        meal planning, 267
        nutritional assessment, 266–267
        plate method, 267
        recommended nutrition visits, 266
    nutritional requirements
        alcohol, 263
        caloric sweeteners, 262
        carbohydrate, 259–261
        cinnamon, 265–266
        fat, 262–263
        fiber, 261–262
        herbal and dietary supplements, 264
        micronutrients, 263–264
        nonnutritive sweeteners, 263–264
        protein, 262
        sucrose, 262

    pathophysiology
        GDM, 257–258
        type 1, 252–255
        type 2, 254–257
    screening and risk factors, 258
    SMBG, 272–273
    staging, 258–259
    surgical treatment options, 285
Diabetic ketoacidosis (DKA), 254
Diabetic ulcers, 199–200
Diagnostic and Statistical Manual of Mental Disorders (DSM-V), 708
Dialectical behavior therapy (DBT), 716
Diarrhea, 107, 324
Diastole, 294
Diastolic blood pressure, 305
Diet assessment, 494
Diet progression
    LAGB, 241, 243–245
    RYGB, 240–243
    sleeve gastrectomy, 240–243
Dietary Approaches to Stop Hypertension (DASH) diet, 307–309, 426–427
Dietary assessment, 187–188, 227, 556–557
Dietary data, 718
Dietary history, obesity, 227
Dietary Reference Intakes (DRIs), 156
Dietary supplements, 264
    antioxidants, 321–322
    B-complex vitamins, 321
    coenzyme Q, 320–321
    fluoride, 339–340
    hawthorne, 321
    vitamin E, 322
Dietary therapy, 515–516
Diet-induced thermogenesis (DIT), 154
Differential count, 48
Digestive system. See Gastrointestinal (GI) maldigestion
Digital clubbing, 488
Direct calorimetry, 158
Disaccharide, 381
Docosahexaenoic acid (DHA), 303
Donation after cardiac death (DCD), 508
Doubly labeled water (DLW), 158–160, 229
Down syndrome (DS)
    anthropometrics, 746
    biochemical and clinical data, 746–747
    child with, 745
    common foods, 746–747
    energy needs, 747
    long-term monitoring/evaluation, 747
Dronabinol (Marinol™), 499
Drug-induced hepatitis, 451–452
Dry weight, 21
Dual energy x-ray absorptiometry (DXA), 26–27, 166–167, 556
Dumping syndrome (DS), 97, 359–360, 703
Duodenal resection, 401
Duodenum, 354

Dysgeusia, 457
Dyslipidemia, 299–301
Dysphagia, 763
Dyspnea, 314, 415, 474

E

Early childhood caries (ECC), 346
Early enteral nutrition (EEN), 107
Early-onset preeclampsia, 590
Eating disorder (ED)
    AN, 708
    ARFID, 711
    BED, 710–711
    BN, 710
    counseling, 723–724
    goals, 719–722
    medical nutrition therapy, 719
    NES, 711
    nutrition assessment, 716–719
        anthropometric assessment, 716
        biochemical assessment, 718–719
        dietary assessment, 716–717
        education, 724
    overview, 708–710
    patient monitoring, 724–725
    Pharmacotherapy, 716
    prevention, 722
    prognosis, 711–715
    psychological treatment, 715–716
    risk factors, 709–710
    unspecified feeding, 711
    vegetarianism, 717
Eating Disorder Examination Questionnaire (EDE-Q), 725
Edentulism
    pathophysiology, 343
    treatment and prevention, 343–344
Eicosapentaenoic acid (EPA), 303
Ejection fraction (EF), 294
Electrical activity, 295, 297
Electrocardiogram (ECG), 295, 297
Electrolyte requirements
    acid–base balance, 623
    calcium and phosphorus, 623
    magnesium, 623–624
    potassium, 622–623
    sodium, 621–622
Electrolytes
    disorders
        classification, 50–51
        extracellular fluid volume, 51
        management, 51
    imbalance of plasma volume, 48
    parenteral nutrition, 126, 134
Elemental formula, 397–398
Elimination diet, 748
Embolism, 138, 297
Enamel hypoplasia, 330
Enamel, oral cavity, 330

Endocardium, 294
Endocrine function, 69–70
Endocrine system, 230–231
Endoscopic nasoenteral technique, 95
Endothelial growth factor (EGF), 196
Endotoxin, 453
End-stage heart failure symptoms, 322
End-stage liver disease (ESLD), 448
End-stage renal disease (ESRD), 422, 506
Energy
    acute posttransplant phase, 511
    AKI, 421
    CKD, 425
    cystic fibrosis, 493–494
    kinetic modeling, 434
    wound healing, 207
Energy expenditure
    direct calorimetry, 158
    indirect calorimetry
        canopy hood, 160
        DLW, 159–160
        measured REE, 160–161
        metabolic cart, 160
        over-and underfeeding, 162
        respiratory quotient, 162–163
        volume of carbon dioxide, 158
        volume of oxygen, 158
    normal and stressed conditions
        components, 154–155
        estimation, 155–158
Energy metabolism, 570
Energy needs, 670
Energy requirements, 616–617
Enteral feeding, 287
Enteral nutrition (EN), 91–112, 121, 323, 391–392, 437–438
    cirrhosis, 463–464
    complication
        abdominal distention, 106
        aspiration, 104
        constipation, 107
        diarrhea, 107
        gastroparesis, 106–107
        nausea and vomiting, 106
    critical illness, acute burn injury, 190–191
    diabetes mellitus, 286–287
    disease-specific formulas
        diabetes, 104
        liver dysfunction, 104
        pulmonary dysfunction, 104
        renal dysfunction, 103
        trauma/wound healing, 104
    EEN, 107
    evolution of, 92
    feeding plan, 104–106
    formula compositions
        carbohydrates, 100–101
        fats, 101
        fiber, 102
        nutrient composition, 100–101

        prebiotics, 102
        probiotics, 102
        protein, 102
        types, 99
        vitamins and minerals, 102
    formula delivery methods
        bolus, 98
        closed tube, 97
        continuous, 98
        hang time, 98
        intermittent, 98
        open tube, 97
    gastric feeding, 96–97
    immunonutrition
        arginine, 109–111
        clinical trials, 110–111
        gastrointestinal tract, 108–109
        glutamine, 109
        gut, 109–110
        omega-3 fatty acids, 110–111
        systemic inflammatory response, 109–110
    site and route
        basic tube placement options, 92, 94
        long-term placement, 95–96
        medical condition/disease state, 92, 94
        short-term placement, 94–95
    small-bowel feeding, 97
    tubes, types of, 96
    wound healing, 212
Enterocytes, 374
Epicardial fat, 687
Epicardium, 294
Episodic abdominal pain, 380
Erythropoietin (EPO), 418
Erythropoietin stimulating agents (ESAs), 430
Esophageal cancer (EC), 533
Essential body fat, 226
Essential fatty acid (EFA), 125, 140–141, 209
Estimated energy requirements (EERs), 156, 661–662
Estimated glomerular filtration rate (eGFR), 419
Euglycemia, 254
European Society for Clinical Nutrition and Metabolism (ESPEN), 6
Euvolemic hypernatremia, 54
Euvolemic hypotonic hyponatremia, 53
Exchange method, 267–268
Exercise
    carbohydrate, 271–272
    type 1 diabetes, 270–271
    type 2 diabetes, 271
Exercise-related activity, 228
Exit site, 117
Express empathy, 700
Extracellular fluid (ECF), 49–50, 417, 619, 620
Extracellular water (ECW), 165
Extraintestinal manifestations, 376, 378
Extravasation, 118
Extremely low birth weight (ELBW), 614

F

Failure to thrive (FTT), 669–670
Familial hypercholesterolemia (FH), 300
Fat
- diabetes mellitus, 262–263
- enteral nutrition, 101
- metabolism, 153–154
- wound healing, 208–209

Fat free mass (FFM), 225, 226
Fat maldigestion, 359
Fat mass, 225
Fat metabolism, 459, 571
Fat requirement, 619
Fat-free mass (FFM), 164–165, 556
Fecal elastase test, 494
Feeding methods
- energy requirements
  - amino acids, 625–626
  - electrolytes, 627
  - glucose, 625
  - lipids, 626–627
  - minerals, 627–628
  - trace elements, 628
  - vitamins, 628
- PN, 624
- vascular access, 625

Feeding selection
- breast milk, 630–631
- breastfeeding, 630–631
- discharge, 632
- donor milk, 630
- transitional formulas, 632

Female athlete triad, 712
Fetal alcohol syndrome, 582
Fetal macrosomia, 574
Fiber
- diabetes mellitus, 261–262
- enteral nutrition, 102

Fibroblast growth factor (FGF), 196
Fibroblast growth factor 23 (FGF23), 427
Fibrosis, 447
Fluids
- acute posttransplant phase, 512
- AKI, 422
- bicarbonate, 64
- calcium, 57–59
- changes in intake, 48
- chloride, 63–64
- CKD, 426–427
- distribution, 49–51
- electrolyte disorders, 50–51
- kinetic modeling, 436
- magnesium, 61–63
- phosphorus, 57, 60–61
- potassium, 55–56
- requirements, 619–621
- sodium, 51–55
- wound healing, 211

Fluoride
- dietary supplements, 339–340
- fluorosis, 338
- foods and beverages, 339
- life cycle, 337
- mechanisms of action, 337–338
- systemic vs. topical, 338
- water, 338–339

Fluoroapatite, 330
Fluoroscopic nasoenteric tube placement, 95
Fluorosis, 338, 340–341
Foam cells, CVD, 296–297
Food and Drug Administration (FDA), 690, 731
Food deserts, 221
Food frequency questionnaire (FFQ), 39
Food insecurity, 548–549
Food records diary, 39
Forced expiratory volume at 1 second (FEV_1), 480, 491
Formula delivery methods
- bolus, 98
- closed tube, 97
- continuous, 98
- hang time, 98
- intermittent, 98
- open tube, 97

Frailty, 758–759
Fulminant liver failure, 452
Functional assay, 48

G

Gamma-aminobutyric acid (GABA) receptors, 742
Gastrectomy, 358
Gastric cancer, 533–534
Gastric residual volume (GRV), 106
Gastric residuals, 104
Gastric surgery
- Billroth I and Billroth II, 357, 358
- Dumping syndrome, 359–360
- fat maldigestion, 359
- gastric stasis, 358–359
- nutrient deficiencies, 359
- nutrition assessment, 360
- nutrition intervention, 360, 361
- postoperative complications, 358
- Roux-en-Y procedure, 357, 358

Gastroenterologic symptoms, 582
Gastroesophageal reflux disease (GERD), 231, 652–653, 743
- esophagus, 368, 370
- medical and surgical treatment, 368–369
- nutrition assessment and intervention, 369–370

Gastrointestinal (GI) complications, cystic fibrosis, 499
Gastrointestinal function, 552, 557
Gastrointestinal (GI) malabsorption, 373–409
- absorption sites, 374–376
- medical nutrition therapy
  - bowel surgery, 400–407
  - celiac disease, 375–379
  - *Helicobacter pylori*, 395
  - IBD, 383–394
  - IBS, 378–382
  - NCGS, 382–383
  - SBS, 404–408
  - SIBO, 396–400

Gastrointestinal (GI) maldigestion
- anatomy, 354–356
- digestion and absorption, 356, 357
- mechanisms, 356–357
- medical nutrition therapy
  - gastric surgery, 357–360
  - GERD, 368–370
  - pancreatitis, 360–368
- pathology, 354

Gastrointestinal (GI) symptoms, 48
Gastrointestinal system, obesity, 231–232
Gastroparesis, 97, 106–107, 279, 358–359
Genetic factors, 694
Geriatric nutrition, 754
Geriatrics, 349–350
- aging process, 756
- body composition
  - frailty, 758–759
  - pressure injury, 759
  - sarcopenia, 757–758
  - sarcopenic obesity, 759–760
- error theory, 756
- immunosenescence, 756
- malnutrition risk, 760
- micronutrient intake
  - calcium, 773
  - vitamin B_{12}, 771
  - vitamin D, 771–773
- nutrient needs
  - dietary fiber intake, 769–770
  - energy requirements, 768
  - fluid requirements, 770
  - protein requirement, 768
- nutrition screening, 765–766
- nutrition support, 774–775
- older adults, 774
- physiologic factors
  - dietary modifications, 764
  - dysphagia, 763–764
  - functional status, 763
  - health status, 762
  - psychological/neurocognitive status, 762–763
  - social factors, 765
- population of, 754
- preprogrammed theory, 756

Gestation, 567
Gestational diabetes mellitus (GDM), 257–258
- blood glucose level, 589–590
- management of, 589–590
- testing and diagnosing, 589

Gestational hypertension, 590

GFR. *See* Glomerular filtration rate
Ghrelin, 224
Gingiva, 341
Gingivitis, 341
Glomerular filtration rate (GFR), 277–278, 415, 419
Glomerulus, 414
Glucagon-like peptide-1 (GLP-1), 225
Gluconeogenesis, 255
Glucose infusion rate (GIR), 134, 625
Glucose intolerance, 557
Glucose-dependent insulinotropic polypeptide (GIP), 225
Glutamine, 109, 176, 209, 539
Glycemic index (GI), 259–260
Glycemic load (GL), 260–261
Glycogenolysis, 255
Glycosylated hemoglobin (HbA1c), 70
Goals, eating disorder
    anorexia nervosa, 719–722
    binge eating disorder, 722
    bulimia nervosa, 722
Graft, solid organ transplantation, 504
Graft thrombosis, 507
Graft *versus* host disease (GVHD), 508–509, 536–539
Gravida, 567
Growth, 638, 639
Growth channels, 638
Growth charts
    CDC, 643, 646, 647
    WHO, 643–645
    z-scores, 648–651
Growth discordance, 616
Growth hormone, 731
Growth reference, 643
Growth standards, 643
Growth velocity, 639–640
Gut hormones, 240
Gut-associated lymphoid tissue (GALT), 108–109
Gut–liver axis, 445

H

Half arm span (HAS), 16–17
Hamwi method, 19–20
Handgrip dynamometer, 35
Handgrip strength, 35–36
Hang time, 98
Harris–Benedict Equation, 461
Hawthorne, 321
Head and neck cancers (HNC), 532
Head circumference (HC), 642
Head-circumference-for-age, 643
Healthy People 2020, 606
Heart disease. *See* Cardiovascular disease
Heart failure (HF)
    blood glucose management, 320, 321
    cardiac cachexia, 317, 319, 322
    chest pain and dyspnea, 313
    classification, 314
    diastolic HF, 314
    dietary supplements
        antioxidants, 321–322
        B-complex vitamins, 321
        coenzyme Q, 320–321
        hawthorne, 321
        vitamin E, 322
    end-stage, 315, 322
    heart-healthy eating, 320
    left-sided HF, 313
    LVAD, 314–316
    medications, 316–317, 319
    MNA, 316, 318
    monitoring and evaluation, 322
    nutrition intervention, 319
    nutritional management, 316
    obesity, 317
    pulmonary edema, 323
    right-sided HF, 313
    risk factors, 312, 314
    SGA, 316, 317
    sodium and fluid restrictions, 319–320
    systolic HF, 313
    VAD, 315
Heart transplantation, 506, 511, 513
Height assessment
    adult height records, 15–16
    knee-height, 16–17
    parameters, 14
    SRH, 16
    stadiometer, 15
    surrogate measures, 15
    total and half arm span, 16–17
Height-for-age, 643
Helicobacter pylori (*H. pylori*)
    medical treatment, 395
    nutrition assessment, 395
    nutrition intervention, 395
HELLP syndrome, 591
Hematocrit (Hct) percentage, 81
Hematologic malignancies, 524
Hematology
    anemia, 78–79
    Hct percentage, 81
    healthy and anemic red blood cells, 79–80
    hemoglobin, 80–81
    MCHC, 82
    MCV, 81–82
    minerals, 80
    primary sites of GI absorption, 80
    RBC count, 81
    RDW, 82–83
    WBC count, 83
Hematopoietic stem cell transplant (HSCT)
    allogeneic HSCT, 536
    alternative medicine, 540
    autologous HSCT, 536
    cancer cachexia
        cytokines, 529, 530
        medical management, 530–531
    cancer treatment
        biotherapy, 527
        chemotherapy, 526
        esophageal cancer, 533
        gastric cancer, 533–534
        HNC, 532
        hormone therapy, 527
        intestinal cancers, 534
        lung cancer, 535
        mucositis, 527
        nutrition impact symptoms, 525–526
        oral mucosa, 532
        pancreatic cancer, 534
        radiation therapy, 525
        risk factors, 522
        surgery, 527
    complementary medicine, 540
    energy needs, 536
    epidemiology, 524
    glutamine, 539
    GVHD, 537–539
    hypermetabolism, 529
    integrative medicine, 540
    low-microbial diet, 539–540
    neutropenia, 536
    nutrition needs, 529
    nutrition screening, 527–528
    nutrition support, 531, 540
    nutritional assessment, 528
    receive EN, 537
    stages of, carcinogenesis, 524
    TNM category, 524, 525
Hemochromatosis, 456
Hemoconcentration, 48
Hemodialysis (HD), 432–433
Hemodilution, 48
Hemodynamic instability, 190
Hemoglobin (Hgb), 80–81
Hepatic decompensation, 448–449
Hepatic encephalopathy (HE)
    classifications, 447, 448
    hepatic decompensation, 449
    pathogenesis, 448
    potential therapies, 449
Hepatic necrosis, 452
Hepatic steatosis, 125, 141
Hepatitis, 451–452
Hepatocellular carcinoma (HCC)
    NAFLD, 455
Hepatocellular liver disease, 446
Hepatorenal syndrome (HRS), 449
Hepatotoxic herbal supplements, 452
Herbal supplements, 264
High anion-gap metabolic acidosis, 68
High-density lipoprotein (HDL), 276
High-density lipoprotein cholesterol (HDL), 77–78
High-fiber diet, 394
Hirschsprung disease, 746
HIV wasting, 558
HIV wasting syndrome, 551

HIV/AIDS infection
    AIDS memorial quilt, 546
    antiretroviral treatment, 548
    breastfeeding, 552
    CD4 cell count, 546
    epidemiology, 547–548
    food insecurity, 548–549
        chronic inflammation, 549
        primary care, 549
    gastrointestinal function, 552, 557
    infection, 546–547
    nutritional management
        bone loss, 559
        gastrointestinal symptoms, 553
        HIV comorbidities, 553–555
        HIV wasting, 558
        lipodystrophy, 559
        micronutrient supplementation, 559
        nutritional assessment, 553–557
        oral problems, 553, 555
        unintentional weight loss, 558
    opportunistic infections, 546
    pathophysiology, physical state
        bone loss, 552
        HIV wasting syndrome, 551
        lipid metabolism, 551–552
        protein metabolism, 550–551
    viral load, 546
Home hemodialysis (HHD), 432
Home parenteral nutrition (HPN), 142–143
Homocysteine (Hcy), 86
Hormonal factors, obesity, 223–224
Hormone therapy, 527
Host, solid organ transplantation, 504
24-hour dietary recall, 37–39
Human energy requirements, 228–229
Human milk fortifiers, 623
Hydroxyapatite, 330
Hyperbaric oxygen therapy (HBOT), 203–204
Hypercalcemia, 59
Hypercapnia, 104
Hyperchloremia, 64
Hyperemesis gravidarum (HG), 586–587
Hyperglycemia, 70, 140, 254, 273–274, 512
Hyperglycemia and Adverse Pregnancy Outcome study (HAPO), 257
Hyperkalemia, 56, 427
Hypermagnesemia, 62
Hypermetabolism, 176, 475, 529
Hypernatremia
    etiology, 54–55
    signs and symptoms, 53–54
    treatment, 54–55
Hyperosmolar hyperglycemic nonketotic coma (HHNC), 274
Hyperphagia, 730
Hyperphosphatemia, 60–61
Hypertension (HTN), 229–230, 301, 517
    alcohol intake, 309–310
    CKD, 423
    clinical course, 305–306
    DASH diet, 307, 308
    energy needs in, 307
    medications in, 307
    monitoring and evaluation, 311
    nutrition assessment, 306
    nutrition intervention, 307
    physical activity, 310
    potassium supplementation, 309
    smoking cessation, 310
    sodium reduction, 307, 309, 310
Hypertonic fluids, 49
Hypertonic hyponatremia, 52
Hypertonic solution, 116
Hypervolemia, 51, 140
Hypervolemic hypernatremia, 54–55
Hypervolemic hypotonic hyponatremia, 53–54
Hypoalbuminemia, 163–164
Hypocalcemia, 58–59
Hypochloremia, 64
Hypoglycemia, 70, 140, 263, 274–275
Hypokalemia
    etiology, 55
    signs and symptoms, 55
    treatment, 55–56
Hypomagnesemia, 61, 185, 512
Hyponatremia
    etiology, 52–54
    signs and symptoms, 51–52
    treatment, 52–54
Hypophosphatemia, 60, 185, 512
Hypotonic hyponatremia, 52–53
Hypovolemia, 51, 140
Hypovolemic hypernatremia, 54
Hypovolemic hypotonic hyponatremia, 53
Hypoxemia, 477

I

IBD. See Inflammatory bowel disease
IBS. See Irritable bowel syndrome
Ileal brake, 402
Ileal resection, 402
Ileocecal (IC) valve, 402
Ileostomy, 403
Ileum, 374
Immune system, obesity, 232
Immunonutrition, 92, 479–480
    arginine, 109–111
    clinical trials, 110–111
    gastrointestinal tract, 108–109
    glutamine, 109
    gut, 109–110
    omega-3 fatty acids, 110–111
    systemic inflammatory response, 109–110
Immunonutrition (IN), 531
Immunosenescence, 756
Immunosuppression, 504, 509, 510
Impaired glucose tolerance (IGT), 690
Implantable cardioverter defibrillators (ICDs), 304

Incretins, 225
Indirect calorimetry (IC)
    canopy hood, 160
    DLW, 159–160
    energy requirements, estimation, 188
    measured REE, 160–161
    metabolic cart, 160
    over-and underfeeding, 162
    respiratory quotient, 162–163
    volume of carbon dioxide, 158
    volume of oxygen, 158
Infancy and early childhood, oral health
    concerns, 345–346
    ECC, 346
    nutritional management, 346–347
Inflammation, 196–198
Inflammatory bowel disease (IBD)
    bone disease, 391
    bottom line, 393
    Crohn's disease, 383–388
    defined diets, 393, 394
    enteral nutrition, 391–392
    etiological factor, 384
    individualized diets, 392–393
    malnutrition, 390
    medical management, 384–385
    micronutrient deficiencies, 390–391
    micronutrient supplementation, 392
    nutrition implications, 389–390
    nutrition intervention, 391
    nutrition support, 391
    parenteral nutrition, 392
    remission
        induction of, 385, 388, 389
        maintenance of, 388–389
    surgical intervention, 389
    ulcerative colitis, 383–388
    weight loss and reduced muscle mass, 390
Inflammatory response
    characteristics, 148
    energy cost, 150
    fat metabolism and lipolysis, 153–154
    glucose metabolism, 151
    protein catabolic state, 152
    stress hyperglycemia, 152
    stress vs. starvation, 150–152
Inherited diseases, 456–457
Insensible water loss, 757
Inspection, 28
Instrumental activities of daily living (IADLs), 763
Insulin, 129
    obesity, 225, 232
    resistance, 255, 557, 689
Insulin to carbohydrate ratio (ICR), 268–270
Integrative medicine, 540
Intensive Behavior Programs (IBT), 233, 235
Intensive care unit (ICU), 38, 121
Interleukin-1 (IL-1), 149
Interleukin-6 (IL-6), 38
Intermediate-density lipoprotein (IDL), 77–78

Intermittent feeding, 98
Intestinal cancers, 534
Intestinal failure, 405
Intra-aortic balloon pump (IABP), 322
Intracellular fluid (ICF), 49–50
Intracellular water (ICW), 166
Intradialytic parenteral nutrition (IDPN), 438
Intramyocellular lipid deposition, 690
Intrauterine growth restriction (IUGR), 569, 614
Intravenous (IV) fluids, 49
Intrinsic AKI, 420
Intrinsic factor, 359
Involution, 596
Iron deficiency, 557, 580
Iron-based binders, 429
Iron-deficiency anemia
    AICD, 84
    clinical signs, 83
    functions, 83
    oral *vs.* intravenous, 86
    serum ferritin, 84
    serum iron, 83–84
    symptoms, 83
    TIBC, 84–85
    transferrin, 84
    treatment, 85
Irritable bowel syndrome (IBS)
    classifications, 378–379
    clinical presentation, 379–380
    factors, 378
    low FODMAP diet, 380–382
    low-fat diet, 380
    probiotics, 381–382
    Rome III Diagnostic Criteria, 379
    treatment, 380
Ischemia-reperfusion model, 110–111
Ischemic cardiomyopathy, 311, 505
Ischemic heart disease, 311
Islet amyloid polypeptide, 225
Isolate, 102
Isotonic fluids, 49
Isotonic hyponatremia, 52
Isotonic saline, 53
Isotope dilution technique, 165

J

Jaundice, 449
Jejunal resection, 401–402
Jejunostomy, 403
Jejunum, 374
Joint Commission (JC), 7
Journal of Clinical Endocrinology and Metabolism, 731

K

Kayser-Fleischer ring, 456
Kidney disease, 413–440
    AKI, 419
        diagnosis, 420, 421
        energy, 421
        etiology, 420
        fluid and sodium, 422
        medical nutrition therapy, 420–421
        medical treatment, 420
        nutrition assessment and intervention, 421
        potassium, 422
        protein, 421
    CKD (*see* Chronic kidney disease (CKD))
    CKD-EPI creatinine equation, 419
    CKD-EPI cystatin C equation, 419–420
    classifications, 419
    during dialysis, 436–437
    end-stage renal disease, 431
    enteral nutrition, 437–438
    functions of, 417–418
    GFR calculation, 419
    IDPN, 438
    kinetic modeling, 433–436
    MDRD study equation, 419
    nephrotic syndrome, 438–439
    parenteral nutrition, 438
    physiology, 414–417
    prevalence, 414
    renal replacement therapy
        hemodialysis, 432–433
        indications, 431–432
Kidney disease improving global outcomes (KDIGO), 419, 421
Kidney transplantation, 506, 512
Kinetic modeling
    CRRT, 434
    energy, 434
    fluid, 436
    nutrition assessment, 434
    peritoneal dialysis, 433–434
    phosphorus, 436
    potassium, 436
    protein, 434, 436
    sodium, 436
    stage 5D, 434–436
Knee-Height measurement, 16–17
Kupffer cells, 444
Kussmaul's respirations, 254
Kwashiorkor, 72

L

Lactate dehydrogenase (LDH), 76
Lactation, 596
    breastfeeding initiation/techniques
        adolescent parenthood, 600–601
        benefits of, 600
        education, 599
        engorgement, 602
        environment, 601
        feeding cues, 600
        frequency, 600
        mastitis, 602–603
        plugged ducts, 602
        preterm births, 601
        pumping breast milk, 600
        RD, 606
        retracted nipples, 602
        solutions, 602
        sore nipples, 602
        tight frenulum, 602
        weight BMI, 601–602
    drug usage, 603
    herpes simplex, 603
    HIV, 603
    human milk composition, 596
    indications, 604
    infant disease, 604
    lead poisoning, 603
    maternal infections, 603
    metabolic disorders, 603
    nutrition assessment, 604
    nutritional composition
        carbohydrates, 597
        energy, 596
        fat, 597
        Iron, 597–598
        minerals, 597
        protein, 596–597
        vitamin D, 597
        vitamins, 597
    nutritional requirements
        Calcium, 605
        Carbohydrate, 605
        fat, 605
        fluid, 605
        Iron, 606
        macronutrient, 605
        micronutrient, 605
        multimineral supplements, 606
        protein, 605
        Vitamin A, 605–606
        Vitamin B_{12}, 605
    physiology
        lactogenesis, 594–596
        mammary gland development, 594
    practices
        environmental benefits, 599
        infant benefits, 598
        long-term benefits, 598
        maternal benefits, 598
        maternal fertility, 599
        maternal morbidities, 598
        maternal weight loss, 599
        microbiome, 598
        uterine contractility, 598
Lactogenesis, 594–596
Lactulose, 449
Lanthanum-based binders, 429
Lanugo, 711
Laparoscopic adjustable gastric banding (LAGB), 241, 243–245
Laparoscopy, 95–96
Larazotide acetate, 395
Large-for-gestational-age (LGA), 567, 614

Latent autoimmune diabetes in adults (LADA), 252
Late-onset preeclampsia, 590
LDL. *See* Low-density lipoprotein
Leaky gut syndrome
    medical diagnosis, 393, 395
    nutrition intervention, 395
Lean body mass (LBM), 148, 202–203, 226, 639
Left ventricular assist device (LVAD), 314
Left ventricular hypertrophy (LVH), 687–688
Leptin, 225
Leptin resistance, 225
Let down, 596
Lipid disorders, 430
Lipid injectable emulsions (ILEs), 125
Lipid lab values, dyslipidemia, 299, 300
Lipid profile, 557
Lipids, parenteral nutrition, 125
Lipodystrophy, 551, 559
Lipolysis, 153–154
Lipomeningocele, 736
Lipoproteins, 299
Liver disease, 443–466
    acute liver disease
        acute liver failure, 452–453
        drug-induced hepatitis, 451–452
        nutrition management, 453
        viral hepatitis, 451
    chronic liver disease
        ALD, 453–454
        inherited diseases, 456–457
        NAFLD, 455–456
    cirrhosis
        energy requirements, 461
        enteral nutrition, 463–464
        hepatic encephalopathy, 447, 448
        oral nutrition, 463
        protein requirements, 461
        tissue scarring, 447
        varices, 447
        vitamin D deficiency, 461–462
        Zinc, 462–463
    malnutrition, 449–450
    metabolic alterations
        carbohydrate, 457
        fat, 459
        protein, 457–458
    NAFLD, 445
    nutrition assessment, 459–460
    overview and pathophysiology, 446–449
    structure and functions, 444–446
Liver dysfunction, 104
Liver transplantation, 506, 513
Long chain triglycerides (LCTs), 125, 480
Loop diuretics, 307
Low birth weight (LBW), 614
Low Calorie Diet (LCD), 233–234
Low FODMAP diet, 380–382
Low-density lipoprotein (LDL), 276, 430, 517
Low-density lipoprotein cholesterol (LDL-C), 77, 296
Low-microbial diet, 516, 539–540

Lung cancer, 535
Lung transplantation, 506, 513
Lungs, cystic fibrosis, 488–490

M

Macrocephaly, 642
Macrocytic anemia, 81–82
Macronutrients, 207–209, 212
    cystic fibrosis, 497
    lactation, 605
    requirements
        calcium, 580
        calories, 575–576
        carbohydrate, 576–577
        dietary fat, 577
        folate, 578
        iodine, 580–581
        AND and the IOM, 581
        iron, 579–580
        protein, 577
        serum level, 578
        vitamin B_{12}, 578–579
        vitamin D, 577–579
Magnesium
    electrolyte, 623–624
    hypermagnesemia, 62
    hypomagnesemia, 61
    pulmonary diseases, 481
    refeeding syndrome, 62–63
    structural component, 61
Magnesium-based binders, 429
Magnetic resonance imaging (MRI), 26, 167
Malabsorption, 356
Malassimilation, 356
Mallory-Weiss tears, 713
Malnutrition
    consequences, 7
    definition, 5–6
    identification, 6–7
    liver disease, 449–450
    pediatrics, 669–670
    vs. screening, 6
    solid organ transplantation, 509
Malnutrition Screening tool (MST), 12–13, 527
Malnutrition Screening Tool for Cancer Patients (MSTC), 527
Malnutrition Universal Screening Tool (MUST), 9–11
Marasmus, 72
Masticatory function, 343
Maternal preeclampsia, 590–591
Matrix metalloproteinases (MMPs), 199
Mature milk, 596
Maturity-onset diabetes of the young (MODY), 252
Maudsley approach, 715
MDRD study equation, 419
Meal planning, 267
Mean arterial pressure (MAP), 294

Mean corpuscular hemoglobin concentration (MCHC), 82
Mean corpuscular volume (MCV), 81–82
Measured REE (MREE), 160–161
Medical and psychosocial history, 227
Medical nutrition therapy (MNT), 295, 319, 320, 322
    AKI, 420–421
    American Diabetes Association, 266
    assessment, 204
    bowel surgery
        bowel resection, 400–401
        colonic involvement, 402
        colostomy, 403
        Crohn's disease, 400
        diet composition, 406, 407
        duodenal resection, 401
        fluid and electrolyte needs, 406–407
        ileal resection, 402
        ileocecal valve, 402
        ileostomy, 403
        intestinal adaptation, 404–405
        Jejunal resection, 401–402
        jejunostomy, 403
        nutritional implications, 403–404
        pathophysiology, 404
        reconstruction, 402–403
    carbohydrate counting, 267–268
    celiac disease
        absorption capacity, 375, 377
        clinical manifestations, 376–378
        nutrition interventions, 376–377, 379
        prolamin, 375
    CKD, 424
    diet and nutrition intervention, 212–214
    exchange method, 267–268
    gastric surgery, 357–360
    GERD, 368–370
    Helicobacter pylori, 395
    IBD
        bone disease, 391
        bottom line, 393
        Crohn's disease, 383–388
        defined diets, 393, 394
        enteral nutrition, 391–392
        etiological factor, 384
        individualized diets, 392–393
        malnutrition, 390
        medical management, 384–385
        micronutrient deficiencies, 390–391
        micronutrient supplementation, 392
        nutrition implications, 389–390
        nutrition intervention, 391
        nutrition support, 391
        parenteral nutrition, 392
        remission, 385, 388–389
        surgical intervention, 389
        ulcerative colitis, 383–388
        weight loss and reduced muscle mass, 390

Medical nutrition therapy (MNT) (continued)
   ICR, 268–270
   irritable bowel syndrome
      classifications, 378–379
      clinical presentation, 379–380
      factors, 378
      low FODMAP diet, 380–382
      low-fat diet, 380
      probiotics, 381–382
      Rome III Diagnostic Criteria, 379
      treatment, 380
   kinetic modeling, kidney disease, 434
   meal planning, 267
   monitoring, 214
   NCGS, 382–383
   nephrotic syndrome, 439
   nutritional assessment, 266–267
   nutritional requirements, 204, 207–211
   pancreatitis (see Pancreatitis)
   plate method, 267
   recommended nutrition visits, 266
   SBS
      bottom line, 408
      diet composition, 406, 407
      home nutrition support, 408
      management, 405
      micronutrient considerations, 407–408
      nutritional implications, 404
      oral diet modifications, 408
      pathophysiology, 404
      secondary nutritional goal, 405–406
   screening, 204–206
   SIBO
      clinical conditions, 396
      clinical presentation, 397
      consequences of overgrowth, 396–397
      definition, 396
      diagnosis, 396
      medical treatment, 397–398
      MMC, 396
      nutrition interventions, 398
      probiotics, 399–400
Medications, parenteral nutrition, 129
Medium chain triglycerides (MCT), 359, 480
Megestrol acetate (Megace™), 499
Metabolic acidosis, 68
Metabolic alkalosis, 68–69
Metabolic stress, 147–169
   BCM, 167–168
   body composition
      anthropometry, 164
      bioelectrical impedance, 165
      catabolic disease, 165–166
      isotope dilution technique, 165
      models, 163–164
      nutritional status, 163–164
      two compartment model, 164–165
   Ebb and flow phases, 148–150
   energy expenditure
      components, 154–155
      direct calorimetry, 157–158
      estimation, 155–158
      indirect calorimetry, 158–163
   inflammatory response
      characteristics, 148
      energy cost, 150
      fat metabolism and lipolysis, 153–154
      glucose metabolism, 151
      protein catabolic state, 152
      stress hyperglycemia, 152
      stress vs. starvation, 150–152
   multi-compartmental models, 166–167
Metabolic surgery, 285
Metabolic syndrome, 231, 688–689
Metal-free binders, 429
Metallothionein, 457
Methylmalonic acid (MMA), 86–87
Micelles, 397
Microalbuminuria, 276, 423
Microcephaly, 642
Microcytic anemia, 81–82
Micronutrients, 209–211, 213, 263–264
   cystic fibrosis, 498
   deficiency, 390–391, 557
   supplementation, 392, 559
Mid-arm muscle circumference (MAMC), 24, 459
Mid-parental height, 641
Mid-upper arm circumference (MUAC), 23–24, 164, 556
Migrating motor complex (MMC), 396
Minerals
   critical illness, acute burn injury, 189–190
   enteral nutrition, 102
   pulmonary diseases, 481
Mini nutritional assessment (MNA), 12, 316, 318, 766
Minnesota experiment, 714
Mixed acid–base disorders, 69
Monosaccharide, 381
Mucolytics, 490
Mucositis, 527
Multi-compartmental models, 166–167
Multivitamins, parenteral nutrition, 126–127, 134
Muscle-strengthening, 700
Musculoskeletal system, obesity, 232
Myelomeningocele, 735
Myocardial infarction (MI), 311
Myocardium, 294, 295, 297
Myocytes, 295

N

NAFLD. See Nonalcoholic fatty liver disease
NASH. See Nonalcoholic steatohepatitis
Nasoduodenal tube, 94
Nasoenteric tube, 92
Nasogastric (NG) tube, 94, 177, 363
Nasojejunal tube, 94
National Eating Disorder Association (NEDA), 584
National Health and Nutrition Examination Survey (NHANES), 19, 475, 574
National Institutes of Health (NIH), 695
National Pressure Ulcer Advisory Panel (NPUAP), 200–201
Nausea, 426
Nausea and vomiting of pregnancy (NVP), 586–587
Nebulizers, 490
Necrotizing enterocolitis (NEC), 628
Negative acute-phase proteins, 72
Neonatal intensive care unit (NICU), 615
Neonatology
   body composition
      carbohydrate requirements, 618–619
      electrolyte requirements, 621–624
      energy requirements, 616–617
      fat requirement, 619
      fluid requirements, 619–621
      protein requirements, 617–618
   classifications, 614
   feeding methods
      energy requirements, 625–628
      enteral nutrition, 628–630
      PN, 624
      vascular access, 625
   feeding selection
      breast milk, 630–631
      breastfeeding, 630–631
      discharge, 632
      donor milk, 630
      transitional formulas, 632
   goals of, growth, 616–622
   overview, 614–615
   preterm infant, 615
Nephrocalcinosis, 623
Nephron, 415, 416
Nephropathy, 276–278
Nephrotic syndrome, 438–439
Net secretory response, 407
Neural tube, 573
Neural tube defect (NTD), 573
Neurogenic bladder, 738
Neurogenic bowel, 738
Neuropathy, 279–280
Neutropenia, 515, 536
New onset diabetes after transplantation (NODAT), 517
New York Heart Association (NYHA), 314
NFPE. See Nutrition-focused physical exam
Night eating syndrome (NES), 711
NIH daily energy, 695, 698
Nil per os (NPO), 363, 450
Nissen fundoplication, 369, 370
Nitric oxide, 110–111
Nitrogen balance, 73–74
Nitrogenous waste, 417
Nonalcoholic fatty liver disease (NAFLD), 231–232, 445, 455–456, 691
Nonalcoholic steatohepatitis (NASH), 231–232, 455

Non-celiac gluten sensitivity (NCGS), 382–383
Nonenteric-coated enzyme, 496–497
Nonexercise-related activity thermogenesis (NEAT)., 228
Nonnutritive sweeteners, 263–264
Nonorganic FTT, 670
Normal anion-gap acidosis, 68
Normal fasting blood glucose, 69
Normalized PNA (nPNA), 437
Normalized protein catabolic rate (nPCR), 437
Normocytic anemia, 81–82
Nutrigenomics, 694
Nutrition assessment, 3–40, 528
  ADA, 4–5
  AKI, 421
  anthropometric measurements
    ABW, 17–18, 21
    BIA, 26–27
    BMI, 21–22
    body composition, 22
    body weight, 21
    circumference measurements, 23
    CT, 26
    dry weight, 21
    DXA, 26–27
    height, 14–16
    height-weight tables, 19
    hip circumference, 25–26
    IBW, 19–20
    Imaging Techniques, 26
    intervention, 14
    knee-height measurement, 16
    MRI, 26
    MUAC, 23–24
    predictive equations, 19–20
    skinfold anthropometry, 22–23
    total and half arm span measurements, 16–17
    TSF, 23
    UBW, 18–19
    waist circumference, 24–25
    %weight change, 18–19
  biochemical values, 27
  body composition, 556
  bone loss, 557
  cardiovascular disease, 300–301
  CKD, 424–425
  client history, 27–28
  critical illness, acute burn injury
    anthropometrics, 183–185
    biochemical assessment, 185–186
    dietary assessment, 187–188
    energy needs, 188–189
    enteral nutrition support, 190–191
    malnutrition, 183
    NFPE, 186–187
    nutrition screen, 183–185
    parenteral nutrition support, 191–192
    protein needs, 188–189
    vitamins/minerals, 189–190
  dietary assessment, 556–557
  eating disorder
    anthropometric assessment, 716
    biochemical assessment, 718–719
    dietary assessment, 716–717
    education, 724
  energy balance, 39
  food and nutrition history
    allergies, intolerances, food avoidances, 37
    calorie counts, 39
    cultural background, 37
    dietary recall methods, 37
    FFQ, 39
    food availability and economics, 37
    food intake, 36–37
    food records diary, 39
    24-hour dietary recall, 37–39
    nutrition and health awareness, 37
    nutrition support, 37
    physical activity and exercise habits, 37
    technological advancements, 39
  gastric surgery, 360
  Helicobacter pylori, 395
  hypertension, 306
  insulin resistance and glucose intolerance, 557
  iron deficiency, 557
  kinetic modeling, 434
  lactation, 604
  lipid profile, 557
  liver disease
    body composition, 459
    functional capacity, 460
    SGA, 459
  malnutrition
    consequences, 7
    definition, 5–6
    identification, 6–7
    vs. screening, 6
  micronutrient deficiency, 557
  NCPM, 5
  nephrotic syndrome, 439
  NFPE
    components, 29–32
    eyes and nose/face, 34
    hands and nails, 33
    head and hair, 33–34
    muscle function and strength, 35–36
    oral cavity, 34
    physical signs, 28
    skin examination, 33
    techniques, 28–29
    trunk and extremities, 34–35
  nutrition-focused physical assessment, 556
  obesity, 226–227
  pediatrics
    BMI, 642–643
    head circumference, 642
    length/height, 641–642
    skinfold thickness, 643
    weight, 642
  renal and liver function, 557
  screening
    in acute care, 7–8, 12–14
    assessment tools, 12
    examples, 8
    MST, 12–13
    MUST, 9–11
    NRS-2002, 8–9
    nutrition risk, 8
    role of, 7
    SNAQ, 11–12
  serum albumin, 557
  weakness and reduced oral intake, 4
Nutrition Care Process and Model (NCPM), 5, 226
Nutrition Care Process Terminology (NCPT), 5
Nutrition impact symptoms, 525
Nutrition intervention
  AKI, 421
  cardiovascular disease, 302–303
  celiac disease, 376–377, 379
  CKD, 424–425
  gastric surgery, 360, 361
  heart failure, 319
  Helicobacter pylori, 395
  hypertension, 307
  IBD, 391
  leaky gut syndrome, 395
  pancreatitis, 368
  pulmonary diseases, 476
  SIBO, 398
  wound healing, 212–214
Nutrition patterns, obesity, 227
Nutrition Risk in the Critically Ill (NUTRIC), 183, 185
NUTrition Risk in the Critically ill (NUTRIC score), 38
Nutrition screening, 527–528
Nutrition support
  enteral nutrition
    administration, 592
    complications, 592
    indications, 592
    monitoring, 592
  parenteral nutrition
    access, 593
    complications, 592
    indications, 592–593
    monitoring, 593
Nutritional composition
  carbohydrates, 597
  energy, 596
  fat, 597
  Iron, 597–598
  minerals, 597
  protein, 596–597
  vitamin D, 597
  vitamins, 597
Nutritional Risk Screening (NRS), 183–184
Nutritional Risk Screening (NRS-2002) tool, 8–9
Nutrition-focused physical assessment, 556

Nutrition-focused physical exam (NFPE), 137, 186–187, 227
   components, 29–32
   eyes and nose/face, 34
   hands and nails, 33
   head and hair, 33–34
   muscle function and strength, 35–36
   oral cavity, 34
   physical signs, 28
   skin examination, 33
   techniques, 28–29
   trunk and extremities, 34–35

O

Obesity, 217–247
   anorexigenic hormones, 225
   bariatric surgery, 234
      inclusion and exclusion criteria, 237, 238
      LAGB, 239
      RYGB, 239, 240
      sleeve gastrectomy, 239
      types, 238
   behavior, 234–235
   biochemical assessment, 227
   biological factors, 222–223
   body composition, 225–226
   cardiovascular disease
      AHA/ACC, 310
      CAD diagnosis and surgical treatment, 311–312
      outcomes, 311
   classification, 220–221
   comorbidity outcomes, 239–245
   comprehensive lifestyle intervention, 233
   cultural and socioeconomic factors, 228
   definition, 218
   developmental factors, 223
   diet, 228
   dietary, 227, 233–234
   energy requirements, 228–229
   environmental factors, 221, 222
   genetic factors, 221
   heart failure, 317
   hormonal factors, 223–224
   micronutrient deficiencies and recommendations, 243, 245–246
   nutrition assessment, 226–227
   orexigenic hormones, 224
   pathophysiology
      cardiovascular system, 229–230
      gastrointestinal system, 231–232
      immune system, 232
      metabolic/endocrine system, 230–231
      musculoskeletal system, 232
      respiratory system, 232–233
      weight-related comorbidities, 229, 230
   pharmacotherapy, 235–236
   physical activity, 227, 235
   prevalence, 218–220
   readiness/motivation, 228
   sleep patterns, 228
   social factors, 221–222
   support system, 228
   treatment options, 241, 246–247
   weight loss and diabetes, 219
Obesity paradox, 317
Obstructive sleep apnea (OSA), 228, 232–233, 691
Odynophagia, 525
Oligohydramnios, 615
Oligosaccharides, 381
Oliguria, 418
Omega-3 fatty acids, 110–111, 303–304
ONS. See Oral nutrition supplements
Open tube feeding system, 97
Open tube placement technique, 96
Opportunistic infections, 546
Oral cavity
   diet and nutrition, 331–332
   overview, 330
   systemic nutrition deficiency, 332–333
Oral glucose tolerance test (OGTT), 257
Oral health, 329–350
   adequate nutrition, 330
   adolescence, 347–348
   adulthood, 348–349
   background, 330
   dental caries (see Dental caries)
   dentures, 343–344
   edentulism, 343–344
   geriatrics, 349–350
   infancy and early childhood
      concerns, 345–346
      ECC, 346
      nutritional management, 346–347
   oral cavity
      diet and nutrition, 331–332
      overview, 330
      systemic nutrition deficiency, 332–333
   oral infections, 344–345
   periodontal disease
      genetic factors, 342
      gingivitis, 341
      pathophysiology, 341–342
      pocket depth, 341
      prevention and management, 342–343
   pregnancy, 345
Oral infections
   pathophysiology, 344
   treatment and prevention, 344–345
Oral nutrition supplements (ONS), 212–213, 463, 775
Oral rehydration solutions (ORS), 407
Orbera intragastric balloon, 246
Orexigenic hormones, 224
Organ donation and matching, 508
Organic FTT, 670
Ornithine transcarbamylase (OTC), 462
Oroenteric tube, 92
Oropharyngeal dysphagia (OD), 763
Orthorexia, 711
Orthostatic hypotension, 569
Orthotopic heart transplantation, 504, 511
OSA. See Obstructive sleep apnea
Osmotic demyelination syndrome (ODS), 52
Osmotic pressure, 49
Osteoarthritis (OA), 232
Osteodystrophy, 518
Osteoporosis, 518
Ostomy, 401
Overweight, 218
Oxalate nephrolithiasis, 406
Oxandrolone, 182–183
Oxidative stress, 474

P

Paleolithic diet, 394
Palpation, 28
Pancreas transplantation, 506, 514
Pancreatic cancer, 534
Pancreatic enzyme preparations (PEP), 365
Pancreatic enzyme replacement therapy (PERT), 365–366, 494–496
Pancreatic exocrine insufficiency (PEI), 365
Pancreatic insufficiency, 488
   fecal elastase test, 494
   nonenteric-coated enzyme, 496–497
   PERT, 494–496
   porcine-derived pancreatic enzymes, 495
   PPIs, 495
   stool pattern, 497
Pancreatitis
   abdominal pain, 364–365
   acute pancreatitis, 361–362
   chronic pancreatitis, 360, 364, 365
   classification, 362–363
   clinical features, 364
   nutrient deficiency and malnutrition, 366–367
   nutrition implications, 367–368
   nutrition interventions, 368
   nutrition support, 363
   pancreatic surgery, 367
   PEI, 365
   PERT, 365–366
   treatment, 363
Paracentesis, 449
Parathyroid hormone (PTH), 57, 430
Parenteral nutrition (PN), 115–143, 324, 363, 392, 438, 538, 624
   amino acids, 123–125
   carbohydrate, 123
   central PN, 118–120
   components, 122
   CRCs
      arterial puncture, 138
      embolism, 138
      infectious mechanical complications, 137–139
      noninfectious mechanical complications, 137

occlusion, 138
phlebitis, 138
pneumothorax, 137
securement, 137
critical illness, acute burn injury, 191–192
diabetes mellitus, 287
early vs. late nutrition, 122
electrolytes, 126, 134
history of, 116
HPN, 142–143
hypertonic solution, 116
indications and contraindications, 120–122
insulin, 129
lipids, 125
macronutrient infusion rates, 134
medications, 129
metabolic complications
    EFAs, 140–141
    electrolyte abnormalities, 140
    hepatobiliary disorders, 141
    hyperglycemia, 140
    hypervolemia, 140
    hypoglycemia, 140
    hypovolemia, 140
    overfeeding, 140
monitoring
    anthropometrics, 136
    biochemistry, 136
    efficiency, 135
    NFPE, 137
    vital signs, 136
multivitamins, 126–127, 134
pediatrics
    additives, 677
    administration of, 677
    carbohydrate, 676
    energy targets, 675–676
    fat, 676
    fluid and electrolytes, 677
    monitoring, 677–678
    parenteral access, 675
    PNALD, 677
    protein, 676–677
peripheral PN, 120
prescription calculation, 130–133, 135
progression, 135
small-bowel feeding, 97
sterile preparation, 122
trace elements, 126–128, 134
transitional feeding, 135
venous access, 116–118
wound healing, 213
Parenteral nutrition associated liver disease (PNALD), 125, 677
Parenteral nutrition–related liver disease (PNALD), 456
Past medical history (PMH), 27–28
Patent ductus arteriosus (PDA), 620
Pediatrics

biochemical data
    bone health markers, 656
    electrolytes, 655
    Iron status, 656
body composition, 639–640
diet history, 652–653
food
    adolescents, 668–669
    preschool-aged children, 666–667
    school-aged children, 667–668
    toddlers, 666
growth charts
    BMI-for-age, 660
    CDC, 643, 646, 647
    height-for-age, 660
    weight-for-age, 657–659
    WHO, 643–645
    z-scores, 648–651
malnutrition
    diagnosis, 670
    etiology and pathophysiology, 670
    FTT, 669–670
    management of, 670
medical history, 656
nutrient requirements
    breast milk, 663–665
    EER, 661–662
    healthy eating, 661
    infant formula, 664–666
    infants, 663
    protein, 662–663
    RDA energy requirements, 662
    vitamins and minerals, 663–665
nutrition assessment
    BMI, 642–643
    head circumference, 642
    length/height, 641–642
    skinfold thickness, 643
    weight, 642
nutrition support
    arginine, 679
    enteral access, 672–673
    enteral formulas, 673
    enteral nutrition, 671–672
    enteral tolerance, 675
    glutamine, 679
    Omega-3 fatty acids, 679
    types of, 674
parenteral nutrition
    additives, 677
    administration of, 677
    carbohydrate, 676
    energy targets, 675–676
    fat, 676
    fluid and electrolytes, 677
    monitoring, 677–678
    parenteral access, 675
    PNALD, 677
    protein, 676–677
physical exam

    abdominal examination, 655
    general inspection, 654
    head and face, 654
    oral cavity, 654–655
    skin and nails, 655
physical growth, 638–639
social history, 656–657
Peptide YY (PYY), 225
Percent ideal body weight (%IBW), 20
Percent usual body weight (%UBW), 18–19
Percent weight change (%weight change), 18–19
Percussion, 28
Percussor, 490
Percutaneous coronary intervention (PCI), 311
Percutaneous endoscopic gastrostomy (PEG), 92, 95–96
Percutaneous endoscopic jejunostomy (PEJ), 95
Periodontal disease
    genetic factors, 342
    gingivitis, 341
    pathophysiology, 341–342
    pocket depth, 341
    prevention and management, 342–343
Peripheral artery disease (PAD), 311
Peripheral parenteral nutrition (PPN), 117, 120, 625
Peripherally inserted central catheter (PICC), 119–120
Peristalsis, 356
Peritoneal dialysis (PD), 278, 433–434
Peritonitis, kidney disease, 434
Pharmacologic therapy
    AKI, 420
    COPD, 474
    obesity, 235–236
Phlebitis, 120, 138
Phosphate binders, 428
Phospholipids, 299
Phosphorus
    CKD, 427–429
    electrolytes, 623
    functions, 60
    homeostasis, 57
    hyperphosphatemia, 60–61
    hypophosphatemia, 60
    kinetic modeling, 436
    mechanisms, 57
    pulmonary diseases, 481
    serum concentration, 60
Physical activity
    carbohydrate, 271–272
    cardiovascular disease, 305
    childhood obesity, 699
    hypertension, 310
    obesity, 235
    type 1 diabetes, 270–271
    type 2 diabetes, 271
Physicochemical incompatibilities, 126
Physiologic anemia, 586

Physiologic factors, geriatrics
    dietary modifications, 764
    dysphagia, 763–764
    functional status, 763
    health status, 762
    psychological/neurocognitive status, 762–763
    social factors, 765
Placenta, 568–569
Placental barrier, 570
Placental insufficiency, 568
Placental preeclampsia, 590–591
Plant stanols, 304–305
Plaque, dental caries, 333
Plate method, 267
Platelet-derived growth factor (PDGF), 196
Pneumothorax, 137
Polycystic kidney disease (PKD), 424
Polydispia, 254
Polyols, 381
Polyphagia, 254
Polyunsaturated fatty acids (PUFA), 303
Polyuria, 254
Porcine-derived pancreatic enzymes, 495
Portal hypertension, 447
Porto-systemic shunting, 447
Positive acute-phase proteins, 72
Postnatal diuresis, 620
Postprandial hyperemic response, 107
Potassium
    AKI, 422
    CKD, 427
    hyperkalemia
        etiology, 56
        signs and symptoms, 56
        treatment goals, 56
    hypokalemia
        etiology, 55
        signs and symptoms, 55
        treatment, 55–56
    kinetic modeling, 436
Prader Willi
    anthropometrics, 730–731
    biochemical and clinical data, 731–734
    energy needs of, 734–735
    long term management, 735
    PWS, 729–730
Prader Willi syndrome (PWS), 729–730
Prealbumin (PAB), 72–73
Prebiotics, enteral nutrition, 102
Preconception health, 572–573
Predicted REE (PREE), 160–161
Preeclampsia, 569
Pregnancy
    bariatric surgery, 584
    biochemical markers, 572
    diabetes, 584–585
    dietary restrictions, 581–582
    enteral nutrition, 592
    folic acid, 573
    food cravings and aversions, 582
    GDM, 257–258
    gestation, 567
    gestational diabetes, 588–590
    gestational weight gain, 575
    gravida, 567
    HbA1c goal, 585
    HIV infection, 585–586
    hyperemesis gravidarum, 586–587
    hypertensive disorders, 590
    iron deficiency, 573–574
    issues, 587–588
    LGA, 567
    macronutrient requirements
        calcium, 580
        calories, 575–576
        carbohydrate, 576–577
        dietary fat, 577
        folate, 578
        iodine, 580–581
        AND and the IOM, 581
        iron, 579–580
        protein, 577
        serum level, 578
        vitamin B_{12}, 578–579
        vitamin D, 577–579
    maternal behavior, 567
    multiple pregnancy, 583–584
    NEDA, 584
    nutritional risk factor, 571–572
    oral health, 345
    overweight and obesity, 574–575
    parenteral nutrition, 592–593
    physical activity, 581
    physiologic anemia, 586
    physiological alterations
        blood volume, 569
        carbohydrate metabolism, 570–571
        cardiovascular and pulmonary, 569
        endocrine, 570
        energy metabolism, 570
        fat metabolism, 571
        gastroenterologic symptoms (see Gastroenterologic symptoms)
        gastrointestinal, 569–570
        IUGR, 569
        metabolic alterations, 570
        orthostatic hypotension, 569
        placenta, 568–569
        preeclampsia, 569
        protein metabolism, 571
    preconception health, 572–573
    preeclampsia, 590–591
    pre-pregnancy weight status, 574
    SGA, 567
    teenage pregnancy, 582–583
Pre-pregnancy weight status, 574
Prerenal AKI, 420
Pressure injury, 759
Pressure ulcers, 200–201
Pretransplant phase, 509

Probiotics
    enteral nutrition, 102
    IBS, 381–382
    SIBO, 399–400
Prolamin, 375
Proliferation, 198
Propranolol, 183
Protein
    acute posttransplant phase, 511–512
    catabolism, 152
    cirrhosis, 461
    critically ill patients, 188–189
    cystic fibrosis, 493–494
    diabetes mellitus, 262
    enteral nutrition, 102
    kinetic modeling, 434, 436
    liver disease, 457–458
    wound healing, 208
Protein equivalent of nitrogen appearance (PNA), 437
Protein metabolism, 571
Protein requirements, 617–618
Proteinenergy malnutrition (PEM), 390
Proteins
    AKI, 421
    cellular growth and metabolism, 70
    CKD, 425–426
    quality, 769
    quantity, 769
    somatic protein, 71, 73–75
    total serum, 71
    visceral protein, 71–73
Proton pump inhibitors (PPIs), 495
Psychological effects, childhood obesity
    cognitive impairment, 693
    depression, 692–693
    family relationship, 693
    health-related quality of life, 693
    peer relationships, 693
Pulmonary diseases, 471–481
    ARDS, 477–478
    asthma, 472
    body composition, 475–476
    COPD
        enteral feeding, 479
        oxidative stress, 474
        pharmacologic therapies, 474
        REE, 475
        spirometry, 472–473
        TEE, 475
        weight status, 476
    diet information, 475
    immunonutrition, 479–480
    micronutrients
        antioxidants, 480
        vitamins and minerals, 481
    nutrition intervention, 476
    nutrition support, 478–479
    oxygen, 472
    psychosocial support, 481

quality of life, 481
respiratory system, 472
Pulmonary dysfunction, 104
Pulmonary edema, 323
Purkinje fibers, 295
Pyloroplasty, 358

Q

Quality of life (QOL), 142, 481

R

Radiation therapy, 525
Randomized controlled trials (RCTs), 303
Recommended Daily Allowance (RDA), 758
Recommended Dietary Allowances (RDAs), 572
Red blood cell (RBC) count, 81
Red blood cell folate (RBC folate), 87
Red cell distribution width (RDW), 82–83
REE. *See* Resting energy expenditure
Refeeding syndrome, 62–63, 721
Refractory ascites, 449
Registered dietitians (RDs), 7, 300, 303, 494
Registered dietitian's role, 606
Remineralization, dental caries, 333–334
Remodeling, 198
Renal and liver function, 557
Renal dysfunction, 103
Renal osteodystrophy, 427
Renal replacement therapy
hemodialysis, 432–433
indications, 431–432
Renal replacement therapy (RRT), 420
Renin-angiotensinaldosterone system (RAAS), 417
Respiratory acidosis, 67
Respiratory alkalosis, 67–68
Respiratory quotient (RQ), 162–163, 459
Respiratory system, obesity, 232–233
Resting energy expenditure (REE), 156–157, 228, 229, 475, 493, 529, 712
Resting metabolic rate (RMR), 221
Restrictive procedures, bariatric surgery, 238, 239
Retinol-binding protein (RBP), 73
Retinopathy, 278–279
Rifaximin, 449
Right ventricular assist devices (RVADs), 315
Roll resistance, 700
Rome III Diagnostic Criteria, 379
Root caries, 348
Roux-en-Y gastric bypass (RYGB), 239–241, 355, 702
Roux-en-Y procedure, 357, 358
Russell's sign, 713

S

Saline resistant metabolic alkalosis, 69
Saline-responsive metabolic alkalosis, 69
Salvage absorption, 406
Sarcomas, 524
Sarcopenia, 756
Sarcopenic obesity, 759–760
Saturated fat intake, 303, 304
SBS. *See* Short bowel syndrome
Selective serotonin reuptake inhibitors (SSRIs), 716
Selective vagotomy, 357
Self-efficacy, 700
Self-monitoring of blood glucose (SMBG), 272–273
Self-reported height (SRH), 16
Sensitivity factor, 268–270
Sepsis, 138
Septic shock, 178
Sequential Organ Failure Assessment scores (SOFA), 38
Serial measures, 641
Serum albumin, 557
Serum cobalamin, 85–86
Serum ferritin, 84
Serum iron, 83–84
Shock liver, 453
Short bowel syndrome (SBS)
bottom line, 408
diet composition, 406, 407
home nutrition support, 408
management, 405
micronutrient considerations, 407–408
nutritional implications, 404
oral diet modifications, 408
pathophysiology, 404
secondary nutritional goal, 405–406
Short chain fatty acids, 190
Short Nutritional Assessment Questionnaire (SNAQ), 11–12
Single-nucleotide polymorphisms (SNPs), 694
SIRS. *See* Systemic inflammatory response syndrome
Skinfold anthropometry
circumference measurements, 23
hip circumference, 25–26
MUAC, 23–24
sites, 22
TSF, 23
waist circumference, 24–25
Skinfold thickness, 643. *See also* Skinfold anthropometry
Sleeve gastrectomy (SG), 239–241, 703
Small intestinal bacterial overgrowth (SIBO)
clinical conditions, 396
clinical presentation, 397
consequences of overgrowth, 396–397
definition, 396
diagnosis, 396
medical treatment, 397–398
MMC, 396
nutrition interventions, 398
probiotics, 399–400
Small intestine, 374, 376
Small-bowel transplantation, 506, 514
Small-for-gestational-age (SGA), 567, 614
Smoking cessation, 305

Sodium
AKI, 422
CKD, 426–427
electrolyte, 621–622
hypernatremia
etiology, 54–55
signs and symptoms, 53–54
treatment, 54–55
hyponatremia
etiology, 52–54
signs and symptoms, 51–52
treatment, 52–54
kinetic modeling, 436
Sodium chloride, 498
Sodium reduction, 307, 309, 310
Solid organ transplantation, 503–518
contraindications, 506–507
heart transplant indications, 506, 511
ischemic cardiomyopathy, 505
kidney transplant indications, 506
liver transplant indications, 506
lung transplant indications, 506
medical treatment
acute posttransplant phase, 511–514
dietary therapy, 515–516
GVHD, 508–509
immunosuppression, 509, 510
malnutrition, 509
organ donation and matching, 508
overview, 504
pretransplant phase, 509
small-bowel transplant indications, 506
Somatic proteins
BUN, 75
CHI, 74–75
nitrogen balance, 73–74
Somatization, 378
Spastic, 740
Specific carbohydrate diet (SCD), 394
Spina bifida (SB), 573
anthropometrics, 736–737
Arnold-Chiari malformation, 739
biochemical and clinical data, 737–738
classifications, 735
club foot, 738
comparison of, 735, 737
digital bed scale, 736, 738
energy needs, 738–739
feeding difficulty, 739
long-term monitoring/evaluation, 739
recommendations, 738
weight challenges, 739
Spirometry, 473
Spontaneous bacterial peritonitis (SBP), 449
Stadiometer, 15
Standard body weight (SBW), 424, 425
Static assay, 48
Steatohepatitis, 231–232, 453, 455
Steatorrhea, 359
Steatosis, 453

Stellate cells, 444
Stent angioplasty, 311, 312
Sterols, 304–305
Stoma, 401
Storage fat, 226
Streptococcus mutans, 334
Stress hyperglycemia, 152, 187
Stroke, 311
Stroke volume, 294
Stunting, 660
Subjective global assessment (SGA), 12, 316, 317, 459
Sucrose, 262
Surgical intervention
    indications, 702
    postoperative care, 705
    weight loss procedures
        adjustable gastric banding, 702–703
        malabsorptive procedures, 702
        sleeve gastrectomy, 703
        vertical banded gastroplasty, 702
Susceptible tooth, 334
Sweat test, 488
Swedish Obese Subjects study, 240
Synbiotic, 399
Syndrome of inappropriate antidiuretic hormone (SIADH), 53
Systemic inflammatory response syndrome (SIRS), 109, 177, 178, 180
Systole, 294
Systolic blood pressure, 305

T

Tacrolimus, 517
Thermic effect of feeding, 154
Thermic effect of food (TEF), 228
Thermogenesis, 226
Thiazide-type diuretics, 307
Third spacing, 50
Thromboembolism, 138
Thrombophlebitis, 118
Thrombosis, 297
Thrombotic occlusion, 138
Total arm span (TAS), 16–17
Total body surface area (TBSA), 180–182
Total cholesterol, 78
Total daily energy expenditure (TEE), 475
Total energy expenditure (TEE), 228
    components, 154–155
        factorial approach
            normal conditions, 155–156
            stressed conditions, 156–158
Total iron binding capacity (TIBC), 73, 84–85
Total nutrient admixture (TNA), 125
Total peripheral resistance, 294
Total serum protein, 72
Total (truncal) vagotomy, 357
Trace elements, 126–128, 134
Transferrin, 73, 84

Transforming growth factor β (TGF-β, 196
Transitional feeding, 135
Transitional milk, 596
Transjugular intrahepatic portosystemic shunt (TIPS), 448
Transthyretin, 72–73
Trauma, 149
    enteral nutrition, 104
Triceps skinfold (TSF), 23
Triceps skinfold thickness (TST), 459
Triglyceride (TG) levels, 153–154
Triglycerides, 78
Troponin, 76–77
Tube feeds (TFs), 92
Tubules, 414
Tumor necrosis factor (TNF), 149
Tumor necrosis factor-alpha (TNF-α), 198, 317, 453
Two compartment model, 164–165
Type 1 diabetes
    diagnostic criteria, 254
    Diamond Project report, 252
    exercise, 270–271
    insulin pump and injection, 254–255
    symptoms, 253–254
    treatment for, 254
    vomiting and abdominal pain, 253
Type 2 diabetes
    beta cell mass, 254
    exercise, 271
    hepatic glucose output, 255
    insulin receptor defects, 255–256
    insulin resistance, 255
    insulin secretion, 255
    loss of postprandial euglycemia, 255
    obesity, 230–231
    treatment of, 257

U

Ulcerative colitis (UC), 383
Ultrafiltrate, 414
Underfill hypothesis, 447
Underweight, 648
Unintentional weight loss, 558
Unsaturated fat intake, 303, 304
Ureters, 415
Urinary system, 415, 416
Urine albumin-to-creatinine ratio (UACR), 425
Urine glucose, 69–70
Urine urea nitrogen (UUN), 73–74
Usual body weight (UBW), 18–19

V

Varices, 447
Vascular access devices (VADs), 117, 118
Vasopressors, 322
Venipuncture, 117
Ventilator-associated pneumonia (VAP), 343
Ventricular assist device (VAD), 314

Ventriculoperitoneal (VP) shunting, 737
Very low birth weight (VLBW), 614
Very Low Calorie Diet (VLCD), 233–234
Very-low-density lipoprotein cholesterol (VLDL), 77, 299
Viokace tablets, 496–497
Viral hepatitis, 451
Viral load, 557
Viral suppression, 557
Visceral hypersensitivity, 378
Visceral protein
    acute-phase proteins, 71
    albumin levels, 72
    inflammation, 72
    negative acute-phase, 72
    non-dietary factors, 72
    PAB, 72–73
    positive acute-phase, 72
    RBP, 73
    transferrin, 73
Vitamin A, wound healing, 211
Vitamin B_{12} deficiency, 359, 578–579
    anemia, 85–88
    folate, 87–88
    metformin, 280
    parameters, 86
    serum cobalamin, 85–86
    subclinical deficiency, 86–87
    supplemental doses, 88
Vitamin B-complex deficiencies, 333
Vitamin C deficiency, 333, 342
Vitamin C, wound healing, 210
Vitamin D deficiency, 57, 330
    cirrhosis, 461–462
    CKD, 429–430
    osteodystrophy, 518
    pregnancy, 577–579
    pulmonary diseases, 481
Vitamins
    critical illness, acute burn injury, 189–190
    enteral nutrition, 102
Vulnerable plaque formation, 297, 298

W

Waist circumference, 24–25, 227
Waist-to-hip ratio (WHR), 25–26, 227, 556
Wasting, 660
Weeks gestational age (WGA), 614
Weight
    ABW, 17–18, 21
    BMI, 21–22
    body composition, 22
    body weight modifications, 21
    dry weight, 21
    height-weight tables, 19
    IBW, 19, 20
    predictive equations, 19–20
    UBW, 18–19
    %weight change, 18–19

Weight gain. *see* Obesity
Weight history, 227
Weight loss medications, 236–237
Weight-for-age, 643
Weight-for-height, 643
Weight-related comorbidities, 229, 230
Wernicke's encephalopathy, 587
Western diet, 384
White blood cell (WBC) count, 83
WHR. *See* Waist-to-hip ratio
Wilson's disease, 456
World Health Organization (WHO), 17, 643
Wound healing, 195–214
    chronic wounds
        chronic venous ulcers, 199
        delayed healing, 199
        diabetic ulcers, 199–200
        factors, 198–199
        pathophysiology, 199
        physiological state and metabolism, alterations, 201–203
        pressure ulcers, 200–201
    defined, 196
    enteral nutrition, 104
    medical treatment
        debridement, 203
        hyperbaric oxygen therapy, 203–204
        vacuum-assisted closure, 203–204
        WOC clinician, 203
    MNT
        assessment, 204
        diet and nutrition intervention, 212–214
        monitoring, 214
        nutritional requirements, 204, 207–211
        screening, 204–206
    pathophysiology
        classification, 196
        inflammation, 196–198
        proliferation, 198
        remodeling, 198
        risk factors, 196

X

Xanthomas, 300
Xerostomia, 333, 349

Z

Zinc
    cirrhosis, 462–463
    wound healing, 209–210
Z-scores, 648–651